DIETARY REFERENCE INTAKES (DRIs): RECOMMENDED INTAKES FOR INDIVIDUALS

LIFE-STAGE GROUP	CALCIUM (mg/day)	CHROMIUM (mcg/day)	COPPER (mcg/day)	FLUORIDE (mg/day)	IODINE (mcg/day)	IRON (mg/day)	MAGNESIUM (mg/day)	MANGANESE (mg/day)	MOLYBDENUM (mcg/day)	PHOSPHORUS (mg/day)	SELENIUM (mcg/day)	ZINC (mg/day)	POTASSIUM (g/day)	SODIUM (g/day)	CHLORIDE (g/day)
Infants															
0-6 mo	210*	0.2*	200*	0.01*	110*	0.27*	30*	0.003*	2*	100*	15*	2*	0.4	0.12	0.18
7-12 mo	270*	5.5*	220*	0.5*	130*	11	75*	0.6*	3*	275*	20*	3*	0.7	0.37	0.57
Children															
1-3 yr	500*	11*	340	0.7*	90	7	80	1.2*	17	460	20	3	3.0	1.0	1.5
4-8 yr	800*	15*	440	1*	90	10	130	1.5*	22	500	30	5	3.8	1.2	1.9
Males															
9-13 yr	1300*	25*	700	2*	120	8	240	1.9*	34	1250	40	8	4.5	1.5	2.3
14-18 yr	1300*	35*	890	3*	150	11	410	2.2*	43	1250	55	11	4.7	1.5	2.3
19-30 yr	1000*	35*	900	4*	150	8	400	2.3*	45	700	55	11	4.7	1.5	2.3
31-50 yr	1000*	35*	900	4*	150	8	420	2.3*	45	700	55	11	4.7	1.5	2.3
50-70 yr	1200*	30*	900	4*	150	8	420	2.3*	45	700	55	11	4.7	1.3	2.0
>70 yr	1200*	30*	900	4*	150	8	420	2.3*	45	700	55	11	4.7	1.2	1.8
Females															
9-13 yr	1300*	21*	700	2*	120	8	240	1.6*	34	1250	40	8	4.5	1.5	2.3
14-18 yr	1300*	24*	890	3*	150	15	360	1.6*	43	1250	55	9	4.7	1.5	2.3
19-30 yr	1000*	25*	900	3*	150	18	310	1.8*	45	700	55	8	4.7	1.5	2.3
31-50 yr	1000*	25*	900	3*	150	18	320	1.8*	45	700	55	8	4.7	1.5	2.3
50-70 yr	1200*	20*	900	3*	150	8	320	1.8*	45	700	55	8	4.7	1.3	2.0
>70 yr	1200*	20*	900	3*	150	8	320	1.8*	45	700	55	8	4.7	1.2	1.8
Pregnant															
≤18 yr	1300*	29*	1000	3*	220	27	400	2.0*	50	1250	60	12	4.7	1.5	2.3
19-30 yr	1000*	30*	1000	3*	220	27	350	2.0*	50	700	60	11	4.7	1.5	2.3
31-50 yr	1000*	30*	1000	3*	220	27	360	2.0*	50	700	60	11	4.7	1.5	2.3
Lactating															
≤18 yr	1300*	44*	1300	3*	290	10	360	2.6*	50	1250	70	13	5.1	1.5	2.3
19-30 yr	1000*	45*	1300	3*	290	9	310	2.6*	50	700	70	12	5.1	1.5	2.3
31-50 yr	1000*	45*	1300	3*	290	9	320	2.6*	50	700	70	12	5.1	1.5	2.3

Data from Food and Nutrition Board, Institute of Medicine: *Dietary reference intakes for calcium, phosphorus, magnesium, vitamin D, and fluoride* (1997); *Dietary reference intakes for thiamin, riboflavin, niacin, vitamin B₆, folate, vitamin B₁₂, pantothenic acid, biotin, and choline* (1998); *Dietary reference intakes for vitamin C, vitamin E, selenium, and carotenoids* (2000); and *Dietary reference intakes for vitamin A, vitamin K, arsenic, boron, chromium, copper, iodine, manganese, molybdenum, nickel, silicon, vanadium, and zinc* (2001), Washington, DC, National Academies Press (www.nap.edu).

NOTE: *This table presents Recommended Dietary Allowances (RDAs) in **bold type** and Adequate Intakes (AIs) in regular type followed by an asterisk (*). RDAs and AIs may both be used as goals for individual intake. RDAs are set to meet the needs of almost all (97%-98%) individuals in a group. For healthy breast-fed infants, the AI is the mean intake. The AI for other life-stage and gender groups is believed to cover needs of all individuals in the group, but lack of data or uncertainty in the data prevent being able to specify with confidence the percentage of individuals covered by this intake.

DIETARY REFERENCE INTAKES (DRIs): TOLERABLE UPPER INTAKE LEVELS (UL[a]), MINERALS

LIFE-STAGE GROUP	ARSENIC[b]	BORON (mg/day)	CALCIUM (g/day)	CHROMIUM	COPPER (mcg/day)	FLUORIDE (mg/day)	IODINE (mcg/day)	IRON (mg/day)	MAGNESIUM (mg/day)[c]	MANGANESE (mg/day)	MOLYBDENUM (mcg/day)	NICKEL (mg/day)	PHOSPHORUS (g/day)	SELENIUM (mcg/day)	SILICON[d]	VANADIUM (mg/day)[e]	ZINC (mg/day)	POTASSIUM	SULFATE	SODIUM (g/day)	CHLORIDE (g/day)
Infants																					
0-6 mo	ND[f]	ND	ND	ND	ND	0.7	ND	40	ND	ND	ND	ND	ND	45	ND	ND	4	ND	ND	ND	ND
7-12 mo	ND	ND	ND	ND	ND	0.9	ND	40	ND	ND	ND	ND	ND	60	ND	ND	5	ND	ND	ND	ND
Children																					
1-3 yr	ND	3	2.5	ND	1000	1.3	200	40	65	2	300	0.2	3	90	ND	ND	7	ND	ND	1.5	2.3
4-8 yr	ND	6	2.5	ND	3000	2.2	300	40	110	3	600	0.3	3	150	ND	ND	12	ND	ND	1.9	2.9
Males, Females																					
9-13 yr	ND	11	2.5	ND	5000	10	600	40	350	6	1100	0.6	4	280	ND	ND	23	ND	ND	2.2	3.4
14-18 yr	ND	17	2.5	ND	8000	10	900	45	350	9	1700	1.0	4	400	ND	ND	34	ND	ND	2.3	3.6
19-70 yr	ND	20	2.5	ND	10,000	10	1100	45	350	11	2000	1.0	4	400	ND	1.8	40	ND	ND	2.3	3.6
>70 yr	ND	20	2.5	ND	10,000	10	1100	45	350	11	2000	1.0	3	400	ND	1.8	40	ND	ND	2.3	3.6
Pregnant																					
≤18 yr	ND	17	2.5	ND	8000	10	900	45	350	9	1700	1.0	3.5	400	ND	ND	34	ND	ND	2.3	3.6
19-50 yr	ND	20	2.5	ND	10,000	10	1100	45	350	11	2000	1.0	3.5	400	ND	ND	40	ND	ND	2.3	3.6
Lactating																					
≤18 yr	ND	17	2.5	ND	8000	10	900	45	350	9	1700	1.0	4	400	ND	ND	34	ND	ND	2.3	3.6
19-50 yr	ND	20	2.5	ND	10,000	10	1100	45	350	11	2000	1.0	4	400	ND	ND	40	ND	ND	2.3	3.6

Data from Food and Nutrition Board, Institute of Medicine: *Dietary reference intakes for calcium, phosphorus, magnesium, vitamin D, and fluoride* (1997); *Dietary reference intakes for thiamine, riboflavin, niacin, vitamin B₆, folate, vitamin B₁₂, pantothenic acid, biotin, and choline* (1998); *Dietary reference intakes for vitamin C, vitamin E, selenium, and carotenoids* (2000); and *Dietary reference intakes for vitamin A, vitamin K, arsenic, boron, chromium, copper, iodine, manganese, molybdenum, nickel, silicon, vanadium, and zinc* (2001), Washington, DC, National Academies Press (www.nap.edu).

[a]UL = The maximum level of daily nutrient intake that is likely to pose no risk of adverse effects. Unless otherwise specified, the UL represents total intake from food, water, and supplements. Due to lack of suitable data, ULs could not be established for arsenic, chromium, and silicon. In the absence of ULs, extra caution may be warranted in consuming levels above recommended intakes.

[b]Although the UL was not determined for arsenic, there is no justification for adding arsenic to food or supplements.

[c]The ULs for magnesium represent intake from a pharmacologic agent only and do not include intake from food or water.

[d]Although silicon has not been shown to cause adverse effects in humans, there is no justification for adding silicon to supplements.

[e]Although vanadium in food has not been shown to cause adverse effects in humans, there is no justification for adding vanadium to food, and vanadium supplements should be used with caution. The UL is based on adverse effects in laboratory animals, and this data could be used to set a UL for adults but not children and adolescents.

[f]ND = Not determinable due to lack of data of adverse effects in this age group and concern with regard to lack of ability to handle excess amounts. Source of intake should be from food only to prevent high levels of intake.

DIETARY REFERENCE INTAKES (DRIs): RECOMMENDED INTAKES FOR INDIVIDUALS, MACRONUTRIENTS

LIFE STAGE GROUP	PROTEIN RDA/AI g/day[A]	AMDR[B]	CARBOHYDRATE RDA/AI g/day	AMDR	FIBER RDA/AI g/day	AMDR	FAT RDA/AI g/day	AMDR	N-6 POLYUNSATURATED FATTY ACIDS (LINOLEIC ACID) RDA/AI g/day	AMDR	N-3 POLYUNSATURATED FATTY ACIDS (α-LINOLENIC ACID) RDA/AI g/day	AMDR[D]	SATURATED AND TRANS FATTY ACIDS AND CHOLESTEROL RDA/AI g/day	AMDR
Infants														
0-6 mo	9.1	ND[c]	60	ND	ND		31		4.4	ND	0.5	ND		
7-12 mo	**11**	ND	95	ND	ND		30		4.6	ND	0.5	ND		
Children														
1-3 yr	**13**	**5-20**	**130**	45-65	19			30-40	7	5-10	0.7	0.6-1.2		
4-8 yr	**19**	**10-30**	**130**	45-65	25			25-35	10	5-10	0.9	0.6-1.2		
Males														
9-13 yr	**34**	**10-30**	**130**	45-65	31			25-35	12	5-10	1.2	0.6-1.2		
14-18 yr	**52**	**10-30**	**130**	45-65	38			25-35	16	5-10	1.6	0.6-1.2		
19-30 yr	**56**	**10-35**	**130**	45-65	38			20-35	17	5-10	1.6	0.6-1.2		
31-50 yr	**56**	**10-35**	**130**	45-65	38			20-35	17	5-10	1.6	0.6-1.2		
50-70 yr	**56**	**10-35**	**130**	45-65	30			20-35	14	5-10	1.6	0.6-1.2		
>70 yr	**56**	**10-35**	**130**	45-65	30			20-35	14	5-10	1.6	0.6-1.2		
Females														
9-13 yr	**34**	**10-30**	**130**	45-65	26			25-35	10	5-10	1.0	0.6-1.2		
14-18 yr	**46**	**10-30**	**130**	45-65	26			25-35	11	5-10	1.1	0.6-1.2		
19-30 yr	**46**	**10-35**	**130**	45-65	25			20-35	12	5-10	1.1	0.6-1.2		
31-50 yr	**46**	**10-35**	**130**	45-65	25			20-35	12	5-10	1.1	0.6-1.2		
50-70 yr	**46**	**10-35**	**130**	45-65	21			20-35	11	5-10	1.1	0.6-1.2		
>70 yr	**46**	**10-35**	**130**	45-65	21			20-35	11	5-10	1.1	0.6-1.2		
Pregnant														
≤18 yr	**71**	**10-35**	**175**	45-65	28			20-35	13	5-10	1.4	0.6-1.2		
19-30 yr	**71**	**10-35**	**175**	45-65	28			20-35	13	5-10	1.4	0.6-1.2		
31-50 yr	**71**	**10-35**		45-65	28			20-35	13	5-10	1.4	0.6-1.2		
Lactating														
≤18 yr	**71**	**10-35**	**210**	45-65	29			20-35	13	5-10	1.3	0.6-1.2		
19-30 yr	**71**	**10-35**	**210**	45-65	29			20-35	13	5-10	1.3	0.6-1.2		
31-50 yr	**71**	**10-35**	**210**	45-65	29			20-35	13	5-10	1.3	0.6-1.2		

Data from *Dietary reference intakes for energy, carbohydrate, fiber, fat, fatty acids, cholesterol, protein, and amino acids*, Washington, DC, 2002, The National Academies Press.

NOTE: *This table presents Recommended Dietary Allowances (RDAs) in **bold type** and Adequate Intakes (AIs) in regular type. RDAs and AIs may both be used as goals for individual intake. RDAs are set to meet the needs of almost all (97%-98%) individuals in a group. For healthy breast-fed infants, the AI is the mean intake. The AI for other life stage and gender groups is believed to cover the needs of all individuals in the group, but lack of data prevents being able to specify with confidence the percentage of individuals covered by this intake.

[a]Based on 1.5 g/kg/day for infants, 1.1 g/kg/day for 1-3 yr, 0.95 g/kg/day for 4-13 yr, 0.85 g/kg/day for 14-18 yr, 0.8 g/kg/day for adults, and 1.1 g/kg/day for pregnant (using pre-pregnancy weight) and lactating women.

[b]Acceptable Macronutrient Distribution Range (AMDR) is the range of intake for a particular energy source that is associated with reduced risk of chronic disease while providing intakes of essential nutrients. If an individual has consumed in excess of the AMDR, there is a potential of increasing the risk of chronic diseases and insufficient intakes of essential nutrients.

[c]ND = Not determinable due to lack of data of adverse effects in this age group and concern with regard to lack of ability to handle excess amounts. Source of intake should be from food only to prevent high levels of intake.

[d]Approximately 10% of the total can come from longer-chain, *n*-3 fatty acids.

Nutritional Foundations and Clinical Applications

A NURSING APPROACH | Fifth Edition

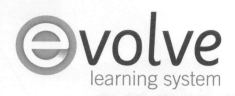
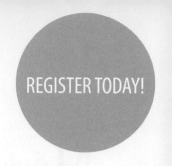

Nutritional Foundations
and Clinical Applications

A NURSING APPROACH | **Fifth Edition**

Michele Grodner, EdD, CHES

Professor
Department of Public Health
William Paterson University
Wayne, New Jersey

Sara Long Roth, PhD, RD

Professor
Department of Animal Science, Food & Nutrition
Southern Illinois University Carbondale
Carbondale, Illinois

Bonnie C. Walkingshaw, MS, RN

Professor of Nursing (retired)
BSN Clinical Coordinator
School of Nursing and Health Sciences
Westminster College
Salt Lake City, Utah

ELSEVIER
MOSBY

3251 Riverport Lane
St. Louis, Missouri 63043

Notice

Knowledge and best practice in this field are constantly changing. As new research and experience broaden our knowledge, changes in practice, treatment and drug therapy may become necessary or appropriate. Readers are advised to check the most current information provided (i) on procedures featured or (ii) by the manufacturer of each product to be administered, to verify the recommended dose or formula, the method and duration of administration, and contraindications. It is the responsibility of the practitioner, relying on their own experience and knowledge of the patient, to make diagnoses, to determine dosages and the best treatment for each individual patient, and to take all appropriate safety precautions. To the fullest extent of the law, neither the Publisher nor the Authors assume any liability for any injury and/or damage to persons or property arising out or related to any use of the material contained in this book.

Previous editions copyrighted 1996, 2000, 2004, 2007

Library of Congress Cataloging-in-Publication Data

Grodner, Michele.
    Nutritional foundations and clinical applications : a nursing approach / Michele Grodner, Sara Long Roth, Bonnie C. Walkingshaw. — 5th ed.
        p. ; cm.
    Rev. ed. of: Foundations and clinical applications of nutrition : a nursing approach / Michele Grodner, Sara Long, Bonnie C. Walkingshaw. 4th ed. c2007.
    Includes bibliographical references and index.
    ISBN 978-0-323-07456-8 (pbk. : alk. paper)   1. Diet therapy.   2. Nutrition.   3. Nursing.   I. Roth, Sara Long.   II. Walkingshaw, Bonnie C.   III. Grodner, Michele. Foundations and clinical applications of nutrition.   IV. Title.
    [DNLM: 1.   Diet Therapy—methods—Nurses' Instruction.   2.   Nutritional Physiological Phenomena—Nurses' Instruction. WB 400]
    RM216.G946 2012
    615.8′54—dc22

                                                            2010035542

Senior Editor: Yvonne Alexopoulos
Senior Developmental Editor: Lisa P. Newton
Publishing Services Manager: Deborah L. Vogel
Project Manager: John W. Gabbert
Design Direction: Paula Catalano

Printed in the United States of America

Last digit is the print number: 9   8   7   6   5   4   3   2

To my mother, Yetta Kaemmer … my role model who always reminds me that a smile, kind words, and compassion make us all feel better!

Michele Grodner

To Kevin … my soul mate, best friend, and so much more!

Sara Long Roth

To my family, friends, and colleagues … thank you for enriching my life through your support and encouragement.

Bonnie C. Walkingshaw

REVIEWERS

Zita Allen, MSN, RN
Professor of Nursing
Alverno College
School of Nursing
Milwaukee, Wisconsin

Bethany M. Derricott, MSN, RN
Assistant Professor of Nursing
Kent State University
Adjunct Faculty
Chamberlain College of Nursing
Kent, Ohio

Daniel G. Graetzer, PhD
Department of Natural Science and Mathematics
Northwest University
Kirkland, Washington

Jane Lucht, MS, RN
Associate Professor
Edgewood College
School of Nursing
Madison, Wisconsin

Never before have we had so much information about the effects of our personal behavior patterns on our level of health. As health care professionals, we need to be concerned with our own nutritional patterns as well as those of our patients. *Nutritional Foundations and Clinical Applications,* fifth edition, continues to recognize the role of nurses to support efforts to realize wellness.

This nutrition text takes into account the personal nutrition needs of nurses to nourish themselves and their families as well as their demanding professional responsibilities to educate patients and clients (and their families) to follow prescribed therapeutic nutrition to maintain or improve health. This approach unites the worlds of nutrition and nursing. The role of nurses expands from the medical clinic and into the community, thereby having a greater influence on the health promotion of individuals and the communities in which they work. Consequently, the need for nurses to have a thorough background in both personal and clinical nutrition applications becomes paramount.

AUDIENCE

Nursing students are the primary audience for this book as they explore and apply nutrition and therapeutic nutrition. Secondary audiences include health education and health science students. Useful in a variety of health care settings, the text provides an excellent reference for nurses, nurse practitioners, and other health care professionals.

The book consists of four parts, allowing for selective use within a one-semester course. For instance, Part I, *Wellness, Nutrition, and the Nursing Role*; Part II, *Nutrients, Food, and Health*; and Part III, *Health Promotion Through Nutrition and Nursing Practice* can be used for a basic, one-semester nutrition course, whereas Part IV, *Overview of Nutrition Therapy*, may be used as a future reference for nutrition therapy. Or all parts may be covered within a one-semester course.

APPROACH

Our focus is on the nursing professional. This concentrated approach allows us to emphasize the nutrition skills applicable to nursing practice. The method of this text tailors nutrition and therapeutic nutrition to the unique perspective of the nursing profession. Most other nutrition texts attempt to meet the needs of dietetic and nutrition majors in addition to nursing majors. Information needed by dietetic majors but not by nurses is omitted. We appreciate that nurses do not prescribe or develop "diets" as nutrition therapy for patients. Instead, skills essential for nursing professionals are emphasized for implementation and education of patients and clients about prescribed dietary patterns.

FEATURES AND CONTENT

The nursing profession is multifaceted. While health promotion and clinical care are primary concerns, nurses have other factors to consider when providing care. These are addressed in every chapter of this fifth edition of *Nutritional Foundations and Clinical Applications*. Consider these features as presented in Chapter 10:

- **Cultural diversity of populations served**
  Food and health customs and concerns are analyzed specific to an array of ethnic groups. Students become sensitized and respectful of culturally defined food differences and are then able to approach, interview, and assess patients from diverse backgrounds. Each **CULTURAL CONSIDERATIONS** box includes a section called, "Application to Nursing," to highlight how to use the knowledge in daily practice. As an added resource, Appendix H provides cultural dietary patterns of different ethnic and religious groups, allowing nurses to focus on the specific population with whom they work.

CULTURAL CONSIDERATIONS
Globesity

More than 300 million adults are obese, while another billion are overweight. Each year about 2.6 million people die from disorders related to being overweight or obese. Globesity, the spread of rising obesity levels throughout the world, seems to be centered on globalization and development tied to poverty. Hunger and malnutrition are no longer leading contributors to mortality; particularly in Latin America, obesity has joined the list. This may be partly due to "nutrition transition" in which traditional local foods and preparation styles are being replaced by highly processed foods that tend to be higher in calories, fat, and sodium and deficient in fiber, iron, and vitamin A—in essence "bad" nutrition or malnutrition.

Another potential factor of globesity is level of development and economy of regions. When incomes rise in poorer countries, people often gain weight and become fatter because more food can be purchased. In developed and transitional economies, greater income is associated with lower body weights. Why are poverty and overweight tied together? Studies show that short stature and growth stunting because of fetal and early life malnutrition are related to obesity in adulthood. It's as if the body is trying to catch up for early damages but cannot be satisfied. In addition, cultural views may represent excess body fat as prosperity to some minority and socioeconomic subgroups. The family has enough wealth to afford sufficient amounts of food to eat well enough to the point of fatness. Higher-educated socioeconomic subgroups, with knowledge of health risk factors, tend not to view overweight in this manner.

Regardless of the cultural and economic reasons that fuel globesity, the health costs of obesity-related disorders are the same, including type 2 diabetes mellitus (DM), coronary artery disease, hypertension, and certain cancers. Developing countries still struggling with the ravages of undernutrition will struggle even more attempting to deal with disorders of overnutrition.

Application to nursing: As we work with populations from varying cultural, economic, and global perspectives, we can be aware that values of excess body fat may have different meanings to others. We may need to initiate discussions about prosperity and the notion of healthy body weight management as being economically "very valuable."

Data from Eberwine D: Globesity: The crisis of growing proportions, *Perspect Health* 7(3):6, 2002; World Health Organization: *10 facts on obesity*, February 2010. Accessed on February 23, 2010, from http://www.who.int/features/factfiles/obesity/facts/en/index1.html.

- **Controversial health issue explorations**
Health care professionals and the public-at-large have access to an abundance of health-related information through the many forms of media. Consequently, differing opinions or controversies about food, nutrition, and health concerns emerge. Students are encouraged to develop their own beliefs. As applicable, some chapters have **HEALTH DEBATE** boxes.

HEALTH DEBATE

Can "Commercial" Diet Programs Teach Healthy Eating Habits?*

With the ever advancing epidemic of obesity in the United States, health professionals are constantly telling the American population, "Don't gain weight! Lose weight!" But at the same time the health professionals are also saying, "Don't go on a diet! Stay away from those dangerous fad diets advertised on television!" So what is the average person suppose to do? How do we expect nondietary experts to lose weight even while we health professionals struggle with our own weight control? Surely there must be some positive aspects of weight loss programs that we can use in our national "battle of the bulge."

This box presents discussion of healthy food aspects of programs like Weight Watchers—focusing on moderation and portion control; and intake of fruits, vegetables, and fiber—and the South Beach Diet—emphasizing whole grains and fruits and vegetables—as helping individuals to normalize eating patterns and food portions, *after* the first 2 weeks of deprivation! Perhaps we need to change our approach to using commercial diet programs. Let's consider how to customize a program whether online or through books. This applies to men and women.

Portion Sizes
Programs that either provide premeasured food *or* have no limit on portion sizes do us a disservice. After years of eating out of control or even just "eating" our usual servings, our portions may be just too large for our caloric needs. It is better to spend a few weeks with measuring cups learning that your favorite cereal bowl actually holds three servings of cereal, not just one.

Cooking Skills
Eating out may be convenient, but it is more nutritious and economical to cook simple meals. Some programs include easy-to-follow recipes that taste good to both dieters and non-dieters. Because more families consist of busy two-career parents, and children have many extracurricular activities, children may grow up without learning basic cooking skills. As young adults they can easily teach themselves by following simple directions. Better healthy eating programs provide recipes for novice cooks.

Personal and Time Management
Goal-oriented individuals succeed. They plan and follow through. These skills are woven into the higher-quality weight management programs. Planning ahead, shopping, and cooking for meals for the week involve time management skills. Consider if a week includes difficult social events involving food and how to cope with them; some programs are flexible enough to educate participants as to strategies for dealing with such situations.

Food Records
Food records or journaling has become an established means for keeping track of foods eaten. It is a diary of all that is consumed including portion sizes and time of day. Studies show more success occurs when written records are kept of food intake when attempting to normalize food consumption. There are now "blogs" or personal diaries online of individuals' food struggles that all can read. A person's food record may be part of an online program of a commercial weight loss program or may be a free program available on the Internet. (See Appendix E for websites.)

Food for Thought?
When a commercial weight loss program advertises that if we do exactly as the program states, we will lose weight, run the other way! A healthy eating plan to manage body weight should be customized to our individual needs. To achieve this, we must take personal responsibility for creating our own strategy for healthy eating.

What is your opinion? Is there a role for commercial weight loss programs? How would you advise your clients who need to manage their body weight?

*This discussion does not advocate the use of any named commercial diet program.

- **Awareness of the personal perspective of individuals**
Content throughout this text is expressed in a human personal way. This approach, which underlies the philosophy of this text, is reflected by first-hand accounts of the ways in which nutrition affects the lives of both nursing professionals and everyday people. Powerful images of patients and their families emerge as individuals describe in their own words their experiences pursuing health and healing. Each chapter offers a **PERSONAL PERSPECTIVES** box on a related experience.

PERSONAL PERSPECTIVES

A Work in Progress

Sometimes it seems as though I've been on a diet all my life, although I can trace my relationship with my weight back to one crucial day during the year I was 8. My father, having noticed that my 12-year-old brother and I were both approaching the top of our age-weight range, decided to take us to a nutritionist. I am sure that she was nice, but all I remember from the meeting was a deep sense of shame rising up from inside me and a chart that hung on our fridge listing the caloric content of common foods. The idea was that my brother and I were to monitor our eating and keep our daily intake between 1200 and 1800 calories. Although I'm sure he had only the best intentions, to this day I'm not sure what my father expected. Thus began my first diet.

During those awkward middle years, I developed a skewed image of myself. I chose to hear only the teasing and none of the praise and began to believe I would be chubby forever. The summer before my freshman year of high school, I discovered the world of sports, however. In order to try out for the field hockey team, I had to be able to run 3 miles. The coach passed out a training guide to those who signed up, and I followed it to the letter. On the first day of tryouts, I found myself keeping pace alongside the team captain, and my baby fat soon disappeared.

But although I was healthy and in shape, I still obsessed about my weight. Over the next 4 years, I became bulimic. When that didn't work, I would put myself on a regimen of 1000 calories a day, even during field hockey season. I developed irritable-bowel syndrome due to the stress I was placing on my body. When I graduated from high school, I weighed 125 pounds, right in the middle of the recommended weight range for my age, gender, and height. Yet I still saw myself as fat.

During college little changed. I was learning about other aspects of my identity, developing my skills and receiving praise for my talents. I exercised regularly and avoided the "freshman 15." Yet when I looked around at the tall, waiflike young women on my campus, I could not shake my insecurities.

During my junior year of college, I went abroad to Spain. I immersed myself in a culture of home-cooked meals, walking, and late nights. There I dropped below 120 pounds for the first time in my life. I wore a size 4 by the time I left, and I was happy with my body. When I returned home, the attention I received for my new figure boosted my confidence even more. Back in New York City my senior year, I spent thousands of dollars on new clothes. But deep down inside, nothing had changed. Those same anxieties were lying buried, waiting for the opportunity to emerge again. When I look at pictures of myself from that time, I am both scared and in awe of the person I see. Behind the shining surface there is nothing but darkness.

Immediately after college I entered a fast-track program for new teachers in the New York City public school system. My first year teaching was exhausting, both physically and emotionally. I was usually broke, and on my third day of teaching, the World Trade Center was attacked. I could see the smoke from the Twin Towers from my bedroom window in Brooklyn. I gained almost 20 pounds in 10 months.

Over the next 4 years my weight increased steadily until, a year before my wedding, I realized I weighed almost 160 pounds. It was then that I turned to a well-respected weight loss program. Since the thought alone of attending meetings embarrassed me, I signed up online. The first time around, it didn't work for me, but I returned. And through the program, I was forced to be aware of what I ate. More important, I learned portion control. I now consider myself a lifetime member.

I have come to see my body as a work in progress. I don't measure my self-worth based on the numbers on a scale, but I do place a great deal of importance on my health. My struggle with my weight is a part of who I am, but it does not define me. My goal is no longer to fit some idea of who I ought to be, but to feel like my true self: healthy and happy in my skin.
Judith Zaft Grodner
Montclair, New Jersey

- **Comprehension of societal issues that impact health status**
  SOCIAL ISSUES boxes emphasize ethical, social, and community concerns on local, national, and international

levels to reveal the various influences on health and wellness. It is imperative for nursing health care professionals to understand the potential effects of societal issues on the lives and health status of populations served.

SOCIAL ISSUES
Dealing With Our Own Prejudices

We live in a world in which fat intolerance or fat phobia (fear of fat) is the last socially acceptable prejudice. "Fatism" even seems to have similarities with racism. As a society, we are committed to self-improvement. Consequently, it may feel wrong to question the directive that all those who deviate from the ideal size and shape should dedicate themselves to rectifying the situation. Our fat intolerance may be motivated by the best intentions to be helpful to ourselves and to others, but like all prejudices, it diminishes the people to whom it is applied.

This prejudice is especially problematic when it exists among health professionals. Obese people often report they feel degraded by their health care encounters and therefore avoid seeking medical help. The traditional medical model holds the patient responsible for the existence of a health problem; this moralistic philosophy tends to justify blaming the patient for choosing to be fat or thin. Although this prejudice could be expected to interfere with their effectiveness, health professionals seem to possess high levels of fat intolerance. Consider these facts from National Association to Advance Fat Acceptance (NAAFA):

Medical Professionals
In a study of 400 doctors, the following was found:
- One out of three listed obesity as a condition to which they respond negatively, ranked behind only *drug addiction, alcoholism,* and *mental illness.*
- Obesity was associated with *noncompliance, hostility, dishonesty,* and *poor hygiene*
- Self-report studies show that doctors view obese patients as *lazy, lacking in self-control, noncompliant, unintelligent, weak-willed,* and *dishonest.*
- Psychologists ascribe more pathology, more negative and severe symptoms, and worse prognosis to obese patients

compared to thinner patients presenting identical psychological profiles.
In a survey of 2449 overweight and obese women, the following was found:
- 69% experienced bias from doctors.
- 52% experienced recurring incidents of bias.
In one survey of nurses, the following was found:
- 31% said they would prefer not to care for obese patients.
- 24% said that obese patients "repulsed them."
- 12% said they would prefer not to touch obese patients.

Consequences
- Avoidance of proper care
- Reluctant to seek medical care
- Cancellation or delay of medical appointments
- Delay important preventative health care
- Doctors seeing overweight patients:
Spend less time with patient
Engage in less discussion
Show reluctance to perform preventive health screenings (i.e., pelvic exams, cancer screenings, mammograms)
Do less intervention
- Appropriate-sized medical equipment not available:
Stretchers
MRIs
Blood pressure cuffs
Patient gowns
Etc.
What about you? Have you been successful in questioning and replacing your own prejudices? Are you able to accept yourself and your body? As a future health professional, are you prepared to empower your patients to work toward total wellness, including the Health At Every Size (HAES) philosophy and habits?

Data from NAAFA: *Healthcare,* 2009. Accessed February 23, 2010, from http://www.naafaonline.com/dev2/the_issues/health.html.

- **Recognition of educative aspects of nursing**
  Nursing professionals often have a primary role to support clients as they strive to achieve compliance of prescribed therapeutic dietary modifications or just attempt to improve their nutrient intake. **TEACHING TOOL** boxes in every chapter provide strategies for teaching clients about optimum dietary patterns and therapeutic nutrition recommendations.

  When appropriate, specific issues of literacy, such as strategies for enhancing patient education for those with low literacy skills, are also presented in **TEACHING TOOL** boxes.

TEACHING TOOL
Mindless Eating

Based on years of studying the psychology of our food choices and quantities consumed, Dr. Wansink, Cornell University professor of psychology, food marketing and nutrition and Director of the Cornell Food and Brand Lab, has revealed some of the cues and influences that govern our mindless consumption of calories. He notes that "The best diet is the one you don't know you are on." The mindful eating approach may be supportive when working with clients needing to improve their dietary intake. Dr. Wansink suggests that rather than trying to "eat right," try to "eat better."

Your Mindful Eating Plan
- **Your Mindless Margin.** By making 100- to 200-calorie changes in your daily intake, you feel deprived and backslide.
- **Mindless Better Eating.** Focus on reengineering small behaviors that will move you from mindless overeating to mindless better eating. Five common places to look (diet danger zones) include meals, snacks, parties, restaurants, and your desk or dashboard.
- **Mindful Reengineering.** To trim your mindless margin, you can use basic diet tips, but a more personalized approach is to use food trade-offs or food polices. Both give you a chance to eat some of what you want without making it a belabored decision.
- **The Power of Three.** Design three easy, doable changes that you can mindlessly make without much sacrifice.
- **Mindless Margin Checklist.** Use this daily checklist to help you move from mindless overeating to mindless better eating.

Data from Wansink B: Mindless eating: Why we eat more than we think, New York, 2006, Bantam Dell; wwwMindlessEating. org.

- **Recognition of psychosocial strategies for behavior change to achieve wellness**
The **TOWARD A POSITIVE NUTRITION LIFESTYLE** section in each chapter within Parts I, II, and III presents psychosocial strategies to support health behavioral changes for individuals wishing to adopt healthier lifestyles. This section recognizes the multidisciplinary skills needed to apply lifestyle changes for oneself and one's clients/patients.

TOWARD A POSITIVE NUTRITION LIFESTYLE: EXPLANATORY STYLE

In his book *Learned Optimism*, Dr. Martin Seligman, a psychologist and professor, explores applications of explanatory styles to everyday life situations.[23] As a component of personal control, *explanatory style* is the way in which a person regularly explains why events happen. An individual with a pessimistic explanatory style spreads learned helplessness by having a pervasive negative view that no matter what he or she does, nothing will change. In contrast, a person with an optimistic explanatory style feels able to stop the reaction of learned helplessness and understands events in a more positive way. An optimistic person feels competent that he or she can change the course of events.

Explanatory style has been studied in relation to health and wellness. A person's approach to dealing with issues of physical health can be helped or hindered by cognitions about personal control over health conditions and maintenance. Seligman notes the following:[32]

- The way we think, especially about health, changes our health.
- Optimists catch fewer infectious diseases than pessimists do.
- Optimists have better health habits than pessimists do.
- Our immune system may work better when we are optimistic.
- Evidence suggests that optimists live longer than pessimists.

How does this information apply to body fat management? Having an optimistic explanatory style may mean accepting one's body as it is and acting in ways to improve health by attempting to eat well and exercise regularly. A pessimistic explanatory style would judge one's body negatively and would not attempt behaviors to improve body composition because physical attributes would be understood to be permanent and thus unchangeable. Consider other ways that explanatory styles affect the approach of our patients toward their illnesses and the effect of our explanatory styles on strategies of nursing care.

- **Focus on the Nursing Process**
THE NURSING APPROACH boxes analyze a realistic nutrition case study from the perspective of the nursing process. By creating situations that may be encountered in clinical practice, the chapter's nutrition subject matter is consistently refocused into a nursing perspective. A **NEW** feature is the addition of discussion questions based on the case study. These can be used for class discussions or as homework assignments. Responses are included for instructors. They are written from a professional nursing perspective and case studies have been revised by author Bonnie C. Walkingshaw, who brings a fresh perspective and years of experience in clinical nursing and patient education.

THE NURSING APPROACH

Low-Fat Project

In preparation for a new wellness and fitness center on the college campus, the new director surveyed students, faculty, and staff about their needs and interests. Results revealed great interest in nutrition. The director met with a committee of students, faculty, and staff to share ideas and plan possible education and communication about nutrition. Ideas included offering nutrition courses, providing speakers for short education sessions, arranging for consulting dietitians, posting nutrition information near the cafeteria menu, disseminating informative posters prepared by various departments on campus, and creating a website to communicate all health- and fitness-related information.

The first nutrition topic chosen by the committee was eating lower-fat foods. Nursing students were assigned to create posters and contributions for the website. Their task was to identify the following important questions for discussion:

1. Why is it beneficial to reduce total fat intake to about 30% of the daily kcal? How many kcal are produced by 1 g of fat? How many grams of fat are in food commonly consumed?
2. Why should saturated fats be limited to 10% or less of daily kcal? What are the potential harmful effects of saturated fats and cholesterol? Which foods contain saturated fats? Which animal products should be limited?
3. What are trans fats, and what are the disadvantages of consuming them? How can they be avoided? Is butter or margarine healthier?
4. What are common food sources of monounsaturated and polyunsaturated fats? What is the best salad oil? What is the best cooking oil?
5. Why are omega-3 fatty acids health promoting? What are food sources of omega-3 fatty acids? Is it more beneficial to eat fish or to take fish oil supplements?
6. How can a consumer purchase healthy low-fat products? How can one interpret the nutrition label?
7. What lower-fat snacks and desserts can be substituted for high-kcal, high-fat and high-sugar snacks and desserts?
8. Which fast foods and restaurant meals are lower in fat?
9. What are the benefits and drawbacks of artificial fat substitutes?
10. What food preparation techniques are best for low-fat eating? How can recipes be modified to make them lower in fat?
11. What is the plate method? How can this method help with portion control?
12. What websites have good information about lowering fat in the diet?

After identifying these questions, the students organized into groups. Questions were divided and assigned to individual groups. Students researched the answers to the questions and then each group created programming for the center. The resulting programs were reviewed by a subcommittee that then compiled all the programs into a coherent project.

Supplementary Materials

The extensive ancillary package accompanying this text contains a wealth of materials for both instructors and students. The instructor materials and student materials are available online only. All online materials can be accessed on the Evolve website: **http://evolve.elsevier.com/Grodner/foundations**.

For Instructors:

- **Instructor's Manual (Online):** Each chapter contains a separate file with Learning Objectives, Key Concepts, a Detailed Chapter Outline, Learning Activities (Application Questions and Issues and Discussion Topics), and Critical Thinking Activities.
- **Test Bank (Online):** Each chapter contains approximately 30 NCLEX-style examination questions with textbook page references, for a total of approximately 670 questions. For this edition, all questions have been reviewed and revised as needed.
- **PowerPoint Presentations (Online):** The authors have developed PowerPoint text slides—approximately 30 per chapter—to guide classroom lectures of each content area within the book.
- **Image Collection (Online):** Approximately 70 photographs, illustrations, and tables from the textbook are provided in an online collection available for download into a variety of instructor materials.
- **Media Resources (Online):** This focused listing of print and electronic resources is provided for instructors seeking to access or direct students to additional sources of nutrition-related information.
- **Answers to Student Activities (Online):** Answers and guidelines to questions posed both in the textbook and online (*Applying Content Knowledge, Critical Thinking: Clinical Applications, Quick Review and The Nursing Approach*) are provided on the instructor portion of the website and can be made available on the student website at the instructor's discretion.

For Students:

- **Additional Virtual Case Studies (Online):** Video clips of six fictitious patients—including one with type 2 diabetes mellitus, one with a respiratory infection, and one with HIV/AIDS wasting syndrome—are accompanied by written case studies; short answer and essay questions; NCLEX-formatted, multiple-choice, examination-style questions; and Internet assignments. This exciting feature provides students with realistic clinical practice.

- *Applying Content Knowledge* **Questions (Online):** One case and question per chapter are provided online, in addition to the cases and questions contained within the foundation and life-cycle chapters of the textbook (Chapters 1-13).
- *Critical Thinking: Clinical Applications* **Questions (Online):** One case study with accompanying application questions is provided online for each of the clinical chapters (Chapters 14-22), in addition to the cases and questions contained within those same textbook chapters.
- *Quick Review* **Questions (Online):** Approximately 5 to 10 short-answer questions per chapter are supplied online.
- **Matching Exercises (Online):** Key terms and definitions within each textbook chapter become fun and interactive practice online. Immediate feedback is provided.
- **Food Composition Table (Online):** This table is again offered online to add a user-friendly search function. It provides a detailed listing of all the nutrients in each of the more than 3700 food items contained within the *Nutritrac Nutrition Analysis Software,* Version IV, CD-ROM (see detailed description below).
- **WebLinks (Online):** A robust listing of online links to relevant nutrition websites is conveniently organized by chapter and updated periodically.
- *Nutritrac Nutrition Analysis Program, Version 5.0* **(Online):** The new edition of this popular tool is designed to allow the user to calculate and analyze food intake and energy expenditure, taking the guesswork out of nutrition planning. The new version features comprehensive databases containing more than 5000 foods organized into 18 different categories and more than 175 common/ daily recreational, sporting, and occupational activities. The *Personal Profile* feature allows users to enter and edit the intake and output of an unlimited number of individuals, and the *Weight Management Planner* helps outline healthy lifestyles tailored to various personal profiles. In addition to foods and activities, new program features include an ideal body weight (IBW) calculator, a Harris-Benedict calculator to estimate total daily energy needs, and the complete *Exchange Lists for Meal Planning*.

Nutrition Concepts Online for Grodner/Roth/Walkingshaw: Nutritional Foundations & Clinical Applications: A Nursing Approach. When this icon appears at the beginning of a chapter, it indicates there is a comparable online module that accompanies the chapter. This is an additional item to use with the text.

ACKNOWLEDGMENTS

To the individuals who shared their stories with us in the *Personal Perspective* boxes, our gratitude for your willingness to educate nursing professionals through your experiences. We acknowledge Gregory Annese, Yetta Kaemmer, Judith Zaft Grodner, and Tanya Popovetsky.

SPECIAL ACKNOWLEDGMENTS

Although this book is quite respectable having reached the fifth edition, it is still young at heart and relevant because of the efforts of the staff of Elsevier. Under the guidance of Yvonne Alexopoulos, Senior Editor, we were motivated to update features and to introduce new technology to support instructors as they enhance the learning experiences of their students. Lisa Newton, Senior Developmental Editor, supervised our progress with great civility when deadlines were unexpectedly missed. Special thanks to John Gabbert, Project Manager, whose production and organizational skills allowed for clarity of process and ease of publication; and to Paula Catalano, Senior Design Manager, for the fresh design concept of this edition.

In addition, we want to acknowledge the work of the Nursing Marketing Department for understanding what's special about our concept and for continuing to communicate this to instructors here in North America and internationally.

Writing is most often a solitary act. With projects such as this continually revised textbook, the process becomes a private aspect of self that cannot be shared. To family, friends, and colleagues who are unavoidably inconvenienced by this lengthy process, our apologies. We vow to discover strategies for easing the burden on others while we proceed with this recurring process.

We symbolize a collaboration of expertise in nutrition education, dietetics, and nursing. As we each become more sensitive to the multilayered responsibilities of nurses, we fine-tune our answers to the questions of "What do nurses need to know about nutrition?" and "How would they apply this knowledge to their patients and clients?" This edition reflects our ever-evolving responses to these questions.

Michele Grodner
Sara Long Roth
Bonnie C. Walkingshaw

CONTENTS

Wellness, Nutrition, and the Nursing Role

Wellness Nutrition

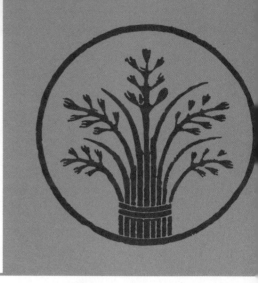

Achieving wellness is a continuous, never-ending journey.

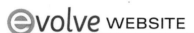 WEBSITE

http://evolve.elsevier.com/Grodner/foundations/

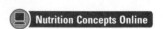 **Nutrition Concepts Online**

ROLE IN WELLNESS

Wellness is a lifestyle through which we continually strive to enhance our level of health. This text provides information, strategies, and techniques about food, nutrition, and health. These tools allow nurses and clients to achieve wellness through personal nutrition lifestyles.

Nutrition is a hot topic that generates interest easily; everyone seems to have opinions about what to eat and concerns about their own eating styles. The public is flooded with information and techniques related to health promotion through nutrition. Health literacy is the ability to acquire and comprehend basic health concepts, such as nutrition, and apply them to one's own health decisions.[1]

So how does health literacy develop? It is not the same as literacy of the printed word, although it is related. Health literacy develops through education on topics related to health promotion and illness. This process of education occurs in three different forms: formal, nonformal, and informal. *Formal education* is purposefully planned for implementation in a school setting. *Nonformal education* takes place through organized teaching and learning events in hospitals, clinics, and community centers. *Informal education* encompasses a variety of educational experiences that occur through daily activities. These informal experiences may include watching television, reading newspapers and magazines, browsing the Internet, and conversing with other people. Health information from many sources becomes part of an individual's database of knowledge. Some information may be valid, some may be partially true, and some may be completely false. Our goal is to ensure that health decisions are based on accurate information.

Health literacy allows for education to be most effective, resulting in behavior changes. Nurses, through formal, nonformal, and informal educational interactions, can introduce knowledge and strategies for personal lifestyle choices that consider the health context of patients' lives.[2] Health context takes into account the influence of cultural, social, and individual factors on the acquisition of health literacy. Cultural factors may encompass ethnic, religious, and racial traditions surrounding health issues. Social factors create the settings for which members of a community receive support or lack support for health-promoting behaviors. Individual factors reflect on the choices people make regarding willingness to acquire and then apply health knowledge. Health literacy actualization means being able to use acquired health knowledge and skills. The extent to which this occurs within health care settings is influenced by the level to which health care providers are supportive of literate health populations seeking greater involvement in their health care (Figure 1-1).

Nurses are involved with the development of client health literacy (see the *Teaching Tool* box Literacy and Health). Formal education may be conducted by school nurses who teach health courses; topics can be approached through the health and nutrition issues of the ethnic and cultural groups of the particular school's population. Nonformal education occurs when associations such as the American Heart Association or hospital wellness programs teach courses on risk-reducing lifestyle changes; these courses are usually open to the community. Informal education takes place when a nurse chats with a patient and his or her family, explaining the purpose of the dietary modifications recommended for the patient's particular disorder.

Never before have we had so much information about the effects of our personal behavior patterns on our level of health. Changing (or maintaining) our patterns of behaviors—and therefore our lifestyles—is the key to achieving wellness. Many social, community, and occupational forces affect our ability to change. Strategies and techniques ease our ability to modify our personal behaviors.

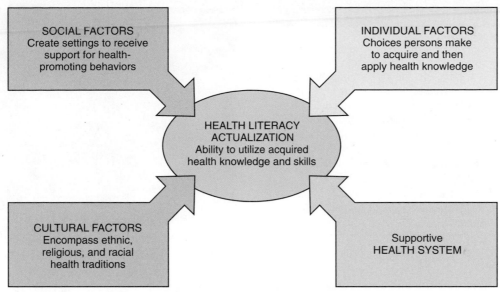

FIG 1-1 Health literacy context.

Modifying behaviors means changing lifestyles. Because this book is about food and nutrition, patterns of behaviors affecting the foods we choose to eat constitute our nutrition lifestyles. Not all of us have the same nutrition lifestyles. Some of us are caught up in extremely hectic work, college, or sports schedules; we're lucky to find time to eat at all. Others find our families of origin still at the center of our eating patterns; our families, however, may not have adopted recent recommendations to decrease the risks of diet-related diseases. Many of us are part of new social settings on campus and need to adjust to rigid schedules and school cafeteria menus. Yet, despite these variances, we have in common the ability to improve wellness through our nutrition lifestyles.

As health care professionals, we need to be concerned with our own nutritional patterns as well as those of our clients. To reflect a health promotion perspective, individuals cared for by health professionals to maintain health are called *clients*. Those who are ill or recuperating from illness are called *patients*.

Enhancing personal health provides the stamina and well-being to fulfill the rigorous demands of the nursing practice. A fundamental responsibility of nursing is client education. When teaching clients about nutritional wellness, nurses also function as role models for the positive effects of enhanced nutrition lifestyles.

DEFINITION OF HEALTH

In the past, *health* was defined as the absence of disease or illness. Modern medicine has conquered many life-threatening diseases, such as smallpox and polio. Public health measures of pasteurization and sanitation have reduced the risk of foodborne and environmental hazards. As concern about the physical status of the human body has lessened, we've been able to consider other aspects of the qualities of health.

One of the first expanded definitions of *health* was provided by the World Health Organization (WHO): "Health is a state of complete physical, mental, and social well-being and not merely the absence of disease and infirmity."[3] Although this definition addresses the concern that health is more than just the absence of disease, health is presented as a static concept that individuals achieve.

A more expanded definition of health was presented by Rene Dubos, biologist and philosopher, who wrote, "Health is a quality of life involving social, emotional, mental, spiritual, and biologic fitness on the part of the individual, which results from adaptations to the environment."[4] This view leads to our present understanding of health as a complex concept best represented by physical and psychologic dimensions, as follows:

- *Physical health:* The efficiency of the body to function appropriately, to maintain immunity to disease, and to meet daily energy requirements
- *Intellectual health:* The use of intellectual abilities to learn and to adapt to changes in one's environment
- *Emotional health:* The capacity to easily express or suppress emotions appropriately
- *Social health:* The ability to interact with people in an acceptable manner and sustain relationships with family members, friends, and colleagues
- *Spiritual health:* The cultural beliefs that give purpose to human existence, found through faith in the teachings of organized religions, in an understanding of nature or science, or in an acceptance of the humanistic view of life

Health is the merging and balancing of the five physical and psychological dimensions of health: physical, mental, emotional, social, and spiritual. This holistic view incorporates many aspects of human existence. Using this definition of health allows more individualized assessment of health status. As our own health and the health of our clients are evaluated in relation to each dimension, some dimensions will be stronger than others (see the *Teaching Tool* box Dimensions of Health).

✴ TEACHING TOOL
Dimensions of Health

To broaden a patient's understanding of health, use the five dimensions of health. Describe the dimensions and then discuss with the patient each that pertains to his or her nutrition and health situation. By exploring aspects of health other than physical health, a person can then use all resources to restore the overall level of well-being.

Wellness through the Five Dimensions of Health
1. *Physical health:* Efficient body functioning
2. *Intellectual health:* Use of intellectual abilities
3. *Emotional health:* Ability to control emotions
4. *Social health:* Interactions and relationships with others
5. *Spiritual health:* Cultural beliefs about the purpose of life

 ## Role of Nutrition

Nutrition is the study of nutrients and the processes by which they are used by the body. **Nutrients** are substances in foods required by the body for energy, growth, maintenance, and repair. Some nutrients are essential; they cannot be made by the human body and must be provided by foods.

Because the primary role of nutrients is to provide the building blocks for efficient functioning and maintenance of the body, nutrition may appear to belong only within the physical health dimension. However, the effects of nutrients and their sources on the other health dimensions are far reaching. Nutrition is the cornerstone of each health dimension.

Physical health is dependent on the quantity and quality of nutrients available to the body. The human body, from skeletal bones to minute amounts of hormones, is composed of nutrients in various combinations.

Intellectual health relies on a well-functioning brain and central nervous system. Nutritional imbalances can affect intellectual health, as occurs with iron deficiency anemia. Although milk is an excellent source of protein, calcium, and phosphorus, it provides a negligible amount of iron. Some young children drink so much milk that it affects their appetite for other foods such as meats, chicken, legumes, and leafy green vegetables, all of which are good sources of iron. As a result, iron deficiency may affect children with nutritional imbalances. The cognitive abilities of iron-deficient children may be affected, which could lead to possible learning problems.

Emotional health may be affected by poor eating habits, resulting in hypoglycemia or low blood glucose levels. Low blood glucose occurs normally in anyone who is physically hungry. When the body's need for food is ignored (e.g., when we miss meals because of poor planning or are too busy to eat), feelings of anxiety and confusion and trembling may occur. Emotions may be harder to control when we feel this way. Although blood glucose levels may affect our emotions, there are, of course, other factors that influence emotional health.

Social health situations often center around food-related occasions, ranging from holiday feasts to everyday meals.

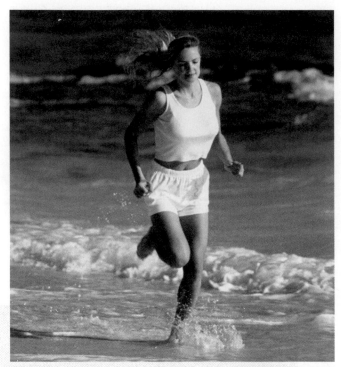

Physical health benefits from a good diet. (From Photos.com.)

Nutritional status is sometimes affected by the quality of our relationships with family and friends. Are family meals an enjoyable experience or a tense ordeal? How might this affect a person's dietary intake?

Spiritual health often has ties to food. Several religions prohibit the consumption of specific foods. Many followers of Islam and Judaism adhere to the dietary laws of their religions. Both forbid consumption of pork products. Seventh Day Adventists follow an ovo-lacto vegetarian diet in which they consume only plant foods and dairy products. In India cows are viewed as sacred, not to be eaten but revered as a source of sustenance (milk), fuel (burning of feces), power (as a work animal), and fertilizer (manure).

HEALTH PROMOTION

Health promotion consists of strategies used to increase the level of the health of individuals, families, groups, and communities. In community and occupational health settings, health promotion strategies implemented by nurses often focus on lifestyle changes that will lead to new, positive health behaviors. Development of positive behaviors may depend on knowledge, techniques, and community supports, as follows (see the *Teaching Tool* box Literacy and Health):

- *Knowledge:* Learning new information about the benefits or risks of health-related behaviors
- *Techniques:* Applying new knowledge to everyday activities; developing ways to modify current lifestyles
- *Community supports:* Availability of environmental or regulatory measures to support new health-promoting behaviors within a social context

Literacy and Health

Although health professionals may take their high level of literacy for granted, many clients do not have command of basic literacy skills. Limited literacy skills often equates with even more limited health literacy (the ability to use health information to make appropriate health decisions) and with limited numeracy (the ability to understand simple math concepts and apply them in everyday life situations). In fact, low reading skills are associated with poor health and increased use of health services. The implications of these limitations are important because a nurse's efforts to educate clients to increase their knowledge and compliance may not be effective.

Health literacy affects patient care in many ways (only a few are mentioned here). Simply filling out medical history and consent forms can leave patients struggling. Patients may also have difficulty explaining their symptoms because of limited vocabulary. They may not understand the medical terminology health care providers use to discuss health conditions but may be too uncomfortable to ask for clarification. Even if understood, the recommendations given to clients may be difficult to implement because their ability to decode or understand food labels is limited. Following cooking directions may be hard, and serving sizes may be misinterpreted. If clients are to track carbohydrate or sodium consumption, reading literacy and numeracy limitations may hinder accuracy and may foster discouragement or worsening of symptoms.

Throughout this textbook, strategies are provided for working with low-literacy clients, discussing the cultural connection, and evaluating and writing health education materials—all with the goal of enhancing health outcomes.

Data from Rothman R: *Health literacy: Communicating effective verbal and written nutrition messages* (presentation), St. Louis, October 23, 2005, American Dietetic Association Food & Nutrition Conference & Expo (FNCE).

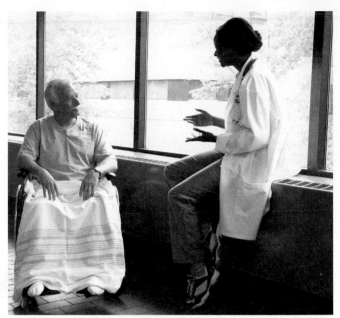

Nutrition is an integral part of health care education. (From Photos.com)

Role of Nutrition

For more than 30 years, national health targets have been set. In 1979 the first initiative, the Surgeon General's report titled *Healthy People*, laid out life-stage targets that continue to be tracked today. Since then, health targets have been updated every 10 years through collaboration among the government, voluntary and professional health associations, businesses, and individuals under the direction of the secretary of the Department of Health and Human Services. The objectives focus on the decisions and policies that affect prevention efforts and create a standard from which to later assess the performance of meeting these goals. In addition, the inter-relatedness of the health of communities and individuals is emphasized. The health status of an individual is dependent on the health supports accessible within the community. (This theme is also discussed in Chapter 2 under the heading "Community Nutrition.")

The target results of the previous report are used to develop the next set of target goals. Data generated by *Healthy People 2010 (HP2010)* are being used to develop the next set of national health targets, *Healthy People 2020 (HP2020)*.

HP2020 is guided by a framework based on the vision of "a society in which all people live long, healthy lives."[5] The mission is "to improve health through strengthening policy and practice."[5] Four overarching goals present pathways to achieve the vision and mission. Details of the *HP2020* framework are listed in Box 1-1.

The Action Model to Achieve *Healthy People 2020* Overarching Goals (Figure 1-2) suggests priorities for change based on determinants of health such as living and working conditions, as well as individual behaviors as affected by the traits of individuals such as age, sex, race, and biological factors. The implementations of strategies are assessed by their outcomes. The outcomes are then evaluated, distributed, and used to create additional interventions.[5] These actions will bring us as a nation closer to achieving the goals by 2020.

Nutrition Monitoring

The nutritional status of the American population is monitored through several ongoing surveys. The National Nutrition Monitoring Act of 1990 provides for collaboration among government organizations that conduct national surveys of the nation's health and nutritional status. This collaboration supports the use of similar standards and research methods so the surveys' findings can be compared.

Two ongoing research projects that focus on nutritional status are the National Health and Nutrition Examination Survey (NHANES) and the National Food Consumption Surveys (NFCS). NHANES focuses on data from the dietary intake, medical history, biochemical evaluation, physical examinations, and measurements of American population groups who are carefully chosen to represent the total

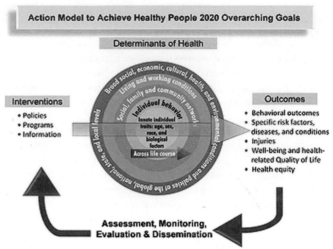

FIG 1-2 Action Model for achieving HP2020 Overarching Goals. To close the gap between where we are now as a nation and where we would like to be by the year 2020, *Healthy People 2020* must provide clear priorities for action (i.e., it should articulate "what" needs to be done) and focused strategies for addressing them (i.e., it should explain "how" this work should be carried out). (From U.S. Department of Health and Human Services, Public Health Service: *Phase 1 Report: Recommendations for the framework and format of Healthy People 2020.* Accessed July 2009 from www.healthypeople.gov/HP2020/advisory/Phase1/summary.htm.

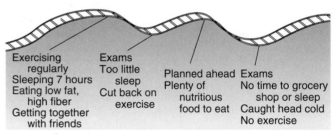

FIG 1-3 Wellness effort roller coaster. (From Rolin Graphics.)

population. Approximately every 10 years, the NFCS surveys subgroups of the American population to monitor nutrient intake. Records of food intake for 2 days are kept. These nutrient values are then compared with recommended dietary standards.

DEFINITION OF *WELLNESS*

Wellness is a lifestyle (pattern of behaviors) that enhances our level of health. This occurs by developing each of the five dimensions of health. Individuals engaged in wellness lifestyles feel a sense of competency and achievement in their ability to modify their behaviors to increase or maintain positive levels of health.

Hectic contemporary schedules may seem to interfere with efforts to achieve wellness. The aim is to strive for wellness even if the path may seem more like a roller coaster than a smooth uphill climb (Figure 1-3). At times, clients may falter in their efforts, but the key is to renew positive behaviors as soon as possible.

Role of Nutrition

"Wellness nutrition" approaches food consumption as a positive way to nourish the body. This approach focuses on ways to organize our lives so we can more easily follow an eating pattern designed to enhance health status. Consuming a diet based on lower fat and higher fiber and moderate caloric consumption is then not a chore but rather an affirmation of our competency to care for ourselves. Conveying this approach to clients is a nursing challenge (see the *Personal Perspectives* box Getting Back to "Great" Again).

DISEASE PREVENTION THROUGH NUTRITION

Disease prevention is the recognition of a danger to health that could be reduced or alleviated through specific actions or changes in lifestyle behaviors. The hazard may be caused by disease, lifestyle, or genetic factors, or an environmental threat. The three classifications of disease prevention are primary, secondary, and tertiary. Disease prevention has strong ties to nutrition (see the *Cultural Considerations* box Healthy People and Culturally Competent Care).

PERSONAL PERSPECTIVES

Getting Back to "Great" Again

This section in each chapter features an individual's viewpoint about a nutrition or health issue. Sometimes the viewpoint may represent a composite of opinions on a topic. Here, a recent university graduate shares his story of getting back to the feeling of "great" again.

I was a very athletic kid in high school. I played sports, worked out, and played drums (my favorite cardio activity) all the time. I wasn't the biggest or best at anything, but I felt great every day. I didn't drink or smoke much; I just liked to have fun and play sports. At the end of my senior year, I was in the greatest shape of my life. I was at my best.

Let's fast-forward to May of my senior year of college. I drank a lot every weekend. I smoked more in a week than most have in a lifetime. I never got up to do anything other than go to class or eat. Now I knew little by little throughout college I was losing that feeling of "great" I had in high school. I was out of it all the time, eating crap food and simply not caring about my body. I'm a thin guy, so it wasn't showing on the outside, but it sure as hell was showing on the inside. I always had a sore throat from smoking, and my stomach was constantly hurting from the munchies and eating junk food. My back actually started to hurt my senior year; it was seriously from sitting on my butt and not moving for hours every day.

By graduation, I felt like crap. How was I ever going to stop? Shortly before graduation, I said to myself, "Self, you can keep this up until you go home. When you go home, it's time to cut the crap. No more smoking and no more eating junk foods every day. You are going to be living with your parents, and you are going to have a job. You have to be at your best again." And it was really weird, too, because that night I had a dream where I looked at myself in the mirror and I was all cut and muscular.

Now I am at my best again. It's August. I made a 100% turnaround since May. I only eat six or seven small meals a day of healthy foods and lift weights exercising almost daily. The feeling of "great" is back.

It takes a lot of mental toughness to change. Just listen to my message. Cut out the negative stuff and bring in the good stuff, and YOU WILL BE AT YOUR BEST, yet again.

Greg Annese
Westwood, N.J.

CULTURAL CONSIDERATIONS

Healthy People *and Culturally Competent Care*

Lifestyle and behavior are central to the maintenance of health and wellness. To influence lifestyle and behavior, health professionals need to take into account the values, attitudes, culture, and life circumstances of individuals. Changes in health status, particularly of minority populations, require professionals to take into account the increasing ethnic/cultural diversity of Americans. There are four recognized minority groups in the United States: Asian/Pacific Islanders, African Americans, Hispanic Americans, and Native Americans. Currently, it is estimated that one in five Americans belongs to a minority group. Minority populations are projected to grow to one third of the population by the year 2050.

Healthy People reports document that the number of premature and excess deaths of ethnic minority populations far outweigh the majority groups. Research shows the factors contributing to this are complex and involve multiple factors. Socioeconomic status among minority groups is generally lower than Caucasian majority groups. Socioeconomic status is measured by the combination of occupation, income, and educational attainment. A second major factor is the use of and access to health care programs by minorities. Many of the available health programs are not culturally relevant or sensitive to the minority populations they serve. There is a paucity of bilingual and bicultural health professionals, and health education materials are generally not culturally specific.

Application to Nursing: Diet and nutrition assessment is imperative to provide culturally competent care. Efforts to understand dietary patterns of clients need to go beyond relying on their membership in a defined group. For example, by learning the assimilative practices of an individual, nurses can assist dietitians in developing the most effective and culturally sensitive medical nutrition therapy recommendations. Together they can develop a treatment regimen that does not conflict with cultural food practices of the client.

(hypertension) are sodium sensitive, and simply reducing the amount of sodium consumed can decrease blood pressure levels and thus bring the disorder under control. Because hypertension is a risk factor for coronary artery disease, stroke, and renal disease, reduction of blood pressure through decreased sodium consumption is a secondary prevention strategy.

Tertiary prevention occurs after a disorder develops. The purpose is to minimize further complications or to assist in the restoration of health. These efforts may involve continued medical care. Often, learning more about the disorder is helpful for patients and their families. Tertiary prevention frequently involves diet therapy. Direct treatments of many disorders have a dietary component. Some of these disorders include ulcers, diverticulitis, and coronary artery disease; they usually occur during the middle and older years of adulthood. Other disorders may affect food intake and the ability of the body to absorb nutrients. For example, chemotherapy for cancer may have the side effects of nausea and loss of

Primary prevention consists of activities to avert the initial development of a disease or poor health. A primary disease prevention approach is to eat a variety of foods to avert nutrient deficiencies. Adopting a low-fat, high-fiber eating style before diet-related health problems develop is a form of primary prevention.

Secondary prevention involves early detection to halt or reduce the effects of a disease or illness. Some diseases cannot be prevented, but early detection can minimize negative health effects. Secondary prevention strategies are useful to reduce the effects of chronic diet-related diseases. Controlling the intake of certain nutrients can decrease the severity of some disorders. Some individuals with high blood pressure appetite. Nutrition counseling during and after these treatments is necessary so patients are as well nourished as possible to aid the healing process. The five dimensions of health can be an excellent teaching tool in promoting health and preventing diseases related to nutrition.

OVERVIEW OF NUTRIENTS WITHIN THE BODY

Which nutrients are the cornerstones of health and disease prevention? What do they do to make them so important? Why can't we just take a nutrient pill?

Nutrient Categories

Nutrients can be divided into the following six categories:
1. Carbohydrates
2. Proteins
3. Lipids (fats)
4. Vitamins
5. Minerals
6. Water

Nutrients may be either essential or nonessential, depending on whether the body can manufacture them. When the body requires a nutrient for growth or maintenance but lacks the ability to manufacture amounts sufficient to meet the body's needs, the nutrient is *essential* and must be supplied by the foods in our diet. Table 1-1 lists the essential nutrients needed in our diet. Other nutrients that the body can make are called *nonessential*. Some nutrients have very specific functions, whereas others are diverse in their impact. Overall the functions of essential nutrients in the body include the following:

- *Providing energy*
  - Carbohydrates, proteins, and lipids provide energy.
  - Vitamins and minerals have indirect roles as catalysts for the body's use of energy nutrients.
- *Regulating body processes*
  - Proteins, lipids, vitamins, minerals, and water are required.
  - Each vitamin serves a specific function related to regulation.
- *Aiding growth and repair of body tissues*
  - Proteins, lipids, minerals, and water are essential for growth and repair.

FOOD, ENERGY, AND NUTRIENTS

Although the discussion to this point has focused on nutrients, we must remember that nutrients are found in foods. Because foods usually contain a mixture of nutrients, we often categorize a food based on the most predominant nutrient found in the food. A bagel is a carbohydrate food and contains mostly complex carbohydrates, although it also contains protein, water, small amounts of vitamins and minerals, and an even smaller amount of lipids or fat (Figure 1-4). The gold mine of nutrients found in whole foods is one of the reasons why taking a nutrient-specific pill will not provide for all the necessities of the human body.

TABLE 1-1	KNOWN ESSENTIAL NUTRIENTS
NUTRIENT	**SOURCE**
Carbohydrates	Glucose
Lipids (fats)	Linoleic acid, linolenic acid
Protein	Amino acids: histidine, isoleucine, leucine, lysine, methionine, phenylalanine, threonine, tryptophan, valine
Vitamins	Fat-soluble vitamins: A (retinol), D (cholecalciferol), E (tocopherol), K
	Water-soluble vitamins: thiamine, riboflavin, niacin, pantothenic acid, biotin, B_6 (pyridoxine), B_{12} (cobalamin), folate, C (ascorbic acid)
Minerals	Major minerals: calcium, phosphorus, sodium, potassium, sulfur, chlorine, magnesium
	Trace minerals: chromium, cobalt, copper, fluorine, iodine, iron, manganese, selenium, zinc
Water	Water

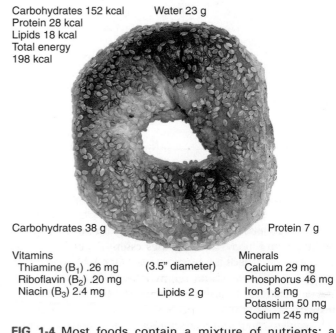

Carbohydrates 152 kcal
Protein 28 kcal
Lipids 18 kcal
Total energy 198 kcal

Water 23 g

Carbohydrates 38 g

Protein 7 g

Vitamins
Thiamine (B_1) .26 mg
Riboflavin (B_2) .20 mg
Niacin (B_3) 2.4 mg

(3.5" diameter)

Lipids 2 g

Minerals
Calcium 29 mg
Phosphorus 46 mg
Iron 1.8 mg
Potassium 50 mg
Sodium 245 mg

FIG 1-4 Most foods contain a mixture of nutrients; a food's kcal content is based on the energy-yielding nutrients it contains. (From Photos.com. Data from U.S. Department of Agriculture, Agricultural Research Service: *USDA national nutrient database for standard reference*, Release 21, Washington, DC, 2008, Nutrient Data Laboratory: www.nal.usda.gov/fnic/foodcomp.)

TABLE 1-2	KCALORIC VALUES
NUTRIENT	**KCAL VALUE PER GRAM**
Carbohydrates	4
Protein	4
Lipids (fats)	9
Alcohol	7

Energy

Let's consider the energy-containing nutrients of carbohydrates, protein, and lipids. These contain energy because they are organic. Being organic means they are composed of a structure that consists of hydrogen, oxygen, and carbon. Living or once-living things, including plants and animals, produce organic compounds. The carbon-containing structure identifies these nutrients as being organic. When these nutrients are oxidized (burned in the body), energy is released and available for use by the cells. Although vitamins are also organic, they do not provide energy for the human body. Only carbohydrates, proteins, and lipids are energy-yielding nutrients.

The energy released from food is measured in kilocalories (thousands of calories) or calories. Technically, a calorie is the amount of heat necessary to raise the temperature of a gram of water by $1°$ C ($0.8°$ F). When someone asks how much energy is in an 8-ounce glass of skim milk, the correct response is 90,000 calories or 90 kilocalories. For numeric simplicity, we commonly refer to the calories in a food rather than the correct term of *kilocalories*. To ensure accuracy, the term *kilocalories* (kcal) is used throughout this text.

Energy-yielding nutrients provide different amounts of energy (Table 1-2). Carbohydrates and protein each provide 4 kcal per gram. Lipids contain more than twice as much energy as carbohydrates or protein by providing 9 kcal per gram. The kcal content of a specific food—for example, a bagel—is based on the amount of carbohydrate, lipid, and protein energy contained in the food (see Figure 1-4). When we consume energy-yielding foods, we usually ingest other nutrients as well, including vitamins, minerals, and water.

Another energy-yielding substance is alcohol. Alcohol provides 7 kcal per gram. Although alcohol provides energy, it is not considered a nutrient because the body does not need it. In fact, when consumed in excess, the body treats alcohol as a toxin. Breaking down or metabolizing alcohol is not only stressful to the body but also uses essential nutrients that could be better used to nourish the body. Moderate consumption of alcohol, however, may be protective for heart disease. The beneficial components of alcohol-containing beverages such as red wine are alcohol plus phytochemicals—nonnutritive plant substances found in the ingredients (red grapes) used to produce the alcoholic beverages.

Moderate use of alcohol is defined as two servings or fewer per day for men and one serving for women. One serving of alcohol equals 12 ounces *beer*, 5 ounces *wine*, or 1.5 ounces 80-proof *spirits*. Alcohol should be avoided if any of the following apply: driving a vehicle, pregnant or breastfeeding, contraindicated while taking certain medications, or contraindicated due to medical conditions.

Although protein, lipids, and carbohydrates provide energy, they—along with the other three nutrient categories of vitamins, minerals, and water—have other important functions. A brief introduction to each nutrient category follows.

Carbohydrates

Carbohydrates are a major source of fuel. They consist of simple carbohydrates, often called sugars, and complex carbohydrates that include starch and most fiber. Simple carbohydrates are found in fruits, milk, and all sweeteners, including white and brown sugar, honey, and high-fructose corn syrup. Complex carbohydrates are found in cereals, grains, pastas, fruits, and vegetables. All, except fiber, are broken down to units of glucose, which is one of the simple carbohydrates. Glucose provides the most efficient form of energy for the body, particularly for muscles and the brain.

Most fiber cannot be broken down by the human digestive system; therefore, it provides little, if any, energy. However, consuming fiber is necessary for good health. Dietary fiber provides several beneficial effects on the digestive and absorptive systems of the body. These effects range from preventing constipation to possibly reducing the risk of colon cancer and heart disease.

Proteins

Proteins, in addition to providing energy, perform an extensive range of functions in the body. Some of these functions include roles in the structure of bones, muscles, enzymes, hormones, blood, the immune system, and cell membranes. The linking of amino acids in various combinations forms proteins. Twenty amino acids are required to create all the necessary proteins to maintain life. Some amino acids are formed by the body, whereas others, called *essential amino acids,* must be consumed in foods. The nine essential amino acids are found in animal and plant sources. Animal sources include meat, fish, poultry, and some dairy products such as milk and cheeses. Plant sources include grains, legumes (peas and beans that contain protein), seeds, nuts, and many vegetables (albeit in small amounts).

Although protein is important nutritionally, eating too much of it can be a problem. Eating substantially more than the recommended amounts of protein does not produce superhumans. Instead, our physical systems can become overworked. Excess protein is broken down to amino acids. The amino acids are then used for energy or broken down further in metabolic processes and either are stored as body fat or excreted through the kidneys in urine.

Lipids (Fats)

Fats are the densest form of energy available in foods and as stored energy in our bodies. Fats, or lipids, serve other purposes, such as functioning as a component of all cell structures, having a role in the production of hormones, and providing padding to protect body organs. Essential fatty acids and the fat-soluble vitamins A, D, E, and K are found in food lipids. It is the fats in certain foods that make them taste so appealing.

Lipids are divided into three categories: triglycerides, phospholipids, and sterols. Triglycerides are called *saturated, monounsaturated,* or *polyunsaturated fats* based on the types of fatty acids they contain. Fatty acids are carbon chains of varying lengths and degrees of hydrogen saturation. The most common phospholipid is lecithin; among sterols, we hear most about cholesterol. Although we consume lecithin and cholesterol in food, our bodies manufacture them as well.

Fats and cholesterol are often in the news. Saturated fats or triglycerides found in some fat-containing foods, *trans* fats from processed fats, and dietary cholesterol are associated with increased blood lipid levels. Elevated blood lipid levels, whether formed by our bodies or consumed in dietary sources, make up a risk factor for the development of coronary artery disease. Saturated fats, and to a certain extent polyunsaturated fats, also have been associated with increased risk for certain cancers. Coronary artery disease and cancer are serious public health diseases that affect millions of North Americans. Consequently, medical and health professionals emphasize the need to reduce intake of foods that contain fats and cholesterol.

Vitamins

Vitamins are compounds that indirectly assist other nutrients through the complete processes of digestion, absorption, metabolism, and excretion. Thirteen vitamins are needed by the body, and each has a specific function. As noted earlier, vitamins provide no energy but assist in the release of energy from carbohydrates, lipids, and proteins.

Vitamins are divided into two classes based on their solubility (i.e., ability to dissolve) in water. The water-soluble vitamins include the B vitamins (thiamine, niacin, riboflavin, folate, cobalamin [B_{12}], pyridoxine [B_6], pantothenic acid, and biotin) and vitamin C. The fat-soluble vitamins, which dissolve in fats, are vitamins A, D, E, and K.

Vitamins are found in many foods; fruits and vegetables are particularly good sources. Because some foods are better sources of specific vitamins, eating a variety of foods is the best way to consume sufficient amounts.

Minerals

Minerals serve structural purposes (e.g., bones and teeth) in the body and are found in body fluids. Minerals in body fluids affect the nature of the fluids, which in turn influence muscle function and the central nervous system. Sixteen essential minerals are divided into two categories: major minerals and trace minerals. Although this distinction is based on the quantity of minerals required by the body, each is equally important.

Minerals are plentiful in fruits, vegetables, dairy products, meats, and legumes. Although minerals are indestructible, some may be lost through food processing. For example, when whole-wheat flour is processed or refined to white flour, minerals such as phosphorus and potassium are lost and not replaced.

Water

Water is a major part of every tissue in the body. We can live only a few days without water. Water functions as a fluid in which substances can be broken down and reformed for use by the body. As a constituent of blood, water also provides a means of transportation for nutrients to and from cells.

Many of us probably do not drink enough water or liquids to best meet the needs of our bodies. We should consume the equivalent of about 9 to 13 cups of water a day from foods and beverages.[6] Awareness of the value of water consumption is growing as bottled water companies heavily advertise their products to the public. Bottled waters have become a fashionable alternative to other beverages. These products seem to offer convenience and status against which tap water cannot compete. Although more money may be spent on bottled water than is necessary, the health benefits are still achieved. Unflavored, plain water, whether purchased bottled or from public water supplies, provides the best value; waters fortified with vitamins, minerals, and herbs are not necessary.

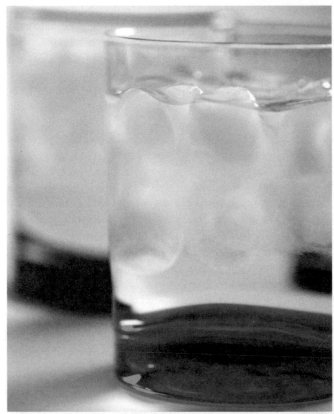

The need for water is more urgent than the need for any other nutrient. (From Photos.com.)

DIETARY STANDARDS

Simply knowing which nutrients are essential to life is not sufficient. We need to know how much of each nutrient to consume to be ensured of basic good health. Similarly, eating foods without awareness of their nutrient value does not ensure an adequate intake of nutrients. Dietary standards provide a bridge between knowledge of essential nutrients and food consumption. They also provide a guide of adequate nutrient intake levels against which to compare the nutrient values of foods consumed.

Dietary Reference Intakes

In the United States, past dietary standards were based on providing nutrients in amounts that would prevent nutritional deficiency diseases. The current set of nutrient standards, Dietary Reference Intakes (DRIs), combines the classic concerns of deficiency diseases that were the original focus of nutrient recommendations with the contemporary interest of reducing the risk of chronic diet-related diseases such as coronary artery disease, cancer, and osteoporosis.[6] The DRIs also take into account the availability of nutrients, food components, and the use of dietary supplements. They are designed to apply to various individuals and population groups.

Responsibility for dietary standards lies with the Standing Committee on the Scientific Evaluation of Dietary Reference Intakes of the Food and Nutrition Board, Institute of Medicine, and National Academy of Sciences, along with the participation of Health Canada. The DRIs are now the nutrient recommendations for the United States and Canada.

The DRIs are based on (1) reviewing the available scientific data about specific nutrient use, (2) assessing the function of these nutrients to reduce the risk of chronic and other diseases and conditions such as coronary artery disease and cancer, and (3) evaluating current data on nutrient consumption levels among U.S. and Canadian populations.

Dietary Reference Intakes Lingo

The DRIs consist of the Estimated Average Requirement (EAR), the Recommended Dietary Allowance (RDA), Adequate Intake (AI), the Tolerable Upper Intake Level (UL), and Acceptable Macronutrient Distribution Ranges (AMDRs).[6]

The Estimated Average Requirement (EAR) is the amount of a nutrient needed to meet the basic requirements of half the individuals in a specific group that represents the needs of a population. The EAR considers issues of deficiency and physiologic functions. Public health nutrition researchers and policymakers primarily use the EARs to determine the basis for setting the RDAs.

The Recommended Dietary Allowance (RDA) is the level of nutrient intake sufficient to meet the needs of almost all healthy individuals of a life-stage and gender group. The aim is to supply an adequate nutrient intake to decrease the risk of chronic disease. The RDA is based on EARs for that nutrient, plus an additional amount to provide for the particular need of each group. Some nutrients do not have an RDA but an AI level.

Adequate Intake (AI) is the approximate level of an average nutrient intake determined by observation of or experimentation with a particular group or population that appears to maintain good health. The AI is used when there is not sufficient data to set an RDA.

The Tolerable Upper Intake Level (UL) is the level of nutrient intake that should not be exceeded to prevent adverse health risks. This amount includes total consumption from foods, fortified foods, and supplements. The UL is not a recommended level of intake but a safety boundary of total consumption. ULs exist only for nutrients of which adverse risks are known.

Acceptable Macronutrient Distribution Ranges (AMDRs) are daily percent energy intake values for the macronutrients of fat, carbohydrate, and protein. For these energy-yielding nutrients, the following daily intake ranges are set to provide adequate energy and nutrients while offering reduced risk of chronic disorders:

- 45% to 65% of kcal intake from carbohydrate
- 20% to 35% of kcal intake from fat
- 10% to 35% of kcal intake from protein

The DRIs are designed to meet the needs of most healthy individuals. Individuals generally use the RDAs and AIs when assessing their nutrient intakes. People with special nutritional needs, such as those suffering from disease, injury, or other medical conditions, may have nutrient needs that are higher than the DRIs.

Use of Dietary Reference Intakes

The DRIs are widely used throughout the U.S. food systems, examples of which follow:

- Planning meals for large groups, such as the military
- Creating dietary standards for governmental food assistance programs, such as the Women, Infants and Children (WIC) and food stamp programs
- Interpreting food consumption information on individuals and populations

Although originally intended only for analysis of the diets of large groups of people, DRIs can be used for individuals if compared with an average intake over a period of time. The intake of a single day does not have to meet the recommended levels. A comparison with the DRIs does not determine nutritional status but is only one of several measurements used to assess nutritional status.

- Meeting national nutrition goals such as those listed in *HP2020*
- Developing new food products, such as imitation products, that duplicate the nutrient values of the original

However, the DRI standards are not the basis of the nutrient information that appears on food and supplement products. The Daily Value (DV) is used for nutrition labeling and is based on dietary standards from 1968—when nutrition labeling was first implemented. When the current food labeling standards were revised in 1994, the U.S. Food and Drug Administration (FDA) did not update the nutrient values. (See Chapter 2, in the section titled "Consumer Information and Wellness," for a detailed discussion of food labeling.)

Additional Standards

The Estimated Energy Requirement (EER) is the DRI for dietary energy intake. The EER aims to maintain good health by providing energy intake levels to maintain individuals' body weights within specific age, gender, height, weight, and physical activity categories. These energy intake recommendations are an average of the need for each category. A margin of safety is not added to avoid recommending potentially excessive intakes of energy; consuming too much energy may be a primary cause of obesity, a major public health issue, which increases chronic disease risk.

Standards around the World

Other countries have developed dietary standards based on energy needs, food supply, or environmental factors that affect their populations. In addition, organizations such as the Food and Agriculture Organization of the United Nations, along with the WHO, have developed dietary standards that meet the practical needs of healthy adults worldwide.

Why aren't nutrient recommendations the same for every country or population? After all, the needs of the human body must be the same around the world. The difference lies in the definitions and purposes of nutrient recommendations.

Standards may be designed to provide the basic amount of a nutrient to prevent deficiency symptoms or to supply sufficient amounts for basic good health. These amounts may differ substantially based on the nature of the nutrient, such as whether it is stored in the body. In addition, health professionals of a nation or organization may interpret the same scientific data differently, arriving at various recommended amounts.

Whether a standard is set to provide for only basic nutrient needs may depend on the availability of food. In the United States, where access to food is easy and the supply plentiful, the setting of nutrient recommendations higher than minimum levels is reasonable; most citizens have access to foods to meet those levels. In parts of the world where the food supply is more limited, the immediate goal is to supply as many individuals as possible with basic needs to prevent deficiencies.

Some values differ from the U.S. standards, based on the most common sources of nutrients worldwide. For example, most of the world relies heavily on plant protein sources, whereas North Americans use mainly animal sources. Recommended protein levels reflect this difference.

Ultimately, all standards are simply guidelines. Standards represent a range of the nutrient requirement, even when set at a specific amount. Individual needs may vary, so consuming enough food to meet the basic amounts should be each person's nutritional goal.

ADEQUATE EATING PATTERNS

Knowing the DRIs makes nutrition seem simple. Just eat enough of the DRI nutrients, and good health seems ensured. However, we don't eat nutrients; we eat foods. For an eating pattern to be considered adequate, the foods we eat must provide all the essential nutrients plus fiber and energy. An adequate eating pattern takes into account assortment, balance, and nutrient density.

Assortment addresses the value of eating a variety of foods from every food group. Eating the same foods every day may be convenient but may not serve health and nutrient needs. The limited selection of foods may not contain sufficient amounts of essential nutrients and dietary fiber or may be high in some nutrients, such as fat, and low in others, such as vitamin A. As shown in Figure 1-5, eating a ham and cheese sandwich every day may seem like a quick lunchtime solution, but an assortment of selections over a 5-day period provides a daily average of fewer calories, less fat, less cholesterol, and less sodium. A good strategy is to adopt a habit of selecting different foods for lunch or, at the least, rotating food choices throughout the week.

An eating pattern exhibiting balance will provide foods from all the food groups in quantities so essential nutrients are consumed in proportion to one another, thus achieving a balance among the levels of nutrients eaten. MyPyramid represents this concept by taking into account different food groups and number of servings. Balance also ensures that energy plus nutrient needs will equal the intake of energy and nutrients to satisfy adequacy (Figure 1-6).

Nutrient density assigns value to a food based on a comparison of its nutrient content with the kcal the food contains. The more nutrients and the fewer kcal a food provides, the higher its nutrient density. Figure 1-7 demonstrates that a 12-ounce glass of orange juice contains many more nutrients than a 12-ounce soda that contains empty kcal. The orange juice is nutrient dense compared with the soda. Although both may quench your thirst and taste sweet, the orange juice supplies so much more for similar kcal.

No single food contains all the nutrients essential for optimum health. An adequate eating pattern incorporates an assortment of foods.

NUTRITIONAL ASSESSMENT

Nutritional assessment is the process of determining nutritional status. The assessment may reveal nutrient deficiencies or excesses. A deficiency may be either a primary nutrient deficiency caused by an inadequate intake of a nutrient or a secondary nutrient deficiency caused by the body's inefficient use of the nutrient once it is absorbed.

There are two levels of nutritional assessment. One level evaluates dietary intake of the foods we eat to determine the quantities of nutrients consumed as compared with the DRI standard. The other level evaluates dietary intake but also considers how the body uses the nutrients for growth and maintenance of health. Several methods of evaluation may be used. Although registered dietitians and nutritionists perform in-depth nutritional assessment, nurses as members of a health team require an awareness of this process as well. Nurses may conduct simple nutritional assessments to

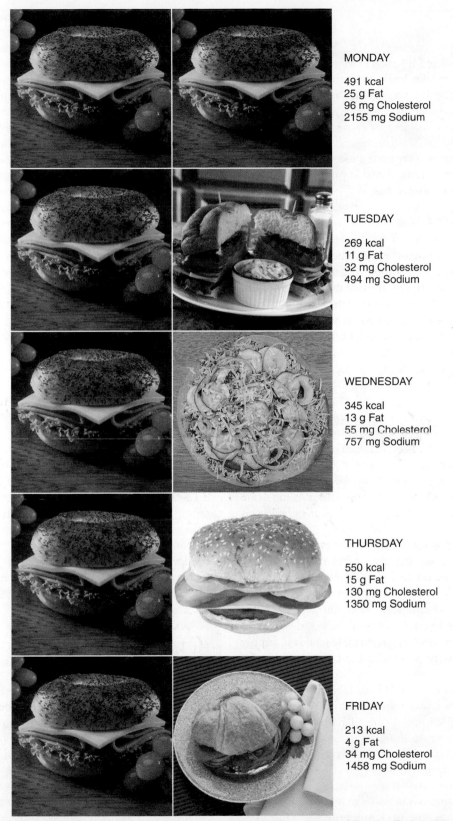

MONDAY

491 kcal
25 g Fat
96 mg Cholesterol
2155 mg Sodium

TUESDAY

269 kcal
11 g Fat
32 mg Cholesterol
494 mg Sodium

WEDNESDAY

345 kcal
13 g Fat
55 mg Cholesterol
757 mg Sodium

THURSDAY

550 kcal
15 g Fat
130 mg Cholesterol
1350 mg Sodium

FRIDAY

213 kcal
4 g Fat
34 mg Cholesterol
1458 mg Sodium

FIG 1-5 An adequate eating pattern incorporates an assortment of foods. Eating the same sandwich every day may be convenient, but an assortment of foods over a 5-day period provides a daily average of fewer calories and a greater variety of nutrients. (From Photos.com. Data from U.S. Department of Agriculture, Agricultural Research Service: *USDA national nutrient database for standard reference,* Release 21, Washington, DC, 2008, Nutrient Data Laboratory: www.nal.usda.gov/fnic/foodcomp.)

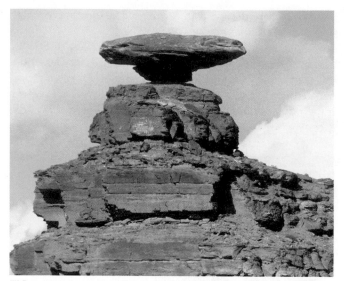

FIG 1-6 A balance of nutrients in the diet helps to ensure adequacy. (From Photos.com.)

provide patient/client information that can be used by nutrition professionals.

A brief introduction to nutritional assessment follows. Chapter 14 (in the section titled "Nutrition Intervention") contains a detailed nursing orientation for comprehensive nutritional assessment to be used as a basis for nutritional therapy.

Nutritional assessment determines nutritional status. The assessment techniques include the following two levels:
1. The quality or range of nutrients consumed
2. The body's use of nutrients for growth and maintenance of health

Assessment of Dietary Intake

The DRIs offer guidelines for safe and appropriate levels of nutrients to be consumed by individuals or provided in the food supply. If a person's intake does not meet DRI levels, however, the diet is not necessarily deficient because the DRIs do not reflect the use of nutrients by individual bodies, nor

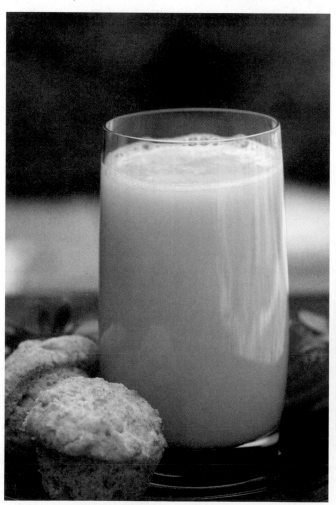

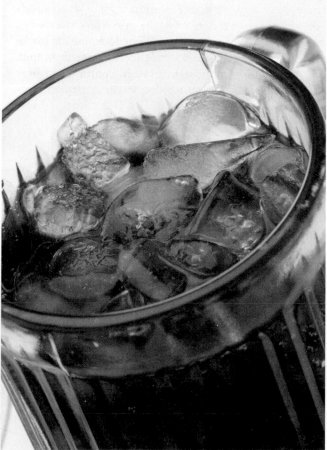

FIG 1-7 The more nutrients and the fewer kcal a food provides, the higher its nutrient density. (From Photos.com. Data from U.S. Department of Agriculture, Agricultural Research Service: *USDA national nutrient database for standard reference*, Release 21, Washington, DC, 2008, Nutrient Data Laboratory: www.nal.usda.gov/fnic/foodcomp.)

do they take into account overconsumption of specific nutrients, health problems, or environmental influences. Therefore, when evaluating nutritional status, a health care worker may note whether a client's dietary intake meets the DRI standard but should not base the evaluation solely on a comparison with the DRIs. A complete nutritional assessment is necessary to evaluate a person's nutritional status.

Estimates of food consumption are often used to determine the nutritional status of individuals and populations. Sometimes if the dietary intake is imbalanced, undernutrition, overnutrition, or malnutrition may be diagnosed.

Undernutrition is the consumption of not enough energy or nutrients based on DRI values. This means either not eating enough food to take in all the essential nutrients or eating enough food for energy but choosing foods that lack certain nutrients. In the United States, some women do not consume enough of the vitamin folate, although the rest of their nutrient intake is adequate.

Overnutrition is consumption of too many nutrients and too much energy compared with DRI levels. North Americans generally overconsume saturated fats, which is a risk factor for the development of heart disease.

Malnutrition is a condition resulting from an imbalanced nutrient and/or energy intake. Malnutrition is both undernutrition *and* overnutrition—undernutrition of too few nutrients or energy intake and overnutrition of excess nutrient or energy consumption. An obese man who consumes an excessive amount of kcal is malnourished because his intake is out of balance. His intake does not equal his energy output. A nutrient overdose is malnutrition. In contrast, a college student who constantly diets for slimness or sports, consuming less than the DRI for nutrients and energy, is also malnourished.

PORTRAITS OF MALNUTRITION

As discussed, not all who are malnourished resemble famine victims. The effects of long-term famines represent extreme forms of malnutrition (see Chapter 6 in the section "Overcoming Barriers: Malnutrition"). Lesser degrees of malnutrition are all around us. Consider the nutritional status of hospital patients, older adults, and chronic excessive alcohol users, for instance.

For hospital patients, the nature of an illness, combined with medications, may affect appetite and the absorption of nutrients. The effects of malnutrition may be caused by the illness rather than by improper nutrient intake. Clinical nurses are trained to detect hospital malnutrition in acute care settings.

Older adults may be at risk for malnutrition. They may be unable to afford fresh fruits and vegetables or may be unable to get to the supermarket regularly because of transportation difficulties. Dental and other health problems may make chewing or digesting foods difficult. Social factors may affect appetite as well. Cooking for one and eating alone are not appealing and may affect food intake. Home health nurses must be alert to the social and economic factors that contribute to malnutrition in older adults.

Individuals who consume alcohol excessively and who may still be functional (e.g., able to work or attend school) are often malnourished because alcohol replaces nutrient-dense foods; alcohol affects the gastrointestinal tract and so impairs absorption of nutrients. The health needs of chronic excessive alcohol abusers may be noticed by nurses in community and occupational health centers.

It is hard to imagine malnutrition happening close to home, especially when we shop in supermarkets that overflow with food products. Although hidden malnutrition among hospital patients, older adults, and chronic alcohol users is not as severe, it still affects their health and productivity.

Diet Evaluation

Ways to gather data on the food a person eats may include the use of the 24-hour recall, usual food intake, a food record, a food frequency checklist, or a diet history. The 24-hour recall is a report on what an individual ate during the previous 24 hours. The information is usually gathered in a personal interview or by telephone. Usual food intake may be obtained by asking what the person usually eats at a typical meal or snack. This helps to develop an eating pattern. The individual who measures and records the amounts and kinds of food and beverages consumed during a certain time period creates a food record.

Maintaining a food record can be somewhat time consuming because the individual needs to keep careful notes on intake and use measuring utensils to provide accuracy. A food frequency checklist records how often a person eats a specific type of food. This helps to focus on groups of foods, which are either deficient or excessive. A diet history is an approximate representation of a person's eating habits over a long period. The data are gathered through interviews or questionnaires. None of these methods is totally accurate. They depend on good memory and recording skills and accurate measurements. Currently, these methods are the most convenient ways to collect data on dietary intake. When possible, it may be helpful to use multiple methods to double-check the accuracy of information collected.

Once the data are collected, they can be analyzed through several computer dietary analysis programs and compared with the DRI for the individual. When this analysis is performed on a group of individuals representative of the larger population, estimates based on the dietary intake analysis can be made of the nutritional status of the population.

Assessment of Nutritional Status

Assessing nutritional status uses several methods of evaluation. Each method provides different data by which to assess nutritional status. See Chapter 14 (in the section "Nutrition Assessment") for specific instructions for implementing these methods.

Because the methods for assessing nutritional status involve dietary, clinical, and biochemical analyses, collaboration by a multidiscipline health team is usually required. In addition to dietary evaluations conducted by dietitians, methods may include the following:

- *A clinical examination performed by a primary health provider, nurse, or dietitian to note outward signs of nutritional health:* This includes physical examination through observation of the eyes, mucous membranes, skin, hair, mouth, teeth, and tongue. Clinical observations are limited in value because overt symptoms of nutrient deficiencies do not become apparent until late stages of deficiencies. In addition, some of the symptoms observed could be caused by conditions other than dietary deficiencies. Therefore, a client's medical history from medical records or through direct interview and a social history is also important to consider.

- *Biochemical analysis of samples of body tissues, such as blood or urine tests, to assess how the body uses nutrients:* If the blood level of a nutrient is low, it could mean the dietary intake was low, the nutrient was consumed but was poorly absorbed, or the individual has a higher than average requirement for the nutrient. Iron is a nutrient assessed through blood levels. Urine analysis can reveal the efficiency with which our bodies use glucose and protein and excrete other nutrients. Although a primary health care provider, nurse, or technician would draw the actual tissue samples, a dietitian would complete the nutritional analysis and interpret the results.

- *Anthropometric measurements, such as measuring the height, weight, and limb circumference of an individual and comparing those dimensions with national standards, to determine healthy growth patterns:* Body composition may also be used to determine percentages of lean body mass and body fat levels. In addition to height, weight, and limb circumference, various techniques are often used to assess body fat composition. These may include skinfold measurements, waist-to-hip ratios, densitometry, and bioelectric impedance analysis. Skill gained through careful practice is necessary to minimize the margin of error in taking body measurements. Before an assessment of this kind of data is completed, a family history should be conducted. Heredity plays a role in the growth patterns and the final height and weight we achieve.

Through consideration of data from clinical, biochemical, and anthropometric measurements, the nutritional status of individuals can be determined. As with dietary assessment, if these analyses are performed on enough individuals who are representative of the total population, the nutritional status of nations can be estimated.

Nurses who provide maintenance health care to nonhospitalized clients may implement a limited form of dietary evaluation as a screening procedure. For example, community and home health nurses who may not have access to computer analysis when conferring with clients can compare the results of the 24-hour recall or food record to the recommended servings of the MyPyramid for the needs of the individual (see Figure 2-2) or, if the client receives nutritional therapy, to a prescribed diet. Clients can then use this form of quick assessment to periodically check the status of their intake. This quick assessment does not, however, provide the same in-depth analysis as the comprehensive nutritional assessment performed by a dietitian who works with a multidisciplinary health team.

The Nutrition Specialist

Who is the nutrition specialist—the dietitian or the nutritionist? The answer is *both*. The difference is in the type of training and credentialing completed after majoring in foods and nutrition at the college or university level. Among health professionals, there has always been a concern that individuals may present themselves as nutritionists based on self-study (a personal interest in nutrition) or from completion of nonaccredited programs. Most states have established licensing for health specialists in nutrition. To be qualified entails years of a specially designed course of study because the ramifications of nutrition therapy and lifestyle counseling are significant. **Nutrition therapy**, the provision of nutrient, dietary, and nutrition education needs based on a comprehensive nutritional assessment to treat an illness, injury, or condition, is a multifaceted process requiring specialized training. Lifestyle counseling concerning the optimum dietary intake for healthy individuals is also complex considering the many factors that impact nutrient consumption and requirements.

Other states defer to the registering process developed by the American Dietetic Association (ADA) that confers the registered dietitian credentials. Nutrition professionals who are not registered dietitians should have graduate degrees in nutrition from accredited university or college nutrition programs.

A **registered dietitian (RD)** is a professional trained in foods and the management of diets (dietetics) who is credentialed by the Commission on Dietetic Registration of the American Dietetic Association. This training includes normal and clinical nutrition, food science, and food service management.

Credentialing is based on completing a bachelor of science degree from an accredited program, receiving clinical and administrative training, and passing a national registration examination. Continuing education is mandatory for continued registration. RDs may also have advanced training in specialized areas of nutritional therapy.

A **nutritionist** is a professional who has earned a master of science (MS), doctorate of education (EdD), or doctorate of philosophy (PhD) degree in foods and nutrition.

In 43 states, "dietitian/nutritionist" is a legally defined and licensed or certified title. Meeting strict requirements allows for the use of designated titles. These may include certified dietitian nutritionist (CDN), licensed dietitian (LD), or licensed medical nutrition therapist (LMNT). These professionals may also be RDs. In some states, it may be illegal to practice dietetics, such as nutrition therapy, without a license.

Similar to nurses, dietitians and nutritionists practice in a variety of health care settings. Clinical dietitians and nutritionists focus on the therapeutic needs of individuals and their families in institutional settings such as hospitals, long-term care facilities, and rehabilitation centers. Others work in community-based practice settings as community nutritionists, dietitians, and educators; they may concentrate on health promotion and disease prevention in addition to therapeutic issues. Public health nutritionists attend to diet-related health issues of the larger community to include state, national, and international nutrition concerns. Dietitians may also work in the food industry conducting research or marketing for the food industry and for pharmaceutical companies.

Toward A Positive Nutrition Lifestyle: Self-Efficacy

Achieving wellness is an ongoing process. We all experience times when meeting our personal dietary goals is easy and other times when it seems as if we will never regain a sense of control over our nutrition lifestyles. These ups and downs are all part of the process of achieving wellness.

To support our pathway toward achieving wellness, this section in each chapter will feature psychosocial strategies to enhance positive self-efficacy. *Self-efficacy* is our perception of our ability to have power over our lives and behaviors. Positive self-efficacy means believing that personal behaviors can be changed and one has control over one's life. Negative self-efficacy refers to feeling as if one is powerless, with little control over circumstances. A sense of positive self-efficacy is essential to attaining and then maintaining nutrition lifestyles for optimum health. These strategies may be applicable in our own life situations and are useful for our clients as they, too, strive for enhanced self-efficacy.

▌ SUMMARY

Health is the merging and balancing of physical, intellectual, emotional, social, and spiritual dimensions. Nutrition, the study of essential nutrients and the ways they are used by the body, is a cornerstone of each health dimension. To improve health and nutrition, health promotion strategies can be implemented. These strategies often rely on knowledge, techniques, and community supports to initiate and maintain lifestyle behaviors to enhance health. Wellness is a lifestyle through which the five dimensions of health are further enhanced. Wellness nutrition approaches food consumption as a positive way to nourish the body.

The essential nutrients obtained from foods are divided into six categories: carbohydrates, proteins, fats, vitamins, minerals, and water. These nutrients aid the growth and repair of body tissues, regulate body processes, and provide energy. Some nutrients are diverse in their effect, whereas others have specific functions. This chapter explores how the recommended daily levels of essential nutrients are determined. To prevent nutrient deficiencies and decrease the risk of the development of chronic disorders, dietary standards have been developed to provide guidelines about sufficient nutrient intakes. The DRIs are the standards for the United States and Canada.

Nutritional assessment determines nutritional status and nutrient deficiency in individuals. The techniques include two levels of assessment: evaluation of the quality of nutrients consumed and the body's use of nutrients for growth and maintenance of health.

THE NURSING APPROACH

Helping with Nutrition—Using Nursing Process

The Nursing Approach section will be found at the end of every chapter of this book. In most *The Nursing Approach* sections you will see a patient case study (an individualized nurse-patient scenario). As you read each case, note how the nurse uses nursing process to help a patient with his/her nutrition. Nursing process is a systematic method of thinking used widely by nurses. Answer the discussion questions at the end of each case, using your critical thinking skills. In a few *The Nursing Approach* sections you will find a student learning activity, such as a nutrition teaching project. In one learning activity you will experience a clinical diet in order to increase your knowledge and empathy for patients who are asked to change their eating patterns.

Nursing process is a systematic method of planning and providing nursing care. It is similar to the problem-solving method. Although ever-changing and not always linear, the nursing process components usually follow the sequence of assessing, diagnosing, planning, implementing, and evaluating. The nurse is legally accountable to assess the patient's health care status, make a judgment about patient responses to actual or potential health problems, design plans to meet identified needs, deliver specific nursing interventions, and evaluate patient outcomes. The steps of the nursing process can be remembered by the acronym **ADPIE**: assessment, diagnosis, planning, implementation, and evaluation. Following is a more detailed explanation of each.

- ***Assessment:*** Collecting, organizing, and recording patient information obtained through interview, physical assessment, and reading patient charts.

EXAMPLE ASSESSMENT

The nurse asks a patient about appetite and how the patient's culture affects his food choices, measures the patient's weight and his fluid intake and urinary output, and monitors his lab results.

Assessment may be comprehensive or focused, depending on the situation. The data recorded may be objective (from the nurse's physical examinations) and/or subjective (from patients'

Continued

THE NURSING APPROACH—cont'd

Helping with Nutrition—Using Nursing Process—cont'd

statements about their history and what they are experiencing). Objective data are sometimes referred to as signs—for example, vomiting, grimacing, and moaning. Subjective data are sometimes referred to as symptoms—for example, nausea and pain.

- ***Diagnosis:*** Identifying and validating nursing diagnoses. A nursing diagnosis is a clinical judgment about patient responses to actual or potential health problems. The North American Nursing Diagnosis Association International (NANDA-I) publishes a list of nursing diagnoses, with common causes and evidences. "A nursing diagnosis provides the basis for selection of nursing interventions to achieve outcomes for which the nurse is accountable" (2009, p. 419). Four types of nursing diagnoses have been developed by NANDA-I: actual, risk, health promotion, and wellness (pp. 419-420). You will find each type of nursing diagnosis in the case studies in this book, especially the actual nursing diagnosis type.

TYPES OF NURSING DIAGNOSES	EXAMPLES OF NURSING DIAGNOSES RELATED TO NUTRITION
Actual nursing diagnosis	Imbalanced nutrition: less than body requirements
	Impaired swallowing
	Excess fluid volume
	Deficient knowledge (specify)
Risk nursing diagnosis	Risk for imbalanced nutrition: more than body requirements
	Risk for constipation
Health promotion nursing diagnosis	Readiness for enhanced nutrition
	Health-seeking behaviors
Wellness nursing diagnosis	Effective breastfeeding

After assessing the patient, the nurse selects a nursing diagnosis from an established NANDA-I list. Then the nurse identifies a nursing diagnosis statement for the specific individual patient. The statement may have two or three parts. You will see examples of these statements in the case studies.

TYPES OF NURSING DIAGNOSES	NURSING DIAGNOSIS STATEMENT		
Actual nursing diagnosis	Nursing diagnosis	*related to* cause(s) or contributing factor(s)	*as evidenced by* patient data
Risk nursing diagnosis	Nursing diagnosis	*related to* risk factor(s)	
Health promotion nursing diagnosis	Nursing diagnosis		*as evidenced by* patient data
Wellness nursing diagnosis	Nursing diagnosis		*as evidenced by* patient data

EXAMPLE RISK NURSING DIAGNOSIS

Risk for aspiration related to impaired swallowing

- ***Planning:*** (1) Establishing priorities; (2) setting realistic, measurable patient outcomes; and (3) deciding which nursing interventions are best.

EXAMPLE PATIENT OUTCOME

The patient will gain one pound by August 31.

The plan of care may be developed by a team composed of health care professionals and the patient. Some nursing interventions are prescribed by the physician or nurse practitioner, some nursing interventions are directed by the dietitian, and some nursing interventions are designed independently by the nurse.

EXAMPLES OF NURSING INTERVENTIONS TO SUPPORT NUTRITION

Providing nourishment through a feeding tube or an intravenous solution

Giving medicine to counteract nausea, vomiting, and/or pain

Teaching a patient the guidelines for following a new diet

Helping a patient choose selections from the hospital menu

Feeding a patient who needs assistance with eating because of weakness or other physical problems

Independent nursing interventions are planned according to the nursing diagnosis and the causes or contributing factors identified. The purpose of the intervention will vary according to the type of nursing diagnosis.

TYPE OF NURSING DIAGNOSIS	PURPOSE OF NURSING INTERVENTION
Actual nursing diagnosis	Correct the problem or minimize the patient response
Risk nursing diagnosis	Reduce vulnerability to prevent the problem
Health promotion nursing diagnosis	Enhance health behaviors of the individual
Wellness nursing diagnosis	Build upon the patient's strengths to enhance wellness

Nurses must understand the principles of nourishment for patients with a variety of health conditions. They must be able to articulate the scientific rationale for interventions they select for individual patients. You will see examples of these rationales in the case studies. Nurses are responsible for evidence-based practice, choosing interventions based upon positive nursing research results.

- ***Implementation:*** Carrying out the plan and documenting the care provided. Although a nurse is less knowledgeable than a dietitian in regard to nutrition, it is usually the nurse who interacts with the patient throughout the day and night. The nurse is in a position to provide care and to coordinate care provided by health care professionals from various disciplines.

EXAMPLE OF AN INTERVENTION COMPLETED

Provided 8 fluid ounces of Ensure (a nutritional supplement) twice a day between meals.

THE NURSING APPROACH—cont'd

Helping with Nutrition—Using Nursing Process—cont'd

- **Evaluation:** Assessing to what extent the patient outcomes were met and revising the care plan as needed.

EXAMPLE EVALUATION OF A PATIENT OUTCOME

The patient gained one-half pound within 5 days. Goal partially met.

The Nursing Approach sections include nurses from a variety of settings: nurse practitioners and nurses from the hospital, the clinic, home health, occupational health, and the school. Regardless of the setting, the nurse is in a unique position to assess an individual's nutritional needs and help the patient to improve his/her nutrition. The nurse who has practical knowledge of basic nutrition will appreciate the importance of dietary intake in maintaining the patient's good health and in facilitating the patient's recovery from disease or injury. By ensuring that the patient receives adequate nutrition, the nurse acts as the patient advocate for health, healing, and well-being.

REFERENCE

NANDA International: Nursing diagnoses: Definition and classifications, 2009-2011, Ames, Iowa, 2009, Wiley-Blackwell.

APPLYING CONTENT KNOWLEDGE

Health promotion strategies often involve lifestyle changes. Bob needs to reduce his dietary fat intake because he is at risk for coronary artery disease. He lives in a suburban community and takes a train into New York City, where he works. Although it is only a half mile to the train station, he usually drives his car there to save time. Breakfast is often coffee, with a mid-morning break that consists of a Danish and more coffee. Lunch is obtained from street vendors who sell hot dogs and sausage sandwiches. Dinner is usually eaten with his family but often features meat and potatoes, his favorites. Because he leaves early in the morning and returns tired in the evening, he says he doesn't know how to change his behavior.

Using the strategies of knowledge, techniques, and community supports, describe the education care plan that could be developed with Bob.

WEBSITES OF INTEREST

American Dietetic Association

www.eatright.org

A resource about nutrition, health, wellness and dietetic professionals.

Healthy People

www.healthypeople.gov

The official website of *Healthy People 2020*.

Nutrient Data Laboratory

www.ars.usda.gov/nutrientdata

A nutrient database of food items commonly consumed in the United States.

REFERENCES

1. Hernandez LM, Rapporteur: *Health Literacy, Health, and Communication: Putting the Consumer First: Workshop Summary,* Washington, DC, 2009, National Academy of Sciences.
2. Nielsen-Bohlman L, et al, editors: *Health literacy: A prescription to end confusion,* Washington, DC, 2004, The National Academies Press.
3. World Health Organization: *Health impact assessment glossary: E-learning modules,* 2009. Accesssd July 14, 2009, from www.who.int/aboutwho/thelexicon.
4. Dubos R: *So human the animal,* New York, 1968, Scribner's.
5. U.S. Department of Health and Human Services, Public Health Service: *Phase 1 Report: Recommendations for the framework and format of Healthy People 2020,* 2008, Accessed July 15, 2009, from www.healthypeople.gov/HP2020/advisory/Phase1/summary.htm
6. Otten JJ, et al, editors: *Dietary DRI References: The essential guide to nutrient requirements,* Washington, DC, 2006, The National Academies Press.

2

Personal and Community Nutrition

A person's food behavior is influenced by personal factors as well as community issues affecting food availability, consumption and expenditure trends, consumer information, and food safety.

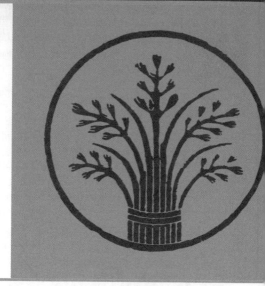

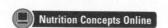

evolve WEBSITE

http://evolve.elsevier.com/Grodner/foundations/

Have you ever thought about who is responsible for your health? Perhaps you thought of your parents, spouse, or significant other. Or possibly you have always taken your health for granted, not as something to actively work toward improving or maintaining. What about the health of the community in which you live or work? Have you ever considered the health status of the residents of your town or college community?

Healthy People 2020 offered the following recommendation:

> *The recommended overarching goals for Healthy People 2020 continue the tradition of earlier Healthy People initiatives of advocating for improvements in the health of every person in our country. They address the environmental factors that contribute to our collective health and illness by placing particular emphasis on the determinants of health. Health determinants are the range of personal, social, economic, and environmental factors that determine the health status of individuals or populations.*[1]

The health of the individual is tied to the overall health of the population or community. Likewise the health status of the community is influenced by the shared attitudes and actions of those who reside in the community. To support promotion of good health, we must take responsibility for our personal health and the health of our communities-at-large. This chapter considers strategies to improve our health by taking charge of our personal nutrition and becoming aware of the nutrition issues of our communities.

ROLE IN WELLNESS

As presented in Chapter 1, wellness is a lifestyle through which we continually strive to enhance our level of health. Health is

the merging and balancing of physical, intellectual, emotional, social, and spiritual dimensions. Considering these dimensions in relation to personal and community nutrition broadens our understanding. The *physical health* dimension is represented by the food guides presented in this chapter. By following the recommendations of the food guides, we may reduce the risk of diet-related diseases. Consumer decisions about food purchases and application of food safety recommendations depend on reasoning abilities that reflect the *intellectual health* dimension. The *emotional health* dimension may affect the ability to be flexible when adopting suggested guideline changes. If we (or our clients) have problems doing so, will we view ourselves as "failures"? *Social health* dimension is tested as we (and our clients) interact with family and friends when we attempt to follow the guidelines. Can we be role models for others without being perceived as threats? Many religions stress personal responsibility for caring for one's body, which embodies the *spiritual health* dimension. Part of that responsibility includes the foods we choose to eat.

The decisions individuals make about the food they eat determine their health and wellness. Health professionals frequently give advice about appropriate foods for clients to consume. Therefore, it is important for nurses in institutional and community settings to understand how personal factors and community issues that affect food availability, consumption and expenditure trends, consumer information, and food safety can influence a person's food behaviors. The effects of these personal and community factors on consumers' food decisions are some of the major topics of this chapter.

PERSONAL NUTRITION

As adults, each of us is ultimately responsible for the quality of our dietary intake. Although external forces may affect our everyday food choices, we can decide to have the internal self-awareness to consciously modify those forces. Being accountable for our nutritional status and health may require adjustment of some personal goals to allow time to work on achieving a wellness lifestyle.

Food Selection

Our food preferences, food choice, and food liking affect the foods we select to eat. Although these terms reflect similar food-related behaviors, they are different.[2] Food preferences are those foods we choose to eat when all foods are available at the same time and in the same quantity. Factors affecting preferences include genetic determinants and environmental effects. Genetic factors include inborn desires for sweet and salty flavors. One study of taste receptors notes that because of genetic taste markers, some people experience the taste of vegetables such as broccoli and Brussels sprouts as bitter and therefore avoid such foods, whereas other people find this flavor enjoyable.[3] Consumption of cruciferous vegetables, such as broccoli and Brussels sprouts, may be associated with a decreased risk of developing certain cancers.[3] If some people avoid them because of perceived bitter taste, will they be more at risk for cancers?

Environmental effects are learned preferences that are the result of cultural and socioeconomic influences. We often adjust our choices to match those around us. Because we are around our families the most, their influence is the most significant factor in the choices we make; therefore, the dietary patterns we experience as children affect us throughout our lives[4] (see the *Cultural Considerations* box, Ethnic Food Preferences and Foodborne Illness). In fact, even the food a mother eats prenatally affects the preferences of her child in the future.[5]

An indirect influence on food preferences is the media. Television advertising in particular is a potent force that influences the foods we prefer and buy. Programs spread messages about the food and lifestyle preferences of different socioeconomic groups. A TV show about a working-class family presents images of food intake associated with those of a lower socioeconomic status; dinner might be hot dogs and beans. In another TV show, an upper socioeconomic family might sit down to a meal of baked salmon and salad. Each unintentionally sends messages about appropriate food intake for individuals belonging to each socioeconomic group.

Health promotion issues are tied to food preferences. If recommendations call for changes in foods for which preference is rooted in genetic determinants, the motivation for change needs to be different from when the food preference is environmentally learned. New preferences can be learned; genetic preferences are more difficult to change.

Food choice concerns the specific foods that are convenient to choose when we are actually ready to eat; rarely are all our preferred foods available at the same time to satisfy our preferences. Food choices are restricted by convenience. As a result of our hectic lifestyles, we tend to avoid foods that take long to prepare. Instead, we often repeatedly choose foods that are easy to prepare and eat, regardless of their nutritional value. Cost is also a factor. We sometimes weigh cost benefits against time benefits. If a food costs more but saves time, we may choose it. We may decide that a food item, even if nutrient dense, costs too much money for the benefits received. Again, nutritional value may not be a prime concern that affects food choice.

Food liking considers which foods we really like to eat. We may want to eat foods that enhance our health, but we like to eat chocolate cake, for example. We constantly weigh all the factors of preference, choice, and liking when we select the foods we eat. Ultimately, these three types of food behaviors greatly affect individual nutritional status.[2]

These three food behaviors may be covertly manipulated when the food industry develops and markets foods that appeal to our possible genetic preferences of sweet and/or salty.[3] These preferences are reinforced by repeated consumption and through advertising promoting the taste and "having fun" when consuming these products.[6] Marketing promotions and product availability may influence selection by consumers because of convenience, including accessibility, cost, or time saving, often with no consideration of nutritional value. Food liking evolves from, and may be the result of, repeated exposures. While some are able to moderate their consumption of less-nutrient-dense food products, others cannot, thereby impacting their nutritional status and health determinants.[6]

It is the small steps we take that eventually lead to cumulative change. As we study different aspects of food and nutrition, we will present suggestions that move us and our clients toward significant change. These suggestions will lead to the formation of new personal food habits.

COMMUNITY NUTRITION

The nutritional status of our communities is a reflection of our individual nutritional health. Perhaps the most significant factor affecting the nutritional status of communities is economics. Having sufficient funds to purchase adequate food supplies is a necessity. Public health nutrition efforts to prevent nutrient deficiencies include the U.S. government's Food Stamp Program. This program provides individuals and families below certain income levels with coupons to purchase nutritious foods. Another such effort is the Special Supplemental Nutrition Program for Women, Infants, and Children (WIC). The WIC program provides nutrition counseling, supplemental foods, and referrals to other health care and social services to women who are pregnant or breastfeeding and to infants and children up to the age of 5 who are at nutritional risk. Both programs have a significant impact on improving the nutritional status of those who participate. Additional government programs are discussed in Chapters 12 and 13.

Another level of public health nutrition is aimed at the nutrient excesses of our dietary intake. In the late 1970s, a new era in nutrition recommendations began in the United States. Rather than focusing on nutrient deficiencies as a cause of poor health, health professionals began to notice that the cause of an increasing amount of chronic illness was possibly tied to excessive intake of certain nutrients such as saturated fats, cholesterol, sodium, and sugars. As knowledge of diet-related diseases (e.g., heart disease, hypertension, cancer, diabetes, osteoporosis, and obesity) increases, sets of dietary recommendations from different government agencies and voluntary health and scientific associations evolve to address this issue.

Each set of recommendations serves a different purpose. For example, recommendations from the American Heart Association focus on lifestyle and dietary factors that affect risk factors of coronary artery disease, whereas those of the American Cancer Society center on issues related to cancer development. Despite differences in the focus of the recommendations, consensus exists on the guidelines for maintaining general good health. These recommendations are incorporated into our national goals. All recommendations suggest reducing intake of saturated fat, trans fat, total fat, cholesterol, sodium, sugar, and excessive kcal and increasing our intake of fiber, complex carbohydrates, fruits, and vegetables. These goals form the basis of health promotion efforts to implement primary, secondary, and tertiary prevention strategies. Education at the community level that reaches as many individuals and families as possible continues to be a challenge for health professionals.

The recommendations are still needed as four of the ten most common leading causes of death in the United States are diet-related disorders including heart disease, cancers, stroke (cerebrovascular disease), and diabetes mellitus.[7]

Dietary Guidelines for Americans

In response to the dietary recommendations, the U.S. Department of Agriculture (USDA) and U.S. Department of Health and Human Services (HHS) developed in 1977 the *Dietary Guidelines for Americans*. These guidelines are updated every 5 years and are intended for healthy Americans older than 2 years of age. The *Dietary Guidelines for Americans* are based on the latest scientific knowledge about diet, physical activity, and other health issues. This knowledge is used to formulate lifestyle and dietary pattern recommendations that will contain adequate nutrients, promote health, maintain active lifestyles, and decrease the risk of chronic diseases. As such, the *Dietary Guidelines* serve as the foundation of federal nutrition policy and education.[8]

The American public consumes insufficient amounts of certain nutrients such as vitamin D, calcium, potassium, and dietary fiber, even though excessive energy intake has led to a majority of Americans being overweight or obese. The current, *Dietary Guidelines for Americans 2010* (hereafter referred to simply as *Dietary Guidelines*), focuses on the goals

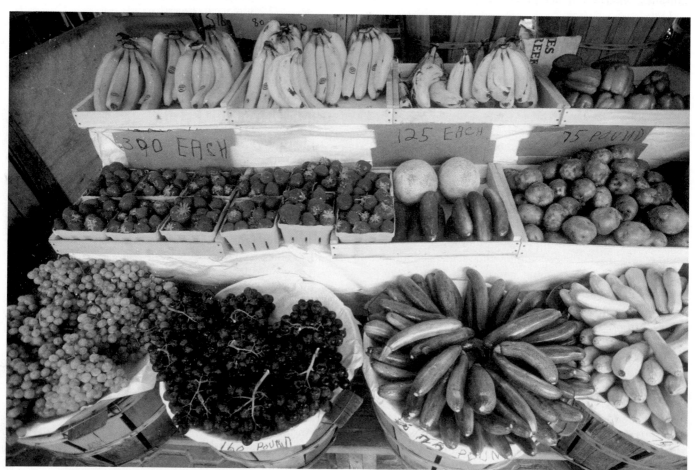

Choose fruits and vegetables each day to reduce the risk of diet-related diseases. (From Photos.com.)

of "good health and optimal functionality across the life span" with consideration of the malnutrition (deficiency of nutrient intake) and weight issues of the population-at-large.[8] Consequently, to attain these goals a lifestyle (behavioral) approach is suggested. This approach centers on a total diet concept. To implement a total diet concept that is balanced in energy and nutrient content, dietary patterns would emphasize portion size and consumption of plant foods such as vegetables, beans, fruits, whole grains, nuts and seeds, and increased intake of low-fat dairy products and moderate amounts of poultry, lean meats, and eggs.[8] In addition, lower intake of foods with added sugars and solid fats supports energy balance goals.

To sustain this endeavor, community support will be critical so that on a population level, individuals and families can adopt these guidelines whether eating at home, at school or work, or in restaurants. Local food availability is a concern to assure that more nutrient dense foods are affordable and accessible in all settings from the neighborhood supermarket to fast food restaurants. The techniques to prepare simple home cooked meals and strategies of food safety are prerequisites for achieving the goals of the *Dietary Guidelines*. These techniques and strategies can be taught in informal and formal educational settings including health care clinics, public health departments, faith-based organization, and print and electronic media.

Listed in Box 2-1 are the four major actions that if implemented would assist everyone to practice health-promoting nutrient consumption and be physically active.

BOX 2-1   MODIFICATIONS TO IMPROVE AMERICAN HEALTH STATUS

Based on a review of scientific evidence from the Nutrition Evidence Library, four significant modifications to our dietary intake patterns and lifestyle habits will significantly improve the overall health status of Americans:

- ***Reduce the incidence and prevalence of overweight and obesity*** *of the U.S. population by reducing overall calorie intake and increasing physical activity.*
- ***Shift food intake patterns to a more plant-based diet*** *that emphasizes vegetables, cooked dry beans and peas, fruits, whole grains, nuts, and seeds. In addition, increase the intake of seafood and fat-free, low-fat milk and milk products and consume only moderate amounts of lean meats, poultry, and eggs.*
- ***Significantly reduce intake of foods containing added sugars and solid fats*** *because these dietary components contribute excess calories and few, if any, nutrients. In addition, reduce sodium intake and lower intake of refined grains, especially refined grains that are coupled with added sugar, solid fat, and sodium.*
- ***Meet the 2008 Physical Activity Guidelines for Americans.***

(From: U.S. Department of Agriculture, U.S. Department of Health and Human Services: Report of the Dietary Guidelines Advisory Committee on the Dietary Guidelines for Americans, 2010, Washington, DC, 2010. Accessed June 16, 2010, from www.dietaryguidelines.gov.)

Additional details of the Dietary Guidelines are available at *www.dietaryguidelines.gov.*

As nurses work within communities and/or hospital settings, the *Dietary Guidelines* provide nutrient and physical health recommendations on which community programming and patient education can be based.

Lifestyle Applications

Your clients and patients would certainly like to follow the *Dietary Guidelines,* but how should they do this? Their busy schedules barely allow time to eat much of anything. Ask them to consider the following nutrition-related suggestions:

- In the morning, choose dry cereals and bread products (e.g., English muffins) that contain whole grains, and alternate or mix these with less-fiber favorites. If no time can be found for breakfast, stock up on portable juices and portable fruit, such as apples or bananas, which can be eaten on the way to class or work. Bring fruit in backpacks or briefcases for a quick snack.
- Be creative with vending machine selections. Choose lower-fat and lower-sugar selections such as raisins, bagel chips, pretzels (rub off the excess salt), popcorn, and even some plain cookies or crackers. Some vending machines stock small cans of tuna fish, yogurt, and fruit. Contact the staff responsible for filling the vending machines to request healthier selections.
- If lunch and dinner are on the run and fast-food drive-throughs are the only option, select lower-fat items such as grilled chicken sandwiches or plain hamburgers without the sauce. Don't order french fries or milkshakes (unless they are low fat) every time, but instead alternate with salads and low-fat milk, juice, or water.
- Perhaps lunch and dinner are in a college or employee cafeteria. Try to select turkey, chicken (without the skin), fish, and lean beef dishes. Include whole grain bread, a grain (rice or pasta), several vegetables, and salad. Try fruit for dessert; it is good with frozen low-fat yogurt, if available.
- Maybe your clients don't really eat "meals" but eat snacks throughout the day. This is called grazing. It is possible to graze and follow the *Dietary Guidelines* by choosing wholesome foods instead of candy bars and soda. High-quality grazing foods often available include bagels (with a little cream cheese), yogurt, fruit, pretzels, pizza (but not daily because of the high-fat content of the cheese), and dry cereals with milk.

The next time your clients are food shopping or grabbing a snack or meal, encourage them to stop a moment and consider the best choices available (Box 2-2).

FOOD GUIDES

When we are armed with the latest nutrient recommendations, we can easily apply this knowledge to the way we eat every day. Because we think about what *food* to eat rather than what *nutrients* we need, these nutrient recommenda-

5), MyPlate for Kids (ages 6 to 11), and MyPlate for Moms (pregnancy and lactating) are also available (available at http://www.choosemyplate.gov). For individuals who do not have a computer or access to one, or don't have computer skills, hard-copy print materials are available.

By following the interrelated recommendations of MyPlate, the following results can be expected:[9]

- Increasing intake of vitamins, minerals, dietary fiber, and other essential nutrients, especially those often low in typical diets
- Lowering intake of saturated fats, trans fats, and cholesterol and increasing intake of fruits, vegetables, and whole grains, decreasing risk for some chronic diseases
- Balancing intake with energy needs, preventing weight gain, and/or promoting a healthy weight

The recommendations represent the following four themes:

1. **Variety:** Eat foods from all food groups and subgroups.
2. **Proportionality:** Eat more of some foods (fruits, vegetables, whole grains, fat-free or low-fat milk products) and less of others (foods high in saturated or trans fats, added sugars, cholesterol salt, and alcohol).
3. **Moderation:** Choose types of foods that limit intake of saturated or trans fats, added sugars, cholesterol, salt, and alcohol.
4. **Activity:** Be physically active every day.

The simple MyPlate symbol reminds us and our clients to make healthy food group choices. The significant concepts of the symbol are highlighted in Figure 2-1.

Other Food Guides

Not all health professionals view the recommendations of MyPlate as the most sound to improve and maintain health. Some cite the increasing incidence of diet-related disorders as evidence that MyPlate recommendations do not meet our health goals. These disorders include type 2 diabetes, obesity, and syndrome X. Syndrome X, or *metabolic syndrome*, is a group of heart disease risk factors including abdominal obesity, glucose intolerance, high blood pressure, and abnormal blood lipid levels. Perhaps the pyramid is not being followed correctly, resulting in continuing diet-related disorders. Research supports that the dietary intake of most Americans is unbalanced when compared with the recommendations of MyPlate. Intake of meats and grains is higher than recommendations, while consumption of dairy, fruits, and vegetables is lower (Figure 2-2).[10] If it is being followed, then the emphasis on complex carbohydrates from grains and the use of animal-derived foods (dairy and protein sources) as the foundation of our dietary intake do not provide the expected health benefits.

One of the first alternative pyramids to address these concerns was developed by Dr. Walter Willett, chairperson of the Department of Nutrition at the Harvard School of Public Health. Based on accumulated scientific research, this pyramid—the Healthy Eating Pyramid—changes the focus of food selection and distinguishes between whole and refined grain foods as well as highlights plant sources of protein, such

tions are most useful when translated into real food. To help us do this, food guides have been developed.

MyPlate Food Guidance System

How do we and our clients implement the recommendations of the *Dietary Guidelines* on an everyday basis? In the past, the Food Guide Pyramid filled this purpose, but it has been replaced by the MyPlate Food Guidance System designed to guide us through our food selections to meet the goals of the *Dietary Guidelines*.[9] The creation of MyPlate took into account the present patterns of consumption of Americans plus the recommendations of the *Dietary Guidelines* and the Dietary Reference Intakes (DRIs). The result is a total diet that meets the nutrient needs from foods while limiting dietary components that are often eaten in excess. A tool to use in conjunction with MyPlate is the Nutrition Facts labels on food products.

MyPlate is an Internet-based interactive tool providing recommendations based on a person's age, sex, and activity level. Individuals can go directly to the website (www.MyPlate.gov) and enter their own data to receive personalized guides to the food group servings to meet their needs. The food groups include grains, vegetables, fruits, milk and dairy products, and meat and beans (Figure 2-1). MyPlate is intended for adults; a MyPlate for Preschoolers (ages 2 to

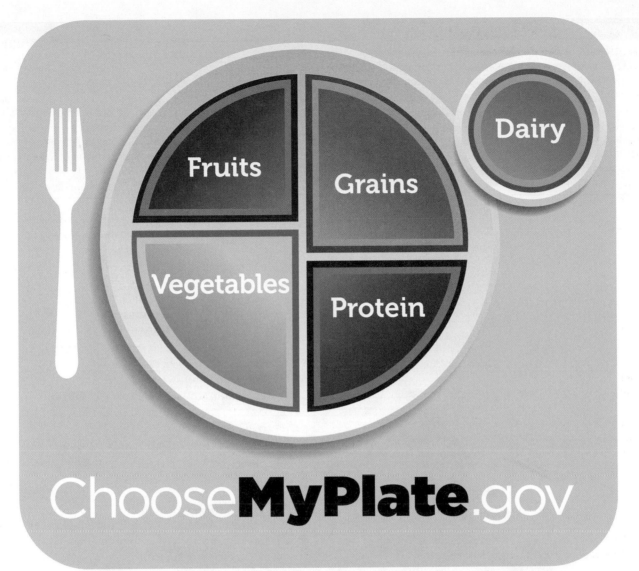

FIG 2-1 MyPlate illustrates the five food groups that are the building blocks for a healthy diet using a familiar image—a place setting for a meal. Before you eat, think about what goes on your plate or in your cup or bowl. **Fruits:** Focus on fruits. **Vegetables:** Vary your veggies. **Grains:** Make at least half your grains whole. **Protein Foods:** Go lean with protein. **Dairy:** Get your calcium-rich foods. (From U.S. Department of Agriculture, The Center for Nutrition Policy and Promotion, 2011, Author. Accessed June 14, 2012, from www.choosemyplate.gov.)

as nuts and legumes, which contain healthful plant oils (Figure 2-3). Animal-derived foods are pushed high up on the Healthy Eating Pyramid to reflect that they are foods to be consumed occasionally. For example, red meat is to be used sparingly or infrequently. Fish, poultry, and eggs are to be consumed zero to two times a day. This is different from the traditional pyramid, which groups animal and plant sources of protein together (meat, poultry, fish, dry beans, eggs, and nuts) with suggested servings of two or three times a day without distinguishing between the nutrient content of these foods. In addition, the Healthy Eating Pyramid includes recommendations for daily exercise and weight control (Figure 2-3).[11]

Alternative (Figure 2-4) and ethnic food pyramids are also available, providing specific food selections conforming to the general pyramid categories. These recognize that traditional dietary patterns of other cultures also offer opportunities to decrease the risk of diet-related disorders. The Asian, Mediterranean, and Latin American Diet Pyramids are accessible from the Oldways Preservation & Exchange Trust website (www.oldwayspt.org). These pyramids differ from MyPyramid in the number of servings of animal foods, legumes, nuts, and seeds recommended.[12] Vegetarian and soul food pyramids have been created as well. Other countries and commonwealths have food guides reflecting their national food supply, food consumption patterns, and nutritional status. Examples of the food guides for Mexico, and Puerto Rico are shown in Figure 2-4. Although the shapes of the guides may differ from MyPyramid of the United States, all recommend similar distributions of food category servings.[13] Ethnic food guides may be useful when caring for clients from other countries.

BOX 2-3 HEALING FOODS PYRAMID

The Healing Foods Pyramid is a softer, kinder food guide to promote mindful nourishment as an aspect of healing and/or to maintain health. Created by Monica Myklebust, MD, director, and Jenna Wunder, MPH, RD, of the University of Michigan Integrative Medicine, the pyramid is based on their extensive experiences with complementary and alternative approaches to health care.

The Healing Foods Pyramid emphasizes foods with restorative benefits and/or essential nutrients in natural forms. The core of dietary intake is primarily plant-based foods, with small amounts of animal foods. Food choices can be varied and balanced by nutrients, colors, and portion sizes. The "healing" aspect of the pyramid also applies to the production of the food supply. We need to heal and renew our environment, since food production affects the earth. Finally, mindful eating, which is eating with awareness of all the senses, keeps us focused on the experience of nourishing our bodies. The Healing Foods Pyramid will continue to evolve as knowledge of food and nutrition expands.

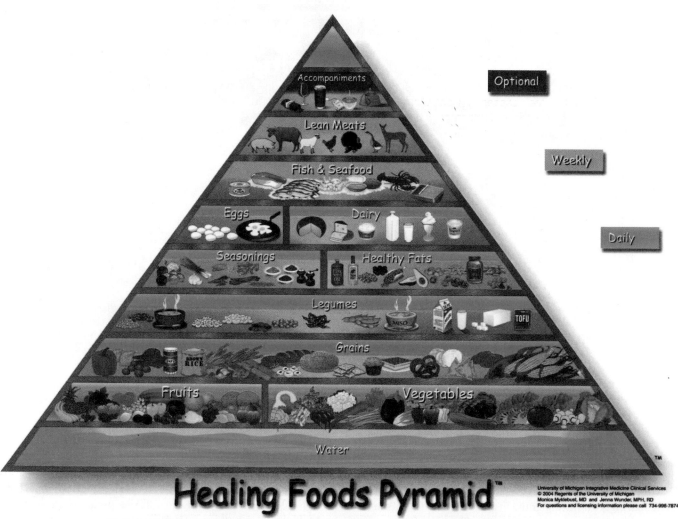

University of Michigan Integrative Medicine Clinical Services
© 2004 Regents of the University of Michigan
Monica Myklebust, MD and Jenna Wunder, MPH, RD
For questions and licensing information please call 734-998-7874

For additional information, or to order your copy, please visit our website at: www.med.umich.edu/umim/clinical/pyramid/.

We emphasize:

- **Healing Foods** — Only foods known to have healing benefits or essential nutrients are included
- **Plant-based choices** — Plant foods create the base and may be accented by animal foods
- **Variety & balance** — Balance and variety of color, nutrients, and portion size celebrate abundance
- **Support of a healthful environment** — Our food, and we in turn, reflect the health of our earth
- **Mindful eating** — Truly savor, enjoy and focus on what you are eating

Healing Foods Pyramid. (Courtesy and copyright 2004 the University of Michigan Integrative Medicine, Ann Arbor. Available for download and purchase at www.med.umich.edu/umim/food-pyramid/index.htm.)

American diets are out of balance with dietary recommendations

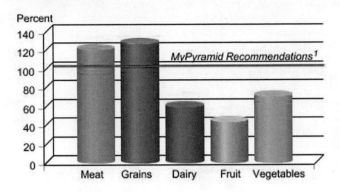

Note: Food availability data serve as proxies for food consumption.
[1]2006 data based on a 2,000-calorie diet.
Source: USDA, ERS.

FIG 2-2 American diets are out of balance with dietary recommendations. (From Centers for Disease Control and Prevention (CDC): *Behavioral Risk Factor Surveillance System Survey Data*. Atlanta, 2008, U.S. Department of Health and Human Services, Centers for Disease Control and Prevention. Accessed January 10, 2010, from www.fruitsandvegetablesmorematters.gov.

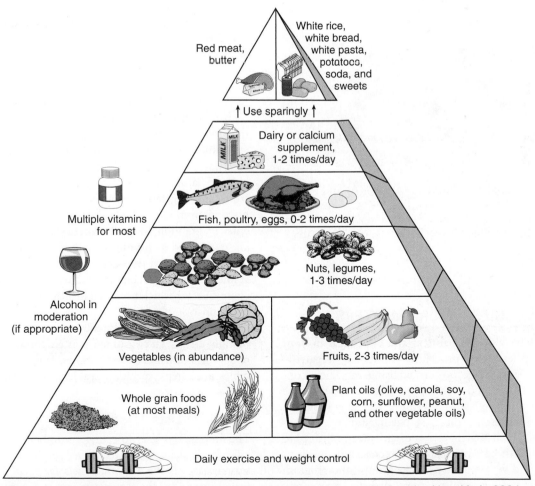

FIG 2-3 Healthy Eating pyramid. (From Willett W: *Eat, drink, and be healthy*, New York, 2004, Simon & Schuster.)

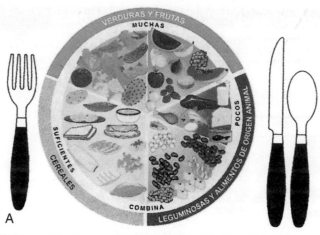

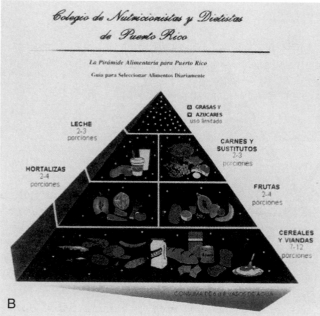

FIG 2-4 International food guides: Mexico **(A)** and Puerto Rico **(B)** (From Painter J, Rah J-H, Lee Y-K: Comparison of international food guide pictorial presentations, *J Am Diet Assoc* 102(4):483-489, 2002, with permission from the American Dietetic Association.)

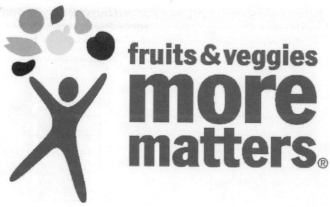

FIG 2-5 Fruits & Veggies—More Matters logo. (Courtesy of Produce for Better Health; www.fruitsandveggiesmore matters.org.)

FRUITS & VEGGIES—MORE MATTERS

Perhaps you have noticed banners and brochures in your local supermarket that proclaim "Fruits & Veggies— More Matters" and other posters advising increased consumption of fruits and vegetables (Figure 2-5). These banners are part of the National Fruit & Vegetable Program. This program represents the first partnership of government, not-for-profit agencies, and private industry to improve the health of Americans. By increasing consumption of fruits and vegetables by all age groups, the program may reduce the risk of certain cancers, diabetes, stroke, and high blood pressure.[14]

The Centers for Disease Control and Prevention (CDC) is the federal agency leading this public health initiative to encourage and motivate consumers to adopt strategies that result in the consumption of 2 to 6½ cups (4 to 13 servings) of fruits and vegetables as recommended daily. By doing so, the goals of the *Dietary Guidelines for Americans, Healthy People,* and other dietary recommendations may be achieved.

Research shows that about 75% of Americans adults do not consume five or more servings of fruits and/or vegetables a day, which means that only 25% are eating the minimum suggestion. Only 10% follow the recommendations of the *Dietary Guidelines* to eat seven or more servings of fruits and/or vegetables a day.[10] Therefore, most Americans do not meet the recommended five servings of fruits and vegetables a day, even though this amount is the minimum number recommended by MyPyramid. By focusing on only fruits and vegetables, the "Fruits & Veggies" campaign becomes an easy way to decrease intake of fats because fruits and vegetables are naturally low in fat. With seven or more servings of fruits and vegetables each day, increased consumption of fiber, vitamin C, and beta carotene will occur. These nutrients, in addition to their functions as essential nutrients, are recognized as having the potential to reduce the risk of developing heart disease and certain cancers. Fruits and vegetables are also excellent sources of antioxidants and phytochemicals, for which potential health benefits are continually being uncovered.

Although it may be difficult to determine the percentage of daily dietary fat consumed, it is easy to count the number of servings of fruits and vegetables. If more fruits and vegetables are eaten every day, cravings for high-fat foods will tend to decrease.

Exchange Lists

The food guides refer to eating a number of servings of specific foods daily. But what is a "serving"? A resource for serving sizes is the *Exchange Lists for Meal Planning,* published jointly by the American Dietetic Association (ADA) and the American Diabetes Association[15] (see Appendix A). Serving sizes may differ by weight or volume from the portion sizes we receive in restaurants or serve ourselves at home.

TABLE 2-1 EXCHANGE GROUP NUTRIENT VALUE

The Following Table Shows the Amount of Nutrients in One Serving from Each List.

GROUPS/LISTS	CARBOHYDRATE (g)	PROTEIN (g)	FAT (g)	CALORIES
Carbohydrates Group				
Starch	15	3	0-1	80
Fruit	15	—	—	60
Milk				
Fat-free	12	8	0-3	90
Reduced-fat	12	8	5	120
Whole	12	8	8	150
Other carbohydrates	15	Varies	Varies	Varies
Vegetables	5	2	—	25
Meat and Meat Substitute Group				
Very lean	—	7	0-1	35
Lean	—	7	3	55
Medium-fat	—	7	5	75
High-fat	—	7	8	100
Fat Group	5	45		

From American Diabetes Association and American Dietetic Association: *Exchange lists for meal planning (revised)*, Alexandria, Va, 1995, American Dietetic Association.

Foods are divided into different groups or lists: carbohydrates, meat and meat substitutes, and fats. Each list or exchange contains sizes of servings for foods of that category, and each serving size provides a similar amount of carbohydrate, protein, fat, and kcal. The carbohydrate group is subdivided into lists of starch, fruit, milk, other carbohydrates, and vegetables. The meat and meat substitute group is sorted by fat content (Table 2-1).

The exchange lists were first developed for use by people with diabetes. A dietitian can create an appropriate dietary program that prescribes the number of kcal and units of each exchange category to be consumed daily, as well as a plan for when foods should be eaten. By using the exchange lists for carbohydrate counting, an individual can choose favorite foods from each list while controlling the amount and kind of carbohydrates consumed throughout the day.

Guidelines for individuals with diabetes, published by the ADA, deemphasize prescribed calculated kcaloric diets only using the exchange lists.[16] The focus is now on adapting dietary intake to meet individual metabolic nutrition and lifestyle requirements (see Chapter 19).

The exchange lists encourage variety and help to control kcal and grams of carbohydrates, protein, and fats. As a tool for dietary instruction, these lists have been adapted to meet the needs of weight reduction programs and nutrition therapy planning. MyPyramid also uses the concept of units of servings by recommending a range of servings for each food category. A difference is that MyPyramid categorizes groups of foods based on the nutrients they contain, whereas the exchange lists categorize groups by proportion of carbohydrate, protein, and fat.

Criteria for Future Recommendations

Although the current recommendations are expected to provide sound advice for a while, other organizations may issue their own guidelines in the future. Which guidelines should we follow? Should we change our eating habits and revise client dietary recommendations for each new study? Or, to avoid confusion, should new recommendations just be ignored?

Following are criteria used to evaluate future dietary guidelines and recommendations:

- *Consider the source of the nutrition advice.* Are the recommendations from a federal government agency? If so, the work of these agencies is usually reviewed by health and nutrition professionals before release to the public. If the advice is from a private nonprofit group, is the group nationally recognized? A number of well-respected organizations are devoted to prevention and treatment of specific diseases, such as the American Heart Association, American Cancer Society, and American Diabetes Association. In addition, there are professional associations, including the ADA and the Society for Nutrition Education, that specialize in the relationship of nutrition and health. *Assess the comprehensiveness of the recommendations.* Do the recommendations address only one health problem? If so, is that a health problem that affects your clients? Would following these recommendations have any negative effects? Would a category of nutrients be underconsumed? Recommendations addressing several health issues are usually more complete and provide an increased level of prevention.

- *Evaluate the basis of the recommendations.* How were the recommendations determined? The current recom-

---

BOX 2-4   TYPES OF RESEARCH

Experimental Study
Consists of an experimental group receiving treatment (or dietary change) and a control group receiving no treatment (or dietary change); differences, if any, are then noted; called *clinical* or *laboratory study.*

Case Study
Analyzes an individual case of a disease or health difference to determine how factors may influence health; a naturalistic study because no manipulation of dietary intake or behaviors occurs.

Epidemiologic Study
Studies populations; tracks the occurrence of health or disease processes among populations; may use historical data, surveys, and/or medical records to determine possible factors influencing the health of a group of people.

---

mendations are based on many research studies on the relationships between diet and diseases. If new recommendations are issued, are they based on the results of new studies? If so, how many and what kinds of studies (Box 2-4)? Collecting this type of information means doing more than just listening to a 2-minute radio announcement or a 5-minute TV report. Some newspapers contain in-depth evaluations of research; others just skim the surface. It may be necessary to read the original study in the library or on the Internet, or to discuss the recommendations with other health professionals.

- *Estimate the ease of application.* Can the recommendations be easily adopted? Are they presented in terms of foods (easier to apply) or nutrients (harder to apply)? Is a degree in nutrition needed to understand the recommendations?

CONSUMER FOOD DECISION MAKING

Community supports can have an impact on the quality of personal nutrition. Most important are the consumer decisions made daily when buying food to be prepared in the home or when eating out.

Food Selection Patterns

Food selection patterns may be estimated from assessing government data gathered through national surveys and programs. One approach is to evaluate information gathered from the online MyPyramid Tracker. Developed as part of the MyPyramid food guidance system, the MyPyramid Tracker measures the dietary quality of an individual's food intake and physical activity based on the extent to which the intake follows the *Dietary Guidelines* and the DRI recommendations.[17]

According to research, those with more healthful dietary intakes have higher levels of nutrition knowledge and advanced education levels. Consequently, the data reveal that higher socioeconomic characteristics are related to a greater understanding of nutrition and the effects of healthy diets in reducing the risks of diet-related disorders.[18] This difference may reflect access to resources (e.g., time and financial means) supporting preparation and consumption of foods that follow the dietary guidelines.

As a nation we need to improve our nutrient intake. An aspect of doing so must take into account our beliefs and attitudes toward our dietary intake. A study using national data reveals that only 23% of the surveyed population is interested in improving their intake, whereas 37% are not interested in doing so, and 40% believe their intake does not need to change. Most view healthy eating as too complicated. In addition, the majority views snacking as an unhealthy practice, and as a result, the majority chooses snacks that are also unhealthy.[19]

Application to nursing: When working with clients, we can be aware of their attitudes toward nutrition and dietary change. Although changing dietary intake is a prime strategy to reduce the risk of diet-related chronic disorders, many Americans are not interested in changing their eating behaviors. In addition, the belief that snacking is unhealthy is unfortunate. Snacks do not have to be high fat, high sodium, or calorie laden. Consuming additional fruits, vegetables, and whole grain foods is often best accomplished through wisely selected additional "mini meals" or snacks. We may need to educate or remind clients about the nutritional benefits of dietary change as a disease-prevention strategy, and we should definitely emphasize the positive value of snacking on wholesome foods. Providing clients with simple techniques for changing food selection habits is crucial.

Food Consumption Trends

Food consumption trends reflect the food decisions Americans made in the past. Tracking these trends is the responsibility of the USDA. Following changes in consumption trends across the years for specific foods reveals information about food substitutions, including food prices or technologic changes that bring new types of food products to the marketplace. Food consumption trends now show that generally Americans eat more food in larger portions with additional snacks, which results in a greater caloric intake than in the past.[20]

Implications of food consumption trends. Food consumption trends affect the nutritional status of the U.S. population. Consumption of fruits and vegetables keeps increasing but still does not meet recommended intakes. This is a concern because fruit and vegetable consumption is ideal to reduce risk factors associated with diet-related chronic diseases.[21] Underconsumption may be related to cost. Income differences may account for the difference in consumption because low-income households consume fewer fruits and vegetables than other households. Generally, however, many of us need to learn how to prepare the wider variety of vegetables available in the supermarkets so they taste and look good and are safe to eat. Teaching how to prepare foods is an adjunct goal of nutrition education. Programs such as Fruits & Veggies—More Matters that provide point-of-purchase preparation techniques and recipes should prove effective. Additionally, the popularity of TV cooking shows, such as those broadcast on the Food Network, increase our knowledge base. Some shows such as *Iron Chef America, Top Chef,* and *Throwdown with Bobby Flay*—through the use of themes and competitions are popular with viewers, including some men who previously had no interest in food preparation.

Although consumption of cereals and grains is increasing, dietary guideline recommendations are to increase the intake of whole grains rather than continue to increase refined grains. A way to accomplish this is to learn new ways to prepare different kinds and forms of grains, such as wheat, rice, buckwheat, and corn, in the forms of pastas, couscous, and tortillas to meet the dietary recommendations of 6 to 11 servings a day. For the best nutrient value, grains and cereals should be consumed as whole grains, not refined, for at least half of the daily servings. Breakfast cereals can be a way to become accustomed to whole grains. These products have qualities in demand by today's consumers; they are convenient, may contain fiber, are good sources of nutrients, and are low in calories.

Animal sources of protein (total meat)—meat, poultry, fish, and shellfish—are increasing.[22] In recent years, within this category, beef consumption decreased while poultry and fish consumption increased. More fish is being consumed because of increased availability of fresh and frozen fish since the development of refrigerated and frozen storage techniques.

The way meat, poultry, and fish are cooked determines the final dietary fat content. The message to reduce dietary fat and cholesterol intake affects how we consume and prepare animal protein. Health benefits are greatest when we choose low-fat cooking methods. Some popular ethnic cuisines extend meat, poultry, or fish by combining protein sources with cereals, grains, vegetables, and sauces.

Dairy product trends reflect dietary recommendations to consume products that are lower in fat. The consumption of whole milk with high amounts of fat is decreasing, while the consumption of low-fat and nonfat milk and other dairy products is increasing because of the wide array of new products in the marketplace. Consumption of yogurt and other fermented dairy products with live cultures continues to increase because of their health benefits. Of concern are the continuing trends that as children and adolescents grow older, consumption of milk and juice declines, while soft drink intake increases.[23] Soft drinks are drunk in larger quantities per serving than either milk or juice products, so they provide more total calories. Such sweetened beverages may be a factor in the increasing obesity rates of American youth.

Caloric sweetener consumption continues to increase.[22] Consumption of cane and beet sugars has decreased, but corn and noncaloric sweetener consumption has increased. These changes occurred because the technologies associated with producing corn sweeteners from cornstarch and manufacturing noncaloric sweeteners reduced their costs, allowing them to compete economically with cane and beet sugars. Sweetener and beverage consumption trends affect the nutritional status, depending on whether the type of sweetener or beverage chosen increases or decreases the intake of energy and other nutrients. Other issues of sweeteners are discussed in Chapter 4.

Although these trends reflect per capita consumption patterns based on the total population, it is our individual food choices that have the greatest influence on our personal level of wellness.

Effective Food-Buying Styles

This chapter is full of information about consumer decisions, but how is it to be applied? How do you and your clients become better shoppers? The first step is to tailor a shopping style to one's particular situation. Consider the following to formulate the most effective approach to food shopping:

- *Food budget:* A food budget should take into account the funds needed to keep a moderate amount of food in the home and the money spent on meals away from home.
- *Consumer diversity:* Buying food for a single young adult is different from buying for a family. Lifestyles of household members affect the number and types of meals served and the kinds and amounts of food served.
- *Dietary preferences:* We all have food preferences based on ethnicity, habits, chronic illness, or ethical views such as vegetarianism. Each preference affects food-buying selections.
- *Shopping frequency:* Each household works best with a shopping plan—perhaps weekly, every 2 weeks, or on the way home from school or work when things are needed.
- *Location and types of food stores:* Different types of food stores provide a range of services and products. Conventional supermarkets, superstores, super centers, and super warehouse stores are valuable for fresh produce, perishables, and basic grocery items; wholesale clubs and limited assortment warehouse stores are good for bulk foods at low prices; specialty stores offer unique foods at high prices; and convenience stores "save the day."

CONSUMER INFORMATION AND WELLNESS

The more information consumers have about the food they eat, the better they can choose foods that contribute to wellness. Nutrition education is necessary for consumers to use the additional information appropriately.

PERSONAL PERSPECTIVES

The LocalHarvest Blog: Local and Organic for $37/week February 24, 2009

LocalHarvest.org, a unique website, is a dynamic public nation-wide directory of small farms, farmers markets, and other local food sources. The site search engine connects consumers with sources of local sustainably grown food and family farms. Products from small farms are accessible through an online store. This entry of the LocalHarvest Blog written by Erin Barnett, director of LocalHarvest.org, gives a perspective of the "home economics" of eating locally.

Last week I was part of a panel at local farm conference, where my assignment was to talk about the "home economics" of eating locally. I spoke about what my family eats and why, and the time and money our diet requires.

I was especially curious about the money part. It should be said that my husband and I put a high value on eating well. We also grow a lot of our own food. It's our sustenance, both physical and spiritual. Turns out, the garden saves us a lot of money, too.

I went through a year's worth of credit card statements, the check book register, and my memory of how much cash I spent at the farmers market and found that on average, our family spent $412 a month on food last year. This is for two adults and one voracious toddler—a 2.5 eater household. Do the math, and it comes out to $37/person per week. If you're broke, or have a big family, $37/person per week is a lot. But if you're lucky enough to have a good job, it might seem like a reasonable number. Did I mention this includes our eating-out budget? It does. We live in a small town with not too many restaurant choices, so that keeps the eating-out impulse in check. So does liking to cook.

After figuring the cash, I made a list of what we're getting for that much money. By intent, and by dint of the bounty of rural Minnesota, all our meat, milk, cheese, and eggs are local and organic. We eat a moderate amount of meat (1-2 chickens a month and a pound or two of beef), but go through a fair amount of eggs and dairy products.

Most of the rest of the food, besides the produce, is not local. Grains, beans, tofu, corn chips, condiments, chocolate—not local, but often organic.

In the summer and fall, 100% of our veggies and fruits are either grown in our gardens or bought at the farmers market. In the winter and spring, about 2/3 of our fruit and 3/4 of our veggies are local because we freeze and can so much food in the summer. Here's a list of the garden produce we are eating this winter.

- Frozen: kale, chard, sweet corn, pesto, red bell peppers, tomato sauce, winter squash, strawberries, plums
- Fresh food, stored in the basement: potatoes, onions, garlic, sweet potatoes, parsnips (also had beets, but they are gone)
- Canned: various tomato products, pickles, salsa, jam, applesauce.

Except the strawberries and apples, which we picked at organic farms near here, all this came out of our large garden.

Another thing that makes our food dollars go farther is that we make a few things we could buy, like bread, yogurt, granola. We do these things because we like the process, the results, and the lack of packaging. Moreover, the food is OURS because we made it. Being so intimately involved with our food brings a lot of soulfulness to our lives, and we love it.

Here is one last thing I have recently realized is key to our family making good use of all this food. Planning ahead. Last month I started spending about an hour a month planning the supper menus for the whole coming month. I cannot tell you what a difference it makes. At our house, if we do not have a plan, the "what's for supper?" question sucks up an unbelievable amount of time and energy. Having it written down makes the actual cooking a snap. It makes trips to the grocery store more efficient and ensures that we don't waste any food because we have a plan for it.

To good food, and happy cooks!

From Barnett E: *The LocalHarvest blog: Local and organic for $37/week, February 24, 2009.* Accessed January 10, 2010, at www.localharvest.org/blog/lh/entry/local_and_organic_for_37.

Food Labeling

Food labels are the best way for consumers to see how individual foods fit their nutritional needs. The function of food labels is twofold. The first is to assist consumers to select foods with the most health-providing qualities. The second is to motivate food companies to enhance the nutritional value of food products because labels reveal ingredient and nutrient content.[24]

Food labeling for processed foods in the United States is based on standards established under authority of the 1990 Nutrition Labeling and Education Act. Although nutrition labeling is mandatory for most processed products, it is voluntary for fresh meat, poultry, fish, milk, eggs, and produce. An example of the label for processed foods is shown in Figure 2-6.

The Nutrition Facts panel must list the quantities of energy (kcal), fat, and the following other specific nutrients in a serving:

- Total food energy
- Food energy from fat
- Total fat
- Saturated fat
- Trans fat
- Cholesterol
- Sodium
- Total carbohydrates
- Dietary fiber
- Sugars
- Protein
- Vitamins A and C
- Calcium
- Iron

The **Daily Values (DVs)** is a system for food labeling composed of two sets of reference values: reference daily intakes (RDIs) and daily reference values. The percent of DVs information, based on a 2000-kcal diet, is intended to show

① Start here
Serving sizes consistent across product lines, stated in household and metric measures, reflecting amounts people actually eat.

② Check calories

③ Limit these nutrients
List of nutrients covers those most important to health of consumers, most of whom need to worry about getting *too much* of certain items (fat, for example) rather than too few vitamins or minerals as in the past

Sugars: Amounts listed include naturally occurring sugars and those added. No Daily Value established.

④ Get enough of these nutrients

⑤ Footnote*
This info must be on all food labels. The remaining info displayed if label is large enough.

Nutrition Facts
Serving Size 1 cup (228g)
Servings Per Container 2

Amount Per Serving

Calories 90   Calories from Fat 30

	% Daily Value*
Total Fat 3g	5%
Saturated Fat 0g	0%
Trans Fat 3g	
Cholesterol 0mg	0%
Sodium 470mg	20%
Total Carbohydrate 13g	4%
Dietary Fiber 2g	10%
Sugars 3g	
Protein 3g	
Vitamin A	80%
Vitamin C	60%
Calcium	4%
Iron	4%

* Percent Daily Values are based on a 2,000 calorie diet. Your Daily Values may be higher or lower depending on your calorie needs.

	Calories:	2,000	2,500
Total Fat	Less than	65g	80g
Sat Fat	Less than	20g	25g
Cholesterol	Less than	300mg	300mg
Sodium	Less than	2,400mg	2,400mg
Total Carbohydrate		300g	375g
Dietary Fiber		25g	30g

Kcals from fat are shown on the label to help consumers meet dietary guidelines that recommend people get no more than 30 percent of their kcals from fat.

⑥ % Daily Value shows how a food fits into the overall daily diet.

Quick guide to % DV based on 2,000 calories

For all nutrients:
• **5% or less is low**

• **20% or more is high**

Some Daily Values are maximums, as with fat (65 grams or *less*): others are minimums, as with carbohydrates (300 grams or *more*). The daily values on the label are based on a daily diet of 2,000 and 2,500 kcals. Individuals should adjust the values to fit their own kcal intake.

FIG 2-6 An example of the food label format that currently is mandatory in the United States. (From U.S. Food and Drug Administration, Washington, DC.)

consumers how much of a day's ideal intake of a particular nutrient they are eating. DVs for selected nutrients and food components based on a 2500-calorie diet are also given at the bottom of the label.

Uses of %DV

The %DV is useful to make comparisons between products, to assess nutrient content claims, and to choose a mix of foods to balance nutrient intake. Making comparisons between the %DV of similar products is possible if the serving sizes are the same. Which brand has the lowest fat content? Which has the highest fiber content? Assessing nutrient content claims is simple when using %DV. By considering the %DV of fiber in two food products, the better source of fiber can be quickly determined. This can be used for any nutrient content claim. Using %DV to balance nutrient intake is accomplished by combining foods high in %DV of a particular nutrient, such as fat, with foods low in %DV of that nutrient. A person's daily intake of fat can still be less than 100%DV.[24]

Uniform definitions for food descriptors, such as light, low fat, and others for nutrient content claims, are now clearly defined and must be consistently used for all foods (Box 2-5). This information helps consumers who try to control their intakes of specific nutrients and food components.

To assist consumers in reaching the *Dietary Guidelines* recommendation to consume at least 3 ounces of whole grains daily, manufacturers have increased whole grain ingredients in many products. The Whole Grains Council, an organization of scientists, manufacturers, and chefs, developed a series of three stamps to appear on packaging that identify the whole grain content of a product (Figure 2-7). A "100% excellent" source stamp signifies a product containing 1 ounce or 1 full serving, and all grains are whole grain. An "excellent" source stamp signifies a product providing 1 ounce or 1 full serving of whole grains. A "good" source stamp represents a product adding ½ ounce or ½ serving of whole grains. (Whole grain content is not the same as dietary fiber content, even though dietary fiber is part of the whole grain.)

Organic Food Standards and Labels

Fresh produce and a variety of foods are labeled "organic." Just what does organic mean? The USDA established national standards for food products to be labeled organic, regardless of where the food is grown or processed. Farmers who produce organic food focus on the use of renewable resources and soil and water conservation to maintain and/or improve the environment for the future. Animal-derived foods such as meat, poultry, eggs, and dairy products are labeled organic when no antibiotics or growth hormones are used in the rearing of the animals. Produce is grown without the use of conventional pesticides, synthetic fertilizers, bioengineering, or radiation. Before a product can be labeled organic, certification by government-approved inspectors is required of farms where foods are grown as well as of companies that

---

BOX 2-5 **FOOD DESCRIPTORS**

Free
Contains only a tiny or insignificant amount of fat, cholesterol, sodium, sugar, and/or calories. For example, a "fat-free" product will contain less than 0.5 g of fat per serving.

Low
"Low" in fat, saturated fat, cholesterol, sodium, and/or calories; can be eaten fairly often without exceeding dietary guidelines. So "low in fat" means no more than 3 g of fat per serving.

Lean
Contains less than 10 g of fat, 4 g of saturated fat, and 95 mg of cholesterol per serving. "Lean" is not as lean as "low." "Lean" and "extra lean" are USDA terms for use on meat and poultry products.

Extra Lean
Contains less than 5 g of fat, 2 g of saturated fat, and 95 mg of cholesterol per serving. Although "extra lean" is leaner than "lean," it is still not as lean as "low."

Reduced, Less, Fewer
Contains 25% less of a nutrient or calories. For example, hot dogs might be labeled "25% less fat than our regular hot dogs."

Light/Lite
Contains one third fewer calories or one half the fat of the original. "Light in sodium" means a product with one half the usual sodium.

More
Contains at least 10% more of the daily value of a vitamin, mineral, or fiber than the usual single serving.

Good Source of ...
Contains 10% to 19% of the daily value for a particular vitamin, mineral, or fiber in a single serving.

From U.S. Food and Drug Administration, Center for Food Safety and Applied Nutrition: *Guidance for Industry A food labeling guide: IX. Appendix A: Definitions of Nutrient Content Claims*, College Park, Md, 2008 (April), Author.

---

process foods to ensure that the USDA organic standards are followed.[25]

Specific labeling rules exist for foods containing organic ingredients. Single-ingredient foods may use the organic seal and the word *organic* on labeling or on display posters. These foods may include fresh fruits, vegetables, cheese, cartons of eggs or milk, meat packages, and other single-ingredient foods. When foods contain more than one ingredient, specific labeling categories are followed (Box 2-6).[25]

The term *natural* may also be used, but it is not the same as organic. *Natural* often signifies that the ingredients of a product are less processed and more wholesome but does not address how the ingredients were grown or the animals reared. *Organic* means that the food is certified as fulfilling

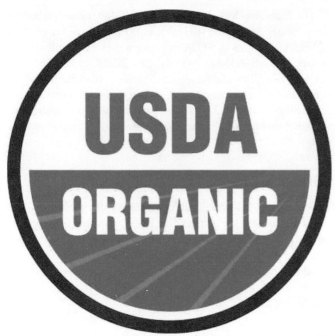

U.S. Organic seal.

BOX 2-6   **LABELING DEFINITIONS FOR ORGANIC FOODS**

The National Organic Program division of the USDA has levels of certification for foods containing organically grown ingredients. A product label may display the following terminology:

"100% Organic": All ingredients meet or exceed USDA specifications for organic foods, which bans the use of synthetic pesticides, herbicides, chemical fertilizers, antibiotics, and hormones.

"Organic": At least 95% of ingredients meet or exceed USDA specifications for organic foods.

"Made with Organic Ingredients": At least 70% of ingredients meet or exceed USDA specifications for organic foods.

If less than 70% of ingredients are organic but one or more ingredients are organic, the specific organic ingredients can be identified as organic but only in the small type on the ingredient panel.

From U.S. Department of Agriculture, Agricultural Marketing Service: *Organic Labeling and Marketing Information,* Washington, DC, 2002 (Updated April 2008), Author. Accessed August 2, 2009, from www.ams.usda.gov/AMSv1.0/nop.

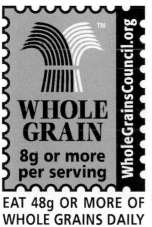 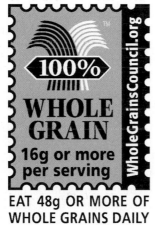

EAT 48g OR MORE OF WHOLE GRAINS DAILY   EAT 48g OR MORE OF WHOLE GRAINS DAILY

FIG 2-7 Whole Grain Stamps. (Whole Grain Stamps are a trademark of Oldways Preservation and Exchange Trust and the Whole Grains Council; www.wholegrainscouncil.org.)

the USDA organic standards for farming and/or rearing of animals, not how the ingredients have been processed during the manufacturing procedures. Organic soda prepared from organically grown sugar/and or high-fructose corn syrup and flavorings is not more nutrient dense or natural than a soda from a national beverage company containing similar ingredients grown under conventional means. Consumers need to be savvy about the nutrient density of the foods chosen regardless of whether the product meets USDA organic standards (see Box 2-6).

Application to nursing: Check the Nutrition Facts panels for products purchased regularly. Ingredients may be changed by manufacturers, and similar products may be created from different formulations. This may result in modifications of

ingredients and serving sizes that affect calories and nutrient content. (See the *Teaching Tool* box Just the Facts: Using Labels to Teach Nutrition Literacy for information on how to help clients evaluate food labels.)

Health Claims

Health claims relating a nutrient or food component to the risk of a disease or health-related condition now appear on food labels. Only health claims approved by the U.S. Food and Drug Administration (FDA) may be on the label. This information helps consumers select those foods that can keep them healthy and well.

So far, the health claims allowed include a relationship among the following:

- Potassium and reduced risk of high blood pressure (hypertension)
- Plant sterol and plant stanol esters and heart disease (Plant sterols and stanols are substances found naturally in certain plant foods that provide health benefits.)
- Whole grains and reduced risk of heart disease and certain cancers
- Soy protein and reduced risk of heart disease
- A diet with enough calcium and a lower risk of osteoporosis
- A diet low in total fat and a reduced risk of some cancers
- A diet low in saturated fat, cholesterol, and trans fat and a reduced risk of coronary heart disease
- A diet rich in fiber-containing grain products, fruits, and vegetables and a reduced risk of some cancers
- A diet rich in fiber-containing grain products, fruits, and vegetables and a reduced risk of coronary heart disease

Just the Facts: Using Labels to Teach Nutrition Literacy

Health care providers view nutrition as a basic component of health education and refer patients to nutritionists for nutrition education. Nurses are in the position to reinforce nutrition concepts first presented by nutritionists. Although physicians may be viewed as the experts on health, patients who have low literacy skills tend to use their social network of family and friends for health and nutrition information. Consequently, for interventions to be successful, members of social networks should be included. The approach should be visual, interactive, and culturally appropriate. This lesson on label comprehension fits these three criteria.

Clients should be presented with three boxes of cereal or Nutrition Facts labels from three cereal products. Choose three different products. For example, include a heavily presweetened cereal, a lightly sweetened cereal, and one with no added sweeteners. Ask the following questions:

- *Which has the most kcal per serving?* This may be affected by weight, volume of the cereal (popped with air), and the density of added ingredients like raisins.
- *Which has the largest serving size?* Serving sizes are the same by weight for all products in a food category.
- *Which contains the most dietary fat?* Fat is not an issue with cereals, except for granola.
- *Which contains the most sodium?* Some cereals contain about 300 mg, which is high for sodium-sensitive clients.
- *Which contains the most added sugars?* Added sugars can range from none to 13 g per serving.
- *How many calories come from sugars?* Multiply the number of grams of sugars by 4 kcal. By dividing this number by the total kcal per serving and multiplying the decimal by 100, you can determine the percentage of sugar content.
- *Which contains the most fiber?* Fiber content can range from none to about 5 g per serving.

As your study of nutrition continues, you may add other questions and be able to relate client responses to preventive health issues of diet-related diseases or to address specific dietary needs of a patient's nutrition therapy.

Data from Lee SY et al.: Health literacy, social support, and health: a research agenda, *Soc Sci Med* 58(7):1309-1321, 2004.

- A diet low in sodium and a reduced risk of high blood pressure
- A diet rich in fruits and vegetables and a reduced risk of some cancers
- Folic acid and a decreased risk of neural tube defect–affected pregnancy
- Dietary sugar alcohols and a reduced risk of dental caries (decay)
- Fluoridated water and reduced risk of dental caries (decay)
- Soluble fiber from certain foods, such as whole oats and psyllium seed husk, as part of a diet low in saturated fat and cholesterol and a reduced risk of heart disease

Food labeling legislation also covers dietary supplements. The Dietary Supplement Health and Education Act of 1994 (DSHEA) requires the FDA to prove a dietary supplement is unsafe or adulterated or has false or misleading labeling. The act does not allow claims about diagnosis, treatment, or prevention of disease but does allow that claims of certain benefits must be truthful. A standard statement is required on the label by the FDA[26] (see Chapter 16).

FOOD SAFETY

Food safety is influenced by community decisions and personal behaviors. We expect the larger community, such as government agencies, to supervise the production and preparation of food products to ensure the safety of the foods we purchase. But once we as consumers purchase food products, we are responsible for the proper handling of foods to prevent foodborne illness.

These concerns apply equally in the nursing setting. Our clients are also consumers. Our recommendations regarding nutritional intake are "translated" by our clients when they become consumers. As we advise about nutrition concerns, public and personal food safety is an issue.

The knowledge, attitudes, perceptions, and concerns that consumers have about food safety affect the food decisions they make. There is enormous concern from consumers and the food industry that the U.S. food supply must be safe. To have a safe food supply, it is essential for each sector of the food chain (producers, manufacturers, wholesalers, food stores, food service outlets, and consumers) to follow correct food-handling procedures. Such procedures, called *Hazard Analysis Critical Control Points (HACCP) programs,* are developed for the various segments of the food system to improve food quality. Regardless of government actions and manufacturing procedures concerning safe food preparation, responsibility ultimately is on the individual consumer who prepares food at home.

Risk Analysis and Food Safety

Setting risk standards involves determining a balance between risk and benefit for those who produce and consume foods. Risks to human health and to the environment are balanced against the economic benefits sustained by the use of insecticides, fungicides, and rodenticides. However, like the other approaches used to set risk standards, risk-benefit estimates for foods are limited by the unavailability of reliable quantitative data to use in the analysis.

Biotechnology: Consumer Risk or Benefit?

Biotechnology has become a common term. But how does it relate to our nutrient intake and food supply? Forms of food biotechnology control the modification of the genetic structure of foods at the molecular level to improve nutrient content, increase crop or animal yield, inhibit spoilage, and otherwise enhance desirable characteristics of food products.

Traditional biotechnology efforts resulted in random mutations from crossbreeding of plants or animals. These changes seem to have shown little risk to consumers or the environment. However, the new molecular biotechnology raises concerns by some consumers and scientists, although risks are decreased compared with traditional biotechnology.

An example of biotechnology involves the transfer of a bacterium gene to corn and cotton plants that allows the plants to create pesticides as part of their natural growth cycle. The created pesticides are harmful only to insects preying on those plants and are harmless to humans and other insects and animals. Consequently, fewer pesticides can be used while maintaining or increasing crops.[27]

Currently, genetically engineered crops are commonly used for feeds for animals. More than half of soybean and a quarter of corn crops are genetically altered forms. This means the poultry and meats we consume most likely were raised on these crops.

To ensure safety, food that has been transformed with genes should be tested to determine whether toxic substances have been unwittingly produced or whether the food produces a protein that may elicit an allergic reaction in susceptive individuals. Routine testing determines whether the modified product now contains an allergen not previously detected. The evaluation process of the FDA meets the international food safety guidelines as set by the Codex Alimentarius Commission. The Codex is an organization of the World Health Organization and the Food and Agriculture Organization of the United Nations. The Codex is the highest international organization overseeing food standards.[27]

Additional questions need to be considered as other food products are genetically modified. Will such changes increase supply and availability, thereby lowering the price of nutritious foods? An example is the increased milk yield from cows treated with recombinant bovine somatotropin (rBST), sometimes called *bovine growth hormone* (BGH) or *bovine hormone somatotropin* (BST). Another change is the use in cheese-making of pure chymosin enzyme from molecular biotechnology rather than the more expensive rennet from calves' stomachs. The FDA has approved both of these products of biotechnology.

How would lower prices affect the farmers who grow the crops or whose cows produce the milk? If these genetic manipulations keep prices high by producing "status" perfect quality produce, who gains? Or are these scientific developments simply a continuation of the food biotechnology time line started when milk was first pasteurized to destroy bacteria? There are no clear answers.

A recent development is the availability of cattle, swine, and goat clones. The clones of these species and their offspring have been declared safe for consumption by humans and animals by the FDA. According to the FDA, special food labels for such cloned and cloned-related products are not necessary because scientifically there is no difference between foodstuff from the cloned animals and traditionally raised animals. Clones are primarily used for breeding rather than as a direct source of food. This means that cloned animals participate in conventional (sexual) breeding and the resulting offspring are a food source. Clones of other animals such as sheep are not recommended for consumption at this time because not much is known as yet about other cloned species.[28]

Food Safety and Manufactured Products

Once produce is grown and ready to be eaten or processed into multi-ingredient products, other issues of food safety arise. Food safety approaches consider *risk* as keeping substances out of the food supply and *benefits* as enhancing the shelf life and maintaining the nutrition quality of food products. This was the basis of the original *Delaney Clause* that addresses food additives and other detailed government regulations. In 1996 the Food Quality Protection Act was passed, which replaced the zero tolerance for cancer-causing agents in foods of the *Delaney Clause* by reforming federal standards for pesticide residues in foods with a standard of "reasonable certainty of no harm."

Additives that are considered safe and were already in use when the food safety acts first went into effect are on a generally recognized as safe (GRAS) list; new additives are added as their safety is established. However, in the years since the original GRAS list was established, methods of analysis have become more sensitive and can detect lower and lower levels of these substances, thus calling into question the safety of additives on the original list. As a result, a comprehensive review of the list and all chemicals added to food is conducted periodically by the Federation of American Societies for Experimental Biology (FASEB).

Additives used for their functional properties in foods during processing—that is, to improve food quality in some way—are called **intentional (direct) food additives**, and those that contaminate or inadvertently become a part of a food at some time as it passes through the food system are called **incidental (indirect) food additives**. Direct additives are used to improve, maintain, and stabilize food quality; to increase availability across the country and lengthen storage time; to increase convenience; to decrease waste; and to stabilize or increase nutrient content. Table 2-2 lists selected intentional GRAS food additives. Indirect additives include pesticide and herbicide residues, animal drugs, processing aids, and packaging constituents that migrate from the package into the food. Regardless of their source, indirect additives seem to be of greatest concern to consumers.

Foodborne Illness

From the practical standpoint of keeping people well, consumers and professionals must acknowledge the importance of microbiologic contaminants; both groups need to work together to help prevent foodborne illness. In addition to discomfort, these illnesses cause greater economic costs in terms of lost time at work and productivity than most people can imagine. Unfortunately, the incidence of foodborne illness in the United States is increasing, according to the CDC, which keeps statistical data on these illnesses. Because

TABLE 2-2   INTENTIONAL FOOD ADDITIVES

TYPE OF ADDITIVE	PURPOSE
Processing Aids	
Anticaking agents	Prevent particles from collecting together in clumps (e.g., keep salt free flowing)
Conditioners	Make dough less sticky and easier to handle
Dough strengtheners	Help dough to withstand mechanical action of automatic processing
Drying agents	Absorb moisture to keep packaged products from becoming soggy or lumpy
Emulsifiers	Prevent oil separation in salad dressings
Enzymes	Speed up reactions that otherwise would be very slow
Firming agents	Stabilize and prevent flow of a dough
Flour treatments	Modify response of flour to mixing, as in making a dough
Leavening agents	Make baked products rise and become light (e.g., yeast baking powder, soda)
Lubricants	Ingredients such as fat in a dough that help keep it pliable and moldable
Propellants	Gases used to make sprays from fluids (e.g., oil spray for coating pans)
Solvents	Fluids in which particles of another compound dissolve (e.g., water is a solvent for sugar)
Stabilizers	Used to keep fat globules small in ice cream or air bubbles small in whipped cream
Texturizers	Contribute to texture in some way (e.g., crunchy)
Thickening agents	Increase thickness (viscosity) of liquids
Preservatives	
Acidulants	Acids that prevent growth of microorganisms in food
Antimicrobials	Control growth of microorganisms in food
Antioxidants	Help prevent or slow down development of "off" flavors and odors of fat-containing foods
Curing and pickling agents	Control microbial growth in meat, pickles, sauerkraut
Fumigants	Chemical control of pests and/or deterioration; usually leave residues in the food
Oxidizing and reducing agents	Influence interactions in food systems that cause deterioration
Appearance and Flavor Enhancers	
Clarifying agents	Combine with and precipitate or disperse compounds that prevent fluids from being clear
Color	Natural or synthetic compounds added to improve the color of food
Flavor enhancers	Improve flavor by strengthening flavors in a product
Flavoring agents	Added to foods to improve flavor or for special effects
Nonnutritive sweeteners	Noncaloric compounds usually with high intensity of sweetness
Nutritive sweeteners	Sweeteners that supply calories

many cases of foodborne illness are not reported, federal agencies must rely on estimates to define the size of the problem. Microorganisms are estimated to be responsible for 76 million cases of foodborne illness, resulting in 325,000 hospitalizations and about 5000 deaths each year.[29]

Food can become contaminated with bacteria, molds, parasites, and viruses during production, processing, transporting, storage, and retailing. It also can become contaminated in the home. Although the entire food distribution system may contribute to foodborne illness, improper handling of food in the home is a commonly overlooked source of contamination and growth of illness-causing microorganisms. The severity of foodborne illness varies with the microorganism, the susceptibility of the person, and the amount of bacteria or enterotoxin ingested. Information about sources, symptoms, and special control recommendations for common bacterial infections and intoxications are identified in Box 2-7.

Some individuals are at greater risk of foodborne illness. These high-risk groups include the elderly, children, pregnant women, individuals with human immunodeficiency

virus/acquired immunodeficiency syndrome (HIV/AIDS), and others whose immune systems are compromised such as individuals undergoing chemotherapy. Individuals living in institutional settings such as nursing homes, assisted living communities, correctional facilities, schools, shelters, or daycare centers are also at greater risk for foodborne illness.[30]

As the palates of Americans become more accustomed to exotic sensations, the Japanese meal of sushi—raw fish with vinegared rice—often is ordered in the growing number of Japanese restaurants. However, the fish must be served fresh and free of parasites; Anisakidae nematode parasites can be a problem when eating raw fish. Although such parasitic infections are usually transient, several cases of more serious parasitic bowel obstruction have occurred, characterized by sudden symptoms of severe nausea and/or vomiting, abdominal pain, and diarrhea.[31]

Therefore, sushi is not a dish to prepare at home. It is safest when prepared by specially trained chefs. Licensing of sushi chefs is not mandatory in the United States; consequently, sushi chefs are not required to meet the strict standards of licensed chefs. As a precaution, people with reduced

BOX 2-7   FOODBORNE ILLNESS: TEN LEAST WANTED FOODBORNE PATHOGENS

Least Wanted Foodborne Pathogens

The U.S. Public Health Service has identified the following microorganisms as being the biggest culprits of foodborne illness, either because of the severity of the sickness or the number of cases of illness they cause. Beware of these pathogens: Fight BAC!

Learn Where They Are and How to Avoid Them

1. *Campylobacter.* Second most common bacterial cause of diarrhea in the United States. Sources: raw and undercooked poultry and other meat, raw milk, and untreated water.
2. *Clostridium botulinum:* This organism produces a toxin that causes botulism, a life-threatening illness that can prevent the breathing muscles from moving air in and out of the lungs. Sources: Improperly prepared home-canned foods; honey should not be fed to children younger than 12 months old.
3. *Escherichia coli 0157:H7:* A bacterium that can produce a deadly toxin and that causes approximately 73,000 cases of foodborne illness each year in the United States. Sources: Beef, especially undercooked or raw hamburger; produce; raw milk; and unpasteurized juices and ciders.
4. *Listeria monocytogenes:* Causes listeriosis, a serious disease for pregnant women, newborns, and adults with a weakened immune system. Sources: Unpasteurized dairy products, including soft cheeses; sliced deli meats; smoked fish; hot dogs; pate; and deli-prepared salads (i.e., egg, ham, seafood, and chicken salads).
5. *Norovirus.* The leading *viral* cause of diarrhea in the United States. Poor hygiene causes Norovirus to be easily passed from person to person and from infected individuals to food items. Sources: Any food contaminated by someone who is infected with this virus.
6. *Salmonella:* Most common *bacterial* cause of diarrhea in the United States and the most common cause of foodborne deaths. Responsible for 1.4 million cases of foodborne illness a year. Sources: Raw and undercooked eggs, undercooked poultry and meat, fresh fruits and vegetables, and unpasteurized dairy products.
7. *Staphylococcus aureus:* This bacterium produces a toxin that causes vomiting shortly after being ingested. Sources: Cooked foods high in protein (e.g., cooked ham, salads, bakery products, dairy products) that are held too long at room temperature.
8. *Shigella:* Causes an estimated 448,000 cases of diarrhea illnesses per year. Poor hygiene causes Shigella to be easily passed from person to person and from infected individuals to food items. Sources: Salads, unclean water, and any food handled by someone who is infected with the bacterium.
9. *Toxoplasma gondii:* A parasite that causes toxoplasmosis, a very severe disease that can produce central nervous system disorders, particularly mental retardation and visual impairment in children. Pregnant women and people with weakened immune systems are at higher risk. Sources: Raw or undercooked pork.
10. *Vibrio vulnificus:* Causes gastroenteritis, wound infection, and severe bloodstream infections. People with liver diseases are especially at high risk. Sources: Raw or undercooked seafood, particularly shellfish.

Chart accessed January 10, 2010, from http://www.fightbac.org/about-foodborne-illness/least-wanted-pathogens. Accessed September 13, 2010.

immune system disorders, liver disorders, and other at-risk people should avoid consuming raw and undercooked fish and animal foods such as sushi and sashimi (raw fish only).[30] Even though such complications are rare, these foods should still not be an everyday treat but can be enjoyed safely in moderation (see the *Cultural Considerations* box, Ethnic Food Preferences and Foodborne Illness).

What could be more wholesome and healthful than fresh cider straight from the cider mill? Unfortunately, a number of people who sipped cider at an apple farm in Massachusetts learned otherwise when they fell victim to a pathogenic type of *Escherichia coli (E. coli)* bacteria and experienced gastrointestinal distress. It seems that apples used for cider are often those that have fallen to the ground and have blemishes. The problem is those apples may come in contact with animal feces and manure fertilizer; unless the apples are washed well or the cider is pasteurized or preserved with sodium benzoate, this contamination can lead to illness.

Consequently, all packaged juices that are not pasteurized or treated to prevent the growth of illness-causing microbes must have warning labels stating the following:

WARNING: This product has not been pasteurized and therefore may contain harmful bacteria that can cause serious illness in children, the elderly, and people with weakened immune systems.

Some types of *E. coli* are normally found in the human intestinal system; they are responsible for producing vitamins B_{12} and K and for limiting the growth of other undesirable bacteria. But we have few defenses against the pathogenic *E. coli* 0157:H7. This form of *E. coli* was found in a batch of meat that had been distributed to restaurants in the northwest United States in 1993. When the cooks at a fast-food restaurant chain undercooked hamburgers containing this *E. coli* organism, 4 children died and about 500 people became ill. The bacteria attacked the intestinal walls, which allowed the effects to spread to other parts of the body, particularly the kidneys. Cooking the meat to a well-done stage with no trace of redness would have destroyed the *E. coli* bacteria.[32] As a result of this outbreak, the USDA now recommends that ground beef and venison be cooked to a minimum internal temperature of 71° C (160° F) and poultry to 82° C (180° F)

⊕ CULTURAL CONSIDERATIONS

Ethnic Food Preferences and Foodborne Illness

America is sometimes described as a "cultural melting pot." This means that the traditions of our many ethnic and racial subgroups are accepted and sometimes adopted by others within the larger American population. Some of these ethnic food preferences may be associated with increased risk of foodborne illness. The following text contains a few examples.

During the Christmas holiday season, chitterlings (cooked swine intestines) are served as part of African American tradition. During this same holiday time frame of November through December, the incidence of *Yersinia enterocolitica* increases and peaks in December among African Americans, particularly among young children. The illness even occurs among infants whose pacifiers test positive for the pathogen. This foodborne illness should be considered when symptoms of fever, abdominal pain, and bloody diarrhea are presented, especially from November through February. The infection may mimic appendicitis. Other symptoms may include joint pain and blood infections. More severe cases may require antibiotic therapy. To prevent infection, boil raw chitterlings for 5 minutes before cleaning and cooking. Care should be taken to avoid cross-contamination through food contact with surfaces and utensils in the cooking area and even through person to person (such as infants and young children) if hands are not washed thoroughly with soap and warm water.

Among Hispanic Americans, a homemade soft cheese prepared from unpasteurized milk, *queso fresco,* has been tied to cases of *Listeriosis*. National data from the CDC indicate that this risk of infection is greater for Hispanic women of childbearing ages and their infants. Other Hispanic food consumption practices potentially linked to greater risk of food-related illness are consumption of unpasteurized fruit juices, undercooked eggs, certain fruits, and vegetables for *Campylobacter* infection as well as salmonellosis and listeriosis.

Application to nursing: Generally, the American minority groups of African Americans, Hispanics, and Asians have higher incidence of foodborne illness than non-Hispanic whites. This may be tied to specific ethnic foods and their preparation and storage. As the differences in rates and types of foodborne illnesses are studied, food safety strategies geared to specific ethnic and racial subgroups will be possible.

We need to ask our clients what they ate the previous day to really determine the cause of their "stomach virus." A response of "some cheese" may not be sufficient, particularly if the client is from a specific ethnic group. Being sensitive to ethnicity does not mean treating everyone as if their diet is the same but treating each individual in a culturally sensitive approach to maintain and/or restore health.

Data from Ray SM et al.: Population-based surveillance for *Yersinia enterocolitica* infections in FoodNet sites, 1996-1999: Higher risk of disease in infants and minority populations, *Clin Infect Dis* 38(Suppl 3):S181-S189, 2004; Taege A: *Food-borne disease, Disease management project*, Cleveland, 2004, The Cleveland Clinic Foundation; U.S. Department of Agriculture, Food Safety and Inspection Service: *Yersiniosis and Chitterlings: Tips to Protect You and Those You Care for from Foodborne Illness,* February 2007. Accessed on January 10, 2010, from www.fsis.usda.gov/PDF/Yersiniosis_and_Chitterlings.pdf.

in restaurants and in the home. *E. coli* 0157:H7 is also thought to have been responsible for illnesses from raw milk, dry cured salami, lettuce, produce from manure-fertilized gardens, potatoes, radish sprouts, alfalfa sprouts, yogurt, sandwiches, and water. The CDC estimates that at least 20,000 cases of *E. coli*–related foodborne illnesses occur each year as additional outbreaks occur.

While these examples of foodborne disease appeared to be locally bound, nationwide outbreaks of *E. coli* and salmonella have occurred and unfortunately may continue as the food sources become more diverse. Green, leafy vegetables, a foundation of a health-promoting dietary pattern, have been determined to be sources of several *E. coli* occurrences due to contamination at various levels of production and processing. Should we still consume green, leafy vegetables? Of course we should but we can take control by practicing appropriate food safety measures in our homes, while federal food-safety agencies which includes the USDA, FDA, and the CDC, work to limit and prevent foodborne illnesses through creation of mechanisms and policies to uncover potential sources of contamination within production and processing of the food supply.[33] Other outbreaks of salmonella include contaminated peppers

and peanut butter that was used as an ingredient of peanut products, including ice cream, snack bars, cereals, and even in pet food.[33] Media-wide announcements of such episodes include specific products that should not be consumed once the source has been identified.

To assist the public in dealing with food and medical related adverse reactions, the following hotlines are available:

Center for Food Safety and Applied Nutrition Outreach and Information Center: (888) SAFE FOOD

FDA Foodborne Illness Reporting Emergency Line: (301) 443-1240

FDA Medical Products Reporting MedWatch Line: (800) FDA-1088

FDA website: www.fda.gov/medwatch/how.htm

USDA Meat and Poultry Food Safety Hotline: (800) 535-4555

Food Preparation Strategies

Although government inspection programs should guard against foodborne illnesses, we must adhere to safe food handling procedures in the home and follow food safety guidelines when we eat away from home as an aspect of personal

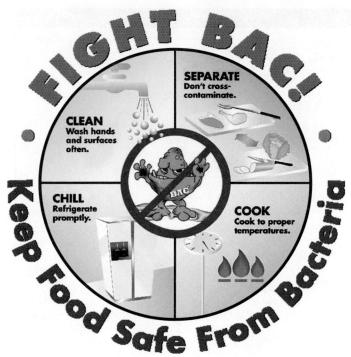

FIG 2-8 Fight BAC! This logo represents the public-private coalition of the Partnership for Food Safety Education, which educates the public about food safety strategies through multiple media approaches. Materials are available at www.fightbac.org. (From Partnership for Food Safety Education, Washington, DC.)

responsibility for our nutrition. Following are some recommendations from FightBAC!, a public-private coalition of the Partnership for Food Safety Education that informs the public about food safety strategies[34] (Figure 2-8):

- To ensure sanitary food handling in the home, make sure the food preparer's hands are clean, that clean equipment is used, and that a clean surrounding is maintained, including cutting boards and countertops.
- Wash hands with soap and hot water before preparing and cooking foods.
- Wash cutting boards, utensils, and countertops that come into contact with uncooked meats, poultry, or fish with hot soapy water and a disinfectant.
- Do not place cooked foods on unwashed surfaces where uncooked foods have been prepared because the cooked foods will become contaminated with the microorganisms on these surfaces. Cooking destroys bacteria, but bacteria from uncooked foods on unwashed surfaces can reinfect any cooked food placed on them.
- Keep foods either colder than 4° C (40° F) or hotter than 60° C (140° F). The danger zone for rapid growth of microorganisms is a temperature inside this range. Foods can easily fall into this zone at a picnic or a potluck meal.
- Use a simple food thermometer to check internal temperatures when cooking meat, poultry, and fish. USDA Recommended Internal Temperatures:

Ground beef/ hamburgers	160° F	Chicken breasts	170° F
Pork	160° F	Whole chicken	180° F
Steaks and roasts	145° F	Fish	145° F
Egg dishes	160° F		

For questions, USDA Meat and Poultry Hotline: 1-888-MPHotline (1-888-674-6854)

- Refrigerate cooked foods *immediately* after meals or after they are cooked. DO NOT cool to room temperature and then refrigerate.
- Boil all home-canned vegetables, meats, poultry, and fish for 10 minutes before tasting.
- Discard or boil marinades used with uncooked meats, poultry, and fish after marinating is completed; bacteria are not destroyed until heated.
- Cook all meat 71° C (160° F), poultry 82° C (180° F), shellfish, and fish to the well-done stage.
- Do not eat or taste any uncooked foods containing raw eggs, including cookie and cake batters. They could contain salmonella.
- NEVER use a recipe that calls for raw eggs and is not cooked or baked after addition of the eggs. When making homemade ice cream, cook the eggs by making soft custard; do not use raw eggs in the mixture to be frozen.
- Microwave cooking can be tricky and dangerous. NEVER store defrosted and/or partially cooked meats and poultry. Cook them completely to the well-done stage first, and then eat or refrigerate.
- When food shopping, choose perishable foods (those from the refrigerator or freezer cases) last and get them home as soon as possible. Don't leave them sitting in the car while doing other errands.
- Never buy or use foods in a bulging can, cracked jar, or bulging lid. Damage to containers may have allowed botulism to develop. Don't taste to determine if spoiled; this toxin is extremely dangerous.

Of course, adhering to these guidelines can become a major challenge in disaster situations. The *Personal Perspectives* box, Surviving Katrina from a Food Perspective, provides some insight into a unique situation in which a medical center was tasked to find safe ways to continue providing meal service to its patients in the aftermath of Hurricane Katrina in 2005, one of the worst natural disasters in the United States.

Additional common food safety mistakes include the following:

- Thawing frozen foods and meats on countertop; *instead, thaw in microwave or refrigerator*
- Cooling leftovers on the counter; *instead, refrigerate in small batches as soon as possible*
- Marinating at room temperature; *instead, refrigerate when marinating*
- Delaying refrigeration of restaurant "doggie bags"; *instead, place in a thermos-cooler bag*
- Tasting stirring spoon; *instead, use a clean spoon for each taste test*

PERSONAL PERSPECTIVES

Surviving Katrina from a Food Perspective

Hurricane Katrina hit the Atlantic basin in August 2005, devastating New Orleans and the coastal regions of Louisiana, Mississippi, and Alabama, which meant that hundreds of thousands of individuals were displaced because their homes and communities were destroyed. Following is a personal account by the director of Food & Nutrition Services, University of South Alabama Medical Center, Mobile, as she and her staff struggled to prepare food for patients and staff during and after the hurricane.*

Despite a good disaster plan in place at the University of South Alabama Medical Center, during Hurricane Katrina we learned there can always be scenarios that plans just do not cover. When that happens, you must improvise!

For example, the ceiling caved in during the lunch service, pouring buckets of water into the cafeteria. We pulled the contents out of our portable salad bar, removed the sneeze guard and used the bar to catch rain and drain through the salad bar floor drain. Then we roped the area surrounding the bar with caution tape. (Always have spare tape stored in your department; you can't wait for the maintenance department, especially during a disaster.)

After the cave-in, we switched dinner to carryout dinners. Each department head preordered the number of meals needed for their staff, and at serving time one person from each department used a cart to pick up meals for their co-workers.

Other issues involved cafeteria transactions. When the cash registers were not functioning due to power outages or leaks, we learned it is a good idea to keep notebooks and pencils in the registers so cashiers can tally and record meal sales.

What do you do when the ice supply keeps getting stolen from the machines? The first night after the theft, I slept next to the ice machine with one eye open. The next night we hooked gauges up to a compressor and posted a sign reading: Contaminated Ice!

Later we had hasp locks installed on the ice machines and secured them when the department was closed. In the future we will also bag ice before a storm and store it in a walk-in freezer with emergency power.

The most important lesson I learned from this experience is to be as prepared as possible, but to be able to think critically and adapt for the numerous unplanned events that occur.

Nancy Brumfield, RD
Director of Food & Nutrition Services
University of South Alabama Medical Center
Mobile, Alabama

The following excerpt is from an FDA bulletin on food safety during and after a hurricane.† For additional information, go to www.fda.gov.

Here's what FDA suggests consumers can do at home to keep their food safe:

Food Safety When the Power Goes Out

- Keep the refrigerator and freezer doors closed as much as possible to maintain the cold temperature. The refrigerator will keep food cold for about 4 hours if it is unopened. A full freezer will keep the temperature for approximately 48 hours (24 hours if it is half full) if the door remains closed. Buy dry or block ice to keep the refrigerator as cold as possible if the power is going to be out for a prolonged period of time. Fifty pounds of dry ice should hold an 18-cubic foot fully stocked freezer cold for two days.
- If you plan to eat refrigerated or frozen meat, poultry, fish, or eggs while they are still at safe temperatures, it's important that the food is thoroughly cooked to the proper temperature to assure that any foodborne bacteria that may be present is destroyed.
- Wash fruits and vegetables with water from a safe source before eating.
- For infants, if possible, use prepared, canned baby formula that requires no added water. When using concentrated or powdered formulas, prepare with bottled water if the local water source is potentially contaminated.

Once the Power Is Restored

- Once the power is restored you will need to evaluate the safety of the food. If an appliance thermometer was kept in the freezer, read the temperature when the power comes back on. If the thermometer stored in the freezer reads 40° F or below the food is safe and may be refrozen. If a thermometer has not been kept in the freezer, check each package of food to determine the safety. Remember, you can't rely on appearance or odor. If the food still contains ice crystals or is 40° F or below, it is safe to refreeze or cook.
- Refrigerated food should be safe as long as the power is out for no more than 4 hours. Keep the door closed as much as possible. Discard any perishable food (such as meat, poultry, fish, eggs or leftovers) that has been above 40° F for two hours or more.

---

*From Brumfield N: "After the theft, I slept next to the ice machine with one eye open," ADA Times, 3(2, Nov/Dec):4, 2005.
†From U.S. Food and Drug Adminstration: Food facts:What consumers need to know about food and water safety during hurricanes, power outages, and floods, December 2009 (updated May 2009), Author, Retrieved September 12, 2010, from www.fda.gov/Food/ResourcesForYou/Consumers/ucm076881.htm.*

- Consuming hide-and-seek Easter eggs; *instead prepare some to be refrigerated*
- Buying foods with expired use dates; *instead, check dates when shopping*

We tend to be casual about food preparation. After all, we eat all the time. However, sometimes being too relaxed allows for these bacterial and viral contaminations to occur. In our homes, we must implement basic food safety procedures when preparing and storing foods; in food retail markets and food service facilities, we count on the expertise and supervision of public health officers to enforce regulations that provide safe food.

As nurses we must recognize our role in providing safe foods to patients. When handling foods for patients, care must be taken to prevent contamination by using the techniques of food handlers, such as hand washing before serving meals or assisting patients with their meals.

Food Preservation to Control Foodborne Illness

Through the years, many methods were developed and used to preserve food for future use by controlling decomposition and microbial growth that could lead to foodborne illness. Besides drying and dehydrating, which limit moisture in the food, methods developed include canning, refrigerating and freezing, pasteurizing, curing and smoking, modified atmosphere packaging, aseptic packaging, and irradiating foods. In canning, heat is used to destroy microorganisms; in pickling, salt, acid (vinegar), and usually heat control microbial growth; and in jellies and jams, sugar is the preservative. Refrigerating and freezing limit the growth of microorganisms by the use of cold temperatures. Pasteurizing uses heat to destroy pathogenic organisms in milk and other undesirable ones in other foods. Salts and different types of smoke cure and preserve meat, poultry, and fish. Modified atmosphere packaging provides an atmosphere of various gases in the package that helps control microbial growth to preserve the food. Aseptic packaging preserves food and prevents contamination by placing food products that are sterilized separately from the packaging into sterilized containers, which are immediately sealed.

Irradiation is a procedure by which food is exposed to radiation that destroys microorganisms, insect growth, and parasites that could spoil food or cause illness. This food preservation technology results in an increase of international and domestic food trade. By decreasing economic losses caused by food spoilage, insects, sprouting, parasites, microorganisms associated with foodborne disease, and changes associated with ripening, irradiated products can be shipped farther and still remain safe to eat. The use of irradiation for poultry products is a specific example of efforts to control *salmonellosis* and *campylobacteriosis*.

Irradiation involves exposure of food to gamma irradiation using cobalt-60 or cesium-137 or to an electron beam from electron accelerators. The machine sources may be the least controversial of the sources of radiation because they are independent of nuclear energy, so there is no radioactive waste. Extensive testing shows irradiated foods as wholesome

FIG 2-9 The radura symbol must be carried by all foods that have been treated with radiation, although it need not be carried by processed foods that include irradiated ingredients.

and nonradioactive and provides consumers with a reduced risk of foods contaminated with micro-organisms that cause foodborne illness.[30]

Irradiated whole foods (as opposed to foods containing irradiated ingredients) in the United States must be labeled as "Treated with Radiation" or "Treated by Irradiation" and must display the international symbol for irradiated foods, radura (Figure 2-9).

As health professionals we can assist other food and nutrition professionals to educate our clients as consumers about the value of this technology as safeguarding our food supply in the marketplace and in our homes.

TOWARD A POSITIVE NUTRITION LIFESTYLE: LOCUS OF CONTROL

Do things just happen to you? Does it seem as if school, family, or society affect what you do without your input? Or do you feel that you have control over what takes place? Do you have a life plan (or weekly plan) that you follow? Locus of control is the perception of one's ability to control life events and experiences. Having an internal locus of control means feeling as if you can influence the forces with which you come into contact. You have an inner sense of your ability to guide life events. An external locus of control is defined as the perception of not being able to control what happens to you and that outside forces have power over what you experience.

Let's apply these concepts to your style of making food choices when shopping. In particular, consider the nutritional implications of locus of control. If you have an internal locus of control, you may develop a basic plan of the types of nutritious foods to be purchased during a shopping trip. You may make a few unplanned purchases, but they would be limited. You feel in control of your choices. Having an external locus of control means you might start out with a shopping list, but you are probably easily swayed by in-store promotions, coupons, and even colorful packaging to select products not on your list. You often buy more than needed because so much "looked good."

Awareness of our type of locus of control allows us to develop strategies to improve our food decisions. Individuals with an internal locus of control tend to develop their own approaches for changing food-related behaviors; those with an external locus of control may need a structured program or group support to provide guidance to modify their food behaviors.

SUMMARY

This chapter considers factors of personal and community nutrition. Food preferences, food choices, and food liking greatly influence the foods we choose and so affect our overall nutritional status. As knowledge of the relationship between diet and disease increases, public health approaches to diet-related disease prevention encourage us to select foods not just for their nutrient and energy content but for their primary disease prevention value as well. Food guides were created to implement the dietary recommendations on a daily basis. These guides address the concerns of nutrient adequacy and primary disease prevention. MyPyramid and the "Fruits & Veggies—More Matters" program are easy to follow to improve our nutritional intake. Food consumption trends in the United States are an indication of changes in the American diet. These trends for fruits and vegetables; cereals and grains; meat, poultry, and fish; dairy products; and sweeteners reflect the availability and food choices of per capita consumption. This information helps us translate nutrients into food categories and attend to consumer needs and issues when advising clients or patients.

Providing health professionals and consumers with more information about foods through food labels increases the probability that decisions made and advice given about which foods to eat will be based on nutrition as well as on taste, thus contributing to health and wellness. Food safety is of concern because of its potential to eliminate or at least substantially decrease foodborne illness as more is learned about the various causes of this illness. Knowledge of how bacteria, molds, parasites, and viruses can be problems in the food supply helps us understand how to control these problems to stay well.

THE NURSING APPROACH

MyPyramid Teaching Project

One of the nurse's main roles in health education is teaching individuals and groups about nutrition. Each learning session is related to assessment of the client's learning needs and goals identified by the nurse and client. The overall objective of teaching/learning is to change behavior.

Factors that contribute to learning include the person's ability to comprehend English, literacy, motivation, readiness, involvement, relevance of the topic, and environment. Obviously, if the person does not speak or understand English, it is important to obtain an interpreter.

Some learning principles include (1) developing appropriate teaching materials that are age specific (e.g., children, older adults), (2) providing information that clients can relate to and covering what is known before proceeding to what is unknown, (3) pacing the learning session, (4) providing teaching aids and materials (e.g., visual handouts), (5) using layperson's terms, and (6) providing feedback and praise when appropriate.

The nurse can implement a variety of teaching methods, such as explanation, discussion, demonstration, group discussion, and role-playing.

Following is an example of a MyPyramid teaching project using the nursing process of ADPIE: assessment, diagnosis, planning, implementation, and evaluation.

ASSESSMENT
Assess Client/Learner Characteristics

- Age
- Language and ability to read
- Readiness to learn
- Learning style preference—visual aids, reading, demonstration, hands-on

DIAGNOSIS
Diagnose the knowledge deficit; determine the learning need
- What is already known about MyPyramid? About the traditional food pyramid?
- What does this person need to know or be able to do?
- What specific aspect of MyPyramid is this individual interested in learning?

THE NURSING APPROACH—cont'd

MyPyramid Teaching Project—cont'd

Example: Deficient knowledge: types and amounts of food recommended

PLANNING

Plan the Teaching

a. Objectives

What measurable behavior changes can result from the learning experience?

Examples:

The client/learner will be able to:

- Explain the symbols and guidelines in MyPyramid.
- Use MyPyramid as a guide for making healthy food choices.
- Seek out the MyPyramid website and obtain personalized guidelines.
- Track eating patterns at www.mypyramid.gov.
- Set a specific goal for improving food choices, based on MyPyramid guidelines.

b. Content

What information is appropriate for a teaching session 15 to 30 minutes long? Consider how long the person can focus and how much depth of information will be appropriate for the age of the person.

Examples:

- Purpose of MyPyramid (why developed, how it helps the individual)
- Meaning of the symbols (figures, colors, etc.)
- MyPyramid's general guidelines for activity and healthy eating
- MyPyramid plan (individualized types and amounts of food)
- Availability of interactive information and MyPyramid Tracker at www.mypyramid.gov

c. Teaching methods

What methods will facilitate change?

Examples:

- Lecture/discussion
- Demonstrate use of MyPyramid interactive site by sitting at a computer guiding the client/learner through the program.
- Provide and interpret a visual handout from www.mypyramid.gov, individualized by age and activity level.

d. Evaluation plan

How can learning be measured to determine if identified goals have been met?

Examples:

- Administer a short verbal quiz about MyPyramid.
- Play a game to sort out different foods and identify best choices to match MyPyramid.
- Assist the client/learner to write a specific measurable goal based on better food choices identified in MyPyramid.
- Observe the individual navigate in the MyPyramid website and obtain a personalized plan.

IMPLEMENTATION

Implement the Teaching Plan

- Choose a time and place where there will be no interruptions.
- Revise your plan as needed to match the knowledge and interest of the client/learner.
- Make the process interactive. Check for understanding frequently through an activity or what the individual states regarding the new information.
- Use understandable, age-appropriate terminology.
- Use visual aids and handouts the client/learner can use later.

EVALUATION

Evaluate

a. Client/learner

- What was the client/learner able to demonstrate at the end of the teaching session?
- Were the behavior change goals met, partially met, or not met?

b. Nurse/teacher

- Was the client/learner engaged in the lesson?
- Which teaching method or activity was effective?
- What was ineffective? What could be implemented differently to improve effectiveness next time?
- Was the teaching experience enjoyable? If not, how could the experience be improved?

Nursing Diagnoses-Definitions and Classification 2009-2011. Copyright © 2009, 1994-2009 by NANDA International. Used by arrangement with Blackwell Publishing Limited, a company of John Wiley & Sons, Inc.

APPLYING CONTENT KNOWLEDGE

Jenny is again visiting her primary health care provider for a "stomach virus." She has been seen several times for the same problem over the past few months. When conducting the intake interview, you wonder if she could have a recurring foodborne illness. What are three assessment questions you might ask her?

WEBSITES OF INTEREST

MyPlate Food Guidance System

www.choosemyplate.gov

The official "home" of MyPlate, the interactive food guidance system.

FoodSafety.gov

www.foodsafety.gov

A gateway linking government food safety-related resources.

U.S. Food and Drug Administration (FDA)

www.fda.gov

Gateway website connecting areas serviced and supervised by the FDA.

REFERENCES

1. U.S. Department of Health and Human Services, Public Health Service: *Executive summary Phase 1 report: Recommendations for the framework and format of Healthy People 2020*, Last revision Dec 11, 2008. Accessed on January 10, 2010, from www.healthypeople.gov/HP2020.

2. Logue AW: *The psychology of eating and drinking: An introduction*, ed 3, New York, 2004, Taylor & Francis Books Inc.

3. Drewrowski A, Henderson SA, Barratt-Fornell A: Genetic taste markers and food preferences, *Drug Metab Dispos* 29(4 pt2, April):535-538, 2001.

4. Birch LL, Fisher JA: The role of experience in the development of children's eating behavior. In Capaldi ED, editor: *Why we eat what we eat: The psychology of eating*, ed 2, Washington, DC, 2001, American Psychological Association.

5. Mennella JA, Beauchamp GK: The early development of human flavor preferences. In Capaldi ED, ed: *Why we eat what we eat: The psychology of eating*, ed 2, Washington, DC, 2001, American Psychological Association.

6. Kessler DA: *The end of overeating: controlling the insatiable American appetite*, New York, 2009, Rodale Inc.

7. Heron M et al: Deaths: Final data for 2006, *Nat Vital Stat Report 57*. Hyattsville, MD: National Center for Health Statistics, 2009.

8. U.S. Department of Agriculture, U.S. Department of Health and Human Services: *Report of the Dietary Guidelines Advisory Committee on the Dietary Guidelines for Americans, 2010*, Washington, DC, 2010, Author. Accessed June 16, 2010, from www.dietaryguidelines.gov.

9. U.S. Department of Agriculture, Center for Nutrition Policy and Promotion: 2011. Author. Accessed June 14, 2012 from www.choosemyplate.gov.

10. Centers for Disease Control and Prevention (CDC): *Behavioral risk factor surveillance system survey data*, Atlanta, 2008, U.S. Department of Health and Human Services, Centers for Disease Control and Prevention. Accessed January 10, 2010, from www.fruitsandveggiesmorematters.gov.

11. Willett WC, Skerrett PJ: *Eat, drink, and be healthy*, New York, 2005, Free Press/Simon & Schuster.

12. Oldways Preservation Trust: *Mediterranean diet pyramid, Latin American diet pyramid, Asian diet pyramid*, Cambridge, Mass, 2009, Author. Accessed January 10, 2010, from www.oldwayspt.org.

13. Painter J, Rah J-H, Lee Y-K: Comparison of international food guide pictorial presentations, *J Am Diet Assoc* 102(4):483-489, 2002.

14. Centers for Disease Control and Prevention: *About the National Fruit & Vegetable Program*, Atlanta, 2009, Author. Accessed January 10, 2010, from www.fruitsandveggiesmorematters.gov.

15. American Diabetes Association, American Dietetic Association: *Exchange lists for meal planning (revised)*, Alexandria, Va/Chicago, 2003, Authors.

16. Wylie-Rosett J, et al: 2006-2007 American Diabetes Association Nutrition Recommendations: Issues for Practice Translation, *J Am Diet Assoc* 107(8):1296-1304, 2007.

17. U.S. Department of Agriculture, Center for Nutrition Policy and Promotion: *MyPyramid Tracker* (OMB 0584-0535), Alexandria, Va, 2005, Author. Accessed January 10, 2010, from www.mypyramidtracker.gov.

18. Beydoun MA, Wang Y: Do nutrition knowledge and beliefs modify the association of socio-economic factors and diet quality among US adults? *Prev Med* 46(2):145-153, 2008.

19. The Hartman Group: Healthy eating trends 2009 *HartBeat* July 29, 2009. Accessed January 10, 2010, from www.hartman-group.com/hartbeat/healthy-eating-connections-to-attitudes-about-aging.

20. Blisard N, et al: *Low-income households' expenditures on fruits and vegetables*, Agricultural Economic Report No. (AER833), Washington, DC, 2004 (May), Economic Research Service, U.S. Department of Agriculture.

21. Wells HF, Buzby JC: *Dietary Assessment of Major Trends in U.S. Food Consumption, 1970-2005*, Economic Information Bulletin No. 33. March 2008, Economic Research Service, U.S. Dept. of Agriculture.

22. Economic Research Service, U.S. Department of Agriculture: *Diet Quality and Food Consumption: Dietary Trends from Food and Nutrient Availability Data*, Washington, DC, 2009 (July), Author. Retrieved January 10, 2010, from www.ers.usda.gov/Briefing/DietQuality/Availability.htm.

23. Rampersaud GC, et al: National survey beverage consumption data for children and adolescents indicate the need to encourage a shift toward more nutritive beverages, *J Am Diet Assoc* 103(1):97-100, 2003.

24. U.S. Food and Drug Administration, Center for Food Safety and Applied Nutrition: *How to understand and use the nutrition facts label*, College Park, Md, 2000 (updated November 2004),

Author. Accessed January 10, 2010, from www.cfsan.fda.gov/~dms/foodlab.html.

25. U.S. Department of Agriculture, Agricultural Marketing Service: *Organic Labeling and Marketing Information*, Washington, DC, 2002 (Updated April 2008), Author. Accessed January 10, 2010, from www.ams.usda.gov/AMSv1.0/nop.

26. U.S. Food and Drug Administration, Center for Food Safety and Applied Nutrition: *Dietary Supplement Health and Education Act of 1994*, College Park, Md, 1995 (December), (Updated June 2009), Author. Accessed January 10, 2010, from www.fda.gov/Food/DietarySupplements/default.htm.

27. Bren L: *FDA Consumer: Genetic engineering: The future of foods?* College Park, Md, 2003 (Nov/Dec), U.S. Food and Drug Administration, Center for Food Safety and Applied Nutrition.

28. U.S. Food and Drug Administration, Center for Food Safety and Applied Nutrition: *FDA Issues Documents on the Safety of Food from Animal Clones* (Press Release). January 15, 2008, (Updated June 2009), Author. Accessed January 10, 2010, from www.fda.gov/NewsEvents/Newsroom/PressAnnouncements/2008/ucm116836.htm.

29. National Digestive Diseases Information Clearinghouse, (NDDIC), National Institute of Diabetes and Digestive and Kidney Diseases (NIDDK), National Institutes of Health: *Bacteria and foodborne illness*, NIH Publication No. 07–4730, 2007 (May). Accessed January 10, 2010, from www.digestive.niddk.nih.gov/ddiseases/pubs/bacteria/.

30. American Dietetic Association: Position of the American Dietetic Association: Food and water safety, *J Am Diet Assoc* 109(8):1449-1460, 2009.

31. Takei H, Powell SZ: Intestinal anisakidosis (anisakiosis), *Ann Diagn Pathol* 11(5):350-352, 2007.

32. Buchanan RL, Doyle MP: Foodborne disease significance of *Escherichia coli* 0157:H7 and other enterohemorrhagic *E. coli*, *Food Technol* 51(10):67-96, 1994.

33. Maki DG: Coming to grips with food borne infection—peanut butter, peppers, and nationwide salmonella outbreaks, *N Engl J Med* 360(10):949-953, 2009.

34. Partnership for Food Safety Education: *FightBAC!* Washington, DC, 2004, Author. Accessed January 10, 2010, from www.fightbac.org.

PART 2

Nutrients, Food, and Health

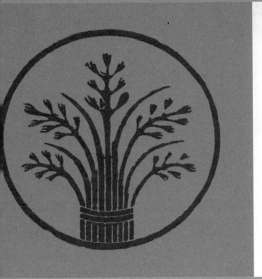

Digestion, Absorption, and Metabolism

The digestive system, which is responsible for processing foods, is itself dependent on our nutrient intake for its maintenance.

evolve WEBSITE

Nutrition Concepts Online

http://evolve.elsevier.com/Grodner/foundations/

ROLE IN WELLNESS

Gulping down breakfast on the way to class or work, skipping lunch, and then eating dinner late may not seem to affect the health status of adults. However, if this kind of eating becomes routine, it characterizes an individual's lifestyle and may negatively influence health status.

The body's health is based on the nutrients available to support growth, maintenance, and energy needs. Inadequate nutritional intake can affect the body's ability to use the foods consumed. The digestive system, which is responsible for processing foods, depends on nutrient intake for its maintenance. Although the body is resilient, we stress our physical limits when we adopt habits that do not support optimal health. A primary way to decrease the risk of future disease and achieve wellness is to use lifestyle choices that support positive health behaviors.

Physical health begins with the gastrointestinal (GI) tract as the first step to maintain body functioning; unless nutrients in foods are digested and absorbed, life cannot continue. The decision and follow-through to change lifestyle behaviors to positively improve health in relation to digestive disorders is an aspect of *intellectual health*. An individual's emotional state and ability to handle stress may increase the risk of several disorders of the GI tract. Consequently, the *emotional health* effects of lifestyle behaviors may be related to constipation, diarrhea, and heartburn. Reducing the causes of intestinal gas helps guard against socially embarrassing moments. Our food choices and styles of eating may affect the level of flatus experienced. Negativity associated with body smells is defined by society and thus affects our *social health* dimension. Respecting the sanctity of the human body, thereby acknowledging our *spiritual health* dimension, may include one's willingness to follow dietary and lifestyle changes to enhance the functioning of the GI tract (see the *Cultural Considerations* box, Wholeness of Body, Mind, and Self). This chapter presents a brief orientation to the processes of digestion, absorption, and metabolism. These processes work together to provide all body cells with energy and nutrients.

DIGESTION

The main organs of the digestion system (Figure 3-1 and Box 3-1) form the **gastrointestinal (GI) tract**, or alimentary canal, which creates an open tube that runs from the mouth to the anus. Everything we eat is processed through the GI tract. The **digestive system** consists of a series of organs that prepare ingested nutrients for **digestion** and absorption and protect against consumed microorganisms and toxic substances. To do this, several processes take place. These processes of ingestion, digestion, absorption, and elimination depend on the motility or movement of the GI wall and the secretions of digestive juices and enzymes.[1]

The Mouth

Are you hungry? Are you thinking about your favorite food? Is your mouth watering? Our mouths really do "water" when we think about or begin to eat foods. However, it is not actually water we sense but a thin mucous-like fluid called **saliva**. Saliva is the term for the secretions of the three salivary glands of the mouth. As **exocrine glands**, each set of salivary glands produces a different type of secretion that is released into the mouth. The parotid glands create watery saliva that supplies enzymes; the submandibular glands produce mucus and enzyme components; and the sublingual glands, the smallest,

🌐 CULTURAL CONSIDERATIONS
Wholeness of Body, Mind, and Self

This text's presentation of digestion and absorption is based on Western perspectives. To most Westerners, body organs tend to be viewed separately from mind and spiritual influences. In contrast, Ayurveda, traditional Indian medicine, meaning "the science of life," is based on living a balanced life. Consequently, Ayurveda treats physical disorders as the body (organs) or life being out of balance. Treatment works to bring balance or harmony back to the individual's life. The wholeness of life is represented by body *(shira),* mind *(manas),* and self *(atman).* All three require attention to achieve and maintain health. Because each component is important, Ayurveda is a holistic approach recognizing the interdependent roles of body, mind, and self. A person is viewed as a combination of three forces or humors called *doshas.* Each person is a different combination of these forces, which are *vata, pitta,* and *kapha. Vata* is a force similar to air; *pitta,* a force similar to fire; and *kapha,* a force like mucus and water. Health occurs when these *doshas* are in balance; otherwise disease occurs. If *pitta* is too strong, fever, ulcers, and liver disorders may occur. An individual would need to strengthen the other *doshas* through (1) changes in behaviors and food choices, (2) use of natural medicines, and (3) yoga and meditation to decrease *pitta* and regain balance.

Application to nursing: This concept may assist clients to understand that their illnesses may be affected by other components of their lives. Sometimes illnesses force us to confront factors that may influence our ability to maintain health or to achieve balance in our lives.

Data from Ninivaggi, FJ: *Ayurveda: A comprehensive guide to traditional Indian medicine for the West,* Westport, Conn, 2008, Praeger Press.

BOX 3-1   DIGESTIVE SYSTEM ORGANS

Segments of the Digestive Tract
Mouth
Oropharynx
Esophagus
Stomach
Small intestine
Duodenum
Jejunum
Ileum
Large intestine
Cecum
Colon
    Ascending colon
    Transverse colon
    Descending colon
    Sigmoid colon
Rectum
Anal canal

Accessory Organs
Salivary glands
Parotid gland
Submandibular gland
Sublingual gland
Tongue
Teeth
Liver
Gallbladder
Pancreas
Vermiform appendix

---

create a mucous type of saliva. A reflex mechanism controls these secretions.

Food in the mouth stimulates chemical and mechanical digestion. **Chemical digestion** occurs through the action of saliva that not only moistens the foods we chew but also contains amylase, an enzyme that begins the digestive process of starches.

Another digestive process that occurs in the mouth is **mechanical digestion**, which depends on teeth. Teeth rhythmically tear and pulverize food. The enamel covering teeth is the hardest substance in the body and therefore protects teeth from the harsh effects of chewing. The tongue assists with mechanical digestion by guiding food into chewing positions and then leading the pulverized food into the esophagus. Another function of the tongue is that of taste. More than 2000 taste buds are responsible for our sensations of sweet, bitter, sour, and salty when tasting foods (Figure 3-2).

As toddlers, we have the highest number of taste buds and a higher degree of taste sensitivity, so bland foods are more appealing. The number of taste buds declines as we grow older, which explains why older adults have diminished taste sensitivity. Older adults may need to be encouraged to avoid the use of too much salt, particularly if they have hypertension or cardiac disorders.

Our sense of smell works along with our taste bud sensations. These two combined senses actually account for the perception (and enjoyment) of the flavors of different foods. Our positive or negative response to specific foods based on our sensory perception affects our food choices.[2]

Portions of the pulverized or masticated food are formed into the shape of a ball called a **bolus.** The tongue effortlessly forms the bolus, which is then swallowed and passed by the epiglottis into the esophagus within about 5 to 7 seconds. The epiglottis is a flap of tissue that closes over the trachea to prevent the bolus from entering the lungs.

The Esophagus

The esophagus is a muscular tube through which the bolus travels from the mouth to the stomach. The process begins at the top of the esophagus when **peristalsis**, the involuntary movements of circular and longitudinal muscles, begins and draws the bolus farther into the GI tract.

This mechanical action further breaks down the size of foodstuff and increases exposure to digestive secretions. Muscular actions depend on the four layers of tissues that form the tube of the GI tract (Figure 3-3). The **mucosa** is composed of mucous membrane and forms the inside layer. Under the mucosa is the **submucosa**, a layer of connective tissue. Digestion depends on the blood vessels and nerves of the submucosa to regulate digestion. Surrounding the submucosa is a thick layer of muscle tissue called the **muscularis**.

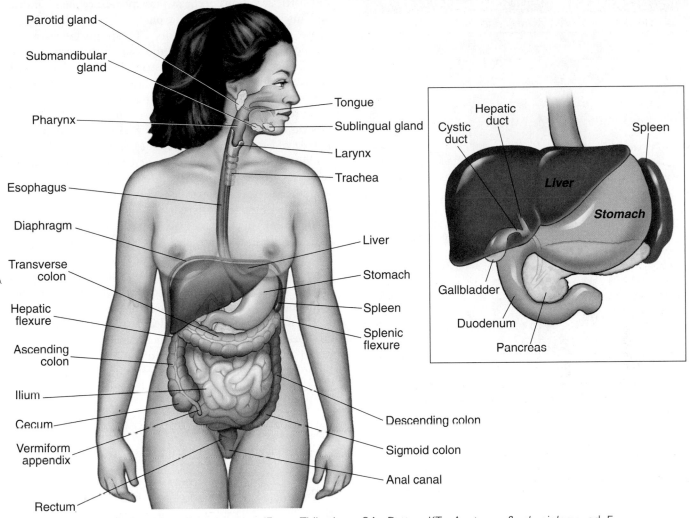

FIG 3-1 Digestive system. (From Thibodeau GA, Patton KT: *Anatomy & physiology*, ed 5, St Louis, 2003, Mosby.)

The outermost layer of the GI wall is made of serous membrane called serosa, which is actually the visceral layer of the peritoneum lining the abdominal pelvic cavity, and covers organs.[1]

The coordination of these layers provides the varied movements required for digestion. Essentially, muscular action controls the movement of the food mass through the GI tract. Churning action within a segment of the GI tract allows secretions to mix with food mass. Circular muscles surround the GI tube. Rhythmic contractions of these muscles cause the wavelike motions of peristalsis, moving food downward. Longitudinal muscles run parallel along the GI tube. The combined effect of the circular and longitudinal muscles causes segmentation as a forward and backward movement that assists in controlling food mass movement through the GI tract.

Sphincter muscles are stronger, circular muscles that act as valves to control the movement of the food mass in a forward direction. In effect, sphincter muscles prevent reflux by forming an opening when relaxed and closing completely when contracted. At the bottom of the esophagus the cardiac sphincter controls the movement of the bolus from the esophagus into the stomach. It also prevents the acidic contents of the stomach from moving upward back through the esophagus.

The Stomach

Functions of the stomach include the following:

- Holding food for partial digestion
- Producing gastric juice
- Providing muscular action that, combined with gastric juice, mixes and tears food into smaller pieces
- Secreting the intrinsic factor for vitamin B_{12} absorption
- Releasing gastrin
- Assisting in the destruction, through its acidity of secretions, of pathogenic bacteria that may have inadvertently been consumed[1]

When the bolus passes through the cardiac sphincter, it enters the fundus, the upper portion of the stomach that connects with the esophagus. The other divisions of the stomach include the body, or center portion, and the pylorus, the lower portion. The stomach wall contains gastric mucosa with gastric pits. At the base of the pits are the gastric glands whose chief cells create gastric juice, a mucous fluid containing digestive enzymes, and parietal cells, which secrete stomach acid called *hydrochloric acid*.

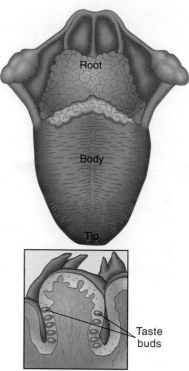

FIG 3-2 **A,** Parts of the tongue. **B,** A detailed site of a taste bud. (From Thibodeau GA, Patton KT: *Anatomy & physiology,* ed 5, St Louis, 2003, Mosby.)

Gastric secretions occur in three phases: cephalic, gastric, and intestinal.[1] The cephalic phase is called the "psychic phase" because mental factors can stimulate gastrin, a hormone secreted by stomach mucosa. In the gastric phase, gastrin increases the release of gastric juices when the stomach is distended by food. The third phase is the intestinal phase in which the gastric secretions change as chyme, a semiliquid mixture of food mass, passes through to the duodenum. Gastric secretions are inhibited by exocrine and nervous reflexes of gastric inhibitory peptides, secretin, and cholecystokinin (CCK) (also called pancreozymin), a hormone secreted by intestinal mucosa.

Some gastric juices provide acidity in the stomach to assist the effective function of certain enzymes. As agents of chemical digestion, enzymes are specific in action, working only on individual classes of nutrients and changing substances from one form to a simpler form. Enzymes are "organic catalysts" formed from protein structures. They function at specific pH and are continually created and destroyed. Specific enzymes are required for energy release and digestion.

Hormones regulate the release of gastric juices and enzymes, acting as messengers between organs to cause the release of needed secretions. In digestion, hormones affect the secretions from the stomach, intestines, and gallbladder. These secretions may slow or speed digestion and affect the

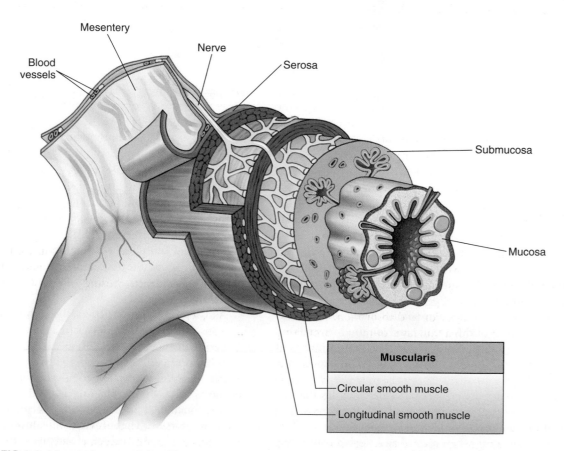

FIG 3-3 Muscle layers of the GI tract. (From Thibodeau GA, Patton KT: *Anatomy & physiology,* ed 5, St Louis, 2003, Mosby.)

pH levels of gastric juice. Overall, the mechanical and chemical actions work together to complete the process of digestion.

Gastric motility, or movement of food mass through the stomach, requires 2 to 6 hours. The churning and mixing of the food mass with gastric juices create a semiliquid mixture called *chyme*. When chyme enters the pylorus section of the stomach, it causes distention and the release of the hormone gastrin. Gastrin sends a message that hydrochloric acid (HCl) is needed to continue the breakdown of chyme. As HCl is released from the stomach lining, thick mucus is also secreted to protect the stomach walls from the harsh HCl.

Every 20 seconds chyme is released into the duodenum, the upper portion of the small intestine; this action is controlled by the hormonal and nervous system mechanism of enterogastric reflex. This consists of duodenal receptors in the mucosa that are sensitive to the presence of acid and distention. The impulses over sensory and motor fiber in the vagus nerve cause a reflex restriction of gastric peristalsis. For example, the gastric inhibitory peptide released in response to fats in the duodenum decreases peristalsis of stomach muscles and slows chyme passage. These result in decreased motility, which is why the stomach empties more slowly when a person eats a high-fat diet.

The combined action of mechanical digestion (the strong muscular movements of peristalsis) and chemical digestion (the effects of the gastric juices) work to prepare nutrients for the process of absorption. Chyme is kept in the stomach by the actions of the pyloric sphincter, which slowly releases it into the duodenum.

The Small Intestine

The chyme entering the duodenum soon moves through to the jejunum and ileum of the small intestine. It takes about 5 hours for chyme to pass through the small intestine because of the action of segmentation and peristalsis. Segmentation in the duodenum and upper jejunum mixes chyme with digestive juices from the pancreas, liver, and intestinal mucosa. Peristalsis is controlled by intrinsic stretch reflexes and is initiated by cholecystokinin (CCK), the hormone secreted by intestinal mucosa.

In the small intestine, the nutrients in chyme are prepared for absorption. The small intestine is the major organ of digestion, and the final stages of the digestive process occur here. Because it is also the site of almost all of the absorption of nutrients, the intestinal lining must be able to accommodate the actions of both digestion and absorption. The intestinal walls are covered with a thin layer of mucus, protecting the walls from digestive juices. The walls are also adapted to enhance the absorption process. Finger-like projections called **villi** greatly increase the amount of mucosal layer available for the absorption of nutrients (Figure 3-4). On the villi are hairlike projections called *microvilli* that also enhance absorption by their structure and movements.

As chyme enters the small intestine, hormones begin sending messages that regulate the release of digestive juices to continue the process of chyme digestion. Some hormones

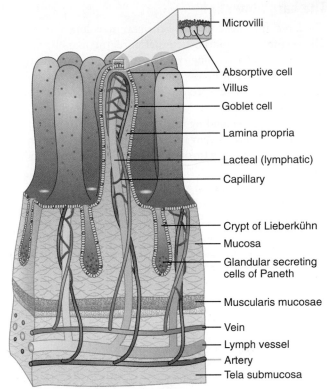

FIG 3-4 Structure of the intestinal wall. The circular folds, villi, and microvilli multiply the surface area and enhance absorption. (From Mahan LK, Escott-Stump S: *Krause's food & nutrition therapy,* ed 12, Philadelphia, 2008, Saunders.)

are provided by the small intestine; several are released by other organs into the small intestine. These secretions include enzymes from the small intestines, bile produced in the liver, and digestive juices from the pancreas.

One of the first hormones released by the small intestine is **secretin**. This hormone causes the pancreas to send bicarbonate to the small intestine to reduce the acidic content of the chyme. As the acidic level decreases, other pancreatic juices enter and begin their work. Another hormone secreted by the small intestine is CCK, or pancreozymin, which initiates pancreatic exocrine secretions; acts against gastrin by inhibiting gastric HCl secretion; and activates the gallbladder to contract, causing bile to be released into the duodenum.

Bile, which is secreted by the liver and stored in the gallbladder, is released to emulsify fats, which aids in the digestion of lipids. The emulsification creates more surface area, allowing lipid enzymes to digest fats to their component parts. The liver continuously secretes bile, and CCK and secretin spur the gallbladder to release bile for the digestion of fats. In addition, the small intestine produces enzymes to assist in the digestive process. Although much of the chyme is absorbed, the rest—which usually consists of fiber, minerals, and water—passes through the next sphincter (ileocecal valve) and into the large intestine (ascending colon).

The Large Intestine

The large intestine consists of the cecum, colon, and rectum. The cecum is a blind pocket; therefore, the mass bypasses it and enters the ascending colon, which leads into the transverse colon running across the abdomen over the small intestine to the descending colon. The descending colon extends down the left of the abdomen into the sigmoid colon and leads into the descending colon, on to the rectum, and into the anal canal. Finally, any remaining mass passes out through the anus. The journey through the large intestine takes about 9 to 16 hours.

In the large intestine or colon, final absorption of any available nutrients, usually water and some minerals, occurs. Bacteria residing in the large intestine produce several vitamins, which are then absorbed. Water is withdrawn from the fibrous mass, forming solidified feces. Mucous glands in the intestinal wall create mucus that lubricates and covers feces as it forms. Again, peristalsis continues to move substances through the GI tract, resulting in the excretion of feces from the colon through the anus, the last sphincter muscle of the GI tract.

The movement of the food mass through the GI tract is controlled to enhance digestion and absorption. During passage through the GI tract, more than 95% of the carbohydrates, fats, and proteins ingested are absorbed. Some minerals, vitamins, and trace elements may be less absorbed.[1] Table 3-1 summarizes the primary mechanisms of the digestive system. Details of carbohydrate, protein, and lipid digestion follow in specific chapters.

ABSORPTION

Although the food mass has possibly spent several hours in the tube of the GI tract, it is not yet actually inside the body until its nutrient components are absorbed. Absorption is the process by which substances pass through the intestinal mucosa into the blood or lymph. Transport processes provide the means for nutrients to actually pass through the wall of the small intestine. These include passive diffusion and osmosis, facilitated diffusion, energy-dependent active transport, and engulfing pinocytosis (Figure 3-5).

Passive diffusion occurs when pressure is greater on one side of the membrane and the substance then moves from the area of greater pressure to less pressure, allowing molecules to travel through capillaries. Facilitated diffusion takes place when, despite positive pressure flow, molecules may be unable to pass through membrane pores unless aided. Specific integral membrane proteins support the movement by bringing the larger nutrient molecules through the capillary membrane.

Energy-dependent active transport happens when fluid pressures work against the passage of nutrients. As an active process, energy is required. This energy is supplied by the cell and a "pumping" mechanism, which are assisted by a special membrane protein carrier. Engulfing pinocytosis takes place when a substance, either a fluid or a nutrient, contacts the villi membrane, which then surrounds the substance and creates a vacuole that encompasses the substance. Passing through the cell cytoplasm, the substance is then released into the circulatory system. The amounts of vitamins and minerals absorbed depend on the body's storage levels and immediate need for these nutrients. Nutrients such as fats, carbohydrates, and protein are easily absorbed regardless of the level of need. The structure of the small intestine, the site of almost all nutrient absorption, allows for efficient absorption to occur. The microvilli are sensitive to the exact nutrient needs of the body. Their wavelike motions, caused by peristalsis, result in the most exposure of the nutrient-laden chyme to the absorbing cells. This exposure allows needed nutrients to leave the GI tract and pass through the microvilli cells. At this point, the nutrients are truly "inside" the body.

Various factors may affect absorption of nutrients. Combinations of naturally occurring substances such as fiber or binders may move nutrients through the GI tract too quickly for optimum absorption to occur. Individual nutrient absorption and other issues of bioavailability are addressed in other chapters. The relationship between food and drug absorption is also an important issue of medical treatment. Ingesting medications with food may decrease the absorption rate of the medication and may interfere with the absorption of other nutrients contained in the food consumed. This issue is explored in depth in Chapter 16.

TABLE 3-1	DIGESTIVE PROCESSES
MECHANISM	**DESCRIPTION**
Ingestion	Process of taking food into the mouth, starting it on its journey through the digestive tract
Digestion	A group of processes that break complex nutrients into simpler ones, thus facilitating their absorption; *mechanical digestion* physically breaks large chunks into small bits; *chemical digestion* breaks molecules apart
Motility	Movement by the muscular components of the digestive tube, including processes of mechanical digestion; examples include *peristalsis* and *segmentation*
Secretion	Release of digestive juices (containing enzymes, acids, bases, mucus, bile, or other products that facilitate digestion); some digestive organs secrete endocrine hormones that regular digestion or metabolism of nutrients
Absorption	Movement of digested nutrients through the GI mucosa and into the internal environment
Elimination	Excretion of the residues of the digestive process (feces) from the rectum, through the anus; defecation

Data from Thibodeau GA, Patton KT: *Anatomy & physiology,* ed 5, St Louis, 2003, Mosby.

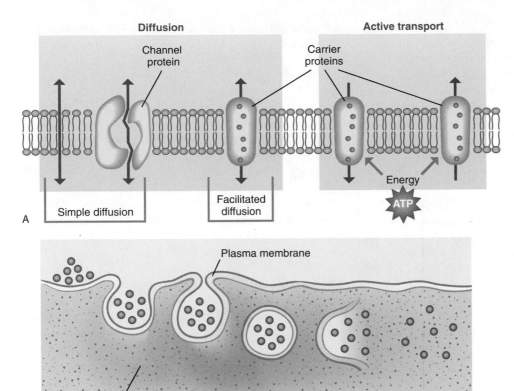

FIG 3-5 A, Methods of absorption. **A,** *Simple diffusion,* the movement of molecules from a region of high concentration to low concentration; *facilitated diffusion,* the movement of molecules by a carrier protein across the cell membrane from a region of high to low concentration; *active transport,* the movement of molecules and ions by means of a carrier protein against fluid pressures that require expenditure of cellular energy. **B,** Pinocytosis. (A, From Mahan LK, Escott-Stump S: *Krause's food & nutrition therapy,* ed 12, Philadelphia, 2008, Saunders. B, From Nix S: *Williams' basic nutrition & diet therapy,* ed 12, St Louis, 2005, Mosby.)

Once "inside" the body, the nutrients enter the circulatory systems of the bloodstream or lymphatic system. The general circulatory or blood system receives absorbed protein, carbohydrates, small parts of broken-down fats, and most vitamins and minerals. This system transports these nutrients throughout the body. The lymphatic system, a secondary circulatory system, receives large lipids and fat-soluble vitamins. The nutrients traveling in the lymphatic system are deposited into the bloodstream near the heart. All nutrients then circulate throughout the body in the blood, providing for the nutrient requirements of cells.

Soon after entering the bloodstream, nutrients pass by the liver. This allows the liver to have "first choice" of the available nutrients. The liver is a powerhouse organ that provides a wide variety of services and substances; thus its nutrient needs are a priority. From there, the bloodstream's journey of nutrients continues to the heart to also give it a prime nutrient selection. The journey then continues through the circulatory system to all cells. Some nutrients end up in nutrient storage sites of the body. These sites include the bones, liver, and kidneys. Other nutrients, if not discarded or used by cells, are filtered out of the blood by the kidneys to be reabsorbed or excreted in urine.

Elimination

The expulsion of feces or body waste products is called *defecation.* When the rectum is distended because of waste accumulation, the reflex to defecate occurs. The residue may include substances such as cellulose and other dietary fibers and connective tissue from meat collagen that are unable to be digested by human enzymes. Undigested fats may combine

with dietary minerals, such as calcium and magnesium, and form residue. Additional residue may include water, bacteria, pigments, and mucus. Figure 3-6 summarizes the functions of the digestive system, and the *Teaching Tool* box, Digesting Food: A Primer for Clients and Patients, provides suggestions for client and patient teaching.

Overall food transit times for nutrients to move from our plate to our cells are as follows:

Chewing and swallowing	Depends on texture and quantity
Esophagus	5-7 seconds
Stomach	2-6 hours
Small intestine	Approximately 5 hours
Large intestine	9-16 hours
Total	16-27 hours ingestion to elimination

✳ TEACHING TOOL

Digesting Food: A Primer for Clients and Patients

As health care professionals, we may assume our clients understand the way the body works as easily as we do. More than likely, however, their knowledge is limited, and even if they studied digestion years ago in a health education class, they may have forgotten or replaced facts with misinformation.

When working with clients for health promotion or with patients recovering from GI disorders, consider using the summary of digestive organ functions (see Figure 3-6) as a teaching tool. By visually reviewing the digestive organs and processes, clients and patients can have a clearer concept of the purposes of dietary recommendations and may therefore find compliance easier.

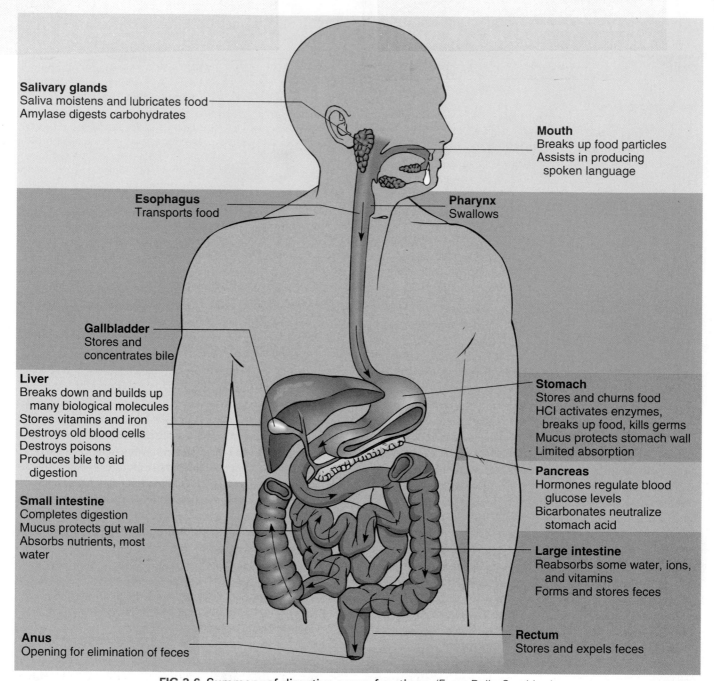

Salivary glands
Saliva moistens and lubricates food
Amylase digests carbohydrates

Mouth
Breaks up food particles
Assists in producing
  spoken language

Esophagus
Transports food

Pharynx
Swallows

Gallbladder
Stores and
concentrates bile

Stomach
Stores and churns food
HCl activates enzymes,
  breaks up food, kills germs
Mucus protects stomach wall
Limited absorption

Liver
Breaks down and builds up
  many biological molecules
Stores vitamins and iron
Destroys old blood cells
Destroys poisons
Produces bile to aid
  digestion

Pancreas
Hormones regulate blood
  glucose levels
Bicarbonates neutralize
  stomach acid

Small intestine
Completes digestion
Mucus protects gut wall
Absorbs nutrients, most
water

Large intestine
Reabsorbs some water, ions,
  and vitamins
Forms and stores feces

Anus
Opening for elimination of feces

Rectum
Stores and expels feces

FIG 3-6 Summary of digestive organ functions. (From Rolin Graphics.)

Digestive Process across the Life Span

Over the course of the life span, the main and accessory organs of digestion develop and change. The immature GI tract, particularly the intestinal mucosa of young infants, may allow intact proteins to be absorbed without complete digestion occurring. This incomplete digestion may result in an allergic response by the immune system and is part of the reason to delay the introduction of solid foods (e.g., cereals) until the GI tract has matured sufficiently. Another age-related condition is lactose intolerance in which the body ceases to produce lactase, the enzyme that breaks down the milk carbohydrate of lactose. For some people, this occurs once the primary growth need for nutrients contained in milk is met. For others, this may not occur until adulthood or not at all (see Chapter 4). Older adults sometimes experience lactose intolerance as the secretion of enzymes, such as lactase, decreases as part of the aging process. Conditions of the middle years include gallbladder disease and peptic ulcers (sores that may occur on the epithelial surfaces of the stomach or small intestine). Older years may be marked by problems of constipation and diverticulosis. These conditions may be associated with age-related reduced peristalsis and decreased physical activity, and may be worsened by a lifelong history of chronic low dietary fiber consumption.[2] Other issues related to aging are discussed in later chapters, particularly in Chapter 13.

METABOLISM

It is hard to imagine that a lunch consisting of tuna on rye bread will actually end up being part of the cells of the body. Fortunately, the human body is able to transform the nutrients of the sandwich into substances usable by cells. Metabolism is a set of processes through which absorbed nutrients are used by the body for energy and to form and maintain body structures and functions. The two main processes of metabolism involve catabolism and anabolism. Catabolism is the breakdown of food components into smaller molecular particles, which causes the release of energy as heat and chemical energy.[1] Anabolism is the process of synthesis from which substances are formed, such as new bone or muscle tissue. Both processes happen within cells at the same time.

When nutrients finally reach individual cells, they may be chemically changed through anabolism to help form new cell structures or to create new substances such as hormones and enzymes. Some vitamins and minerals assist in the use of other nutrients within the cell. They act as catalysts or coenzymes to initiate and support the transformation and use of carbohydrates, proteins, and lipids. Other nutrients may be used as energy to continue life-supporting processes. These processes include the energy needed to support deoxyribonucleic acid (DNA) reproduction and create proteins and other molecules, nerve impulses, and muscle contractions. Some energy is stored in a ready-to-use state. Specific metabolic functions of individual nutrients are discussed in Chapters 4 to 8.

Waste products from metabolism are discarded by the cells and wind up circulating in the blood. They are then excreted through the lungs, kidneys, or large intestine. The lungs release excess water and carbon dioxide. The kidneys filter and excrete metabolic waste and excess vitamins and minerals but reabsorb nutrients that the body needs to retain. Waste products may also be discarded through the large intestine in feces. Fortunately, we do not have to consciously control these processes. Our responsibility is to provide an adequate selection of nutrients through the foods we choose to eat and to eat those foods in a way that enhances the functioning of the GI tract.

Metabolism across the Life Span

Metabolic changes are most noticeable later in life as the amount of food energy required decreases in relation to lowered metabolic rates. Nutrient needs, however, remain constant. As we (and our clients) enter the middle years and beyond, our challenge is to meet nutrient needs while maintaining or reducing our kcal needs to equal actual metabolic use. Recognition of this change can forestall the unexpected weight gain that appears to accompany aging in the United States.

OVERCOMING BARRIERS

Some of our lifestyle behaviors affect the functioning and health of our GI tracts and therefore influence our nutritional status (see the *Social Issues* box, Hunger vs. Appetite vs. Time). Some common GI tract health problems are caused by the everyday decisions that we make but that can be changed. Prevention suggestions and treatment strategies for some common GI tract health problems follow.

Heartburn

Heartburn fortunately has nothing to do with the health of the heart. Instead, it is a burning sensation felt in the esophagus when food that has already been passed to the stomach refluxes or passes back up through the cardiac sphincter into the esophagus. The esophagus is not lined with acid-resistant mucus, as is the stomach, so the acidic mixture of food burns the walls of the esophagus and causes pain. Heartburn, or gastroesophageal reflux (GER), is a common experience. Depending on the frequency and severity of heartburn, including symptoms such as severe burning sensation under the sternum; asthma; chronic cough; and other ear, nose, and throat ailments, a diagnosis of either gastroesophageal reflux disease (GERD) or laryngopharyngeal reflux (LPR) (in which reflux affects the larynx or pharynx) may occur. (See Chapter 17 for a detailed discussion of GERD.)

Prevention and treatment strategies attempt to reduce the amount of pressure in the stomach so that the cardiac sphincter is not opened by excess pressure from stomach contents. A primary approach is to avoid overeating so the stomach can easily accommodate its contents. Other strategies include the following:[3]

- *Preventing constipation:* Straining to defecate affects the contents of the stomach by creating additional pressure.
- *Lying down shortly after eating:* Resting or sleeping with a full stomach may push contents against the cardiac sphincter. Wait several hours after a meal before lying flat or keep head and shoulders elevated when reclining.
- *Avoiding high-fat meals:* Slow emptying of the stomach from eating high-fat food increases sphincter relaxation, leading to potential reflux.
- *Avoiding tight clothing:* Wearing restrictive clothing around the waist and midriff affects the functioning of the stomach and may increase stomach pressure.
- *Eating "on the run":* Eating meals while under stress or trying to do other activities at the same time may cause food to not be chewed enough. Big clumps of foods in the stomach force the stomach muscles to react strongly, which may cause reflux (see the *Health Debate* box, Are Advertisers Leading Us Astray?).
- *Staying away from certain foods and drinks:* Consuming chocolate, alcohol, peppermints, spearmints, liqueurs, caffeine, and high-acid foods, such as tomatoes, vinegar-based foods, citrus fruits and juices, may irritate the esophagus and cause heartburn.
- *Avoiding some medications:* Taking certain medications regularly may initiate heartburn. If heartburn often occurs

SOCIAL ISSUES
Hunger vs. Appetite vs. Time

Our daily schedules often determine our responses to hunger. Ever notice how differently you eat during the week compared with the weekend? The weekday mosaic of classes, studying, work, and possibly sports training often makes fitting in time to get to the campus cafeteria a Herculean feat. Or, if you prepare your own meals, time must be set aside for buying and cooking foods. Weekends may be more leisurely without classes or work, or perhaps we find time for socializing.

Yet somehow we manage. Although fewer meals may be eaten during the week, we are not any less hungry nor are energy needs lower. Sometimes, chaotic schedules may be accommodated by telling ourselves we are not really hungry or we just do not have time to eat.

How can we do that? Isn't hunger a physiologic need for energy and nutrients? Can we just think ourselves through the hunger sensation? To understand this process, we need to explore the feeding regulating mechanism of the body.

Our sense of hunger and satiety is governed by the hypothalamus, a small portion of the brain. Its purpose is to maintain homeostasis (a state of balance) by regulating food intake through a feeding (hunger) center and a satiety center. The response of the hypothalamus, which initiates the hunger sensation, is thought to be related to either low blood glucose levels or to the lack of chyme in the stomach.

When we eat, blood glucose levels rise and chyme is once again in the stomach. The hypothalamus responds by providing a feeling of satiety or satisfaction, and we stop eating.

When we "feel" hungry, we are recognizing the internal stimuli of hunger. Perhaps our stomach seems to be rumbling or "empty" or we are "starving." These sensations are tied to physical events in our bodies. When we act on this, we eat. However, we can also choose to ignore these signals. This means we cognitively override the sensation and do not respond. There are physical mechanisms to cope with the lack of new energy sources, but it is still stressful to our bodies.

External stimuli also affect our desire or appetite for eating. Referred to as *environmental cues*, these include the smell and sight of food, which may artificially increase our hunger. Simply seeing a food commercial on television or talking about food can excite the feeding center even if the stomach is not actually "empty." We also associate eating with specific social settings and time of day, regardless of our physical need for food. How can a birthday be celebrated without a cake? Religious holidays are often associated with special foods or meals. Throughout our elementary school experience, we ate lunch when we were scheduled, not necessarily when we were hungry.

All those years of eating by schedules and events have led us to adapt by overriding our cognitive cues about our real sense of hunger. Now, when personal schedules are more individualized, we may find that the external stimuli supporting our appropriate intake of food are gone; we must develop our own cues to ensure optimal nutritional intakes.

Data from Logue AW: *The psychology of eating and drinking: An introduction,* ed 3, New York, 2004, Freeman; and Mahan LK, Escott-Stump S: *Krause's food & nutrition therapy,* ed 12, Philadelphia, 2008, Saunders.

when taking birth control pills, antihistamines, tranquilizers (e.g., diazepam [Valium]), or any drug taken often, check with the primary care provider. Heartburn could be caused by these medications.

If these strategies do not help and heartburn remains, consult a primary care provider. Chronic heartburn or GER may result in esophagitis, which is inflammation of the lower esophagus or may be caused by hiatal hernia. Hiatal hernia, which requires medical intervention, is the herniation of a portion of the stomach into the chest through the esophageal hiatus of the diaphragm.

HEALTH DEBATE
Are Advertisers Leading Us Astray?

A TV commercial begins with a man and his adult daughter shopping in a gourmet deli. The daughter displays a spicy sausage she has just selected for their dinner; he protests that it will upset his stomach and cause him bad heartburn. Allaying his fears, she presents him with an over-the-counter (OTC) drug product that will prevent his painful symptoms if taken in advance. Everyone is happy!

What's wrong with this picture? Advertisers paint a false picture of the appropriate use of OTC histamine receptor antagonists such as Tagamet, Axid, Zantac, and Pepcid. These drugs were originally developed to treat peptic ulcers. Because it is now known that most ulcers are caused by the bacterium *Helicobacter pylori* and can be cured with antibiotics, pharmaceutical companies whose sales of histamine receptor antagonist drugs would diminish are attempting to expand the use of these medications to other somewhat-related conditions. In lower doses, these drugs can relieve heartburn symptoms but cannot treat the cause of the discomfort. By promoting the use of these drugs to alleviate symptoms caused by hard to digest foods or overeating, underlying conditions such as gastroesophageal reflux (GER) and esophagitis, for which heartburn is a symptom may be overlooked. Although immediate reflux discomfort may be eased, the dosage in these OTC drugs is not high enough to prevent damage to the esophagus. Rather than emphasizing lifestyle and dietary changes, this approach encourages abuse of medication and disregard for dietary common sense.

Should these drugs be advertised as a premeal cure-all for heartburn, or should OTC advertisements be restricted?

Data from *USP DI-Volume II advice for the patient: Drug information in lay language,* ed 25, Rockville, Md, 2005, U.S. Pharmacopeial Convention, Inc; and Yuan Y, Hunt RH: Evolving issues in the management of reflux disease? *Curr Opin Gastroenterol* 25(4):342-351, 2009.

Vomiting

Although vomiting is not usually related to lifestyle behaviors, it is a common digestive disorder worthy of review. Vomiting is reverse peristalsis. Instead of food moving down the GI tract, the peristalsis muscles move the contents of the stomach back through the esophagus and forcefully out the mouth. It is an involuntary muscular action that we cannot easily control. Often it is painful; the contents of the stomach already consist of a mixture of food and acidic gastric juices that burns the unprotected esophagus.

Vomiting is a way of the body protecting itself. Perhaps an intruding virus or toxin has entered the GI tract; vomiting removes the offending substance. Mixed messages regarding the body's sense of equilibrium during air or sea travel can result in motion sickness, of which vomiting may be a symptom. Dehydration is a concern when vomiting is continual. Vomiting causes a loss of fluid and electrolytes, such as magnesium, potassium, and sodium, which stresses the functioning of the body. Infants are at particular risk for dehydration because their bodies consist mostly of fluids.[3] A primary health care provider should be consulted to determine the cause of vomiting and to recommend treatment.

Also at medical risk are individuals who vomit as a way to control their weight and suffer from eating disorders such as anorexia nervosa and bulimia. Repetitive self-induced vomiting can injure the esophagus and wear away tooth enamel. Anyone practicing this self-destructive behavior should consult a primary care provider or mental health professional as soon as possible (see Chapter 12).

Intestinal Gas

Annoying, embarrassing, and offensive are all terms that come to mind when intestinal gas, or *flatus*, is the subject. Actually, everyone's body produces and releases gas from the lower intestinal tract. Most gas leaves the GI tract without our awareness because it is odorless. Sometimes if the gas passes through too quickly, it is quite noticeable!

Bacteria in the large intestine may cause gas formation when specific indigestible carbohydrates ferment. These may include some of the carbohydrates found in legumes (dried beans) such as soybeans and black beans. Another cause may be lactose intolerance, which is the inability to break down lactose, the carbohydrate in milk. The lactose then begins to ferment, causing gas buildup, bloating, and diarrhea (see Chapter 4). The longer any undigested substances linger in the large intestine, the more likely it is that fermentation will occur, leading to gas formation. This may result from constipation that slows the passage of chyme through the GI tract. Another factor contributing to flatulence may be eating so quickly that food is swallowed in large clumps, which thereby requires more time to sufficiently process the chyme before it is excreted.[3]

Generally, however, intestinal gas can probably be decreased through some simple changes of food-related behaviors. Following are some suggestions:

- If making dietary changes to increase fiber intake, gradually add more fibrous foods such as legumes to allow the system to adjust.
- Notice the effects of drinking milk. Drink fluid milk in small quantities over several weeks, working up to an 8-ounce glass. Note at what level gas may develop. If a problem occurs, consider eating other milk-related products such as yogurt, cheese, or lactose-reduced milk.
- Increase fluid intake and consume sufficient amounts of fiber to prevent constipation.

- Take the time to consider which foods may be problematic. Each person's cause of flatulence may be different.
- Eat slower and chew foods more thoroughly.

Constipation

There is no clear definition of constipation. It is usually considered as difficulty and discomfort associated with defecation probably because of slow movement of feces through colon. Individuals may interpret these terms differently and may vary in their natural urge to defecate. Not everyone needs to pass a bowel movement daily. Normal functioning ranges from once a day to every 3 days. Generally, constipation is recognized as straining to pass hard, dry stools.

The causes of constipation are usually related to lifestyle behaviors that can easily be changed. The following strategies address these behaviors:

- *Choose foods that are high in fiber, particularly insoluble fiber such as wheat bran.* Whole grain breads, fruits, and vegetables are important foods to consume. Fiber provides bulk that softens the stool and makes elimination easier.
- *Listen to body signals and follow a schedule that allows time for a bowel movement to occur.* Ignoring the natural urge to defecate causes feces to remain in the colon longer. This allows more water to be withdrawn, resulting in harder, drier feces.
- *Exercise regularly.* Lack of exercise can lead to a loss of tone in the muscles of the lower GI tract.
- *Drink enough liquids.* Fluid intake should be approximately 8 to 10 glasses a day. Most of us need to consciously remember to drink water or other liquids to fulfill this need.
- *Relax.* Stress tightens muscles throughout the body and may inhibit proper bowel functioning.
- *Consume regular meals.* The body works best with an intake of nutrients and fiber throughout the day.

Constipation caused by lifestyle behaviors should respond to these strategies. If these strategies do not relieve constipation, consult a primary care provider to rule out more serious disorders (see the *Personal Perspectives* box, Constipation as a Warning? and the *Health Debate* box, Are Specialty Yogurts the Key to "Regularity"?)

Diarrhea

Diarrhea is the passing of loose, watery bowel movements that result when the contents of the GI tract move through too quickly to allow water to be absorbed in the large intestine. Diarrhea may be caused by bacterial or viral infections (e.g., stomach virus or intestinal flu), lactose intolerance, spoiled foods, or even stress.[1,3] An occasional bout is not a problem. However, if diarrhea continues, too much fluid and electrolytes may be lost, and dehydration is possible. Efforts should be made to drink enough fluids to replace those lost. This is particularly a concern for infants and older adults, who are most at risk for dehydration; their fluid levels are delicately maintained. Infants cannot easily communicate their thirst, and a greater proportion of their bodies consist of fluid; the excessive loss of fluid has serious consequences of electrolyte imbalance and a distorted ability to maintain body temperature and functions.

Among older adults the ability to detect thirst may be diminished; disorientation, sometimes assigned to senility, may actually be a sign of dehydration that if not diagnosed may further deteriorate health. Because it is a symptom of illness, diarrhea that lasts more than 2 days should be discussed with a primary care provider to uncover the actual cause.

TOWARD A POSITIVE NUTRITION LIFESTYLE: CONTRACTING

Have you ever made a bet? Contracting is similar to making a bet with a friend, except the object of the bet is a health behavior. A contract is a specific agreement with oneself or between you and a friend, spouse, or other relative. The agreement represents your willingness to attempt to change a health-related behavior. The advantage to contracting is that the goal or behavior change is clearly defined and observable. You also decide on a specific period within which to achieve the goal. As with a bet, you determine a reward or penalty for not completing the contract. (Yes, contracts with oneself are much easier to break.) By practicing a new health-related behavior for a specific period, the expectation is that the change will be permanent.

A contract with oneself might be to drink 8 glasses of water a day for a week to relieve constipation. The change to increase fluid intake is a behavior you can directly control and observe. Although the aim is to alleviate constipation, which may not be a behavior you can consciously change, its risk factors can be reduced. At the end of the week, your reward could be to see a movie with a friend, whereas the penalty might be to clean out your messy bedroom closet.

Perhaps you have noticed that you regularly work through lunch and eat at your desk. The result is that heartburn has become a regular discomfort, and a discussion of remedies is often the topic of work breaks. A co-worker complains that she seems unable to break her habit of buying a high-calorie Danish pastry with her coffee each morning. You could contract with her that for the next 2 weeks you will eat lunch away from your desk, either in the employee cafeteria or at a local restaurant. She contracts with you that she will buy fruit instead of a Danish pastry for her morning snack. If you both complete the contracts, a reward could be to lunch together at a special restaurant. If only one person completes a contract, the penalty could be for the "loser" to pack a brown bag lunch for a week for the "winner." Contracting is applicable to many aspects of contemporary lifestyles and is limited only by our imagination.

SUMMARY

The processes of digestion, absorption, and metabolism work together to provide all body cells with energy and nutrients. Within the digestive system, all foods are digested. The organs forming the GI tract include the mouth, esophagus, stomach, small intestine, and large intestine and colon. Peristalsis, segmentation, and the action of sphincter muscles regulate the movement of foodstuff through one organ to the next. Other structures support the digestive system, including the teeth, tongue, salivary glands, liver, gallbladder, and pancreas. They assist with mechanical digestion (chewing) and chemical digestion (producing or storing secretions).

The main site of nutrient digestion and absorption is the small intestine. Once absorbed, nutrients are truly "inside" the body. Nutrients then enter the circulatory system of the bloodstream or lymphatic system and become available to all cells. When the nutrients reach the cells, they may be metabolized. The metabolic changes allow the nutrients to fulfill many cell functions.

Some common GI tract health problems are caused by lifestyle behaviors that can be changed. Prevention suggestions and treatment strategies for heartburn, intestinal gas, and constipation consider the effect of lifestyle behaviors. Although vomiting and diarrhea are not usually related to lifestyle, each has an impact on the functioning of the GI tract.

THE NURSING APPROACH

Case Study: Gastroesophageal Reflux Disease (GERD)

Sally is a 35-year-old who came to the nurse practitioner's clinic with complaints of recurring heartburn and lack of sleep. Her medical record indicated she had problems with heartburn during her pregnancy and then again 6 months ago. Endoscopy revealed no hiatal hernia and no esophageal pathology. The medical diagnosis was gastroesophageal reflux disease (GERD), and the doctor prescribed a medication to reduce acid production.

ASSESSMENT
Subjective (from Patient Statements)

When interviewed, Sally said, "The medicine that the doctor prescribed for me was really expensive, so I stopped taking it. The last two weeks I have been getting burning chest pain nearly every night, and it has kept me from sleeping well. I'm really tired. I usually am OK during the day, but I get heartburn in the evening whenever I eat a big dinner. The doctor told me I should avoid spicy foods, and I have been doing that, so why am I still having pain?"

With further questioning, Sally reported, "I worked late last night, so I got some fast food. I ate a large hamburger with cheese, tomato, and onions; french fries with ketchup; and a diet cola. While traveling home in the car, I ate a chocolate milkshake. I was so tired that I went straight to bed. One hour later I woke up with awful heartburn. I took some antacid, but it didn't help very much, and I couldn't go back to sleep."

Objective (from Physical Examination)

Height: 5 feet 6 inches; Weight: 160 pounds
Dark circles under Sally's eyes
Abdomen nontender, without distension
Throat pink, without evidence of irritation

DIAGNOSIS (NURSING)

Disturbed sleep pattern related to esophageal reflux and heartburn as evidenced by dark circles under Sally's eyes and "The last two weeks I have been getting burning chest pain nearly every night, and it has kept me from sleeping well. I'm really tired."

PLANNING
Patient Outcomes

Short term (at the end of this visit):
- Sally will verbalize ways she can change her diet and lifestyle to prevent heartburn.
- Long term (at follow-up visit in 2 weeks):
  - Sally will report dietary and lifestyle changes that she made.
  - Sally will report she slept through the night, without any heartburn.

Nursing Interventions

- Teach Sally the causes of heartburn and measures to reduce heartburn.
- Explore possible medications that are cheaper.

IMPLEMENTATION (Also see Chapter 17.)

1. Using a drawing, the nurse showed Sally how acids and food can back up into the esophagus from the stomach through the cardiac (lower esophageal) sphincter, causing heartburn.
2. The nurse identified physiologic causes of reflux and how Sally's actions had contributed to the problems.

CAUSES OF HEARTBURN	SALLY'S CONTRIBUTING FACTORS
Large volume	Large meal, carbonated beverage
Pressure from stomach when reclining	Went straight to bed after eating, overweight
Cardiac sphincter relaxation	High-fat foods: french fries, cheese on fried hamburger, and chocolate milkshake; caffeinated and carbonated cola; and onion
Esophageal irritation	Very cold cola and milkshake, tomato products

3. The nurse listed the following recommended changes to prevent heartburn:
   - Small frequent meals
   - Sit up for two to three hours after eating

Continued

THE NURSING APPROACH—cont'd

Case Study: Gastroesophageal Reflux Disease (GERD)—cont'd

- Nonfat milk instead of carbonated drinks and caffeine
- Beverages mostly between meals
- Less fat—broil hamburger; omit cheese, french fries and milkshake
- Choose noncitrus fruit for dessert
- Eat fewer calories and exercise to lose weight
4. The nurse discussed possible alternate medications that might be cheaper, such as antacids.

EVALUATION

Short term (at the end of the visit):

- Sally wrote down specific goals for changes in diet and lifestyle.
- Changes to make right away: small, frequent meals; no carbonated drinks; eat several hours before going to bed; no fast food
- Changes to make gradually, starting next week: nonfat milk, smaller portions of food, fewer high-fat foods, exercise

- Changes not willing to make: giving up chocolate
- Sally set up an appointment for follow-up in 2 weeks
- Short-term outcome achieved

DISCUSSION QUESTIONS

When Sally returned to see the nurse practitioner in 2 weeks, she reported that she was still having some difficulty with heartburn and not being able to sleep. She said she had forgotten much of the nurse's instructions, and she had felt overwhelmed by too many suggestions for changing her diet and lifestyle.

1. Had the nurse and patient set realistic goals at the first visit? What assessment questions should the nurse ask now?
2. How could the nurse simplify her teaching and help Sally to remember the recommendations?
3. What would be the three most important suggestions to emphasize?

Nursing Diagnoses-Definitions and Classification 2009-2011. Copyright © 2009, 1994-2009 by NANDA International. Used by arrangement with Blackwell Publishing Limited, a company of John Wiley & Sons, Inc.

❓ APPLYING CONTENT KNOWLEDGE

James, a senior at the local university, is completing his internship at the rock radio station while continuing to work at his part-time job. Without any time to spare, he has been eating meals whenever he can, often from fast-food restaurants. These meals are usually gobbled quickly in his car. Lately, though, he is feeling stressed and is experiencing heartburn. List three lifestyle behaviors that James could change to possibly reduce heartburn.

▎ WEBSITES OF INTEREST

American College of Gastroenterology

www.acg.gi.org

Focuses on GI tract disorders including latest information on GERD for consumers and health professionals.

American Dental Association

www.ada.org

Source of health knowledge about our teeth and mouths through up-to-date news items and search tools.

American Medical Association

www.ama-assn.org

Under the *Physician Resources* is the *Patients Education Materials* section that includes *Atlas of the Human Body*, a good resource for patient education.

REFERENCES

1. Klein S, Cohn SM, Alpers DH: Alimentary tract in nutrition. In Shils ME, et al, editors: *Modern nutrition in health and disease*, ed 10, Philadelphia, 2006, Lippincott Williams & Wilkins.
2. Logue AW: *The psychology of eating and drinking: An introduction*, ed 3, New York, 2004, Taylor & Francis Books Inc.
3. Mahan LK, Escott-Stump S: *Krause's food and nutrition therapy*, ed 12, Philadelphia, 2008, Saunders.

Carbohydrates

*All carbohydrates are organic compounds composed of carbon, hydrogen,
and oxygen in the form of simple carbohydrates or sugars.*

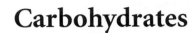

 Nutrition Concepts Online

WEBSITE

http://evolve.elsevier.com/Grodner/foundations/

ROLE IN WELLNESS

Nature has provided us with an excellent source of energy: carbohydrates. Found primarily in plants, carbohydrates are a convenient and economical source of calories for people throughout the world. Carbohydrates are organic compounds composed of carbon, hydrogen, and oxygen. These compounds consist of simple carbohydrates, such as glucose and sucrose, and complex carbohydrates, which include starch and dietary fiber. Each type of carbohydrate serves a distinct role in nourishing the body.

In addition to serving as an energy source, some carbohydrates are also used as sweetening agents. When carbohydrate sweeteners are found naturally in foods, such as in fruits, they are accompanied by essential nutrients. The sweetness makes eating nutrient-dense foods even more enjoyable. Some carbohydrates also supply dietary fiber.

The energy value of carbohydrates was discovered in 1844.[1] Recognition that increasing our consumption of carbohydrates from grains, vegetables, and fruits provides preventive health benefits is more recent. Increased levels of complex carbohydrates, particularly dietary fiber, appear to reduce the risk factors associated with chronic diet-related disorders such as heart disease, diabetes, and some cancers.[2] The *Acceptable Macronutrient Distribution Range (AMDR)* for carbohydrate is 45% to 65% of kcal intake per day as primarily complex carbohydrates.[2] The *Dietary Guidelines* concur, recommending that we emphasize a plant-based diet including fruits, vegetables, cooked dried beans and peas, whole grains, and seeds.[3] This advice is reflected in MyPyramid. Although recommendations vary based on individual needs, average suggestions of two cups of fruits, two and one half cups of vegetables, and 6 ounces of grains (bread, cereal, rice, and pasta) provide adequate amounts of complex carbohydrates (Box 4-1).

Considering carbohydrates through the health dimensions provides perspective on their role in wellness. The *physical health* dimension depends on our ability to provide our bodies with enough carbohydrate kcal for energy and enough complex carbohydrates and fiber consumption for optimum body functioning. Issues related to the role of carbohydrates are often in the headlines. Our ability to process research findings and make decisions about our food choices reflects our level of *intellectual*, or reasoning, *health* dimension. For some of us, *emotional health* may depend on the ability to distinguish hypoglycemic (low blood glucose) symptoms. If we are aware of our personal response to normal hypoglycemia, can we then distinguish real emotional issues from those caused by hypoglycemia? The *social health* dimension also may be tested. Social groups can support change or make changes more difficult to achieve. Will you or your client feel comfortable snacking on a banana (a good fiber source) while chocolate bars are unwrapped? The *spiritual health* dimension has ties to carbohydrates because several religions view bread, a carbohydrate, as the "staff of life."

FOOD SOURCES

The carbohydrates we consume are primarily from plant sources. As plants grow, they capture energy from the sun and chemically store it as carbohydrates. This process, called *photosynthesis*, depends on water from the earth, carbon dioxide from the atmosphere, and chlorophyll in the plant leaves to form carbohydrates.

All carbohydrates are organic compounds composed of carbon, hydrogen, and oxygen in the form of simple carbohydrates or sugars (Figure 4-1). When linked together, these simple sugars form three sizes of carbohydrates: monosaccharides, disaccharides, and polysaccharides (Figure 4-2).

BOX 4-1   MYPLATE: CARBOHYDRATES

www.choosemyplate.gov provides a wealth of resources about nutrients, foods, portions sizes, and activity levels related to caloric needs. Highlights of carbohydrate food sources are listed here, but do explore the MyPlate site at www.choosemyplate.gov to customize the information to individual needs.

Carbohydrate food sources include the following:

- *Grains:* Cereals, breads, crackers, rice, or pasta, at least half as whole grains (see following chart)
- *Vegetables:* Fiber-rich vegetables, starchy vegetables such as carrots, sweet potatoes, white potatoes, peas; legumes or dry beans such as kidney beans, chickpeas, and black-eyed peas

- *Fruits:* Fiber-rich fruits, most fruits especially bananas, grapes, pears, apples
- *Milk:* Fat-free or low fat milk, yogurt, and other milk products containing lactose (does not include most cheeses)
- *Meats and beans:* Replace animal sources with servings of legumes or dry beans

For each of the nutrient categories studied, a MyPlate section will be included to emphasize the importance of portion sizes for the five food categories. For carbohydrates, the focus is on portions of grains.

What Counts as an Ounce-Equivalent of Grains?*

In general, 1 slice of bread; 1 cup of ready-to-eat cereal; or $\frac{1}{2}$ cup of cooked rice, cooked pasta, or cooked cereal can be considered 1 ounce-equivalent from the grains group.

The following table lists specific amounts that count as 1 ounce-equivalent of grains toward your daily recommended intake. In some cases, the number of ounce-equivalents for common portions also is shown.

GRAIN	TYPES AND EXAMPLES	AMOUNT THAT COUNTS AS 1 OUNCE-EQUIVALENT OF GRAINS	COMMON PORTIONS AND OUNCE-EQUIVALENTS
Bagel	WG: whole wheat RG: plain, egg	1 mini bagel	1 large bagel = 4 ounce-equivalents
Biscuit	RG: baking powder/buttermilk	1 small (2-inch diameter)	1 large (3-inch diameter) = 2 ounce-equivalents
Bread	WG: 100% whole wheat RG: white, wheat, French, sourdough	1 regular slice 1 small slice French 4 snack-size slices rye	2 regular slices = 2 ounce-equivalents
Crackers	WG: 100% whole wheat, rye RG: saltines, snack crackers	5 whole wheat crackers 2 rye crispbreads 7 square or round crackers	
English muffin	WG: whole wheat RG: plain, raisin	$\frac{1}{2}$ muffin	1 muffin = 2 ounce-equivalents
Muffin	WG: whole wheat RG: bran, corn, plain	1 small (2$\frac{1}{2}$-inch diameter)	1 large (3$\frac{1}{2}$-inch diameter) = 3 ounce-equivalents
Oatmeal	WG	$\frac{1}{2}$ cup cooked 1 packet instant 1 ounce dry (regular or quick)	
Pancakes	WG: whole wheat, buckwheat RG: buttermilk, plain	1 pancake (4$\frac{1}{2}$-inch diameter) 2 small pancakes (3-inch diameter)	3 pancakes (4$\frac{1}{2}$-inch diameter) = 3 ounce-equivalents
Popcorn	WG	3 cups, popped	1 microwave bag, popped = 4 ounce-equivalents
Ready-to-eat breakfast cereal	WG: toasted oat, whole-wheat flakes RG: corn flakes, puffed rice	1 cup flakes or rounds 1$\frac{1}{4}$ cups puffed	
Rice	WG: brown, wild RG: enriched, white, polished	$\frac{1}{2}$ cup cooked 1 ounce dry	1 cup cooked = 2 ounce-equivalents
Pasta (spaghetti, macaroni, noodles)	WG: whole wheat RG: enriched, durum	$\frac{1}{2}$ cup cooked 1 ounce dry	1 cup cooked = 2 ounce-equivalents
Tortillas	WG: whole wheat, whole grain corn RG: flour, corn	1 small flour tortilla (6-inch diameter) 1 corn tortilla (6-inch diameter)	1 large tortilla (12-inch diameter) = 4 ounce-equivalents

RG, Refined grains; *WG,* whole grains. This is shown when products are available both in whole grain and refined grain forms.
*Accessed June 14, 2012, from www.choosemyplate.gov/food-groups/carbohydrates-count.html.

Monosaccharides are composed of a single carbohydrate unit. Glucose, fructose, and galactose are monosaccharides. Disaccharides consist of two single carbohydrates bound together. Sucrose, maltose, and lactose are disaccharides.

Polysaccharides consist of many units of monosaccharides joined together. Starch and fiber are food sources of polysaccharides, whereas glycogen is a storage form in the liver and muscles.

The three sizes of carbohydrates are divided into two classifications: *simple carbohydrates* (monosaccharides and disaccharides) and *complex carbohydrates* (polysaccharides) (Table 4-1). Both are valuable sources of carbohydrate energy. There are differences, however, between the health values of simple and complex carbohydrates found in the foods we consume. Although simple carbohydrates primarily provide energy in the form of glucose, fructose, and galactose, complex carbohydrates also may provide fiber in addition to glucose.

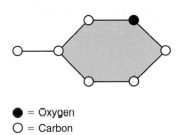

● = Oxygen
○ = Carbon

FIG 4-1 Structure of a molecule of carbohydrate.

CARBOHYDRATE AS A NUTRIENT WITHIN THE BODY

Function

Carbohydrates provide energy, fiber, and naturally occurring sweeteners (sucrose and fructose). Energy is the only real nutrient function of carbohydrates; the roles of fiber and carbohydrate sweeteners are discussed later in this chapter. Carbohydrates supply energy in the most efficient form for use by our bodies. If enough carbohydrate is provided to meet the energy needs of the body, protein can be spared or saved to use for specific protein functions. This service of carbohydrates is called the *protein-sparing effect.*

When adequate amounts of carbohydrates are available, both carbohydrates and small amounts of fats are used for energy. When there are not enough carbohydrates available, fat is metabolized, which results in the formation of ketones, intermediate products of fat metabolism. The body without distress easily disposes of low levels of ketones. If carbohydrate levels continue to be insufficient to meet energy demands, increased levels of ketones overwhelm the physiologic system and ketoacidosis develops; ketoacidosis affects the pH balance of the body, which can be lethal if uncontrolled. Although lipids and proteins can, if necessary, provide energy for most bodily needs, the brain and nerve tissues function best on glucose from carbohydrates.

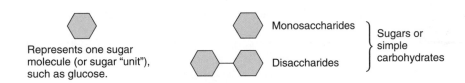

Represents one sugar molecule (or sugar "unit"), such as glucose.

Monosaccharides

Disaccharides

Sugars or simple carbohydrates

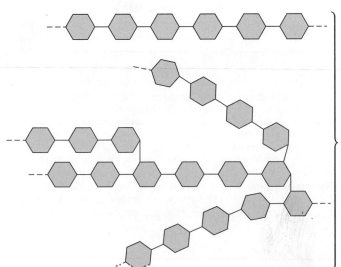

FIG 4-2 Structure of monosaccharides, disaccharides, and polysaccharides.

Complex carbohydrates or polysaccharides

TABLE 4-1	DIETARY CARBOHYDRATES	
CARBOHYDRATE TYPE	COMMON NAMES	NATURALLY OCCURRING FOOD SOURCES
Simple		
Monosaccharides		
Glucose	Blood sugar	Fruits, sweeteners
Fructose	Fruit sugar	Fruits, honey, syrups, vegetables
Galactose	—	Part of lactose, found in milk
Disaccharides		
Sucrose (glucose + fructose)	Table sugar	Sugarcane, sugar beets, fruits, vegetables
Lactose (glucose + galactose)	Milk sugar	Milk and milk products
Maltose (glucose + glucose)	Malt sugar	Germinating grains
Complex		
Polysaccharides		
Starches (strings of glucose)	Complex carbohydrates	Grains, legumes, potatoes
Fiber (strings of monosaccharides, usually glucose)	Roughage	Legumes, whole grains, fruits, vegetables

Digestion and Absorption

Our food sources of carbohydrates tend to be disaccharides (sugars) and polysaccharides (starches). The gastrointestinal (GI) tract has the role of digesting carbohydrates into monosaccharides for easy absorption. The digestive process begins in the mouth. Mechanical digestion breaks food into smaller pieces and mixes the carbohydrate-containing food with saliva, which contains amylase, called *ptyalin*. This begins the hydrolysis of starch into the simpler carbohydrate intermediary forms of dextrin and maltose. In the small intestine, intestinal enzymes and specific pancreatic amylase work on starch intermediary products to continue the breakdown to monosaccharides.

Enzymes specific for disaccharides (lactase for lactose, sucrase for sucrose, maltase for maltose) are secreted by the small intestine's brush border cells, which then hydrolyze disaccharides into monosaccharides. (For more information, see the *Cultural Considerations* box, The Missing Enzyme, and the *Teaching Tool* box, Lacking Lactose? No Problem!) After an active absorption process (i.e., one that requires energy input), absorptive cells in the small intestine take up these monosaccharides. Once glucose, fructose, and galactose enter the villi, the portal blood circulatory system transports them to the liver. The liver removes fructose and galactose

⊕ CULTURAL CONSIDERATIONS

The Missing Enzyme

Many adults throughout the world are unable to easily digest the lactose found in milk. Approximately 75% of the adult world population and 25% of the U.S. population are lactose maldigesters. This condition, lactose intolerance, occurs when the body does not produce enough lactase, a digestive enzyme that breaks lactose into glucose and galactose. When the lactose sits in the large intestine, bacteria begin to ferment the undigested lactose, causing diarrhea, bloating, and increased gas formation.

Lactase deficiency may be the result of a primary or secondary cause. Primary lactose intolerance is caused by a genetic factor that limits the ability to produce lactase. Although small amounts of lactose can often be tolerated, the level of lactase produced cannot be enhanced. The condition is common among Asian/Pacific Islanders (Asian Americans), Africans (African Americans), Hispanics (Hispanic Americans), Latinos, and Native Americans. In the United States the prevalence of lactose intolerance caused by maldigestion or low lactose levels is approximately 75% in African Americans and Native Americans, 90% in Asian/Pacific Islanders, 50% in Hispanic Americans, and least common among whites.

One explanation for primary lactose intolerance is that the ability to digest milk is an age-related ability. Consider that the milk of mammals, including humans, was intended for the young to consume during periods of major growth. The ability to digest milk may diminish because the biologic need is lessened as maturity is reached. Older adults may also develop lactose intolerance as the aging process diminishes the production of some digestive enzymes such as lactase. The recent identification of a genetic variation is valuable for future diagnostic testing to determine risk for and severity of lactose intolerance earlier in life.

Sometimes secondary lactose intolerance occurs when a chronic gastrointestinal illness affects the intestinal tract, reducing the amount of lactase produced (see Chapter 17). Even a bout of an intestinal virus or flu can cause temporary lactose intolerance. Most of these individuals recover and are again able to digest lactose.

Application to nursing: Health professionals can guide clients to determine what amounts of lactose-containing foods can be tolerated despite low lactase levels. Fine-tuning eating styles may require the assistance of a registered dietitian (RD) to ensure adequate consumption of calcium-containing foods. Depending on the severity of the sensitivity, advice to clients may include additional label reading for lactose-containing foods and medications especially for clients dealing with conditions such as irritable bowel syndrome.

Data from Matthews SB et al: Systemic lactose intolerance: A new perspective on an old problem, *Postgrad Med J* 81(953):167-173, 2003; National Institutes of Health: *Lactose intolerance,* National Institutes of Health Pub No 03-2751, Washington, DC, 2003, National Digestive Diseases Information Clearinghouse; and Ridefelt P, Hakansson LD: Lactose intolerance: Lactose tolerance test versus genotyping, *Scan J Gastroenterol* 40(7):822-826, 2005.

Lacking Lactose? No Problem!

Lactose intolerance is not an illness and should not undermine a person's sense of wellness. To ensure that clients receive an adequate supply of nutrients usually consumed in lactose-containing dairy products—especially calcium, riboflavin, and vitamin D—without the use of supplements, consider suggesting the following to clients:

- Experiment with different portion sizes of lactose-containing foods to determine individual levels of tolerance; small amounts up to ½ cup consumed throughout the day can often be tolerated.
- Use over-the-counter lactase-enzyme tablets when consuming dairy products (presently available as Lactaid, Lactrase, Dairy Ease, and others).
- If available, purchase lactose-reduced dairy products such as milk, ice cream, and soft cheeses.
- Consume foods high in nutrients found in lactose-containing foods; high-calcium foods include broccoli, eggs, kale, spinach, tofu, shrimp, canned salmon, sardines with bones, and calcium-fortified orange juice.
- Consume hard cheeses (in moderate amounts because of fat content) that contain lower lactose levels such as Swiss, cheddar, Muenster, Parmesan, Monterey, and provolone.
- Avoid softer cheeses (or experiment to learn level of tolerance), including ricotta, cottage cheese, mozzarella, Neufchatel, and cream cheese (see Appendix L for lactose content of foods).
- Test tolerance of different brands of yogurt; lactose levels may vary according to processing variations. Generally, lactase bacteria in yogurt culture hydrolyse some of the lactose.
- Consider supplementation if these dietary modifications are not achieved; consult with a nutritionist for an appropriate supplement.

and converts them to glucose. This glucose may be used immediately for energy or for glycogen formation, a storage form of carbohydrate providing an always-ready source of energy. Figure 4-3 summarizes carbohydrate digestion.

Glycogen: Storing Carbohydrates

Glycogen is carbohydrate energy stored in the liver and in muscles. The amount held in the muscles of an adult is 150 g (600 kcal); 90 g (360 kcal) is stored in the liver. Retrieved as needed for energy, glycogen is quickly broken down by enzymes to produce a surge of energy. The process of converting glucose to glycogen is glycogenesis.

Glycogen levels can be significantly increased through physical training and dietary manipulations (see Chapter 9). It is still considered a relatively limited source of energy compared with the amounts of energy stored in body fat.

Metabolism

A primary aspect of carbohydrate metabolism is the maintenance of blood glucose homeostasis at a level of between 70 and 100 mg/dL. Sources of blood glucose, the most common sugar in the blood, may be carbohydrate and noncarbohydrate. Dietary starches and simple carbohydrates provide blood glucose after digestion and absorption; glycogen stored in the liver and muscle tissue is converted back to glucose in a process called glycogenolysis. Intermediate carbohydrate metabolites are also a source of blood glucose. The metabolites include lactic acid and pyruvic acid, which occur when muscle glycogen is used for energy.

Noncarbohydrates can also provide blood glucose. Gluconeogenesis is the process of producing glucose from fat. It is not as efficient as using carbohydrate directly for glucose. As fat is metabolized into fatty acids and glycerol (see Chapter 5), the smaller glycerol portion can be converted by the liver into glycogen, which is then available for glucose needs through glycogenolysis. Protein, which is composed of numerous combinations of amino acids, also may be a source of glucose. Some of these amino acids are glucogenic; if they are not used for protein structures, they can be metabolized to form glucose. Carbohydrate as an energy source is also discussed in Figure 9-2.

Blood glucose is a source of energy to all cells. Glucose may be used immediately as energy or converted to glycogen or fat; both conversions provide energy for the future. Although glycogen can be converted back to glucose, the conversion of glucose to fat is irreversible. Glucose cannot be formed again but is stored as fat and, if needed, is metabolized later as fat, although its original source was carbohydrate.

Glucose is essential for brain function and cell formation, particularly during pregnancy and growth. Because the body can form glucose through gluconeogenesis from protein and fat, glucose technically is not an essential nutrient. Gluconeogenesis can provide some glucose but not enough to meet essential needs if dietary carbohydrate is insufficient. To compensate (as previously discussed), ketone bodies can be used for energy. Ketone bodies are created when fatty acids are broken down for energy when sufficient carbohydrates are unavailable; this process of fat metabolism, however, is incomplete. If dietary carbohydrate continues to be insufficient, a buildup of ketones results, which causes ketosis, possibly leading to acid-base imbalances in the body.

Blood Glucose Regulation

Metabolism of glucose and regulation of blood glucose levels are controlled by a sophisticated hormonal system. Insulin, a hormone produced by the beta cells of the islets of Langerhans, lowers blood glucose levels by enhancing the conversion of excess glucose to glycogen through glycogenesis or to fat stored in adipose tissue. Insulin also eases the absorption of glucose into the cells so the use of glucose as energy is increased.

Whereas insulin lowers blood glucose levels, other hormones raise glucose levels. The pancreas produces two hormones with this function: glucagon and somatostatin. Glucagon stimulates conversion of liver glycogen to glucose, assisting the regulation of glucose levels during the night;

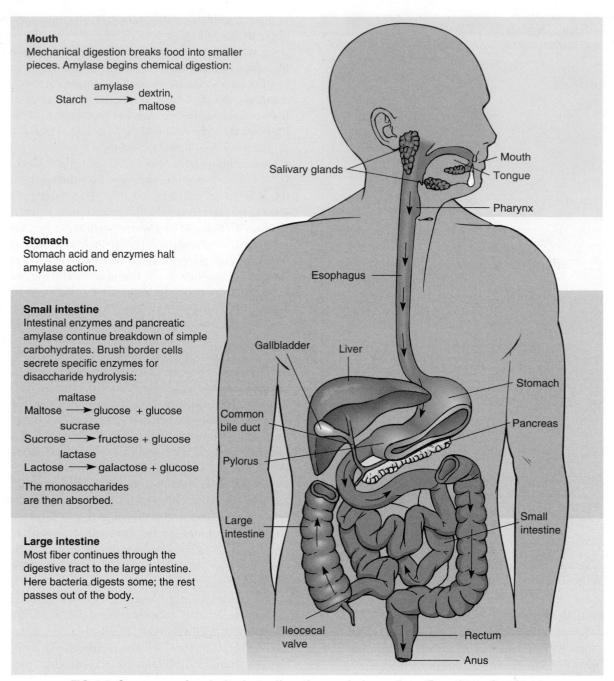

Mouth
Mechanical digestion breaks food into smaller pieces. Amylase begins chemical digestion:

$$Starch \xrightarrow{amylase} dextrin, maltose$$

Stomach
Stomach acid and enzymes halt amylase action.

Small intestine
Intestinal enzymes and pancreatic amylase continue breakdown of simple carbohydrates. Brush border cells secrete specific enzymes for disaccharide hydrolysis:

$$Maltose \xrightarrow{maltase} glucose + glucose$$

$$Sucrose \xrightarrow{sucrase} fructose + glucose$$

$$Lactose \xrightarrow{lactase} galactose + glucose$$

The monosaccharides are then absorbed.

Large intestine
Most fiber continues through the digestive tract to the large intestine. Here bacteria digests some; the rest passes out of the body.

Salivary glands — Mouth — Tongue — Pharynx — Esophagus — Gallbladder — Liver — Stomach — Common bile duct — Pancreas — Pylorus — Large intestine — Small intestine — Ileocecal valve — Rectum — Anus

FIG 4-3 Summary of carbohydrate digestion and absorption. (From Rolin Graphics.)

somatostatin, secreted from the hypothalamus and pancreas, inhibits the functions of insulin and glucagon. Several adrenal gland hormones also have a role in raising blood glucose levels. Epinephrine enhances the fast conversion of liver glycogen to glucose. Steroid hormones function against insulin and promote glucose formation from protein. Produced by the pituitary gland, growth hormone and adrenocorticotropic hormone (ACTH) function as insulin inhibitors. The thyroid hormone thyroxine affects blood glucose levels by enhancing intestinal absorption of glucose and releasing epinephrine.

Glycemic Index and Glycemic Load

Although the sophisticated hormonal system controls the metabolism and regulation of blood glucose levels, most likely the composition of foods we consume may differ significantly in their effect on blood glucose levels. To account for this, the concepts of glycemic index and glycemic load are used. Glycemic index is the ranking of foods based on the level to which a food raises blood glucose levels compared with a reference food such a 50-g glucose load or white bread containing 50 g carbohydrate.[4,5] A ranking of 100 is the highest glycemic index level—that is, it raises blood glucose

BOX 4-2 GLYCEMIC INDEX COMPARISONS OF COMMONLY CONSUMED FOODS

GLYCEMIC INDEX	FOOD
60	Mini-wheat cereal (WG)
60	Raisin bran cereal (WG)
92	Corn flake cereal (RG)
60	Whole grain bread (WG)
72	White bread (RG)
72	Bagel (RG)
30	Spaghetti/whole wheat (WG)
60	Spaghetti (RG)
50	Brown rice (WG)
60	White rice (RG)
30	Skim milk
40	Apple juice
50	Orange juice
63	Cola
70	Sports drinks
33	Pear
40	Apple
48	Orange
50	Banana
50	Sweet potato
90	Potato (baked, no fat)
14	Peanuts
22	Cashews
30	Legumes (lentils, chickpeas)

GI, Glycemic index; *RG,* refined grains; *WG,* whole grains.
Data from Foster-Powell K et al: International table of glycemic index and glycemic load values: 2002, *Am J Clin Nutr* 76:5-56, 2002.

levels the highest. Note the glycemic index rankings of commonly consumed foods listed Box 4-2.

The glycemic index of a food is affected by the following factors:[4]

- The physical form such as a baked potato compared with a mashed potato
- The fat and protein content in addition to carbohydrate, which slows digestion
- The ripeness such as in fruits and vegetables, which increases glucose content
- The fiber content, which slows digestion
- The botanic variety of a food, such as the different glycemic indexes of rice species

Because the glycemic index assesses only one food item, another measurement tool is needed because we usually eat several foods at the same time. This is accounted for by the glycemic load, which considers the total glycemic index effect of a mixed meal or dietary plan. It is calculated by the sum of the products of the glycemic index for each of the foods multiplied by the amount of carbohydrate in each food.[5] Given that glycemic load accounts for the mixed consumption of foods, it measures the quantity and quality of the effect of carbohydrate on blood glucose and the resulting effect on insulin release.[4]

Recent epidemiologic work notes associations between glycemic index and glycemic load with risk of chronic diseases such as type 2 diabetes mellitus, cardiovascular disease, and diet-related cancers of the colon and breast. Seemingly limiting consumption of foods producing a high glycemic index and overall high glycemic load would seem prudent to reduce risk. Public health recommendations, however, will most likely not be forthcoming until long-term clinical trials demonstrate a clear role of these diet-related effects. Regardless, the concept of glycemic index is controversial—in relation to health and disease—because it measures individual foods, not mixed meals within which the carbohydrate effect might vary.[5]

Nonetheless, consider its potential value in the following situations. The glycemic index of a food may affect a person's blood glucose level, but that same food as part of a meal of several foods (a mix of high and low glycemic indexes) will have a different effect or glycemic load. If a person's dietary goal is to have an even blood glucose level, one could choose foods that provide an even response and by consuming foods throughout the day avoid a feasting or fasting experience. Certainly this is what individuals with diabetes (abnormally high blood glucose levels) accomplish through carbohydrate counting and planning nourishment within intentional intervals. For those of us who are prone to hypoglycemia (abnormally low blood glucose level), consuming low glycemic index foods or meals with moderate glycemic loads may maintain adequate blood glucose levels. For the rest of us, having a stable level of blood glucose for energy from the foods we consume provides much-needed stamina. The bottom line to this issue for most of us is that we struggle enough with just preparing and finding time to eat adequate meals. Adding the layer of assessing glycemic index and glycemic loads to foods and meals may be more than can be expected within our contemporary lifestyles (Box 4-3).

SIMPLE CARBOHYDRATES

Monosaccharides

Glucose, often called *blood sugar,* is the form of carbohydrate most easily used by the body. It is the simple carbohydrate that circulates in the blood and is the main source of energy for the central nervous system and brain. Glucose is rapidly absorbed into the bloodstream from the intestine, but it needs insulin to be taken into the cells, where energy is released.

Fructose is the sweetest of the sugars. Although fruits and honey contain a mixture of sugars, including sucrose, fructose provides the characteristic taste of fruits and honey. After absorption from the small intestine, fructose circulates in the bloodstream. When it passes through to the liver, liver cells rearrange fructose into glucose.

Galactose is rarely found in nature by itself but is part of the disaccharide lactose, the sugar found in milk. Absorbed like fructose, galactose is converted to glucose by the liver.

"Carbs" are a part of everyday food talk, much as "fat" used to be. We thought if only "fat" intake was lower we would be at healthy weights and free of heart disease and other chronic diseases. Not so. As a nation, we gained weight instead. Now, just replace "fat" with "carbs," and the myth continues.

Can Eating Fewer Carbs Lead to Weight Loss?

Yes, it can, but only if total caloric intake is lower. Weight will return, though, if calories and carbohydrate intake are again elevated. Reducing intake to very low levels such as 20 g a day is not a long-term weight-loss approach. Our bodies function best when we consume some carbohydrates because daily we must use about 100 g of carbohydrates as glucose for brain function.

Isn't Eliminating Carbs Such as Doughnuts and Sweets a Healthy Approach to Weight Loss?

This depends on how carbs are decreased. If carbohydrate calories are replaced with saturated fats found in animal proteins, it is not health promoting. But if nutrient-empty caloric carbohydrate foods are replaced by low-carbohydrate salad greens and vegetables, health benefits may accrue. The key is portion size and calorie control. Moderate intake of all nutrient groups is best. Some of us may feel better with a higher carbohydrate intake, whereas others feel best with a greater proportion of protein (lean, of course) consumption.

What About Lower-Carb Products Such as Breads, Tortillas, and Pasta?

This too depends on how many calories of carbohydrates a person tends to consume and what kinds of carbohydrates. Whole grain foods provide more health benefits than refined grain products. Lower-carb products may be labeled as reduced in carbohydrate content because of added dietary fiber to the ingredient formulation of the product. The label statement of reduced carbohydrate content is based on "net carbs," which are not defined by U.S. Food and Drug Administration (FDA). Manufacturers often present net carbs as equaling total carbohydrates minus dietary fiber and sugar alcohols (which do not quickly raise blood glucose levels). Consuming such products may increase fiber intake, but 100% whole grain products are the best choice by most likely containing dietary fiber and less-processed ingredients.

For each of the nutrient categories studied, an "Inside the Pyramid" section will be included to emphasize the importance of portion sizes for the five food categories. For carbohydrates, the focus is on portions of grains.

Disaccharides

Sucrose is formed from the pairing of units of glucose and fructose. We know it as *table sugar*. Sugarcane and sugar beets are two sources of sucrose, and it is found naturally in fruits. Because it contains fructose, sucrose is quite sweet. Sucrose has a special place in our history of food consumption and is further explored in the following section.

Maltose is created when two units of glucose are linked. It is available when cereal grains are about to germinate and the plant starch is broken down into maltose. The majority of maltose in human nutrition is created from the breakdown of starch in the small intestine. Maltose is of particular value in the production of beer and other malt beverages. When maltose ferments, alcohol is formed.

Lactose is composed of glucose and galactose. It is sometimes called *milk sugar* because it is the primary carbohydrate in milk.

Sugar—A Special Disaccharide

The term *sugar* is a word with many meanings. Sugar may refer to the simple carbohydrates (monosaccharides and disaccharides). Sucrose, the disaccharide naturally found in many fruits, is also called sugar. White table sugar refers to sucrose extracted from sugarcane and sugar beets. Sugar may also be an umbrella term used to cover numerous kcal-sweetening agents used in our food production system, although U.S. commercial law defines sugar as "sucrose." There is a distinction between how the term *sugar* is used on a label versus its use by a biologist, chemist, or nutritionist. Often, blood glucose levels are called *blood sugar levels*. It is important that we, as health professionals, be aware that our clinical use of the term may confuse clients. Concerns about sugar focus on the following three issues: sources in the food supply, consumption levels, and health effects.

Sources in the Food Supply. Sugar in our food supply may include the following nutritive sweeteners: refined white sugar, brown sugar, dextrose, crystalline fructose, **high fructose corn syrup (HFCS)**, glucose, corn sweeteners, lactose, concentrated fruit juice, honey, maple syrup, molasses, and reduced energy polyols or sugar alcohols (e.g., sorbitol, mannitol, xylitol)[6] (Table 4-2). All forms of sugar are chemically similar; each provides kcal and most do not contain any other nutrients. Blackstrap molasses does contain iron, but other more nutrient-dense sources of iron are easily available. Honey, which seems less processed than other sweeteners, provides only a trace of minerals and therefore is as nonnutritious as any other sweetener.

The U.S. Food and Drug Administration (FDA) categorizes some sweeteners as generally recognized as safe (GRAS) ingredients and others as food additives (see Chapter 2). For food additives, an acceptable daily intake (ADI) is determined as the amount that a person can safely consume daily over one's life without risk. Table 4-2 lists descriptions, regulatory status, and energy amounts provided by sweeteners.

Consumption Levels. Our national intake of refined white sugar has declined, whereas consumption of high fructose corn syrup (HFCS) has greatly increased since the 1970s. In the 1970s, a process was perfected in which HFCS, very sweet-tasting syrup, could be made from corn syrup. HFCS is less expensive to produce than refined sugar and is sweeter. Used extensively in food manufacturing, it has replaced refined white sugar in many products, such as soft drinks.

TABLE 4-2 NUTRITIVE AND NONNUTRITIVE SWEETENERS

SWEETENER	KCAL/g	REGULATORY STATUS	OTHER NAMES	DESCRIPTION
Sucrose	4	GRAS	Granulated: coarse, regular, fine; powdered; confectioners'; brown; turbinado, Demerara; liquid: molasses	Sweetens; enhances flavor; tenderizes, allows browning, and enhances appearance in baking; adds characteristic flavor with unrefined sugar
Fructose	4	GRAS	High-fructose corn syrups: 42%, 55%, 90% fructose; crystalline fructose: 99% fructose	Sweetens; functions like sucrose in baking. Some people experience a laxative response from a load of fructose ≥20 g. May produce lower glycemic response than sucrose
Polyols-monosaccharide				
Sorbitol	2.6	GRAS (label must warn about a laxative effect)	Same as chemical name	50%-70% as sweet as sucrose. Some people may experience a laxative effect from a load of sorbitol ≥50 g.
Mannitol	1.6	Permitted for use on an interim basis (label must warn about a laxative effect)	Same as chemical name	50%-70% as sweet as sucrose. Some people may experience a laxative effect from a load of mannitol ≥20 g
Xylitol	2.4	GRAS	Same as chemical name	As sweet as sucrose
Saccharin	0	Permitted for use on interim basis (label must contain cancer warning and amount of saccharin in the product)	Sweet'N Low	200%-700% sweeter than sucrose. Noncariogenic and produces no glycemic response. Synergizes the sweetening power of nutritive and nonnutritive sweeteners. Sweetening power is not reduced with heating
Aspartame	4*	Approved as a general purpose sweetener	NutraSweet, Equal	160%-220% sweeter than sucrose. Noncariogenic and produces limited glycemic response. New forms can increase its sweetening power in cooking and baking
Acesulfame K	0	Approved for use as a tabletop sweetener and as an additive in a variety of desserts, confections, and alcoholic beverages	Sunette[†]	200% sweeter than sucrose. Noncariogenic and produces no glycemic response. Sweetening power is not reduced with heating. Can synergize the sweetening power of other nutritive and nonnutritive sweeteners
Sucralose	0	Approved for use as a tabletop sweetener and as an additive in a variety of desserts, confections, and nonalcoholic beverages	Splenda[‡]	600% sweeter than sucrose. Noncariogenic and produces no glycemic response. Sweetening power is not reduced with heating

*Provides limited energy to products because of its sweetening power.
[†]Hoechst Food Ingredients, Edison, N.J.
[‡]McNeil Specialty Products Company, New Brunswick, N.J.
GRAS, Generally recognized as safe by the U.S. Food and Drug Administration.
From Position of the American Dietetic Association: Use of nutritive and nonnutritive sweeteners, *J Am Diet Assoc* 104:255-275, 2004.

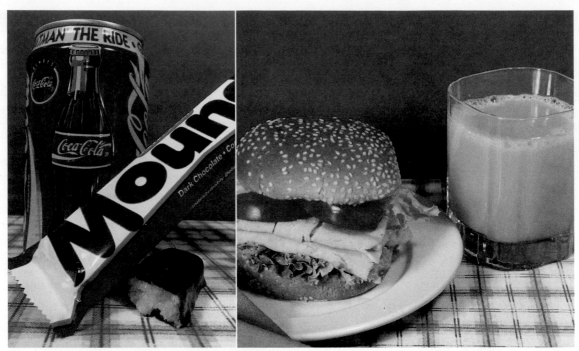

FIG 4-4 Consuming products with added sugars can displace more nutrient-dense foods. (From Joanne Scott/Tracy McCalla.)

Health Effects. The health concerns regarding sugar consumption include nutrient displacement, dental caries, and the related issues of obesity and diabetes.

Does it matter to our bodies what the source of the sweet taste is? That depends. A major health concern is nutrient displacement. Displacement occurs when whole foods, which are minimally processed, are not eaten and are replaced by foods containing added sugars. If we eat candy, soda, and other sweet snack foods instead of a sandwich and juice for lunch, we lose a number of important nutrients (Figure 4-4).

Foods and drinks with added sugars often contain empty kcal that provide few nutrients. Because all forms of sugar are chemically similar, the sucrose in fruits is actually the same as the sucrose in a cream-filled doughnut. The difference, however, is that naturally occurring vitamins, minerals, and fiber available in the fruit are not available in the doughnut. The doughnut's empty kcal can replace kcal from other foods that might contain a natural sweetener and also provide vitamins, minerals, protein, complex carbohydrates, and fiber. Consumption of excessively sugared food does not support wellness goals because it probably replaces other more nutrient-dense foods.

Dental caries are related to eating concentrated sweets and sticky carbohydrates. Sugar supports the growth of bacteria, which promotes the formation of plaque. Plaque leads to tooth decay. Ways to decrease the development of caries are to eat sweets at the end of meals—rather than between meals—and to monitor the quantity and frequency of sugar intake. Sticky, sugary foods are more cariogenic than sweet liquids. Optimal dental hygiene reduces plaque formation and promotes dental health.

A misconception is that obesity is caused by high sugar intake only. In fact, obesity may be caused by an excess intake of kcal from any of the energy nutrients, which is then stored as body fat. Many sugared foods are also high in fat. Because fat is the most energy-dense nutrient, fat intake may be more of a risk factor for obesity than sugar intake.

There is no confirmed relationship between the level of sugar intake and increased risk of developing type 2 diabetes mellitus.[2] People with diabetes are counseled to restrict their intake of concentrated sweets to assist the regulation of insulin needs once the disorder is confirmed. However, consumption of sweets does not cause the disorder. These issues become complicated because obesity is a risk factor for type 2 diabetes mellitus. Health concerns related to obesity and type 2 diabetes mellitus are explored in Chapters 10 and 19.

A myth that sugar consumption by children produces hyperactivity or attention deficient/hyperactivity disorder (ADHD) continues to be perpetuated. Controlled research studies have consistently failed to support this assertion.[6] More than likely, excessively active behavior is related to the occasions at which sugared foods such as cake and candy are ingested. If children regularly consume excessive amounts of refined sugar, their overall dietary intake may be nutritionally deficient, possibly resulting in altered behaviors.

So how much sugar is acceptable? Moderate amounts are okay when our diets are low in fat and high in fiber. The *Dietary Guidelines for Americans* suggests consuming sugars in moderation (see Chapter 2). The Dietary Reference Intake (DRI) report on carbohydrates suggests that added sugars be kept to 25% or less of energy intake on a daily basis. Less added sugar intake ensures a dietary intake that is adequate in complex carbohydrates.[2] Following recommendations to increase consumption of fruits and vegetables to at least five servings or four and one half cups a day and grains to 6 ounces a day, we can reduce our intake of simple sugars.

Other Sweeteners

Other available sweeteners are sugar alcohols (polyols) and alternative sweeteners. Sugar alcohols, also called *sugar replacers* to avoid confusion with noncarbohydrate alcohol, are nutritive sweeteners because they provide 2 to 3 kcal/g but fewer than the 4 kcal/g of carbohydrates. They occur naturally in fruits and berries. Sorbitol, mannitol, and xylitol are the most commonly used sugar alcohols. Alternative sweeteners are nonnutritive substances produced to be sweet-tasting; however, they provide no nutrients and few, if any, kcal. For food production purposes, sugar alcohols are synthesized rather than derived from natural sources.[6] Aspartame and saccharin are commonly used alternative sweeteners.

Products containing these sweeteners may be labeled as "sugar free," but this does not mean "calorie free." Consumers still need to be aware of calories per serving as well as trans and saturated fat content. Sometimes when "sugar" is removed, fats are added to improve the taste and texture of the product. This may be problematic for individuals with diabetes who monitor their carbohydrate and dietary fat intake.

Sugar alcohols have several advantages when replacing sugar. They are less cariogenic than sucrose. In contrast to carbohydrate sugars, sugar alcohols do not encourage the growth of bacteria in the mouth that leads to tooth decay. In fact, xylitol may actually prevent cavity formation and be protective when used in chewing gum. Although chemically related to carbohydrates, sugar alcohols are absorbed more slowly and incompletely than carbohydrates. The longer absorption time leads to a slower rise in blood glucose levels or reduced glycemic response. People with diabetes may be able to consume moderate amounts of these sweeteners and still control their blood glucose levels.

A disadvantage of sugar alcohols is that if large quantities are consumed, they may ferment in the intestinal tract because of their slower absorption rate. This fermentation may cause gas and diarrhea. The incomplete absorption results in a lower caloric value per gram, and thus less energy is available. Therefore the sugar alcohols are called *reduced-energy* or *low-energy sweeteners*.[6]

Alternative sweeteners, also called *artificial sweeteners,* are manufactured to be used as sweetening agents in food products. Their function is to replace naturally sweet substances such as sugar, honey, and other sucrose-containing substances. Alternative sweeteners most commonly used in the United States and approved by the FDA are aspartame, saccharin, acesulfame potassium (K), and sucralose. Often, a combination of alternative sweeteners is used that results in an increased sweetness.[6]

Aspartame is formed by the bonding of the amino acids phenylalanine and aspartic acid. When consumed, aspartame is digested and absorbed as two separate amino acids.

Although aspartame contains the same kcal as sucrose, much less aspartame is needed to get the same sweet taste because it is 180 to 200 times sweeter than sucrose. This provides so few kcal that aspartame can be considered a noncaloric sweetener. Approved in 1981 and used in a wide variety of products such as soft drinks, cereals, chewing gum, frozen snacks, and puddings, aspartame is consumed in more than 100 countries. In 1996, aspartame was approved as a general purpose sweetener for all foods and beverages.

Several studies have shown aspartame to be safe, yet some individuals have reported side effects thought attributable to its consumption. These included allergic reactions such as rashes; edema of the lips, tongue, and throat; and respiratory difficulties. However, within controlled settings, these reactions were not replicated; this means that aspartame consumption was not responsible for the allergic reactions.[6] The Internet has been used by some individuals to spread false information about aspartame, linking its consumption to disorders that range from multiple sclerosis to brain tumors to arthritis. Logically, one substance would not cause an array of serious disorders. Investigation of the authors of the e-mails revealed sources that were not credible, and therefore the FDA maintains its approval of aspartame.

Individuals with the genetic disorder phenylketonuria (PKU) should not consume aspartame because their bodies cannot break down excess phenylalanine, which results in a buildup that causes medical problems. All products containing aspartame have a warning label to alert individuals with PKU. This warning should apply to pregnant women as well. Because the fetus would be exposed to excess phenylalanine before the presence of PKU could be determined, the safest approach is to restrict consumption of aspartame during pregnancy.

The general adult population (for a 132-pound person) is advised to keep daily aspartame consumption at or less than 50 mg/kg body weight (the equivalent of 83 packets of Equal, an aspartame product) or 14 12-ounce cans of aspartame-sweetened soda.[6] Aspartame, when added to products, is most often listed by its original brand name of NutraSweet or Equal.

Saccharin has had a stormy history since it was accidentally discovered more than 100 years ago. The storm began when some animal studies indicated an association between excessive saccharin consumption and the development of bladder cancer. In 1977 the FDA proposed a ban of saccharin. Many Americans were upset that the only available noncaloric sweetener was to be banned. The public outcry was so great that Congress, in an unusual move, created a moratorium to prevent the ban. In addition, Congress passed legislation requiring all products containing saccharin to clearly state a warning that the consumption of saccharin may be hazardous to health.

The danger from saccharin is probably minimal. The risk of bladder cancer does not appear to apply to humans because no noticeable increase of bladder cancer has occurred. In addition, an association between cancers and saccharin is not supported by studies of individuals with diabetes who tend to consume high amounts of saccharin.[6] Consequently, the moratorium is no longer in effect because the FDA is not pursuing the ban on saccharin. Saccharin is now considered an interim food additive to be used in cosmetics, pharmaceuticals, and foods and beverages.[6] For food products, the amount of saccharin contained must be identified on the product label. Restrictions include that beverages may contain no more than 12 mg/ounce or less than 30 mg per food serving.[7]

Compared with other alternative sweeteners, saccharin has a bitter aftertaste. To mask this, it is often used in combination with other alternative sweeteners. Saccharin is still valuable because it is extremely sweet—300 to 700 times sweeter than sucrose.[6] Trade names for saccharin include Sweet'N Low and Sugar Twin.

Acesulfame K received FDA approval in 1988. Synthetically produced, it tastes 200 times sweeter than sucrose, but it is not digestible by the human body and therefore provides no kcal. Acesulfame K is approved for use in a variety of products, from chewing gum to nondairy creamers, but so far its use has been limited. One advantage of this product over aspartame is that it can be used for baking. Heat does not affect its sweetening ability, whereas heat destroys the sweet taste of aspartame. People who must severely limit potassium intake because of nutritional therapy for renal disorders should consult a registered dietitian about acceptable levels of acesulfame K. The consumer brand name for acesulfame K is Sunette.

Sucralose (trichlorogalactosucrose) was approved by the FDA in April 1998 for use in desserts, candies, and nonalcoholic beverages, and as a tabletop sweetener. Made from chemically altered sucrose, sucralose provides no energy but is 600 times sweeter than sucrose. Because the body poorly absorbs it, sucralose passes through the digestive tract and is excreted in urine. An advantage of sucralose is that it can be used in baking and cooking.[6] Sucralose is presently sold as Splenda.

A recent addition is stevia, which is created from the leaves of a South American shrub. Stevia has been approved as a GRAS food additive. Rebiana may be extracted from the stevia leaves and combined with other ingredients to create sweetening products such as Truvia and Sun Crystals. Because it is used in very small quantities and has no caloric value (depending on other ingredients), individuals with diabetes may use stevia as another sweetener alternative.

Sweet Decisions

Should you consume foods with real sugar or artificial sugar? Which is the best? Which is the worst? There are no clear answers, but here is a way to decide. A concept used with food safety issues is a benefit-risk analysis. Does the benefit of consuming a substance outweigh the risk? This analysis can be applied to the decision of whether to consume artificial sweeteners.

Benefits of consuming artificial sweeteners include experiencing a sweet taste with fewer kcal and a less cariogenic effect than sucrose. Many people believe these sweeteners are

an important part of their weight reduction effort. For most, though, the saved kcal are often replaced by consuming other kcal foods, thereby undermining their weight-loss efforts. However, within a formal multidiscipline weight control program, aspartame-sweetened foods and beverages supported long-term weight-loss maintenance among obese women.[8] In other words, individuals who successfully lose weight and maintain that weight loss do not depend solely on alternative sweeteners. Instead, changes in exercise and food selection behaviors are the basis of the weight change.

Risks associated with the use of alternative sweeteners may involve safety concerns. This is a difficult issue to sort out. Because sucrose in the form of white table sugar has been used for thousands of years, we essentially have a large-scale study of its safety for humans. In contrast, alternative sweeteners have existed only for a century or less. Because alternative sweeteners are not naturally formed in plants or animals, their safety must be determined through research studies.

The research process is difficult. Rather than use humans as test subjects, researchers use animals. The test animals are given extremely large doses of the artificial sweeteners and are followed by researchers for several generations of their species. If the physiology of the animals is affected, particularly in regard to cancerous tumors, the substance may be regarded as too dangerous for consumption by humans. The difficulty is that the extremely large doses given to the animals do not replicate the amounts that would be typically consumed by humans. Concerns raised include whether the substance caused the tumor or whether the excessive quantity interfered with normal cell function. Also, how many animals need to be affected for a substance to be considered dangerous and in what animal generation of the experiment? Attention should also be paid to who funds such studies. If the company manufacturing the substance pays for the research, does that affect the interpretation of the results? These are difficult questions with which health scientists and FDA officials grapple.

This is an area, however, in which we can make a personal decision whether to consume products that contain alternative sweeteners. Based on our analysis of the benefits and risks, we can decide if our wellness goals are better met by consuming a moderate amount of sucrose or a reasonable intake of alternative sweetened products.

COMPLEX CARBOHYDRATES: POLYSACCHARIDES

Polysaccharides are many units of monosaccharides held together by different kinds of chemical bonds. These types of bonds affect the ability of the body to digest polysaccharides and therefore account for the classification of polysaccharides as **complex carbohydrates**.

Starch

All starchy foods are plant foods. Starch is the storage form of plant carbohydrate. The strings of glucose that form starch are broken down by the digestive tract to provide glucose.

Food sources of starch include grains, legumes, and some vegetables and fruits. Grains are the best source of starch. Grains provide more carbohydrates than any other food category.[2] Grains are consumed in many forms and include wheat, oats, barley, rice, corn, and rye. The overall health value of processed grain products differs based on their sugar, fat, and fiber content.

Breads, bagels, breakfast cereals, pasta, pancakes, grits, oatmeal, and other cooked cereals provide high-quality complex carbohydrates. These grain products may also contain fiber if made with whole grains. Depending on the spreads and toppings served, they may also be low in fat. Main dish items such as pizza, rice casseroles, and pasta mixtures create another category of complex carbohydrate foods. Other foods such as crackers, cakes, pies, cookies, and pastries also provide carbohydrates but often contain considerable amounts of added sugar and fats; they should be eaten in moderation.

Legumes (beans and peas) are another significant source of complex carbohydrates. They are low in fat and are an excellent source of fiber, iron, and protein. Available dried, canned, or frozen, beans easily can be incorporated into commonly eaten foods.

Multicultural influences have expanded our exposure to inexpensive and versatile legumes. Mexican foods feature kidney beans as an ingredient of taco fillings and chili. Puerto Rican and Caribbean meals highlight rice and beans in savory sauces. Hearty Italian-style soups often depend on white and kidney beans combined with pasta. An African influence is reflected in dishes that combine black-eyed peas with meats or green vegetables. Hummus, a chickpea paste dip of Middle Eastern heritage, is often served with pita bread or vegetables.

Among vegetable sources of starch, potatoes lead the way. We consume potatoes in so many ways that we sometimes forget their humble "roots." As a root vegetable, the potato is a powerhouse of complex carbohydrates, fiber, vitamins, and even some protein. Unfortunately, some of the ways we prepare potatoes undo their positive health benefits. Most potatoes are processed into products loaded with fat and sodium. Nutritionally, potato chips have little in common with baked potatoes. The best health value is to eat potatoes in the least-processed form. Instead of french fries, choose a baked potato, or prepare mashed potatoes with skim milk and a small amount of margarine.

Other starchy root vegetables include parsnips, sweet potatoes, and yams. Sweet potatoes and yams provide the same nutrients as white potatoes plus significant amounts of beta carotene. Carrots and some varieties of squash such as acorn and butternut also provide starch and beta carotene. Beta carotene, a substance the body can convert into vitamin A, may have a protective effect against some forms of cancer.

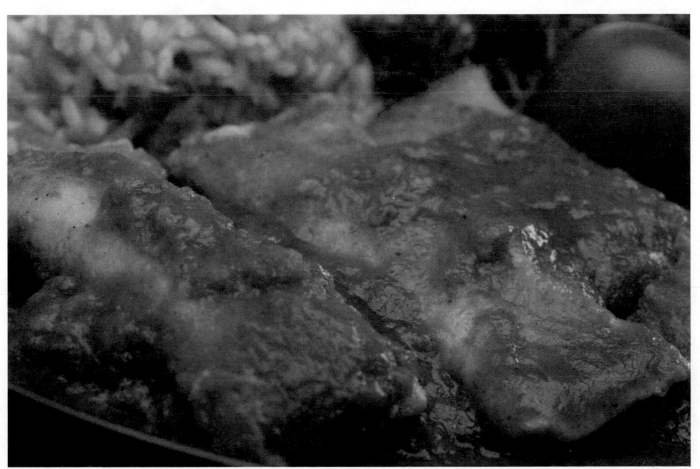

Ethnic cuisine can provide a source of complex carbohydrates and variety in the diet.

Fiber

Fiber, like starch, also consists of strings of simple sugars. Unlike starch, however, human digestive enzymes cannot break down fiber. Dietary fiber consists of substances in plant foods including carbohydrates and lignin that, for the most part, cannot be digested by humans.[2] We do not produce digestive juices strong enough to break down the bonds that hold the simple carbohydrates of most plant fibers, so fiber "passes through" our bodies without providing kcal or nutrients. Its texture provides bulk that thickens chyme and eases the work of the GI muscles that regulate movement of the food mass.

Although human digestive juices cannot digest fiber, microflora that normally reside in the colon use fiber as a medium for microbial fermentation, resulting in the synthesis of vitamins and the formation of short-chain fatty acids (SCFAs). The bacteria that reside in the colon synthesize several vitamins, including vitamin K, biotin, B_{12}, folate, and thiamine. Only vitamin K and biotin can be absorbed in sufficient amounts from the colon to be significant; the other vitamins are absorbed from the small intestine so that the synthesized vitamins are not bioavailable. The SCFAs that are produced can be absorbed and used for energy by the mucosa of the colon, thereby maintaining the health of the colon epithelial cells.[9] The effects of SCFAs also increase fecal matter bulk.

Dietary fiber actually refers to several kinds of carbohydrate substances from different plant sources; all serve similar functions in the human body. Dietary fibers are divided into two categories based on their solubility in fluids. Soluble dietary fibers, which dissolve in fluids, include pectin, mucilage, psyllium seed husk, guar gum, and other related gums. Soluble fiber thickens substances. Insoluble dietary fibers do not dissolve in fluids and therefore provide structure and protection for plants. Some insoluble dietary fibers are cellulose and hemicellulose. Lignin, considered a dietary fiber, is composed of chains of alcohol rather than carbohydrate.

Foods are sometimes classified based on the predominant type of fiber they contain. Oatmeal is a good source of soluble fiber because oat bran, part of the whole oatmeal grain, is particularly high in soluble fiber. But the whole grain is a good source of insoluble fiber as well. Although Table 4-3 specifically lists foods containing soluble and insoluble dietary fiber, many fiber-rich foods contain some of each kind of fiber. For example, an apple is a source of the soluble dietary fiber pectin, which is part of the inside "stuff" of the apple. An apple also provides cellulose, an insoluble dietary fiber that forms the structure of the apple and gives it its characteristic shape (Figure 4-5). Popcorn is another source of insoluble dietary fiber that has been with us for a long time (see the *Cultural Considerations* box, The "Pop" Heard through the Centuries).

Health Effects

All the health benefits of fiber improve the physical functioning of the human body. The benefits are not directly nutri-

TABLE 4-3	DIETARY FIBERS AND FOOD SOURCES
FIBERS	**FOOD SOURCES**
Insoluble	
Cellulose	Whole grains, brown rice, buckwheat
Hemicellulose	groats, whole wheat flour, whole-wheat
Lignin	pasta, oatmeal, unrefined cereals,
	vegetables, wheat bran, seeds,
	popcorn, nuts, peanut butter, leafy
	green vegetables such as broccoli
Soluble	
Pectin	Kidney beans, split peas, lentils,
Mucilage	chickpeas (garbanzo beans), navy
Guar and other	beans, soybeans, apples, pears,
gums	bananas, grapes, citrus fruits (oranges
	and grapefruits), oat bran, oatmeal,
	barley, corn, carrots, white potatoes

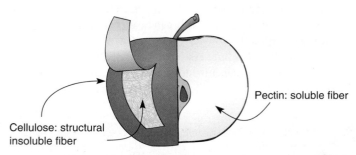

Pectin: soluble fiber

Cellulose: structural insoluble fiber

FIG 4-5 In an apple, insoluble fiber (cellulose) inside and in the skin provides structure, and soluble fiber (pectin) inside adds substance.

tional but instead allow the body to function at a more efficient level. Each of the following disorders listed may develop because of genetic predisposition, environmental factors, or lifestyle behaviors. However, the risk of developing these disorders seems to increase when consumption of dietary fiber is low. Because eating sufficient fiber appears to be a preventive factor, we consider the benefits of fiber on primary disease prevention. Primary prevention aims to avert the initial development of a disorder or health problem. The risk of developing obesity, constipation, hemorrhoids, diverticular disease, and colon cancer may be decreased by regularly consuming sufficient amounts of fiber.

Obesity. Eating high-fiber foods seems to make weight control easier. The volume of fibrous foods makes us feel fuller, so less food is consumed. Often, fibrous foods replace those that are higher in fat and kcal. Regularly eating foods high in fiber and low in fat may reduce or prevent obesity.

Constipation. Fiber, particularly insoluble fiber such as wheat bran and whole grains, prevents the dry, hard stools of constipation (see Chapter 3). A sufficient fiber intake plus adequate fluid intake ensures larger, softer stools that are

The "Pop" Heard through the Centuries

The next time you're at the movies digging into a giant tub of popcorn, be sure to appreciate one of the tastier contributions of Native Americans to our food supply: popping corn, first created over an open fire 5000 years ago. The delectable popcorn added variety to ways to prepare corn, a mainstay of the Native American diet. Gifts of popcorn necklaces and popcorn beer were made by the Indians of the Caribbean in the 1500s, and the Aztecs used popcorn in religious ceremonies. And what would Thanksgiving have been without some popped corn—compliments of the Wampanoag tribe?

Popcorn most likely originated in Mexico, but it was also grown in India, Sumatra, and China years before Columbus "discovered" America. Biblical stories of "corn" in Egypt were not entirely true. The term *corn* meant the most commonly used grain of a region. In Scotland and Ireland, corn referred to oats; in England, corn was wheat. In the Americas, the common corn was maize, and the two terms, *corn* and *maize*, became synonymous.

Today special varieties of corn have been developed for their "popping" characteristics. When heated, water in the corn kernel creates steam. This steam, unable to escape through the heavy skin of the kernel, causes an explosion that exposes the white starchy center. Fortunately, the skin remains attached to the starch, which makes popcorn an excellent source of dietary fiber.

Although all popcorn provides dietary fiber, some of the ways it is prepared negate this health benefit. Popcorn laden with butter and covered with salt is not a healthful snack. Nor is a batch popped with the aid of oil, even if vegetable oil is used. Microwaveable packets of popcorn are equally deceiving because they contain oil and other additives. We also may easily be misled into eating more than we should because each bag contains four servings, which most of us devour singlehandedly.

Instead, return to the native style—fresh air-popped corn. Air-popping appliances and microwave containers eliminate the need for oil. Better toppings include sodium-reduced salt, garlic powder, or Cajun spices. While devouring your wholesome snack, remember to acknowledge the inventiveness of Native Americans.

Data from Popcorn Institute: *Early popcorn history,* Chicago, 1996, Author; National Agricultural Library, Special Collections: *Popcorn: Ingrained in America's Agricultural History,* February 2002. Accessed October 1, 2009, from www.nal.usda.gov/speccoll/images1/popcorn.html.

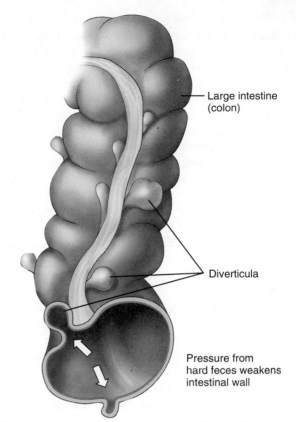

FIG 4-6 Diverticulosis in the colon. A low-fiber diet may increase the risk for this disorder.

easier to eliminate. Less straining during elimination also reduces the risk of developing hemorrhoids (enlarged veins in the anus) and diverticular disease.

Diverticular Disease. Diverticular disease is a disorder that primarily afflicts people in their 50s and 60s. Some 30% of Americans older than the age of 50 are estimated to have the disorder.[10] It begins, however, earlier in life because of a consistently low intake of dietary fiber.

Diverticular disease affects the large intestine. Pockets (diverticula) develop on the outside walls of the intestine, as shown in Figure 4-6. Low-fiber diets may create increased internal pressure from segmentation muscles attempting to move the food mass because the bulk of fiber is not available. This pressure may then weaken intestinal muscles. Weakened muscles are more at risk for the formation of diverticula. If feces get caught in the pockets, bacteria may develop, multiply, and cause serious and painful inflammation (diverticulitis). Medical treatment and nutritional therapy are necessary and are discussed in Chapter 17.

Colon Cancer. Eating enough dietary fiber may also reduce the risk of developing colon cancer. Two potential risk factors for colon cancer related to fiber intake are a high dietary fat intake and exposure to carcinogenic substances in the GI tract.[5] The higher our fat intake, the more at risk we are for colon cancer. By eating more fiber, we tend to eat less fat. Fiber foods tend to replace foods that are high in fat. Because foods containing fiber are bulkier, they seem to fill the stomach quicker, providing satiety sooner and with fewer kcal than foods containing fat. Fiber-containing foods such as fruits and vegetables may contain other substances that may be protective for the colon.

Consumption of sufficient fiber also speeds the movement of substances through the GI tract, potentially reducing exposure of the colon to carcinogens.[2,9] In particular, the longer feces sit in the large intestine or colon, the greater the chance for carcinogenic substances to form and affect the colon. A direct mechanism of dietary fiber occurs when dietary fiber absorbs potential carcinogens that then leave the body in feces. Wheat bran has been shown to provide this benefit.[11]

Ongoing laboratory research has led to speculation that the SCFAs (also called *volatile fatty acids*) produced by the fermentation of fiber in the colon may have a role in protecting colon cells from cancer and may inhibit cholesterol synthesis. These roles, although still being explored, may reveal further physiologic benefits of dietary fiber.[9]

Heart Disease. Two heart disease risk factors are high blood cholesterol and increased lipid levels (see Chapter 5 for recommended levels). Increasing dietary fiber consumption can lower blood cholesterol and lipid levels in two ways: (1) fiber foods replace higher-fat foods, particularly those containing dietary cholesterol and saturated fats; (2) soluble fiber such as pectin (citrus fruits and apples), guar gum (legumes), and oat gum (oat bran) binds lipids and cholesterol as they move through the intestinal tract.[12] Because fiber is not digested, neither are the bound lipids and cholesterol, which make less cholesterol and lipids available to the bloodstream.

Diabetes Control. Dietary fiber intake may help people with diabetes to stabilize blood glucose levels. Diabetes mellitus affects the body's ability to regulate blood glucose levels. When fiber is consumed, particularly soluble fiber, glucose may be absorbed more slowly. The slower absorption rate of glucose may keep blood glucose within acceptable levels.[12]

Consuming increased amounts of dietary fiber may seem to decrease the risk for developing certain diseases; however, reduced risk may not be caused by the increased dietary fiber but by other dietary changes. By eating more foods that contain fiber, we may reduce our intake of high-fat foods. It may be the lower fat intake that reduces the risk, not the higher dietary fiber intake.

When the recommended increase of dietary fiber intake is fulfilled by fiber-containing foods, there tend to be few health risks. Problems may develop when fiber supplements or other forms of processed or purified fiber, such as oat or wheat bran, are consumed in large quantities. When used as a supplement, excessive quantities of purified fiber can overwhelm the GI tract and lead to blockages in the small intestine and colon.[12] This is a serious medical condition that fortunately is rare.

Bioavailability of minerals may be lowered by the presence of fiber-containing foods. Some fibers and substances in whole grains, such as phytates and oxalates, may bind minerals, making them unable to be absorbed. However, higher fiber dietary patterns tend also to be higher in mineral content; therefore, absorption of minerals remains adequate.[12]

As fiber passes through the GI tract, it provides several health-promoting services that are still being analyzed. Some foods that contain fiber also contain an assortment of essential nutrients. That is why it is best to get fiber from real foods rather than from supplements.

Because some benefits do vary between soluble and insoluble fiber, should daily intakes of each kind of fiber be

---

✳ TEACHING TOOL

What's Your Fiber Score Today?

Although the following foods are particularly good sources of dietary fiber, many other foods—all fruits and vegetables—contain smaller amounts that add up by the day's end. Does your typical intake meet the recommended levels of about 20 to 38 g per day?

APPROXIMATELY 2 g PER SERVING

Apricot	Carrot	Pineapple
Banana	Cauliflower	Rye crackers
Blueberries	Grapefruit	Whole-wheat bread
Broccoli	Oatmeal	Whole-wheat cereals
Cantaloupe	Peach	

APPROXIMATELY 3 g PER SERVING

Apple with skin	Pear	Raisins
Corn	Peas	Shredded wheat cereal
Orange	Potato with skin	Strawberries

APPROXIMATELY 4 g OR MORE PER SERVING

Baked beans	Kidney beans	Navy beans
Bran cereals	Lentils	Whole-wheat spaghetti

Data from Pennington JAT, Douglass JS: *Bowes & Church's food values of portions commonly used*, ed 19, Philadelphia, 2009, Lippincott Williams & Wilkins.

---

calculated? Not at all. Increase total dietary fiber to recommended levels slowly by gradually substituting whole grain foods, fresh fruits, and vegetables for some lower-fiber foods (see the *Teaching Tool* box, What's Your Fiber Score Today?). This allows the body to adjust to the additional fiber, reducing the possible formation of intestinal gas.

Food Sources and Issues

Although dietary fiber is not absorbed and does not serve a nutrient function in the body, the effects of fiber are important for optimum health. An Adequate Intake (AI) of dietary fiber is about 20 to 38 g per day, depending on age and gender.[2,12] Most Americans consume much lower levels of fiber; adults often average only 14 to 15 g of fiber per day, whereas children and young adults average 12 g.[13] This is because of several factors. First, many Americans do not consume enough fruits and vegetables on a daily basis. Somehow, high protein and fat dietary intakes have pushed fruits and vegetables out of our meal patterns. Also, possibly the most significant factor is that many Americans regularly eat foods made with refined grains from which dietary fiber has been removed. Consumption of legumes and high-fiber cereal foods provides considerably more fiber.

Unrefined versus Refined Grains

Unrefined grains are prepared for consumption containing their original components. These grains are really seeds or kernels that include all the nutrients necessary to support plant growth and are segmented inside the kernel to be used

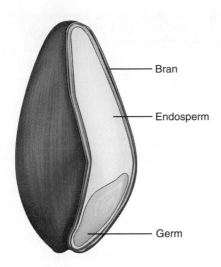

FIG 4-7 Inside a wheat kernel.

when needed. **Whole grain products** refer to food items made using all the edible portions of kernels.

In contrast, **refined grains** have been taken apart. Only portions of the edible kernel are included in refined grain products. Although both unrefined and refined grain products are good sources of complex carbohydrates, other nutritional qualities of the whole grain are lost when grains are refined. Grains most often refined are wheat, rice, oats, corn, and rye.

To better understand how the nutrients are lost, consider the wheat kernel shown in Figure 4-7. The kernel consists of three nutrient-containing components. The outer layer, bran, is an excellent source of cellulose dietary fiber and contains magnesium, riboflavin, niacin, thiamine, vitamin B_6, and some protein.

The germ found in the base of the kernel contains a wealth of nutrients to support the sprouting of the plant. Some of these include thiamine, riboflavin, vitamin B_6, vitamin E, zinc, protein, and wheat oil (polyunsaturated vegetable oil). The endosperm, the largest component of the kernel, contains starch, the prime energy source for the sprouting plant. It also contains protein and riboflavin but much smaller amounts of niacin, thiamine, and B_6.

When flour is refined, the bran and germ are removed; the bran affects the physical lightness of the flour, and the oil in the germ may become rancid, reducing the shelf life of the flour. Only the starchy endosperm is used to mill refined flour. Because flour is the mainstay of grain products, the loss of nutrients to the population is significant. In the 1940s it was determined that deficiencies of thiamine, riboflavin, niacin, and iron occurred because of the refining process. To counteract this loss, those four nutrients were added back to flour. Now, flour with these specific nutrient additives is called *enriched flour.*

Enrichment is the replacement of nutrients to the level that was present before processing. Although the four lost nutrients are replaced, other vitamins, minerals, and fiber originally in whole wheat are not. Zinc, magnesium, vitamin

E, and dietary fiber are not returned to the refined white flour. Consequently, any product made with enriched white flour is still nutritionally inferior to whole-wheat flour (see the *Health Debate* box, If Dietary Fiber Is So Important, Should Grain Products Be Allowed to Be Refined?).

HEALTH DEBATE

If Dietary Fiber Is So Important, Should Grain Products Be Allowed to Be Refined?

This chapter highlights the health benefits of eating the recommended levels of fiber. Also emphasized are nutrition losses that occur when fruits, vegetables, and grains are processed or refined. The process of refining can lead to the extensive loss of fiber and various nutrients. Although some nutrients are replaced, some, such as dietary fiber, are not.

If health benefits of dietary fiber and nutrients are so valuable, should there be government regulations to restrict or prohibit the removal of valuable nutrients and dietary fiber? Several of the diseases associated with low-fiber intake are chronic diseases. Treating these long-term diseases places a burden on the entire U.S. health care system.

Is it fair for all of us to bear the financial burden for those not consuming the most healthful form of foods available? Should there be a law against the processing of whole grains? Should white flour production be restricted? Or is the availability of white (or wheat) and whole wheat products sufficient? Is it our "freedom of choice" to be able to select among different food products although some are more beneficial to health than others?

What do you think?

The preference for refined complex carbohydrates may be changing. The health benefits of dietary fiber have been so newsworthy and the focus of such intensive advertising that consumer perception of fiber has evolved from a negative selling point to a positive one. Twenty years ago, if products claimed to be high in fiber or made from whole grains, sales would decline. Today, high-fiber food items are among the better sellers in categories such as cereals and breads (see the *Cultural Considerations* box, Cereals around the World).

OVERCOMING BARRIERS

As we eat throughout the day, our bodies respond to the available glucose and easily adjust to provide glucose during the hours between food intakes. For some of us, however, these regulating mechanisms malfunction. When this happens, the effect of food consumption on blood glucose levels needs to be considered to avoid sudden rises and falls in blood glucose levels. The two conditions most related to carbohydrate metabolism are hypoglycemia and diabetes mellitus. These conditions are introduced here; nutritional therapy for diabetes mellitus is detailed in Chapter 19.

🌐 CULTURAL CONSIDERATIONS
Cereals around the World

Hot cereals have been the mainstay of carbohydrate break-fast calories among cultures in colder climates. The old adage of "stick to the ribs" foods refers to the warming and filling effects of freshly cooked cereals such as oatmeal, cream of wheat, and oat bran. Just as the Inuit have many words for snow to reflect its many variations in a climate often characterized by snow, Norway, another cold country, has many kinds of porridge or hot cereal. In Norway, porridges may include oats, wheat, barley, rye, and rice. It is often eaten as a winter dinner and can be served cold as dessert pudding topped with fruit sauce. Porridge also has social significance. Extra-creamy porridge is served to women who just gave birth as a way to boost their nutrition. A lucky individual may refer to good luck as being "in the middle of a butter island," meaning the kind of melting butter found in a bowl of steaming porridge.

Consider your own cultural background. Is there a grain or carbohydrate food that has special significance to your family because of its ethnic or regional influence?

Data from The Norwegian Table: *Some like it hot,* Norway, 2001, fromnorway.net. Accessed October 1, 2009, www.fromnorway.net/norwegian_food/199910/foodcultureone.htm.

Hypoglycemia

Hypoglycemia, or low blood glucose level, is a symptom of an underlying disorder; it is not a disease. We may all experience hypoglycemia when we haven't eaten for a few hours and begin to feel hungry. If we don't eat, our bodies switch to an alternative source of energy. This causes the release of epinephrine and glucagon, which act to make the liver glycogen release glucose to be available for energy. For some individuals, the transition to this energy source or the experience of hypoglycemia may be uncomfortable, causing rapid heartbeat, sweating, weakness, anxiety, and hunger.

If these symptoms occur regularly, even when an individual eats well, a primary health care provider should be consulted. The underlying cause of hypoglycemia needs to be determined. Some health problems for which hypoglycemia may be a symptom are overproduction of insulin by the pancreas, which excessively lowers blood glucose levels, and intestinal malabsorption of glucose or insufficient glucose storage (glycogen) in the liver.

Other disorders may have symptoms similar to hypoglycemia. A tumor on the adrenal gland may cause excessive amounts of epinephrine to be released, or a circulatory problem may affect blood flow to the brain, thus causing the confusion, headaches, and other symptoms often associated with hypoglycemia.[5]

Symptoms similar to chronic hypoglycemia may also occur when patterns of food intake are erratic or when we simply don't eat enough. True hypoglycemia is rare.[5] If hypoglycemia is suspected, dietary intake patterns are analyzed. Is the day's food intake full of concentrated sweets and sodas? This would cause an excessive release of insulin that could then lead to a low blood glucose response. That is not true hypoglycemia. Instead, a mix of carbohydrate and protein foods should be eaten throughout the day and hypoglycemic symptoms will probably decrease. However, if the best efforts at diet control do not eliminate hypoglycemic episodes, medical advice should be sought.

Diabetes Mellitus

Whereas hypoglycemia involves low blood sugar, diabetes is concerned with very high blood glucose levels, or hyperglycemia. Diabetes mellitus is a disorder of carbohydrate metabolism characterized by hyperglycemia caused by insulin that is either ineffective or deficient. The impact of diabetes is that the energy supply of glucose keeps circulating in the bloodstream; it is not available in sufficient quantities to support the energy needs of the cells. There are several types of diabetes: type 1, type 2, and gestational.

Type 1 Diabetes Mellitus

In type 1 diabetes mellitus (DM), the pancreas produces insufficient amounts of insulin. Insulin must be provided through daily insulin injections to control blood glucose levels. Type 1 DM tends to occur early in life, caused by viral or autoimmune destruction of the area of the pancreas responsible for insulin production; genetic factors may also be associated with type 1 DM. This disorder is not risk related. We cannot prevent or develop type 1 DM by our dietary intake or lifestyle behaviors. When the disorder occurs, lifelong treatment depends on dietary intake that balances food intake with insulin injection and on lifestyle behaviors to reduce the complications of type 1 DM. Individuals with type 1 DM are at more risk for heart disease, kidney disorders, and retinal damage.

Type 2 Diabetes Mellitus

In type 2 diabetes mellitus (DM), the pancreas produces some insulin, but it is ineffective and unable to meet the body's needs. Risk is related to genetic, environmental, and lifestyle factors. The risk of developing type 2 DM increases with family history, age, weight, and caloric intake. Type 2 DM is associated with advancing age, being overweight and consuming excess kcal. If family members have type 2 DM, relatives can adopt preventive lifestyle behaviors as young adults, reducing the risk of developing this disorder later in life. Preventive lifestyle behaviors include exercising regularly and eating a moderate kcal, high-fiber, low-fat diet to avoid weight gain, as we grow older. Both of these behaviors also work to treat type 2 DM as well.

As a nation we are becoming more concerned as the prevalence of type 2 DM is increasing rapidly—even among children and young adults. Health professionals are recognizing prediabetic disorders, and efforts to begin prevention earlier are becoming public health goals. A panel of experts from the American Diabetes Association and the U.S. Department of Health and Human Services recommends screening adults younger than 45 if they are seriously overweight and have one or more of the following risk factors:

- Family history of diabetes
- Low high-density lipoprotein (HDL) cholesterol and high triglycerides
- High blood pressure
- History of gestational diabetes or gave birth to an infant that weighed more than 9 pounds
- Minority group heritage (e.g., African Americans, Native Americans, Hispanic Americans, and Asian/Pacific Islanders are at increased risk for type 2 diabetes)[14]

Gestational Diabetes Mellitus

Gestational diabetes mellitus (GDM) may occur during pregnancy when blood glucose levels remain abnormally high. This form of diabetes may affect the health and development of the fetus as well as the health of the mother. Although it seems as if the pregnancy triggers the diabetic response in some women, studies show that women who develop gestational diabetes tend to develop type 2 DM later in life. Many exhibit several of the risk factors of type 2 DM before pregnancy and thus are predisposed to develop diabetes.[15] To limit the negative effects of GDM that, if not controlled, can lead to pregnancy-induced hypertension, premature birth, large fetus size, congenital abnormalities, future obesity, and diabetes in the infant, as well as other birth complications, routine screening for diabetes must be part of quality prenatal care.

Dietary modifications are an important part of controlling diabetes. This is accomplished through individually developed dietary prescriptions based on metabolic nutrition and lifestyle requirements. Basic changes include reduced intake of simple sugars such as white table sugar and syrups. These are replaced by more complex carbohydrates and a balanced intake of nutrients, particularly carbohydrates, throughout the day. To make implementation of the treatment plan easier, registered dietitians (RD) use the *Exchange Lists for Meal Planning* to assist clients with diabetes with meal

PERSONAL PERSPECTIVES

"Eat Food, Not Too Much, Mostly Plants"

"Eat food. Not too much. Mostly plants," is the succinct nutrition/food consumption advice of author Michael Pollan for eating wisely. These seven words sum up his many years of extensive journalistic research about "What should I eat?" His results are in two of his bestsellers: *The Omnivore's Dilemma* and *In Defense of Food: An Eater's Manifesto*. Mark Bittman, a journalist, a researcher, and a food lover also influences attitudes towards what to eat and how to prepare foods through his numerous bestselling cookbooks and writings. His most recent book, *Food Matters: A Guide to Conscious Eating*, provides doable strategies for consuming "more plants, fewer animals, and as little highly processed food as possible." Here are simple suggestions based on his writings that pertain to ecologically, mindful, healthful, and satisfying consumption of carbohydrates and plants.

Eat fewer animal-derived foods. Eat more plant foods.
Why: Production of animal-derived foods substantially affects the global environment, particularly climate change. For example, livestock production releases greenhouse gases into the atmosphere. The amount created accounts for 20% of all greenhouse gases produced. Animal-derived foods tend to be energy intensive. More energy is used to create these foods from animals than their actual food energy value. And finally, animal-derived foods tend to provide more saturated fats, dietary cholesterol, and energy than plant-based foods; these are potential risk factors for diet-related chronic disorders.

How: If less meat is eaten, more plant food easily takes its place. Smaller portion sizes are a good way to start. Rather than filling half the dinner plate with meat (beef, pork, chicken, fish, cheese, or eggs), restructure proportions to one part (a quarter of the plate) meat; two parts vegetables (half of the plate); and one part grains (quarter of the plate). Legumes (such as chickpeas, kidney beans, and black beans) can be added replacing some or all of the meat or added to the vegetables or grains.

Eat real food.
Why: Real food is closest to the form found in nature. Foodstuff may be cleaned of outer inedible parts, eaten raw or cooked, eaten alone or with other ingredients. But the plant or animal source is whole, not taken apart and put back together again with some parts containing nutrients removed (and not returned).

Avoid heavily processed foods. Why? The energy cost to create and package processed foods is substantial. Nutrients are lost during manufacturing. Often, these nutrients are not returned to the product. Preservatives are added to maintain "freshness" so products can have a long shelf life allowing processed foods to be shipped worldwide. The energy used for transportation adds to the actual cost of processed foods. Real food products, though, should not last forever!

How: We lost the connection between the means of producing our food and our level of health. Just because a food product exists, it does not mean that it is worth consuming or is sufficiently valuable to expend our planet's limited energy and resources for its production.

We can take responsibility for our food intake. Michael Pollan, as described in *The Omnivore's Dilemma*, set out to procure all the ingredients for a meal including participating in a hunt for a wild pig that he then helped eviscerate and cook as well as foraging for wild mushrooms in secretive forest areas in California. His intent was to realize the effect of his consumption on the earth in a very concrete manner.

While we don't need to repeat his experience, we can take action by learning how to cook simple meals from scratch. Return to our kitchens (and to simple cookbooks or Internet recipes) and begin planning and preparing real food. Bittman's advice is that with a little planning, we can alter our lifestyles to nourish our bodies while reducing our impact on the environment.

From: Bittman M: *Food Matters: A Guide to Conscious Eating*, New York, 2009, Simon & Schuster; Pollan M: *The Omnivore's Dilemma: A Natural History of Four Meals*, New York, 2007, Penguin Group (USA) Inc.; Pollan M: *In Defense of Food: An Eater's Manifesto*, New York, 2008, Penguin Group (USA) Inc.

planning. The *Exchange Lists* (see Appendix A) was first developed for diabetic meal planning but has become a basic tool for almost all food guides and dietary recommendations. Another system to control diabetes, carbohydrate counting, recently has been introduced. This system allows the client to keep track of carbohydrate intake during the course of the day. Chapter 19 provides more details on this approach. Overall management of GDM takes into account the physical, psychosocial, and educational requirements. Whereas an RD has primary responsibility for developing and teaching the individualized dietary prescriptions, nurses reinforce these dietary modifications and teach the skills of blood glucose monitoring, insulin therapy, and exercise. Health professionals can develop a supportive relationship with clients by consideration of cultural orientation and learning styles.

TOWARD A POSITIVE NUTRITION LIFESTYLE: TAILORING

Consider what a tailor does. A tailor takes a bolt of cloth and by cutting, shaping, and sewing, fits a garment to a person's exact measurements. Tailoring as a behavior-change technique takes a health recommendation and by "cutting," "shaping," and "sewing," fits the recommendation to the limitations or requirements of our individual lifestyles.

Strong recommendations to increase our fiber intake are made in this chapter. Ideally, fiber intake should be about 20 to 38 g a day. The most efficient means of intake would be to replace all refined grain products with whole grain products. But is that possible considering contemporary lifestyles? Often we are not able to control available food choices, and thus we have difficulty changing our behavior to implement this type of recommendation. By tailoring the recommendation or goal to our individual lifestyles, we can succeed. Following are some recommendations for "tailoring" in practice:

- Overwhelmed by the thought of eating only whole grain foods? Decide to eat more whole grain products for breakfast and dinner, which are eaten at home when control is easier.
- No time to cook vegetables? Prepare or order salads and keep fresh fruits of any kind handy.
- Needing to add fiber to your diet? When possible, choose fiber-rich foods for lunch. Be realistic, however, because foods available at the cafeteria or coffee shop are limited.
- Attending a family holiday dinner or special event or going on vacation? Enjoy what's served. Then resume a regular fiber-rich dietary pattern when back at work or school.

Although the goal is to increase fiber intake, the objective is to fit positive dietary choices and habits to the shape of our nutrition lifestyles.

■ SUMMARY

Carbohydrates are composed of carbon, hydrogen, and oxygen. There are three sizes of carbohydrates: monosaccharides (glucose, fructose, and galactose), disaccharides (sucrose, maltose, and lactose), and polysaccharides (starch and dietary fiber). These three sizes are divided into the two categories of simple carbohydrates (monosaccharides and disaccharides) and complex carbohydrates (polysaccharides).

Primarily found in plant foods, carbohydrates are an abundant food source of energy and dietary fiber. Glucose is the carbohydrate form through which energy circulates in the bloodstream. Blood glucose levels are naturally regulated through hormonal systems that aim to keep the body in balance. Hypoglycemia and diabetes mellitus may occur when these systems cannot regulate glucose within normal levels. In contrast to glucose, dietary fiber does not provide energy. Although dietary fiber is a carbohydrate, it is not digestible by humans. The health benefits of consuming sufficient quantities of dietary fiber, however, are significant.

The best food energy sources of carbohydrates are grains, legumes, and starchy root vegetables. Dietary fiber is available in many foods such as fruits, vegetables, and whole grain products. Dietary fiber and other nutrients are often lost when foods, particularly grains, are processed.

The most recent dietary guidelines recommend the increased consumption of complex carbohydrates. MyPyramid suggests 6 ounces of grains (with at least 3 ounces whole grain) and $4\frac{1}{2}$ cups of fruits and vegetables. The intent is to reduce our fat intake by increasing intake of starch and dietary fiber. By following these guidelines, our risk of developing diet-related diseases will be decreased.

THE NURSING APPROACH

Case Study: Fiber (Constipation)

Mary, age 62, is in the nurse practitioner's (NP) office for a routine annual physical examination. When collecting the health history, the NP finds that Mary frequently has had abdominal discomfort and constipation. The health record indicates a medical diagnosis of diverticulosis. The NP interviews Mary and does an abdominal examination.

ASSESSMENT
Subjective (from Patient Statements)

- Small, hard, pebble-like stools, usually two times a day
- Uncomfortable straining with bowel movements
- Bloating and gas, especially after drinking milk
- Usually avoids milk, drinks four to six glasses of water per day

THE NURSING APPROACH—cont'd

Case Study: Fiber (Constipation)—cont'd

- Prefers white bread, usually skips breakfast because she doesn't want milk with cereal
- Eats few fruits and vegetables and peels those she does eat
- Has no regular exercise

Objective (from Physical Examination)

- Abdomen distended, nontender
- Bowel sounds hypoactive

DIAGNOSIS (NURSING)

Constipation related to low fiber and fluid intake, lactose intolerance, and no regular exercise as evidenced by hypoactive bowel sounds and patient statements about small, hard stools and uncomfortable straining with bowel movements

PLANNING

Patient Outcomes

Short term (at the end of this visit):

- Mary will identify foods high in fiber and develop plans to gradually include them in her diet.
- Mary will verbalize intention to drink at least eight glasses of water and walk at least 15 minutes per day.

Long term (at the follow-up visit in 1 month):

- Mary will report she was able to follow her plan.
- Mary will report regular soft bowel movements with no discomfort or straining.

Nursing Interventions

- Teach Mary about the causes of constipation and diverticulosis.
- Teach Mary about lifestyle changes that will prevent constipation.

IMPLEMENTATION (Also see Chapter 17.)

1. Explained causes of constipation and how constipation can lead to diverticulosis and diverticulitis.

   Common causes of constipation are insufficient fiber, fluids, and activity. Strained defecation increases intracolonic pressure and can weaken the muscles in the bowel, allowing outpouching of the intestinal wall (diverticulosis). If fecal matter gets caught in the diverticula, infection can result (diverticulitis). For diverticulosis, a high-fiber diet is prescribed. For diverticulitis, the patient may receive nothing by mouth temporarily or receive only low-fiber foods and fluids, in order to allow healing of the irritated bowel.

2. Encouraged Mary to add fiber gradually until she is eating at least six servings of whole grain breads and cereals and legumes and five servings of fruits and vegetables per day.

   Fiber adds bulk to stools and stimulates peristalsis. Fiber increased too quickly can lead to bloating, gas, cramps, abdominal discomfort, and diarrhea. Generally, one high-fiber food can be added every 2 weeks, until the client is eating 25 to 38 g of fiber per day.

3. Provided written information on types and sources of fiber and explored food likes and preferences to determine high-fiber foods acceptable to Mary.

   Substituting high-fiber foods for low-fiber foods can prevent constipation, but the diet needs to be individualized. Examples of high-fiber foods are whole-wheat bread, bran cereal, kidney beans, prunes and other fruits with peelings, and broccoli.

4. Encouraged Mary to drink 8 to 12 glasses of fluid per day, especially water and fruit juices.

   Fluid softens stools and increases bulk, promoting peristalsis. As fiber is increased, fluids must be increased to prevent further constipation, intestinal blockage, and abdominal pain.

5. Discussed possible substitutions for milk.

   With lactose intolerance, residual undigested lactose draws water into the bowel by osmosis. If excessive, this can cause abdominal pain, flatulence, and diarrhea. Cheese and yogurt may be tolerated more easily than milk when a person has lactose intolerance. Lactase can be added to milk, or soy milk can be substituted for cow's milk.

6. Encouraged Mary to exercise regularly—for example, walking for at least 15 minutes five times a week.

   Activity promotes peristalsis.

EVALUATION

Short term (at the end of the visit):

Mary wrote down specific goals for lifestyle changes to correct constipation.

- Changes to make right away:
  - Substitute whole-wheat bread for white bread.
  - Eat three fruits per day.
  - Drink eight glasses of water per day.
  - Walk for 15 minutes three times a week.
- Changes to make gradually, starting in 2 weeks:
  - Replace one low-fiber food with one new high-fiber food every 2 weeks.
  - Try drinking calcium-fortified soy milk.
  - Increase walking to 20 minutes five times a week.
- Changes not willing to make: drinking prune juice

Short-term outcomes achieved.

Mary set up an appointment for follow-up in 1 month.

DISCUSSION QUESTIONS

At her follow-up appointment, Mary said her stools had been softer, better formed, and more comfortable to eliminate. She said she had eaten whole-wheat bread three days per week, had eaten three fruits per day, had drunk about five glasses of water per day, and had walked for 15 minutes twice a week. Last week she began eating raisin bran cereal four days per week.

1. How would you judge Mary's goal achievement—met, partially met, or not met at all? What was the basis for your answer?
2. If you were the nurse, what would you say to Mary about her report? What questions would you ask?
4. What other high-fiber foods could you recommend?

Nursing Diagnoses-Definitions and Classification 2009-2011. Copyright © 2009, 1994-2009 by NANDA International. Used by arrangement with Blackwell Publishing Limited, a company of John Wiley & Sons, Inc.

❓ APPLYING CONTENT KNOWLEDGE

You are at a restaurant having lunch with friends. After a friend hears you order a sandwich on whole-wheat bread, the friend comments, "Whole-wheat bread, white bread, what's the big deal? They're all complex carbohydrates." How would you respond?

■ WEBSITES OF INTEREST

American Diabetes Association

www.diabetes.org

Presents health professionals and the public with diabetes Internet resources, research updates as well as volunteer opportunities.

Wheat Foods Council

www.wheatfoods.org

Provides nutrition and food preparation resources for incorporating more grains into the American diet.

USA Rice Federation

www.usarice.com

Offers information about rice production and preparation, research, and environmental issues.

REFERENCES

1. Dolan JP, Adams-Smith WN: *Health and society: A documentary history of medicine*, New York, 1978, The Seabury Press.
2. Otten JJ, et al, editors, Institute of Medicine of the National Academies: *Dietary (DRI) reference intakes: The essential guide to nutrient requirements*, Washington, DC, 2006, National Academies Press.
3. U.S. Department of Agriculture, U.S. Department of Health and Human Services: *Report of the Dietary Guidelines Advisory Committee on the Dietary Guidelines for Americans, 2010*, Washington, DC, 2010, Author. Accessed June 16, 2010, from www.dietaryguidelines.gov.
4. Gallagher ML: The nutrients and their metabolism. In Mahan K, Escott-Stump S, editors: *Krause's food & nutrition therapy*, ed 12, St. Louis, 2008, Saunders/Elsevier.
5. Keim NL et al: Carbohydrates. In Shils ME, et al, editors: *Modern nutrition in health and disease*, ed 10, Philadelphia, 2006, Lippincott Williams & Wilkins.
6. American Dietetic Association: Position of the American Dietetic Association: Use of nutritive and nonnutritive sweeteners, *J Am Diet Assoc* 104:255-275, 2004.
7. U.S. Food and Drug Administration: *Code of federal regulations: Food and drugs*, Parts 10 to 199, Washington, DC, 1996 (April 1), The Office of the Federal Register.
8. Blackburn G et al: The effect of aspartame as part of a multidisciplinary weight-control program on short- and long-term control of body weight, *Am J Clin Nutr* 65:409-418, 1997.
9. Klein S, Cohn SM, Alpers DH: The alimentary tract in nutrition. In Shils ME, et al, editors: *Modern nutrition in health and disease*, ed 10, Philadelphia, 2006, Lippincott Williams & Wilkins.
10. Simmang CL, Shires FT: Diverticular disease of the colon. In Feldman M, Sleisenger MH, Scharschmidt BF, editors: *Gastrointestinal and liver disease*, ed 6, Philadelphia, 1998, Saunders.
11. Willett WD, Giovannucci E: Epidemiology of diet and cancer risk. In Shils ME, et al, editors: *Modern nutrition in health and disease*, ed 10, Philadelphia, 2006, Lippincott Williams & Wilkins.
12. American Dietetic Association: Position of the American Dietetic Association: Health implications of dietary fiber, *J Am Diet Assoc* 108:1716-1731, 2008.
13. Lupton JR, Trumbo PR: Dietary fiber. In Shils ME, et al, editors: *Modern nutrition in health and disease*, ed 10, Philadelphia, 2006, Lippincott Williams & Wilkins.
14. National Diabetes Information Clearinghouse, National Institute of Diabetes and Digestive and Kidney Diseases (NIDDK): *Pre-diabetes What you need to know* NIH Publication No. 08–6236 November 2007. Accessed October 2009 from http://diabetes.niddk.nih.gov/dm/pubs/prediabetes_ES/index.htm#3.
15. Metzger BE: Long-term outcomes in mothers diagnosed with gestational diabetes mellitus and their offspring, *Clin Obstet Gynecol* 50(4):972-979, 2007.

The term fats *actually refers to the chemical group called lipids. Lipids are divided into three classifications: fats (or triglycerides) and the fat-related substances of phospholipids and sterols.*

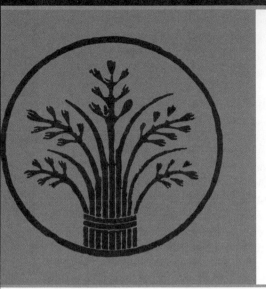

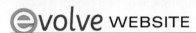

http://evolve.elsevier.com/Grodner/foundations/

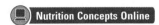 Nutrition Concepts Online

ROLE IN WELLNESS

It may be time for a truce about the consumption of dietary fat. Since the 1970s consumption of fats gained a negative reputation as a possible source of diet-related disorders and a factor in the increasing waistlines of Americans. We are now recognizing that the types and amount of fats being consumed determine the impact on our bodies. Some dietary fats are essential, while others are not. Some actually confer additional benefits for health, and a few, when eaten in large amounts, may increase the risk of certain diseases. This chapter explores these issues.

Fat is valuable and necessary to health. It is important to learn about fat in food, what the fat we eat does in our bodies, and how it can be both helpful and harmful to our health. Individual preference for fat is developed either in infancy or early childhood; innate preferences for sweet taste are observed at birth.[1] Thus children learn to prefer tastes, flavors, and textures that are associated with foods that are rich in fat, sweet, or both. Aging may be associated with increasing acceptance of bitter tastes and consumption of more fruits, vegetables, and whole grains.[1] Nonetheless, decreasing fat consumption takes time and effort, perhaps because of food selection habits, symbolic meaning associated with certain foods, and sensory values of fats in foods.

The five dimensions of health provide ways to think about the effects of changing dietary fat consumption. *Physical health* is maintained by consuming dietary fats that are necessary for essential fatty acids, for energy, and for fat-soluble vitamins. Excessive intake of fats, though, may increase the risk of obesity and diet-related diseases. The *intellectual health* dimension encompasses the skills necessary to assess the type of dietary fat modification most appropriate for our clients' and our own health needs. How we emotionally approach nutritional lifestyle changes for our clients and ourselves

affects success, which reflects the *emotional health* dimension. Can these emotions be expressed, or are changes simply disregarded because they make us feel uncomfortable? The *social dimension* is tested as change is initiated. Are relationships of family and friends based on sharing high-fat meals? Can you or your clients refuse to take part in social situations without jeopardizing relationships or making others feel defensive? Can food preparation suggestions to lower the fat content be made without seeming overly critical? Some religions maintain that taking care of one's body is necessary to achieve spiritual goals. Adopting a healthier fat intake supports these *spiritual health* dimension goals.

Fat actually refers to the chemical group called *lipids.* Lipids are divided into three classifications: fats (or triglycerides), and the fat-related substances of phospholipids and sterols. Triglycerides are the largest class of lipids and may be in the form of fats (somewhat solid) or oils (liquids). Approximately 95% of the lipids in foods and in our bodies are in the triglyceride form of fat. The other two lipid classifications are the fat-related substances of phospholipids and sterols. Lecithin is the best-known phospholipid; cholesterol is the best-known sterol. All are organic—composed of carbon, hydrogen, and oxygen—and cannot dissolve in water.

FUNCTIONS

The functions of lipids may be divided into two categories: (1) specific characteristics of foods caused by lipids and (2) maintenance of the physiologic health of our bodies.

Food Functions
Source of Energy

Fat is the densest form of stored energy in food and our bodies. This means that gram for gram, food fat—in the form of triglycerides—can produce more than twice the energy in kcal as carbohydrate or protein. For example, a gram of nearly pure fat (9 kcal), such as butter, provides more than twice the kcal as a gram of nearly pure carbohydrate (4 kcal), such as sugar, or a gram of nearly pure protein (4 kcal) such as dried, lean fish.

Palatability

Fat makes food smell and taste good. Deep-fat fried potatoes outrank all other vegetable choices among North Americans. Whether it's bread with butter (or margarine), salad with dressing, or desserts with cream, fat makes these foods taste pleasant for many people. For patients who are anorectic because of illness, strategically adding small amounts of fats to meals may increase their nutrient intake.

Satiety and Satiation

Fat helps prevent hunger between meals. Fat slows down digestion because of the hormones released in response to its presence in the gastrointestinal (GI) tract, causing us to feel full and satisfied; we call this feeling *satiety*. *Satiation* is another, different aspect of fat consumption that occurs during, not after, eating. In contrast to satiety, satiation tends to increase our desire to eat additional fatty foods, not less. The effect of fat on satiation is likely to be more important than its effect on satiety and may lead to overeating.[2] A situation that often occurs with the last slice of pizza provides a good example: You want it, you eat it, and half an hour later, you feel too full.

Food Processing

Certain qualities of lipids, besides their nutritional purposes, make them a valuable resource for the processing of foods. The use of processed hydrogenated fats helps keep the fat in food products from turning rancid. Lecithin, a phospholipid, has an extensive role as an emulsifier. An emulsifier is a substance that works by being soluble in water and fat at the same time. These functions, which will be described in more detail, also increase our overall intake of lipids by allowing their use in numerous processed foods.

Nutrient Source

Some fats contain or transport the fat-soluble nutrients of vitamins A, D, E, and K and the essential fatty acids of linoleic and linolenic fatty acids.

These essential fatty acids (EFAs), components of fat triglycerides, are polyunsaturated fatty acids that cannot be made in the body and must be consumed in the diet. EFAs are necessary materials for making compounds, such as prostaglandins, that regulate many body functions, including blood pressure, blood clotting through platelet aggregation, gastric acid secretions, and muscle secretions. The overall strength of cell membranes depends on EFAs.

Overt deficiency symptoms of EFAs include skin lesions and scaliness (eczema) caused by increased permeability, which leads to membrane breakdown throughout the body (Figure 5-1). Inflammation of epithelial tissue and increased susceptibility to infections throughout the body are also possible. Because the minimum amount of EFA required is contained in only about 2 teaspoons of polyunsaturated vegetable oil, deficiencies of EFAs were thought to be rare. However, deficiencies have been noted in (1) older patients with peripheral vascular disease (a potential complication of diabetes mellitus); (2) patients with fat malabsorption, such as cystic fibrosis; and (3) patients receiving treatment for protein malnutrition with low-fat, high-protein diets. Individuals recovering from serious accidents and burns are also at risk.[3] It is possible that individuals who strive to achieve extremely low dietary fat intake for health reasons or from disordered eating could develop EFA deficiencies.

Physiologic Functions
Stored Energy

Body fat cells contain nearly pure fat, also in the form of triglycerides. This means a pound of adipose tissue, the storage depot of body fat, could produce about 3500 kcal as energy. Because glucose stored in our bodies as glycogen is stored with water, carbohydrate is a bulkier form of stored energy than body fat. Adipose tissue provides important fuel

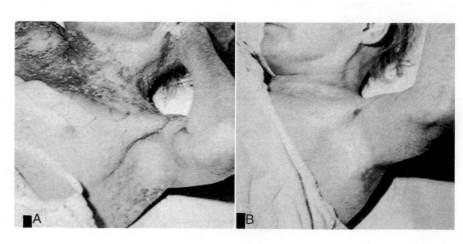

FIG 5-1 A, Essential fatty acid deficiency. **A,** A patient receiving fat-free parenteral nutrition has developed biochemical abnormalities and skin lesions as shown here. **B,** Resolution in same patient after 2 weeks of treatment. (Courtesy Dr. M.C. Riella. From McLaren DS: *A colour atlas and text of diet-related disorders*, ed 2, London, 1992, Mosby.)

during illness or times of food restriction and is a major energy source for muscle work.

Organ Protection

Stored fat safely cushions and protects body organs during bumpy activities, such as participating in impact aerobics or snowboarding.

Temperature Regulation

The fat layer just under our skin serves as insulation to regulate body temperature by minimizing the loss of heat.

Insulation

A substance composed largely of fatty tissue, called *myelin*, covers nerve cells. This covering provides electrical insulation that allows for transmission of nerve impulses.

Functions of Phospholipids and Sterols

So far, we have discussed the major roles of triglycerides. Phospholipids are also important as a part of all cell membrane structure and serve as emulsifiers to keep fats dispersed in body fluids.

Lecithins are the main phospholipids. Lecithin is a constituent of lipoproteins—carriers or transporters of lipids—including fats and cholesterol in the body. This characteristic has earned lecithin a reputation for carrying fat and cholesterol away from plaque deposits in the arteries. Although lecithin does play a role in transporting fat and cholesterol, supplementary lecithin from sources outside the body does not help make the body's transportation system more efficient. Instead, dietary lecithin is simply digested and used by the body as any other lipid.

As a lipid group, sterols are critical components of complex regulatory compounds in our bodies and provide basic material to make bile, vitamin D, sex hormones, and cells in brain and nerve tissue. Cholesterol in particular is a vital part of all cell membranes and nerve tissues and serves as a building block for hormones. When exposed to ultraviolet light, a cholesterol substance in our skin can be converted to vitamin D by the kidneys and liver. The liver synthesizes cholesterol to make bile, the emulsifying substance necessary to absorb dietary lipids.

STRUCTURE AND SOURCES OF LIPIDS

Fats: Saturated and Unsaturated

Triglyceride is the largest class of lipids found in food and body fat. **Triglycerides** are compounds consisting of three fatty acids and one glycerol molecule (Figure 5-2). The glycerol portion is derived from carbohydrate, but it is a small part compared with the fatty acids that may be alike or different from each other. Fatty acids can be made of long or short chains of carbon atoms. Each carbon atom has four bonding sites or imaginary arms where it can attach to other atoms. To form a carbon chain, one site on each side of the carbon bonds to a neighboring carbon, as if one arm on each side were outstretched to form a chain. Because these atoms

Three fatty acids join to glycerol in a condensation reaction to form a triglyceride.

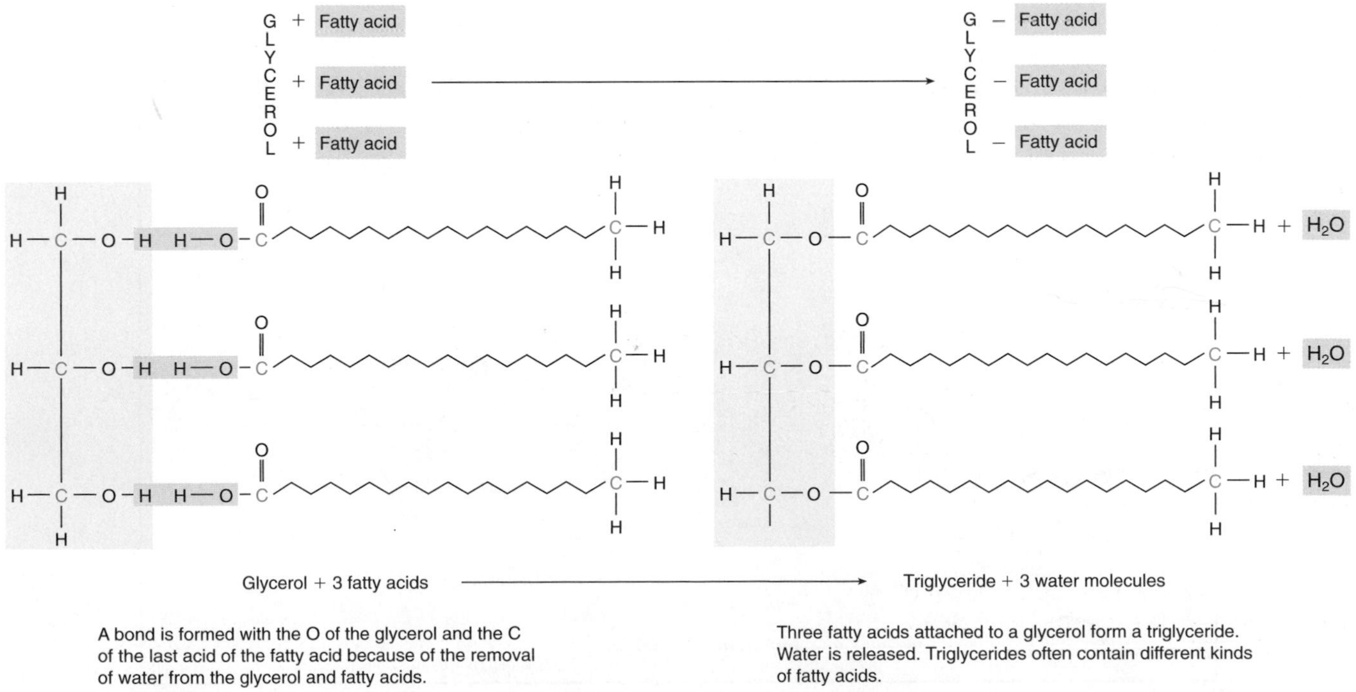

Glycerol + 3 fatty acids ⟶ Triglyceride + 3 water molecules

A bond is formed with the O of the glycerol and the C of the last acid of the fatty acid because of the removal of water from the glycerol and fatty acids.

Three fatty acids attached to a glycerol form a triglyceride. Water is released. Triglycerides often contain different kinds of fatty acids.

FIG 5-2 Formation and structure of a triglyceride.

have four arms, the two extra arms each attach to a hydrogen atom, which makes the chain saturated with hydrogen.

If a hydrogen atom is removed from two neighbor carbons, freeing the extra arm on each, the carbons are bonded to each other at two sites. The two arms on the same side both clasp the two arms of the neighboring carbon, forming a double bond. We call this an *unsaturated carbon chain* because there is a possibility that hydrogen could come along and saturate the chain by breaking one set of clasped arms and attaching to them. In foods, this is sometimes done artificially through the process of hydrogenation, which forces hydrogen atoms to break a double bond and attach to the carbons, creating a saturated fat (Figure 5-3). Hydrogenation is discussed in the section on processed fats.

All natural fats are mixtures of different types of fatty acids. Plants contain mostly polyunsaturated fats, but most plant oils contain some saturated fatty acids (Figure 5-4). Animal fats, though high in saturated fats, contain amounts of polyunsaturated fats. The predominant type of fat in a food determines its category.

FIG 5-3 Process of hydrogenation.

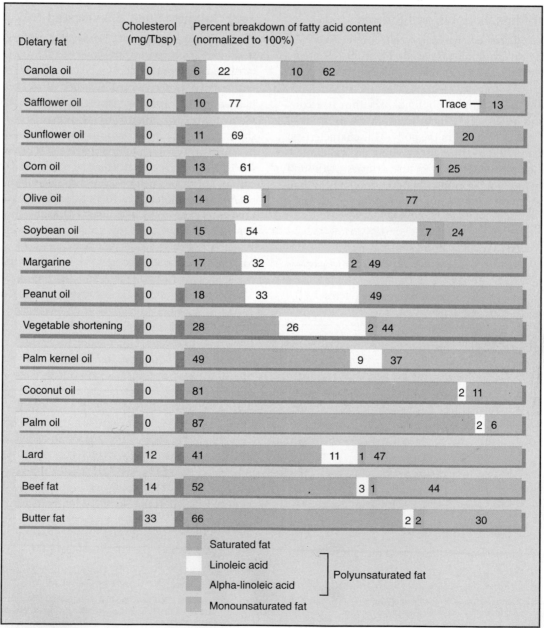

FIG 5-4 Comparison of dietary fats in terms of cholesterol, saturated fat, and the most common unsaturated fats.

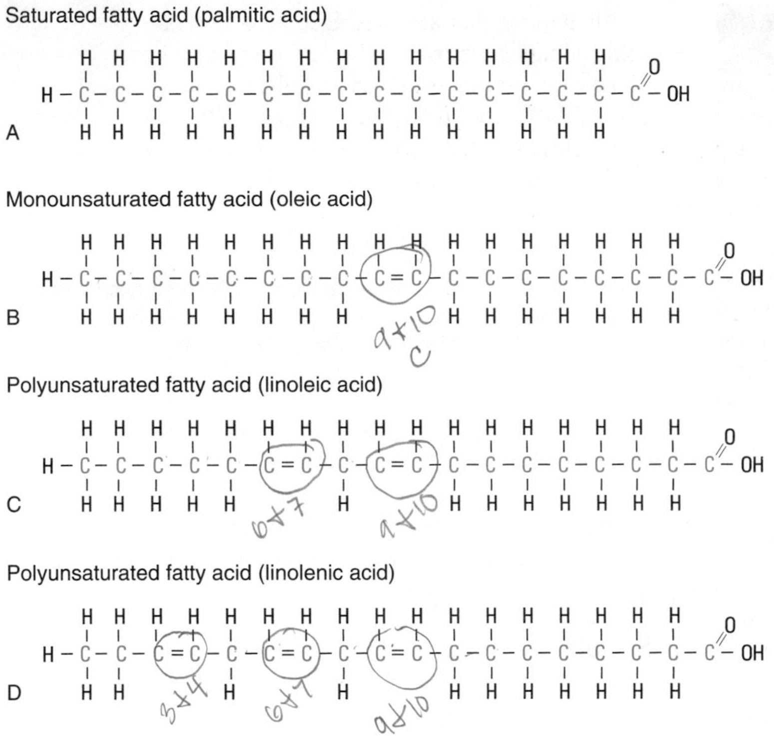

Saturated fatty acid (palmitic acid)

Monounsaturated fatty acid (oleic acid)

Polyunsaturated fatty acid (linoleic acid)

Polyunsaturated fatty acid (linolenic acid)

FIG 5-5 Examples of fatty acids found in foods. Foods with these fatty acids include **(A)** animal-derived foods (beef, poultry, lamb, pork, eggs, dairy, tropical oils); **(B)** olive oil, peanuts (butter and oil), canola oil; **(C)** vegetable oils (margarine and salad dressings), some animal fats, prepared foods; and **(D)** fatty fish (bluefish, tuna, salmon, etc.), fish, canola oil.

A **saturated fatty acid** has a single-bonded carbon chain that is fully saturated because hydrogen atoms are attached to all available bonding sites. Palmitic acid (16 carbon atoms) (Figure 5-5, A), a saturated fatty acid, is contained in meats, butterfat, shortening, and vegetable oils. Other saturated fatty acids include stearic acid (18 carbon atoms), myristic acid (14 carbon atoms), and lauric acid (12 carbon atoms).[2] Additional food sources of saturated fatty acids are primarily animal, including beef, poultry, pork, lamb, luncheon meats, egg yolks, and dairy products (milk, butter, and cheeses); the only major plant sources are palm and coconut oils (often called *tropical oils*) and cocoa butter.

Unsaturated fatty acids have one or more unsaturated double bonds along the carbon chain. If a carbon chain has only one unsaturated double bond, it is a **monounsaturated fatty acid**. Oleic acid (see Figure 5-5, B) is the main monounsaturated fatty acid in foods. Dietary sources include olive oil, peanuts (peanut butter and peanut oil), and canola oil.

If a carbon chain has two or more unsaturated double bonds, it is a **polyunsaturated fatty acid (PUFA)**. Food sources include vegetable oils (corn, safflower, wheat germ, canola, sesame, and sunflower), fish, and margarine.

PUFAs are categorized by the location of the unsaturation in the molecular structure of the fatty acid. Two categories of polyunsaturated fatty acids, omega-6 and omega-3, contain two fatty acids (linoleic and linolenic) that our bodies cannot manufacture; these acids are EFAs and must be provided by dietary intake. The characteristic that distinguishes them from other PUFAs is the position of the final double bond in relation to the end of the carbon chain. The final double bond is at the sixth carbon from the omega end of the chain in linoleic acid (see Figure 5-5, C), the main member of the omega-6 family. The first double bond is at the third carbon atom from the omega end in linolenic acid (see Figure 5-5, D), the main member of the omega-3 family.

Americans consume an abundance of linoleic acid from consumption of large amounts of vegetable oils, such as margarine and salad dressing, and large amounts of prepared foods. Another source of linoleic acid may be animal foods; for example, although poultry fat is predominantly saturated, it also contains some PUFA, including linoleic acid.

In contrast, American consumption of linolenic acid is not abundant at all. Linolenic acid is associated with fish consumption because that is how it was first recognized as important in health. A low incidence of heart disease among the native people of Greenland and Alaska, in spite of a very high-fat diet, was traced to the oils in deep-water fish, the staple in their diet.[4] One of the main omega-3 fatty acids in fish is **eicosapentaenoic acid (EPA)**, which is derived from linolenic acid. Fish are more efficient in this conversion of fatty acids than humans. Omega-3 fatty acids appear to lower the risk of heart disease by reducing the blood clotting process; clots can cause blockages in the arteries if plaques exist. Although consuming extra omega-3 fatty acids is likely to have little effect on blood cholesterol levels, it may reduce the risk of clots that may cause a myocardial infarction (heart attack) and possible sudden death.[3] According to prospective studies, reduced risk of coronary artery disease (CAD), because of higher consumption of fish or omega-3 fatty acids, appears applicable to men and women.[3,4]

Certain fish provide more omega-3 fatty acids than others. Good sources include tuna, salmon, bluefish, halibut, sardines, and rainbow trout. Table 5-1 lists additional sources. Eating fish twice a week or using canola oil, another source

TABLE 5-1	**FOOD SOURCES OF OMEGA-3 FATTY ACIDS**
FISH SOURCES	**PLANT SOURCES**
Salmon	Canola oil
Mackerel	Walnuts and walnut oil
Herring	Soybean and soybean oil
Tuna	Flaxseed ground and oil
Rainbow trout	Wheat germ and oat germ
Sardines	Green leafy vegetables

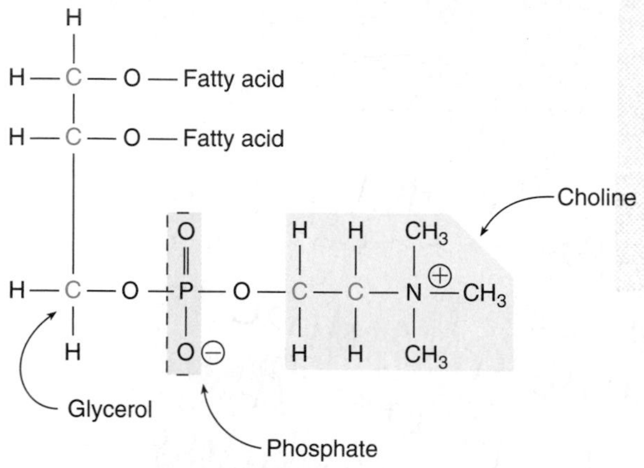

FIG 5-6 A phospholipid: lecithin.

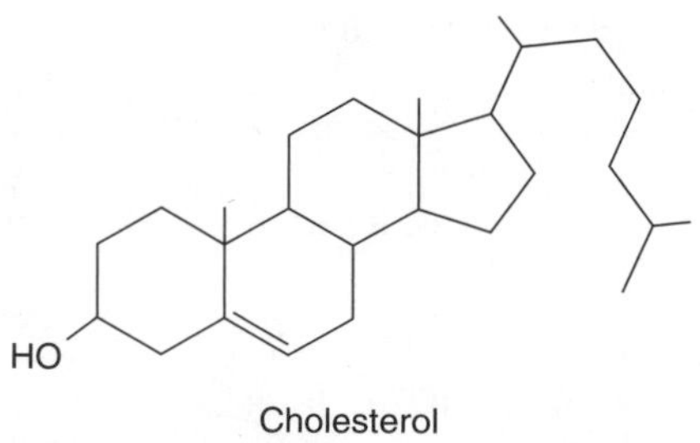

Cholesterol

FIG 5-7 A sterol: cholesterol. Foods containing cholesterol include animal-derived foods such as beef, pork, chicken, bacon, luncheon meats, eggs, fish, and dairy products.

of linolenic acid, should provide an adequate balance between sources of omega-6 and omega-3 fatty acids, although the best balance is still unknown.

Inuits consume 4 to 5 g of EPAs daily,[5] about the amount in 1.5 to 3 pounds of certain deep-water fish. Because it is unlikely that most Americans will consume this quantity of fish, fish oil supplements of these fatty acids are manufactured. However, questions about proper dosages, safety, and side effects are still being researched. Symptoms that may potentially occur from high intakes of omega-3 fatty acids include infections and increased bleeding time, and may affect blood glucose levels of individuals with diabetes.[3] For now, the best approach is to increase consumption of foods containing these potentially important fatty acids, unless a health care professional prescribes fish oil supplements, indicating dose levels.

Phospholipids

Phospholipids are lipid compounds that form part of cell walls and act as a fat emulsifier. Similar to triglycerides, phospholipids contain fatty acids, but they have only two fatty acids; the third spot contains a phosphate group. The body manufactures phospholipids, found in every cell; therefore, they are not essential nutrients. Lecithin, the main phospholipid, contains two fatty acids, with the third spot filled by a molecule of chloline plus phosphorus (Figure 5-6). In the body, lecithin's function as an emulsifier is to work by being soluble in water and fat at the same time.

Lecithin from soybeans is used in food processing to perform an emulsification role. Lecithin, naturally found in egg yolks, is the versatile ingredient in mayonnaise that prevents separation of vinegar and oil. Lecithin is also used in manufacturing chocolates to keep the cocoa butter and other ingredients combined and in cakes and other bakery products to maintain freshness.

Sterols

Sterols, a fatlike class of lipids, serve vital functions in the body. Sterol structures, including cholesterol, are carbon rings intermeshed with side chains of carbon, hydrogen, and oxygen, which make them more complex than triglycerides (Figure 5-7). Like phospholipids, sterols are synthesized by the body and are not essential nutrients. For example, if dietary cholesterol is not consumed, the liver will produce the amount required for body functions.

Generally, dietary cholesterol accounts for about 25% of the cholesterol in the body. The rest, which is made in the liver, seems to be produced in relation to how much is needed. The only food sources of cholesterol are animal and include beef, pork (bacon), chicken, luncheon meats, eggs, fish, and dairy products (milk, butter, and cheeses); plant foods do not contain cholesterol.

FATS AS A NUTRIENT IN THE BODY

Digestion

Mouth

The mouth's primary fat digestive process is mechanical, as teeth masticate fatty foods. The glands of the tongue produce a fat-splitting enzyme (lingual lipase) released with saliva that begins digestion of long-chain fatty acids such as those found in milk.

Stomach

Mechanical digestion continues through the strong actions of peristalsis. Fat-splitting enzymes such as gastric lipase hydrolyze some fatty acids from triglycerides.

Small Intestine

Fats entering the duodenum initiate the release of cholecystokinin (CCK) hormone from the duodenum walls. CCK, as described in Chapter 3, then sparks the gallbladder to release

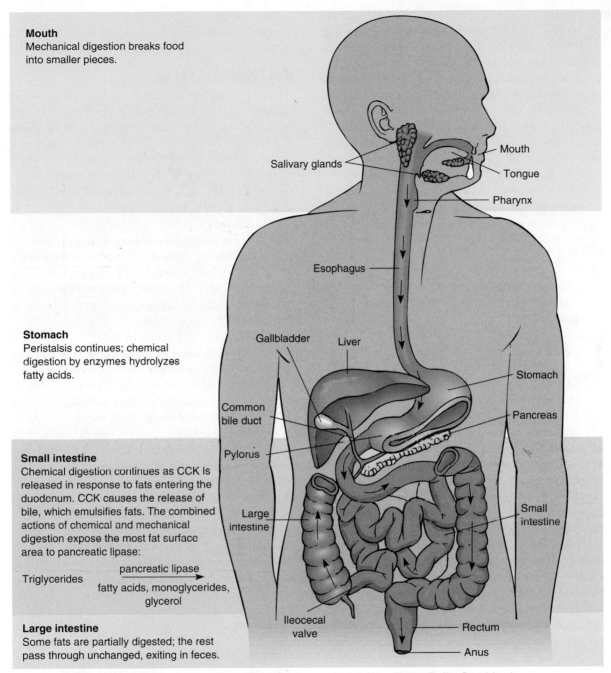

Mouth
Mechanical digestion breaks food into smaller pieces.

Stomach
Peristalsis continues; chemical digestion by enzymes hydrolyzes fatty acids.

Small intestine
Chemical digestion continues as CCK is released in response to fats entering the duodenum. CCK causes the release of bile, which emulsifies fats. The combined actions of chemical and mechanical digestion expose the most fat surface area to pancreatic lipase:

Triglycerides $\xrightarrow{\text{pancreatic lipase}}$ fatty acids, monoglycerides, glycerol

Large intestine
Some fats are partially digested; the rest pass through unchanged, exiting in feces.

FIG 5-8 Summary of fat digestion and absorption. (From Rolin Graphics.)

bile into the small intestine. The bile emulsifies fats to facilitate digestion. Mechanical digestion through muscular action allows for increased exposure of the emulsified fat globules to pancreatic lipase. This enzyme is the primary digestive enzyme that breaks triglycerides into fatty acids, monoglycerides, and glycerol molecules. Note that fats may not be completely broken down. Some may also pass through without being digested or absorbed. Figure 5-8 summarizes digestion of triglycerides.

Use of Medium-Chain Triglycerides

Triglycerides are composed of long chains of fatty acids. To aid fat digestion in those patients with malabsorption, synthetically manufactured medium-chain triglycerides (MCTs) may be incorporated into a patient's dietary intake. MCTs should not be used to completely replace dietary fats because they do not contain EFAs.

Absorption

Fatty acids, monoglycerides, and cholesterol are assisted by bile salts in moving from the lumen to the villi for absorption. Micelles, created by bile salts encircling lipids, aid diffusion through the membrane wall. When through the membrane wall, fatty acids and glycerol combine back into triglycerides. These triglycerides are incorporated into chylomicrons, which are the first lipoproteins formed after absorption of lipids from food. They contain fats and cholesterol and are coated with protein. The protein coating allows travel through the lymph system to the blood circulatory system toward the hepatic portal system and the liver. Some glycerol and any short- and medium-chain fatty acids are absorbed directly into the blood capillaries leading to the portal vein and liver.

At the cell membranes, the triglycerides in the chylomicrons are broken down into fatty acids and glycerol with assistance from an enzyme called *lipoprotein lipase.* Muscle cells, adipose cells, and other cells in the vicinity take up most of the fatty acids released by the breakdown of chylomicrons. Cells can use the absorbed fatty acids immediately as fuel, or they can reform them into triglycerides to be stored as reserve energy supplies.

Metabolism

Lipid metabolism consists of several processes. Catabolism (breakdown) of lipids for energy involves the hydrolysis of triglycerides into two-carbon units that become part of acetyl coenzyme A (acetyl CoA). Acetyl CoA is an important intermediate byproduct in metabolism formed from the breakdown of glucose, fatty acids, and certain amino acids. The acetyl CoA then enters the series of reactions called the TCA cycle, eventually leading to the oxidation of the carbon and hydrogen atoms derived from fatty acids (or carbohydrates or amino acids) to carbon dioxide and water with the release of energy as adenosine triphosphate (ATP) (see Figure 9-2). If fat catabolizes quickly because of a lack of carbohydrate (glucose) for energy, the liver cells form intermediate products from the partial oxidation of fatty acids called *ketone bodies.* These ketone bodies may excessively accumulate in the blood, causing a condition called ketosis.

Anabolism (synthesis) of lipids, or lipogenesis, results in the formation of triglycerides, phospholipids, cholesterol, and prostaglandins for use throughout the body. Triglycerides and phosphates form from fatty acids and glycerol or from excess glucose or amino acids. Extra carbon, hydrogen, and oxygen from any source can be converted to and stored as triglycerides in adipose tissues, so we can gain fat from foods other than fat.

Lipid metabolism is regulated mainly by insulin, growth hormone, and the adrenal cortex hormones; adrenocorticotropic hormone (ACTH), which stimulates secretion of more hormones; and glucocorticoids, which affect food metabolism.

FAT INTAKE AND ISSUES

Awareness of the fat content of foods is steadily growing. Whether we are consuming a sophisticated gourmet feast or chowing down on hot dogs and hamburgers at a summer barbecue, the fat levels of our meals may be of interest. Concerns about fat in our diets center around health issues of excessive intake of energy, excessive fat intake that replaces other nutrients, and the relationship between dietary fat intake and the development of chronic diet-related diseases. Some lipids consumed in foods are essential to our bodies to achieve wellness.

Fat Content of Foods

High-fat foods are almost always high-calorie foods. This is because fats are the most concentrated source of food energy, supplying 9 kcal/g; carbohydrates and proteins supply 4 kcal/g. Because most foods contain a mixture of nutrients, we can identify the fat content of food by the number of fat grams in a serving or the percent of daily value of recommended fat intake in a serving. Nutritional labels on packaged food contain this information.

The Dietary Reference Intakes (DRIs), based on Acceptable Macronutrient Distribution Ranges (AMDRs), recommend that we eat 20% to 35% of our kcal intakes from fats, with 10% or less of kcal from saturated fats.[6] Based on the daily values, total fat intake for an average daily kcal intake of 2000 to 2500 kcal should range from about 40 to 97 g or less (400 to 875 kcal or less). Saturated fat should be 25 to 20 g or less (225 to 180 kcal or less).

There is evidence that diets with fat levels of 18% to 22% may have undesirable effects, including lower high-density lipoprotein (HDL) levels and higher triglyceride levels.[7] The evidence does not support reducing fat much below 26% kcal as fat—not a problem for most Americans, who have a long way to go toward lower-fat diets. In fact, most Americans are still within the 30% to 40% of total energy intake as fat, even though many believe they are avoiding or limiting high-fat foods.[3] One reason may be because high-fat foods have both potent sensory qualities and high-energy density; overeating is then often more passive than active. Another reason is that people who eat a lot of high-fat foods are unsure whether their diets are high in fat because home cooking has fallen sharply; the cook no longer knows exactly what goes into each dish. Also, portion

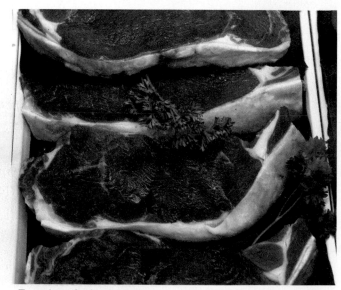

To reduce fat intake, trim meat before cooking. (Photos.com.)

Calculating Your Daily Fat Intake

Use the following steps to calculate your daily grams of fat:
1. Use the Recommended Energy Intake chart in Chapter 9 to determine your appropriate energy needs for the day. Multiply that number of kcal by 0.25 for 25% fat intake or by 0.30 for 30% fat intake.
2. Divide that number by 9, because each gram of fat has 9 kcal. For example, if you consume 1800 kcal a day and want to get 25% of those kcal from fat: 0.25 × 1800 = 450. Then divide 450 by 9 to get 50 g of fat. Energy needs for the day kcal × 0.30 = kcal fat intake/day. Kcal fat intake a day/9 kcal = g of fat/day.
3. Next, check food labels and/or use food composition tables (see Appendix A) for the grams of fat per food serving. You then can compare the sum of the fat grams consumed with the recommended levels for your particular energy needs.

sizes at restaurants are often twice the size of that recommended for good health by MyPyramid. Then there is the "less fat, more carbs" message that has been incorrectly translated into sweet, kcal-dense, low-fiber carbohydrate foods, so the low-fat diet has become a high-calorie, processed-carbohydrate diet. It is also likely that people are misled by labels of "reduced fat" foods and thus actually *increase* the total intake of such foods. The individual foods we eat daily may have a higher or lower fat content, but overall we should generally average 25% to 30% of kcal fat intake from all the foods we eat each day (see the *Teaching Tool* box, Calculating Your Daily Fat Intake).

How do we measure the fat in foods without labels, such as fresh foods, home-cooked recipes, and restaurant items? One way is to classify foods into groups according to fat content. The Exchange List uses this system by listing protein foods based on their "leanness" (see Chapter 2 or Appendix A). In contrast, MyPyramid devotes a section to oils (fats that are liquid at room temperature) and provides information on the dietary fat content of foods in the oil category as well as foods in fruit, meats, and bean categories that contain oils. Oils are not considered a food group but *are* recognized as needed for good health. MyPyramid emphasizes the health-promoting oils from plants and fish, rather than the solid, more saturated fats from palm kernel oil and coconut oil and many animal foods and from hydrogenation of vegetable oils. As shown in Box 5-1, frequently consumed oils are canola, corn, olive, cottonseed, safflower, and soybean. Foods listed as good sources of oils consist of nuts, certain fish, avocado, and olives. Table 5-2 provides examples of fat in servings from different foods. Common solid fats include butter, lard (pork fat), shortening, beef fat (suet, tallow), stick margarine, and chicken fat.

Detecting Dietary Fat

Some fats are visible; others are invisible. Visible fat is fairly easy to find and control; just cut off the white fat on the outside of a steak and measure the butter or sour cream on the baked potato. Invisible fat is harder to measure. Fat in milk, cheese, and yogurt is nearly impossible to see, but many people learn to taste the difference between whole- and low-fat dairy products. In addition, dairy foods are all labeled so fat content is known. Some foods give other clues that they contain fat. Press a napkin on a slice of pizza, a Danish pastry, or an egg roll. Look for oil around the edge of stir-fried Chinese food.

Be aware of general characteristics that signal the level of fat in foods. Some cooking methods, such as deep-frying, add fat. The way a prepared food is usually eaten may also increase fat intake, such as spreading butter or oil on bread rather than just dipping it in soup. Whether eating in or dining out, the amount of food regularly selected from high-fat animal sources such as meat and cheese compared with the amount of food consumed from low-fat grains, vegetables, and fruit affects total dietary fat consumption levels.

Government and consumer groups have encouraged restaurants and institutional food service operations to offer identifiable low-fat, low-calorie food choices. These choices allow clients to meet health promotion goals while maintaining social interactions. Encourage clients to identify healthy menu choices when eating away from home.

The cuisines of China and Italy are based on rice, pasta, and bread. When prepared with small amounts of fat and eaten with little fatty meat and plenty of vegetables, these cultural food patterns are excellent examples of healthful diets. Yet, when Chinese and Italian foods are prepared to please the American palate, large amounts of fat are used in cooking the food, and portion sizes are larger than usual for specific ethnic tradition (see the *Cultural Considerations* box, Choosing Lower-Fat Ethnic Dishes).

Fast but High-Fat Foods

Contemporary lifestyles sometimes leave little room for meal planning and preparation. Often we may find ourselves heading for the nearest fast-food restaurant or snack bar as we dash off to school or work. What impact do these meals have on our nutritional status? A positive trend among fast-food chains is the use of less saturated fat in fried potatoes and the addition of items such as salads and skim milk to the menu. On the negative side, between 40% and 50% of fast-food kcal comes from fat—far higher than the recommended 30%.

When we study the major food contributors of fat in the American diet, hamburgers, cheeseburgers, meat loaf, and hot dogs top the list. Whole-milk beverages including shakes are next, followed by cheese and salad dressings. Doughnuts, cookies, and cake tie with fried potatoes.[8] It is no surprise that the majority of fat in the American diet happens to appear in menu favorites served in fast-food restaurants and sporting events. In addition, the majority of fat in these foods tends to be saturated, with hamburgers and cheeseburgers leading the pack.

BOX 5-1   MYPLATE: OILS

MyPlate focuses on oils, which are fats that are liquid at room temperature. Oils come from plant sources and fish. Common plant oils that do not contain cholesterol or saturated fats include canola, corn, olive, cottonseed, safflower, soybean, and sunflower. A few plant oils such as palm kernel oil and coconut oil contain saturated fats, making them more similar in function to solid fats such as those found in animal-derived foods.

Some foods that are naturally high in oils contain monounsaturated and/or polyunsaturated fat. These include nuts, avocado, olives, salmon, and tuna.

Solid fats are solid at room temperature. Solid fats primarily come from animal foods and can be made from plant oils when hydrogenated. Solid fats include butter, beef fat (tallow, suet), chicken fat, pork fat (lard), and processed hydrogenated stick margarine and vegetable shortening. Hydrogenated fats usually contain trans fat, which are identified on nutrition labels.

The focus of this MyPlate box is on portions of oils.

How Do I Count the Oils I Eat?*

The following table gives a quick guide to the amount of oils in some common foods.

FAT	AMOUNT OF FOOD	AMOUNT OF OIL (TEASPOONS/GRAMS)	KCAL FROM OIL (APPROXIMATE)	TOTAL KCAL (APPROXIMATE)
Oils				
Vegetable oils (such as canola, corn, cottonseed, olive, peanut, safflower, soybean, and sunflower)	1 Tbsp	3 tsp/14 g	120	120
Foods Rich in Oils				
Margarine, soft (trans fat-free)	1 Tbsp	2½ tsp/11 g	100	100
Mayonnaise	1 Tbsp	2½ tsp/11 g	100	100
Mayonnaise-type salad dressing	1 Tbsp	1 tsp/5 g	45	55
Italian dressing	2 Tbsp	2 tsp/8 g	75	85
Thousand Island dressing	2 Tbsp	2½ tsp/11 g	100	120
Olives, ripe, canned	4 large	½ tsp/2 g	15	20
Avocado[†]	½ medium	3 tsp/15 g	130	160
Peanut butter[†]	2 Tbsp	4 tsp/16 g	140	190
Peanuts, dry-roasted[†]	1 oz	3 tsp/14 g	120	165
Mixed nuts, dry-roasted[†]	1 oz	3 tsp/15 g	130	170
Cashews, dry-roasted[†]	1 oz	3 tsp/13 g	115	165
Almonds, dry-roasted[†]	1 oz	3 tsp/15 g	130	170
Hazelnuts[†]	1 oz	4 tsp/18 g	160	185
Sunflower seeds[†]	1 oz	3 tsp/14 g	120	165

*Accessed June 14, 2012, from www.choosemyplate.gov/food-groups/oils_count.html.
[†]Avocados are part of the fruit group; nuts and seeds are part of the meat and beans group.

One may wonder why some foods that are fast to fix, such as apples, oranges, and bananas, are not considered fast foods, nor are they sold in fast-food restaurants. The answer probably has to do with the fact that fat lends a seductive flavor to fast-food favorites (see the *Teaching Tool* box, But Fast Foods Are So Convenient).

How can fat intake be lowered? First, start early to include children and the whole family in buying food, preparing it, and having low-fat foods on hand. Many people prefer fast food because they don't have fresh or partly prepared foods ready to cook. Teaching children cooking skills from simple recipes, videos, and friends establishes low-fat food preferences early. Individuals are more likely to adopt low-fat diets if eating partners or families do the same by modeling healthy eating patterns.

Second, most major secondary and tertiary health care settings have an active dietetic department, often geared to pediatrics and family practice. Programs offered may include healthy cooking classes for children and their parents or nutrition and wellness classes. Providing lists of such programs is a valuable resource for clients.

Third, never say never. It is okay to include some high-fat foods in food plans because they taste good. If a mixture of low-fat and high-fat foods is eaten, preferences for both are developed; this automatically controls overdoing the fatty foods. The *Teaching Tool* that discusses fast foods is packed with other strategies for fast-food, low-fat eating patterns.

Preserving Fats in Food
Processed Fats and Oils: Hydrogenated and Emulsified

A problem with unsaturated fats in foods is that oxygen attacks the unsaturated double bonds (oxidation), causing

TABLE 5-2	FAT IN FOOD SERVINGS	
FOOD	**SERVING SIZE**	**FAT CONTENT**
Butter/margarine	1 Tbsp	11 g
Salad dressing	1 Tbsp	7 g
Mayonnaise	1 Tbsp	11 g
Cream cheese	1 Tbsp	10 g
Carrots	½ cup	Trace
Broccoli	½ cup	Trace
Potato, baked	1	Trace
French fries	1 cup	8 g
Apple	1	Trace
Orange	1	Trace
Banana	1	Trace
Fruit juice	1 cup	Trace
Rice or pasta	½ cup	Trace
Bagel	1	Trace
Muffin	1 medium	6 g
Danish pastry	1 medium	13 g
Skim milk	1 cup	Trace
Low-fat milk	1 cup	5 g
Whole milk	1 cup	8 g
American cheese	2 oz	18 g
Cheddar cheese	1½ oz	14 g
Frozen yogurt	½ cup	2 g
Ice milk	⅓ cup	3 g
Ice cream	⅓ cup	7 g
Lean beef	3 oz	6 g
Poultry	3 oz	6 g
Fish	3 oz	6 g
Ground beef	3 oz	16 g
Bologna (2 slices)	1 oz	16 g
Egg	1	5 g
Nuts (⅓ cup)	1 oz	22 g

CULTURAL CONSIDERATIONS

Choosing Lower-Fat Ethnic Dishes

Perhaps you've grown up eating rice and beans, homemade lasagna, or Chinese takeout. Regardless of who prepares the food, Americans are consuming more international foods than ever before. We have a smorgasbord of ethnic foods from which to choose. Chinese, Indian, Mexican, and Greek dishes have become commonplace.

We may assume, however, that because these foods are different and exotic, they are healthier for us. After all, aren't hamburgers and hot dogs—all-American favorites—the worst offenders for our health? However, although some ethnic dishes are lower in fat and higher in dietary fibers, others aren't much better than traditional American favorites.

The Chinese foods eaten in America would be considered far too rich (and high in fat) by the Chinese; they are reserved for banquets and even then are eaten in moderation. To enhance the healthfulness of prepared Chinese foods, avoid fried dishes, especially egg rolls, and make rice the centerpiece of your meal. Top the rice with moderate portions of entrées of chicken or seafood mixed with vegetables.

Italian dishes of pasta and gravy (i.e., tomato sauce) are healthful but become problematic when teamed with sausage, meatballs, fried breaded meats, and layers of cheeses or when tomato sauce is replaced by a cream Alfredo sauce. Each adds substantial amounts of saturated fats. Be aware of portion sizes and focus on large portions of pasta served with smaller servings of the high-fat foods.

Mexican and Latino foods are sometimes made with lard, a heavily saturated animal fat, and with fatty portions of pork. These negatives, however, are somewhat offset by the generous (and delicious) use of beans, rice, and soft tortillas made from corn or wheat. When possible, avoid or reduce the use of lard; vegetable oils are a good substitute. Generally the less fat used, the healthier the entrée. For example, a taco made with a soft tortilla contains less fat than one made with a hard fried tortilla. And be sure to pile on lots of lettuce, tomatoes, and salsa!

Application to nursing: Become familiar with the exotic tastes of international cuisines. By doing so, you'll be able to assist clients in understanding the fat content of their ethnic favorites. Just remember that the palatability of fat is a worldwide phenomenon, so choose wisely.

---

damage that makes them rancid; rancid fats have an odor and bad flavor and may cause illness. One way to reduce vulnerability to oxidation is to artificially saturate the fatty acids by adding hydrogen at the double bonds. This process of *hydrogenation* makes the fat solid and more stable, which provides cooking benefits. When vegetable oil, which is polyunsaturated, is completely hydrogenated, it becomes a white, waxy, or plastic-like substance called *vegetable shortening*. Because it is saturated with hydrogens, the body processes it as if it were a saturated fat.

The ingredient list on a product label can truthfully state that the product contains more unsaturated liquid oil, although it is mixed with the partially hydrogenated fat. Partially hydrogenated fats are used in a variety of food products.

Sometimes the solution to one problem causes another problem. Although it stabilizes fat, hydrogenation changes the structure of some of the fatty acids, from cis fatty acids to *trans* fatty acids (Figure 5-9). Most fatty acid double bonds in natural foods are in the *cis* form, but margarine and vegetable shortening may contain high concentrations of *trans* fatty acids (*trans* fats). *Trans* fatty acids have unusual double-bond structures cause by hydrogenated unsaturated

oils. Some margarines are now processed to contain no *trans* fatty acids. Often manufacturers will note if their margarine products are free of *trans* fatty acids. Controversy over the effect of *trans* fats in relation to cancer vulnerability and elevated blood cholesterol levels has confused the public.

Before completely deciding butter is better, consider that although some margarines are fairly high in *trans* fats, they usually have less than many commercially made foods such as french fries, potato chips, and bakery products made from partially hydrogenated vegetable oils. Many margarines and other products are now offered as "*trans* free." On the other hand, of the average 35% of kcal consumed as fat by Americans, only about 3% of total kcal comes from *trans* fats.[3]

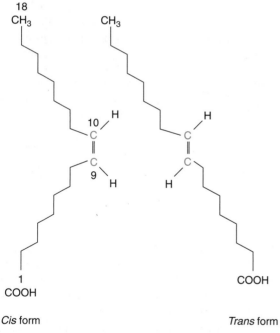

FIG 5-9 *Cis* bond to *trans* bonds.

Nonetheless, *trans* fat consumption appears to increase risk for CAD. Risk is increased because the *trans* fat raises the blood cholesterol component (low-density lipoproteins [LDLs]), which delivers cholesterol throughout the body and, while doing so, may contribute to plaque formation in arteries. *Trans* fat also decreases the blood cholesterol component (high-density lipoproteins [HDLs]) that removes excess and used cholesterol from the body. Maintaining higher levels of this component decreases risk of CAD. Considering these effects on blood cholesterol, consumption of *trans* fatty acids formed from partially hydrogenated oils should be limited.[9]

Since January 2006, listing *trans* fatty acid content on nutrition labels has been mandatory.[10] This recent requirement led manufacturers to reformulate products without *trans* fats. "Partially hydrogenated fat or oil" as an ingredient is another clue that *trans* fat is present in a product. When possible, *trans* fat should be replaced by a monounsaturated fat such as canola oil. Guidelines currently suggest as a priority to reduce overall food fat to 30% of total kcal; less fat means less *trans* fats as well. Depending on product formulation, this may mean eating less margarine, french fries, potato chips, cakes, and cookies, as well as less fried chicken, fried fish, fatty meat, and ice cream.

Antioxidants

Another way to preserve polyunsaturated fats without hydrogenation is through the use of antioxidant additives. These substances block oxidation, or the breakdown of double bonds by oxygen. Food manufacturers can use either natural or synthetic forms of antioxidants. Natural sources include vitamin E (tocopherol) and vitamin C (ascorbic acid). Their use not only helps to preserve foods but also adds essential vitamins. Synthetic forms consist of the food additives of butylated hydroxyanisole (BHA) and butylated hydroxytoluene (BHT). These forms are used in packaging as well to help prevent oxidation of the foods.

Food Cholesterol versus Blood Cholesterol

Cholesterol is a waxy substance found in all tissues in humans and other animals; thus all foods from animal sources, such as meat, eggs, fish, poultry, and dairy products, contain cholesterol. The highest sources of cholesterol are egg yolks and organ meats (liver and kidney). No plant-derived food

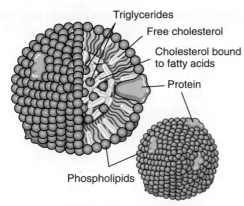

Triglycerides
Free cholesterol
Cholesterol bound
to fatty acids
Protein
Phospholipids

FIG 5-10 Lipoprotein.

TABLE 5-3	**BLOOD CHOLESTEROL LEVELS**	
RISK CLASSIFICATION	**TOTAL CHOLESTEROL**	**LDL CHOLESTEROL**
Desirable	<200 mg/dL	<130 mg/dL
Borderline-high	200-239 mg/dL	130-159 mg/dL
High	≥240 mg/dL	≥160 mg/dL

Modified from National Cholesterol Education Program: *ATP III guidelines at-a-glance quick desk reference*, NIH Pub No 01-3305, Washington, DC, 2001, U.S. Department of Health and Human Services; Public Health Service; National Institutes of Health; National Heart, Lung, and Blood Institute.

TABLE 5-4	**CHOLESTEROL CONTENT OF SELECTED FOODS***	
FOOD	**AMOUNT**	**CHOLESTEROL (mg)**
Milk, nonfat/skim	1 cup	4
Mayonnaise	1 Tbsp	8
Cottage cheese, lowfat 2%	½ cup	10
Milk, lowfat/2%	1 cup	18
Cream cheese	1 oz	28
Hot dog[†]	1	29
Ice cream, 10% fat	½ cup	30
Cheddar cheese	1 oz	30
Butter	1 Tbsp	31
Milk, whole	1 cup	33
Clams, fish fillets, oysters	3 oz	50-60
Beef,[†] pork,[†] poultry	3 oz	70-85
Shrimp	3 oz	166
Egg yolk[†]	1	213
Beef liver	3 oz	410

*In ascending order.
[†]Leading contributors of cholesterol to U.S. diet.

contains cholesterol, not even avocado or peanut butter, which are very high in fat. People often misunderstand this because they confuse food (dietary) cholesterol with blood cholesterol.

A high level of cholesterol in the blood is a risk factor for CAD. (Refer to Table 5-3 Blood cholesterol levels.) To understand blood cholesterol levels, the role of lipoproteins—specialized transporting compounds—needs clarification. Lipoproteins are compounds that contain a mix of lipids—including triglycerides, fatty acids, phospholipids, cholesterol, and small amounts of other steroids and fat-soluble vitamins—that are covered with a protein outer layer (Figure 5-10). The outer layer of protein allows the compound to move through a watery substance, such as blood. Lipoproteins transport fats in the circulatory system.

The amount of fat and protein determines the density or weight of the lipoprotein. The more fat and lipid substances present, the lower the density (or lighter) of the compound. Four forms of these compounds are most important for understanding the route of cholesterol in the body; they are chylomicrons, very low-density lipoproteins, LDLs, and HDLs.

Chylomicrons transport absorbed fats from the intestinal wall to the liver cells. Fats are then used for synthesis of lipoproteins. **Very low-density lipoproteins (VLDLs)** leave the liver cells full of fats and lipid components to transfer newly made (endogenous) triglycerides to the cells. **Low-density lipoproteins (LDLs)** form from VLDLs because density is reduced as fats and lipids are released on their journey through the body. LDLs carry cholesterol throughout the body to tissue cells for various functions.

In contrast to the delivery functions of the first three lipoproteins, **high-density lipoproteins (HDLs)** are formed within cells to remove cholesterol from the cell, bringing it to the liver for disposal.

A total blood cholesterol reading reflects the level of cholesterol contained in LDL and HDL. To get a clearer assessment of cholesterol activity in the body, the individual levels of LDL and HDL are valuable. The risk of CAD associated with blood cholesterol levels is presented in Table 5-4. LDL levels reflect the amount of cholesterol brought to cells that have the potential to be dropped off along the way to clog

vessels and arteries, contributing to plaque formation. **Plaques** are deposits of fatty substances, including cholesterol, that attach to arterial walls. As this happens, HDLs remove cholesterol from the circulatory system. Removal of cholesterol is a positive action that reduces CAD risk.

Health guidelines generally recommend a dietary cholesterol intake of 300 mg or less per day. However, if LDL cholesterol is elevated, dietary cholesterol intake should be less than 200 mg.[11] Table 5-4 lists the cholesterol content of selected foods. However, the major culprit that raises blood cholesterol is not dietary food cholesterol but too much *food fat* (dietary triglycerides), particularly saturated fats; food cholesterol alone makes a minor difference for most people. Too much food cholesterol becomes a problem when it is eaten in conjunction with very high-fat diets. Sometimes, this extra cholesterol in the blood may be dropped off, staying in the vessels and arteries. It is a factor involved in the accumulation of plaques that result in blockage in the arteries call **atherosclerosis**, or CAD (Figure 5-11).

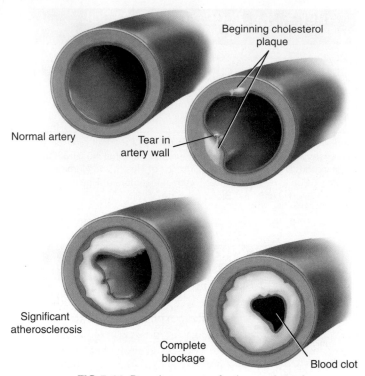

FIG 5-11 Development of atherosclerosis.

One reason for the confusion is the way food is cooked and eaten. Eggs, for example, are high in cholesterol and are often cooked and served with high-fat bacon or sausage. The combined meal of eggs and bacon then gets a bad reputation for raising blood cholesterol. The fact is that the large amount of fat in bacon and sausage is more likely to raise blood cholesterol than the food cholesterol in eggs. Shrimp are high in cholesterol but low in fat—that is, low in fat if the shrimp are steamed or broiled, not encased in a deep fat–fried coating. Of course, moderation is recommended when eating eggs or shrimp.

Another source of confusion is that cooking oils made from corn, safflower, and soybeans are often labeled as cholesterol free. Of course, they are cholesterol free; only foods from animals contain cholesterol. Yet vegetable oils are virtually 100% food fat, and large amounts of dietary fat can also raise blood cholesterol.

To be a savvy consumer (and teach your clients), read ingredient labels and be aware of some finer points of fat education:

- Hydrogenated vegetable oils—corn, soybean, and cottonseed—contain *trans* fatty acids and cholesterol-forming saturated fats often used to prepare potato and corn chips.
- Tropical oils of palm, palm kernel, and coconut are the only naturally saturated fat plant source. Found in many food products, they should be consumed only occasionally. (Popcorn popped in tropical oils came under fire; many movie theater chains now offer air-popped popcorn in addition to traditionally prepared popcorn.)

- Margarines are cholesterol free if made from vegetable oils but still contain the same number of calories as butter; both are about 100% lipid. Margarines, however, contain unsaturated fatty acids. Note that the level of hydrogenation used to form the margarine affects the amount of trans and saturated fatty acids contained. Use label information to select the least saturated product.
- Advise clients to check the labels of foods regularly eaten; a cholesterol-free product might not be as healthy as it seems.

In addition to the amount of fat, another characteristic of food fat that causes it to affect blood cholesterol differently is whether the fat is saturated or unsaturated—that is, whether the fat contains mostly saturated or unsaturated fatty acids. Saturated fatty acids generally raise blood cholesterol by providing the liver with the best building blocks for making cholesterol.

A simple guideline followed by many people is that blood cholesterol is *raised* by eating solid saturated fats and *lowered* by unsaturated and monounsaturated liquid fats. However, this rule is oversimplified for two reasons. First, food fats are a mixture of the three types. Second, although saturated fatty acids as a group raise cholesterol, some individual ones do not. Therefore, although we classify food fats as cholesterol raising (butter/saturated) and cholesterol lowering (corn oil/PUFA and olive oil/monounsaturated), these guidelines are based on the proportion of specific fatty acids in each food and how much each individual fatty acid affects blood cholesterol. Total fat intake can also influence blood cholesterol levels regard–less of the source. Table 5-2 and Figure 5-5 clear up some confusion over the finer points of fat.

Researchers have studied individual fatty acids as well as combinations regarding their effects on blood cholesterol[7] and other mechanisms including cancer.[12] We discussed these effects in the "Fats as a Nutrient in the Body" section.

Synthetic Fats and Fat Replacers

Many people dream about eating brownies and ice cream that are magically stripped of fat but still richly satisfying in taste and texture. Although surveys show that sugar substitutes have not reduced the amount of sugar we consume, optimists hope fat substitutes will reduce fat in our diets. Scientists are working to develop reduced-fat or fat-free substances that replace fat yet retain the taste and mouth-feel of fat in foods.[13]

Fat replacers, as they are called, are generally classified two ways: already existing in nature or synthesized in the laboratory. The naturally occurring ones do not change chemically and thus require less rigorous testing before the U.S. Food and Drug Administration (FDA) allows them to be used in foods. Heating and then blending protein from milk or eggs in a process called *microparticulation* produces one type of fat replacer. Simplesse is an example. Food applications include ice cream, frozen yogurt, and salad dressings—but not baked or deep-fried foods.

Carrageenan, a carbohydrate extracted from seaweed, has been used for centuries to thicken foods. Added to lean ground beef, carrageenan yields moist, juicy cooked meat with the texture of higher-fat beef. Similar gumlike products from oats, corn, and potatoes are under development and would provide lower kcal fatlike properties in food.

Salatrim, which stands for *short- and long-chain triglyceride molecules,* is made in the laboratory and provides sensory qualities with reduced energy content (5 kcal/g vs. 9 kcal/g). Olestra is a fat replacer made in the laboratory that binds fatty acids to sugar in a nontraditional way so that enzymes in the digestive tract are not able to break away the fatty acids. Olestra resembles standard fats and oils in many ways, including the ability to withstand frying and baking at high temperatures. Several characteristics of olestra are attractive to manufacturers and consumers, including the sensory properties of taste and texture, the no-kcal value because of the body's inability to digest it, and the reduced absorption of fat and cholesterol from the intestine. Potato chips cooked in olestra have 75 kcal/oz—half that of regular chips. A disadvantage is that olestra passes through the gut swiftly, possibly causing abdominal cramping and loose stools and loss of fat-soluble nutrients such as vitamins and carotenoids.

As the story of fat replacers continues to unfold, we need to study their effect on people's food choices. Will we be misled into thinking that low- or no-fat foods automatically are low kcal? Many fat-reduced foods will increase the amounts of other ingredients, such as carbohydrates, and do not result in low-kcal items.

To what degree will products containing fat replacers stimulate mechanisms to compensate for reduction in fat? Some studies suggest that incorporating reduced-fat products into the diet results in total fat reduction. Yet diets reduced in fat may not result in a reduction of total kcal. Thus fat-free foods help some people consume fewer kcal overall; other times people eat a fat-free food at one meal and then make up the kcal by eating more at the next. What about appetite guiding what we eat? If mouth-feel is maintained in reduced-fat foods, we may not distinguish between high- and reduced-fat foods. Then there is the "bargain" appeal. In studies in which people did not know which chips were regular and which were olestra, they ate similar amounts of each. When they did know, they ate significantly more olestra chips, thus mistakenly thinking they got two for the "fat price" of one.

Although fat replacers are widely available, the most prudent and health-promoting approach is for products to be reformulated or developed without the use of fat replacers so products contain lower-fat ingredients without added sugars and still taste good. Consistently consuming a low-fat diet can lead to a decrease in the preference for fat. Is it possible that fat replacers could undermine this healthful change? Nutritionists and scientists undoubtedly will continue to seek answers to make our fat-free brownie and ice cream dreams come true—without side effects.

OVERCOMING BARRIERS

Health concerns about our dietary fat intake fall into several categories: energy intake, reduced intake of other nutrients because of dietary fat consumption, and the relationship between dietary fat intake and diet-related diseases.

Energy Intake

Foods containing significant amounts of dietary fat will naturally provide more kcal than other lower-fat foods. Although high-fat treats are fine occasionally, indulging too often or not even realizing which foods are fat laden can result in consumption of too many kcal that may end up stored as body fat in adipose tissues.

Fat is even more efficient at being stored than are carbohydrate and protein, which means that we may gain more body fat from eating fat kcal than eating the same number of carbohydrate kcal (see Figure 9-2). The evidence for this comes from studying people who eat low-fat, high-calorie diets, as discussed earlier. A likely explanation for this is that the energy cost to convert dietary fat to body fat requires only 3% of the kcal consumed, whereas carbohydrate requires 23% of the energy consumed to be converted to body fat. Both fat storage and fat oxidation differ from that of carbohydrates and fat.

Diets high in fat are not the primary cause for the high prevalence of excess body fat in our society. We have an "all-food-all-the-time" lifestyle coupled with an aversion to physical activity. Overeating and underactivity are likely reasons for the steady increase in overweight and obese Americans (see the *Personal Perspectives* box, End of Overeating?). Another reason may be the ability to be aware of internal cues of hunger. Consider if we mistake fatigue as a cue of hunger. Consumption of food becomes a way to relieve tiredness, which of course does not work. Still, for many individuals struggling with moderate or even excessive weight, awareness of their dietary fat intake sources can make a difference. By gradually reducing fat intake—without increasing carbohydrate intake—energy intake decreases and weight maintenance becomes easier.

Extreme Dietary Fat Restrictions

Dietary intake of fat also can get too low. Although general population recommendations are for fat consumption to be 30% or less of our kcal intake, Dr. Dean Ornish developed a regimen to reverse CAD that is based on a dietary fat intake of 10% or less of kcal intake. The Ornish program has been successful in reducing cardiac risk factors, slowing the advance of CAD, and supporting continuation of lifestyle behaviors such as dietary modifications, regular exercise, and relaxation techniques.[14] However, an intake this low, based on a primarily vegetarian dietary pattern, may be difficult for most Americans to maintain. Adequate intake of EFAs also must be provided. There also is concern that a low-fat, high-carbohydrate diet may lower HDL cholesterol and raise triglycerides.[15]

PERSONAL PERSPECTIVES

End of Overeating?

David A. Kessler, MD, is a former FDA commissioner. The following is an excerpt from his book *The End of Overeating—Taking Control of the Insatiable American Appetite*, which explores why we are often unable to resist particular foods and eat too much of them. Dr. Kessler is concerned about the relationship between uncontrollable overeating of foods containing sugar, fat, and salt and the resulting public health dilemma of increased obesity and poor health status.

To understand how eating promotes more eating—and why homeostasis is under sustained assault—we must first understand the concept of *palatability* as the term is used scientifically. In everyday language, we call food "palatable" if it has an agreeable taste. But when scientists say a food is palatable, they are referring primarily to its capacity to stimulate the appetite and prompt us to eat more. Palatability does involve taste, of course, but, crucially, it also involves the motivation to pursue that taste. It is the reason we want more.

Palatability is largely based on how food engages the full range of our senses. Usually the most palatable foods contain some combination of sugar, fat, and salt. The sensory properties of palatable foods—the cold, creamy pleasure of a milkshake, the aroma of chocolate cake, the texture of crispy chicken wings sweetened with a honey-mustard dipping sauce—all stimulate the appetite. And it's that stimulation, or the anticipation of that stimulation, rather than genuine hunger that makes us put food into our months long after our caloric needs are satisfied.

"Palatable foods arouse our appetite," said Peter Rogers, a biological psychologist at the University of Bristol in England. "They act as an incentive to eat."

Our preference for sweetness is no surprise. Newborns who are given drops of a solution of sucrose and water exhibit pleasure with their facial expressions. And the sweeter the solution, the more they prefer it.

Adam Drewnowski of the University of Washington in Seattle has spent 30 years studying human taste, food preferences, and dietary choices. Like many of his colleagues, he initially focused on sugar, but he soon became convinced that sugar itself is not the only reason we're so partial to sweet foods. If nothing else mattered, more of us would just open a packet of sugar and eat it.

No one had looked closely at fat until the 1980s. "The focus was on the pleasure response to sugar, as though sugar were the only sensation in food that people responded to," said Drewnowski. Certain there was more to the story, he set out to prove it. He found what that we like is not sugar alone but sugar in combination with fat. Fat, he wrote, "is responsible for the characteristic texture, flavor, and aroma of many foods and largely determines the palatability of the diet."

Because fat provides so many different sensations in the mouth, we can't always tell which foods contain the most fat or why we prefer one sugar-fat mixture to another. But we can certainly point to what we like best. ...

The combination of sugar and fat is what people prefer, and it's what they'll eat most. The art of pleasing the palate is in large part a matter of combining them in optimal amounts. That can do more than make food palatable. It can make food "hyperpalatable."

From Kessler DA: *The end of overeating—taking control of the insatiable American appetite*, New York, 2009, Rodale.

Our health warnings about fat intake can be taken too seriously and interpreted too intensely, creating health hazards throughout the life span. Infants and young children depend on dietary fats and cholesterol for the formation of brain and nerve tissue and to provide adequate kcal for growth. Cases of failure to thrive have been reported when parents restricted the intake of dietary fats of their infants.[16] Dietary fats should not be restricted for children younger than 2 years of age.[7] After that, a prudent diet with recommended levels of fats can be followed.[7]

People afflicted with the eating disorder of anorexia nervosa envision their bodies as being fat, and although they are emaciated, they often focus on their dietary fat consumption. They may reduce dietary fat intake to dangerously low levels through the erroneous belief that fat consumption at *any* kcal level would make them fat.

Among older adults, fear of dietary fat and cholesterol may cause malnutrition. Some older adults have become so focused on the potential negative effects of cholesterol on the health of their hearts that their food intake is overly restrictive of all nutrients. Although our dietary fat and cholesterol intake affects the course of CAD, it is most potent during the early and middle years of adulthood, rather than in the later years of life.

Reduced Intake of Other Nutrients

Even if dietary fat consumption does not result in weight gain, foods high in fat tend not to contain much dietary fiber and may be low in other nutrients. Not consuming enough dietary fiber, as noted in Chapter 4, is a risk factor for several chronic conditions. The seductive nature of foods containing fats may lead us to crave these foods and neglect others. The best guarantee toward achieving the goal of nutritional wellness is to consume a balanced intake of nutrients, based on recommended guidelines, through consumption of at least five to seven servings of naturally low-fat fruits and vegetables per day.

Dietary Fat Intake and Diet-Related Diseases

The presence in the American diet of too much fat is directly related to several chronic diseases such as CAD and certain types of cancer. High-fat diets are indirectly related to type 2 diabetes mellitus and hypertension. Health guidelines to prevent and treat these diseases call for less dietary fat than the average American eats. The Dietary Reference Intake daily recommendations are to eat a total fat intake of 30% or less of kcal, saturated fatty acid less than 10% of kcal, and less than 300 mg of cholesterol.[1] The average intakes of Americans are actually above those levels. Consider how this affects our risk for these diet-related diseases.

Coronary Artery Disease

The relationship between CAD and dietary fat intake, particularly of saturated fats, seems strong. Based on the effects of saturated fat and cholesterol intake on blood cholesterol levels, a high-fat diet is a risk factor for the development of CAD.

Compared with recommended guidelines (see Table 5-3), more than 50% of Americans have high or borderline high blood cholesterol levels.[11] Although a downward trend in blood cholesterol levels is evident, according to National Health and Nutrition Examination Survey III (NHANES III) data collected between 1978 and 1991, an elevated blood cholesterol count is considered a signal for risk of CAD and a potential heart attack, especially when the ratio of LDL to HDL is high.[11] There is good evidence that eating a lot of saturated fat is related to high blood cholesterol and, conversely, eating mostly monounsaturated and polyunsaturated fats is related to low blood cholesterol and low rate of heart disease deaths. Consequently, the National Cholesterol Education Program, Adult Treatment Panel III report focuses on therapeutic lifestyle changes (TLCs) for those most at risk for CAD. Although the general recommendations are to keep saturated fat intake to 10% or less of daily kcal intake, the TLC suggests 7% or less; instead of 300 mg of dietary cholesterol a day, the TLC recommends less than 200 mg.[11] Yet what exactly is the connection between saturated fat and heart disease? Following are suggested steps in the theory linking saturated fat to heart disease:

1. Large amounts of saturated fat produce more LDL to circulate in the blood.
2. The cholesterol carried in the LDL is more likely to be attacked by oxygen, which in turn attracts big scavenger cells called **macrophages**. These cells are able to surround, engulf, and digest microorganisms and cellular debris.
3. The macrophages consume the oxidized material that accumulates in a modified form, called *foam cells.*
4. The foam cells cluster under the lining of the artery wall, forming bulges that cause fatty streaks, which is the first event in plaque formation.
5. The foam cells produce chemicals that further damage the artery wall and cause changes that produce artery-clogging plaque.

Saturated fat started this entire process by requiring too many LDL buses to carry it around.

To reduce the amount of LDL, we should eat less saturated fat. If we eat more saturated fat than we need, the gradual buildup of plaque as atherosclerosis is likely to follow. In addition, some people seem to be more disposed than others to this series of events that lead to atherosclerosis.

An active area of research is whether the oxidation of LDLs can be inhibited or retarded by antioxidants, particularly those derived from diet. Vitamin E, beta carotene, and vitamin C are antioxidants in fruits and vegetables. Because the optimal amount to prevent oxidative damage is unknown and there is evidence that high doses of some antioxidants, particular carotenoids, may be harmful, the safest source is fruits and vegetables rather than supplements. The same goes for reducing homocysteine in the blood. Homocysteine is a compound linked to increased risk of CAD and stroke. High homocysteine levels may be related to low folate and vitamins B_6 and B_{12}. Fruits, vegetables, and low-fat animal products are safe sources of these nutrients.

There is growing evidence that genetic factors may determine who will—and who won't—benefit from dietary changes designed to lower cholesterol. Geneticists have claimed discovery of a gene that could account for the characteristics of what is called an *atherogenic profile,* which describes an estimated 30% of the U.S. population. These characteristics include upper-body obesity, low concentration of HDL, and a preponderance of LDL fatty compounds in the blood.[17] This finding suggests that some people may indeed be predisposed to atherosclerosis and heart disease.

Because we cannot control our heredity, prevention is the main goal for everyone, regardless of genes, to lower the risk factors for atherosclerosis and heart disease that are within our control. High blood cholesterol, especially LDL cholesterol, is one risk factor affected by diet, mainly by reducing total fat intake and particularly saturated fatty acids. Blood cholesterol level is just one of several risk factors. Other widely known risk factors are tobacco, sedentary lifestyle, stress, overweight, alcohol, and hypertension. Experts stress the importance of reducing each risk factor to prevent or reduce the symptoms of heart disease.

Cancer

Since the 1960s a connection between consumption of dietary fat and the development of various cancers was thought to exist. This assumption was based on international comparison studies, which produced incomplete findings because important factors related to cancer initiation were not considered. The relationship between dietary fat intake and cancer development continues to be explored.

Within the past decade, epidemiologic studies have investigated the role of dietary fat and risk of breast cancer development. Overall, the studies did not support a strong positive association between intake of specific types of dietary fat and breast cancer risk, but positive associations of alcohol intake, being overweight, and gaining weight with risk of breast cancer development do appear to exist.[18] Consistent consumption of too many calories tends to result in excess weight. Since dietary fat is higher in calories than other macronutrients, excess caloric intake from any source may explain the inconsistent findings relating dietary fat intake with breast cancer risk.

Although previous view of total dietary fat and saturated fatty acids was thought to increase risk for colorectal cancer

(CRC), review of recent epidemiological studies does not reveal a relationship between animal fat intake and/or animal protein intake and increased risk of CRC.[19]

In the case of prostate cancer, based on international comparisons, genetic factors—rather than diet—appear strong. The different rates of prostate cancer when individuals switch, for example, from an Asian dietary pattern (low in fat) to a Western pattern (higher in animal fat) still supports genetic factors but does show the influence of animal fat or meat-related effects on cancer rates. Although dietary factors such as excessive intake of total calories, meat, dairy products and calcium intake may increase risk, tomatoes/lycopene, cruciferous vegetables (such as broccoli and Brussels sprouts), and fish/marine omega-3 fatty acids may reduce the risk of prostate cancer.[20]

Continued research is needed to accurately determine the association between dietary fat intake and cancer. Recommendations for heart-healthy dietary fat intake (increase PUFAs and monounsaturated fats) should not affect cancer risk but will decrease the risk of heart disease.

Age-Related Macular Degeneration

Age-related macular degeneration (AMD) is a disorder of aging that affects vision. A growing body of evidence from the Women's Health Initiative supports the theory that diets high in total fat and saturated fatty acids may increase the risk of AMD. In contrast, an increased intake of monounsaturated fatty acids may be protective or decrease the risk of AMD.[21]

Type 2 Diabetes Mellitus and Hypertension

Type 2 diabetes mellitus (DM) and hypertension are indirectly related to dietary fat intake. Both of these disorders may stress the circulatory system; a high dietary fat intake may further limit the functioning of the circulatory system through the potential development of atherosclerosis. In addition, these disorders are managed better when weight moderation is achieved; dietary fat reduction may enhance this process. Medical nutritional therapy for these disorders is detailed in Chapters 19, 20, and 22.

TOWARD A POSITIVE NUTRITION LIFESTYLE: GRADUAL REDUCTION

It's the subject of TV situation comedies. One member of the family becomes a health food fanatic, serving blades of grass, sprouts, and weird mixtures of soybeans, nuts, and who knows what. And what is the immediate response of the sitcom family? Disgust and rebellion, of course.

As we make recommendations to our clients to reduce or modify the type of fat intake consumed (and perhaps for ourselves and our families), consider that often the most effective way to achieve permanent change is through gradual reduction. That's the mistake made by the TV character: too many changes made too quickly. An action plan for gradual reduction of dietary fat intake could include the following steps:

1. For 1 week, record all food and beverages consumed.
2. Based on reading this chapter, assess which foods are likely to be high in fat. Particularly note if one high-fat food item, such as whole milk, is consumed often or if a certain meal or snack regularly includes fatty foods. Perhaps scrambled eggs and bacon are eaten almost every morning for breakfast, and an afternoon coffee break always includes either a sweet Danish pastry or a huge, buttery muffin.
3. The next week, choose one item and either reduce consumption or replace it with a lower-fat substitute. Instead of whole milk, use 2% or 1% fat milk, or replace the coffee break treat with an English muffin with a bit of butter or margarine and jelly.
4. The following week, select another food item or meal and make a simple substitution.

This process can continue with small changes—gradual reductions—resulting in major reductions in dietary fat intake.

▮ SUMMARY

Lipids are organic and are composed of carbon, hydrogen, and oxygen. They include fats and fat-related substances divided into three classifications. About 95% of the lipids in foods and in our bodies are in the form of fat as triglycerides, the largest class of lipids. The other two lipid classifications are the fat-related substances of phospholipids and sterols. Lecithin is the best-known phospholipid; cholesterol is the best-known sterol.

The functions of lipids fall into two categories: their food value and their physiologic purposes in the body. Food value functions take into consideration that fat is the densest form of stored energy in both food and in our bodies. Foods containing fat smell and taste good and provide satiety. Fat-soluble nutrients—vitamins A, D, E, K, and linoleic and linolenic fatty acids, the EFAs—are available through foods.

Physiologic functions of stored fat include providing a backup energy supply, cushioning body organs, and serving to regulate body temperature.

Phospholipids are part of body cell membrane structure and serve as emulsifiers. Cholesterol, a sterol, has a role in the formation of bile, vitamin D, sex hormones, and cells in brain and nerve tissue.

Triglycerides are compounds made of three fatty acids and one glycerol molecule. The fatty acids may be saturated, monounsaturated, or polyunsaturated, depending on their number of double bonds. Phospholipids are similar to triglycerides except they have only two fatty acids; the third spot contains a phosphate group. Sterol structures, including cholesterol, are carbon rings intermeshed with side chains of carbon, hydrogen, and oxygen. All three types of lipids can be manufactured in our bodies. The only exceptions are two fatty acids, linolenic and linoleic fatty acids, found in triglycerides; these cannot be formed by the body and are essential nutrients.

Digestion of lipids occurs mainly in the small intestine; absorption depends on the transportation of lipids through the lymph and blood circulatory systems. Lipids travel through the body in lipoprotein packages containing triglycerides, protein, phospholipids, and cholesterol. Lipoproteins differ according to the proportions or ratio of these ingredients. VLDLs, LDLs, and HDLs are found in the blood. Because they contain cholesterol, the levels of LDLs and HDLs may serve as medical markers of one of the risks of CAD.

Health concerns about our dietary fat intake fall into several categories, including appropriate energy intake, reduced intake of other nutrients because of excessive dietary fat consumption, and the relationship between dietary fat intake and diet-related diseases.

THE NURSING APPROACH

Low-Fat Project

In preparation for a new wellness and fitness center on the college campus, the new director surveyed students, faculty, and staff about their needs and interests. Results revealed great interest in nutrition. The director met with a committee of students, faculty, and staff to share ideas and plan possible education and communication about nutrition. Ideas included offering nutrition courses, providing speakers for short education sessions, arranging for consulting dietitians, posting nutrition information near the cafeteria menu, disseminating informative posters prepared by various departments on campus, and creating a website to communicate all health- and fitness-related information.

The first nutrition topic chosen by the committee was eating lower-fat foods. Nursing students were assigned to create posters and contributions for the website. Their task was to identify the following important questions for discussion:

1. Why is it beneficial to reduce total fat intake to about 30% of the daily kcal? How many kcal are produced by 1 g of fat? How many grams of fat are in food commonly consumed?
2. Why should saturated fats be limited to 10% or less of daily kcal? What are the potential harmful effects of saturated fats and cholesterol? Which foods contain saturated fats? Which animal products should be limited?
3. What are trans fats, and what are the disadvantages of consuming them? How can they be avoided? Is butter or margarine healthier?
4. What are common food sources of monounsaturated and polyunsaturated fats? What is the best salad oil? What is the best cooking oil?
5. Why are omega-3 fatty acids health promoting? What are food sources of omega-3 fatty acids? Is it more beneficial to eat fish or to take fish oil supplements?
6. How can a consumer purchase healthy low-fat products? How can one interpret the nutrition label?
7. What lower-fat snacks and desserts can be substituted for high-kcal, high-fat and high-sugar snacks and desserts?
8. Which fast foods and restaurant meals are lower in fat?
9. What are the benefits and drawbacks of artificial fat substitutes?
10. What food preparation techniques are best for low-fat eating? How can recipes be modified to make them lower in fat?
11. What is the plate method? How can this method help with portion control?
12. What websites have good information about lowering fat in the diet?

After identifying these questions, the students organized into groups. Questions were divided and assigned to individual groups. Students researched the answers to the questions and then each group created programming for the center. The resulting programs were reviewed by a subcommittee that then compiled all the programs into a coherent project.

Nursing Diagnoses-Definitions and Classification 2009-2011. Copyright © 2009, 1994-2009 by NANDA International. Used by arrangement with Blackwell Publishing Limited, a company of John Wiley & Sons, Inc.

APPLYING CONTENT KNOWLEDGE

Disease prevention for chronic diet-related diseases depends on changes in lifestyle behaviors. Consider the lifestyle behaviors John Mason could adopt based on his personal history. John Mason is a 20-year-old white male; his mother and father both have high cholesterol levels and family history of CAD. Although John's cholesterol level is average for his age, what three disease prevention strategies could he pursue? Would these strategies be primary, secondary, or tertiary?

WEBSITES OF INTEREST

Center for Science in the Public Interest (CSPI)
www.cspinet.org
Improving the American food supply through educative, legislative, regulatory, and judicial advocacy and by publication of the monthly Nutrition Action Healthletter.

Drive thru Diet
www.wfubmc.edu/Nutrition/Count+Your+Calories/dtd.htm

Provides the nutrient content of menu items from seven fast-food restaurants.

Eating Well On-Line
www.eatingwell.com
Online version of Eating Well: The Magazine of Food and Health on nutrition, food, and low-fat cooking.

REFERENCES

1. Drewnowski A: Sensory control of energy density at different lifestages, *Proc Nutr Soc* 59(2):239-244, 2000.

2. Tso P, Liu M: Ingested fat and satiety, *Physiol Behav* 81(2):275-287, 2004.

3. Jones PJH, Kubow S: Lipids, sterols and their metabolites. In Shils ME, et al, editors: *Modern nutrition in health and disease,* ed 10, Philadelphia, 2006, Lippincott Williams & Wilkins.

4. Harris WS: Fish oils and plasma lipid and lipoprotein metabolism in humans: A critical review, *J Lipid Res* 30:785-807, 1989.

5. Harper CR, Jacobson TA: Usefulness of omega-3 fatty acids and the prevention of coronary heart disease, *Am J Cardiol* 96(11):1521-1529, 2005.

6. Otten JJ, et al, editors: *Dietary DRI References: The essential guide to nutrient requirements,* Washington, DC, 2006, The National Academies Press.

7. Knopp RH, et al: Long-term cholesterol-lowering effects of 4 fat-restricted diets in hypercholesterolemic and combined hyperlipidemic men, *J Am Med Assoc* 278:1509-1515, 1997.

8. Cotton PA, et al: Dietary sources of nutrients among U.S. adults, 1994 to 1996, *J Am Diet Assoc* 104(6):921-930, 2004.

9. Mozaffarian D, Willett WC: Health effects of trans-fatty acids: Experimental and observational evidence, *Eur J Clin Nutr* 63(Suppl 2):s21-s33, 2009.

10. U.S. Food and Drug Administration, CFSAN/Office of Nutritional Products, Labeling, and Dietary Supplements: *Trans fat now listed with saturated fat and cholesterol on the nutrition facts label,* College Park, Md, Updated November 10, 2009, Author. Accessed November 17, 2009, from www.cfsan.fda.gov/~dms/transfat.html.

11. Stone NJ, et al: Recent National Cholesterol Education Program Adult Treatment Panel III update: Adjustments and options, *Am J Cardiol* 96(4A):53E-59E, 2005.

12. Ruxton CH, et al: The impact of long-chain n-3 polyunsaturated fatty acids on human health, *Nutr Res Rev* 18(1 June):113-129, 2005.

13. Position of the American Dietetic Association: Fat replacers, *J Am Diet Assoc* 105:266-275, 2005.

14. Dansinger ML, et al: Comparison of the Atkins, Ornish, Weight Watchers, and Zone diets for weight loss and heart disease risk reduction: A randomized trial, *JAMA* 293(1):43-53, 2005.

15. Antman EM, Sabatine MS: *Cardiovascular Therapeutics—A Companion to Braunwald's Heart Disease,* ed 3, Philadelphia, 2006, Saunders.

16. Krugman SD, Dubowitz H.: Failure to thrive, *Am Fam Physician* 68(5):879-884, 2003.

17. Doney AS, et al: The *FTO* gene is associated with an atherogenic lipid profile and myocardial infarction in patients with Type 2 diabetes, *Circ Cardiovasc Genet* 2:255-259, 2009.

18. Lof M, Weiderpass E: Impact of diet on breast cancer risk, *Curr Opin Obstet Gynecol* 21 (1):80-85, 2009.

19. Ryan-Harshman M, Aldoori W: Diet and colorectal cancer: Review of the evidence, *Can Fam Physician* 53(11):1913-1920, 2007.

20. Alexander DD, et al: Meta-analysis of animal fat or animal protein intake and colorectal cancer, *Am J Clin Nutr* 89(5):1402-1409, 2009.

21. Parekh N, et al: Association between dietary fat intake and age-related macular degeneration in the Carotenoids in Age-Related Eye Disease Study (CAREDS): an ancillary study of the Women's Health Initiative, *Arch Ophthalmol* 127(11):1483-1493, 2009

Protein

*Protein in food is our only source of amino acids, which are absolutely necessary to
make the thousands of proteins that form every aspect of the human body.*

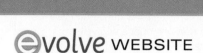 **WEBSITE**

http://evolve.elsevier.com/Grodner/foundations/

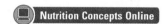 Nutrition Concepts Online

ROLE IN WELLNESS

In 1928 a political slogan promised "a chicken in every pot!"
At that time, being able to afford animal protein on a daily
basis was the mark of a high standard of living and an assurance of good health. Today the phrase might be "Rice and
beans for all of us!" We now know that there are many sources
of protein available in our food supply. Some offer advantages
over others by being lower in fat and higher in other nutrients
such as complex carbohydrates and fiber.

Protein in food is our only source of amino acids, which
are absolutely necessary to make the thousands of proteins
that form every aspect of the human body. No wonder
protein, which is plentiful in our food supply, has gained the
status of a super nutrient for Americans. A common but
inaccurate belief is that we expect that the more protein we
eat, the stronger our immune system will be, the less we will
weigh, and the more muscles we will develop.

Although proteins formed by our bodies do have a role in
those functions, the amounts we consume are often greater
than we need. Awareness of protein sources and portion
sizes is important as we work toward achieving health promotion goals to decrease our risk of diet-related diseases
(Box 6-1).

The five dimensions of health provide ways to think about
the effects of protein consumption. Our overall *physical
health* and well-being depend on our eating enough essential
amino acids for body protein synthesis. The ability to comprehend and apply new approaches to protein consumption
by adapting to different protein sources (e.g., legumes and
grains) and reducing portion sizes depends on our *intellectual
health* capacity to implement change. Protein is a super-
status food for some Americans; favorite sources may provide
emotional health security. Clients needing to make dietary

changes, such as changing to lower-fat sources of protein
(e.g., cutting back on sausages), may need our advice on
coping strategies. Because we and our clients follow different
eating patterns, such as practicing vegetarianism or reducing
consumption of animal protein, family and social dynamics
may be affected when one member changes and thereby tests
our level of *social health*. Religious and *spiritual health* beliefs
lead individuals to nourish their bodies through a harmless
philosophy that views humans as civilized enough to nourish
their bodies without taking life.

STRUCTURE OF PROTEIN

Proteins are organic compounds formed by the linking of
many smaller molecules of amino acids. Amino acids, like
glucose, are organic compounds made of carbon, hydrogen,
and oxygen. However, amino acids also contain nitrogen,
which clearly distinguishes protein from other nutrients.

There are 20 amino acids from which all the proteins that
are required by plants and animals are made. The human
body is able to manufacture some of the amino acids for its
own protein-building function; however, 9 amino acids
cannot be made by the cells of the body. Therefore, these
essential amino acids (EAAs) must be eaten in food, digested,
absorbed, and then brought to cells by circulating blood. The
remaining 11 are non-essential amino acids (NEAAs) (Box
6-2). The liver can create NEAAs as long as structural components, including nitrogen, from other amino acids are
available.

Each cell constructs or synthesizes the proteins it needs.
To build proteins, the cell must have access to all 20 amino
acids. This available supply of amino acids is in the metabolic
amino acid pool. The amino acid pool is a collection of
amino acids that is constantly resupplied with EAAs (from

BOX 6-1   MYPLATE: PROTEN FOODS

The protein group includes not only meat and dry beans or peas but also poultry, fish, eggs, nuts, and seeds, all of which provide protein. Choose lean or low-fat cuts of meat and poultry, trimming fat and removing skin. Some fish (such as tuna, salmon, and trout), nuts, and seeds (walnuts and flax) contain healthy oils and are good sources of omega-3 fatty acids, which may reduce the risk for cardiovascular disease. Other nuts and seeds (almonds, hazelnuts, and sunflower seeds) provide vitamin E. Eating an assortment of protein sources means consuming other valuable nutrients as well.

What Counts as an Ounce?*

The focus of this MyPlate box is on portions of the protein foods group.

In general, 1 ounce of meat, poultry, or fish; $\frac{1}{4}$ cup of cooked dry beans; 1 egg; 1 tbsp of peanut butter; or $\frac{1}{2}$ ounce of nuts or seeds can be considered as 1 ounce-equivalent from the meat and beans group.

PROTEIN SOURCE	AMOUNT THAT COUNTS AS 1 OUNCE-EQUIVALENT IN THE MEAT AND BEANS GROUP	COMMON PORTIONS AND OUNCE-EQUIVALENTS
Meats	1 ounce cooked lean beef 1 ounce cooked lean pork or ham	1 small steak (eye of round, filet) = $3\frac{1}{2}$ to 4 ounce-equivalents 1 small lean hamburger = 2 to 3 ounce-equivalents
Poultry	1 ounce cooked chicken or turkey, without skin 1 sandwich slice of turkey ($4\frac{1}{2} \times 2\frac{1}{2} \times \frac{1}{8}$ inches)	1 small chicken breast half = 3 ounce-equivalents $\frac{1}{2}$ Cornish game hen = 4 ounce-equivalents
Fish	1 ounce cooked fish or shellfish	1 can of tuna, drained = 3 to 4 ounce-equivalents 1 salmon steak = 4 to 6 ounce-equivalents 1 small trout = 3 ounce-equivalents
Eggs	1 egg	
Nuts and seeds	$\frac{1}{2}$ ounce of nuts (12 almonds, 24 pistachios, 7 walnut halves) $\frac{1}{2}$ ounce of seeds (pumpkin, sunflower, or squash seeds, hulled, roasted) 1 Tbsp of peanut butter or almond butter	1 ounce of nuts or seeds = 2 ounce-equivalents
Dry beans and peas	$\frac{1}{4}$ cup of cooked dry beans (such as black, kidney, pinto, or white beans) $\frac{1}{4}$ cup of cooked dry peas (such as chickpeas, cowpeas, lentils, or split peas) $\frac{1}{4}$ cup of baked beans, refried beans $\frac{1}{4}$ cup (~2 ounces) of tofu 1 ounce tempeh, cooked $\frac{1}{4}$ cup of roasted soybeans 1 falafel patty ($2\frac{1}{4}$ inches, 4 ounces) 2 Tbsp hummus	1 cup split pea soup = 2 ounce-equivalents 1 cup lentil soup = 2 ounce-equivalents 1 cup bean soup = 2 ounce-equivalents 1 soy or bean burger patty = 2 ounce-equivalents

*Accessed June 14, 2012, from www.choosemyplate.gov/food-groups/protein-foods-counts.html.

BOX 6-2   AMINO ACIDS

ESSENTIAL AMINO ACIDS	NONESSENTIAL AMINO ACIDS
Histidine	Alanine
Isoleucine	Arginine
Leucine	Aspartic acid
Lysine	Cysteine
Methionine	Cystine
Phenylalanine	Glutamic acid
Threonine	Glutamine
Tryptophan	Glycine
Valine	Proline
	Serine
	Tyrosine

dietary intake) and NEAAs (synthesized in the liver). The pool allows the cell to build proteins easily.

Protein Composition

The functions of proteins are closely related to their structures. The complex composition of proteins is best understood through four structural levels: primary, secondary, tertiary, and quaternary[1] (Figure 6-1).

The primary structure of protein composition is determined by the number, assortment, and sequence of amino acids in polypeptide chains. Amino acids are linked together by peptide bonds to form a practically unlimited number of proteins. The peptide bond occurs at the point at which the carboxyl group of one amino acid is bound to the amino group of another amino acid (Figure 6-2).

The 20 amino acids form chains that may contain any combination or assortment of amino acids. This allows for

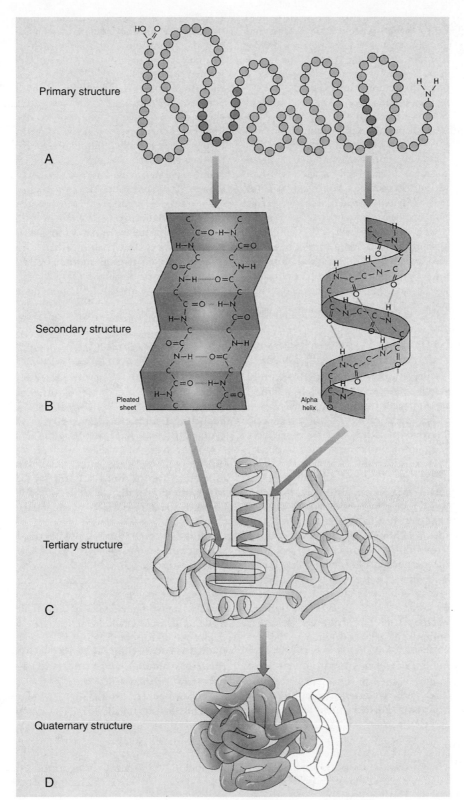

FIG 6-1 Structural levels of protein. A, Primary structure: determined by number, kind, and sequence of amino acids in the chain. **B,** Secondary structure: hydrogen bonds stabilize folds of helical spirals. **C,** Tertiary structure: globular shape maintained by strong intramolecular bonding and by stabilizing hydrogen bonds. **D,** Quaternary structure: results from bonding between more than one polypeptide unit. (Courtesy Bill Ober. In Thibodeau GA, Patton KT: *Anatomy & physiology,* ed 4, St Louis, 1999, Mosby.)

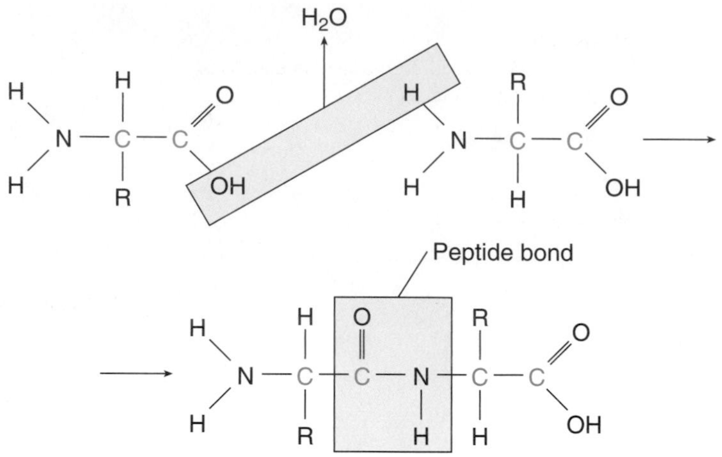

FIG 6-2 Peptide bonds.

thousands of different proteins to be formed. Two proteins may contain the same assortment and number of amino acids yet still have different functions because of the sequencing or order of the amino acids.

The secondary structure level of proteins affects the shape of the chain of amino acids; they may be straight, folded, or coiled. The tertiary structure results when the polypeptide chain is so coiled that the loops of the coil touch, forming strong bonds within the chain itself. The quaternary structural level is proteins containing more than one polypeptide chain.

A protein may not be able to perform its original function if its structure or shape changes. The shape may be changed by heat (cooking), ultraviolet light (exposure to sunlight), acids (vinegar), alcohol, and mechanical action. A protein has been denatured and physically changed when the shape of a protein is affected (e.g., a folded chain unfolding).

An example of denaturing a food protein is the change that occurs when the white of an uncooked egg (a clear liquid) is beaten. The clear liquid turns white, foamy, and stiff. Although the protein in the egg has been denatured, it is still a valuable source of amino acids. The amino acids are not affected; only the shape of the chain has been changed.

Inside the body, denaturing of proteins is controlled by mechanisms that keep the internal body environment from getting too basic or too acidic. Either extreme can lead to the denaturation of vital proteins within the body. Body temperature also affects the protein structure of the body. High fevers can become lethal when protein structures within the body become denatured. When body proteins are denatured, they cannot perform their original functions.

Although uncontrolled denaturation can be dangerous, it is helpful for digestion. Denaturing changes the three-dimensional structure of a protein, providing more surface area on which digestive juices act to release the amino acids of the food proteins.

PROTEIN AS A NUTRIENT IN THE BODY

The proteins we consume in foods are not the same proteins used by our bodies. Actually, the only nutrient role protein

in foods serves is to provide amino acids, the building blocks of all proteins.

Digestion and Absorption

Because of the complex structure of proteins, a number of protein enzymes, or **proteases**, produced by the stomach and pancreas are required to hydrolyze proteins into smaller and smaller peptides until individual amino acids are ready for absorption (Figure 6-3).

Mouth

Only mechanical digestion of protein occurs in the mouth. Mastication breaks protein-containing food into smaller pieces that mix with saliva passing through to the stomach.

Stomach

Pepsinogen, an inactive form of the gastric protease **pepsin,** is secreted by the stomach mucosa. Pepsin becomes activated when it mixes with hydrochloric acid (HCl), also produced by stomach secretions. Pepsin then begins the process of protein hydrolysis, breaking the bonds linking the amino acids of the protein peptide bonds. The result is smaller-sized polypeptides rather than single amino acids or dipeptides. The polypeptides pass through to the small intestine for further hydrolysis.

Rennin, an important gastric protease, is produced only during infancy. It functions with calcium to thicken or coagulate the milk protein casein; this slows the movement of milk nutrients from the stomach, allowing additional digestion time.[2]

Small Intestine

In the small intestine, pancreatic and intestinal proteases continue the hydrolysis of polypeptides. As these smaller peptides touch the intestinal walls, peptidases are released that complete the hydrolysis of protein into absorbable units of individual amino acids and dipeptides.

The primary pancreatic enzyme is **trypsin**. It is first secreted as trypsinogen, an inactive form. The intestinal hormone enteropeptidase activates trypsinogen into trypsin,

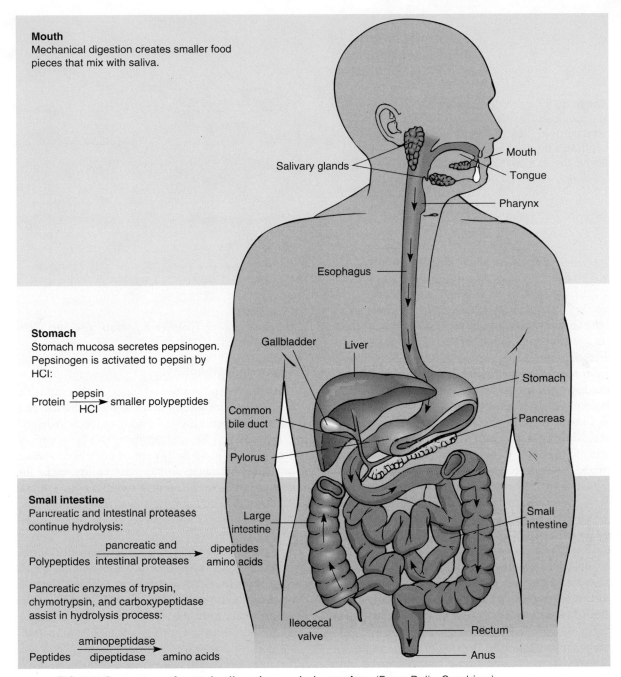

Mouth
Mechanical digestion creates smaller food pieces that mix with saliva.

Stomach
Stomach mucosa secretes pepsinogen. Pepsinogen is activated to pepsin by HCl:

$$\text{Protein} \xrightarrow[\text{HCl}]{\text{pepsin}} \text{smaller polypeptides}$$

Small intestine
Pancreatic and intestinal proteases continue hydrolysis:

$$\text{Polypeptides} \xrightarrow[\text{intestinal proteases}]{\text{pancreatic and}} \begin{array}{c}\text{dipeptides}\\\text{amino acids}\end{array}$$

Pancreatic enzymes of trypsin, chymotrypsin, and carboxypeptidase assist in hydrolysis process:

$$\text{Peptides} \xrightarrow[\text{dipeptidase}]{\text{aminopeptidase}} \text{amino acids}$$

Salivary glands — Mouth
Tongue
Pharynx
Esophagus
Gallbladder   Liver
Stomach
Common bile duct
Pancreas
Pylorus
Large intestine
Small intestine
Ileocecal valve
Rectum
Anus

FIG 6-3 Summary of protein digestion and absorption. (From Rolin Graphics.)

which continues the hydrolysis of polypeptides. Two other pancreatic enzymes assist in the hydrolysis process: **chymotrypsin** hydrolyzes polypeptides into dipeptides, and **carboxypeptidase** breaks polypeptides and dipeptides into amino acids. Two intestinal peptidases are **aminopeptidase**, which releases free amino acids from the amino end of short-chain peptides, and **dipeptidase**, which completes the hydrolysis of proteins to amino acids.

Absorption of amino acids occurs through the intestinal walls by means of competitive active transport that requires vitamin B_6 (pyridoxine) as a carrier. Because amino acids are water soluble, they easily pass into the bloodstream.

Metabolism

To understand the importance of protein metabolism in the growth and maintenance of the body, consider that most protein functions are a result of protein anabolism (synthesis) in cells. Hormones have a major role in the regulation of protein metabolism. Anabolism is enhanced by the effect of growth hormone (from the pituitary gland) and the male hormone testosterone. Hormones affecting the catabolism (break down) of proteins are the glucocorticoids that are enhanced by adrenocorticotropic hormone (ACTH); these hormones are secreted from the adrenal cortex. This process releases proteins in the cells to break down to amino acids,

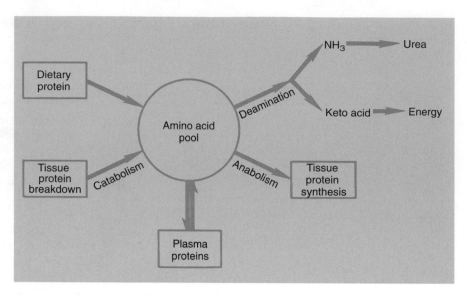

FIG 6-4 The body's equilibrium depends on a balance between the rates of protein breakdown (catabolism) and protein synthesis (anabolism). (Modified from Williams SR: *Essentials of nutrition and diet therapy,* ed 7, St Louis, 1999, Mosby.)

and then the amino acids travel in the bloodstream, contributing to an available pool of amino acids (Figure 6-4).

The liver cells begin the process of catabolism through deamination. **Deamination** results in an amino acid (NH_2) group breaking off from an amino acid molecule, resulting in one molecule each of ammonia (NH_3) and a keto acid. Liver cells convert most of the ammonia to urea, which is later excreted in urine. The keto acid may enter the tricarboxylic acid (TCA) cycle to be used for energy (see Figure 9-2) or, through gluconeogenesis and lipogenesis, be converted to glucose and fat[1] (see Figure 6-4).

Protein Excess

An excessive intake of protein results in increased deamination by the liver. The increased deamination may result in high levels of keto acids, possibly putting the body into a state of ketosis. The increased urea is excreted by the kidneys. Because the liver and kidneys are involved with the deamination process, the increased stress on the organs could initiate an underlying disorder of these organs. Because there are no definitive benefits of excessive protein intake, the general recommendation is to consume no more than twice the Recommended Dietary Allowance (RDA) for protein.

In fact, the source of excess protein may be a health concern. Animal-derived protein sources such as meats may also be high in saturated fat and cholesterol. This may increase the risk of coronary artery disease (CAD) and some cancers. The relationship between protein intake and osteoporosis also has been considered. When protein intake is high, there is a slight increase of calcium excretion from the body, but calcium absorption is not affected. Studies have yielded mixed results about this effect on the risk of osteoporosis. Because osteoporosis is multifactorial, this specific relationship is difficult to determine. Recommendations to consume moderate amounts of protein and to meet the new Dietary Reference Intake (DRI) levels for calcium are the best dietary approaches to decrease the risk of CAD

and cancer. (See Chapter 8 for an in-depth discussion of osteoporosis.)

Nitrogen Balance

Nitrogen-balance studies are used to determine the protein requirements of the body throughout the life cycle and to assign value to the protein quality of foods to determine their biologic value.[2] Because nitrogen (N) is a primary component of protein, the body's use of protein can be determined by nitrogen-balance studies that compare the amount of nitrogen entering the body in food protein with the nitrogen lost from the body in feces and urine.

Nitrogen lost or excreted from the body may be endogenous nitrogen (from catabolism of body protein), metabolic nitrogen (from intestinal cells), or exogenous nitrogen (from dietary proteins). Nitrogen in feces may be metabolic and exogenous (from cells and dietary proteins) and in urine may be endogenous (catabolism of body protein) and exogenous (from dietary proteins).

An individual is in nitrogen equilibrium or zero nitrogen balance if the amount of nitrogen consumed in foods equals the amount excreted. This occurs in normal, healthy adults when nitrogen in food protein entering (input) the body equals the nitrogen leaving the body (output). Because adults are no longer growing, the nitrogen that enters the body is not needed to build new tissue but is used simply to maintain the body.

Positive nitrogen balance occurs when more nitrogen is retained in the body than excreted. The nitrogen is used to form new cells for growth or healing. This occurs in growing children and in pregnant women who require additional nitrogen (and protein) for the growth of the fetus. Individuals recovering from illness or injury may be in positive nitrogen balance as the body heals. Negative nitrogen balance happens when more nitrogen is excreted from the body than is retained from dietary protein sources. This occurs when there is a breakdown of proteins within the body, such as in muscles and organs. Negative nitrogen balance may be caused by aging, physical illness, extreme stress, starvation, surgery, or eating disorders.

FUNCTIONS

Proteins created in our bodies perform numerous functions, including the following:

- Growth and maintenance
- Creation of communicators and catalysts
- Immune system response
- Fluid and electrolyte regulation
- Acid-base balance
- Transportation

Growth and Maintenance

Each body cell contains proteins. All growth depends on a sufficient supply of amino acids. The amino acids are needed to make the proteins required to support muscle, tissue, bone formation, and the cells themselves.

Maintaining our bodies also requires a constant supply of amino acids. There is a continual turnover of body cells, which are composed of protein. The cells break down and must immediately be replaced. Each replacement cell requires the formation of additional protein.

Also needed for growth and maintenance is the protein collagen, found throughout the body. Collagen forms connective tissues such as ligaments and tendons and acts as a glue to keep the walls of the arteries intact. In addition, collagen has a role in bone and tooth formation by forming the framework structure that is then filled with minerals such as calcium and phosphorus. Synthesis of scar tissue also depends on collagen. Other structures such as hair, nails, and skin are composed of similar protein substances.

Creation of Communicators and Catalysts

Many vital substances produced by our bodies are formed of protein. Some hormones are proteins. Hormones act as communicators to alert different parts of the body to changes or to regulate functions of organs. Insulin, a hormone that directs cells to take in glucose, is a protein. Enzymes are also proteins. Enzymes are catalysts that enable chemical reactions or biologic changes to occur within the body. Each enzyme has a specific target; consequently, numerous enzymes are continually formed.

Blood clotting depends on protein substances as well. Twelve blood clotting factors must be in place for blood to clot when injury has occurred; several of the factors, such as fibrogen, are composed of protein.

Immune System Response

The defense system of our bodies depends on proteins produced in response to foreign viruses and bacteria that invade our bodies. The proteins, or antibodies, are specific to each intruder. If sufficient levels of amino acids are not available to form these antibodies, we may have difficulties maintaining our health. Our overall immunologic response—our resistance to disease—depends on proteins formed within our bodies.

Fluid and Electrolyte Regulation

Water is balanced among three compartments in the body: intravascular (within veins and arteries), intracellular (inside cells), and interstitial (between cells). Proteins and minerals attract water, creating osmotic pressure. As proteins circulate through our bodies, they maintain body fluid and electrolyte balance by keeping water appropriately divided among the three compartments.

Acid-Base Balance

Some reactions occurring within the body lead to the release of acidic substances; others cause basic matter to enter the fluids of the body. Blood proteins can buffer the effects of fluids to maintain a safe acidic level in body fluids. The ability of protein to regulate the balance between the acidic and base characteristics of fluids is called the *buffering effect* of protein. Because the chemical structure of amino acids combines an acid (the carboxyl group [COOH]) and base (amine), an amino acid can function either as an acid or a base depending on the pH of its medium. This is why the buffering effect of blood proteins is possible. This function is crucial to protect all proteins in the body. If fluids become either too acidic or too basic, the shape of proteins is altered or denatured. Denatured proteins are not able to perform their usual functions.

Many of the constituents of blood are protein based, and if protein functions are affected, the result can be lethal. Therefore proteins maintain a delicate pH level to ensure the proper functioning of all body systems (Box 6-3).

Transportation

Throughout our bodies, proteins are able to transport nutrients and other vital substances. For individual cells, proteins act as pumps, assisting the movement of nutrients in and out of cells. Many nutrients, including lipids, minerals, vitamins, and electrolytes, are carried in the blood by proteins such as lipoproteins. This allows the nutrients to be available to all parts of the body. Hemoglobin, a special carrier composed of protein, transports oxygen in the blood. Oxygen is stored in our muscles in another protein carrier, myoglobin. These protein carriers, hemoglobin and myoglobin, are essential for a well-functioning body.

FOOD SOURCES

Quality of Protein Foods

The proteins in foods are categorized by the EAAs they contain. **Complete protein** contains all nine EAAs in sufficient quantities that best support growth and maintenance of our bodies. Animal-derived foods, including meat, poultry, fish, eggs, and most dairy products, contain complete protein. (A notable exception is gelatin, which is incomplete.) Soybeans are the only plant source that provide all nine essential

---

BOX 6-3   GENETIC DISORDERS

Phenylketonuria (PKU) is a genetic disorder with a protein link. This disorder is characterized by the inability to use or break down excess phenylalanine, an essential amino acid. The excess phenylalanine circulating inside the body can cause various health problems. Infants with this disorder consume low-phenylalanine formulas, whereas children and adults follow a limited protein diet to control the intake of phenylalanine.

Another genetic protein disorder is sickle cell disease, which affects the shape of red blood cells. Because of abnormalities of the hemoglobin molecule, the red blood cell is curved or sickle shaped rather than round. The sickle shape can cause these blood cells to clog small blood vessels. This can be painful, may cause damage to internal organs such as the kidneys and heart, and may lead to frequent infections throughout the body. Early screening followed by long-term penicillin treatment can prevent secondary infections.

Having the sickle cell disease trait is not the same as having the disease itself. Both parents have to have the trait for a child to be at risk. Even then, there is only a 25% chance of developing the disorder. Sickle cell disease may occur in any ethnic group, but it is more common among Africans and African Americans; some states screen all infants to determine susceptibility.

BOX 6-4   SOURCES OF COMPLETE AND INCOMPLETE PROTEINS

Foods Containing Complete Proteins
Fish
Shellfish
Chicken
Turkey
Duck*
Beef*
Lamb*
Pork*
Eggs*
Soybeans (tofu)
Cheese
   Hard cheeses
      Cheddar
      Muenster
      Swiss
   Soft cheeses
      Cottage cheese[†]
      Ricotta[†]
Milk[†]
Ice milk/reduced-fat ice cream
Yogurt[†]
Frozen yogurt

Foods Containing Incomplete Proteins
Cereals
   Ready-to-eat
   Oatmeal
   Wheatena
Grains
   Wheat
   Rice
   Corn
   Oats/oatmeal
   Barley
   Spaghetti/pasta
   Bagels
   Bread
Legumes
   Black-eyed peas
   Lentils
   Beans
   Peanuts/peanut butter
   Chickpeas
   Split peas
Broccoli
Potatoes
Green peas
Leafy green vegetables

*Possible high-fat source of protein.
[†]Protein in skim, 2%, and whole-milk products.

---

amino acids. Foods that contribute the best balance of EAAs and the best assortment of NEAAs for protein synthesis and are easily digestible are **high-quality protein** foods. The two highest-quality protein foods are eggs and human milk. The egg is of high quality because it contains all the necessary nutrients to support life. Human breast milk is the perfect food; its nutrient profile is ideal for human growth.

Incomplete protein lacks one or more of the nine essential amino acids. These proteins will not provide a sufficient supply of amino acids and will not support life (Box 6-4). Many plant foods contain considerable amounts of incomplete proteins. Some of the better sources are grains and legumes.

The EAAs that those incomplete proteins lack are called **limiting amino acids.** The limiting amino acid reduces the value of the protein contained in the food. Unless the limiting amino acid is consumed in other foods, the amino acid pools inside the cells would be missing some of the essential amino acids. Protein production within the cell would be affected, and fewer proteins could be formed. Consequently, limiting amino acids reduces the number of proteins our bodies can make. Generally, we consume a sufficient mix of complete and incomplete proteins; therefore, this is not a health problem. Only those who adopt a dietary pattern restricting certain types of protein foods are at risk for an imbalanced intake.

Complementary Proteins

By eating different kinds of plant foods throughout the day, the total protein intake will equal that of complete proteins found in animal-related products. The advantages to complementary proteins are that plant foods cost less and tend to contain less fat; consuming less dietary fat is a prevention strategy for several chronic diet-related diseases.

A balance of amino acids is required throughout the day for protein synthesis. A sufficient assortment of EAAs is

BOX 6-5	FOOD COMBINATIONS THAT PROVIDE COMPLETE PROTEINS

Grains + Legumes = Complete Protein
Peanut butter sandwich
Tacos with refried beans
Rice and beans
Split pea soup with croutons
Falafel (chickpea balls) on pita bread
Lentil soup with rye bread
Baked beans with bread

Grains or Legumes + Animal Protein (Small Amount) = Complete Protein
Chili with beans and cornbread
Ready-to-eat cereal with skim milk
Cheese sandwich
Pasta with cheese
Rice pudding
French toast
Pancakes (made with milk and/or eggs)
Tuna casserole

$$PER = \frac{\text{Weight gain}}{\text{Protein intake}}$$

Protein RDA

The RDA for protein provides for sufficient intake of the EAAs and enough total protein to provide the amino groups needed to build new NEAAs. Other factors that affect the RDA for protein are age, gender, physiologic state, and sources of protein.[3]

Age affects protein requirements because when growth occurs, such as during childhood, a greater percentage of dietary intake of protein is needed compared with adulthood. Growth results in additional muscle and tissues, all of which require the amino acids contained in dietary protein. Theoretically, older adults may require lower levels of protein because muscle mass is reduced as we age; protein use may also be affected by variables of decreased physical activity, illness, and chronic use of medications. However, few studies exist to confirm a lower requirement, so the protein RDA for adults aged 50 and over is the same as for younger adults.[3] Gender differences also affect protein needs. Men tend to have more lean body mass or muscle than women. Lean body mass requires more protein for maintenance (see the *Health Debate* box, Amino Acid Supplements).

Certain physiologic states, such as pregnancy and lactation, require different amounts of nutrients. Pregnant women should consume additional protein to meet the needs of the growing fetus, as well as those of their own bodies. RDA recommendations for protein are 25 g protein/day higher for pregnant women (71 g). Lactation, the production of breast milk, also requires consumption of additional protein. Breast milk contains high-quality protein that is formed from amino acids provided by the woman. The protein RDA for lactation is the same as for pregnancy (71 g). Special circumstances of serious physical illness, wound healing, fevers (increased metabolic rate), or unusual stress may also increase protein needs.

The type of food source also affects the amount of protein needed. In the United States most of the protein eaten is complete protein from animal sources. These sources are considered when the RDA for protein is set. Other countries rely on more plant sources of incomplete proteins, so worldwide recommendations, such as those of the World Health Organization, differ from the U.S. guidelines.

The RDA for protein is 0.8 g/kg (or 2.2 pounds). For an average adult man, the RDA is 58 to 63 g; for an average adult woman, the RDA is 46 to 50 g (see the RDA table inside the front cover). Recent research suggests that recommended levels for athletes are 1.2 to 1.7 g protein/kg body weight, depending on whether a sport requires endurance or strength.[4] Because most Americans eat more protein than recommended, even athletes tend to easily meet protein recommendations.[4] Determine your recommended protein intake using the formula in the *Teaching Tool* box, Calculating Your Recommended Protein Intake.

provided without planning if both animal and plant protein foods are eaten. If animal foods are not eaten, more care is required to ensure that limiting amino acids are consumed. Combinations of plant foods that provide all the EAAs are grains (e.g., wheat or rice) with legumes (e.g., kidney beans or chickpeas) and grains or legumes with small amounts of animal protein from dairy, meat, poultry, or fish (Box 6-5).

Measures of Food Protein Quality

Many foods contain protein, but the value of specific foods as protein sources varies. Perhaps the protein contained is incomplete or is difficult to digest (bound tightly to fiber). If food proteins are not digested, the amino acids can't be absorbed to nourish our bodies.

Several methods are used to analyze the quality of proteins in food, including biologic value, amino acid score, and protein efficiency ratio. Biologic value measures how much nitrogen from a protein food is retained by the body after digestion, absorption, and excretion. This measurement of nitrogen balance reveals how available the protein of that food is to the human body. An egg has the highest reference protein score of 100; all of the egg protein can be used. It has become a standard against which all other food proteins are judged. Fish has a score of 75 to 90, and corn, which contains protein but also has lower amino acid ratios, has a score of 40.[2]

The amino acid score is a simple measure of the amino acid composition of a food as compared with a reference protein. The score is based on the limiting amino acid of the food. Digestibility of the protein is not considered.

A third method for assessing protein quality is protein efficiency ratio (PER). Using this method, rats are fed a set amount of protein and then, based on weight gain, the physiologic value of the food protein consumed is determined:[2]

HEALTH DEBATE

Amino Acid Supplements

Bodybuilders focus on muscles, muscles, muscles! Unfortunately, many believe that because protein loss occurs during strength and endurance exercise and muscles are composed of protein, excessive amounts of protein must be eaten. However, a moderate increase of dietary protein is indicated. Because most Americans eat significantly higher amounts of protein than the RDA, this additional need is most likely consumed. In any event, simply eating extra protein does not build muscles. It is only working a muscle that will cause it to develop and strengthen, along with the provision of adequate protein.

There is also a mistaken belief that certain NEAAs, such as arginine and ornithine, should be taken as supplements. The perception is that they have special abilities to enhance muscle development. However, studies show that amino acids taken as supplements are ineffective for increasing lean body mass.

When ingested, these supplements are treated as any other protein source of amino acids. Too much of any one may prevent absorption—and result in a deficiency—of another because they compete for the same absorption sites. Once a supplement is absorbed, the liver views any protein supplement as a source of amino acids. The supplemental amino acids will not necessarily be directed to muscle development. They may just be converted to other NEAAs. Or if too much protein or too few kcal are consumed, amino acids will be used for energy immediately or stored as body fat.

Some bodybuilders also use drugs illegally to pump up muscles. These drugs, such as anabolic steroids, produce dangerous emotional and physical side effects. Amino acid supplements that are perceived to build muscles, although ineffective, are less dangerous than steroids. Should this misperception continue to be fostered as a safer option? Should bodybuilders use drugs at all? What do you think?

Data from: Armsey TD, Green GA: Nutrition supplements: Science vs. hype, *Physician Sportsmed* 25(6):1, 77-92. 1997. Lambert CP et al: Macronutrient considerations for the sport of bodybuilding, *Sports Med* 34(5):317-327, 2004; and Williams MH: Facts and fallacies of purported ergogenic amino acids supplements, *Clin Sports Med* 18(3):633-649, 1999.

TEACHING TOOL

Calculating Your Recommended Protein Intake

To determine your personal protein recommendation, compute the following:
1. Divide your body weight by 2.2 to determine your weight in kilograms (kg).
2. Weight in lb ÷ 2.2 = Weight in kg
Example:
   140 ÷ 2.2 = 63.63 kg
3. Multiply the kilogram weight by 0.8 g/kg to determine your protein RDA (i.e., weight in kg × 0.8 g/kg = g of protein/RDA).
Example:
   63.5 kg × 0.8 g/kg = 50.9 g protein/RDA

TABLE 6-1	VEGETARIAN CATEGORIES	
Vegan	Includes all plant foods (grains, legumes, fruits, vegetables, seeds, and nuts)	Excludes all animal-derived foods
Lacto-vegetarian	Includes all plant foods plus dairy products (milk, cheese, yogurt, and butter)	Excludes animal meat (meat, fowl, and fish) and eggs
Ovo-lacto vegetarian	Includes all plant foods, dairy products, and eggs	Excludes animal meat
Pescetarian	Includes all plant foods, dairy products, eggs, and fish	Excludes meat and fowl
Flexitarian	Includes all plant foods, dairy, and eggs with occasional consumption of meat, fowl, or fish	No exclusions but minimal consumption of animal meat

The Acceptable Macronutrient Distribution Ranges (AMDRs) suggest that protein consumption range between 10% and 35% of energy intake. Depending on the percentage of protein energy consumed, consumption of energy from carbohydrates and lipids should be adjusted accordingly.[3]

VEGETARIANISM

Vegetarianism, particularly veganism, has recently gained more acceptance as awareness grows of the values resulting from plant-based food plans. Advantages include health benefits such as reduced risk of diet-related disorders, protection of environmental resources, and recognition for the ethical treatment of animals, including avoiding the use of hormones and antibiotics to enhance animal food production.[5] Instead of animal protein sources, vegetarian dietary categories focus on plant proteins to provide EAAs (Table 6-1). The **vegan dietary pattern** consists of only plant foods, including grains, legumes, fruits, vegetables, seeds, and nuts; no animal-derived products are eaten. The **lacto-vegetarian dietary pattern** is a food plan composed of only plant foods plus dairy products. It contains all the vegan foods plus dairy products such as milk, cheese, yogurt, and butter. The **ovo-lacto vegetarian dietary pattern** or food plan is comprised of plant foods plus dairy products and eggs. This pattern incorporates eggs into the lacto-vegetarian assortment of foods.

The Benefits of Vegetarianism

Vegetarian dietary patterns may be followed to achieve health, spiritual, economic, and/or environmental benefits. When well planned, vegetarian dietary patterns result in health benefits that are similar to those of a low-fat, high-fiber diet and consist of reduced risk of obesity, CAD, type 2 diabetes mellitus, hypertension, gastrointestinal disorders, and certain cancers such as lung and colorectal cancers.[6]

Because animal foods are our primary source of saturated fat and our only source of cholesterol, plant-based vegetarian dietary patterns tend to be lower in total fat and cholesterol. This reduced intake, combined with the high fiber content of plant foods, often results in lower blood cholesterol levels. Other nutrients that are usually higher in vegan diets are magnesium, folic acid, vitamins C and E iron, and phytochemicals.[5] In addition, the body weight of individuals following vegetarian dietary patterns is generally lower. This also reduces the risk of developing hypertension and diabetes.

The spiritual rationale for some individuals who are vegetarians is based on the belief in nonharming. Several religions, including Hinduism and Seventh-Day Adventists, see the consumption of animal flesh as being unhealthy or polluting to the body. Other vegetarians do not follow a formal religion but believe strongly in the protection of animal rights and are opposed to the slaughter of animals for human consumption. Information about the treatment of animals before and during the slaughtering process is now more available to the public because of increased exposure through Internet videos and websites.

The economic approach addresses the belief that animal-related products cost more than plant protein foods, not only financially but in terms of costs to our natural environment as well. Livestock and other domesticated animals are inefficient producers of protein. Although protein foods from cattle and chicken are of high quality, many pounds of grains are used by these animals to produce one pound of edible food. Some people maintain that by eating from lower on the food chain—that is, eating more plant foods—there will be less waste and limited environmental impact on our natural resources.

The Drawbacks of Vegetarianism

The vegetarian dietary pattern has several drawbacks. The most critical affects vegans. The vegan dietary pattern can provide all the essential nutrients except vitamins D and B_{12}, calcium, and omega-3 fatty acids. These will need to be consumed through carefully selected fortified foods or consumption of supplements as needed.[5]

Most dietary vitamin D is consumed through milk fortified with the vitamin. Because vegans do not consume any dairy products, this source of vitamin D is diminished. However, vitamin D is available through synthesis during exposure of the skin to direct sunlight, but many individuals (even those consuming a traditional animal-derived intake) have inadequate levels of vitamin D and should rely on vitamin D–fortified foods or supplements. Factors such as regional limitation to sun exposure, darker skin pigmentation, elderly, cultural clothing customs that conceal the body, and regular use of sunscreen increase the risk of vitamin D deficiency for children and adults vegans.[5]

Worldwide, vitamin D deficiency and increased incidences of rickets are occurring; vegetarianism is a potential risk factor.[7] In the United States, a disproportionate number of cases of nutrition-related rickets occurs among young breast-fed African American children. When transition from breast milk to solid foods takes place, emphasis should be on good food sources of vitamin D and calcium.[8]

Reliable sources of vitamin B_{12} are all animal related. By excluding animal-derived foods, including milk, sources of B_{12} are simply not available. Even ovo-lacto vegetarians may have low levels of vitamin B_{12}. Symptoms of vitamin B_{12} deficiency take years to appear and may cause permanent damage to the central nervous system. Individuals who restrict their intake or exclude animal foods should take B_{12} supplements or consume foods fortified with vitamin B_{12} such as fortified soy milk to ensure adequate intake.[6]

Other nutrients for which vegans could be deficient are iron and zinc, minerals usually consumed in meat, fish, and poultry. Calcium levels may also be low if dairy products are excluded; few plants are good sources of calcium. These nutrients are available in a well-planned vegan diet of whole foods. Nonetheless, care must be taken to consume sufficient amounts of calcium during pregnancy and growth periods; supplements will be necessary. If the vegan dietary pattern is poorly implemented and depends on refined and processed foods, nutrients may be lacking.

Another drawback pertains to the dimension of social health. Social health is the ability to interact with people in an acceptable manner and to sustain relationships with family members, friends, and colleagues. Those following a vegetarian dietary pattern often find themselves rationalizing their behaviors to others. It can sometimes be tricky to do so without alienating others—especially while seated at a steak dinner. Perhaps the simplest approach is to emphasize the health benefits gained by adopting a vegetarian dietary pattern.

Ensuring that a vegetarian dietary pattern is healthful necessitates learning about protein complementing and new ways of preparing meatless dishes. Simply replacing meat with a lot of cheese won't result in any health benefits. In fact, the fat content of a cheese dish is probably higher than a lean meat dish. The most helpful approach is to read vegetarian cookbooks that not only provide recipes but also include vegetarian nutrition information. MyPyramid includes support for vegetarian dietary patterns. The food group recommendations for age, sex, and activity levels provide adequate energy and nutrient intake for vegetarianism if a variety of nutrient-dense foods are chosen. Guidance is available at the MyPyramid website (www.mypyramid.gov).

Contemporary Vegetarianism

Other terms have evolved to describe semivegetarian dietary patterns. The most inclusive term is the *flexitarianism* approach. Flexitarians primarily consume vegetarian foods with occasional meat, chicken, or fish consumption. This pattern enables an individual to decrease meat consumption without total elimination. Another approach is *pescetarian,*

🌐 CULTURAL CONSIDERATIONS

Rituals for Animal-Derived Protein

Most religions identify foods with specific holidays and rules regarding consumption. Two predominantly Western religions, Judaism and Islam, have rules regarding the daily preparation and consumption of foods; most of these directions focus on consumption of animal-derived protein foods.

Kashrut, Jewish Dietary Laws

The rules of *kashrut* were presented in the Torah, or bible of the Jewish people. *Kosher* means "fit" and is the concept referring to the Jewish dietary laws. Although most of the rules can be explained on the basis of physical health benefits, the foundation and observance of the restrictions are because of spiritual health rather than physical. By observing the kosher dietary laws, one is respecting God, oneself, and other Jews. There are about eight laws regarding consumption of animal-derived protein. They are briefly described as follows:

1. Only certain animals may be eaten. Only mammals with cloven hooves that chew the cud may be eaten and their milk consumed; this allows cattle, deer, goats, and sheep to be consumed but not pigs. Birds must also meet specific criteria; acceptable birds (and their eggs) include chickens, ducks, geese, and turkey. In addition, fish must have fins and scales to be consumed; therefore all shellfish, eel, and catfish are not permitted. Acceptable foods are viewed as coming from "clean" animals and unacceptable foods are viewed as "unclean."

2. Animals must be slaughtered in a specific manner that is quick and painless and that causes most blood to drain from the carcass.

3. Slaughtered animals must be free of any bruises or diseases to be consumed.

4. Only certain parts of permitted animals may be consumed. Animal blood from any animal and layers of solid fat may not be consumed.

5. Meat must be prepared for consumption in specific procedures. Blood must be completely drained and cuts of meat must avoid certain nerves and animal parts. Specially trained "kosher" butchers prepare animals foods according to kashrut.

6. Meat and dairy are not consumed together. Consequently, separate cooking utensils, plates, and eating utensils are maintained for meat consumption and dairy consumption. Some foods are considered neither meat nor dairy and may be eaten with either category. These foods are called *pareve*.

7. Products from unclean animals may not be consumed. The exception is honey. Although bees may not be consumed, honey is acceptable.

8. Foods are examined for insects and worms that may not be consumed but may be on vegetables, fruits, and grains.

To ensure that these rules are followed, food preparation is supervised by rabbis (spiritual teachers), after which point the product may then display special logos to that effect. Most often it is a "K" that appears on product packaging.

Halal, Islamic Dietary Laws

The Islamic rules of *halal* or permitted foods, presented in the Koran (bible of Islam), consider food consumption as an aspect of worship. Consequently, eating is viewed as a way to keep one's body healthy. Food should not be consumed excessively and is to be shared with others. All food is permitted unless specifically prohibited. Specific rules concerning foods that may not be consumed include the following:

- Swine (pigs) and birds of prey may not be consumed.
- Animals that are not slaughtered according to specific Muslim procedures may not be consumed. These are similar to those of Jewish laws that regard the exact means of slaughter and blood drainage.
- Alcoholic beverages and drugs that affect consciousness, unless required for medicinal purposes, may not be consumed. Coffee and tea, because they contain the stimulant caffeine, are discouraged.

Application to nursing: In nursing practice it is valuable to be knowledgeable and thereby respectful of the possible dietary restrictions of clients. Assistance can then be given as to the best dietary pattern to ensure wholesome nutrient intakes and the alternative medications or treatment available. For example, because observant Jews and Muslims do not consume pigs or products derived from pigs, the source of insulin (usually from pigs) may be problematic for patients with diabetes.

---

which includes fish in addition to vegetarian selections. These concepts do not reflect the original ideals of vegetarianism. Instead, they represent new contemporary dietary patterns evolving in response to current health issues. These health issues center on the risk of developing one or more of the chronic diet-related diseases: CAD, cancer, type 2 diabetes mellitus, and hypertension. Risk is reduced as dietary fat intake is lowered. A major source of fat in our diets is our consumption of animal protein foods. Reducing levels of this category of dietary fat lowers risk for chronic diet-related diseases. By doing so, the health promotion goals of *Healthy People 2020* recommendations may be achieved.

DIETARY PATTERNS OF PROTEIN

So what should we eat for protein? No longer do we need to be confined to a meat and potatoes mentality when it comes to protein. The healthiest approach is to eat mixed sources of protein—animal and plant sources. (See the *Cultural Considerations* box, Rituals for Animal-Derived Protein, for a discussion of the religious aspects of protein consumption.) The mix provides an excellent assortment of EAAs plus sufficient building block materials for constructing NEAAs. By eating fewer animal protein foods, dietary fat intake is reduced. By eating more plant protein foods, dietary fiber is increased.

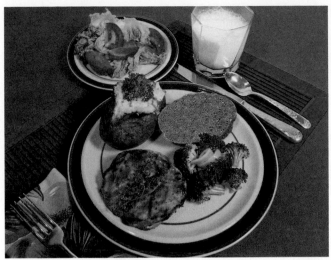

FIG 6-5 A balanced meal. (From Joanne Scott/Tracy McCalla.)

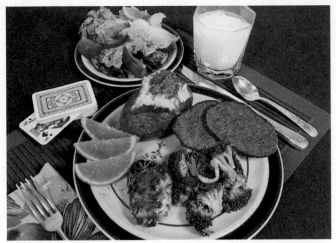

FIG 6-6 A restructured meal. (From Joanne Scott/Tracy McCalla.)

Restructuring the Dinner Plate

If asked to plan a balanced meal, what would the plate look like? Perhaps it would have animal protein (meat, fish, or poultry), vegetables (broccoli, potato, and a salad), and a grain (bread). But how much room on the plate would each portion take?

Before reading this chapter, a person's plate would most likely look like that in Figure 6-5. Notice how meat is the centerpiece that takes up the most space on the plate. Such a large portion of chicken, however, is not necessary. A 6-ounce serving of chicken provides about 53 g of protein. Add to that amount the protein in the bread (3 g), potato (4 g), broccoli (2 g), salad (1 g), and skim milk (8 g), and the total protein intake from one meal alone is 71 g. Because we eat protein throughout the day, no one meal needs to provide all our protein. Instead, the balance of the meal needs to be restructured. Because each component of the meal contains protein, whether from animal or plant sources, portion quantities can shift and still provide plenty of protein. An adequate serving of meat is about the size of a deck of cards or the size of your palm. Notice in Figure 6-6 how the chicken, now reduced to 3 ounces, is no longer the focus of the plate. Each item occupies a more equal space on the plate. The protein total is still high at 48 g.

By spreading protein intake throughout the food groups, the objectives of MyPyramid are met. The first plate (see Figure 6-5) provides the following:
- 1 ounce (whole) grains
- 3 cups vegetables
- 0 cups fruit
- 1 cup milk (low-fat or fat-free)
- 6 ounces meat and beans

The second plate (see Figure 6-6) provides the following:
- 2 ounces (whole) grains
- 4 cups vegetables
- ½ cup fruit
- 1 cup milk (low-fat or fat-free)
- 3 ounces meat and beans

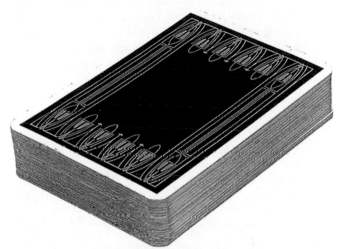

FIG 6-7 A deck of cards is a simple visual tool to judge the size of a protein food.

The new plate provides more complex carbohydrates from grains, fruits, and vegetables while still providing sufficient amounts of protein.

Use the concept of the deck of cards and the restructured meal to visually display to clients appropriate animal-protein portion sizes (Figure 6-7).

OVERCOMING BARRIERS

Malnutrition

Malnutrition, the imbalance of nutrient intake, encompasses conditions that range from overconsumption of nutrients to extreme underconsumption. This discussion concerns the conditions related to underconsumption of nutrients. Underconsumption can result in nutrient deficiencies that range from marginal to severe starvation. Marginal deficiencies occur when lower than recommended levels of nutrients are regularly consumed. Although obvious signs of specific nutrient deficiencies may not be visible, the level of wellness and ability to function at an optimum level are compromised. As the other nutrient categories of vitamins and minerals are studied, specific symptoms of deficiencies will be explored.

Starvation has become a catch-all term. Although we may say "I'm starving" when we've missed a meal, our starvation in no way compares with that experienced by those who truly do not have access to sufficient quantities of high-quality food. The technical term for starvation is **protein energy malnutrition (PEM)**. PEM is an umbrella term for malnutrition caused by the lack of protein, energy, or both.

PEM affects populations around the world. This form of malnutrition is responsible for about half of the 10.9 million child deaths per year. Of children with PEM, 70% are found in Asia, 26% in Africa, and 4% in Latin America and the Caribbean Islands.[9] In young children, PEM can cause permanent disabilities because most brain growth occurs during the early years of life. Extreme PEM results in the conditions of *marasmus* and *kwashiorkor* (Figure 6-8). These disorders can be fatal because of decreased resistance to infections; the body, lacking protein, is unable to create sufficient quantities of antibodies to support the immune system.

Marasmus is malnutrition caused by a lack of sufficient energy (kcal) intake. An individual with marasmus is extremely thin; skin seems to hang on the skeletal bones. Fat stores that normally fill out the skin have been used for energy to maintain minimum body functioning. Muscle mass is also reduced, having also been used for energy, and nutrients are not available to rebuild it. If the condition continues, damage may occur to major organs such as the heart, lungs, and kidneys. Marasmic children will not grow. If the condition occurs between 6 and 18 months of age, the time during which the most brain development occurs, permanent brain damage may result.

In contrast to marasmus, the symptoms of kwashiorkor give the appearance of more than sufficient fat stores in the stomach and face. **Kwashiorkor** is malnutrition caused by a lack of protein while consuming adequate energy. The swollen belly and full cheeks of kwashiorkor are caused by edema (water retention). Edema occurs because protein levels in the body are so low that protein is not available to maintain adequate water balance in the cells, and fluid accumulates unevenly. When adequate nutrition is provided, the fluid is no longer retained. Instead of a full belly and round cheeks, the loss of fat stores becomes apparent and the skin hangs loosely, similar to marasmus. An individual with kwashiorkor is apathetic and experiences muscle weakness and poor growth.

Without sufficient protein, lipids produced by the liver are unable to leave and thus accumulate there. The liver becomes fatty and unable to function well. Even hair quality is affected because protein is the main constituent of hair. Curly hair becomes straight, hair falls out easily, and the pigmentation changes. Skin develops a scaly dermatitis (rash).

The definition of kwashiorkor is evolving. Kwashiorkor was identified as a disorder that develops when very young children are switched from breast milk to solid foods. Although they are consuming enough kcal, it seems that their protein intake is too low for the needs of their growing bodies.[10] Based on these observations, kwashiorkor is defined as malnutrition caused by protein deficiency even though adequate energy is consumed.

This definition, however, does not explain why other children and adults in the same community develop marasmus instead of kwashiorkor. As researchers continue to study the disorder, they have noticed similarities between the locations where kwashiorkor is prevalent and where exposure to dietary aflatoxin occurs. They also have noted that the symptoms of kwashiorkor are similar to those of aflatoxin poisoning. Aflatoxin is a mold that develops when grains are stored under poor conditions of heat and humidity. Eating grains affected by aflatoxin can affect liver function, even leading to liver cancer.[11]

The liver produces NEAAs, without which protein synthesis throughout the body is limited. If liver function is reduced, as with aflatoxin poisoning, production of protein-related structures and substances is decreased. Compared with healthier children and adults, it appears that when malnourished children consume aflatoxin-tainted grains, their weakened immune systems are not able to fight off the effects of aflatoxin. Aflatoxin also induces immunosuppression,

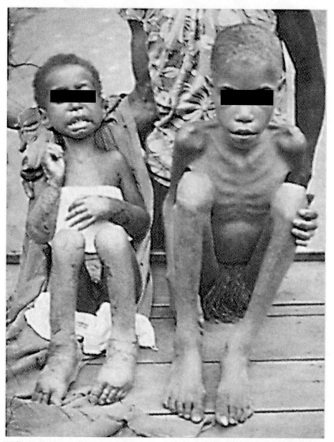

FIG 6-8 Children suffering from kwashiorkor (left) and marasmus (right) as a result of inadequate energy intake. (Courtesy Professor R. Hendricksen. In McLaren DS: *A colour atlas and text of diet-related disorders,* ed 2, London, 1992, Mosby Europe Limited.)

creating a cumulative effect that may lead to the development of kwashiorkor.[11]

Kwashiorkor does not only occur where protein foods are scarce. Two Philadelphian infants whose intake consisted almost entirely of a rice-based protein-poor beverage (Rice Dream) developed kwashiorkor.[12] "Milks" made from nuts, rice, and other grains do not contain complete protein values. Only human breast milk and infant formulas provide adequate levels of protein and other nutrients for infant growth and development.

Malnutrition Factors

Malnutrition is often caused by several factors that affect food availability. Although poverty tends to be a dominant influence, other forces also affect the development of malnutrition. These include biologic, social, economic, and environmental factors (Box 6-6).

Biologic factors affect the ability of the body to use nutrients. Economic effects encompass the ability to purchase food and also consider the structure of a country's economy and access to employment. Environmental factors directly affect the availability of food as related to crop production

and food safety. Lack of education, social isolation, and the rippling effects of underemployment seem to be malnutrition factors throughout the world, regardless of the overall wealth of nations. Health and economic support systems provided throughout the life cycle may prevent the development of factors affecting food availability.

Groups at Risk in North America

Most people in North America are well nourished, although growing numbers of homeless individuals living in shelters or other temporary sites are at risk for varying levels of malnutrition.[13] Without access to cooking facilities or the funds to purchase adequate quantities of foods, these individuals are at nutritional risk. In response to this crisis, food pantries and soup kitchens have been established by nonprofit and charitable groups to distribute food and meals (see the *Social Issues* box, Hunger All Around: How to Help). Also at risk are the working poor, whose incomes barely cover the basic

---

BOX 6-6 MALNUTRITION FACTORS

Biologic Factors
- Maternal malnutrition before or during pregnancy and/or lactation
- Infections that may affect nutrient absorption
- Chronic diarrhea as both a cause and effect of malnutrition
- Toxins such as aflatoxin
- Lack of food, particularly protein

Social Factors
- Ignorance of nutrient needs of children, resulting in inappropriate weaning foods
- Child abuse and neglect
- Eating disorders, particularly anorexia nervosa
- Drug abuse affecting the ability to care for oneself appropriately
- Social isolation of older adults, leading to an inability to purchase and prepare adequate quantities of food
- Alcoholism (kcal from alcohol replace consumption of nutrient-dense foods)
- Wars/civil strife disrupting normal social and food production systems

Economic Factors
- Poverty and socioeconomic status
- Unemployment
- Little education
- Political strife affecting distribution of wealth and land ownership

Environmental Factors
- Polluted water, which reduces food production and directly affects the health of populations
- Famine caused by droughts or crop failures
- Improper farming techniques

SOCIAL ISSUES

Hunger All Around: How to Help

"Finish all that food on your plate. Children in India are starving." Parents often said this to their children at the dinner table, causing countless numbers of children to try to figure out how finishing their own vegetables would help feed the children in a faraway land. Of course, parents wanted their children not to waste food and to appreciate their good fortune. However, many children probably believed that by finishing their food they were somehow helping those hungry children.

Because of today's technology, we can have no illusions about the plight of others. We get complete, immediate reports of devastation caused by wars and famines. Reports of hunger among the homeless and older adults are televised. If only finishing the food on our plates would help.

So what can we do? Here are some ideas:

As Individuals
- Be well informed. Learn about hunger in your neighborhood. All communities have people who are in need.
- Volunteer to help in a local soup kitchen.
- Create a food drive at holidays; donate foods to a food bank.
- Let local politicians know of your concerns; give a voice to the voiceless. Send an e-mail to local and state officials.

Campus Organizations (Political, Social, and Religious)
- Include a service component to the group's mission.
- Support World Food Day sponsored by the United Nations and other organizations.
- Ask local antihunger agency representatives to speak to campus groups.
- Incorporate volunteer time as part of an initiation process or as a commitment of all members of sororities, fraternities, and social clubs.

Data from Food First, Institute for Food and Development Policy: *Hunger at Home: The growing epidemic,* Oakland, Calif, Author. Accessed April 12, 2006, from www.foodfirst.org/progs/humanrts/hungerhome.html.

expenses of housing, utilities, and health care and leave little for food purchases. Programs providing support services to these populations also can arrange nutrition education on healthier choices when buying and preparing economical meals. Societal and personal changes may interrupt family ties, causing the loss of recipes and opportunities to share skills of preparation of low-cost, nutritious meals.

Older adults also are at risk. Although their nutritional concerns are covered in depth in Chapter 13, consider that the physical and financial limitations of older adults may reduce their ability to purchase and prepare wholesome meal. When these issues are also compounded by social isolation, the situation of older adults becomes serious.

Hospital patients and those with chronic illnesses such as acquired immunodeficiency syndrome (AIDS) and cancer are also at risk for PEM, even while under medical care. Depending on their illness, 25% of hospital patients may experience treatable malnutrition.[14] This is called *hospital malnutrition* or *iatrogenic* malnutrition. Iatrogenic malnutrition is inadvertently caused by treatment or diagnostic procedures. This condition may be due to not consuming enough food, side effects from an illness, prolonged liquid diet (as a result of extended diagnostic testing), or medications that reduce the body's ability to absorb nutrients. An extended hospital stay also may increase the risk of poor nutritional status.[15] Weight loss associated with an extended hospital stay may be attributed to the illness rather than to lack of nutrients. The patient seems sicker but is actually malnourished and not absorbing the nutrients needed to heal and recover.

Primary care providers, nurses, and dietitians all play a collaborative role in preventing, identifying, and treating hospital malnutrition. Astute nursing assessment may uncover early signs of malnutrition or factors predisposing a patient to it. Some patients may enter the hospital already malnourished. Dietitians work not only with individual patients but also with the health care industry to develop new products and technologies designed to either prevent or reduce the incidents of PEM among hospital patients. Clinical guidelines, coupled with nutrition support teams, can enhance nutritional adequacy.

Chronic Hunger

Although famines and wars affect the nutritional status of people throughout the world, the population of North America has not experienced these extremes of deprivation. Instead, chronic hunger, defined as a continual experience of undernutrition (not enough food to eat), has become the

---

PERSONAL PERSPECTIVE

An Unexpected Kitchen: The George Foreman Grill

The Hidden Kitchens project, created by The Kitchen Sisters—Nikki Silva and Davia Nelson—finds hidden makeshift kitchens across the country. To broaden their search, they began a National Public Radio hotline asking listeners, "What food traditions are disappearing from your life? Who glues your community together through food? What should be captured and documented before it disappears or changes beyond recognition?" The responses were overwhelming. The following story, about the George Foreman grill, was passed on through the Chicago Coalition for the Homeless and is one of several Personal Perspectives boxes throughout this textbook that chronicle some of the responses.

Jeffrey Newton is 57 years old. Until recently, he lived in a refrigerator box, part of a makeshift cardboard community tucked in around trash cans and restaurant loading docks hidden under Chicago's Wacker Drive.

"Me and Smokey found the George Foreman grill at the shelter," Jeffrey remembers. Someone had donated one, broken, without a plug, so the two guys jury-rigged it. "Then you just get you a long extension cord and hookup. There's a lot of electrical plugs on the poles down there. You'd come home in the evening, and you'd fire up your Foreman. Some of us had jobs. Some of us had food stamp Link cards. You put anything in that thing: bologna, hamburgers, grilled cheese sandwiches. We used to take an iron and do that, too, press down, hot on the bread and cheese. You'd be inventive like that."

[At a later time ...] George Foreman, two-time heavyweight champion of the world, Olympic gold medalist, former street preacher, and "King of the Grills," is in a radio studio in Houston, Texas ... we tell George what we've been hearing about his grill. The story hits a nerve.

"Whoa ... what a story! I've never considered it all," he says, "how homeless people and low-income people, wanting to cook but not being able to, how that little grill afforded them a kitchen. I'm just happy that it's helped so many people. It helped me, of course.

"Growing up in Houston, my whole life was spent trying to get enough to eat. Having seven kids, and my mother raising all of us by herself, there just was never enough food for me. I always dreamed not about a car, not about a beautiful home, but about having enough to eat." Sometimes George's mother would come home with a cheeseburger and try to divide it among her seven kids. "I remember the taste of the mustard. It was the most supreme thing in our family when she'd come home with a burger."

The grill lets Americans grill indoors on a rainy day or in a college dorm, and it gives the homeless a way to have hot bologna and cheese. It gave George and his brother Roy the means to open the George Foreman Youth Center. Foreman has never forgotten the central lesson of the Job Corps (the federal program that saved him from a life of crime): All that most kids need is a chance. He still imagines what his life might have become, and so he holds out the same chance he got to kids who are hungry, and angry.

From Silva N, Nelson D: *Hidden kitchens: Stories, recipes, and more from NPR's The Kitchen Sisters*, New York, 2005, Rodale Books.

norm for a subset of our population. This subset is growing as the economies of North America tighten, causing government food and welfare programs to be unable to provide an appropriate safety net to prevent and alleviate chronic hunger. Instead, more individuals and families are faced with a consistent lack of opportunities to improve their standard of living and, most important, their health. (See the *Personal Perspectives* box, An Unexpected Kitchen: The George Foreman Grill for a unique and interesting story about dealing with chronic hunger.)

TOWARD A POSITIVE NUTRITION LIFESTYLE: CHAINING

Chaining refers to the linking of two behaviors. If two actions consistently occur together, they often become linked or tied to each other. They become one behavior and a habit. Many of us already practice chaining; unfortunately, the results often have a negative impact on our dietary intake patterns. Frequently eating potato chips while studying can link these two actions—eating chips and studying. The chain requires that whenever studying takes place, chips need to be eaten. Chaining, however, can also be used to improve nutritional status.

Consider the following chains:
- When you eat a sandwich, eat a fruit, too. Instead of linking chips and a sandwich (or hoagie, grinder, or sub), this links a sandwich to a fruit.
- Have a glass of skim milk with the midday meal regularly to increase calcium intake. Skim milk becomes chained to lunch.
- At home, weigh portions of meat, fish, and poultry. Compare the size of an appropriate portion to the size of a deck of cards. Are they similar in size? Weigh portions regularly and consciously compare sizes. Animal protein portion sizes will be linked to the deck of cards, and portion control can be achieved without weighing.

These are just a few chains related to protein consumption. Chaining can be applied to other nutrition and wellness situations of our clients as well.

SUMMARY

Proteins consist of chains of amino acids. Amino acids are organic compounds made of carbon, hydrogen, oxygen, and nitrogen. There are 20 amino acids from which all proteins are made. The body can manufacture some, but not all, of the amino acids. EAAs cannot be made by the body; these 9 amino acids are needed from food. The other 11 NEAAs can be created by the liver. All are available to the cells through the amino acid pool to allow proteins to be synthesized.

The proteins in foods are categorized by the EAAs they contain. Complete proteins contain all nine essential amino acids, whereas incomplete proteins lack one or more of the essential amino acids.

The proteins in foods are not the same as those used by our bodies. During digestion, food protein is broken down to amino acids. Once absorbed, the amino acids circulate in the blood to build new proteins. The new proteins are used to perform numerous functions, including growth and maintenance, creation of essential substances, immune system response, fluid regulation, acid-base balance, and transportation of nutrients and other substances in the body. Malnutrition resulting in PEM, marasmus, and kwashiorkor is a worldwide concern.

THE NURSING APPROACH

Case Study: Protein (Wound Healing)

Roy, a 69-year-old homeless man, came to a neighborhood mobile van health clinic with a leg ulcer. Roy said the ulcer had been there for several months, and it had gradually gotten bigger. He was obviously poorly nourished. He said he ate what he could find on the street and sometimes went to the city food center for a hot meal. The nurse cleaned Roy's leg ulcer, and the physician ordered laboratory tests.

ASSESSMENT

Subjective (from patient statements)
- Minimal intake of meat, eggs, or other protein foods
- Fatigue

Objective (from physical examination)
- Height 6'2", weight 140 pounds
- Muscle atrophy in extremities bilaterally

- Decreased muscle strength
- Poor skin turgor
- Hair is dull and thin
- Slight ankle edema bilaterally
- Left lower leg ulcer 4 cm in diameter, stage II
- Serum albumin 2.7 g/dL (norm 3.4 to 4.8 g/dL)

DIAGNOSES (NURSING)

1. Imbalanced nutrition: less than body requirements related to lack of food availability as evidenced by minimal intake of protein foods, 74% ideal body weight (IBW), albumin 2.7 g/dL, delayed healing of lower left leg ulcer
2. Impaired skin integrity related to inadequate nutrition as evidenced by stage II left lower leg ulcer 4 cm, present for several months and increasing in size

Continued

THE NURSING APPROACH—cont'd

Case Study: Protein (Wound Healing)—cont'd

PLANNING

Patient Outcomes

Short term (at the end of this visit):

- Roy will identify foods high in protein, appropriate portion sizes (such as a deck of cards), and state the importance of protein in healing wounds.
- Roy will verbalize intention to eat high-protein foods at least once each day.
- He will agree to come to clinic for follow-up twice a week.

Long term (after two months):

- Roy will report he ate several appropriate portions of high-protein foods each day.
- Roy's ulcer will heal within two months.
- He will gain four pounds in two months

Nursing Interventions

1. Teach Roy about the importance of protein in wound healing.
2. Discuss resources for obtaining high-protein food.
3. Provide wound care as ordered by the physician.

IMPLEMENTATION (Also see Chapter 15.)

1. Discussed with Roy the role of protein in wound healing.

Protein is needed for tissue repair and resistance to infection. Sufficient kcal are needed to spare use of proteins for energy.

2. Discussed dietary sources of protein.

Soy and foods from animals contain complete proteins. Plant foods must be combined in order to have complete proteins.

3. Supplied Roy with cans of high-protein and vitamin supplements at each clinic visit.

Adequate protein, calories, water, and vitamins are needed for tissue repair. Vitamins A and C and zinc are particularly helpful in wound healing. Vitamin C is needed for collagen formation. Vitamin A is an antioxidant and an important helper in wound healing. Zinc increases tensile strength of the healing wound.

4. Applied wet-to-damp dressing and antibiotic ointment to leg ulcers during clinic visits twice a week.

Wet-to-damp dressings maintain moisture for healing and help débride wounds. Antibiotics help prevent infection.

5. Encouraged Roy to move into a homeless shelter affiliated with the clinic until the leg ulcer heals.

A shelter can provide cleanliness, rest, and nutritious food, an environment conducive to healing.

6. Encouraged Roy to eat at least one meal per day in the shelter.

Nutritious food can help an individual heal wounds and regain weight.

EVALUATION

Short term (at the end of the first visit):

- Roy identified several foods high in protein and thanked the nurse for the supplements to help his ulcer heal.
- He said he would try to eat at least one meal per day at the shelter.
- Roy said he would return to the clinic twice a week for follow-up.
- Short-term goal met.

Long term (in one month):

- Roy said he had eaten at least one meal each day at the shelter on most of the days and was thinking about moving to the shelter.
- His leg ulcer measured 2 cm.
- He had gained two pounds.
- Goal partially met.

DISCUSSION QUESTIONS

1. What resources are available in your community to help the homeless and hungry?
2. If Roy has little money for food, what should he buy? Consider nutrient density, food preparation needed, and cost.
3. Role play how you would teach Roy about complementary proteins.

ⓐ APPLYING CONTENT KNOWLEDGE

Karen and her husband, Roger, want to reduce their intake of fat and increase their fiber intake. Both grew up in families that prided themselves as being the "meat and potatoes" type. Suggest three strategies they could adopt to restructure their dinner plates.

Want more practice? Visit http://evolve.elsevier.com/Grodner/foundations.

WEBSITES OF INTEREST

Healthfinder

www.healthfinder.gov

Links to consumer health and human services information through online publications, clearinghouses, databases, government agencies, and nonprofit organizations.

The Sickle Cell Information Center

www.scinfo.org

Provides education, counseling, research updates, and international resources for patients and health professionals.

The Vegetarian Resource Group

www.vrg.org

Offers a comprehensive guide to vegetarian information, cookbooks, journals, and related links.

REFERENCES

1. Thibodeau GA, Patton KT: *Anatomy & physiology*, ed 5, St Louis, 2003, Mosby.
2. Matthews DE: Proteins and amino acids. In Shils ME et al, editors: *Modern nutrition in health and disease*, ed 10, Philadelphia, 2006, Lippincott Williams & Wilkins.
3. Otten JJ, et al, editors: *Dietary DRI References: The essential guide to nutrient requirements*, Washington, DC, 2006, The National Academies Press.
4. Position paper of the American Dietetic Association, Dietitians of Canada, and the American College of Sports Medicine: Nutrition and athletic performance, *J Am Diet Assoc* 109:509-527, 2009.
5. Craig WJ: Health effects of vegan diets, *Am J Clin Nutr* 89(Suppl):1627S-1633S, 2009.
6. Position of the American Dietetic Association: Vegetarian diets, *J Am Diet Assoc* 109:1266-1282, 2009.
7. Calvo MS et al: Vitamin D intake: A global perspective of current status, *J Nutr* 135(2):310-316, 2005.
8. Weisberg P et al: Nutritional rickets among children in the United States: Review of cases reported between 1986 and 2003, *Am J Clin Nutr* 80(6 Suppl):1697S-1705S, 2004.
9. World Health Organization: *Nutrition: Alleviating protein-energy malnutrition*, Geneva, 2002 (March 13), Author.
10. Krawinkel M: Kwashiorkor is still not fully understood, *Bull World Health Org* 81(12):910-911, 2003.
11. Hendricksen RG: Of sick turkeys, kwashiorkor, malaria, perinatal mortality, heroin addicts and food poisoning: research on the influence of aflatoxins on child health in the tropics, *Ann Trop Med Parasitol* 91(7):787-793, 1997.
12. Katz KA et al: Rice nightmare: Kwashiorkor in two Philadelphia-area infants fed Rice Dream beverage, *J Am Acad Dermatol* 52(5 Suppl 1):S69-S72, 2005.
13. Struble MB, Aomari LL: Addressing world hunger, malnutrition, and food insecurity: Position of the American Dietetic Association, *J Am Diet Assoc* 103:1046-1057, 2003.
14. Kruizenga HM et al: Effectiveness and cost-effectiveness of early screening and treatment of malnourished patients, *Am J Clin Nutr* 82(5):1082-1089, 2005.
15. Braunschweig C et al: Impact of declines in nutritional status on outcomes in adult patients hospitalized for more than 7 days, *J Am Diet Assoc* 100(11):1316-1322. quiz 1323-1324, 2000.

CHAPTER

7

Vitamins

Vitamins are organic molecules that are required in very small amounts.

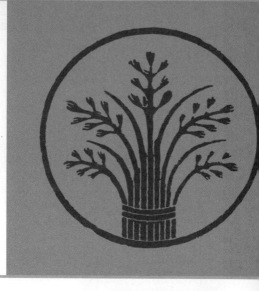

evolve WEBSITE

http://evolve.elsevier.com/Grodner/foundations/

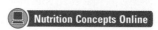
Nutrition Concepts Online

ROLE IN WELLNESS

Vitamins seem to have a magical aura. Take enough and you'll have more energy and be healthier, smarter, and even better looking. If only it were that easy. Although vitamins are essential for life, they are only one of many factors required for wellness.

Knowledge of the existence of vitamins is recent; the discovery of vitamins slowly evolved, beginning in the early part of the twentieth century. The focus of research was to discover the amounts of vitamins needed to prevent deficiency symptoms and diseases that undermine the health and well-being of populations throughout the world.

The scientific view of vitamins, however, is in flux. Additional effects of vitamin use are surfacing as more is learned about the functions of vitamins as antioxidants and hormone-like substances. Some vitamins and related substances such as carotenoids may reduce the risk of developing certain chronic diseases. New information points to relationships between consuming foods high in vitamins and a lower incidence of developing diseases.

The Dietary Reference Intake (DRI) considers the concern of providing nutrient requirements necessary to prevent deficiencies and toxicity from overdoses and accounting for the value of nutrient intake as a means of reducing disease risk.[1] Recommendations within the DRI documents include the use of fortified foods or supplements for particular nutrients, such as folic acid for women of childbearing age to ensure proper neural tube formation of the fetus during pregnancy.

Vitamins are organic molecules required in very small amounts for cellular metabolism. Each vitamin performs a specific metabolic function. Vitamins, except for vitamin D, are not synthesized by our bodies and thus are essential nutri-ents that must be provided through dietary intake (see the *Personal Perspectives* box, Joseph Aguilar's Mercado [San Antonio]: A Street Kitchen Vision). Vitamin D is the only vitamin created by the human body.

Vitamins are vital to life and therefore to the physical, intellectual, emotional, social, and spiritual dimensions of health. Vitamins are essential nutrients without which the body cannot continue functioning within the *physical dimension*. Dietary recommendations to eat at least five fruits and vegetables per day throughout the life span are made to reduce the risk of diet-related diseases in the future. *Intellectual health* skills are used to envision future benefits that accrue from food choices today. Deficiencies of several B vitamins can produce irritability, confusion, and paranoia, thereby affecting the *emotional health* dimension. Older adults may be at risk for deficiencies because of their inability to get to the store to buy fruits and vegetables; the physical health of older adults may depend on their *social health* in relation to neighbors who may provide assistance with shopping needs. Sometimes following religious teachings may jeopardize health, as noted by the development of rickets, the vitamin D deficiency disorder, among some African American children of families following the dietary and dress customs of the Islamic faith. *Spiritual health* is interdependent on the other dimensions of health.

As vitamins are discussed, note that some are referred to by specific names or by letters and numbers. Each vitamin has a history that affects how we refer to it today. In 1929 Henrik Dam in Copenhagen, Denmark, discovered vitamin K. It was the only substance capable of halting a hemorrhagic disease in which blood does not coagulate. Dam named the vitamin *K* for the Danish word *koagulation*.

In another case, several B vitamins were isolated into the same test tube labeled B, and we therefore have vitamins

Joseph Aguilar's Mercado (San Antonio): A Street Kitchen Vision

Following is another excerpt from the Hidden Kitchens project. The Kitchen Sisters, Nikki Silva and Davia Nelson, are visiting San Antonio, Texas. Most of us buy our fruits and vegetables in large supermarkets, but not everyone finds these markets to be convenient. In the midst of a drab urban area, The Kitchen Sisters find a small shop bursting with colorful produce.

We were walking … to find some remnant of what had once been San Antonio's vital commercial hub. … But there's not much commerce on West Commerce anymore. It's one way with no parking on the street, blocks of mostly empty buildings with no shop windows to look in, and no people, except the homeless and those standing at a bus stop waiting to go someplace else.

Then, amid the endless gray, a beacon of bananas glows in a doorway. A tiny storefront with a scale hanging out front surrounded by a basket of ripe mangoes, nopales cactus, deep green chillies, brilliant red tomatoes. We pick up our pace, pulled in by the life force.

As we approach, a horn honks. A middle-aged man darts out of the store, runs up to a car idling out front, hands off a plastic bag, grabs a bill, and runs back inside as the car pulls out into the fast-moving traffic. The man is Joseph Aguilar, owner of West Commerce Mercado.

"Everything we do here is illegal," he tells us. "But it's not bad illegal. I don't sell beer. I don't sell cigarettes—just produce. A little produce stand. A family thing.

"I just delivered a snack bag. That's what we call them. A bag with a banana, apple, orange, and a pear for a dollar. Cars come up and just honk. They don't even get out of their seats. We already know who they are and what they want. It's illegal because this is a bus line in front of our store. It's kind of exciting."

A handsome man with salt-and-pepper hair and a thick mustache, 57-year-old Joseph Aguilar proudly takes us through his tiny market. It has everything "from salsa to sweet peaches." Old-fashioned wooden shelves display hot sauce with lemon and dry pepper that he's selling for a friend who lives in Mexico; crisp tortillas wrapped the old traditional way in paper, imported from a family in Chicago; beautifully packaged species and herbs. …

"My customers are downtown working people, senior citizens, and 'the criminal element' who are coming in for food. The courthouse and probation office are nearby. A lot of them are pretty good people; it's just that they had bad luck and got caught."

When Joseph started up his little business, he spent $2,000 to have the windows in his market set back off the sidewalk so he could display his produce outside "so people could see the beauty of how produce looks outside your little store."

From Silva N, Nelson D: *Hidden Kitchens: Stories, recipes, and more from NPR's The Kitchen Sisters*, New York, 2005, Rodale Books.

---

numbered B_1, B_2, and B_3. In the 1970s the science community decreed that all vitamins should be called by their formal biochemical titles. The public and many health professionals still refer to the simpler letter and number names for vitamins. Both the formal and informal names are used in this chapter.

This chapter lists vitamin DRI. Because *DRI* is an umbrella term that includes Recommended Dietary Allowance (RDA), Adequate Intake (AI), and Tolerable Upper Intake Level (UL), applicable standards will be identified. Because there are different RDAs and AIs based on age, gender, and physiologic need, only those for men and women ages 19 to 30 are included for each vitamin, unless special circumstances surrounding the need for a vitamin warrant discussion. The DRI tables are located inside the front cover of this book.

A primary deficiency of a vitamin occurs when the vitamin is not consumed in sufficient amounts to meet physiologic needs. A secondary deficiency develops when absorption is impaired or excess excretion occurs, limiting bioavailability. Most deficiencies are detected through clinical and biochemical assessment; specific diagnostic and laboratory procedures are beyond the scope of this text and are available elsewhere.[2]

Although vitamin deficiencies are no longer common among Americans, subgroups are at risk. Because of their increased needs, pregnant women are often at risk for marginal deficiencies of essential vitamins. Older adults may also be at risk because of decreased absorptive ability and limited economic and physical resources for food availability. Poverty is an overwhelming factor that affects the nutritional status of children and adults. Chronic alcohol and drug abuse not only alters psychologic and mental capacities but also limits the body's ability to absorb and use essential vitamins.

Health professionals can also take into account other special circumstances that may initiate vitamin deficiencies. Individuals dealing with long-term chronic disorders that affect the total body response, such as acquired immunodeficiency syndrome (AIDS) or liver or kidney disorders, have special vitamin concerns because the metabolic processes of the body may be compromised by these disorders and by the medications prescribed. Deficiencies have been documented that were possibly caused by the effects of cancer treatment, use of multiple alternative therapies, and lifestyle behaviors. These deficiencies were at first misdiagnosed because vitamin deficiencies were no longer thought to occur.[3-5]

Toxicities of vitamins rarely occur naturally from food consumption. Instead, inappropriate use of supplements may be toxic to our bodies. Vitamins have been studied for their physiologic effect or basic need for health maintenance (Box 7-1). The recommended levels reflect this knowledge. Use of vitamin supplements at megadose levels is equivalent to a pharmacologic effect, with potential druglike physical responses. Some vitamins have UL; for others, a megadose (i.e., 10 times the RDA for a specific nutrient) of a vitamin

BOX 7-1 CONSIDERING VITAMINS AND MINERALS THROUGH FUNCTION

Vitamins and minerals are discussed as two separate nutrient categories in Chapters 7 and 8. Although each is discussed individually, they are not grouped based on their functions in the body. Following are the vitamins and minerals required for specific body functions of blood health, bone health, energy metabolism, and fluid and electrolyte balance. Additional functions of individual vitamins and minerals may be found in Tables 7-3, 7-6, 8-2, and 8-3.

Blood Health

Blood is *the* body fluid, supplying tissues with oxygen, nutrients, and energy through circulation within the cardiovascular system. It is composed of water, red and white blood cells, oxygen, nutrients, and other formed substances. Always moving, blood gathers and distributes nutrients and oxygen to all cells and disposes of waste products. Deficiency of any of these nutrients will affect overall blood health. Only the blood-related functions of the vitamins and minerals are listed.

VITAMIN*	FUNCTION	MINERAL†	FUNCTION
Vitamin B$_{12}$	Transport/storage of folate needed for heme and cell formation and other functions	Iron	Distributes oxygen in hemoglobin and myoglobin
Folate *Folic acid, folacin*	Coenzyme metabolism (synthesis of amino acid, heme, deoxyribonucleic acid [DNA], ribonucleic acid [RNA]) and other functions	Zinc	Cofactor for more than 200 enzymes including enzymes to make heme in hemoglobin, genetic material, and proteins
Vitamin B$_6$ *Pyridoxine*	Hemoglobin synthesis and other functions	Copper	Helps with iron use
Vitamin K	Cofactor in synthesis of blood clotting factors; protein formation		

Bone Health

As living tissue, bone requires nutrients to maintain cellular structure. Blood circulates through bone capillaries, delivering nutrients while removing waste materials no longer needed by cells. Hormones regulate the use of minerals either for storage and structural purposes in bone or for regulating body processes. Specific vitamins and minerals are indispensable for these functions to occur.

VITAMIN*	FUNCTION	MINERAL†	FUNCTION
Vitamin D	Bone mineralization	Calcium	Bone and tooth formation
Vitamin K	Protein formation for bone mineralization; cofactor for blood-clotting factors	Phosphorus	Bone and tooth formation (component of hydroxyapatite)
Vitamin A	Bone growth; maintains epithelial cells; regulation of gene expression	Magnesium	Bone structure
Precursor: beta carotene		Fluoride	Bone and tooth formation; increases stability of bone

Energy Metabolism

In order to metabolize carbohydrates, lipids, and protein for energy and other needs, the body depends on many nutrients to support the process, create new cells, and implement various related functions.

VITAMIN*	FUNCTION	MINERAL†	FUNCTION
Thiamine *Vitamin B$_1$*	Coenzyme energy metabolism; muscle nerve action	Iodine	Thyroxine synthesis (thyroid hormone) regulates growth and development; basal metabolic rate (BMR) regulation
Riboflavin *Vitamin B$_2$*	Coenzyme energy metabolism	Chromium	Carbohydrate metabolism, part of glucose tolerance factor
Niacin *Vitamin B$_3$, nicotinic acid, nicotinamide, niacinamide*	Cofactor to enzymes involved in energy metabolism; glycolysis and tricarboxylic acid (TCA) cycle synthesis	Phosphorus Sulfur	Energy metabolism (enzymes) Component of protein structures
Vitamin B$_6$ *Pyridoxine*	Forms coenzyme pyridoxal phosphate (PLP) for energy metabolism	Iron	Distributes oxygen in hemoglobin and myoglobin
Folate *Folic acid, folacin*	Coenzyme metabolism (synthesis of amino acid, heme, DNA, RNA)		

*See text for additional information on vitamins.
†See Chapter 8 for additional information on minerals.

BOX 7-1	CONSIDERING VITAMINS AND MINERALS THROUGH FUNCTION—cont'd		
VITAMIN*	**FUNCTION**	**MINERAL†**	**FUNCTION**
Vitamin B$_{12}$ *Cyanocobalamin*	Metabolism of fatty acids/amino acids	Zinc	Carbohydrate metabolism (insulin function); cofactor to more than 200 enzymes
Pantothenic acid	Part of coenzyme A		
Biotin	Metabolism of carbohydrate, fat, and protein		

Fluid and Electrolyte Balance

Life systems are dependent on fluid and electrolyte balance within the body. Electrolytes consist of mineral salts that maintain cellular fluid balance. The acid-base balance of body fluids is buffered by other minerals.

MINERAL†	**FUNCTION**
Sodium	Major extracellular electrolyte for fluid regulation; body fluid levels; acid-base balance; nerve impulse and contraction; blood pressure/volume
Potassium	With sodium and chloride, major intracellular electrolyte for fluid regulation; muscle function
Chloride	Acid-base balance
Phosphorus	Acid-base balance

DNA, Deoxyribonucleic acid; *RNA*, ribonucleic acid.

is considered the highest amount of the nutrient that will not cause adverse health effects. Because most vitamins have not been studied to determine function and safety at these megadose levels, extensive use without guidance can be problematic.

VITAMIN CATEGORIES

Vitamins are divided into two categories based on their solubility in solutions. *Water-soluble vitamins* dissolve or disperse in water; they are the B complex vitamins (thiamine, riboflavin, niacin, pyridoxine, folate, vitamin B$_{12}$, biotin, and pantothenic acid), choline, and vitamin C. *Fat-soluble vitamins* dissolve in fatty tissues or substances; they are vitamins A, D, E, and K.

Solubility characteristics affect how vitamins are absorbed and transported in the body. Water-soluble vitamins are easily absorbed in the small intestine and then pass into the bloodstream for circulation throughout the body. Fat-soluble vitamins follow the more complicated route of other fat-containing substances; bile is required for absorption from the small intestine. Fat malabsorption problems may also lead to potential deficiencies of fat-soluble vitamins.

The water solubility of the B vitamins and vitamin C allows for minimal storage of any excess vitamin consumed; tissues may be saturated with these vitamins, but they usually are not stored. Deficiencies can develop quickly—within weeks—so we need to consume these vitamins on a daily basis. Excesses are generally not toxic and are simply excreted in urine. However, damage may result if vitamin levels are chronically high because of supplementation.

If we consume more than the daily requirement of a fat-soluble vitamin, our bodies store the excess rather than excrete it (Box 7-2). The DRI for fat-soluble vitamins takes into account this storage capacity. Although storage is expected in organs such as the liver and spleen, other fatty

tissues in the body can also retain excessive amounts of fat-soluble vitamins. Overloading the storage capabilities can be toxic and produce illness; toxicity rarely comes from excessive dietary intake but rather from improper use of vitamin supplements.

FOOD SOURCES

Vitamins are in almost all foods, yet no one food group is a good source of all vitamins. Fresh fruits and vegetables are particularly rich sources. Others include legumes, whole grains, and animal foods of meat, fish, poultry, eggs, and dairy products. Even the almost pure fats of vegetable oils and butter provide vitamins E and A, respectively. Although this does not mean we should consume these products for their vitamin content, it does mean we have a wide range of foods from which to choose for our vitamin nutrition.

It is always best to consume vitamins from food sources. Although synthetic forms of vitamins will perform vitamin functions, there may be other factors in foods that provide benefits. For instance, broccoli and other cruciferous vegetables contain a wide variety of chemicals, including sulforaphane, which is a phytochemical (Box 7-3). Phytochemicals are nonnutritive substances in plant-based foods that appear to have disease-fighting properties Sulforaphane appears to block the growth of tumors in animals. Broccoli, along with onions and grapes, also contains flavonols, which seems to reduce the risk of coronary artery disease (CAD) and cancer while having an anti-inflammatory effect.[6]

WATER–SOLUBLE VITAMINS

Thiamine (B$_1$)

For centuries, a mysterious disease afflicted people of all ages and status throughout Asia. The disease so wasted muscles that Thai sufferers who tried to stand would cry out, "*Beri,*

BOX 7-2   MYPLATE: FRUITS

The health benefits of eating fruits overlap with those of eating vegetables. Both the fruit and vegetable categories of MyPlate provide rich sources of vitamins and are valuable components of an overall healthy diet, providing nutrients essential for the health and maintenance of our bodies (see also Boxes 8-5 and 8-6). Health benefits of eating fruits and vegetables as part of an overall health diet include reduced risk for stroke, coronary artery disease, and type 2 diabetes mellitus; protection against some cancers (mouth, stomach, colorectal cancer); and, as an excellent source of fiber, possible decreased risk of several chronic diet-related disorders. The recommendation is to eat at least 2 cups of fruits every day.

What Counts as a Cup of Fruit?*

The focus of this MyPlate box is on portions of the fruits group.

In general, 1 cup of fruit or 100% fruit juice, or $\frac{1}{2}$ cup of dried fruit can be considered as 1 cup from the fruit group. The specific amounts outlined in the following table count as 1 cup of fruit (in some cases equivalents for $\frac{1}{2}$ cup are also shown) toward your daily recommended intake.

FRUIT	AMOUNT THAT COUNTS AS 1 CUP OF FRUIT	AMOUNT THAT COUNTS AS $\frac{1}{2}$ CUP OF FRUIT
Apple	$\frac{1}{2}$ large (3$\frac{1}{4}$-inch diameter) 1 small (2$\frac{1}{2}$-inch diameter) 1 cup sliced or chopped, raw or cooked	$\frac{1}{2}$ cup sliced or chopped, raw or cooked
Applesauce	1 cup	1 snack container (4 oz)
Banana	1 cup sliced 1 large (8-9 inches long)	1 small (less than 6 inches long)
Cantaloupe	1 cup diced or melon balls	1 medium wedge ($\frac{1}{8}$ of a medium melon)
Grapes	1 cup whole or cut up 32 seedless grapes	16 seedless grapes
Grapefruit	1 medium (4-inch diameter) 1 cup sections	$\frac{1}{2}$ medium (4-inch diameter)
Mixed fruit (fruit cocktail)	1 cup diced or sliced, raw or canned, drained	1 snack container (4 oz), drained = $\frac{3}{8}$ cup
Orange	1 large (3$\frac{1}{16}$-inch diameter) 1 cup sections	1 small 2$\frac{3}{8}$-inch diameter)
Orange, mandarin	1 cup canned, drained	
Peach	1 large (2$\frac{3}{4}$-inch diameter) 1 cup sliced or diced; raw, cooked, or canned; drained 2 halves, canned	1 small (2-inch diameter) 1 snack container (4oz), drained = $\frac{3}{8}$ cup
Pear	1 medium (2$\frac{1}{2}$ per lb) 1 cup sliced or diced; raw, cooked, or canned; drained	1 snack container (4 oz), drained = $\frac{3}{8}$ cup
Pineapple	1 cup chunks; sliced or crushed; raw, cooked, or canned; drained	1 snack container (4 oz), drained = $\frac{3}{8}$ cup
Plum	1 cup sliced, raw or cooked 3 medium or 2 large	1 large
Strawberries	Approximately 8 large 1 cup whole, halved, or sliced; fresh or frozen	$\frac{1}{2}$ cup whole, halved, or sliced
Watermelon	1 small wedge (1 inch thick) 1 cup diced or balls	6 melon balls
Dried fruit (raisins, prunes, apricots, etc.)	$\frac{1}{2}$ cup dried fruit is equivalent to 1 cup fruit ($\frac{1}{2}$ cup raisins, $\frac{1}{2}$ cup prunes, $\frac{1}{2}$ cup dried apricots)	$\frac{1}{4}$ cup dried fruit is equivalent to $\frac{1}{2}$ cup fruit (1 small box raisins [1$\frac{1}{2}$ oz])
100% fruit juice (orange, apple, grape, grapefruit, etc.)	1 cup	$\frac{1}{2}$ cup

*Accessed June 14, 2012, from www.choosemyplate.gov/food-groups/fruits-counts.html.

PHYTOCHEMICALS AND FUNCTIONAL FOODS: THE VALUE OF FOOD

Nutrition tends to focus on the nutrients required for the health and well-being of the human body. Other food components exist that may have other health benefits but do not qualify as a nutrient.

Phytochemicals are nonnutritive substances in plant-based foods that appear to have disease-fighting properties. The health-promoting value of these substances is best obtained by eating a diverse assortment of vegetables, fruits, legumes, grains, and seeds. Green tea, soy, and licorice also contain phytochemicals with healthful qualities. *Functional foods* provide physiological health benefits beyond the nutrients they contain. Phytochemicals and functional foods are of great interest because they may assist in preventing or treating chronic diseases such as diabetes, coronary artery disease, cancer, and hypertension. Even osteoporosis, arthritis, and neural tube defects may be reduced by adequate consumption of these substances. Onions and garlic not only taste good but also contain allylic sulfides—phytochemicals—that enhance immune function, enhance excretion of cancer-inducing substances, decrease blood cholesterol levels, and reduce spread of tumor cells—quite a long list of benefits for foods that taste so good. Tomatoes provide lycopene, which appears to have the ability to halt cancer cells from spreading. Consequently, consumption of cooked tomatoes has been related to a decreased risk of certain cancers. Soy contains isoflavones, which also decrease blood cholesterol levels and flavonoids that may reduce menopausal symptoms.

A number of products already use soy-derived ingredients and others are in development. Consumers can gain health benefits while consuming familiar foods that have added soy ingredients (see also the *Health Debate* box in Chapter 22). The availability of other functional food products continues to expand. Factors influencing this expansion consist of: increasing health care costs; aging population; changing food regulations; increasing sense of self-efficacy and health care autonomy; and enhancing personal health among the general population.

Perhaps a significant means for disease prevention has always been available for us: consumption of adequate amounts of whole foods such as fruits and vegetables, along with less-processed grains and legumes, possibly topped off with a few cups of green tea.

Data from Position of The American Dietetic Association: Functional foods, *J Am Diet Assoc* 109:735-746, 2009.

beri," meaning "I can't! I can't!" This phrase, beriberi, became the name of a serious disease resulting from thiamine deficiency. In the 1890s it was discovered that beriberi resulted from consumption of hulled (white) rice and that unhulled (brown) rice prevented or cured this disease. Later, researchers found that the thiamine in the hulls of whole grains prevents or cures beriberi.

Function

The main function of thiamine is to serve as a coenzyme, a substance that activates an enzyme, in energy metabolism;

it also has a role in nerve functioning related to muscle actions.

Recommended Intake and Sources

The RDA for thiamine is 1.2 mg per day for men and 1.1 mg for women. The amount of thiamine required increases as the metabolic rate rises. Those engaged in rigorous physical activity burn more energy, so they require more thiamine.

Lean pork, whole or enriched grains and flours, legumes, seeds, and nuts are good sources of thiamine. As a water-soluble vitamin, some thiamine can be lost in food processing or when foods are cooked at home.[2] Thiamine may be leaked into cooking fluid or destroyed by heat. Generally, however, most of us consume sufficient amounts of thiamine.

Deficiency

Thiamine deficiency alters the nervous, muscular, gastrointestinal (GI), and cardiovascular systems.[7] In beriberi, a severe, chronic deficiency results, characterized by ataxia (muscle weakness and loss of coordination), pain, anorexia, mental disorientation, and tachycardia (rapid beating of the heart). Wet beriberi manifests with edema, affecting cardiac function by weakening the heart muscle and vascular system. Dry beriberi affects the nervous system, producing paralysis and extreme muscle wasting. Marginal deficiencies may occur, producing psychologic disturbances, recurrent headaches, extreme tiredness, and irritability.[7]

Beriberi still occurs in areas of the world, such as Asia, where the staple food is highly polished rice, which is low in thiamine. The practice of repeatedly washing the milled rice results in further loss of thiamine. Very high intakes of raw fish can also produce beriberi. Raw fish naturally contains an enzyme, thiaminase, that destroys thiamine. This does not affect those of us who occasionally enjoy sushi or sashimi, Japanese specialties of raw fish.

In the United States, enrichment of refined flour has virtually eliminated thiamine deficiency. However, people who are chronic alcohol users may develop thiamine deficiency because of decreased food intake and reduced intestinal absorption coupled with an additional need for thiamine by the liver to detoxify alcohol (see the *Cultural Considerations* box, Cuban Crisis).

A severe deficiency of thiamine may cause a cerebral form of beriberi called Wernicke-Korsakoff syndrome. It is the most common disorder of the central nervous system as a neuropsychiatric affect of chronic excessive alcohol intake on nutritional status.[8] Others at risk for this syndrome include individuals with severe GI disease, human immunodeficiency virus (HIV), and improper parenteral glucose solutions.[7] The effects of this thiamine deficiency syndrome may cause the loss of memory, extreme mental confusion, and ataxia exhibited by people with chronic excessive alcohol ingestion. Clinically, care must be taken when a malnourished person is given parenteral fluids containing dextrose. Parenteral fluids should contain a mix of B vitamins; otherwise, the marginal thiamine levels of nutritionally depleted individuals, combined with a sudden increase of glucose to the brain, can

Cuban Crisis

In the spring of 1993 a harsh economy and natural disasters played havoc with Cuba's food supply. The breakup of the Soviet Union dissipated a valuable trade network for Cuba. This, combined with the devastating effects of a tropical storm, severely limited the variety of foods available. The consequence? A disease resulting in vision loss and a numbness caused by nerve damage spread primarily among men. The *New York Times* headlines were startling: "26,000 Cubans partly blinded."

There is speculation that the epidemic was caused by nutritional deficiencies of thiamine and/or folate. These deficits were exacerbated by consumption of home-brewed rum. The rum required thiamine to detoxify the alcohol, further decreasing the available thiamine for body functions. Folate levels declined as supplies of folate-containing foods diminished. Increased reliance on naturally available foods, such as cassava root, and the popularity of cigarettes among 95% of Cuban men further affected folate availability. Both are high in cyanide, which uses up folate stores in the body. The epidemic was eventually brought under control when the Cuban government distributed vitamin supplements to provide the missing nutrients.

A follow-up epidemiologic study reveals that the Cuban male population is still at risk for vitamin B deficiencies, suggesting the need to continue recommendation of preventive vitamin supplementation and increased consumption of fruits and vegetables containing an assortment of B vitamins.

Application to nursing: Unusual circumstances may precipitate unexpected conditions. We often expect disorders to be the result of new variations of bacteria or viruses, but sometimes simple deficiencies may be the cause. Note that this chapter also discusses instances of rickets (vitamin D deficiency disorder) and pellagra (niacin deficiency disorder) unexpectedly occurring. All factors affecting health should be considered to determine the true cause of symptoms.

Data from Altman LK: 26,000 Cubans partly blinded; cause is unclear, *New York Times*, May 21, 1993, A7; Arnaud J et al: Vitamin B intake and status in healthy Havanan men, 2 years after the Cuban neuropathy epidemic, *Br J Nutr* 85(6):741-748, 2001; and Community Nutrition Institute: Epidemic, *Nutrition Week Newspaper* 22:8 (June 11), 1993.

initiate Wernicke-Korsakoff syndrome, regardless of the level of alcohol intake.

Others at risk for thiamine deficiency include renal patients who are undergoing dialysis, are receiving parenteral nutrition, have HIV-AIDS, have persistent vomiting (hyperemesis gravidarum), have anorexia nervosa, have gastrectomy, and have genetic disorders that affect thiamine use.[7] As gastric bypass surgeries increase, instances of peripheral neuropathy from thiamine deficiency may increase as well.

Toxicity

Excess thiamine is excreted in urine. Although thiamine is nontoxic, there is no rationale for supplementation in healthy people. In acute care settings, supplemental thiamine and other B vitamins may be recommended for individuals with chronic excessive alcohol consumption. In general, the best advice is to take a daily multivitamin containing B vitamins.

Riboflavin (B₂)

Have you ever wondered why milk is sold in opaque cardboard or nontransparent plastic containers? These containers protect riboflavin from exposure to light. Riboflavin is sensitive to ultraviolet rays in sunlight and artificial light; much of the riboflavin is destroyed if milk, an excellent source of riboflavin, is sold in clear glass or clear plastic receptacles. Why risk loss of a valuable vitamin?

Function

Like thiamine, riboflavin's main function is as a coenzyme in the release of energy from nutrients in every cell of the body.

Recommended Intake and Sources

The RDA for riboflavin is 1.3 mg per day for men and 1.1 mg for women. The body's need is related to total kcal intake, energy needs, body size, metabolic rate, and growth rate. Conditions requiring increased protein also require increased riboflavin, such as during wound healing or the growth periods of childhood, pregnancy, and lactation.

Riboflavin is found in both plant and animal foods. In the United States, however, milk is a major source, with small amounts coming from other foods such as enriched grain. Good plant sources are broccoli, asparagus, dark leafy greens, whole grains, and enriched breads and cereals. Rich sources of animal origin include dairy products, meats, fish, poultry, and eggs.

As mentioned, riboflavin is sensitive to light and irradiation. It also can be lost in cooking water but is heat stable.

Deficiency

Ariboflavinosis is the name for a group of symptoms associated with riboflavin deficiency. The lips become swollen, and cracks develop in the corners of the mouth (cheilosis). The tongue becomes inflamed, swollen, and purplish red (glossitis), a common symptom of riboflavin and other B vitamins. Seborrheic dermatitis, a skin condition characterized by greasy scales, may occur in the regions of the ears, nose, and mouth. Riboflavin deficiency may also affect the availability and use of pyridoxine and niacin.

Nutritional deficiencies tend to be multiple rather than single, and it is difficult to separate symptoms. If an individual is deficient in a nutrient such as riboflavin, more than likely a deficiency of other nutrients also will be present. For example, esophageal cancer is associated with deficiencies of riboflavin and zinc, particularly in Africa, Iran, and China. In the United States, riboflavin deficiency may be related to anorexia nervosa, inadequate intake when active individuals restrict caloric intake, and lactose intolerance[9]—all of which are associated with potential multiple nutritional deficiencies.

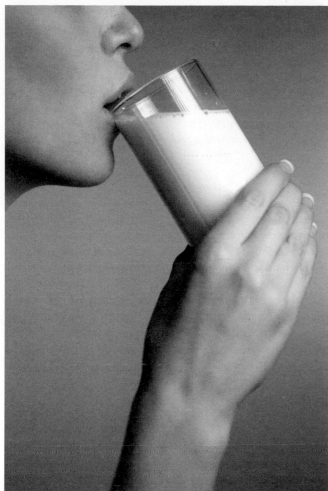

Milk is the major source of riboflavin in the United States. (Photos.com.)

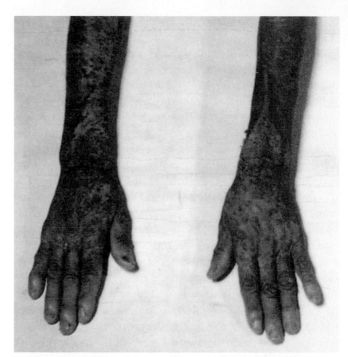

FIG 7-1 Dermatitis in a patient suffering from pellagra. (From McLaren DS: *A colour atlas and text of diet-related disorders,* ed 2, London, 1992, Mosby.)

Toxicity

Toxicity to riboflavin has not been reported. Absorption of riboflavin tends to be limited under normal circumstances; excessive absorption is extremely unlikely.[9]

Niacin (B₃)

Niacin occurs naturally in two forms: nicotinic acid and niacinamide. It's hard to imagine, but before niacin was identified, people who were actually suffering from niacin deficiency were so psychologically disoriented that they were sent to mental institutions for treatment. Niacin deficiency can bring on a psychosis that dissipates once sufficient quantities are consumed.

Function

Niacin is involved as a coenzyme for many enzymes, especially those involved in energy metabolism; it is critical for glycolysis and the tricarboxylic acid (TCA) cycle.

Recommended Intake and Sources

Niacin is available in foods as the active vitamin or as its precursor, the amino acid tryptophan. That is, tryptophan can be converted to niacin, and some niacin can be provided this way. Diets adequate in protein tend to be adequate in niacin.

Niacin requirements are measured in niacin equivalents (NE), reflecting the body's ability to convert tryptophan to niacin. To form 1 mg of niacin, 60 mg of tryptophan is needed, both of which equal 1 mg NE. The RDA recommends that men and women consume 16 mg NE and 14 mg NE per day, respectively. The DRI for niacin includes a UL of 35 mg NE per day because of the adverse reactions experienced when excess amounts are taken in supplement form (see the section titled "Toxicity").

Protein-containing foods are good sources of both niacin and tryptophan. Meats, poultry, fish, legumes, enriched cereals, milk, and even coffee and tea are sources of niacin.

Deficiency

Pellagra, the niacin deficiency disorder, is characterized by the three D's, as follows:[10]

1. *Diarrhea:* Damage to the GI tract affects digestion, absorption, and excretion of food, leading to glossitis, vomiting, and diarrhea.
2. *Dermatitis:* A symmetric scaly rash occurs only on skin exposed to the sun (Figure 7-1).
3. *Dementia:* As the central nervous system becomes affected in severe deficiencies, confusion, anxiety, insomnia, and paranoia develop.

In the early 1900s, pellagra was common in the southern United States among the poor who subsisted on corn-based diets. The niacin in corn is in a bound form unavailable for absorption, and many people subsisting on low incomes had such a limited intake of protein food that neither tryptophan nor preformed niacin was available. Since the discovery of the cause of pellagra, flours have been enriched with niacin, and the incidence of pellagra has decreased dramatically.

In the United States, health professionals need to be vigilant to recognize the symptoms of vitamin deficiencies among patients undergoing specialized treatments or experiencing disorders that may negatively affect their nutritional status. For example, pellagra may develop among people with chronic excessive alcohol ingestion, particularly if combined with homelessness and failure to eat regularly (not using shelter-based meal programs).[11] Several cases have been reported in which the symptom of dermatitis was not recognized as pellagra. In one situation, the simultaneous use of several alternative remedies initiated pellagra, although the individual consumed sufficient dietary niacin.[4] Another report discusses pellagra dermatitis possibly caused by cancer treatment (5-fluorouracil) exacerbating the low niacin levels of the patient.[1] Pellagra may even occur, as a secondary condition to anorexia nervosa.[12] In contrast, in Africa and Asia, pellagra still occurs among the general population.

Toxicity

The UL for niacin is 35 mg NE per day. When preformed niacin and nicotinic acid (but not niacinamide) are consumed in levels greater than the UL, the vascular system is affected, producing a flushing effect throughout the body. A pharmacologic dose is 3 to 9 g of niacin, compared with the RDA of 16 mg NE. Niacin has been used therapeutically because megadoses may lower total cholesterol and low-density lipoprotein (LDL) and increase high-density lipoprotein (HDL).[10] These therapeutic doses, however, must be medically administered to guard against liver damage and related gout and arthritic reactions.

Pyridoxine (B₆)

Vitamin B_6 and pyridoxine are generic terms representing a group of related chemicals. The three main members are pyridoxine, pyridoxal, and pyridoxamine. All three forms can be converted to the coenzyme pyridoxal phosphate (PLP) for use in the body.

Function

The major function of vitamin B_6, in the form of PLP, is to act as a coenzyme in the metabolism of amino acids and proteins. These reactions are involved in the formation of neurotransmitters and are essential for proper functioning of the nervous system. PLP is essential for hemoglobin synthesis. It is required for the conversion of tryptophan to niacin. It also serves as a coenzyme for fatty acid and carbohydrate metabolism.

Supplements of B_6, folate, and B_{12} may reduce risk of CAD by lowering homocysteine levels (see also "Overcoming Barriers" later in this chapter). Several epidemiologic studies suggest that the greater the *dietary* intake of B_6, the lower the risk of colorectal cancer in women.[13,14]

Recommended Intake and Sources

The RDA for vitamin B_6 is 1.3 mg per day for men and women. These amounts are based on protein intake. Vitamin B_6 is found in a wide variety of foods. Particularly good sources include whole grains and cereals, legumes, and chicken, fish, pork, and eggs.

Deficiency

A deficiency of vitamin B_6 rarely occurs alone; it normally accompanies low intakes of other B vitamins. Symptoms include dermatitis, altered nerve function, weakness, poor growth, convulsions, and microcytic anemia (small red blood cells deficient in hemoglobin).

Of the numerous drugs affecting the bioavailability and metabolism of vitamin B_6, oral contraceptive agents (OCAs) may be among the most widely used. Prolonged use of such drugs as isoniazid (for tuberculosis), penicillamine (for lead poisoning, cystinuria, Wilson's disease, sclerosis, and rheumatoid arthritis), cycloserine (for tuberculosis), and hydralazine (for hypertension) may require vitamin B_6 supplements to reduce neurologic side effects and prevent deficiency during treatment.[15]

Toxicity

Vitamin B_6 has sometimes been prescribed to relieve the symptoms associated with premenstrual syndrome (PMS); however, there are no adequate data to support this treatment. Although doses of 10 mg, an amount often prescribed, are most likely not harmful (even considering the RDA of 1.3 mg), long-term supplementation in megadose gram quantities has been reported to cause ataxia and sensory neuropathy. The UL of B_6 is 100 mg/day.

Folate

Folate, like other B vitamins, actually consists of several similar compounds. One of these compounds was originally extracted from spinach and was given the name folic acid, from the Latin word *folium*, meaning "leaf." Folic acid was discovered in 1945 during the search for the nutritional factor responsible for control of pernicious anemia. We now know that vitamin B_{12}, rather than folate, is the nutrient that cures pernicious anemia. Folate and its related compounds, however, play a role in other essential biologic processes. The terms *folate, folic acid, folacin,* and *pteroylglutamic acid (PGA)* are often used interchangeably. Folate is the form of this vitamin found naturally in foods. Folic acid is a synthetic form used in vitamin supplements and for food fortification. Folic acid is actually more available for absorption by the body.

Function

Folate acts as a coenzyme in reactions involving the transfer of one-carbon units during metabolism. As such, it is required for the synthesis of amino acids, which are the building

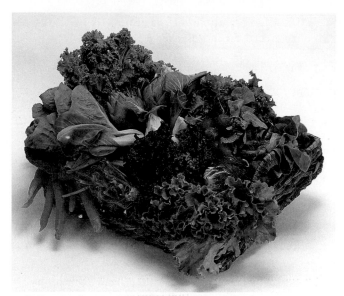

Leafy green vegetables are rich in folate. (Photos.com.)

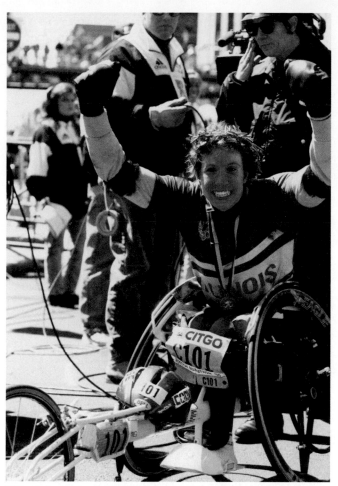

FIG 7-2 Jean Driscoll is an Olympian, Paralympian, author, and advocate for persons with disabilities around the world who happened to be born with spina bifida. (More information about Jean Driscoll can be found on her website: www.jeandriscoll.com.) (Copyright 1995 PVA Publications, Sports 'N Spokes, Phoenix.)

blocks of protein, and for the synthesis of deoxyribonucleic acid (DNA) and ribonucleic acid (RNA). Blood health also depends on folate to form the heme portion of hemoglobin. For the active form of folate to be maintained for use in the body, vitamin B_{12} must be available.

Folate has a role in the proper formation of fetal neural tubes. Neural tube birth defects affect brain and spinal cord development, resulting in the disorders of spina bifida and anencephaly. Spina bifida is a congenital neural tube defect caused by the incomplete closure of the fetus's spine during early pregnancy. It may involve incomplete development of the brain, spinal cord, and/or their protective coverings. This results in a range of disabilities, including paralysis and incontinence (Figure 7-2). In cases of anencephaly, a congenital defect in which the brain does not develop, death may occur shortly after birth. Although these disorders result from a combination of genetics and environment, adequate folate levels during the first month after conception appear to greatly reduce the incidence of these serious birth defects. Unfortunately, women of childbearing age are sometimes marginally deficient in folate. They may not know they are pregnant during the first few crucial weeks when the neural tube of the fetus forms.

Recommended Intake and Sources

The RDA reflects that some folate is stored in the liver, but generally daily supplies are needed. The RDA is 400 mcg per day for men and women. Physiologic state greatly affects folate need. During pregnancy, a woman's blood supply increases. This increase of blood and the growth of other tissues necessitate a greater need for folate. Consequently, the RDA jumps to 600 mcg during pregnancy. While lactating, nutrient needs are elevated because of the nutrient content of the human milk being produced. Therefore, the RDA for folate is 500 mcg for lactation needs.

It is recommended that women of childbearing age increase their folate intake to include 400 mcg of synthetic folic acid to reduce the risks of birth defects, including spina bifida. The increased levels could be provided by natural sources, fortified foods, or supplements (Table 7-1). To ensure adequate access to folic acid, the U.S. Food and Drug Administration (FDA) mandates that cereal-grain products be fortified with 140 mcg/100 g folic acid. This means that manufacturers of enriched breads, flours, cornmeals, rice, pastas, and other grain products are required to add folate to their products.[16] Fortified product labels may include the claim that adequate intake of folic acid may reduce the risk of neural tube defects.[17]

Although this folic acid fortification assists in meeting the recommended levels for women of childbearing age, health care professionals must be prepared to individualize nutrition guidance to ensure daily optimal consumption of folate and folic acid. Clients and patients need to understand that simply consuming fortified cereals and grains does not necessarily provide sufficient amounts of folate. Dietitians should be consulted to ensure the appropriateness of dietary recommendations.

TABLE 7-1   FOOD SOURCES OF FOLATE

FOOD	SERVING SIZE	AMOUNT (MICROGRAMS)	% DAILY VALUE*
Chicken liver	3.5 oz	770	193
Breakfast cereals	½ to 1½ cups	100-400	25-100
Braised beef liver	3.5 oz	217	54
Lentils, cooked	½ cup	180	45
Chickpeas	½ cup	141	35
Asparagus	½ cup	132	33
Spinach, cooked	½ cup	131	33
Black beans	½ cup	128	32
Burrito with beans	2	118	30
Kidney beans	½ cup	115	29
Baked beans with pork	1 cup	92	23
Lima beans	½ cup	78	20
Tomato juice	1 cup	48	12
Brussels sprouts	½ cup	47	12
Orange	1 medium	47	12
Broccoli, cooked	½ cup	39	10
Fast-food french fries	Large order	38	10
Wheat germ	2 tbsp	38	10
Fortified white bread	1 slice	38	10

*Based on daily value for folate of 400 mcg.
Data from Pennington JAT, Douglass JS: *Bowes & Church's food values of portions commonly used,* ed 19, Philadelphia, 2010, Lippincott Williams & Wilkins.

BOX 7-4   HOMOCYSTEINE, VITAMINS, AND HEART HEALTH

Homocysteine is a compound found in blood formed during the metabolism of the essential amino acid methionine. An elevated level of homocysteine (hyperhomocysteinemia) is an inflammation marker associated with an increased risk of coronary artery disease (CAD). There may also be a relationship between elevated homocysteine, low folate levels, and increased risk of Alzheimer's disease and/or dementia. The risk of CAD may be caused by increased clotting and damage to the vascular system because of excess homocysteine. Lowering blood homocysteine levels after an acute myocardial infarction may not reduce risk of future cardiovascular events because the vascular damage has already occurred. The mechanism of Alzheimer's disease and homocysteine levels has not been determined.

Individuals at high risk for CAD should be screened for hyperhomocysteinemia. High levels of homocysteine have been associated with low consumption of foods containing folate, vitamin B_6, and vitamin B_{12} that results in low serum levels of these vitamins. Treatment recommendations to lower blood homocysteine levels are based on this association between homocysteine levels and intake of the three B vitamins. One treatment approach consists of pharmacologic doses of folic acid (400-1000 mcg/day) and a vitamin supplement containing the Dietary Reference Intake (DRI) for pyridoxine (B_6) and vitamin B_{12}. Another treatment strategy focuses only on levels of folic acid (100% of the DRI) and vitamin B_6 (150% of the DRI). In addition to supplements, consumption of foods high in these vitamins is strongly recommended. Refer to Table 7-1 for specific food sources containing these nutrients. Studies have found that either approach significantly reduces blood homocysteine levels and reduces risk of CAD. A registered dietitian or health care provider should determine levels of supplementation.

Concern has been expressed regarding the risks and benefits of this fortification to other age groups. In particular, the effects on older adults may be an issue because an excess of folate can mask a B_{12} deficiency for which older adults are at risk. Requiring vitamin supplements that contain folic acid to also contain vitamin B_{12} can reduce this risk. This decreases the risk of the larger folate intakes overshadowing possible deficiencies of B_{12}. Overall, the benefits appear to outweigh the risk because the increase in folic acid intake from fortification should also cause decreases in homocysteine blood levels, thereby decreasing the risk of heart disease and possibly strokes (in men) (Box 7-4). The actual risk, though, will need to be studied as the fortification program progresses.[18] Higher intakes of folate, along with B_6, may also reduce the risk of colorectal cancer in women.[14,18]

Folate is widely available in foods, particularly in leafy green vegetables, legumes, ready-to-eat cereals, and some fruits and juices. Folate is affected by heat, oxidation, and ultraviolet light; processing and cooking of fresh foods reduce the amount of folate available. Folate is found in many foods that contain ascorbic acid (vitamin C), such as oranges and orange juice. Ascorbic acid protects folate from oxidation. Diets deficient in folate often are deficient in vitamin C, and vice versa.

Deficiency

Cells whose normal activities require rapid cell growth and division are particularly sensitive to folate deficiency. Examples include red blood cells and the cells that line the GI tract. Folate deficiency results in megaloblastic anemia. This is a form of anemia characterized by large red blood cells that cannot carry oxygen properly. Other deficiency symptoms include glossitis, diarrhea, irritability, absentmindedness, depression, and anxiety.[19]

Deficiency may result from any condition that requires cell division to speed up, including infection, cancer, burns, blood loss, GI damage, growth, and pregnancy. Currently about one-third of pregnant women worldwide are affected by folate deficiency. Other groups at risk include those with a limited intake and variety of food, including older adults with low incomes and those with chronic excessive alcohol ingestion. Alcoholic cirrhosis often results in both liver damage (which interferes with storage and metabolism of folate) and excessive losses of the vitamin in feces and urine.[19]

Numerous medications may affect folate absorption or be antagonistic to folate. These drugs include anticonvulsants, oral contraceptives, aspirin, cancer chemotherapy agents, sulfasalazine, nonsteroidal anti-inflammatory drugs, and antacids. Long-term use of any medication may affect the body's use of nutrients; folate is one that is particularly vulnerable.

Before folic acid supplementation is administered, the absence of vitamin B_{12} deficiency must be established. Therapy with folic acid in the presence of vitamin B_{12} deficiency will favorably improve blood profiles, decreasing megaloblastic anemia, while damage to the central nervous system from lack of B_{12} continues.

Toxicity

Excess folate or folic acid intake is not recommended or warranted. Consuming amounts beyond the UL of 1000 mcg folic acid (for men and women) has not been studied. Such high levels may mask the presence of pernicious anemia, discussed under the following section on cobalamin.

Cobalamin (B_{12})

Cobalamin and vitamin B_{12} are used as generic terms to refer to a group of cobalt-containing compounds. The common pharmaceutical name, used widely in supplements, is *cyanocobalamin*.

Function

Two cobalamins function as vitamin B_{12} coenzymes in humans. B_{12} has a role in folate metabolism by modifying folate coenzymes to active forms to support metabolic functions, including the synthesis of DNA and RNA. The metabolism of fatty acids and amino acids also requires vitamin B_{12}. In addition, B_{12} develops and maintains the myelin sheaths that surround and protect nerve fibers.

Vitamin B_{12}, in conjunction with consumption of vitamin B_6 and folate, appears to reduce the levels of homocysteine, thereby decreasing the risk of CAD (see Box 7-4).

Recommended Intake and Sources

Absorption of vitamin B_{12} relies on an intrinsic factor. The intrinsic factor is produced by stomach mucosa. Both vitamin B_{12} and the intrinsic factor must be present for absorption. Recommended B_{12} levels take into account that some vitamin B_{12} is stored in the liver. The RDA for young adults is 2.4 mcg daily. Foods of animal origin are the only reliable sources of vitamin B_{12}; meat, fish, poultry, eggs, and dairy products are all good sources. For example, one glass of skim milk provides 0.93 mcg of vitamin B_{12}. The vitamin has been reported to be found in legumes (nodules on roots) because of bacteria formation in soil, but they are not a reliable source. Vegans must supplement their intake with vitamin B_{12} supplements or use fortified products.

Deficiency

Deficiencies of B_{12} are usually secondary. Pernicious anemia (from lack of intrinsic factor for B_{12} absorption) or megaloblastic anemia (from related folate dysfunction) occurs. Additional neurologic effects develop because of damage to the spinal cord as the breakdown of myelin sheath synthesis affects brain, optic, and peripheral nerves.[20]

Older adults are more at risk for deficiency because of a naturally occurring reduction in production of the intrinsic factor by the stomach mucosa. Most older adults, however, remain within normal range. For those who do become deficient, injections to bypass intestinal absorption are warranted. Particularly noted among this population are neuropsychiatric symptoms, including delusions and hallucinations, that may occur in the absence of anemia.[21] These symptoms can be misdiagnosed as senility or other illnesses. To alleviate this risk, the recommendations include that adults older than age 50 consume foods fortified with vitamin B_{12} or take a B_{12} supplement to ensure adequacy of the RDA for B_{12}. Vitamin B_{12} is more absorbable in this form because it is already separated from food.

As discussed, folate levels may disguise a B_{12} deficiency. Blood hematologic damage is masked by folate, but neurologic damage continues.

Toxicity

Toxicity to vitamin B_{12} has not been noted, but there are no benefits to large doses unless deficiency exists.

Biotin

Humans need biotin, a member of the B vitamin complex, in tiny amounts.

Function

Biotin assists in the transfer of carbon dioxide from one compound to another, playing an important role in carbohydrate, fat, and protein metabolism.

Recommended Intake and Sources

Biotin is synthesized in the lower GI tract by bacterial microorganisms. However, the amount produced and its bioavailability is unknown. Although biotin is produced in the body, it is still an essential nutrient. (The human body does not produce biotin, but bacteria hosted in the gut do.) It must also be consumed in foods.

The AI for biotin is 30 mcg per day. Biotin is widespread in foods. The richest sources are liver, kidney, peanut butter, egg yolks, and yeast.

Deficiency

Deficiency of biotin is unknown among people eating a typical North American diet. When experimentally produced, symptoms of biotin deficiency include a scaly red skin rash, hair loss, loss of appetite, depression, and glossitis.[22]

Biotin deficiency has been produced by consumption of large amounts of avidin, a protein in raw egg whites that binds biotin. A person would need to consume many raw egg whites for this to occur; salmonella poisoning would probably strike first. Avidin is denatured by heat, so cooked egg whites pose no problem to biotin status.

Antibiotics are known to reduce the number of biotin-producing bacteria. In addition, clients receiving long-term intravenous feeding are prone to biotin deficiency; therefore, their feeding mixtures should contain biotin.

Toxicity

There is no known toxicity for biotin.

Pantothenic Acid

Pantothenic acid gets its name from its presence in all living things (from the Greek *pantothen*, meaning "from all sides").

Function

The principal active form of pantothenic acid functions as part of coenzyme A (CoA for short); therefore, it is required for the metabolism of carbohydrates, fats, and protein.

Recommended Intake and Sources

The AI for pantothenic acid is 5 mg per day. Pantothenic acid is widespread in foods and easily consumed in whole grain cereals, legumes, meat, fish, and poultry.

Deficiency

Deficiencies in pantothenic acid do not naturally occur in humans.

Toxicity

Doses of up to 10 g daily have been administered with no ill effects. Researchers have reported that daily doses of 10 to 20 g may produce diarrhea or water retention.

Choline
Function

Choline is needed for the synthesis of acetylcholine, a neurotransmitter, and lecithin, the phospholipid.

Recommended Intake and Sources

The body can actually make choline from the amino acid methionine, but this process does not produce enough choline to meet the needs of the body. Consequently, food sources are still required. This requirement qualifies choline as an essential nutrient. The AI is 550 mg/day for men and 425 mg/day for women with a UL of 3500 mg/day for adults.[1]

Food sources include many commonly consumed foods with rich sources including milk, eggs, and peanuts.

Deficiency

Deficiency of choline is rare.

Toxicity

Toxicity symptoms include sweating, fishy body odor, vomiting, liver damage, reduced growth, and low blood pressure (hypotension).

Vitamin C

Vitamin C is almost a household word. It's hard to believe that it was isolated as a nutrient only around 1930. The discovery of vitamin C is associated with the search for the cause of **scurvy**, a potentially fatal disease that weakens the body's connective tissues and causes inflammation to them. As early as the eighteenth century, it was known that eating certain foods, particularly citrus fruits, could control scurvy, but the actual substance responsible for gluing the cells together was not determined until Albert Szent-Gyorgyi and Glen King isolated it in 1928 and 1930, respectively.[23] One of the two active forms of vitamin C is ascorbic acid (*ascorbic* meaning "without scurvy").

Function

Vitamin C functions as an antioxidant and as a coenzyme. It can perform different functions in various situations. Collagen formation for bone matrix, teeth, cartilage, and connective tissue depends on ascorbic acid. Vitamin C provides the cement that holds structures together. Wound healing, which necessitates the formation of new tissue, also requires vitamin C.

As an antioxidant, vitamin C protects folate, vitamin E, and polyunsaturated substances from destruction by oxygen as they move throughout the body. An **antioxidant** is a compound that guards others from damaging oxidation by being oxidized itself. Vitamins C and E also work together as antioxidants to destroy substances released as cells age, are oxidized, or become damaged. Their work may prevent damage by free radicals to vascular walls, thereby limiting the development of atherosclerotic plaques.

Among its other functions, vitamin C enhances the absorption of nonheme iron, found in plant foods. Thyroid and adrenal hormone synthesis requires vitamin C. Several conversion processes depend on vitamin C; these include tryptophan to serotonin, cholesterol to bile, and folate to its active form.

Vitamin C may have a role in reducing the risk of cancer development. Epidemiologic studies have uncovered an association between levels of dietary intake of vitamin C and incidence of cancer in the stomach, esophagus, and colon. Because these studies are of dietary intakes of populations, it is not yet known whether the effects are caused by vitamin C or to other, as yet unidentified, components of foods containing vitamin C.

It is a common myth that vitamin C can prevent the common cold. Unfortunately, the bulk of evidence does not support the theory that vitamin C reduces the incidence of

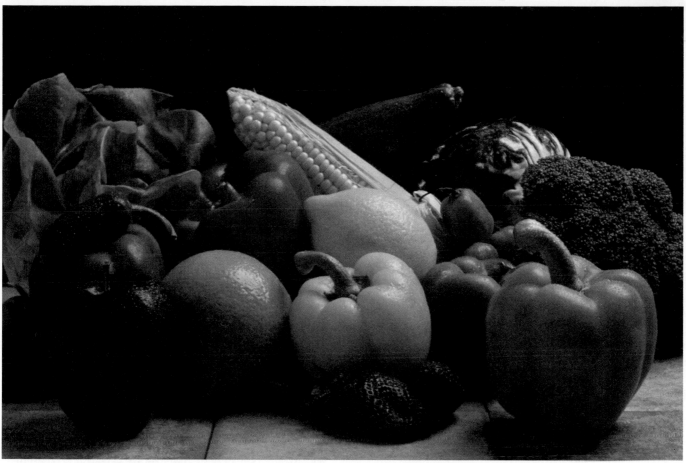

Although citrus fruits are well known for being rich in vitamin C, vegetables such as cauliflower, broccoli, and red, yellow, and green peppers are also nutrient-dense sources. (Photos.com.)

the common cold. Taking supplemental vitamin C for a limited period of time, however, can decrease the duration and reduce the severity of the symptoms. UL, though, should always be observed.

Recommended Intake and Sources

The RDA for vitamin C has varied from 45 mg to 60 mg per day for adults. Currently, the RDA is 90 mg for men and 75 mg for women. Recommendations vary worldwide; the minimum daily requirement to prevent symptoms of scurvy is 10 mg. However, the amount recommended daily to provide enough circulating vitamin C for tissue saturation for good health is open to interpretation.

As more is learned about vitamin C functions, recommendations customized to specific disease and lifestyle behaviors will be determined. For example, cigarette smokers have lower circulating levels of vitamin C compared with nonsmokers, regardless of their dietary intake of vitamin C. The metabolic use of vitamin C by smokers is twice that of nonsmokers. Recognizing this deficit, smokers are advised to increase their vitamin C intake from the 90 mg RDA to 125 mg daily.[1]

Fruits and vegetables provide 95% of the vitamin C we consume. Many foods are excellent sources; some of them include citrus fruits, red and green peppers, strawberries, tomatoes, potatoes, broccoli, and other green leafy vegetables. Serving sizes to meet the RDA are listed in Table 7-2.

Some foods and drinks are fortified with vitamin C. Ready-to-eat cereals have added vitamin C (about 25% of the daily values) and other vitamins not naturally found in grains. Additional vitamin C, often 100% of the daily values, is added to the small amounts naturally found in apple and grape juice.

Vitamin C is destroyed by air, light, and heat. Fruit juices should be stored in an airtight container that holds only the amount that can be consumed in a short time. The vitamin C content of cooked foods can be maximized by cooking in the minimal amount of water or, even better, by microwaving (see the *Teaching Tool* box, Vegetable Victories).

Deficiency

Although vitamin C deficiency is rare in developed countries in the West, it may still occur among chronic alcohol and drug users, smokers, and those whose dietary intakes are poor. Older adults may have marginal intake because of difficulty in obtaining and preparing fresh foods. Low maternal dietary intake of vitamin C may increase risk of gestational diabetes mellitus.[24] These at-risk groups may experience other vitamin and mineral deficiencies as well.

TABLE 7-2	**RECOMMENDED DIETARY ALLOWANCE SERVING SIZES OF VITAMIN C***	

FOOD	SERVING SIZE	VITAMIN C (mg)
Orange juice	¾ cup	93
Orange	1 medium	80
Kiwifruit	1 medium	75
Cantaloupe	1¼ cups	68
Peppers, green or red	¾ cup	64
Strawberries	1 cup	64
Broccoli	¾ cup	58
Brussels sprouts	¾ cup	48
Grapefruit	½ fruit	47

*RDA = 75-90 mg.
Data from Pennington JAT, Douglass JS: *Bowes & Church's food values of portions commonly used*, ed 19, Philadelphia, 2010, Lippincott Williams & Wilkins.

✳ TEACHING TOOL

Vegetable Victories

We may focus on teaching clients what vitamins do in their bodies, but this education is pointless unless they relate the information to the foods they actually eat. Some of our clients, who may be willing to experiment with preparing foods (particularly vegetables) in a more nutrient-retaining manner, may be at a loss as to how to proceed. We cannot assume that everyone has grown up naturally knowing how to steam broccoli.

Clients need assistance in achieving vegetable victories. What is a vegetable victory? This is a situation in which individuals learn to prepare the vegetable they most enjoy in a way that still retains the most nutrients possible. With vegetables, most of those nutrients are vitamins, mainly water-soluble vitamins. Because water-soluble vitamins are in the liquid parts of vegetables, if vegetables are cooked or boiled (please don't), the vitamins are either leached into the cooking water or may even be destroyed by the heat. What to do? Nutritional value is reduced by air, heat, water, and light. The following are some preparation pointers to provide to clients, especially younger inexperienced food preparers:

- To prevent loss from air exposure, use plastic containers to store vegetables and cook with lids.
- To limit vitamin forfeiture from water-related preparation, cook vegetables with as little water as possible or use vegetable cooking water in soups or sauces.
- To reduce destruction from light, keep vegetables in dark places; most should be stored in the refrigerator.
- To reduce heat damage to vitamins, keep vegetables cool and cook only until they are crisp by microwaving, stir-frying, or lightly steaming.

Data from Clark N: *Nancy Clark's sports nutrition guidebook*, ed 3, Champaign, Ill, 2003, Human Kinetics.

Scurvy represents the extreme result of vitamin C deficiency. The symptoms are tied to the functions of vitamin C in the body. When the glue-like substance of collagen is not replaced, tissues throughout the body degenerate. Gingivitis causes gums to bleed, and teeth come loose; joints and limbs ache from muscle degeneration and lack of new connective tissue formation; bruising and hemorrhages occur as the vascular system weakens; and plaques form as a result of the vascular damage. Death ultimately occurs as functioning of all body systems disintegrates.

Marginal deficiency symptoms may manifest as gingivitis with soreness and ulcerations of the mouth, poor wound healing, inadequate tooth and bone growth or maintenance, and increased risk of infection as the integrity of tissues throughout the body becomes compromised.

Toxicity

Toxicity from foods high in vitamin C does not occur even if we consume cups of fresh strawberries washed down with a quart of orange juice. Chronic supplement intakes of megadoses from 1 to 15 g may result in cramps, diarrhea, nausea, kidney stone formation, and gout. The effects of anticlotting medication also may be affected.[1]

Taking supplements of vitamin C seems benign, but the body adapts to protect itself from harm. If continually inundated with excessive vitamin C, the body develops a mechanism that destroys much of the extra vitamin C circulating in the body. A rebound effect may occur if, after taking megadoses for several months or more, an individual abruptly stops supplementation and consumes a quantity closer to the RDA. The protective mechanism of the body is still in gear and continues to destroy vitamin C. An individual may develop symptoms of scurvy even though the RDA is consumed. A newborn exposed to vitamin C megadoses in utero may experience this rebound effect. Although the rebound effect may not occur in every case, withdrawal from vitamin C megadoses should be gradual, over a period of 2 to 4 weeks. Consequently, there is an UL of 2000 mg for adults and 400 to 1800 mg for children and adolescents.

Table 7-3 provides a quick reference to water-soluble vitamins.

FAT-SOLUBLE VITAMINS

Vitamin A

Each year approximately 250,000 children enter a world of permanent darkness. The cause? Vitamin A deficiency. Extreme vitamin A deficiency is so damaging to corneas that blindness occurs. Although this could be prevented with just a few cents' worth of vitamin A per year, there is little money for preventive health measures in areas of the world where food is scarce.

Function

Vitamin A is a group of compounds that function to maintain skin and mucous membranes throughout the body. Specific activities depending on vitamin A are vision, bone growth, functioning of the immune system, and normal reproduction. Our eyes depend on visual purple, technically

TABLE 7-3 WATER-SOLUBLE VITAMINS

VITAMIN	FUNCTION	CLINICAL ISSUES (DEFICIENCY/TOXICITY)	RECOMMENDED DAILY INTAKES	FOOD SOURCES
Thiamine (B₁)	Coenzyme energy metabolism; muscle nerve action	Deficiency: beriberi (ataxia, disorientation, tachycardia); marginal (headaches, tiredness); wet beriberi (edema); dry beriberi (nervous system): Wernicke-Korsakoff syndrome (alcoholism)	Men: 1.2 mg Women: 1.1 mg	Lean pork, whole or enriched grains and flours, legumes, seeds, and nuts
Riboflavin (B₂)	Coenzyme energy metabolism	Deficiency: ariboflavinosis with cheilosis, glossitis, seborrheic dermatitis	Men: 1.3 mg Women: 1.1 mg	Milk/dairy products; meat, fish, poultry, and eggs, dark leafy greens (broccoli); whole and enriched breads and cereals
Niacin (B₃) (nicotinic acid and niacinamide) precursor: tryptophan	Cofactor to enzymes involved in energy metabolism; glycolysis and TCA cycle	Deficiency: pellagra Toxicity: vasodilation, liver damage, gout, and arthritic reactions	Men: 16 mg NE Women: 14 mg NE (UL 35 mg NE)	Meats, poultry, and fish; legumes; whole and enriched cereals; milk
Pyridoxine (B₆)	Forms coenzyme pyridoxal phosphate (PLP) for energy metabolism; CNS; hemoglobin synthesis	Deficiency: dermatitis, altered nerve function, weakness, anemia; OCAs decrease B₆ levels Toxicity: ataxia, sensory neuropathy	Men: 1.3 mg Women: 1.3 mg (UL 100 mg)	Whole grains/cereals legumes, poultry, fish, pork, eggs
Folate (folic acid, folacin, PGA)	Coenzyme metabolism (synthesis of amino acid, heme, DNA RNA); fetal neural tube formation	Deficiency: megaloblastic anemia; many drugs affect folate use Toxicity: megadoses may mask pernicious anemia	Men: 400 mcg Women: 400 mcg Pregnancy: 600 mcg Lactation: 500 mcg (UL 1000 mcg)	Widely available leafy green vegetables, legumes, ascorbic acid-containing foods
Cobalamin (B₁₂)	Transport/storage of folate; metabolism of fatty acids/amino acids	Deficiency: pernicious anemia, CNS damage	Adults: 2.4 mcg	Animal sources
Biotin	Metabolism of carbohydrate, fat, and protein	Deficiency: produced by avidin and long-term antibiotics	Adults: 30 mcg AI	Liver, kidney, peanut butter, egg yolks, intestinal synthesis
Pantothenic acid	Part of coenzyme A	Deficiency: not possible	Adults: 5 mg AI	Widespread in foods
Choline	Synthesis of acetylcholine and lecithin	Deficiency: rare Toxicity: body odor, liver damage, hypotension	Men: 550 mg Women: 425 mg (UL 3500 mg)	Widespread—milk, eggs, peanuts
Vitamin C	Antioxidant, coenzyme, collagen formation, wound healing, iron absorption, hormone synthesis	Deficiency: scurvy Toxicity: cramps, nausea, kidney stone formation, gout (1-15 g), rebound scurvy	Men: 90 mg Women: 75 mg (UL 2000)	Fruits/vegetables (citrus fruits, tomatoes, peppers, strawberries, broccoli)

AI, Adequate Intake; *CNS,* central nervous system; *DNA,* deoxyribonucleic acid; *NE,* niacin equivalent; *OCAs,* oral contraceptive agents; *PGA,* pteroylglutamic acid; *RNA,* ribonucleic acid; *TCA,* tricarboxylic acid; *UL,* Tolerable Upper Intake Level.

called *rhodopsin,* to be able to adjust to light variations. Rhodopsin is formed from retinal, a vitamin A substance, and opsin, a protein. Without enough vitamin A, rhodopsin cannot be formed, and the retina cannot easily respond to light changes. As a result, night blindness develops (Figure 7-3). Bone growth involves a process of remodeling that reshapes and enlarges the skeleton. Reshaping requires vitamin A to undo existing bone. Vitamin A maintains integrity of epithelial tissues throughout the body, providing protection against infections and ensuring optimum function. Hormone-like effects of vitamin A appear to be tied to cell synthesis for reproductive purposes.

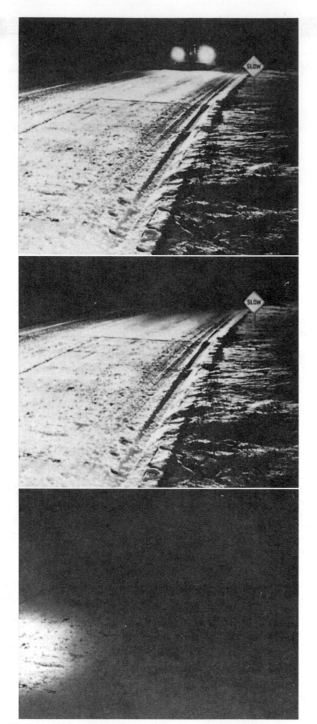

TABLE 7-4	VITAMIN A/BETA CAROTENE SOURCES*	
FOOD	**SERVING SIZE**	**CAROTENE (RAE)**
Liver (beef)	3 ½ oz	10,000
Sweet potato	1 whole, baked	2488
Carrots	1 whole, raw	2025
	½ cup, cooked	1915
Spinach	½ cup, cooked	737
Butternut squash	½ cup, cooked	714
Cantaloupe	1 cup	516
Red pepper	1 whole	422
Apricots	3 medium	277

*RDA = 900 RAE for men; 700 RAE for women.
RAE, Retinol activity equivalent.
Data from Pennington JAT, Douglass JS: *Bowes & Church's food values of portions commonly used*, ed 19, Philadelphia, 2010, Lippincott Williams & Wilkins.

FIG 7-3 Night blindness. These photographs simulate the eyes' slow response to a flash of light at night. (From Pharmacia and Upjohn.)

Recommended Intake and Sources

Vitamin A is measured as retinol activity equivalents (RAE). The RDA, based on providing optimum storage of vitamin A in the liver, is 900 mcg RAE for men and 700 mcg RAE for women.[1] RAE incorporates both the preformed, active forms of vitamin A called *retinoids* (found in animal foods) and the precursor forms of vitamin A called *carotenoids* (found in plant foods). The carotenoid beta carotene is the primary source of vitamin A from plant foods.

Because vitamin A (a fat-soluble vitamin) is stored in the body, daily doses are not necessary, but they are desirable. Deficiency of other nutrients affects the absorption and use of vitamin A.[25] Nutrients are interdependent, and imbalances of specific nutrients affect the functioning of others.

Natural preformed vitamin A is found only in the fat of animal-related foods; these include whole milk, butter, liver, egg yolks, and fatty fish. Carotenoids are found in deep green, yellow, and orange fruits and vegetables. The best sources include broccoli, cantaloupe, sweet potatoes, carrots, tomatoes, and spinach (Table 7-4). High consumption of carotenoids has been associated with decreased risk of certain cancers and other chronic diseases.

When fats are removed from animal-related foods, preformed vitamin A is also lost. To maintain traditional sources of the vitamin, low-fat, skim, and nonfat milks are fortified with vitamin A. Other fortified products include margarine (which often replaces butter, a natural source of vitamin A), and ready-to-eat cereal, a staple food product commonly fortified with many nutrients.

Deficiency

Vitamin A deficiency is either primary, caused by lack of dietary intake, or secondary, the result of chronic fat malabsorption. As liver storage becomes depleted, symptoms develop. The effects are closely tied to vitamin A functions. Ocularly, xerophthalmia incorporates a range of symptoms manifested by night blindness (the inability of the eyes to readjust from bright to dim light) progressing to a hard, dry cornea (keratinization) or keratomalacia, resulting in complete blindness. The degeneration of the epithelial tissues protecting the eye itself leads to the effects of xerophthalmia. Compromised epithelial tissues also result in hair follicles developing hard white lumps of keratin (hyperkeratosis), respiratory infections, diarrhea, and other GI disturbances. Overall, the immune system is endangered; for children especially, a minor illness or a bout of measles may be deadly.

| | ANTIOXIDANT | | | DAILY RECOMMENDED |
ANTIOXIDANT	FUNCTIONS	MAJOR FOOD SOURCES	ADULT RDA	SUPPLEMENTATION
Beta carotene (pre–vitamin A)	May decrease risk of some cancers and CAD	Sweet potatoes, winter squash, carrots, red bell peppers, dark green vegetables, apricots, mangos, cantaloupe	No RDA (1 sweet potato = 15 mg, 1 carrot = 10 mg)	6-15 mg, nontoxic, higher doses may give skin a harmless orange cast (not recommended for smokers)
Vitamin C	May decrease risk of certain cancers and CAD	Kiwi, citrus fruits, berries, cantaloupe, honeydew, bell peppers, tomatoes, cabbage family vegetables	75-90 mg (1 kiwi = 150 mg, 1 cup broccoli = 115 mg, 1 orange = 70 mg)	250-500 mg, more may cause diarrhea (UL 2000 mg)
Vitamin E	May decrease risk of cancer; may also prevent or delay cataracts	Vegetable oil, nuts, seeds, margarine, wheat germ, olives, leafy greens, avocado, asparagus	15 mg α-TE (1 Tbsp oil = 9 mg, 1 Tbsp margarine or 1 oz nuts = 2 mg)	300-600 mg (200-400 international units) daily* for all adults, higher doses may cause headaches and diarrhea (UL 1000 mg)
Selenium	Prevents cell and lipid membrane damage	Meat, fish, eggs, whole grains	55 mcg	Same as RDA; not more than 200 mcg; higher very toxic with severe liver damage, vomiting, diarrhea, metallic aftertaste (UL 400 mcg)

*Contraindicated for those with hypertension or who take warfarin (Coumadin) and other drugs to inhibit blood clots.
α-TE, Alpha-tocopherol; CAD, coronary artery disease; RDA, Recommended Dietary Allowance; UL, Tolerable Upper Intake Level.

Growth is inhibited because of lack of vitamin A–dependent proteins for bone growth.

In the United States, individuals experiencing chronic fat malabsorption are at risk for vitamin A deficiency and deficiencies of other fat-soluble vitamins. These nutrients are incorporated into their overall medical nutrition therapy plans. Although marginal vitamin A deficiency is possible, overt deficiencies are rare.

Deficiency is a health threat in parts of the world where food availability is limited. To counteract this in areas where rice is a staple food, "Golden Rice" has been genetically transformed to accumulate increased amounts of provitamin A. Public health efforts to distribute Golden Rice to farmers and to further increase the nutrient value of the grain (Table 7-5).[26]

Toxicity

Hypervitaminosis A occurs only from preformed vitamin A from either an acute or chronic intake of supplements. Most food sources of preformed A do not contain high enough levels to ever result in toxicity. The only exception noted is polar bear liver and the livers of other large animals. Explorers who feasted on polar bear liver developed hypervitaminosis A; in fact, the way we learned about the toxic effects of vitamin A was through their misfortune. Apparently, the livers of hibernating animals store an extraordinary quantity of vitamin A to provide sufficient amounts for a long winter without nourishment. When humans consume the preformed vitamin A of these livers, the quantity is toxic.

Toxicity does not occur from the carotenoid precursor in foods. If carotenoids are consumed in excess, either from foods or supplements, the skin takes on an orange hue, which dissipates when carotenoid consumption is reduced.

Immediate symptoms of vitamin A toxicity include blistered skin, weakness, anorexia, vomiting, headache, joint pain, irritability, and enlargement of the spleen and liver; long-term effects include bone abnormalities and liver damage.[25]

Vitamin A supplements taken internally will not cure or improve acne and are toxic in excess. Even prescription medications can be problematic. The acne medications sotretinoin (Accutane) and isotretinoin (oral forms) are nonnutritive sources of vitamin A that cause birth defects when used by pregnant women. Advise women who take either of these drugs to use a highly reliable birth control method.

Vitamin D

With sufficient exposure to ultraviolet light or sunshine, the body can manufacture its own supply of vitamin D. The exposure of skin to ultraviolet light begins the conversion process of the vitamin D precursor 7-dehydro-cholesterol (found in our skin) to cholecalciferol, the active form of vitamin D. Because the body can produce vitamin D, it is technically a hormone. However, when vitamin D is supplied by the diet, it is technically a vitamin. Regardless of how it is classified, vitamin D is a substance necessary for a variety of the body's regulating processes as well as normal development of bones and teeth.

Function

Intestinal absorption of calcium and phosphorus depends on the action of vitamin D. This vitamin also affects bone mineralization and mineral homeostasis by helping to regulate blood calcium levels.

Recommended Intake and Sources

The AI for vitamin D is 5 mcg per day. The DRI includes AI recommendations for vitamin D for people ages 51 through 70; the suggested level jumps from 5 mcg (200 international units) a day to 10 mcg (400 international units). After age 70, the recommended levels jump again to 15 mcg (600 international units). These levels reflect that older adults are less efficient at synthesizing vitamin D from sun exposure. If these amounts are not consumed from foods or obtained from sunlight, supplement use may be appropriate. Before beginning supplementation, a dietitian should be consulted; these amounts may already be contained in multivitamin mineral supplements formulated for individuals older than 51 years of age. The UL for vitamin D is 50 mcg (2000 international units). The effects of intakes higher than the UL are discussed in the section on toxicity.

The present recommendations for vitamin D intakes are based on preventing bone disease. Recommendations may be revised as higher levels may reduce the risk of type 1 diabetes, multiple sclerosis, and cancer.[27]

Vitamin D is available through body synthesis or from dietary sources. Cholecalciferol, the active form of vitamin D, can be synthesized. Ultraviolet irradiation from sunlight affects the vitamin D precursor 7-dehydrocholesterol in our skin, and this cholesterol derivative is transformed by the liver and kidneys into cholecalciferol. The amount of vitamin D produced depends on length of exposure to ultraviolet irradiation, atmospheric conditions, and skin pigmentation. Geographic regions and seasons that are particularly cloudy and rainy diminish the quantity of vitamin D synthesized. Darker skin pigmentation also reduces the effect of radiation on the skin, as does sunscreen and concealing clothing. Aging may lessen the amount of vitamin D to be formed from sunlight exposure.

The few sources of natural preformed vitamin D are the fat of the animal-related foods of butter, egg yolks, fatty fish, and liver. Milk, although containing fat, is not a good source; it is, however, a good vehicle for vitamin D fortification because it contains calcium and phosphorus, which need vitamin D for absorption. Because vegans consume no animal foods, they may require supplements or regular sunlight exposure to ensure formation of cholecalciferol. Appropriate guidance should be sought from a primary health care provider or dietitian.

Deficiency

A deficiency of vitamin D can lead to the disorders of rickets (Figure 7-4) and osteomalacia; the extent of vitamin

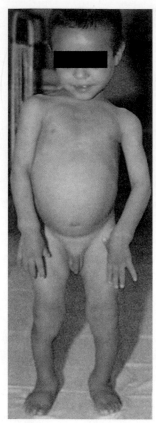

FIG 7-4 Rickets. This child has characteristic bowed legs. (From McLaren DS: *A colour atlas and text of diet-related disorders,* ed 2, London, 1992, Mosby.)

D deficiency among children and adults in the United States may be more widespread than previously suspected.[27] Because of insufficient mineralization of bone and tooth matrix, rickets in children leads to malformed skeletons, characterized by bowed legs unable to bear body weight, oddly angled rib bones and chests, and abnormal tooth formation. In adults, osteomalacia, or bad bones, is characterized by soft demineralized bones that are at risk for fractures. This may be due to vitamin D or calcium deficiency.

It has been thought that rickets occur rarely among well-nourished populations. However, recent reports reveal the risk of rickets has increased among breastfed infants and toddlers, particularly African American children. Other documented instances in Alaska are among breastfed African American and Native Alaskan children between the ages of 11 and 20 months. The increased risk for these children is caused by several factors, including darker pigmentation, use of heavier clothing by children that limits exposure of the skin to vitamin D synthesis, and limited consumption of dietary sources of fortified vitamin D dairy products by children or women who are breastfeeding infants. Use of rice milk or soy milk, not fortified with vitamin D and other nutrients found in human breast milk from well-nourished mothers and from infant formulas, may lead to severe nutrient deficiencies such as rickets. Health care providers initially misdiagnosed cases of rickets among these children because the disease is more common in instances of famine, neglect, malabsorption, or restricted dietary intakes.[5,28]

Children are also at risk for rickets as a result of chronic lipid malabsorption or continuous anticonvulsive therapy.[28]

Among older adults who may have a diminished ability to produce vitamin D, osteomalacia may develop when marginal intakes of vitamin D or calcium exist for a number of years. Calcium absorption may also be affected by the aging process and contribute to osteomalacia risk. Older women are more at risk than men because of the effects of repeated pregnancies and lactation on bone density. Symptoms of osteomalacia include weakness, rheumatic-like pain, and an awkward gait. Because bones are weakened, fractures of the spine, hips, and limbs may occur.

Another disorder of the skeleton is osteoporosis. Osteoporosis is a condition in which bone density is reduced, and the remaining bone is brittle and breaks easily. Because vitamin D is crucial for absorption of calcium and the mineralization of bone, chronic vitamin D deficiency may be one of the risk factors of this disorder. Osteoporosis is discussed in detail in Chapter 8.

Vitamin D deficiency is associated with increased risk of CAD, rheumatoid arthritis, cancers, type 1 diabetes, and multiple sclerosis.[27]

Outright deficiency of vitamin D is thought to be rare in the United States because milk and related food products are fortified. But the amounts recommended for dietary consumption assume a greater amount being produced by our bodies. Deficiency, though, is a concern when a lack of exposure to sunlight occurs as a result of (1) environmental limitations, (2) cultural clothing customs that conceal the body, or (3) the inability of older adults or people with disabilities to get outdoors or to the store, resulting in malnourishment. These conditions may require vigilance in the consumption of fortified dietary sources, or supplements may be appropriate. When dietary intake and blood levels of vitamin D are assessed, many more Americans have marginal levels of vitamin D status.

Toxicity

High intakes of vitamin D can result in hypercalcemia (high blood levels of calcium) and hypercalciuria (high calcium level in urine), which affect kidneys and may cause cardiovascular damage. Toxicity symptoms occur when dietary intake of vitamin D is just above the UL of 50 mcg or 2000 international units.

Vitamin E

During the 1970s, vitamin E supplements were a popular aphrodisiac. Male virility, in particular, was thought to be enhanced by taking extra vitamin E. There was only one problem. Vitamin E increased the libido of male rats, not of humans. Research conducted on rats about the effects of vitamin E noted that the rats were able to reproduce better with additional intake of vitamin E. Although research conducted on rats is often applicable to humans, in this instance the results could not be generalized to humans. However, vitamin E is an essential nutrient that performs vital functions; we are still learning about its role in relation to disease prevention.

Function

Vitamin E acts as an antioxidant, protecting polyunsaturated fatty acids and vitamin A in cell membranes from oxidative damage by being oxidized itself. This function is particularly important in protecting the integrity of lung and red blood cell membranes, which are exposed to large amounts of oxygen. Other antioxidative functions of vitamin E are performed as part of a system in conjunction with selenium and ascorbic acid (vitamin C).

Recommended Intake and Sources

Vitamin E is the name given to a family of compounds called *tocopherols*, which are found in plants. Alpha-tocopherol is the most widely occurring form and the most active. Vitamin E is measured in terms of alpha-tocopherol equivalents (α-TE). The RDA for vitamin E is 15 mg α-TE for men and women (the older measurement, international units, may still be in use on dietary supplements: one mg α-TE equals 1.49 international units). A positive relationship exists between dietary intake of polyunsaturated fats and vitamin E requirements. As our dietary intake of polyunsaturated fats increases, we need more vitamin E to protect the integrity of these fats from oxidation.

For vitamin E to function as an antioxidant protecting against heart disease and possible reduced risk of prostate cancer, higher levels—30 to 70 mg α-TE (50 to 100 international units)—are recommended. These amounts cannot be consumed through dietary means and suggest the use of supplements. These amounts are most often measured as international units. Although a number of studies support the use of vitamin E in this manner, use of vitamin E at these levels for antioxidant function is not part of the RDA.[1] Some of the studies used levels of 400 to 800 international units. The optimum level is still being studied. Vitamin E may increase the risk of stroke for those with hypertension.[29]

The best sources of vitamin E are vegetable oils (e.g., corn, soy, safflower, canola, and cottonseed) and margarine. Whole grains, seeds, nuts, wheat germ, and green leafy vegetables also provide adequate amounts of vitamin E. Processing of these foods may decrease the final vitamin E content.

Deficiency

A primary deficiency of vitamin E is rare. Secondary deficiencies occur in premature infants and others who are unable to absorb fat normally. Some chronic fat absorption disorders in which deficiencies may occur are cystic fibrosis, biliary atresia (blocked bile duct), other disorders of the hepatobiliary system, or liver transport problems. Symptoms of vitamin E deficiency include neurologic disorders resulting from cell damage and anemia caused by hemolysis of red blood cells (hemolytic anemia).[28]

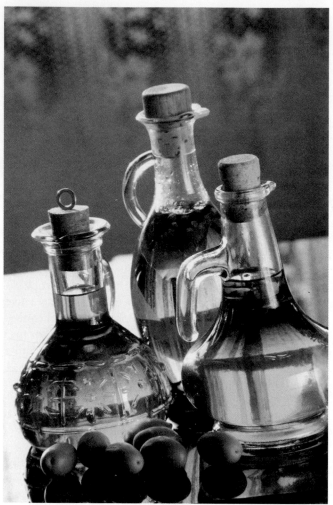

Vegetable oils provide vitamin E. (Photos.com.)

Toxicity

There is no evidence of toxicity associated with excessive intake of vitamin E. Intakes of about 70 to 530 mg α-TE (100 to 800 international units) per day appear to be tolerated, but the value of such doses has not been determined. Megadoses of vitamin E can exacerbate the anticoagulant effect of drugs taken to reduce blood clotting; vitamin E supplementation is not recommended in people who receive anticoagulant therapy, have a coagulation disorder, or have a vitamin K deficiency. A UL of 1000 mg α-TE has been set.[29]

Vitamin K

Discovered by a Danish scientist, vitamin K was called *koagulationsvitamin* for its blood clotting properties. Later research revealed that vitamin K is several related compounds with similar functions in the body.

Function

Vitamin K's main function is as a cofactor in the synthesis of blood clotting factors, including prothrombin. Protein formation in bone, kidney, and plasma also depends on the actions of vitamin K.

Recommended Intake and Sources

The AI for vitamin K is 120 mcg per day for men and 90 mcg for women. This amount provides for sufficient storage of vitamin K in the liver. Vitamin K actually consists of compounds in different forms in plant and animal tissues. All are converted by the liver to the biologically active form of menaquinone called vitamin K.

Vitamin K is available through dietary sources and can be synthesized by microflora in the jejunum and ileum of the digestive tract. From plants, vitamin K is consumed as phylloquinone; bacterial synthesis produces vitamin K homologues as forms of menaquinones. As noted, phylloquinone and vitamin K homologues are converted to the active form of menaquinone—vitamin K—by the liver.

Vitamin K is still an essential nutrient, although bacteria residing in the intestinal tract can synthesize it. The key distinction is that bacteria hosted by the human body produce the vitamin. Additionally, not enough vitamin K is produced by the microflora to ensure adequate levels for total blood clotting needs; dietary intake is still required.[30]

Primary food sources for vitamin K are dark green leafy vegetables. Lesser amounts are found in dairy products, cereals, meats, and fruits.

Deficiency

Deficiency of vitamin K inhibits blood coagulation. Deficiencies may be observed in clinical settings related to malabsorption disorders or medication interactions. Long-term intensive antibiotic therapy destroys the intestinal microflora that produce vitamin K. As with the other fat-soluble vitamins, any barrier to absorption affects the quantity of fat-soluble vitamin absorbed.

Premature infants and newborns are unable to immediately produce vitamin K; their guts are too sterile, free from the microflora necessary to produce vitamin K. Hospitals in the United States routinely give newborns an intramuscular dose of vitamin K to prevent hemorrhagic disease. Infants born in nonhospital settings (such as at home) may not receive the recommended dose of vitamin K. Intracranial bleeding and other symptoms consistent with abuse may present but be due to vitamin K deficiency.[31]

Because vitamin K also has a role in bone metabolism, research is considering whether vitamin K has a function in the treatment of osteoporosis. Although insufficient data exist to support vitamin K as a formal treatment component for osteoporosis,[30] they do highlight the need to regularly consume at least the RDA.

Toxicity

Consumption of foods containing vitamin K produces no problems of toxicity. Certain medications may be affected by vitamin K. The effectiveness of anticoagulant medications such as warfarin (Coumadin) and other blood-thinning drugs can be reduced by high intakes of vitamin K from either foods or supplements. Clients should be advised to moderate their consumption of foods containing vitamin K. Therapeutic administration of vitamin K in the menadione form has caused reactions in neonates, including hemolytic anemia and hyperbilirubinemia (excessively high levels of bilirubin, leading to jaundice). Phylloquinone administration has been acceptable.[11]

Vitamin K supplements should be used only if advised by a registered dietitian or primary health care provider. Because vitamin K has a role in blood clotting, excess amounts may decrease clotting time, thereby increasing the potential risk for stroke.

Table 7-6 provides a summary of fat-soluble vitamins.

OVERCOMING BARRIERS

Just Swallowing a Pill

Why do vitamins capture the attention of Americans? We generally do not suffer from vitamin deficiencies, and any problems of vitamin toxicity tend to be self-imposed. Considered through a wellness perspective, vitamin consumption is just one of many factors for achieving optimum health. Yet sales of dietary supplements continue to significantly increase. More than half the adult American population uses these products.[32]

TABLE 7-6   FAT-SOLUBLE VITAMINS

VITAMIN	FUNCTION	CLINICAL ISSUES DEFICIENCY/TOXICITY	REQUIREMENTS	FOOD SOURCES
Vitamin A Precursor: carotenoids Preformed vitamin: retinoids	Maintains epithelial tissues (skin and mucous membranes); rhodopsin formation for vision; bone growth; reproduction	Deficiency: xerophthalmia; night blindness; keratomalacia; degeneration of epithelial tissue; inhibited growth (respiratory and gastrointestinal disturbances) Toxicity: hypervitaminosis A (from supplements) with blistered skin, weakness, anorexia, vomiting, enlarged spleen and liver	Men: 900 mcg RAE Women: 700 mcg RAE UL 3000 mcg RAE	Deep green, yellow, and orange fruits and vegetables; animal fat sources: whole milk, fortified skim, and low-fat milk; butter; liver; egg yolks, fatty fish
Vitamin D Precursor: 7-dehydrocholesterol Active form: cholecalciferol	Calcium and phosphorus absorption; bone mineralization	Deficiency: bone malformation, rickets (children), osteomalacia (adults) Toxicity: hypercalcemia, hypercalciuria	Adults: 5 mcg AI (<51 yr 10 mcg) (<70 yr 15 mcg) UL 50 mcg	Animal (fat) sources: butter, egg yolks, fatty fish, liver, fortified milk; body synthesis
Vitamin E α-tocopherol	Antioxidant for PUFA and vitamin A; antioxidant with selenium and ascorbic acid	Deficiency: primary deficiency rare; secondary deficiency (caused by fat absorption) neurologic disorders Toxicity: none, but supplements contraindicated with anticoagulation drugs	Adults: 15 mg α-TE UL 1000 mg α-TE	Vegetable oil, whole grains, seeds, nuts, green leafy vegetables
Vitamin K Active form: menaquinones	Cofactor in synthesis of blood clotting factors; protein formation	Deficiency: blood coagulation inhibited; hemorrhagic disease (infants) Toxicity: therapeutic vitamin K (menadione form) reactions in neonates, causing hemolytic anemia and hyperbilirubinemia	Men: 120 mcg AI Women: 90 mcg AI	Green leafy vegetables, intestinal synthesis

α-TE, Alpha-tocopherol equivalent; AI, Adequate Intake; RAE, retinol activity equivalent; UL, Tolerable Upper Intake Level; PUFA, polyunsaturated fatty acid.

Perhaps vitamins are an easier target on which to focus when emphasizing good health. If a person is concerned about vitamin intake, a vitamin pill can always be taken. That's a lot easier than the dietary and behavior modifications required to meet other health factors, such as decreasing fat intake or increasing physical activities. There are, though, circumstances that may warrant supplementation.

Rethinking Vitamin Supplementation

Recommendations for vitamin supplementation intend to improve the nutritional status of at-risk groups of the population. These have included adolescent girls, pregnant and lactating women, individuals with limited economic resources, older persons, alcohol-dependent individuals, and possibly those following vegetarian or vegan food patterns. Additionally individuals with increased nutrient needs due to medication interaction with nutrients and/or as an effect of chronic health conditions may require vitamin supplementation. Another subgroup at risk are people experiencing food insecurity whose intake may have nutrient gaps.[32] Folate, vitamins A and C, and the minerals iron, calcium, and zinc tend to be consumed in inadequate amounts by these at-risk groups.

The purpose of recommendations for these groups is to address basic deficiency issues. If the adequate levels are not consumed as a result of social, cultural, or economic reasons,[32] then it is the role of health professionals to provide guidance as to how to meet these levels.

Recommendations are beginning to move beyond the level of nutrient adequacy to issues of health promotion and prevention of disease. For example, folate requirements are vitally important for the development of a healthy fetus. Should the whole population receive folic acid through fortification when only potentially pregnant women have the additional requirement? Is this supplementation of folic acid acceptable if increased folic acid intake is associated with lowering homocysteine levels (see Box 7-4)?

The DRI addresses the issue of availability of vitamin B_{12} and older adults. It recommends that adults older than age 50 use a vitamin B_{12} supplement or foods fortified with the vitamin to ensure adequate bioavailability to prevent potential deficiencies. But what foods should be fortified that older adults are sure to eat? The DRI has also recommended that the level of vitamin D be increased above the levels usually consumed, suggesting the use of vitamin D supplements. This marks a significant change in philosophy, because supplements of vitamin D had been discouraged because of toxicity issues. An important question for health professionals to consider is, how will older adults know of these vitamin B_{12} and vitamin D recommendations, and how should they be implemented?

Nutrition education regarding the use of functional (fortified) foods and appropriate use of supplements is one means of teaching a target population about nutrient needs. When implemented on a broad scale to the public-at-large, other segments of the population learn of the nutrient value. For example, women should be taught the value of folic acid during pregnancy, but men can also be aware of this value so that they can support the implementation of the folic acid goal by the women in their lives. In addition, younger women can become aware of the special nutrient needs of the pregnancy years before they enter them so that the importance of nutrition during pregnancy is not something new or an afterthought when they are older.

Functional foods may increase the amount of a nutrient in the food supply. By careful selection of the foods to which specific nutrients are added, increased consumption of the nutrient can be achieved with little effort by the target group. This is a public health approach that affects the community-at-large. The newly approved folic acid fortification begins to provide a safety net for women of childbearing age but only if foods containing the additional folic acid are consumed. Supplements may still be warranted.

A third approach toward nutrient supplements is an individualized approach. Individuals take the supplements on their own. Ideally, a qualified health professional such as a registered dietitian, licensed nutritionist, or primary health care provider guides the individual as to the need and quantity of the nutrient supplements to be regularly taken. This approach requires the individual to take the responsibility for continued consumption, if appropriate, of the supplement.

The optimal approach is the use of all three approaches to achieve nutrient adequacy that takes into account the special needs of subgroups.

Role of the Health Practitioner

Recommendations for use of nutrient supplements should be determined by dietetic professionals such as registered dietitians or by informed primary health care providers. Their counseling evaluates the client's current nutrient intake and assesses his or her dietary supplementation practices and possible interactions with prescribed medical treatments and medications. Foremost in importance is that dietary adequacy should first be met by eating a diverse selection of whole foods, while following the basic dietary guidelines of MyPyramid with awareness of portion (moderation) sizes.

The role of other health professionals, such as nurses, is to guide clients to the appropriate nutritional counseling to determine the client's actual nutrient status. After counseling has been completed, nurses can support the recommendations of the dietitian through teaching strategies such as how to incorporate more fruits and vegetables into one's diet and how to reinforce the understanding of potential drug-nutrient interactions.

TOWARD A POSITIVE NUTRITION LIFESTYLE: SOCIAL SUPPORT

Social support extends throughout the life span; it goes beyond having friends and family with whom to socialize. For families with young children, social support may be cooperative meals when illness strikes (e.g., during a flu epidemic) and cooking time becomes compromised. The term *cooperative* may mean cooking double portions to feed a friend's family during bouts of chicken pox or childhood ear infections. The kindness would then be reciprocated in the future. Both families gain nutritious meals at times when merely thinking about cooking seems overwhelming.

Support for older adults, as mentioned earlier in this chapter, may mean assistance with food shopping or food delivery. Neighbors or relatives may provide this social support. In some communities, local Red Cross chapters and other charitable organizations have developed car or bus services specifically to provide transportation for older residents. This enables individuals to safely shop in food stores and have the convenience of being driven to their homes and assisted with carrying groceries into their kitchens. Health care professionals working with older clients should be aware of these services or perhaps help community organizations initiate similar programs.

SUMMARY

Vitamins are organic molecules that perform specific metabolic functions and are required in very small amounts. As essential nutrients, they must be provided through dietary intake. Vitamins are divided into the two categories of water soluble and fat soluble. Solubility of vitamins affects the processes of their absorption, transportation, and storage in our bodies.

Water-soluble vitamins are vitamin C, choline, and the B complex vitamins (thiamine, riboflavin, niacin, folate, pyridoxine [B_6], vitamin B_{12}, pantothenic acid, and biotin). The B vitamins function as coenzymes. Choline is part of a neurotransmitter and lecithin. Vitamin C serves as an antioxidant in addition to its coenzyme ability. Water-soluble vitamins are easily absorbed into blood circulation. Because excesses are excreted, toxicity is less likely; however, they may occur with pyridoxine and vitamin C.

Fat-soluble vitamins are vitamins A, D, E, and K. These vitamins serve structural and regulatory functions throughout the body. Fat-soluble vitamins are absorbed the same as lipids; bile is required, and the nutrients enter the lymphatic system. Because they are retained in fatty substances in the body, toxicity from supplemental intakes is possible.

THE NURSING APPROACH

Case Study: Vitamins and Chronic Alcohol Use

Brad, age 24, worked in a manufacturing plant. His supervisor had been concerned about his frequent absences from work, declining productivity, and noticeable weight loss. When Brad came to work today, he looked unkempt and thin. With alcohol on his breath, he was slurring his words and having difficulty with balance. His co-worker reported that Brad had a longtime drinking problem. His supervisor, worried about safety, took Brad to the occupational nurse on site.

ASSESSMENT
Subjective (from patient statements)

- "Maybe I drank a little too much last night, but I am not an alcoholic."
- "I can't remember how long I have worked here. Am I in trouble because I was late today? Where am I anyway?"
- Complained of headache
- Said he has lost weight, is not interested in eating because food doesn't taste good and his mouth is sore

Objective (from physical examination)

- Height 5'10", weight 135 pounds
- Blood pressure 110/70, temperature 98° F, pulse 92, respirations 21
- Ataxia (muscle weakness and loss of coordination)
- Alcohol on breath, speech slurred
- Stomatitis (inflamed mouth and gingiva)
- Pale conjunctiva

DIAGNOSES (NURSING)
1. Imbalanced nutrition: less than body requirements related to probable chronic alcohol use and inadequate food intake as evidenced by alcohol on breath, reported weight loss, 81% ideal body weight (IBW), ataxia, stomatitis, and pale conjunctiva
2. Probable ineffective coping related to chronic alcohol use

PLANNING
Patient Outcomes

Short term (at the end of this visit):
- Brad will eat at least two meals per day and take a multiple vitamin with minerals each day.
- He will identify foods he can eat without irritation to his mouth.

Long term (at follow-up visit in one month):
- Brad will report he took a multiple vitamin every day, and he will participate in a more thorough nutrition assessment.
- He will weigh at least two more pounds.
- No alcohol on breath, stable balance, less inflammation in mouth, conjunctiva pink

Nursing Interventions

1. Encourage Brad to decrease or avoid alcohol intake.
2. Encourage him to increase food intake and take a multiple vitamin with minerals every day.

IMPLEMENTATION
1. Sent a blood sample to the lab for complete blood count, hemoglobin and hematocrit, ferritin, and albumin.
Pale conjunctiva could indicate anemia. Weight loss and muscle weakness could be a result of inadequate food intake and toxicity from alcohol.
2. Recommended that Brad stop drinking alcohol and start taking a multiple vitamin with minerals every day.

Continued

THE NURSING APPROACH—cont'd
Case Study: Vitamins and Chronic Alcohol Use—cont'd

Alcohol inhibits the absorption of thiamine while increasing the need for thiamine. Insufficient thiamine can lead to decreased mental alertness, short-term memory loss, and ataxia (muscle weakness and loss of coordination). Lack of riboflavin can cause stomatitis. Lack of vitamin B_6, folate, and iron can cause anemia. Vitamin supplements ensure adequate intake of vitamins when diets are not consistently well balanced.

3. Encouraged him to eat small frequent meals high in protein, vitamins, and calories.

Small, frequent meals are more easily absorbed than large meals and are easier to tolerate when a person has anorexia. Protein, vitamins, and sufficient calories are needed for healing and weight gain.

4. Gave him a list of nonirritating dietary sources of protein and vitamins (especially B vitamins).

Milk products are high in protein. Cold, smooth foods are soothing to a sore mouth: puddings, eggnog, milkshakes, ice cream, yogurt, cottage cheese, instant breakfast drinks, and supplements like Ensure. Soy milk could be substituted if Brad has lactose intolerance. Other foods that would help provide vitamins include bland fruits without peelings, soft cooked vegetables; refined enriched breads, cereals and pasta; and tender pork, tuna, and chicken.

5. Set up an appointment for a follow-up visit in one month.
Follow-up is needed to evaluate health status and changes made.
6. Encouraged Brad to see a counselor to help him reduce his alcohol intake.
An alcohol rehabilitation program is likely indicated.

EVALUATION
Short term (at the end of the visit):
- Brad said he could take a vitamin each day and eat ice cream more often. He couldn't remember any other dietary recommendations but did take the list of foods.
- He declined to see a counselor about his alcohol intake but said he would come back in a month to see the nurse again.
- Short-term goals partially met.

DISCUSSION QUESTIONS
Brad did not return for a follow-up visit in the nurse's office.
1. How could the nurse encourage Brad to come to the nurse's office for follow-up?
2. What additional information would the nurse need to obtain in order to confirm or rule out her nursing diagnoses?
3. How does alcoholism contribute to malnutrition? What food could provide the vitamins that Brad may be lacking?

Nursing Diagnoses-Definitions and Classification 2009-2011. Copyright © 2009, 1994-2009 by NANDA International. Used by arrangement with Blackwell Publishing Limited, a company of John Wiley & Sons, Inc.

❓ APPLYING CONTENT KNOWLEDGE

Mark, age 3, is having his yearly health examination. His mom, rather proudly, tells you that Mark eats one apple and carrot sticks every day. She says that means he gets all the vitamins he needs. How do you respond?

WEBSITES OF INTEREST

Nutrition.gov
www.nutrition.gov
Offers resources about life span nutrition, consumer dietary concerns, and nutrition education programs.

Aetna InteliHealth
www.intelihealth.com
Partners with Harvard Medical School for content on vitamin supplements, nutrition for specific health problems, interactive tools and more.

U.S. Food and Drug Administration Center for Food Safety and Applied Nutrition
www.cfsan.fda.gov
Supplies FDA policies, rules, and FDA Talk Papers pertaining to supplements and health claims on foods.

REFERENCES

1. Otten JJ, et al, editors: *Dietary DRI References: The essential guide to nutrient requirements*, Washington, DC, 2006, The National Academies Press.
2. Pagana KD, Pagana JT: *Mosby's diagnostic and laboratory test reference*, ed 7, St Louis, 2004, Mosby.
3. Fain O, Mathieu E, Thomas M: Scurvy in patients with cancer, *BMJ* 316:1661-1662, 1998.
4. Wood B, et al: Pellagra in a woman using alternative remedies, *Australas J Dermatol* 39(1):42-44, Feb 1998.
5. Gessner BD, et al: Nutritional rickets among breast-fed black and Alaska Native children, *Alaska Med* 39(3):72-74, 1997.
6. Bidlack WR, Wang W: Designing functional foods. In Shils ME, et al, editors: *Modern nutrition in health and disease*, ed 10, Philadelphia, 2006, Lippincott Williams & Wilkins.
7. Butterworth RF: Thiamin. In Shils ME, et al, editors: *Modern nutrition in health and disease*, ed 10, Philadelphia, 2006, Lippincott Williams & Wilkins.

8. Roman GC: Nutritional disorders of the nervous system. In Shils ME, et al, editors: *Modern nutrition in health and disease*, ed 10, Philadelphia, 2006, Lippincott Williams & Wilkins.

9. McCormick DB: Riboflavin. In Shils ME, et al, editors: *Modern nutrition in health and disease*, ed 10, Philadelphia, 2006, Lippincott Williams & Wilkins.

10. Bourgeois C, et al: Niacin. In Shils ME, et al, editors: *Modern nutrition in health and disease*, ed 10, Philadelphia, 2006, Lippincott Williams & Wilkins.

11. Kertesz SG: Pellagra in 2 homeless men, *Mayo Clin Proc* 76(3):315-318, 2001.

12. Prousky JE: Pellagra may be a rare secondary complication of anorexia nervosa: a systematic review of the literature, *Altern Med Rev* 8(2):180-185, 2003.

13. Wei EK, et al: Plasma vitamin B_6 and the risk of colorectal cancer and adenoma in women, *J Natl Cancer Inst* 97(9): 684-692, 2005.

14. Zhang SM, et al: Folate, vitamin B_6, multivitamin supplements, and colorectal cancer risk in women, *Am J Epidemiol* 163(2):108-115, 2006.

15. Morgan SL, Weinsier RL: *Fundamentals of clinical nutrition*, ed 2, St Louis, 1998, Mosby.

16. U.S. Department of Health and Human Services: FDA announces name changes for lower-fat milks and folic acid fortification for bakery products, HHS News, Dec 31, 1997. Retrieved April 18, 2006, from www.fda.gov.

17. U.S. Food and Drug Administration, Office of Public Affairs: *Fact sheet: Folic acid fortification*, Rockville, Md, 1996 (February 29), Author. Accessed April 18, 2006, from www.ods.od.nih.gov/factsheets/folate.asp.

18. He K, et al: Folate, vitamin B_6 and B_{12} intakes in relation to risk of stroke among men, *Stroke* 35(1):169-174, 2004.

19. Carmel R: Folic acid. In Shils ME, et al, editors: *Modern nutrition in health and disease*, ed 10, Philadelphia, 2006, Lippincott Williams & Wilkins.

20. Carmel R: Cobalamin (vitamin B_{12}). In Shils ME, et al, editors: *Modern nutrition in health and disease*, ed 10, Philadelphia, 2006, Lippincott Williams & Wilkins.

21. Lindenbaum J, et al: Neuropsychiatric disorders caused by cobalamin deficiency in the absence of anemia or macrocytosis, *N Engl J Med* 318:1720-1728, 1988.

22. Marshall MW, et al: Effect of low and high fat diets varying in ratios of polyunsaturated to saturated fatty acids on biotin intakes and biotin in serum, red cells and urine of adult men, *Nutr Res* 5:801-814, 1985.

23. Levine M, et al: Vitamin C. In Shils ME, et al, editors: *Modern nutrition in health and disease*, ed 10, Philadelphia, 2006, Lippincott Williams & Wilkins.

24. Zhang C, et al: Vitamin C and the risk of gestational diabetes mellitus: a case-control study, *J Reprod Med* 49(4):257-266, 2004.

25. Ross AC: Vitamin A and carotenoids. In Shils ME, et al, editors: *Modern nutrition in health and disease*, ed 10, Philadelphia, 2006, Lippincott Williams & Wilkins.

26. Tang G, et al: Golden Rice is an effective source of vitamin A, *Am J Clin Nutr* 89(6): 1776-1783, 2009.

27. Hathcock JN, et al: Risk assessment for vitamin D, *Am J Clin Nutr* 85-86, 2007.

28. Hollick MF: Resurrection of vitamin D deficiency and rickets, *J Clin Invest* 116(8): 2062-2072, 2006.

29. Traber MG: Vitamin E. In Shils ME, et al, editors: *Modern nutrition in health and disease*, ed 10, Philadelphia, 2006, Lippincott Williams & Wilkins.

30. Suttie JW: Vitamin K. In Shils ME, et al, editors: *Modern nutrition in health and disease*, ed 10, Philadelphia, 2006, Lippincott Williams & Wilkins.

31. Brousseau TJ, et al: Vitamin K deficiency mimicking child abuse, *J Emerg Med* 29(3):283-288, 2005.

32. American Dietetic Association: Position of the American Dietetic Association: Nutrient supplementation, *J Am Diet Assoc* 109:2073-2085, 2009.

CHAPTER

8

Water and Minerals

An ever-circulating ocean of fluid bathes all the cells in our bodies; this fluid allows for chemical reactions, transmission of nerve impulses, and transportation of nutrients and waste products throughout the body.

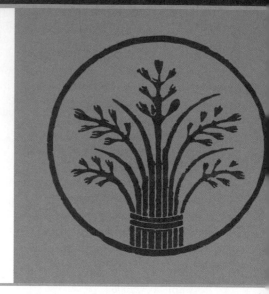

evolve WEBSITE

http://evolve.elsevier.com/Grodner/foundations/

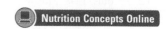

ROLE IN WELLNESS

An ever-circulating ocean of fluid bathes all the cells in our bodies; this fluid allows for chemical reactions, transmission of nerve impulses, and transportation of nutrients and waste products throughout the body. The fluid is not simply water, although water is its primary constituent. Some fluid in the body is used to form blood, lymph, and structure for cells. Minerals circulating in our body fluids create the setting for biochemical reactions to occur.

Water and minerals affect every system of our bodies, as well as our five dimensions of health. *Physical dimension* of health depends on adequate levels of these nutrients. *Intellectual health dimension* is compromised when iron levels are low; iron deficiency affects cognitive abilities and thus diminishes the ability to learn. *Emotional health* may rely on our being sufficiently hydrated with fluids; cases of fluid volume deficit or dehydration have been mistaken for senility when the thirst acuity of older adults diminishes. *Social health dimension* may be affected if older adults become debilitated by bone fractures or osteoporosis caused by chronic calcium deficiencies; social mobility may be limited as their physical movement is inhibited. Vegans who consume no animal-derived foods because of *spiritual health* beliefs need carefully designed eating plans to provide adequate levels of zinc, iron, and calcium to avoid deficiencies.

Although water and minerals are primary components of body fluids, they perform other functions as well. This chapter explores water and minerals in the context of their nutritional requirements and physiologic roles for achieving nutritional wellness.

WATER

We can live several weeks without food but can survive only a few days without water or fluids. Although our bodies use stored nutrients to fuel energy needs, a minimum intake of water is required for cell function and as a solution through which waste products of the body are excreted in urine.

Food Sources

If we drank only water and no other liquids, we could meet our body's need for fluid. Most of us, however, consume fluids in addition to water throughout the day. Some fluids also contain other nutrients. Consider the wealth of nutrients found in milk (skim or whole), fruit juices, and soups. Some fruits and vegetables contain as much as 85% to 95% water. Watermelon, grapes, oranges, lettuce, tomatoes, and zucchini have high water content. Most foods contain water, but some are better sources of fluids than others. Generally, we depend on beverages as our main source of fluids.

The Adequate Intake (AI) recommendations for water are about 13 cups a day for men and 9 cups a day for women. This amount is in addition to fluids from foods consumed throughout the day, such as fruits and vegetables.[1] Although the minimum amount needed by healthy adults may be about 4 cups, higher amounts are optimum considering an individual's physiologic status and energy output.

Our primary source of water should be the liquids we drink (Table 8-1). Notice that coffee, tea, alcohol, and soft drinks are not listed as primary sources. Although they do contain water, coffee, tea, and alcohol act as diuretics, which cause an increase in water loss via the kidneys as urine. Soft

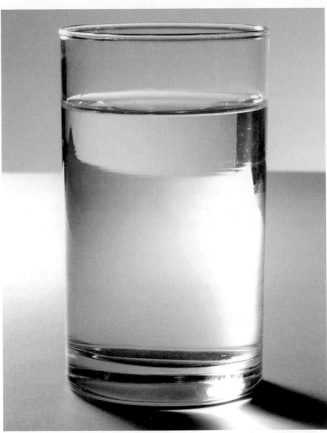

We need water in our diets every day. (Photos.com.)

TABLE 8-1	FOODS AS SOURCES OF WATER (BY PERCENTAGE)
FOOD	PERCENT WATER
Dairy Products	
Milk	88-91
Cheddar cheese	37
Cottage cheese	79
Ice cream, ice milk	61-66
Fruits	
Apples	84
Grapefruit (whole or juice)	90
Grapes	81
Melons	90
Oranges (whole or juice)	88
Vegetables	
Asparagus	91
Carrots	88
Cucumber	96
Lettuce	96
Potato	75
Spinach	90
Sweet potato	73
Tomatoes	94
Miscellaneous	
Beans (cooked)	60-70
Bread	30-40
Fruit punch	88
Gelatin	84
Meats	50-60
Oatmeal (cooked)	85
Poultry	65
Soups	85-98

Data from U.S. Department of Agriculture, Agricultural Research Service: *Nutrient data laboratory,* Washington, DC, Authors. Accessed February 12, 2010, from www.ars.usda.gov/ba/bhnrc/ndl.

drinks add fluid to the body, but they contain solutes (sugar, salt, various chemicals) that must be diluted as they enter the bloodstream. Drinking a soda increases the concentration of these solutes in the blood. The body responds by pulling fluid from the cells into the bloodstream to dilute the sugar and salt. The body loses the increased fluid in the bloodstream when it is excreted as urine. In addition, the body responds to the increased solutes and decreased fluid content by once again triggering the thirst mechanism.

Bottled water has become a mainstay in U.S. beverage selections and an economic force. Sales of bottled water have reached to more than $11 billion.[2] Products range from imported sparkling mineral waters to spring waters to waters treated from nearby reservoirs. Although the price range is equally broad, the common denominator is that Americans enjoy the convenience of water as a beverage when available in portable containers and single portions.

Water Quality

The minerals found naturally in water vary. Hard water refers to water that contains high amounts of minerals such as calcium and magnesium. Drinking this water can provide a significant amount of these nutrients. Non-nutrition-related problems from hard water can develop; mineral deposits may damage appliances and other machinery that interacts with water, and soap suds are reduced. To reduce these problems, a filtration process can be installed to soften water by replacing some minerals with sodium chloride

(salt). Soft water containing sodium, however, can be a problem for sodium-sensitive individuals, such as those at risk for hypertension. To prevent health problems, water softeners may be used on only the hot tap in kitchens, leaving the cold tap unsoftened for consumption.

Another aspect of water quality is contamination. For example, many older buildings have pipes with lead solder joints that can release lead into the water that sits in or runs through them. If the level of lead in water is more than 15 parts per billion (ppb), pregnant women, infants, and children are advised to drink bottled water because even low levels of lead can seriously impair normal development. The local health department can recommend a competent laboratory that tests household water quality.

To reduce the chance of lead leaking into drinking and cooking water, do the following:

- Run the water for 2 minutes after it has been standing in the pipes.

- Use only cold water for drinking, cooking, and preparing baby formula (cold water absorbs less lead than hot).

Water treatment processes can remedy some contamination concerns. Others, such as industrial pollution, can be difficult to identify. Complications of bacterial contamination or inadvertent exposure of water to carcinogenic industrial substances can lead to health problems that range from simple gastroenteritis to cancer. Municipal and regional water processing plants take great care to ensure the safest water supply possible. Some water sources (private wells, surface water, springs, and cisterns), however, may exceed the maximum contaminant levels set by the Environmental Protection Agency (EPA).

The most severe water-related threats such as cholera and typhoid are no longer public health hazards in North America. Other potential industrial and environmental pollutants, however, can enter our water supply and endanger our health. Small suppliers may not have the financial means to improve technologic surveillance.

Poorer countries throughout the world continue to struggle with unsafe water supplies (see the *Cultural Considerations* box, Who Will Bring Water to the Bolivian Poor?). Without the financial and technologic knowledge and resources, many people become ill by consuming bacteria-contaminated water. Increased incidence of stomach cancer is associated with exposure to *Helicobacter pylori*, which is sometimes found in contaminated waters.

Water as a Nutrient in the Body
Structure

The structure of water—two hydrogen atoms bonded to one oxygen atom—allows it to provide a base for biochemical reactions in the body and to easily move through the various compartments of cells and body systems. As the basis of body fluids, water can host other substances of different electrical charges and characteristics. Intracellular fluids (within the cell) are composed of water plus concentrations of potassium and phosphates. Interstitial fluids (between the cells) contain concentrations of sodium and chloride. Extracellular fluids include interstitial fluid and encompass all fluids outside cells, including plasma and the watery components of body organs and substances (Box 8-1).

🌐 CULTURAL CONSIDERATIONS

Who Will Bring Water to the Bolivian Poor?

In Cochabamba, Bolivia, water for many is a scarce commodity. Ten years ago, an American multinational company, Bechtel, operated the waterworks of Bolivia. Rates charged continually increased. The company was forced out of Bolivia after significant social protest. A community group now runs the waterworks company, Semapa, and prices are cheap again. But only half the city's population of 600,000 receives water service. Service for some though is irregular, consisting of water availability for only 2 hours a day to at most 14 hours. No one has 24-hour availability. The other 300,000 remain without water. There is much social unrest.

The lack of a continual water supply is indicative of the struggles in Latin America to come to terms with international marketing forces that seem unable to alleviate the plight of poverty-stricken populations such as that of Bolivia. Privatizing utilities as attempted with the American multinational company to lead to economic restructuring as recommended by the World Bank and the International Monetary Fund did not result in sustained growth or any growth at all. Perhaps more problematic is that when efforts such as the private water supply was disbanded, community water supply companies such as that in Cochabamba are unable to provide resources effectively because the economic structures to build and support expansion of a modern waterworks supply system are not available. Adequate funding is not available within Bolivia. To request foreign investment means acquiescing to requirements that leads to issues of social unrest still affecting the general population.

Semapa, the community-controlled water company, is hindered by the lack of money to update and expand service. Many people of Cochabamba, who do not have any water service, obtain water from pipes extending from community wells. Others, especially the poor, are unable to participate in community wells and have freelance water dealers deliver water two or three times a week. Service is erratic. Water quality varies significantly. One man reports that sometimes the delivered water contains tiny worms. His children request piped water, but there is little that he can do. The multinational corporation could not provide his family with water, nor can the community run company, Semapa. "Who will bring water to the Bolivian poor?"

Application to nursing: It is hard to imagine that a nutrient, *water*, which we take for granted is hardly available to some Bolivian citizens. Direct application to nursing in a setting of limited access to water, especially clean water, includes the hygienic conditions under which much of the population lives. Sanitation systems like indoor plumbing would probably be crude or nonexistent. Health care services would be burdened by water- and food-related illness precipitated by contaminated water used for cooking, consumption, and cleansing.

An indirect application to nursing is our assumptions about the living conditions and resources of our clients and patients. Care needs to be taken not to assume that individuals have equal knowledge and the wherewithal to provide themselves and their families with basic needs. For example, the appropriately dressed and well-spoken elderly female patient with breathing problems may not tell you she is overwhelmed trying to keep up with repairs of her large, old home. When her bathroom began to fill with black mold because of a water leak behind the walls and the faucet stopped working, she just continued to use the toilet and the shower. She was unaware of health ramifications. A casual chat may elicit valuable information.

Data from Forero J: Who will bring water to the Bolivian poor? *The New York Times*, Dec 15, 2005, pp. C1, C7; Olivera O, Lewis T: *Cochabamba! Water Rebellion in Bolivia*, New York, 2008, South End Press.

BOX 8-1 BODY FLUID COMPARTMENTS

Intracellular Fluid (65% of Body Water)
Enzymes
Hemoglobin
Magnesium
Minerals
Phosphorus
Potassium
Proteins

Extracellular Fluid (35% of Body Water)
Antibodies
Bicarbonate ions
Blood proteins
Carbohydrates
Chloride
Glucose
Minerals
Proteins
Lipids
Lipoproteins
Sodium

BOX 8-2 FUNCTIONS OF WATER

Provides shape and rigidity to cells
Helps to regulate body temperature
Acts as a lubricant
Cushions body tissues
Transports nutrients and waste products
Acts as a solvent
Provides a source of trace minerals
Participates in chemical reactions

Digestion and Absorption

Because water is inorganic, it is not digested. It passes quickly to the small intestine. Once there, most water is absorbed; the rest is regulated by the colon and is either absorbed or excreted with feces.

Metabolism

Although not metabolized or broken down by the gastrointestinal (GI) tract processes, water is an integral component of metabolic processes. In some reactions, the water of metabolism is water released as a byproduct of oxidative reactions; in others, water may be a part of the process to release energy from adenosine triphosphate (ATP), which is discussed in greater detail in Chapter 9. The released water may be excreted as waste or used elsewhere in the body. Glycogen in muscle and the liver contains water in the structure of glycogen molecules. When glycogen is used for energy, the water becomes available for body functions.

Functions

Water performs a variety of vital functions in the body (Box 8-2). It is an important structural component of the body, giving shape and rigidity to cells. It assists in regulating body temperature. Water conducts heat, absorbing and distribut-

ing it throughout the body, keeping body temperature stable from day to day. Water also helps cool the body by evaporating invisibly from the lungs and the surface of the skin, carrying off excess heat. This type of water loss is called **insensible perspiration**.

Water acts as a lubricant in the form of joint fluid and mucous secretions. It forms a shock-absorbing fluid cushion for body tissues such as the amniotic sac, spinal cord, and eyes.

Water is a major component of blood, lymph, saliva, and urine. As such, it delivers nutrients and removes waste products. Acting as a **solvent**, it enables minerals, vitamins, glucose, and other small molecules to be moved throughout the body.

Water may also supply trace minerals such as fluoride, zinc, and copper. Sometimes it is a source of too many minerals, including potentially toxic metals such as lead, cadmium, and incidental substances from pesticides and industrial waste products.

In addition to serving as a medium for biochemical reactions, water also participates as a reactant. A **reactant** is a substance that enters into and is altered during a chemical reaction. For example, large molecules such as polysaccharides, fats, and protein are split into smaller molecules in which water participates and is changed by the process.

Ultimately, no growth or cell renewal occurs without water; it is part of every cell and is necessary as a medium for reactions and transporter of supplies.

Regulation of Fluid and Water in the Body

Our bodies have delicate but efficient mechanisms for maintaining appropriate fluid levels. The intake of fluids is balanced with the output through urine, sweat, feces, and insensible perspiration (Figure 8-1). Regulation of fluid in the body is of physiologic importance because water makes up 50% to 60% of the weight of an average adult; the percentages are even higher for infants, whose body weight is 75% to 80% water (Figure 8-2). Fortunately, all we need to do is take in enough fluids and our bodies' natural systems take care of the rest.

Homeostasis (physiological equilibrium) is maintained by electrolytes that include minerals and blood proteins. Two of the most important minerals are sodium and potassium. The extracellular distribution of fluid depends on sodium, and potassium influences intracellular water. Water moves within and between the cells in interstitial fluids in response to the levels of these minerals. An imbalance is corrected by mechanisms that cause thirst and regulate the ability of the kidneys to release or retain fluids.

Thirst, a dryness in the mouth, stimulates the desire to drink liquids. We often ignore our thirst until mealtimes. The thirst mechanism is controlled by the hypothalamus and involves several steps. The sodium and **solute** levels in blood increase as the water level in the body gets low. This causes water to be drawn from the salivary glands to provide more fluid for the blood. The mouth then feels dry because less saliva, which keeps the mouth moist, is produced. This

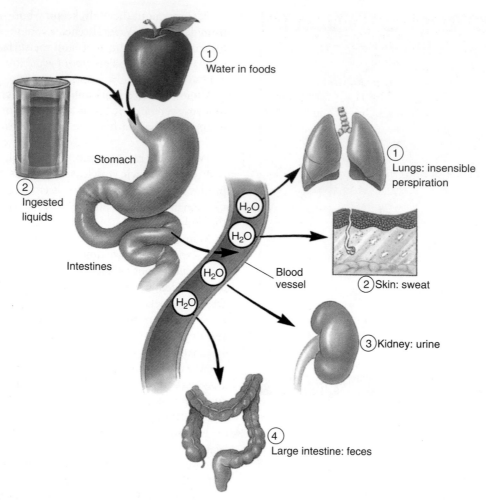

FIG 8-1 Intake of fluids is balanced with output. (Courtesy Joan Beck. Modified from Thibodeau GA, Patton KT: *The human body in health and disease,* ed 2, St Louis, 1997, Mosby.)

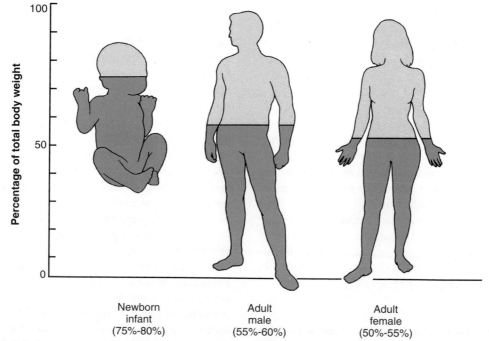

FIG 8-2 Percentage of body weight represented by water in infants compared with adults. (From Rolin Graphics. In Thibodeau GA, Patton KT: *Structure and function of the body,* ed 10, St Louis, 1997, Mosby.)

sensation, thirst, stimulates the drinking process. If the thirst mechanism is faulty, as it may be during illness, physical exertion, or aging, hormonal mechanisms also help conserve water by reducing urine output.

The mechanisms of the kidneys regulate the amounts of water excreted. Obligatory water excretion of at least 500 mL (1 pint) must be excreted daily, regardless of the amount ingested, to clear the body of waste products. The mechanism relies on the combined actions of the brain, kidneys, pituitary gland, and adrenal gland. When fluid in the body becomes low, the hypothalamus stimulates the pituitary gland to release antidiuretic hormone (ADH). ADH is secreted in response to high sodium levels in the body or too low blood pressure or blood volume. The target organ of the hormone is the kidney. The kidneys then conserve water by decreasing excretion of water, and the retained fluid is recycled for use throughout the body.

When the sodium concentration in the kidneys gets high (too much fluid excreted), another process kicks in to counteract the lowered blood volume and pressure. The kidneys release renin, an enzyme that activates the blood protein angiotensin. Angiotensin raises blood pressure by narrowing blood vessels; it is a vasoconstrictor. Angiotensin also prompts the adrenal gland to release the hormone aldosterone. The target organ of aldosterone is the kidney. The effect is to decrease excretion of sodium, causing the kidneys to respond by retaining fluid in the body.

Fluid and Electrolytes

Dissolved in body fluids are minerals and other organic molecules required for the regulation of both intracellular and extracellular fluid distribution. Fluids follow salt concentrations; this means that cells can control fluid balance by directing the movement of mineral salts.

Electrolytes are minerals that carry electrical charges or ions (particles) when dissolved in water. These minerals separate into positively charged ions (cations) or negatively charged ions (anions). The primary extracellular electrolytes in body fluids are sodium (Na^+/cation) and chloride (Cl^-/anion), and the primary intracellular electrolyte is potassium (K^+/cation). To maintain fluid balance, cells control the movement of electrolytes. Water will follow sodium concentration. Moving electrolytes in and out of the cell membrane requires transport proteins. The sodium/potassium pump is a transport protein that works to exchange sodium from within the cells for potassium. Other ions are also exchanged.

In addition to water regulation, the kidneys also regulate electrolyte levels. If body levels of sodium are low, aldosterone directs the kidneys to reabsorb or retain more sodium. This in turn results in potassium being excreted so the balance of electrolytes is maintained.

Imbalances

What happens when our regulatory mechanisms are unable to maintain the balance? Abnormal shifts in fluid balance may cause a deficit or excess in fluid volume.

Fluid volume deficit. In fluid volume deficit (FVD), a person experiences vascular, cellular, or intracellular dehydration. Severe FVD, when body fluid levels fall by 10% of body weight, is a medical emergency.[3]

FVD can occur from diarrhea, vomiting, or high fever—symptoms often experienced with stomach and intestinal viral infections or influenza. Other causes of excessive fluid loss may be sweating, diuretics, or polyuria (excessive urination). Whenever we lose fluid and have difficulty taking in additional fluids, we are at risk for FVD.

Determining whether symptoms are caused by dehydration or illness can be difficult. Characteristics of FVD include infrequent urination, decreased skin elasticity, dry mucous membranes, dry mouth, unusual drowsiness, lightheadedness or disorientation, extreme thirst, nausea, slow or rapid breathing, and sudden weight loss. The person will be less able to maintain blood pressure immediately after rising from a sitting or lying position (called *orthostatic hypotension*). A primary health care provider should be consulted for any illness that lasts more than a few days and causes loss of body fluids. In moderate or severe FVD, intravenous (IV) therapy is indicated to replace fluids.

FVD can also happen when we are not ill. Strenuous physical activity, either athletic or work-related, that causes excessive sweating can lead to FVD. Hot, dry weather also can overwork the body's cooling mechanisms. Drinking fluids throughout the day despite a low level of thirst sensation can alleviate these risks.

Older adults and infants are the groups most at risk for FVD. Older adults have decreased fluid reserves and diminished thirst mechanism acuity. FVD symptoms may be misdiagnosed as senility. Reminding older clients to drink even when thirst is not experienced is appropriate to ensure adequate intake of fluids. In infants, water makes up a larger percentage of body weight than in adults, and a greater percentage is extracellular fluid; dehydration from fluid loss can occur rapidly. In addition to other signs of FVD, infants may have a depressed fontanelle (soft spot) in the skull.

Fluid volume excess. Fluid volume excess is a condition in which a person experiences increased fluid retention and edema. It is associated with a compromised regulatory mechanism, excess fluid intake, or excess sodium intake.

Edema is excess accumulation of fluid in interstitial spaces caused by seepage from the circulatory system, which results in the retention of about 10% more water than normal. Some of us may notice that when we eat meals that are particularly high in sodium, we feel bloated, and our weight may even rise a few pounds the next day. This weight gain is not true weight gain but simply water retention that occurs in response to the excess intake of sodium. Within a few days, weight and water levels in the body return to their usual levels.

Edema can be a symptom of a health risk in certain situations. Sodium-sensitive individuals not only retain fluid when consuming high levels of sodium but also experience an increase in blood pressure, leading to hypertension.

Reducing excess water retention through a reduction in sodium consumption is a first step in treating this type of hypertension. A more serious form of edema occurs in victims of kwashiorkor when the protein levels in the body are so low that cellular fluid levels are imbalanced. Inappropriate levels of interstitial fluid accumulate in the stomach, face, and extremities.

Water intoxication refers to the consumption of large volumes of water within a short time, which results in a dilution of electrolytes in body fluids. It causes muscle cramps, decreased blood pressure, and weakness. Water intoxication is also possible if there is extensive loss of electrolytes because of dehydration, and rehydration is accomplished using only water, without the addition of replacement electrolytes. This condition is relatively rare but tends to occur when athletes continually hydrate without equivalent loss of fluid while participating in slower-paced events such as runs lasting longer than 4 hours or extend triathlons or rehydrate after a strenuous event with excessive amounts of water. Nonetheless, fluid volume deficit, dehydration, is much more common and more dangerous for athletes.[4]

MINERALS

Minerals serve a variety of functions in our bodies (Box 8-3). Structurally, minerals provide rigidity and strength to the teeth and skeleton; the skeletal mineral components also serve as a storage depot for other needs of the body. Minerals, allowing for proper muscle contraction and release, influence nerve and muscle functions. Other functions of minerals include acting as cofactors for enzymes and maintaining proper acid-base balance of body fluids. Minerals are also required for blood clotting and for tissue repair and growth.

Mineral Categories

Based on the amount of each mineral in the composition of our bodies, the 16 essential minerals are divided into two categories: major and trace minerals. To maintain body levels of **major minerals**, these minerals are needed daily from dietary sources in amounts of 100 mg or higher. In contrast, **trace minerals** are required daily in amounts less than or equal to 20 mg (Box 8-4). Although the required amounts

---

BOX 8-3   CONSIDERING VITAMINS AND MINERALS THROUGH FUNCTION

Vitamins and minerals are discussed as two separate nutrient categories in Chapter 7 and this chapter. Although each essential vitamin and mineral is discussed individually, they are not grouped together based on their functions for the body. The information here provides vitamins and minerals required for specific body functions of blood health, bone health, energy metabolism, and fluid and electrolyte balance. Additional functions of individual vitamins and minerals may be found in Table 7-3, Table 7-6, Table 8-1, and Table 8-2.

Blood Health

Blood is *the* body fluid, supplying tissues with oxygen, nutrients, and energy through circulation within the cardiovascular system. It is composed of water, red and white blood cells, oxygen, nutrients, and other formed substances. Always moving, blood gathers and distributes nutrients and oxygen to all cells and disposes of waste products. Deficiency of any of these nutrients will affect overall blood health. Only the blood-related functions of the vitamins and minerals are listed.

VITAMIN*	FUNCTION	MINERAL†	FUNCTION
Vitamin B$_{12}$	Transport/storage of folate needed for heme and cell formation and other functions	Iron	Distributes oxygen in hemoglobin and myoglobin
Folate *Folic acid, folacin*	Coenzyme metabolism (synthesis of amino acid, heme, DNA, RNA) and other functions	Zinc	Cofactor for more than 200 enzymes including enzymes to make heme in hemoglobin, genetic material and proteins
Vitamin B$_6$ *Pyridoxine*	Hemoglobin synthesis and other functions	Copper	Helps with iron use
Vitamin K	Cofactor in synthesis of blood clotting factors; protein formation		

Bone Health

As living tissue, bone requires nutrients to maintain cellular structure. Blood circulates through bone capillaries, delivering nutrients while removing waste materials no longer needed by cells. Hormones regulate the use of minerals either for storage and structural purposes in bone or for regulating body processes. Specific vitamins and minerals are indispensable for these functions to occur.

VITAMIN*	FUNCTION	MINERAL†	FUNCTION
Vitamin D	Bone mineralization	Calcium	Bone and tooth formation
Vitamin K	Protein formation for bone mineralization; cofactor for blood-clotting factors	Phosphorus	Bone and tooth formation (component of hydroxyapatite)
Vitamin A	Bone growth; maintains epithelial cells; regulation of gene expression	Magnesium	Bone structure
Precursor: beta carotene		Fluoride	Bone and tooth formation; increases stability of bone

BOX 8-3   CONSIDERING VITAMINS AND MINERALS THROUGH FUNCTION—cont'd

Energy Metabolism

In order to metabolize carbohydrates, lipids, and protein for energy and other needs, the body depends on many nutrients to support the process, create new cells, and implement various related functions.

VITAMIN*	FUNCTION	MINERAL†	FUNCTION
Thiamine *Vitamin B₁*	Coenzyme energy metabolism; muscle nerve action	Iodine	Thyroxine synthesis (thyroid hormone) regulates growth and development; basal metabolic rate (BMR) regulation
Riboflavin *Vitamin B₂*	Coenzyme energy metabolism	Chromium	Carbohydrate metabolism, part of glucose tolerance factor

Niacin
  Vitamin B₃, nicotinic acid,
  nicotinamide, niacinamide
	Cofactor to enzymes involved in energy metabolism; glycolysis and TCA cycle synthesis	Phosphorus	Energy metabolism (enzymes)

Vitamin B₆ *Pyridoxine*	Forms coenzyme pyridoxal phosphate (PLP) for energy metabolism	Sulfur Iron	Component of protein structures Distributed oxygen in hemoglobin and myoglobin
Folate *Folic acid, folacin*	Coenzyme metabolism (synthesis of amino acid, heme, DNA, RNA)	Zinc	Carbohydrate metabolism (insulin function); cofactor to more than 200 enzymes
Vitamin B₁₂ *Cyanocobalamin*	Metabolism of fatty acids/amino acids		
Pantothenic acid	Part of coenzyme A		
Biotin	Metabolism of carbohydrate, fat, and protein		

DNA, Deoxyribonucleic acid; *RNA*, ribonucleic acid; *TCA*, tricarboxylic acid.

Fluid and Electrolyte Balance

Life systems are dependent on fluid and electrolyte balance within the body. Electrolytes consist of mineral salts that maintain cellular fluid balance. The acid-base balance of body fluids is buffered by other minerals.

MINERAL†	FUNCTION
Sodium	Major extracellular electrolyte for fluid regulation; body fluid levels; acid-base balance; nerve impulse and contraction; blood pressure/volume
Potassium	With sodium and chloride, major intracellular electrolyte for fluid regulation; muscle function
Chloride	Acid-base balance
Phosphorus	Acid-base balance

*See Chapter 7 for additional information on vitamins.
†See text for additional information on water and minerals.

differ greatly between the major and trace minerals, each is absolutely necessary for good health.

The Dietary Reference Intakes (DRIs) listed in this chapter for minerals are those for young adults ages 19 to 24.[1] Levels for other groups are noted when special mention is needed. Keep in mind that because nutrition is a relatively young science, new functions of minerals as nutrients in the human body are still being discovered.

Food Sources

The prime sources of minerals include both plant and animal foods. Valuable sources of plant foods include most fruits, vegetables, legumes, and whole grains. Animal sources consist of beef, chicken, eggs, fish, and milk products. The discussions of individual minerals highlight the best food choices (Box 8-5).

In contrast to vitamins, minerals are stable when foods containing them are cooked. As inorganic substances, they are indestructible. Minerals may leach into cooking fluids but are still able to be absorbed if the fluid is consumed.

Although plants may contain an abundance of various minerals, some minerals in plants are not easily available to the human body. *Bioavailability* refers to the level of absorption of a consumed nutrient and is of nutritional concern. Binders such as phytic and oxalic acids may bind some minerals to the plant fiber structures. Binders are substances in plant foods that combine with minerals to form indigestible compounds, making them unavailable for our use. The amount of plant minerals available for absorption may depend on minerals in soils in which the plants are grown.

Minerals from animal foods do not have the same bioavailability issues. In fact, minerals from animal foods can be absorbed more easily than those from plants. However, fat content may be an issue for some animal foods. Lower fat sources of dairy and meat products are usually available and provide the same levels of minerals at a higher nutrient

BOX 8-4 ESSENTIAL MINERALS IN THE HUMAN BODY

Major
Calcium
Chloride
Magnesium
Phosphorus
Potassium
Sodium
Sulfur

Trace
Chromium
Copper
Fluoride
Iodine
Iron
Manganese
Molybdenum
Selenium
Zinc

density. Liver is often cited as a good source of minerals, such as iron and zinc. But liver is also high in cholesterol and saturated fats and may contain toxins to which the animal may have been exposed. These factors, combined with liver's somewhat unusual taste, often leaves the impression that good nutrient intake depends on eating healthy food that tastes bad. Other sources of each nutrient may be more appealing and equally as nutritious.

Food processing may reduce the amount of minerals available for absorption. Processing oranges into orange juice does not affect potassium levels naturally contained in oranges. However, processing whole-wheat flour into white flour does cause significant loss of minerals because the whole grain is not used. Iron is the only mineral returned to white flour through enrichment; zinc, selenium, copper, and other minerals are permanently lost.

Because we have difficulty obtaining high enough levels of some minerals naturally, fortification of manufactured foods has become commonplace. It is in this manner that food processing can serve the nutrient needs of consumers while

BOX 8-5 MYPLATE: VEGETABLES

As noted in Chapter 7 (Vitamins), the health benefits of eating vegetables overlap with those of eating fruits. Both fruit and vegetable MyPlate categories provide rich sources of minerals and are valuable components of an overall healthy diet providing nutrients essential for the health and maintenance of our bodies (also see Box 7-2). Health benefits of eating vegetables and fruits as part of an overall health diet include reduced risk for stroke, coronary artery disease, and type 2 diabetes mellitus; protection against some cancers (mouth, stomach, colorectal); and, as an excellent source of fiber, may decrease risk of several chronic diet-related disorders. The recommendation is to eat at least 2½ cups of vegetables every day.

What Counts as a Cup?*
The focus of this MyPlate box is on portions of the vegetables group.

In general, 1 cup of raw or cooked vegetables or vegetable juice, or 2 cups of raw leafy greens can be considered as 1 cup from the vegetable group. The following lists specific amounts count as 1 cup of vegetables (in some cases equivalents for ½ cup are also shown) toward your recommended intake.

VEGETABLE	AMOUNT THAT COUNTS AS 1 CUP OF VEGETABLES	AMOUNT THAT COUNTS AS ½ CUP OF VEGETABLES
Dark Green Vegetables		
Broccoli	1 cup, chopped or florets	
	3 spears, 5 inches long, raw or cooked	
Greens (collards, mustard greens, turnip greens, kale)	1 cup cooked	
Spinach	1 cup cooked	
	2 cups raw = 1 cup	1 cup raw = ½ cup
Raw, leafy greens: spinach, romaine, watercress, dark green leafy lettuce, endive, escarole	2 cups raw = 1 cup	1 cup raw = ½ cup
Orange Vegetables		
Carrots	1 cup; strips, slices, or chopped; raw or cooked	1 medium
	2 medium	Approximately 6 baby carrots
	1 cup baby carrots (approximately 12)	
Sweet potato	1 large, baked (2¼ inches or more in diameter)	
	1 cup sliced or mashed, cooked	

BOX 8-5	MYPLATE: VEGETABLES—cont'd	
VEGETABLE	**AMOUNT THAT COUNTS AS 1 CUP OF VEGETABLES**	**AMOUNT THAT COUNTS AS ½ CUP OF VEGETABLES**
Winter squash (acorn, butternut, hubbard)	1 cup cubed, cooked	½ acorn squash, baked = ¾ cup
Dry Beans and Peas		
Dry beans and peas (such as black, garbanzo, kidney, pinto, soybeans, black-eyed, split peas)	1 cup whole or mashed, cooked	
Tofu	1 cup ½-inch cubes (approximately 8 oz)	1 piece, 2 ½ inches × 2¾ inches × 1 inch (approximately 4 oz)
Starchy Vegetables		
Corn, yellow or white	1 cup 1 large ear (8-9 inches long)	1 small ear (approximately 6 inches long)
Green peas	1 cup	
White potatoes	1 cup diced, mashed 1 medium boiled or baked potato (2 ½ to 3 inches in diameter) French-fried: 20 medium to long strips (2 ½ to 4 inches long) (contains *discretionary calories*)	
Other Vegetables		
Bean sprouts	1 cup cooked	
Cabbage, green	1 cup, chopped or shredded, raw or cooked	
Cauliflower	1 cup, pieces or florets, raw or cooked	
Celery	1 cup, diced or sliced, raw or cooked 2 large stalks (11-12 inches long)	1 large stalk (11-12 inches long)
Cucumbers	1 cup raw, sliced or chopped	
Green or wax beans	1 cup cooked	
Green or red peppers	1 cup chopped, raw, or cooked 1 large pepper (3 inches in diameter, 3¾ inches long)	1 small pepper
Lettuce, iceberg or head	2 cups raw, shredded or chopped = 1 cup	1 cup raw, shredded or chopped = ½ cup
Mushrooms	1 cup raw or cooked	
Onions	1 cup chopped, raw or cooked	
Tomatoes	1 large raw, whole (3 inches) 1 cup chopped or sliced; raw, canned, or cooked	1 small raw, whole (2 ¼ inches) 1 medium, canned
Tomato or mixed vegetable juice	1 cup	½ cup
Summer squash or zucchini	1 cup cooked, sliced or diced	

*Accessed June 14, 2012, from www.choosemyplate.gov/food-groups/vegetables-counts.html.

still addressing the issues of convenience and taste appeal. Salt fortified with iodine is available; dry cereals have added minerals such as iron and an assortment of vitamins and other minerals.

Minerals as Nutrients in the Body
Structure

Minerals are inorganic substances. As elements, they are found in the rocks of the earth. Their tendency to gain or lose electrons makes them electrically charged. Thus they have special affinities for water, which itself carries positive and negative charges. As we consume plant and animal foods containing minerals, we can incorporate them into our body structures (bones), organs, and fluids.

Digestion and Absorption

During the process of digestion, minerals (as inorganic substances) are separated from the foodstuffs in which they entered our bodies. Digestion does change the valence states of some minerals, which changes their ability to be absorbed. However, their structure is not changed so they can be absorbed.

As noted, bioavailability affects the level of minerals we actually absorb. Generally, consuming a variety of whole foods ensures an adequate intake of minerals. Mineral deficiencies for which Americans tend to be at risk are iron, calcium, and zinc. Concerns and strategies for consuming appropriate amounts of these nutrients are discussed later in this chapter.

Metabolism

Because minerals are inorganic and do not provide energy, they are not metabolized by the human body. Instead some minerals assist as cofactors of metabolic processes.

MAJOR MINERALS

Calcium

Function

Calcium is the most abundant mineral in the body. Almost all of the calcium in the body, about 99%, is found in our bones, serving structural and storage functions. The other 1% of body calcium is released into body fluids when blood passes through bones; this constant interaction of blood with bone allows calcium to be distributed throughout the body. Other functions that depend on calcium include (1) the central nervous system, particularly nerve impulses; (2) muscle contraction and relaxation, when needed; (3) formation of blood clots; and (4) blood pressure regulation. Continuing research supports that increased levels of calcium (and vitamin D) intakes may be protective for colorectal cancer.[5]

Regulation

Our dietary intake of calcium influences the deposition of calcium in our bones. Blood calcium levels, however, do not depend on a daily dietary calcium intake. Instead the skeletal supply of calcium provides the source of calcium to be distributed throughout the body through the circulatory system. If calcium blood levels get too low, three actions can occur to reestablish calcium homeostasis: bones release calcium, intestines absorb more calcium, and kidneys retain more calcium.

Hormones that regulate the level of calcium in body fluids control the release of calcium from bones. Hormones affecting blood levels include parathormone (parathyroid hormone), calcitriol (active vitamin D hormone), and calcitonin. Parathormone is secreted by the parathyroid gland in response to low blood calcium levels. It raises blood calcium levels by stimulating all three ways of providing calcium to body fluids. Vitamin D has a hormone-like effect as calcitriol and increases blood calcium levels by acting on all three systems. The third hormone involved, calcitonin, is released by the Special C cells of the thyroid gland. Calcitonin reacts in response to high blood levels of calcium by lowering both calcium and phosphate in the blood.

Reactions of very low or extremely high blood levels can occur if regulatory mechanisms are hindered by a lack of vitamin D or hormone malfunction. If calcium blood levels get too high, calcium rigor (with symptoms of hardness or stiffness of muscles) may occur. Conversely, if levels are too low, a person may experience calcium tetany, with spasms caused by muscle and nerve excitability.

Recommended Intake and Sources

Calcium AI for men and women ranges from 1300 mg per day (ages 9 through 13) to 1000 mg (ages 19 through 50). Levels increase to 1200 mg for men and women older than 50 years. The AI during pregnancy and lactation is 1000 mg.

Concerns have been raised regarding the calcium intake of those most at risk for deficiency: youths age 11 through 24 and pregnant and lactating women. During these times, calcium needs are still high, although actual consumption of calcium may decrease. For many Americans, meeting these recommendations means increasing their number of servings of calcium-rich foods to at least three or more a day (Box 8-6). Other issues surrounding calcium intake and children are discussed in Chapter 12.

Primary sources of calcium are dairy products, mainly milk (whole, low-fat, and skim) and milk-based products such as ice cream, ice milk, yogurt, frozen yogurt, cheeses, and puddings (Figure 8-3). Although butter, cream cheese, and cottage cheese are dairy products, they are not good sources of calcium; butter and cream cheese are predominantly fat, and cottage cheese loses calcium through processing. Nondairy sources include green leafy vegetables (broccoli, kale, and mustard greens), small fish with bones (sardines and salmon canned with processed edible bones), legumes, and tofu processed with calcium. In addition, a variety of calcium-fortified foods are available, ranging from fortified orange juice to bread products. Box 8-7 gives examples of foods that boost calcium intake, and the *Teaching Tool* box, Visualizing the Calcium Values of Foods, provides education strategies for working with clients with low literacy skills.

Some leafy green vegetables—in particular, spinach, collards, Swiss chard, and escarole—contain oxalic acid, a binder that reduces the calcium absorbed. Plant foods containing oxalic acid cannot be considered a trustworthy source of calcium. Tea contains oxalic acid as well as tannins (also found in coffee), both of which may affect the absorption of calcium in foods consumed with tea. With the increased consumption of iced tea beverages, this effect should be considered, particularly for female adolescents and young adults.

Many adults are lactose intolerant. Lactose intolerance occurs when the body does not produce enough lactase, an enzyme necessary for the digestion of lactose, the carbohydrate found in milk. (Lactose intolerance is detailed in Chapter 4.) People experiencing lactose intolerance need to regularly incorporate sources of calcium other than dairy products into their dietary patterns. For some people, calcium supplements may be indicated; a registered dietitian or qualified nutritionist may be consulted.

Some calcium supplements are poorly absorbed because they don't dissolve in the stomach. If a calcium tablet doesn't

BOX 8-6   MYPLATE: MILK

MyPlate focuses on the milk group of foods as a source of the minerals calcium and potassium and vitamin D and protein. These nutrients can also be obtained from non-milk-derived foods, but milk products are rich sources and are a traditional part of the dietary intake of most Americans.

Health benefits of consuming foods in the milk group include assisting the building and maintaining of bone mass during the life span, particularly during childhood and adolescence; possible reduced risk of osteoporosis; and overall higher quality of nutritional intake. The recommendation is to consume 3 cups or servings daily of milk or milk products. If milk products are not consumed because of lactose intolerance, lactose-reduced products, calcium-fortified foods, and other naturally good sources of calcium can be chosen instead.

What Counts as a Cup?[*]
The focus of this MyPlate box is on portions of the dairy group.
The following lists specific amounts that count as 1 cup in the milk group toward your daily recommended intake.

DAIRY PRODUCT	AMOUNT THAT COUNTS AS 1 CUP IN THE MILK GROUP	COMMON PORTIONS AND EQUIVALENTS
Milk [choose fat-free or low-fat milk most often]	1 cup 1 half-pint container ½ cup evaporated milk	
Yogurt [choose fat-free or low-fat yogurt most often]	1 regular container (8 fluid oz) 1 cup	1 small container (6 oz) = ¾ cup 1 snack-size container (4 oz) = ½ cup
Cheese [choose low-fat cheeses most often]	1½ ounces hard cheese (cheddar, mozzarella, Swiss, Parmesan) ⅓ cup shredded cheese 2 oz processed cheese (American) ½ cup ricotta cheese 2 cups cottage cheese	1 slice hard cheese = ½ cup milk 1 slice processed cheese = ⅓ cup milk ½ cup cottage cheese = ¼ cup milk
Milk-based desserts [choose fat-free or low-fat types most often]	1 cup pudding made with milk 1 cup frozen yogurt 1½ cups ice cream	1 scoop ice cream = ⅓ cup milk

[*]Accessed June 14, 2012, from http://www.choosemyplate.gov/food-groups/dairy-counts.html.

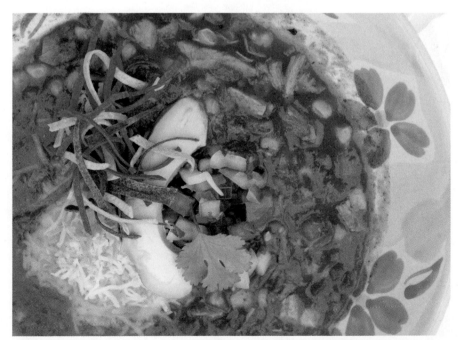

FIG 8-3 Calcium can be consumed in many different foods. (Photos.com.)

Continued

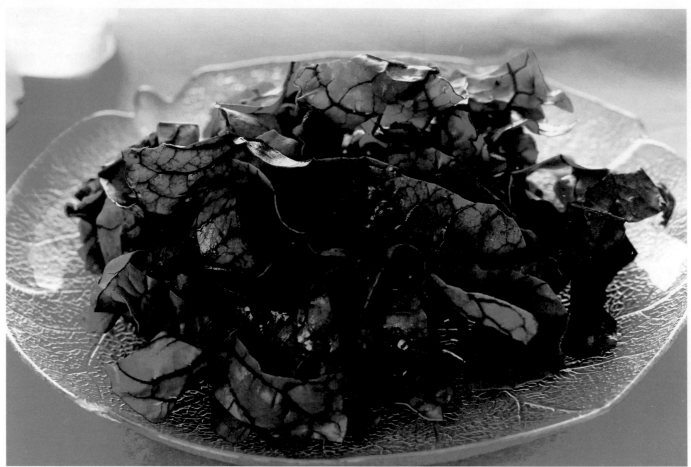

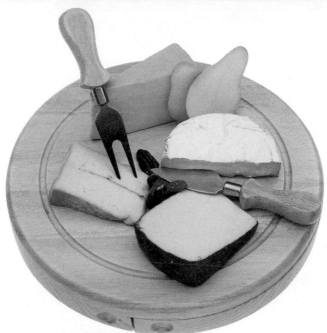

FIG 8-3 cont'd

BOX 8-7 SUGGESTIONS FOR BOOSTING CALCIUM INTAKE

Dairy

Broccoli with melted cheese

Calcium-fortified milk and cottage cheese

Powdered milk added to baking mixes, soups, puddings, gravies, hamburgers, and meat loaves

Sliced apples and pears with cheese wedges

Smoothies (fruit drinks made with milk, yogurt, and fruits)

Soups made with low-fat or skim milk

Nondairy

Bean burritos

Bean soups (split pea or lentil soup)

Breads fortified with calcium

Chicken cacciatore (chicken with bones cooked in tomato sauce; acid of tomatoes pulls calcium from bones)

Juices fortified with calcium

Soy milk and soy products fortified with calcium

Tofu (made with calcium carbonate), fresh or in frozen meals and desserts

BOX 8-8 FACTORS FAVORING AND HINDERING CALCIUM ABSORPTION

Factors Favoring Calcium Absorption
- Acidity of digestive mass
- Body's need for higher amounts (as in pregnancy)
- Lactose
- Sufficient vitamin D

Factors Hindering Calcium Absorption
- Aging
- Binders such as phytic acid and oxalic acid
- Dietary fat
- Dietary fiber
- Drug use
- Excessive phosphorus intake
- Laxative use
- Sedentary lifestyle

TEACHING TOOL

Visualizing the Calcium Values of Foods

Food charts that show the calcium values of different foods may be helpful to most people, but they may be meaningless to clients who cannot read English or have minimal literacy skills. Consider this innovative teaching strategy for visualizing the calcium content of commonly consumed foods (e.g., skim milk, yogurt, hard cheese), as follows:

1. Select four calcium-rich foods and four low-calcium foods (e.g., cottage cheese, broccoli, pinto beans).
2. Fill plastic resealable bags with small marshmallows to represent the calcium content of each of the selected foods. Each marshmallow can represent 10 mg of calcium. In addition, fill a large plastic resealable bag with 100 marshmallows (1000 mg or 100% Daily Value) as a reference.
3. Match the bag of "calcium" with the appropriate food model (or picture). Have the participants do the matching.
4. Distribute a pictorial representation of this activity with additional foods along with their bag of "calcium."

Courtesy Gayle Coleman, MS, RD, Michigan State University Extension, East Lansing.

readily dissolve when stirred into cider vinegar, it probably will not dissolve in the body.

Absorption Factors

Our bodies absorb calcium based on physiologic need. During childhood growth phases, we may absorb up to 75% of calcium consumed, compared with absorption rates of 30% to 60% once we complete our prime growth years. Similarly, during pregnancy and lactation, percentages of absorption are higher based on physiologic need.[6] In addition to physiologic need, other factors also seem to enhance the levels of calcium absorbed, including the following (Box 8-8):

- *Lactose:* Found naturally in milk (an excellent source of calcium), lactose appears to increase calcium absorption.
- *Sufficient vitamin D:* Vitamin D is involved in the synthesis of a protein that allows calcium to pass through the intestinal wall into the bloodstream.
- *Acidity of digestive mass:* Calcium is more soluble in acidic substances, so it is better absorbed when ingested as part of a meal. Generally, enough hydrochloric acid passes from the stomach to the intestine for calcium absorption. As we age, the amount of hydrochloric acid in digestive juices may decrease, causing less calcium to be absorbed.
- *Binders:* Naturally occurring substances in plant foods may bind with calcium in plant foods; two common calcium binders are phytic and oxalic acids (also called *phytates* and *oxalates*). Human digestive processes may be unable to separate calcium from the binder; both are then excreted, reducing the calcium available for absorption.
- *Dietary fat:* Dietary fat can form insoluble soaps with calcium; the insoluble soaps are harder to digest, making calcium less accessible for absorption. Moderate and low dietary fat intakes discourage the formation of this insoluble mass.
- *High-fiber intake and laxatives:* Excessive fiber consumption or laxative abuse results in food stuff moving through the GI tract too quickly for minerals, particularly calcium, to be absorbed.
- *Excessively high intakes of phosphorus or magnesium:* Excessively high intakes of these minerals disturb the balance of calcium in the body. Calcium is best absorbed when moderate or recommended levels of phosphorus and magnesium are ingested in proportion to calcium intake.

- *Sedentary lifestyle:* Being a couch potato has its consequences. A physically inactive lifestyle leads to less bone density. In contrast, weight-bearing exercise that pulls the muscle against the bone enhances calcium deposits in the bone matrix. This action occurs during running, brisk walking, biking, and strength training.
- *Drugs:* Some medications, including anticonvulsants, tetracycline, cortisone, thyroxine, and aluminum-containing antacids, are associated with reduced calcium absorption.

Deficiency

Deficiency of calcium primarily affects bone health. During the growing years, inadequate intake of calcium reduces the density of bone mass and, if severe, can stunt growth. For adults, long-term calcium deficiency may be one of the risk factors of *osteoporosis,* a multifactorial systemic skeletal disorder. This condition takes many years to develop, and overt symptoms appear late in life. Osteoporosis is a condition in which bone density is reduced and the remaining bone is brittle and breaks easily.

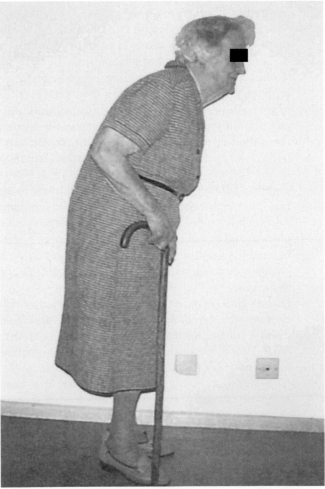

Typical posture in osteoporosis. (From Shipley M: *A colour atlas of rheumatology,* ed 3, London, 1993, Mosby-Year Book Europe Limited. By permission of Mosby International Ltd.)

One of the most recognizable characteristics of osteoporosis is the dowager's hump; as vertebrae in the spine collapse from weakness, the spine is no longer able to support the weight of the head. The back bows and the head angles down. Most significantly, the internal organs affected by the curvature are unable to function efficiently, and other health difficulties develop.

In contrast to *osteomalacia,* osteoporosis is multifactorial, and all the factors are tied to bone mineral density. These factors include genetics, diet, and lifestyle determinants. Bone density builds through early adulthood. Peak bone density is reached by about age 20, although some additional bone mineralization continues into the 30s. The more density built early in life, the less potential risk encountered. Factors that affect bone density but cannot be modified include genetic determinants of race and gender and family history, as follows:[7]

- *Race:* Osteoporosis is more common in white and Asian women than among African and African American women. This is because of racial differences in the skeletal density, possibly caused by hormonal differences.
- *Gender:* Men have greater bone density than women. They enter the later years when bone demineralization begins with a larger storage of calcium. The fact that men have more lean body mass or muscularity may cause more calcium to be deposited and retained in comparison with women. Women lose greater amounts of bone calcium during the first few years after menopause. The drop in estrogen levels appears to initiate the calcium loss. To slow the loss and to provide additional protection against heart disease, many primary health care providers prescribe hormone (estrogen) replacement therapy for postmenopausal women.
- *Family history:* A predisposition to lower bone density may be genetically passed between generations, particularly from mother to daughter. If a close family member develops osteoporosis, care should be taken to reduce the effects of other risk factors.

Osteoporosis, however, does occur in men and women. For men, osteoporosis tends to be a result of secondary causes that affect peak bone mass development or speed the loss of bone density. These causes may include steroid therapy, chronic alcoholism, hypogonadism, skeletal metastasis, multiple myeloma, gastric surgery, and anticonvulsant treatment.[8] Men and women who undergo organ transplantation are more at risk for osteoporosis, particularly during the first year after surgery. The loss of bone density is probably caused by the medications used to prevent organ rejection, such as glucocorticoids, that disturb bone and mineral homeostasis.

Osteoporosis prevention can begin before transplantation if bone density is marginal, or therapy can be implemented immediately following transplantation. Rates are lowest among patients receiving kidney transplants and highest among those receiving liver transplants.[9]

Factors related to development of osteoporosis that can be adjusted include nutrition, particularly calcium intake, and lifestyle determinants, as follows:

- *Nutrition/calcium intake:* Dietary calcium intake is of concern throughout the life span. In particular, the growth years (when calcium is deposited in the bone matrix) and the postmenopausal years of bone mineralization loss are periods when calcium intake appears crucial. Although the AI for calcium provides sufficient amounts, many individuals consume less than these levels. Female adolescents often consume levels of kcal and nutrients well below the AI while attempting to control body weight. These eating patterns often continue through adulthood. This long-term marginal deficiency of calcium may set the stage for future bone disorders. The issue is even more complicated for older adults. When they consume calcium-containing foods, less calcium may be absorbed because of decreased gastric acidity and reduced levels of available vitamin D.
- *Alcohol:* Long-term excessive intake of alcohol appears to reduce bone density. Alcohol may directly depress bone formation or may take the place of more nutritious foods, producing marginal deficiencies.
- *Smoking:* Cigarette smoking has been associated with a higher risk of osteoporosis. Smokers tend to be of lower weight (less bone density) than nonsmokers and appear to lose more bone mineralization after menopause.
- *Caffeine:* Caffeine consumption has been tied to urinary excretion of calcium. Reasonable use of caffeinated beverages, however, may be acceptable. More than likely, the relationship of caffeine to lower levels of body calcium concerns caffeinated beverages replacing those containing calcium such as skim milk. Although caffeinated coffee consumption may affect bone density of postmenopausal women, one glass of skim milk per day can overcome the effects of the coffee.[10] Another study showed consuming dietary caffeine regularly did not affect bone mineral density of the hip or of the total body.[11]
- *Sedentary lifestyle:* A physically active lifestyle not only enhances calcium absorption but also helps to maintain bone matrix mineralization. However, excessive exercise that results in extremely low body fat levels for women may be detrimental to bone density. If amenorrhea (abnormal cessation of menses) occurs because of excessive exercise, the resulting premature drop in estrogen may limit or decrease bone mineralization during the prime growth periods. Similarly, women with a smaller body size, including those experiencing anorexia nervosa, may have a greater risk of hip fracture later in life compared with those of larger body size.[12] Although no standards have been determined, it is likely that a body mass index (BMI) greater than 26 to 28 may provide reduced risk, whereas a lower BMI of less than 22 to 24 increases the risk of osteoporosis.[13]

Although the risk factors for osteoporosis may seem overwhelming, several can be reduced by following basic recommendations for achieving wellness. By consuming the

---

✴ TEACHING TOOL
Calcium: By Any Means Possible

The adequate intake (AI) for calcium ranges from 1000 to 1300 mg per day, depending on a person's age. The best sources are calcium-rich foods. But what if a client is lactose-intolerant or just doesn't like many calcium-containing foods?

Because the potential ramifications of chronic calcium deficiency are serious—fractures and other complications of osteoporosis—calcium supplementation may be appropriate. Following are some suggestions and cautions for client education:

- Calcium supplementation may increase the dietary intake of calcium, but it does not alleviate other risk factors associated with osteoporosis. Other nutrients and lifestyle behaviors also affect the level of risk. Popping a calcium pill does not mean a person is osteoporosis-free.
- Many people have problems with compliance; the regularity of calcium intake, not an occasional dose, builds dense bones. It is better to rely on food sources.
- The source of calcium affects the amount of actual calcium available. Tablets composed of calcium carbonate contain more elemental calcium (often 500-600 mg) than those made of calcium citrate or lactate (usually 200 mg per tablet), and it takes fewer pills to achieve the AI. Calcium citrate, however, is more easily absorbed by the digestive tract, even if more pills are needed.
- Be aware that calcium is always combined with another substance to form the tablet. A tablet may contain 1200 mg of calcium carbonate but only 500 mg of elemental calcium. The supplements to avoid are those made from dolomite, bone meal, and oyster shell; they may be contaminated with lead and other toxic metals.
- Although the tablets are supplementing dietary intake, it's best to take them with meals. The acid of the digestive process also helps in the breakdown and absorption of the calcium tablet(s), and tying the supplement to meals works as a reminder system. This also helps to spread supplementation throughout the day. One large dose will not be absorbed as well as two or three smaller doses.
- Calcium supplements often contain added vitamin D. The new vitamin D recommendation doubles after age 50 and triples after age 70, so the added vitamin D may be age appropriate. If other sources provide sufficient amounts of vitamin D, such as from multivitamin/mineral supplements or from foods or cereals fortified with 100% of the daily value for vitamin D, then the added D is not necessary.
- Before supplementing, keep track of sources and amounts of dietary calcium for several days. Intake may be adequate. If not, first contemplate ways to increase intake with foods, then consider supplementation.

---

serving amounts recommended by MyPyramid and engaging in regular physical exercise, most of the risk can be minimized. The *Teaching Tool* box, Calcium: By Any Means Possible, provides tips on educating clients on appropriate calcium intake.

Low levels of calcium intake are also associated with an increased risk of colon cancer and hypertension.

Toxicity

Calcium toxicity from consuming foods that contain calcium is not a concern. Problems may occur when supplements of calcium and other nutrients are used instead of foods. Over-supplementation may cause constipation, urinary stone formation affecting kidney function, and reduced absorption of iron, zinc, and other minerals.[6] The general guideline for calcium supplements is that levels should not exceed the AI for calcium. In addition, a UL of 2500 mg has been established.

Phosphorus

Function

Most of the phosphorus in the body (85%) is in our bones and teeth as a component of hydroxyapatite, a natural mineral structure. The other 15% of body phosphorus has functions (1) in energy transfer; (2) as part of the genetic material of deoxyribonucleic acid (DNA) and ribonucleic acid (RNA); (3) as a buffer in the form of phosphoric acid, which balances body acid-base levels; and (4) as a component of phospholipids used for transportation and structural functions.

Recommended Intake and Sources

The Recommended Dietary Allowance (RDA) for phosphorus is 700 mg per day for men and women aged 19 years and older. Phosphorus is widely available in foods. Particularly good sources are protein-rich foods such as dairy foods, eggs, meat, fish, poultry, and cereal grains. Because of the processing of convenience foods and soft drinks, both are also sources of phosphorus.

Deficiency

Deficiency of phosphorus is unknown. It is part of the genetic material of every cell of the body.

Toxicity

Excessive amounts of phosphorus, usually only possible from phosphorus supplements, cause calcium excretion from the body. Very high phosphorus intakes could affect the calcium/phosphorus ratio, possibly reducing the amount of calcium absorbed. This is a problem only if calcium intake is inadequate. Because phosphorus-containing soft drinks and convenience foods have replaced milk beverages and less-processed foods for many American teens and adult women, this may be a dietary concern. A UL of 4000 mg has been determined for phosphorus.

Magnesium

Function

As with calcium and phosphorus, most of the magnesium in the body is found in our bones, providing structural and storage functions. Magnesium assists hundreds of enzymes throughout the body. It also regulates nerve and muscle function, including the actions of the heart, and has a role in the blood clotting process and in the immune system.

Recommended Intake and Sources

The RDAs for magnesium are 420 mg per day for men and 320 mg for women. Many commonly eaten foods contain magnesium. Particularly good sources are most unprocessed foods, including whole grains, legumes, broccoli, leafy green vegetables, and other vegetables. Hard water can be a significant source of magnesium.

Deficiency

Magnesium deficiency tends to be related to secondary causes, rather than from a primary lack of magnesium consumption. These secondary causes may include excessive vomiting and diarrhea caused by pathologic conditions. A GI tract disorder may affect magnesium absorption, or kidney disease may inhibit retention of the mineral. Malnutrition and alcoholism also may have a negative impact on magnesium levels in the body. Similarly, drug interference or artificial feeding solutions deficient in magnesium may influence total body levels of magnesium. Whenever body fluids are lost, so is magnesium. Individuals on long-term regimens of diuretics are also at risk for deficiency.

In addition, if magnesium intake levels are borderline and intake of calcium is high, such as from calcium supplements, magnesium absorption may be limited.

Symptoms of magnesium deficiency include twitching of muscles, muscle weakness, and convulsions. In children, magnesium deficiency also may be associated with growth failure.

Toxicity

Toxic effects of magnesium are rare but serious and are due to nondietary sources such as supplements or mineral salts. A tolerable upper intake level (UL) of 350 mg pertains to nonfood sources. Self-supplementation with calcium tablets containing magnesium while also taking magnesium supplements adds up to an excess that is not seriously toxic but is excessive enough to cause long-term diarrhea and deficient fluid volume (dehydration). This is an example of why all medications and dietary supplements should be reported to health care providers before invasive and/or costly procedures are conducted to determine the cause of symptoms. Simply stopping the magnesium supplementation will most likely restore proper function of the large intestine.

Sulfur

Function

Sulfur is a component of protein structures. It is present in every cell of the body and is part of several amino acids, thiamine, and biotin. Sulfur is also involved with maintaining the acid-base balance of the body.

Recommended Intake and Sources

No DRI has been established for sulfur. Diets adequate in protein provide sufficient amounts of sulfur. Sulfur is found in all protein-containing foods.

Deficiency

Deficiencies of sulfur do not occur; sulfur is so basic to the structure of the human cell that deficiencies cannot develop.

Toxicity

Toxicity to sulfur is not a health issue.

ELECTROLYTES: SODIUM, POTASSIUM, AND CHLORIDE

Electrolytes are minerals circulating in blood and other body fluids that carry an electrical charge. Maintaining a balance of these minerals is important because of their effect on body processes such as the amount of water in the body, blood pH, and muscle action. Electrolytes travel in blood as acids, bases, and salts and include sodium, calcium, potassium, chlorine, magnesium, and bicarbonate. Laboratory studies of blood serum determine electrolyte values.

Sodium, potassium, and chloride are major electrolytes of the body. As electrolytes, these minerals serve specific functions. The acid-base balance of body fluids depends on regulated distribution of these minerals, proteins, and other electrolytes. Electrolytes also have a role in the normal functioning of nerves and muscles. In addition, each mineral serves other specific functions in the body.

Sodium

Function

Sodium performs a variety of important functions in the body. Blood pressure and volume are maintained by the characteristics of sodium as the major cation in extracellular fluid. Transmission of nerve impulses relies on body sodium levels. As the major extracellular electrolyte, sodium has a role in the regulation of body fluid levels in and out of cells. This movement affects blood volume as well, which is tied to the thirst mechanism and total body fluid levels. The blood proteins, such as albumin, that prevent the development of some types of edema also regulate blood volume.

Recommended Intake and Sources

The AI for sodium is 1500 mg per day for adults or about ¾ teaspoon of salt (sodium chloride).This dietary recommendation is based on the known adequate intake required for good health.

Health-related associations have set guidelines for appropriate and safe levels of sodium. The National Research Council Recommendations suggest limiting daily salt intake to less than 6 g; this equals 2400 mg of sodium (Figure 8-4).[1] The American Heart Association advises sodium limits of 2300 mg daily, or about 1 teaspoon of salt.

Most sodium enters our diet as sodium chloride (table salt). Sodium occurs naturally in many foods. It is also added to foods as salt during the cooking process and right before consumption (see *Cultural Considerations* box, A [Cooking] History of Salt). Processing of foods, particularly quick-serve foods, often adds substantial amounts of sodium, as dis-

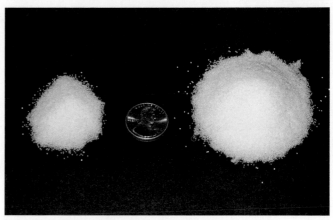

FIG 8-4 Daily salt intakes: Adequate Intake of sodium (1500 mg) equals ¾ tsp salt (on the left); typical intake of sodium (6000 mg) equals 3 tsp salt (on the right).

🌐 CULTURAL CONSIDERATIONS
A (Cooking) History of Salt

The course of history has been influenced by salt. Nations explored the world in search of salt because of its value in preserving foods. Bacterial and mold cells are inhibited from growing when placed in a concentrated salt solution. This decreases food spoilage. Though salt is no longer needed to preserve foods, we continue to value its ability to transform the taste of a dish from bland to sublime. Salt's importance to the human body cannot be denied because we have specialized taste buds to identify its consumption. Salt as a compound of sodium chloride contains two essential minerals without which the human body cannot survive.

Recognition of the importance of salt to human life began early. In the Old Testament of the Bible, salt was identified as an offering to God. Later on, Roman soldiers were given a stipend, called *salarium,* to buy salt. Today we can buy salt with our "salaries," a term that is derived from *salarium.* "Salt of the earth" was a phrase used by Jesus to describe his followers who were pure and of the earth.

Application to nursing: Although salt has its virtues, it also has drawbacks. Health professionals continue to recommend moderate intakes of sodium to reduce the risk of hypertension. The amounts recommended for cooking vary because an amount that is pleasing to one person may vary for another. Amounts of salt listed in a recipe can usually be modified to suit the health and taste requirements of the cook and the eaters.

Data from McGee H: *On food and cooking: The science and lore of the kitchen,* New York, 1997, Firestone; O'Neill M: Let it pour, *New York Times Magazine,* Oct 22, 1995, p. 77.

cussed in Box 8-9. Processed foods are carriers for other additives that often contain sodium. The sodium adds flavor that may be lost in processing.

Do you salt your food first, and then taste it? Some habits are hard to break but are worth the effort. However, breaking the saltshaker habit will reduce sodium intake only 15% for most Americans; most of the sodium eaten comes from processed foods.

BOX 8-9	PROCESSING EFFECTS ON FOOD SODIUM CONTENT

FOOD PRODUCT	TOTAL SODIUM CONTENT
Potatoes	
Baked potato (1)	16 mg
French-fried potatoes (10 strips)	108 mg
Scalloped potatoes from dry mix (1 cup)	835 mg
Chicken	
Baked chicken (3 oz)	64 mg
Batter-fried chicken (3 oz)	231 mg
Chicken nuggets (6 pieces)	542 mg
Oats	
Oatmeal prepared with water (1 cup)	2 mg
Oatmeal bread (1 slice)	124 mg
Ready-to-eat cereal (1 cup)	307 mg
Apples	
Apple (1)	Trace
Applesauce (1 cup)	8 mg
Apple pie (1 slice)	476 mg

Data from Pennington JAT, et al: *Bowes & Church's food values of portions commonly used*, ed 19, Philadelphia, 2010, Lippincott Williams & Wilkins; U.S. Department of Agriculture, Agricultural Research Service: *USDA national nutrient database for standard reference*, Release 18, Washington, DC, 2005, Nutrient Data Laboratory Home Page. Accessed February 12, 2010, from www.ars.usda.gov/ba/bhnrc/ndl.

The more a foodstuff is processed, the higher the sodium content becomes (see Box 8-9). More nutrients are also lost along the way. Which is saltier or, to be more exact, which contains more sodium—a bowl of corn flakes or a large order of fast-food fries? The corn flakes win, containing 290 mg of sodium compared with 200 mg for the fries. Of course, the fries contain a lot more fat and calories.

Consider the potato. A plain baked potato contains only 16 mg of sodium. Fixed up at a local fast-food restaurant, a baked potato with cheese sauce and broccoli skyrockets to more than 400 mg of sodium and lots of fat. A cheese or sour cream mix prepared at home is even higher in sodium—close to 600 mg. The sodium in plain mashed potatoes from a mix (dehydrated and then reconstituted) jumps from 8 mg in its original whole form to more than 300 mg, and that's without butter or gravy. The point is that processing foods adds invisible sodium as sodium chloride; in fact, it's so invisible that we can no longer taste the saltiness.

Sodium enjoys widespread use in the American diet as a flavoring agent (sodium chloride, monosodium glutamate [MSG], sodium saccharin), dough conditioner (baking powder, baking soda), and preservative (sodium sulfite). Because of consumer demand, lower-sodium versions of many products are available. Nutrition labeling information must include sodium content. This is powerful information that allows for comparing the sodium content of similar products.

Deficiency

Depletion of sodium can develop through dehydration or excessive diarrhea. Because of concern over the relationship between sodium and hypertension, some people may overly restrict sodium and thus be at risk. Typical athletic activity or physical labor that produces excessive sweating may cause dehydration and sodium loss, but drinking fluids and consuming foods containing sodium soon restore body levels of sodium. Salt tablets, once a common remedy, are not recommended and may be dangerous.

Symptoms of sodium deficiency include headache, muscle cramps, weakness, reduced ability to concentrate, and loss of memory and appetite. For most people, sodium deficiency is unlikely to occur because we get enough sodium naturally from foods. These symptoms are similar to those of fluid volume deficit, which is more common.

Hyponatremia, or low blood sodium, may occur. The symptoms are the same as for sodium intake deficiency. Hyponatremia may be acute as a one-time episode due to specific factors or chronic—that is, a recurring condition. Acute hyponatremia is of concern for endurance athletes. Athletes completing endurance events or slower runners in marathon races who continually drink fluid without an equivalent loss of fluid through sweat or urination may so overhydrate as to experience hyponatremia.[4] Even though this is rare, awareness is important because medical treatment is different if fluid volume deficit or acute hyponatremia is present because the symptoms are the same. Blood testing determines the cause of the symptoms. Chronic hyponatremia may occur because of secondary disorders such as neurologic and kidney disorders that affect the fluid regulatory mechanisms of the body. Blood levels of sodium decrease as excess fluid is retained, which dilutes blood sodium levels or too much sodium is excreted by the kidneys. Drug and dietary treatment may address chronic hyponatremia.[3]

Toxicity

An excess sodium intake is difficult for the body to handle. The kidneys have the primary responsibility to flush out the excess sodium. Some individuals are sodium sensitive and may develop hypertension and edema in response to high intake of sodium. Levels consumed in diets based on highly processed foods and high-sodium foods may be enough to initiate hypertension in sodium-sensitive individuals. Although others may not experience negative ramifications from high-sodium intakes, there are no benefits either. This is one of the few nutrients that we can overdose on from foods consumed.

An occasional very salty meal may produce edema but not hypertension. The best remedy for occasional edema is simply to drink more water to equalize the sodium concentration of body fluids. The kidneys take care of the rest by filtering out the excess sodium.

Potassium
Function

Although sodium as a cation maintains the fluid levels extracellularly, potassium, as the primary intercellular cation, maintains fluid levels inside the cells. Potassium is also crucial for normal functioning of nerves and muscles, including the heart.

Recommended Intake and Sources

The AI for potassium is 4700 mg per day. Even though the AI is higher than most Americans consume now, it should lower blood pressure, decrease the negative effects of sodium chloride on blood pressure, reduce the risk of kidney stones, and possibly reduce bone loss. The best sources for potassium for these purposes are the forms found naturally in fruits and vegetables.[1]

Sources of potassium include whole unprocessed foods, white potatoes with skin, sweet potatoes, tomatoes, bananas, oranges, other fruits and vegetables, dairy products, and legumes.

Deficiency

Similar to magnesium deficiency, potassium deficiency may be caused by dehydration from vomiting or diarrhea, diuretics, and misuse of laxatives. If long-term use of diuretics is warranted to reduce edema associated with hypertension, particular attention should be paid to consuming adequate levels of potassium from foods. Some diuretics are potassium wasting; some are potassium sparing. Supplementation when using a potassium-sparing diuretic could be dangerous. Potassium supplements should be taken only when prescribed by a primary health care provider.

Most often, bananas and oranges are suggested to patients at risk for potassium deficiency. These fruits may not be the best sources based on nutrient content, satiety, and economy. Whereas an *edentulous* (toothless) older person with congestive heart failure who is taking potassium-wasting diuretics and is on a low-income budget can make a meal out of a whole baked potato, he or she cannot be equivalently satisfied with a banana. A baked potato eaten with the skin contains 844 mg of potassium, whereas a whole banana contains 891 mg. A whole orange yields only 326 mg. A potato stores easily without refrigeration for much longer than a banana, and somewhat longer than an orange, and fits better into a tight budget. Yet foods like a simple potato may not be suggested to patients. Nurses can create patient education nutrient/food lists that consider factors such as satiety and economy to enhance compliance.

Symptoms associated with potassium deficiency include muscle weakness, confusion, loss of appetite and, in severe cases, cardiac dysrhythmias.

Toxicity

In general, potassium toxicity occurs only from supplements, not from consuming excess from foods. Toxicity doesn't usually occur with foods as long as a person has properly functioning kidneys. For individuals with renal disease, high-potassium foods are toxic. Even patients on dialysis may still be at risk for potassium toxicity. Symptoms of toxicity are similar to those of a deficiency. They include muscle weakness, vomiting and, at excessively high levels, cardiac arrest.

Chloride
Function

As the key anion of extracellular fluids, chloride assists in maintaining fluid balance inside and outside cells. In addition, chloride is a component of hydrochloric acid, an indispensable gastric juice produced by the stomach.

Recommended Intake and Sources

The AI for chloride is 2300 mg per day for adults. This requirement is easily met by consumption of sodium chloride; foods containing sodium usually provide chloride as well.

Deficiency

Deficiency of chloride is rare; adequate amounts are easily consumed. Although deficiency is possible, it would occur from the same circumstances as sodium deficiency or from excessive vomiting.

Toxicity

Chloride toxicity may occur because of dehydration, causing an imbalance of chloride to the other electrolytes. However, the other effects of dehydration are more severe than those of chloride toxicity.

Table 8-2 provides a summary of the major minerals.

TRACE MINERALS

Trace minerals as a group of nutrients function primarily as cofactors by performing metabolic and transport functions.

Iron
Function

Iron is responsible for distributing oxygen throughout our bodies. Oxygen depends on the iron in hemoglobin (an oxygen-transporting protein) of red blood cells (erythrocytes) to bring oxygen to all cells. Myoglobin (an oxygen-transporting protein) holds oxygen in the muscle cells for quick use when needed. Because of its ability to change ionic charges, iron also assists enzymes in the use of oxygen by all cells of the body.

Iron is conserved and recycled by the body. When red blood cells are old or damaged, the spleen removes their iron component. Some iron is kept in the spleen for later use, and the rest is sent to the liver for processing. From the liver, iron is transported as transferrin to bone marrow and recycled for use in new red blood cells. Some iron is lost through the shedding of tissue cells in urine and sweat and when bleeding occurs; this lost iron must be replaced by dietary sources.

Recommended Intake and Sources

When red blood cells break down, the iron in the hemoglobin is recycled to the liver and used to form new red blood cells. Whenever blood is lost from the body, iron is lost as well and cannot be recycled. Internal bleeding, such as from acute ulcers, can be a deceptive cause of iron loss. More obvious is

TABLE 8-2   MAJOR MINERALS

MINERAL	FUNCTION	CLINICAL ISSUES DEFICIENCY/ TOXICITY	RECOMMENDED DAILY INTAKES*	FOOD SOURCES	ABSORPTION ISSUES
Calcium (Ca)	Bone and tooth formation; blood clotting; muscle contraction/ relaxation; CNS; blood pressure	Deficiency: reduced bone density; osteoporosis Toxicity: constipation; urinary stones; reduced iron and zinc absorption	AI Adults: 1000-1200 mg Pregnancy/lactation 1000 mg UL 2500 mg	Milk (whole, low-fat, skim), milk-based products, green leafy vegetables legumes	Absorption based on need: increased by vitamin D; decreased by binders, inactivity, coffee/tea
Phosphorus (P)	Bone and tooth formation (component of hydroxyapatite); energy metabolism (enzymes); acid-base balance	Deficiency: rare Toxicity: increased calcium excretion	RDA Adults: 700 mg Pregnancy/ lactation: 700 mg UL 4000 mg	Dairy foods, egg, meat, fish, poultry	Absorbed with calcium
Magnesium (Mg)	Structure/storage; cofactor; nerve and muscle function; blood clotting	Deficiency: secondary with muscle twitching, weakness, convulsions from FVD	RDA Men: 420 mg Women: 320 mg Pregnancy/ lactation: 320-360 mg UL 350 mg	Whole grains, legumes, green leafy vegetables (broccoli), hard water	
Sulfur (S)	Component of protein structures	Deficiency: only if protein malnourished	Protein-adequate diets contain adequate levels	Protein-containing foods	
Sodium (Na)	Major extracellular electrolyte for fluid regulation; body fluid levels; acid-base balance; nerve impulse and contraction; blood pressure/volume	Deficiency: FVD with headache; muscle cramps, weakness, decreased concentration, memory and appetite loss Toxicity: sodium sensitive hypertension	AI Adults: 1200-1500 mg	Table salt; naturally in many foods; processed foods	
Potassium (K)	Major intracellular electrolyte for fluid regulation; muscle function	Deficiency: muscle weakness, confusion, decreased appetite, cardiac dysrhythmias caused by FVD from vomiting/diarrhea or diuretics Toxicity: from diet or supplements if renal disease present	AI Adults: 4700 mg	Unprocessed foods, fruits, vegetables, dairy products, meats, legumes	
Chloride (Cl)	Acid-base balance; gastric hydrochloric acid for digestion	Deficiency: FVD caused by vomiting/ diarrhea	AI Adults: 1800-2300 mg	Table salt	

*Ages 19-30.
AI, Adequate Intake; *CNS,* central nervous system; *EMR,* estimated minimum requirement; *FVD,* fluid volume deficit; *RDA,* Recommended Dietary Allowance; *UL,* Tolerable Upper Intake Level.

the loss of blood by women from menstruation. Based on this monthly loss and the increased iron demands of pregnancy, women's overall need for iron is higher than men's. The RDA for men is 8 mg and is 18 mg for women. During pregnancy the requirement is 27 mg; the blood supply of a pregnant woman is 1.5 times greater than her normal level.

The RDA allows for the unusual absorption rate of dietary iron. Only about 10% to 15% of dietary iron consumed is absorbed; this amount increases up to 20% if body levels are deficient. Higher percentages are absorbed during pregnancy and during periods of growth.

Intestinal mucosal cells contain two proteins that assist in absorption of dietary iron. One protein, *mucosal transferrin*, moves iron to a protein carrier in blood transferrin. This allows for the movement of iron through blood to bone marrow and tissues as needed. The second, *mucosal ferritin*, stores iron in the mucosal cells as a reserve if iron is needed. If not used, mucosal cells are replaced every few days so a continuous short-term supply of iron is available.

The RDA is also set to provide adequate storage levels of iron in the liver; iron is also stored in the spleen and bone marrow. In these organs, iron is contained in the proteins ferritin and hemosiderin. Ferritin is always being made and is easily available as an iron source. Hemosiderin is made when iron levels are high. Although it is a source of iron, its availability from storage to be used by the body takes longer than ferritin.

Iron is found in both plant and animal sources (Figure 8-5). **Heme iron**, found in animal sources of meat, fish, and poultry, is more easily absorbed than nonheme iron found in plant foods. Animal sources of iron also contain nonheme iron in addition to heme iron. Although egg yolks contain iron, the iron is not absorbed as well as other heme sources. **Nonheme iron** plant sources include vegetables, legumes, dried fruits, whole grain cereals, and enriched grain products, especially iron-fortified dry cereals.

Increased absorption of iron occurs when dietary sources are consumed with foods containing ascorbic acid (vitamin C). For example, drinking orange juice or eating slices of cantaloupe with meals increases the amount of nonheme iron absorbed. Absorption of nonheme iron increases in the presence of heme iron. This means that consuming iron from several sources improves absorption of the total iron amounts of heme and nonheme iron.

Another way to increase dietary iron intake is to cook foods in cast-iron skillets. Iron in the skillet leaches into the foods, providing an easy means for boosting iron intake.

Factors that inhibit iron absorption include consumption of foods that contain binders (e.g., phytates) and oxalates that keep the dietary iron from separating from plant sources. Tannins in plants, most notably in teas and coffee, can also interfere with iron absorption. Continual use of antacids and excessive intake of other minerals competes with the absorption sites for iron. Pica, the consumption of nonnutritive substances, creates health problems. When the nonnutritive substances are excreted from the body, minerals are also excreted, which decreases mineral absorption. Pica is discussed in the next section.

Deficiency

Iron deficiency has been a public health problem for many years. Although the incidence has decreased in the United States, most likely because of increased fortification, it is still common for iron deficiency and iron deficiency anemia to occur among young children, teenage girls, and women of childbearing age. These disorders are more common among minority women of low income who have had many children. In other parts of the world it is still the most widespread nutrient deficiency, primarily in the developing world. Children and women of childbearing age are most at risk. The effects of iron deficiency can be subtle and may be assigned to other causes. A range of symptoms accompanies different degrees of deficiency. All levels of iron deficiency affect the availability of oxygen throughout the body.[14]

Iron deficiency occurs when there is reduced supply of iron stores available in the liver. If neither the diet nor body stores can supply the iron needed for hemoglobin synthesis, the number of red blood cells will decrease in the bloodstream. The blood hemoglobin concentration also falls. When both the percentage of red blood cells (called *hematocrit*) and the hemoglobin level fall, a health care provider should suspect iron deficiency.

In severe deficiency, the hemoglobin and hematocrit levels fall so low that the amount of oxygen carried in the blood is decreased and the person is pale, tired, and anemic. Iron deficiency anemia is characterized by microcytes or small, pale red blood cells. Physical activity or work may be difficult to perform because not enough oxygen is available for use by the muscles. Cognitive functioning is compromised. For children, developmental delays and learning problems may develop; an iron-deficient child is easily distracted and unable to focus on learning tasks. A person may have a sensation of always feeling cold, as if body temperature cannot be regulated appropriately. The immune system is compromised as well, reflected in decreased wound-healing ability. During pregnancy, iron deficiency anemia caused by inadequate dietary intake is associated with greater risk of premature delivery and low birth weight.

Because infants have received more iron during the past 3 years, a decline in iron deficiency anemia among American children has occurred. However, prevalence has remained constant among women of childbearing age. The Centers for Disease Control and Prevention (CDC) recommendations exist for use by primary health care providers to prevent, detect, and treat iron deficiency. The guidelines focus on adequate iron nutrition for infants and young children, screening for anemia among women of childbearing age, and the value of low-dose iron supplements for pregnant women.

A form of anemia called *sports anemia* occurs among endurance athletes. As the body adapts to aerobic development from intense exercise, the individual's volume of blood expands. This expansion lowers hemoglobin concentration,

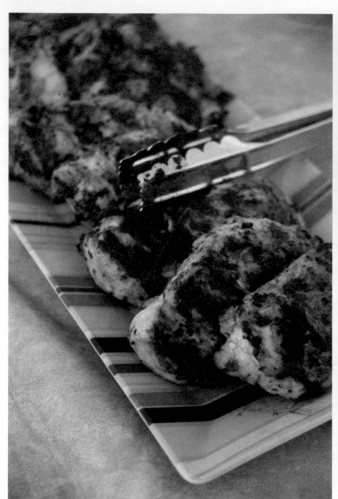

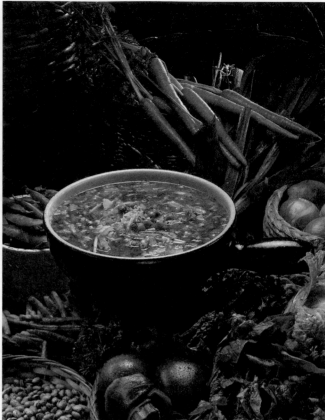

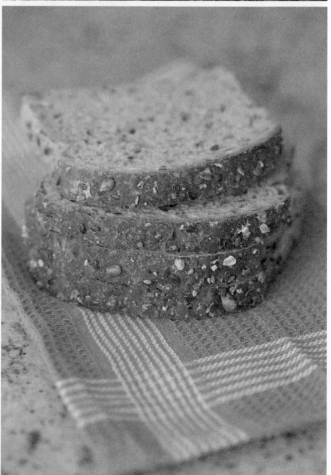

FIG 8-5 An assortment of foods containing iron. (Photos. com.)

producing an appearance of anemia. This condition, however, is not an illness but a positive adaptation of the body.

To alleviate iron deficiency, the cause of the deficiency (either internal loss of blood or lack of dietary intake) needs to be addressed. Children may lack sufficient intake of iron foods. Toddlers may develop iron deficiency anemia from drinking too much milk, a poor source of iron, which fills them up and keeps them from eating other iron-containing foods. Women tend to be doubly at risk because of dieting habits and female physiology. Chronic dieting may affect the intake of iron-rich foods; loss of blood through menses and the high iron demands of pregnancy combine to greatly increase female iron requirements. The recent increased consumption of iced tea as a popular soft drink may also affect women's iron levels. The tannin in tea reduces iron absorption. For adults in the United States, iron deficiency is rarely caused by dietary deficiency; instead it usually results from the blood loss of menstrual bleeding or internal bleeding in the GI tract, perhaps from bleeding ulcers or hemorrhoids.

An unusual behavior associated with iron deficiency is pica. Pica is characterized by a hunger and appetite for nonfood substances including ice, cornstarch, clay, and even dirt. These substances contain no iron and may even lead to loss of additional minerals, particularly when clay and dirt are consumed. Although *geophagia* (pica of clay or dirt) and *amylophagia* (pica of cornstarch and laundry starch) are primarily recognized among women of rural lower socioeconomic groups, *pagophagia* (excessive ice consumption) has been noted among all socioeconomic levels.[14] Of particular concern is the practice of pica during pregnancy, when the risk and implications of iron deficiency anemia are most severe. A challenge to obstetric nurses is to elicit information about this type of dietary behavior when assessing clients.

If increases in dietary sources of iron-rich foods do not raise hematocrit levels, supplements may be prescribed. Determination of dose is made based on physiologic requirements as assessed by primary health care providers. Long-term compliance is necessary to adequately restore iron storage levels in the body. Client education and support by nurses are advantageous.

Strategies to enhance absorption of iron supplements are simple. Drinking a glass of orange juice when taking an iron supplement will maximize iron absorption. Avoid taking iron supplements with milk because the calcium in milk interferes with absorption. Use of iron supplements may cause stools to turn black and constipation to result.

Toxicity

Hemosiderosis, storing too much iron in the body, is a health concern. This condition may be caused either by hemochromatosis, a genetic disorder that allows more dietary iron to be absorbed than usual, or by consumption of very high levels of iron-containing foods, perhaps through iron fortification. The resulting iron overload can damage tissue cells when storing excess iron. Bacterial microorganisms may thrive on the excessive amounts of iron circulating in the blood. These effects are manifested in vague symptoms of weakness and fatigue. More specific symptoms include liver and heart damage, diabetes, arthritis, and discoloration of skin.[15]

Those at risk include men, people with chronic excessive alcohol consumption, and individuals who are genetically at risk for hemochromatosis. Because men lose no iron through menstruation or childbirth and may consume more foods fortified with iron, their bodies can potentially store more iron than needed. Excessive consumption of alcohol puts people at risk because their livers are affected by alcohol and may malfunction, absorbing too much iron. Individuals with diabetes may also be at higher risk.[15]

Hemochromatosis alters iron metabolism, allowing excess iron to be absorbed from food and supplements. Treatment for hemochromatosis is blood removal by giving blood regularly and by decreasing dietary intake of iron-containing foods. This disorder is sometimes misdiagnosed as diabetes or as liver disorders. Although they are caused by hemochromatosis, these disorders are treated as individual ailments rather than addressing the underlying iron overload. However, awareness of hemochromatosis is increasing among primary health care providers and other health professionals. Screening during regular checkups is recommended for those older than age 30, particularly if they have diabetes. Screening is conducted by a blood test to assess transferrin saturation.

A final concern about iron toxicity is less a nutritional issue and more of a public health and safety issue. Accidental iron poisoning of children who consume iron supplements or vitamin or mineral supplements containing iron is a medical emergency. As few as 6 to 12 pills can be lethal, depending on the dose and the age of the child. All supplements, even the fruit-flavored shapes formulated for children, should be treated as medicinal drugs and be kept out of the reach of children.

Zinc
Function

More than 200 enzymes throughout the body depend on zinc. Zinc affects our growth process, taste and smell ability, healing process, immune system, and carbohydrate metabolism by assisting insulin function.

Recommended Intake and Sources

The zinc RDA for men and women is 11 and 8 mg per day, respectively. During pregnancy and lactation, suggested levels for women increase to 11 to 12 mg.

Zinc-containing foods include meat, fish, poultry, whole grains, legumes, and eggs. In the United States, a variety of zinc sources are easily available. In parts of the world where animal foods are not regularly consumed and grains are a primary zinc source, deficiencies may develop because of the low bioavailability of zinc from fibrous whole grain plant foods. Grains contain phytic acid that remains bound to zinc in the intestinal tract; human digestive juices cannot break this bond. Use of leavening agents such as yeast to prepare whole grain food products breaks this bond, making zinc available. Zinc deficiency still occurs in parts of the world where food sources may be limited and whole grains are consistently consumed as unleavened breads.

Deficiency

Deficiency symptoms are related to zinc's functions in the body. Symptoms include impaired growth, reduced appetite, and immunologic disorders. Severe zinc deficiency during the growth years may result in dwarfism and hypogonadism (reduced function of gonads), leading to delayed sexual development. Reduced appetite is most likely related to a reduced ability to taste (hypogeusia) and smell foods (hyposmia). The difficulty is that once appetite is reduced, fewer potential sources of zinc may be consumed, which causes the zinc deficiency to worsen. Marginal deficiencies among children categorized as picky eaters have been noted to negatively affect height status. Among older adults, inadequate dietary intake resulting in reduced zinc intake appears to affect wound healing, taste and scent ability, and immune functions.

Toxicity

Zinc toxicity from inappropriate supplementation produces GI distress, leading to vomiting and diarrhea, fever, and exhaustion. The symptoms appear similar to those of the flu. Continual use of supplements decreases iron and copper levels in the body and reduces levels of high-density lipoprotein (HDL), thereby increasing risk of coronary artery disease. Intake should be no higher than the RDA unless directed by a primary health care provider; individuals should not self-medicate. Consequently, the UL of 40 mg should be observed.

Iodine
Function

Iodine is part of the hormone thyroxin produced by the thyroid gland. Thyroxin is involved with regulating growth and development, basal metabolic rate, and body temperature.

Recommended Intake and Sources

The RDA for iodine is 150 mcg per day for both men and women. Many sources of iodine provide inconsistent amounts. Water may contain some iodine, but the amounts vary. Seafood is a good source, and dairy products and eggs may contain some iodine depending on the feed the animals consumed. Surprisingly, sea salt does not contain iodine; the iodine is lost in processing. The amount of iodine in plant foods depends on the amount in the soil in which the food is grown. Incidental sources of iodine are cleaning products whose residues adhere to cooking and baking equipment and dough conditioners. To ensure the population receives adequate amounts of this nutrient, salt in the United States may be purchased fortified with iodine.

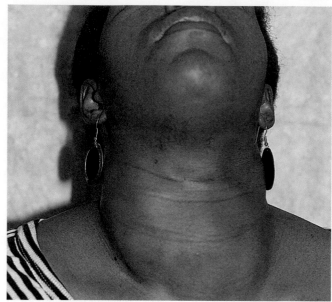

FIG 8-6 Goiter caused by iodine deficiency. (From Swartz MH: *Textbook of physical diagnosis history and examination,* ed 3, Philadelphia, 1998, Saunders.)

Deficiency

Iodine deficiency reduces the amount of thyroxine produced. Symptoms of iodine deficiency then reflect the effects of reduced thyroxine, including sluggishness and weight gain. Severe iodine deficiency during pregnancy causes cretinism of the fetus, resulting in permanent mental and physical retardation.

Goiter, enlargement of the thyroid gland, occurs during extended iodine deficiency (Figure 8-6). The thyroid gland works to compensate for the low iodine levels and expands; the goiter frequently remains even after iodine intake is again sufficient.

The incidence of goiter in certain populations is endemic or regionally defined. In the past, a goiter belt existed in the Midwestern states. Iodine was unavailable in the soil and water of the area because this region is untouched by oceans; oceans provide a natural source of iodine. Since then, fortification of salt with iodine and the wider availability of seafood because of improved refrigeration and transportation systems reduced this deficiency. Goiter, although extremely rare in North America, may still occur in parts of Europe, Africa, and South and Central America. To eliminate iodine deficiency globally, the United Nations Joint Commission on Health Policy recommends universal salt iodization in countries in which iodine deficiency is a public health concern.

Goiter may also be caused by the action of goitrogens. When consumed as a staple component of dietary intake, goitrogens (substances in the root vegetable cassava and in cabbage) suppress the actions of the thyroid gland. Although the thyroid gland swells as in iodine deficiency goiter, the iodine level is not the initiating agent; instead, substances in these vegetables suppress the actions of the thyroid gland. To control these iodine deficiency disorders (IDDs) in areas such as southern Ethiopia, programs are conducted to teach villagers how to prepare cassava using safer methods.

Toxicity

Too much iodine can cause iodine-induced goiter called **thyrotoxicosis**; therefore, the UL is set at 1100 mcg per day.

Fluoride

Function

Fluoride increases resistance to tooth decay and is part of tooth formation. Skeletal health also depends on fluoride for bone mineralization.

Recommended Intake and Sources

The AI for fluoride is 4 mg per day for men and 3 mg for women.

Sources of fluoride vary. The most consistent is fortified water to which fluoride has been added. Tea, seafood, and seaweed are other reliable sources. Unfortunately, these are not regularly consumed, particularly by children during tooth formation years.

An inadvertent source of fluoride is toothpaste. Most toothpaste has fluoride added as a topical agent to strengthen tooth enamel. However, some fluoride is ingested during the rinsing process, providing a kind of dietary source of fluoride. Children can ingest a lethal dose of fluoride if a tube of toothpaste is consumed.

Deficiency

Low levels of fluoride increase the risk of dental caries. Factors such as hygiene, food choices, and possibly genetics also affect plaque and subsequent dental caries.

Toxicity

Too much fluoride causes **fluorosis**. Fluorosis consists of mottling or brown spotting of the tooth enamel; severe fluorosis may also cause pitting of the teeth. A UL of 10 mg per day reduces the risk of toxicity.

Selenium

Function

Selenium is part of an enzyme that acts as an antioxidant. Vitamin E and selenium work together to prevent cell and lipid membrane damage from oxidizing substances. Selenium is also associated with thyroid function. It is found extensively throughout the body.

Recommended Intake and Sources

The RDA for selenium ranges from 55 to 70 mcg per day. Meats, fish, eggs, and whole grains are good sources of selenium. It is a nutrient for which the RDA is easily met.

Deficiency

Deficiency of selenium may predispose individuals to heart disease, particularly Keshan disease. Keshan disease was first noted in China, primarily in children and women of childbearing age. The symptoms of the disease include cardiomyopathy and other features common to selenium deficiency, including muscle pain and tenderness. It is difficult, however, to separate other environmental factors specific to China that may also affect long-term nutritional status. Deficiencies of nutrients other than selenium may have a role in the etiology of Keshan disease. Keshan disease differs from the form of heart disease common in the United States because the myocardium of the heart is affected. In the United States most heart disease is coronary artery disease. Therefore, selenium deficiency is probably not a factor affecting the American incidence of heart disease.

However, low dietary levels of selenium or reduced blood levels of selenium may be associated with an increased risk of cancer among Americans. The relationship of cancer to selenium consumption is probably caused by selenium's antioxidant functions combined with other antioxidants in the body. This relationship continues to be explored.

Toxicity

Selenium can be toxic at levels as low as five times the RDA of 55 mcg per day. The most frequent symptoms of chronic toxicity are hair and nail brittleness and loss. Other effects include severe liver damage, vomiting, and diarrhea. Additional symptoms include metallic aftertaste, respiratory distress with lung edema and bronchopneumonia, and garlic-scented breath and sweat. Chronic toxicity is not likely to occur in the U.S. population, because food consumed from many regional areas. This dilutes consumption of food grown in naturally occurring high selenium areas.[1]

The toxicity of selenium highlights the delicate nature of the body's use of trace minerals. Although selenium is proposed as an antioxidant supplement, the amounts suggested are those of the RDA for selenium. To avoid toxicity, a UL of 400 mcg per day is established.

Copper

Function

Although the body requires minute amounts, copper performs many functions. Some roles of copper include action as (1) a coenzyme involving antioxidant reactions and energy metabolism, (2) a component of wound healing, (3) a constituent of nerve fiber protection, and (4) a required element for iron use.

Recommended Intake and Sources

The RDA for copper is 900 mcg per day for adults. Good sources include organ meats (liver), seafood, green leafy vegetables, legumes, whole grains, dried fruits, and water, if it flows through copper pipes.

Deficiency

Copper deficiency causes bone demineralization and anemia; this form of anemia also can be caused by zinc toxicity

PERSONAL PERSPECTIVES

"Wilson" Joins the Family

I've never heard the whole story, but apparently my sister Natalie begged my parents for a sibling. Nine and a half years later, I came along. To me, Natalie was a mother, sister, and friend all rolled into one. When my sister was 39 years old—a full-time IT manager, wife, and mother—I was 30, a stay-at-home mom with a daughter and a newborn baby boy. Everything seemed perfect, until my sister started feeling tired and came down with a fever.

Everyone assumed she was run-down and tired. This was in September 2005. She was diagnosed with bronchitis. After 2 weeks of antibiotics, her fever had not gone down and she felt worse.

Natalie consulted my husband, Gary, an emergency room (ER) doctor, who ran a battery of tests. In the next few weeks, she met with an infectious disease specialist, as well as her own doctor, all of whom ordered test after test. From bloodwork to CT scans to ultrasounds, all her tests were negative. She did not have mononucleosis or Epstein-Barr virus. Her blood was negative for hepatitis and a host of other diseases. She was told to stop taking her birth control pills and not to take Tylenol or other medications in case she was having a weird reaction to medications.

By mid-October, my sister's stomach swelled like she was 4 months pregnant. Gary suggested she come for another CT scan even though she just had one 2 weeks prior. [*The results were shocking.*] In the space of 2 weeks, my sister's liver started to go into failure. She already reached the point at which she would need a liver transplant!

Natalie was immediately transported from Jersey Shore Medical Center in New Jersey to the Hospital of the University of Pennsylvania, [*Philadelphia, Pennsylvania*], known for its liver transplant teams. Natalie spent 4 days in a general room, waiting for some news as to what was wrong. Her skin was yellow and her stomach grew to enormous proportions. This was a woman who up until 2 months ago was young, vibrant, and beautiful. Now she was deteriorating.

Finally, on the fourth day, an important liver biopsy was performed. The biopsy results came back. Apparently, my sister has *Wilson's* disease. What is Wilson's disease? Why had no one thought of this? What disease changed all of us forever?

Now five years later, my family is well versed on Wilson's disease. This [*genetic*] disease releases excess copper into the liver [*also brain and cornea of the eye*], eventually leading to hepatic failure. But this is not the whole story. The way my sister presented with this disease only affects 5% of Wilson's disease patients. Most have extreme symptoms, such as neurologic disturbances (psychotic episodes, seizures) and other obvious physical ailments. Natalie did not. She did have obsessive-compulsive disorder, difficulty conceiving, and periods of mood swings. At times, her liver functions were elevated, but not too serious. During the battery of tests performed at the beginning of her illness, Natalie's blood was tested for Wilson's disease but was negative. Now we know there is a point when the copper leaves the blood and travels into the liver, becoming undetectable in simple blood tests. A urine test would have showed the excess copper in her body but was never ordered. The signs were there but not obvious enough.

Wilson's disease is a genetic disorder. Natalie has had it her *whole* life, dormant. What set it off at this point is still not known. Because Wilson's is a genetic disorder, I was tested as well.

I collected a urine sample for 24 hours, to be tested for copper level. I also gave blood for a genetic test as well. What would my results show?

The test results were borderline normal. However, to the Wilson's disease specialist we consulted in New York City, the results predicted that my genetic test would be the same as my sister's—detecting the identical genetic defects. Sure enough, he was right. I, too, have this disease. It has been diagnosed so early that the simple treatment is to take zinc pills three times a day for the rest of my life. I can take what is essentially a mineral and be a healthy person. The zinc will counteract the copper. [*The zinc competes with the copper for absorption receptor sites.*] Unfortunately, Wilson's experts are very few, and genetic testing is new and very expensive. There is simply not enough education about this disease.

Little did my parents know that when my sister begged to have a sibling, she would end up saving her sibling's life. If my sister had not gone into hepatic failure, I would have at some point. It was only a matter of time. If more was known about this disease and its abstract symptoms, maybe my sister would have been diagnosed earlier and able to take zinc, just as I am.

Tanya Popovetsky
Marlboro, N.J.

Tanya's sister received a liver transplant within a few days of diagnosis and continues her recovery while on many medications, adjusting to a life much different from the one she knew.

reducing body levels of copper. Copper deficiency does not occur in the United States.

Toxicity

Toxicity occurs from supplementation. Common toxic response consists of vomiting and diarrhea. Wilson's disease, an inherited disorder, results in the excessive accumulation of copper in the liver, brain, and cornea of the eye (see the *Personal Perspectives* box, "Wilson" Joins the Family). Eventually the disorder can lead to cirrhosis, chronic hepatitis, liver failure, and neurologic disorders. Worldwide, the incidence of copper toxicity appears tied to the use of brass and copper pots to prepare and store foods. Nutritional treatment for copper toxicity, whether caused by Wilson's disease or dietary sources, is through dietary restrictions and chelation therapy that initiates excretion of excess copper from the body.[16] In addition, 10,000 mcg per day is the UL for copper.

Chromium

Function

Chromium has a role in carbohydrate metabolism as a constituent of the glucose tolerance factor (GTF) that facilitates the reaction of insulin.

Recommended Intake and Sources

The AI of chromium is 35 mcg per day for men and 25 mcg for women. Found in animal-related foods, eggs, and whole grains, chromium is lost in food processing, particularly when wheat is refined to white flour.

Studies are exploring the effects of chromium supplementation on increasing HDL and decreasing glucose and insulin levels. The findings may have implications for populations who consume refined foods and for those who are exposed to stressors that increase the need for chromium; these may include infections, trauma, and diets high in simple sugars.

Deficiency

Although chromium is lost through food processing, outright deficiencies of chromium are unusual. Inadequate chromium status may be responsible in part for some cases of impaired glucose tolerance, hyperglycemia, hypoglycemia, and unresponsiveness to insulin.

Toxicity

Toxicity has been noted from environmental contaminants in industrial settings rather than from excessive dietary intakes.

Other Trace Minerals

The amount needed of the following trace minerals is so low that it is easy to meet these amounts through ordinary consumption of foods. All are problematic in large doses; supplements are contraindicated.

Manganese is a component of enzymes involved in metabolic reactions. The AI for manganese is 2.3 mg per day for men and 1.8 mg for women. Found in whole grains, green vegetables, legumes, and other foods, manganese deficiency in humans is unknown. A UL of 11 mg for manganese exists.

Molybdenum functions as a coenzyme. The RDA of 45 mcg per day is easily consumed through typical dietary selections. Deficiencies have not been recorded except under medical circumstances in which dietary intakes have been greatly altered. The UL for molybdenum is 2000 mcg per day.

Other trace minerals found in our bodies that may have a role in human health include *silicon, boron, nickel, vanadium, lithium, tin,* and *cadmium.* The amounts required are so small that we naturally consume enough and are never deficient in these nutrients.

Table 8-3 provides a quick reference to the trace minerals.

OVERCOMING BARRIERS

Hypertension

Overcoming barriers to wellness pertaining to individual mineral status has already been addressed in this chapter.

TABLE 8-3   TRACE MINERALS

MINERAL	FUNCTION	CLINICAL ISSUES DEFICIENT/ TOXICITY	RECOMMENDED DAILY INTAKES	FOOD SOURCES	ABSORPTION ISSUES
Iron (Fe)	Distributes oxygen in hemoglobin and myoglobin; growth	Deficiency: microcytic anemia (children and women at risk) Toxicity: hemosiderosis; hemochromatosis	RDA Men: 8 mg Women: 18 mg Pregnancy: 27 mg Lactation: 9 mg UL 45 mg	Heme sources: meat, fish, poultry, egg yolks Nonheme sources: vegetables, legumes, whole grains, enriched grains	Conserved and recycled; absorption 10%-15% of dietary iron consumed
Zinc (Zn)	Cofactor for more than 200 enzymes; carbohydrate metabolism (insulin function)	Deficiency: decreases wound healing; decreases taste and smell; impaired sexual and physical development; immune disorders Toxicity: similar to flu with vomiting/ diarrhea/fever/ exhaustion	RDA Men: 11 mg Women: 8 mg UL 40 mg	Meat, fish, poultry, whole grains, legumes, eggs	Binders may decrease absorption in whole grains

Continued

TABLE 8-3   TRACE MINERALS—cont'd

MINERAL	FUNCTION	CLINICAL ISSUES DEFICIENT/ TOXICITY	RECOMMENDED DAILY INTAKES	FOOD SOURCES	ABSORPTION ISSUES
Iodine (I)	Thyroxine synthesis (thyroid hormone) regulates growth and development; BMR regulation	Deficiency: decreases thyroxine, causing sluggishness and weight gain, goiter, cretinism (if during pregnancy) Toxicity: thyrotoxicosis	RDA Adults: 150 mcg UL 1100 mcg	Iodized salt, seafood	
Fluoride (Fl)	Bone and tooth formation; increases resistance to decay; increases mineralization	Deficiency: increases dental caries Toxicity: fluorosis	AI Men: 4 mg Women: 3 mg UL 10 mg	Fluoridated water, tea, seafood, seaweed	
Selenium (Se)	Antioxidant cofactor with vitamin E; prevents cell and lipid membrane damage	Deficiency: possible Keshan disease/ cancer Toxicity: liver damage, vomiting, diarrhea	RDA Adults: 55 mcg UL 400 mcg	Meat, fish, eggs, whole grains	
Copper (C)	Coenzyme in antioxidant reactions and energy metabolism; wound healing; nerve fiber protection; iron use	Deficiency: bone demineralization and anemia (not in U.S.) Toxicity: Wilson's disease or with supplements producing vomiting/ diarrhea	RDA Adults: 900 mcg UL 10,000 mcg	Organ meats (liver), seafood, green leafy vegetables	
Chromium (Cr)	Carbohydrate metabolism, part of glucose tolerance factor	Deficiency: possible link with cardiovascular disorders; hypoglycemia, hyperglycemia, and unresponsive insulin	AI Men: 35 mcg Women: 25 mcg	Animal food, whole grains	
Manganese (Mn)	Part of metabolic reaction enzymes	Deficiency: unknown	AI Men: 2.3 mg Women: 1.8 mg UL 11 mg	Whole grains, green leafy vegetables, legume	
Molybdenum (Mo)	Coenzyme	Deficiency: unknown	RDA Adults: 45 mcg UL 2000 mcg	Many foods	

AI, Adequate Intake; *BMR,* basal metabolic rate; *CNS,* central nervous system; *FVD,* fluid volume deficit; *RDA,* Recommended Dietary Allowance; *UL,* Tolerable Upper Intake Level.

Hypertension appears to be affected by the actions of several minerals and therefore is explored here.

Continuing research appears to suggest that adequate levels of calcium and magnesium have roles in the maintenance of appropriate blood pressure levels. Population studies point to lower intakes of these nutrients among individuals who are hypertensive. Marginal intake of these nutrients, combined with other lifestyle factors such as lack of exercise, excessive weight, cigarette smoking, and sodium sensitivity, sets the stage for hypertension to occur. Sodium sensitivity reflects the need to avoid excesses even if marginally higher intakes than recommended are consumed safely by most of the population.

Consumption levels of calcium, magnesium, and sodium are based on recommendations to consume foods as whole as possible. It is through processing that minerals are lost and sodium levels in foods escalate.

Reclassification of blood pressure levels supports the value of long-term lifestyle changes to reduce blood pressure among individuals with hypertension. The Seventh Report of

BOX 8-10 BLOOD PRESSURE CLASSIFICATION

CATEGORY	SYSTOLIC BLOOD PRESSURE (mm Hg)		DIASTOLIC BLOOD PRESSURE (mm Hg)
Normal	<120	and	<80
Prehypertension	120-139	or	80-89
Hypertension, stage 1	140-159	or	90-99
Hypertension, stage 2	160	or	100

From the National High Blood Pressure Education Program, National Heart, Lung, and Blood Institute, National Institutes of Health: *Reference card from the Seventh Report of the Joint National Committee on Prevention, Detection, Evaluation, and Treatment of High Blood Pressure (JNC7)*, NIH Publication No. 03-5231, Bethesda, Md, 2003 (May; reprinted January 2005), U.S. Department of Health and Human Services.

the Joint National Committee on Prevention, Detection, Evaluation, and Treatment of High Blood Pressure created guidelines as listed in Box 8-10. A category of "prehypertension" has been created. It is not a disease category but an identification of high risk for developing hypertension. This is to alert individuals and health care providers to implement lifestyle modifications such as increased exercise and dietary changes, rather than drug therapy, to decrease the risk of developing hypertension and its related disorders.[17]

The Dietary Approaches to Stop Hypertension (DASH) is a complete eating plan proven to reduce blood pressure. Consisting of dietary selections of whole foods lower in fat and higher in fruits, vegetables, and low-fat dairy foods without salt control, DASH may reduce blood pressure levels ranging from normal to slightly elevated. Additional analysis has continued to affirm the value of the DASH program as an effective foundation for the reduction and prevention of hypertension.[17]

TOWARD A POSITIVE NUTRITION LIFESTYLE: PROJECTING

Projection is placing responsibility for our own unacceptable feelings or behaviors on others. In relation to health, we may attribute our poor eating patterns to hectic schedules and possibly to roommates or family members who don't want to shop for food or prepare meals. We project our unacceptable behaviors on others, rather than take responsibility for our own health.

One mineral for which projection sometimes occurs is iron. Because iron deficiency is often manifested with tiredness, paleness, and frequent infections, it is frequently self-diagnosed as the pathologic cause of poor health. Accurate diagnosis of iron deficiency is based on blood analysis, not on self-reporting. As an aspect of client education, we can help clients clarify the actual cause of their symptoms if they are not clinically iron deficient. Often these symptoms are caused by poor health habits: not enough sleep, irregular meals, and too little exercise. Rather than projecting ill health on the mineral iron, clients can take responsibility and modify their own health behaviors.

SUMMARY

In this chapter, water and minerals are explored through their nutritional requirements and physiologic roles for achieving nutritional wellness. Although water and minerals are primary components of body fluids, each performs other functions as well.

Water supports a variety of functions, including acting as a structural component of the body, a temperature regulator, a lubricant, a fluid cushion, a transportation vehicle, a trace mineral source, and a medium for and participant in biochemical reactions. Sources may include beverages and foods with high water content, although the best source is water in its pure form.

Minerals also fill diverse roles. Structurally, minerals provide rigidity and strength to the teeth and skeleton; the skeletal mineral components also serve as a storage depot for other needs of the body. Minerals allowing for proper muscle contraction and release influence nerve function. Minerals also assist enzymes, maintain proper acid-base balance of body fluids, and are required for blood clotting and wound healing.

The 16 essential minerals are divided into two categories: major and trace minerals. Major minerals, needed daily in amounts of 100 mg or higher, include calcium, phosphorus, magnesium, sulfur, and the electrolytes of sodium, potassium, and chloride. Trace minerals, required daily in amounts less than or equal to 20 mg, include iron, zinc, iodine, fluoride, selenium, copper, chromium, manganese, and molybdenum.

Prime food sources of minerals include both plants and animals. Valuable plant sources include most fruits, vegetables, legumes, and whole grains. Animal sources consist of beef, chicken, eggs, fish, and milk products. Although minerals are stable when cooked, the bioavailability of some minerals may be limited, depending on the source. Some plant minerals are not easily available to the human body because of binders inhibiting absorption. Generally, minerals from animal foods are able to be absorbed more easily than those from plants. Whatever the specific food source, dietary patterns consisting primarily of whole foods provide an adequate supply of minerals.

THE NURSING APPROACH
Case Study: Deficient Fluid Volume

Ben, an 8-month-old infant, developed a rectal temperature of 101.2° F. His mother suspected he had a viral infection and brought him to the emergency department, worried he might be getting dehydrated.

It was November, and the nurse suspected Ben had rotavirus. After interviewing the infant's mother, the nurse did a physical examination, and Ben was admitted to the rapid treatment unit. The physician ordered lab tests, including a stool culture, white blood count, hematocrit, and electrolytes. Prescriptions were written for acetaminophen per rectum every 6 hours, Pedialyte by mouth as tolerated, and lactated Ringer's intravenously.

ASSESSMENT
Subjective (from mother's statements)

- For 24 hours Ben vomited whenever his mother attempted to give him a bottle of formula.
- Ben had been crying and seemed weak.
- Ben had several loose brown stools in his diaper and probably urinated less than usual.
- One of his brothers also has had diarrhea and vomiting.

Objective (from physical examination)

- Dry skin and oral mucous membranes
- Sunken fontanelle
- Skin flushed and warm
- Temperature of 101.2° F (rectal)
- Rapid pulse and respirations
- Abdomen soft
- Bowel sounds hyperactive
- Urine concentrated

DIAGNOSES (NURSING)

- Deficient fluid volume related to diarrhea and vomiting as evidenced by report of mother, dry mucous membranes, sunken fontanelle, and concentrated urine
- Hyperthermia related to infection and dehydration as evidenced by temperature 101.2° F, skin flushed and warm

PLANNING
Patient Outcomes

Short term (within 24 hours):
1. No further fluid loss, and fluid balance restored
2. Temperature of 100° F or less

Nursing Interventions

1. Carry out physician's orders.
2. Monitor health status hourly.

IMPLEMENTATION

1. Sent a stool specimen from the diaper to the lab.
   A stool culture can lead to identification of microorganisms, a correct diagnosis, and appropriate treatment.

2. Gave acetaminophen per rectum as ordered.
   Acetaminophen (Tylenol) can lower the temperature. Aspirin is not given to children because of its association with Reye's syndrome (an uncommon but potentially lethal complication).
3. Offered sips of Pedialyte in a baby bottle every hour.
   Pedialyte, containing glucose, water, and electrolytes, helps replace fluids and electrolytes lost through diarrhea and vomiting. Clear liquids minimize peristalsis and are better tolerated than formula when diarrhea and vomiting are present.
4. Administered intravenous fluids (IV), regulated by an IV pump.
   Intravenous fluids can immediately replace lost fluids. Rate must be carefully controlled to prevent fluid overload.
5. Checked vital signs hourly.
   Monitoring vital signs frequently aids early detection of complications and evaluation of health status.
6. Recorded intake and output and monitored for signs of dehydration.
   Once stabilized, intake (IVs and fluids by mouth) should be approximately equal to output (vomitus, diarrhea, urine). Diapers are weighed to determine amounts of urine.
7. Monitored lab reports.
   White blood count is commonly elevated by infections. Increased hematocrit can indicate a loss of fluids. Electrolytes are diminished by vomiting and diarrhea.

EVALUATION

Short term (within 24 hours):
1. A stool was sent to the lab. Ben drank two ounces of Pedialyte, but then vomited. An IV was administered, and urination increased. Oral mucous membranes were moist, and fontanelle was flat.
   - Goal partially met. Plan: Continue to offer Pedialyte hourly. Continue IVs until Ben is taking fluids well by mouth.
2. Temperature dropped to 100.8° F after acetaminophen was given. Pulse rate and respirations decreased.
   - Goal partially met.

DISCUSSION QUESTIONS

1. Why is it important to keep Ben hydrated?
2. How does Pedialyte help balance electrolytes as well as fluids? At what temperature should it be given?
3. What drinks and/or foods would be best for decreasing diarrhea in Ben's older brother?

❓ APPLYING CONTENT KNOWLEDGE

The camp nurse gives a talk to the camp staff about the signs of fluid volume deficit. She encourages the counselors to be sure the campers drink fluids throughout the day. One counselor responds, "Oh, that's no problem. The kids guzzle flavored iced tea all day long." How should she respond?

WEBSITES OF INTEREST

American Hemochromatosis Society (AHS)

www.americanhs.org

Supplies information about hereditary hemochromatosis such as genetic testing, diagnosis, and research.

Dietary Approaches to Stop Hypertension (DASH)

www.nhlbi.nih.gov/hbp/prevent/h_eating/h_eating.htm

Presents a comprehensive guide to implementing DASH dietary plans.

National Osteoporosis Foundation (NOF)

www.nof.org

Offers resources on causes, prevention, detection, and treatment of osteoporosis.

REFERENCES

1. Institute of Medicine, Food and Nutrition Board: *Dietary DRI References: The essential guide to nutrient requirements*, Washington, DC, 2006, The National Academies Press.

2. Beverage Marketing Corporation: *Bottled water perseveres in a difficult year, new data from BMC show*, New York, 2009, Beverage Marketing Corporation. Accessed February 12, 2010, at www.beveragemarketing.com.

3. Mans OH, Uribarri J: Electrolyte, water, and acid-base balance. In Shils ME, et al, editors: *Modern nutrition in health and disease*, ed 10, Philadelphia, 2006, Lippincott Williams & Wilkins.

4. Position paper of the American Dietetic Association, Dietitians of Canada, and the American College of Sports Medicine: Nutrition and athletic performance, *J Am Diet Assoc* 109:509-527, 2009.

5. Mazda J, et al: Vitamin D receptor and calcium sensing receptor polymorphisms and the risk of colorectal cancer in European populations, *Cancer Epidemiol Biomarkers Prev* 18(9):2485-2491, 2009.

6. Weaver CM, Heaney RP: Calcium. In Shils ME, et al, editors: *Modern nutrition in health and disease*, ed 10, Philadelphia, 2006, Lippincott Williams & Wilkins.

7. NIH Consensus Development Panel on Osteoporosis Prevention, Diagnosis, and Therapy: Osteoporosis prevention, diagnosis, and therapy, *JAMA* 285(6):785-795, 2001.

8. Jacobs-Kosmin D, et al: Osteoporosis (updated September 30, 2009), eMedicine/WebMD. Accessed February 12, 2009, from www.emedicine.medscape.com/article/330598-overview.

9. Rodino MA, Shane E: Osteoporosis after organ transplantation, *Am J Med* 104(5):459-469, 1998.

10. Barrett-Connor E, et al: Coffee-associated osteoporosis onset by daily milk consumption: The Rancho Bernardo Study, *J Am Med Assoc* 271(4):280-283, 1994.

11. Delaney MF: Strategies for the prevention and treatment of osteoporosis during early postmenopause, *Am J Obstet Gynecol* 194(2 Suppl):S12-S23, 2006.

12. Gass M, et al: Preventing osteoporosis-related fractures: an overview, *Am J Med* 119(4 Suppl 1):S3-S11, 2006.

13. Korpelainen R, et al: Lifestyle factors are associated with osteoporosis in lean women but not in normal and overweight women: A population-based cohort study of 1222 women, *Osteoporos Int* 14(1):34-43, 2003.

14. Kushner RF, Shanta RV: Emergence of pica (ingestion of non-food substances) accompanying iron deficiency anemia after gastric bypass surgery, *Obes Surg* 15(10):1491-1495, 2005.

15. Needs S, George DK: Haemachromatosis: Testing and management, *Gastrointest Nurs* 4(1):27-31, 2006.

16. Turnland JR: Copper. In Shils ME, et al, editors: *Modern nutrition in health and disease*, ed 10, Philadelphia, 2006, Lippincott Williams & Wilkins.

17. National Institutes of Health, National Heart, Lung, and Blood Institute: *Seventh report of the Joint National Committee on Prevention, Detection, Evaluation, and Treatment of High Blood Pressure (JNC7)*, NIH Publication No. 04-5230, Bethesda, Md, 2004 (August), Author.

PART 3

Health Promotion Through Nutrition and Nursing Practice

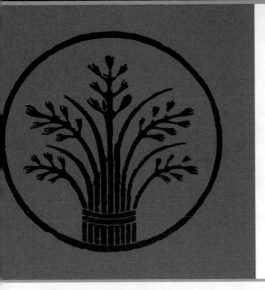

Energy Supply and Fitness

The abilities to perform work, produce change, and maintain life all require energy.

evolve WEBSITE

http://evolve.elsevier.com/Grodner/foundations/

 Nutrition Concepts Online

ROLE IN WELLNESS

Consideration of the physical, intellectual, emotional, social, and spiritual dimensions of health guides our understanding of the value of energy supply and fitness. To achieve optimal *physical health* and fitness, dietary intake and regular physical activity are essential. Exercise affects all muscles; even the muscles of our gastrointestinal tract function better when we regularly exercise. To strengthen our *intellectual health* dimension, the old saying "A sound body makes for a sound mind" still holds true.

By being physically fit, we may be able to devote our full intellectual capacity to our work. The *emotional health* dimension may be supported by fitness because for some people, depression seems to lift if they regularly engage in sustained aerobic activities. Even if we are not depressed, our general state of mind improves with daily physical exercise. Group sports provide an excellent opportunity for social activity while pursuing healthful goals that enhance *social health*. A sense of belonging and sharing occurs whether the group is a formal organization, such as a running club, or consists of friends who bike together. Respecting and caring for our bodies by engaging in regular physical activity reflects the understanding of the unique nature of the human body, which reflects *spiritual health* (see the *Personal Perspectives* box, Detecting a Deficiency).

Physical activity has always been recognized as a component of health. Within the past decade this importance has increased because an inverse relationship between level of fitness and risk of development of chronic degenerative disorders is becoming better understood. This means that the less physical activity a person experiences, the greater the risk of developing disorders such as diabetes, coronary artery disease (CAD), cancer, and hypertension. This chapter addresses the health benefits of exercise as complementing optimum nutrition to decrease risk factors and as improving quality of life. In the nursing profession, we may also work with athletes of all ages who will benefit from our knowledge of their physical requirements. Consequently, this chapter discusses specific nutrient issues that affect the *athlete*, defined as "a person who is trained or skilled in exercises, sports, or games requiring physical strength, agility, or stamina."[1] Finally, as nurses we have a responsibility to maintain our own fitness levels as role models for our clients and for our own benefits to function comfortably in our sometimes physically demanding profession.

ENERGY

The abilities to perform work, produce change, and maintain life all require energy. Energy exists in many forms, such as mechanical, chemical, heat, electrical, light, and nuclear energies. The laws of thermodynamics tell us that each type of energy can be converted from one form to another. As our bodies function, chemical energy from food is converted to mechanical energy and heat.

The ultimate source of energy is the sun. Sunlight is used by plants to produce chemical energy in the form of carbohydrates, proteins, or fats. These foods possess stored energy. People are not capable of doing this. We must convert the chemical energy from the foods we eat into forms usable by the human body.

The energy released from food is measured in kcal (thousands of calories), or Calories. Technically, a calorie is the amount of heat necessary to raise the temperature of a gram of water by 1° C (0.8° F). As first noted in Chapter 1, to ensure accuracy, the term *kilocalories* is used throughout this text, abbreviated as *kcal*.

Two methods are used to determine the energy a food contains. One is through the use of a bomb calorimeter

PERSONAL PERSPECTIVES

Detecting a Deficiency

George Sheehan, MD, was as comfortable writing articles as medical editor for *Runner's World* magazine as he was practicing medicine. His running habit began at age 45, "a decisive age, an age for change." He was responsible for inspiring many to find the athlete within themselves to achieve their own personal best. His message was that physical excellence leads to achievements in other arenas of life. Here is an excerpt from his book *Personal Best*.

Are you feeling run-down, sluggish, low in energy? Is simply getting to school or work becoming too much for you? Are you exhausted by three o'clock in the afternoon? Do you feel depressed? Have you lost your initiative?

If you answer yes, you may be suffering from a lifestyle disease that, surveys tell us, affects about one-half of all Americans. It is called exercise deficiency, it is undoubtedly a leading cause of ill health, and no household is exempt.

Exercise deficiency—the sweat deficit—is a self-inflicted disease. It is an old and familiar story: Our greatest tendency is to cheat on ourselves. We think we can enjoy the fullness of life without paying for it. But that is not the way the world works—or the human machine, either: Nothing is free.

Full-blown exercise deficiency states are evident to the most inexperienced observer—sufferers are manifestly out of shape. These extreme cases usually fatigue easily and early and spend most of the day in physical and mental torpor. They are much too tired when they get home at night to even consider taking any physical exercise. For them, repose is the natural state, and any activity is an effort.

Many people with exercise deficiency are unaware that they have it. They expect no more from their bodies than they are getting. They believe their lack of energy and enthusiasm goes with age. They think they are normal. The reality: They are average, because it's average to slow down, average to become less productive, average to have less energy—and since that's exactly what happens to most of us, we confuse the two. But average is not normal. Normal is the best you can be.

The notion that loss of physical vigor is inevitable usually comes in the mid-thirties. At the FBI Academy, where recruits are placed in a fitness program to get them back in condition, one aspirant complained to the director, "I'm 35; I'm too old for this stuff."

But we are never too old to be fit, and never too young to start preserving fitness. We need to be physically fit whether we are 20 or 35 or even 70. Being unfit at any age is settling for less than your best and is a classic example of the sort of thinking that is behind the widespread incidence of exercise deficiency.

Fortunately, the movement toward fitness is equally widespread. Half the people in this country now realize the need for physical exercise. They know there is no need to lose the gleam in their eye, the bloom in their cheek, the lift in their walk, and the life in their day.

And all it takes is sweat.

From Sheehan G: *Personal best: The foremost philosopher of fitness shares techniques and tactics for success and self-liberation,* Emmaus, Pa, 1989, Rodale Press.

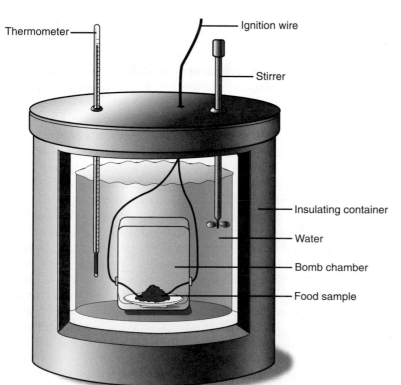

FIG 9-1 Cross section of a bomb calorimeter. To determine energy, a dried portion of food is burned inside a chamber charged with oxygen that is surrounded by water. As the food is burned, it gives off heat. This raises the temperature of the water surrounding the chamber. The increase in water temperature indicates the number of kcal contained in the food. One kcal equals the amount of heat needed to raise the temperature of 1 kilogram of water by 1° C (0.8° F).

(Figure 9-1). This instrument is designed to burn a food while measuring the amount of heat or energy released. This provides an estimate of the energy available to humans. Because the bomb calorimeter method is more efficient than the human body, the kcal value assigned to a food item is adjusted to reflect the limitations of the human system. Amounts listed in food tables reflect this adjustment.

The other method of assessing food energy is proximate composition, which determines the grams of carbohydrates, proteins, and fats of a food item. The grams are then multiplied by the energy value of each (carbohydrates 4 kcal/g; proteins 4 kcal/g; fats 9 kcal/g). The sum of these calculations equals the total energy content of a specific food.

Energy Pathways

The processes of digestion, absorption, and metabolism for each of the three energy-supplying nutrients—carbohydrates, fats, and proteins—have been presented in previous chapters. (Alcohol also provides energy but is not considered a nutrient category.) Carbohydrate digests to glucose, triglycerides (fats) to fatty acids and glycerol, and protein to amino acids. Here we continue to follow their journey as they are used for energy in individual cells.

The nutrients release energy when they are catabolized (broken down), forming carbon dioxide and water. The released energy becomes caught within adenosine triphosphate (ATP), the fuel for all energy-requiring processes in the body (Figure 9-2).

Carbohydrate as a Source of Energy

Glucose releases energy and is converted to carbon dioxide and water through three processes: glycolysis, tricarboxylic acid (TCA) cycle, and oxidative phosphorylation. These complicated processes are reviewed in general here; the intricate details are beyond the scope of this text.

Through glycolysis, which results in the conversion of glucose to carbon compounds, a glucose molecule produces pyruvic acid and ATP. Part of this process depends on niacin and other B-complex vitamins. Oxygen is not needed for glycolysis to occur because it is an anaerobic pathway. The anaerobic pathway provides energy for sprint or speed-type exercise such as soccer, basketball, and football. We also depend on this energy source to run for the train, chase after toddlers, or bound across the room to answer the phone. This type of exertion is limited because oxygen is not available quickly enough to continue its support. Instead, the incomplete use of glucose causes the pyruvic acid to be converted to lactic acid. As lactic acid builds up, the muscles become sore and stiff. Consequently, the exertion ceases because of pain. Within a few minutes, enough oxygen is available to break down the lactic aid, relieving the physical discomfort. The effect is called oxygen debt.

Anaerobic glycolysis takes place in the cell cytoplasm, but oxygen-dependent aerobic glycolysis (the aerobic pathway) occurs in the mitochondria of the cell. In the mitochondria, pyruvic acid (made without oxygen) reacts with coenzyme A (CoA) creating acetyl CoA. The energy process continues as acetyl CoA reaches the TCA cycle. The reactions that are part of that cycle lead to the formation of additional ATP and carbon dioxide. The aerobic pathway is the primary energy source for exercise that is low enough in intensity to be carried on for at least 5 minutes or longer. This includes endurance-type exercise (e.g., swimming, bicycling, running), as well as walking and most of our daily activities.

The last process of glucose conversion to energy is oxidative phosphorylation. A number of actions lead to the release of hydrogens in the forms of water and additional energy that is captured in ATP. The term oxidative reflects the combination of hydrogen with oxygen to form water; phosphorylation is the creation of the phosphate bond to form ATP.

Fat as a Source of Energy

The first step in the use of fat for energy is the hydrolysis into glycerol and three fatty acids. Glycerol is changed into pyruvic acid and is used for energy. The fatty acids undergo a process known as beta-oxidation, which involves the breakdown of the fatty acids into acetyl CoA molecules that enter the TCA cycle and proceed like the acetyl CoA from carbohydrate (glucose).

Protein as a Source of Energy

Amino acids are first catabolized through deamination, as described in Chapter 6. Whereas the liver and kidneys process the nitrogen-containing amino acid groups, the other amino acid components enter the energy metabolism pathway, with each component entering at a different location. Some of the amino acid components are converted to pyruvic acid; others become intermediaries of the TCA cycle or part of the acetyl groups. If sufficient energy is available, amino acids are used for protein synthesis rather than for energy.

It is important to note that just as all three nutrients (carbohydrate, protein, and fat) can be used for energy when consumed in excess, they can also be stored as fat in the body. Likewise, when too little energy is consumed, these processes reverse. Energy that is consumed is used immediately, regardless of its source. The first stored energy used is glycogen, followed by the energy reserve of body fat in adipose cells. Glucose must be available to the brain. Only a small portion of triglycerides (glycerol) can yield glucose, and continuous use of this source results in a buildup of ketones and the potential imbalance of the body pH (see Chapter 6). The body prefers to spare protein for its more important function: building and repairing cells and tissues.

Anaerobic and Aerobic Pathways

How do anaerobic and aerobic energy pathways work together to supply energy? For the first minute or two of exertion, oxygen has not arrived at the muscles, and therefore energy must come from anaerobic sources. After several minutes the aerobic pathway takes over. However, as the exertion or exercise continues, there is a constant interchange or use of energy sources.

The energy source that muscles use during exercise depends on the intensity and length of exercise, the person's fitness level, and the foods eaten. Short-term, high-intensity activities such as sprinting rely mostly on the anaerobic

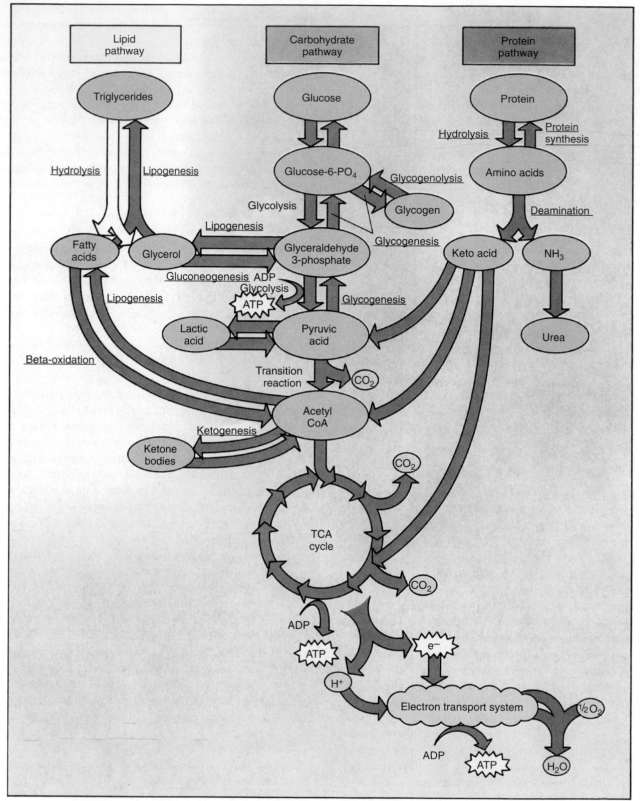

FIG 9-2 Summary of key steps in the metabolism of glucose, fatty acids, glycerol, and amino acids. *ADP*, Adenosine diphosphate; *ATP*, adenosine triphosphate; *TCA*, tricarboxylic acid cycle. (From Thibodeau GA, Patton KT: *Anatomy and physiology*, ed 4, St Louis, 1999, Mosby.)

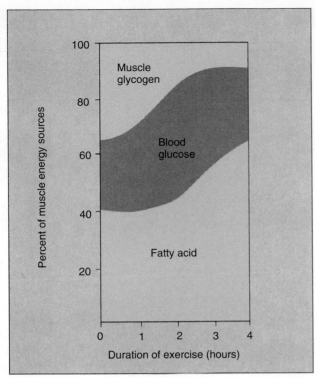

FIG 9-3 Relative use made of energy sources in the body as exercise continues. (From Guthrie HA, Picciano MF: *Human nutrition,* New York, 1995, McGraw-Hill, with permission from Helen A. Guthrie.)

pathway for energy, and only carbohydrates (primarily from muscle glycogen) can be used. On the other hand, exercise of low to moderate intensity is supported primarily by the aerobic system, and both carbohydrate and fats are used. Fats are an important energy source during exercise because, unlike carbohydrates, fatty acids are abundant in the body and their use spares muscle glycogen.

The length of activity also determines what type of fuel the muscles will use during exercise. As the duration of exercise increases, glycogen stores become depleted and fat becomes the primary source of energy (Figure 9-3). A sedentary person breaks down glycogen faster and as a result accumulates more lactic acid in the tissues. The lactic acid causes muscle fatigue. A physically fit person has a higher aerobic capacity (the ability of the heart to supply oxygen) so that oxygen is available sooner and in greater quantity; this allows use of the aerobic pathway of energy, avoiding lactic acid buildup. This also means that more fat than glycogen can be used for fuel.

If we eat a diet high in carbohydrates, more glycogen can be stored as energy. The amount of carbohydrate stored in the body depends on how much carbohydrate we consume and our level of fitness. Endurance training increases the capacity of the muscles to store glycogen, but there is still a limit to the total amount of energy that can be stored. The more glycogen that we store, the more energy we have available for all kinds of activities, not just for marathons.

ENERGY BALANCE

To maintain a healthy weight, our energy intake should equal energy expended. Because of our sedentary lifestyles, some of us may need less energy than standard energy requirement charts recommend. In contrast, the serious competitive athlete's energy intake must support a training and competition schedule that allows the athlete to achieve his or her personal best.

Individuals who are acutely ill and hospitalized or adapting to chronic disorders may require energy intake levels specifically calculated to meet their changing physiologic needs. Consultation with a registered dietitian may be warranted for patients, their family members, and other caregivers. Misconceptions about energy needs can be eliminated by nutrition counseling regardless of the nature of the health disorder.

Estimating Daily Energy Needs

The recommended energy allowances published by the National Research Council appear in Table 9-1. These energy values are based on individuals with a light to moderate activity level. The average daily energy intake for the referenced 19- to 24-year-old man is 2900 kcal, or 40 kcal/kg. It is 2200 kcal or 38 kcal/kg for the same age-referenced woman. If a person is more active or of a larger or smaller body size, further adjustments must be made. Most important, these levels are simply guidelines; the only accurate recommendation for individuals is one that supports healthy weight levels.

Many different formulas have been developed to estimate energy expenditure, some of which are complicated. An easy way to determine kcal need is to multiply weight by one of the numbers in Table 9-2. For example, a 77-kg (170-pound) man who participates in moderate exercise needs about 3060 kcal a day. Remember that these numbers represent averages. Some people need fewer kcal; others need more.

Components of Total Energy Expenditure

Our daily energy requirement depends on many variables, including basal metabolism, physical activity, and the thermic effect of food. **Basal metabolism** represents the amount of energy required to maintain life-sustaining activities (e.g., breathing, circulation, heartbeat, secretion of hormones) for a specific period. Basal metabolic rate (BMR) is the rate at which the body spends energy to keep all these life-sustaining processes going. BMR is measured in the morning on awakening, before any physical activity, and again at 12 to 18 hours after the last meal. Two methods are used. One consists of human subjects being placed in a chamber; the body heat given off changes the temperature of the chamber, reflecting the energy used by their bodies for the most basic functions. The second method, *indirect calorimetry,* uses a calorimeter. The calorimeter measures the respiratory quotient or exchanges of gases as a person breathes into the mouthpiece of the machine. This determines the amount of oxygen used and carbon dioxide (CO_2) expired.

| TABLE 9-1 | MEDIAN HEIGHTS AND WEIGHTS AND RECOMMENDED ENERGY INTAKE | | | | | | | | |

CATEGORY	AGE (YEARS) OR CONDITION	WEIGHT (kg)	WEIGHT (lb)	HEIGHT (cm)	HEIGHT (in)	REE* (kcal/day)	AVERAGE ENERGY ALLOWANCE (kcal)[†] MULTIPLES OF REE	AVERAGE ENERGY ALLOWANCE (kcal)[†] PER kg	AVERAGE ENERGY ALLOWANCE (kcal)[†] PER DAY[‡]
Infants	0-0.5	6	13	60	24	320		108	650
	0.5-1	9	20	71	28	500		98	850
Children	1-3	13	29	90	35	740		102	1300
	4-6	20	44	112	44	950		90	1800
	7-10	28	62	132	52	1130		70	2000
Men	11-14	45	99	157	62	1440	1.70	55	2500
	15-18	66	145	176	69	1760	1.67	45	3000
	19-24	72	160	177	70	1780	1.67	40	2900
	25-50	79	174	176	70	1800	1.60	37	2900
	51+	77	170	173	68	1530	1.50	30	2300
Women	11-14	46	101	157	62	1310	1.67	47	2200
	15-18	55	120	163	64	1370	1.60	40	2200
	19-24	58	128	164	65	1350	1.60	38	2200
	25-50	63	138	163	64	1380	1.55	36	2200
	51+	65	143	160	63	1280	1.50	30	1900
Pregnant	1st trimester								+0
	2nd trimester								+300
	3rd trimester								+300
Lactating	1st 6 months								+500
	2nd 6 months								+500

From National Academies of Sciences, Food and Nutrition Board, National Research Council: *Recommended dietary allowances*, ed 10, Washington, DC, 1989, National Academies Press.

*REE, Resting energy expenditure; calculation based on Food and Agriculture Organizations (FAO) equations, then rounded.
[†]In the range of light to moderate activity, the coefficient of variation is ± 20%.
[‡]Figure is rounded.

Several factors affect BMR, including age, body size, sex, body temperature, fasting/starvation, stress, menstruation, and thyroid function. BMR varies with the amount of lean tissue in the body; higher levels of lean body mass increase BMR. For example, men have higher BMRs than women because of larger body size and more lean body tissue. The BMR of adults slowly lowers after age 35 because of decreases in lean body tissue associated with aging. As a physically fit person ages, the BMR may not slow down as much as that of a person who is physically unfit. The process of sustaining fitness maintains the muscle mass of lean body tissue and slows the loss caused by aging. It is never too late to develop fitness; with the approval of a primary health care provider, exercise is appropriate at any age.

BMR also depends on thyroid function. The thyroid hormone *thyroxine* is a key BMR regulator; the more thyroxine produced in the body, the higher the BMR. Of course, production of too much thyroxine is not desirable either.

Many scientists, however, prefer to use a more practical measurement called *resting energy expenditure (REE)*. REE is the energy a person expends in a normal life situation while at rest, and it includes some energy the body uses following meals and exercise. It accounts for approximately 60% to 75% of our total energy needs, similar percentages to those of BMR (Figure 9-4).

Physical Activity

The second largest component of energy expenditure after REE (or BMR) is physical activity. **Physical activity** is any body movement produced by skeletal muscles that results in energy expenditure. It demands about 20% to 30% of our total energy needs. Of all the components, it varies the most among people. The amount of energy we expend depends on the intensity and duration of the activity. Walking requires more energy than sitting, and walking for 60 minutes uses more energy than walking for 15 minutes. Thus even a moderate activity can become one of high energy if it is carried on for a long time.

Body size affects energy expenditure more than any other single factor. A heavier person uses more energy to perform a given task than does a lighter person. Table 9-3 shows the number of kcal burned per hour for two individuals, one weighing 205 pounds and the other 125 pounds, as they engage in various activities.

Thermic Effect of Food

The third component of energy output is the energy required for our body to digest, absorb, metabolize, and store food. When we eat, the body's cells increase their activities. This increase in cellular activity is called the **thermic effect of food (TEF)**, or **diet-induced thermogenesis**. The thermic effect is

TABLE 9-2	FACTORS FOR ESTIMATING DAILY ENERGY ALLOWANCES AT VARIOUS LEVELS OF PHYSICAL ACTIVITY FOR MEN AND WOMEN (AGES 19 TO 50)	
LEVEL OF ACTIVITY	**ACTIVITY FACTOR*** (× REE)	**ENERGY EXPENDITURE†** (kcal/kg per day)
Very light		
Men	1.3	31
Women	1.3	30
Light		
Men	1.6	38
Women	1.5	35
Moderate		
Men	1.7	41
Women	1.6	37
Heavy		
Men	2.1	50
Women	1.9	44
Exceptional		
Men	2.4	58
Women	2.2	51

*Based on examples presented by World Health Organization (1985).
†Resting energy expenditure (REE) is the average of values for median weights of people ages 19 to 24 and 25 to 74 years: men, 24 kcal/kg; women, 23.2 kcal/kg.

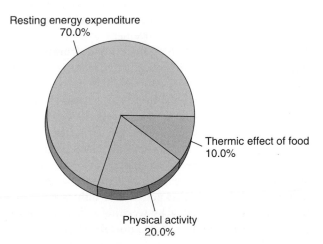

FIG 9-4 Breakdown of human energy expenditure. (From Rolin Graphics.)

Resting energy expenditure 70.0%
Thermic effect of food 10.0%
Physical activity 20.0%

relatively small, accounting for approximately 7% to 10% of a person's total energy needs.

Adaptive Thermogenesis

Adaptive thermogenesis is the energy used by our bodies to adjust to changing physical and biologic environmental

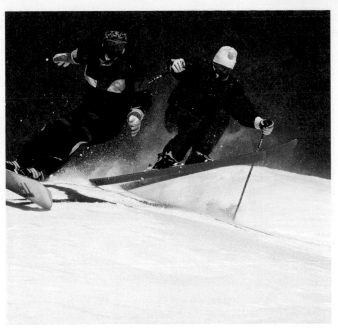

Physical fitness consists of flexibility, muscular strength and endurance, and cardiovascular endurance. (Photos. com.)

situations. This includes energy used to adapt to coldness, extreme changes in kcal intake (of several days' duration), and physical and emotional trauma. This category of energy need incorporates additional demands caused by illness and the process of recovery. Because the expenditure depends on individualized variables, it is not calculated into average energy requirements.

FITNESS

Major advances in technology have made the lives of our clients and our own more comfortable and simple. We drive instead of walk, take the elevator instead of the stairs, and ride the lawn mower instead of pushing it. The amount of physical activity at work and in the home has declined steadily. How important is physical activity to health, fitness, and total well-being? Let's take a closer look.

Physical activity is defined as any body movement produced by skeletal muscles that requires energy expenditure. It varies by day, time of year, and stage of life. Physical activity is similar to yet different from physical fitness. Physical activity describes the actions or movements that we make, whereas physical fitness describes the limits on the actions that we are capable of making.

Being physically fit is more than just being fast or strong. True physical fitness consists of three major components: flexibility, muscular strength and endurance, and cardiovascular endurance. **Flexibility** is the ability to move the muscles to their full extent without injury. **Muscular strength and endurance** describes the ability of the muscles to perform hard or prolonged work. **Cardiovascular endurance** is the ability of the body to take in, deliver, and use oxygen for physical work. Although flexibility and muscular strength

TABLE 9-3	**APPROXIMATE CALORIES USED PER HOUR**	
125-lb PERSON	**ACTIVITY**	**205-lb PERSON**
234	Baseball—infield or outfield	382
299	—pitching	488
352	Basketball—moderate	575
495	—vigorous	807
251	Bicycling—on level ground, 5.5 mph	409
537	13 mph	877
209	Dancing—moderate	341
284	—vigorous	464
416	Football	678
271	Golf—twosome	443
165	Horseback riding—walk	270
338	—trot	551
503	Mountain climbing	820
251	Rowing—pleasure	409
684	—rowing machine or sculling 20 strokes/min	1116
537	Running—5.5 mph	887
669	—7 mph	1141
777	—9 mph level	1269
285	Skating—moderate	465
513	—vigorous	837
483	Skiing—downhill	789
586	—level, 5 mph	956
447	Soccer	730
194	Swimming—backstroke—20 yd/min	316
418	—40 yd/min	682
241	—breaststroke—20 yd/min	392
482	—40 yd/min	786
586	—butterfly	956
241	—crawl—20 yd/min	392
532	—50 yd/min	869
347	Tennis—moderate	565
488	—vigorous	797
285	Volleyball—moderate	565
488	—vigorous	797
176	Walking—2 mph	286
331	—4.5 mph	540
643	Wrestling, judo, or karate	1049

and endurance are important components of health and well-being, cardiovascular endurance is the best physiologic index of total body endurance. Life depends on the strength of the heart and lungs to deliver nutrients and oxygen to the cells.

Health Benefits of Physical Exercise

Much of what we do today will affect our future health. We have many choices to make regarding health behaviors. These choices have positive and negative consequences. The choices include using seat belts, smoking cigarettes, consuming alcohol, nutrition, and frequency of exercise. Our choices reflect our lifestyles; we are responsible for those choices.

Exercise is one of the many lifestyle factors that can be controlled. Increased physical activity leads to improved physical fitness and to other physiologic changes (Box 9-1). It is the combination of these changes that leads to better

health. People who exercise regularly often adopt a healthier lifestyle; they may stop smoking, have more energy, handle stress better, and make wise food choices—all of which improve the quality of life.

Most Americans have little or no physical activity in their daily lives. National surveys indicate that approximately one in four adults have sedentary lifestyles. Inactivity increases with age and is more common among women than men.

Physical inactivity is a major risk factor for CAD, the leading cause of death in the United States. This disease begins in early childhood and progresses in severity over a period of decades. Coronary artery disease is about twice as likely to occur in sedentary persons as in those who exercise, independent of other risk factors such as smoking and obesity.

Regular exercise can reduce the risk of heart disease in several ways. It can improve cardiovascular fitness, decrease blood pressure, aid in losing and maintaining weight, and alter blood lipid and lipoprotein levels. However, individuals with CAD and related conditions should discuss proposed exercise programs with their primary health care providers.

In addition to preventing heart disease, exercise may decrease the risk of colon cancer, stroke, and hypertension. It can also delay the onset of or help treat type 2 diabetes mellitus, depression, osteoporosis, and obesity. Increasing the activity level and consuming a low-fat diet are probably two of the most effective ways to attain a healthy body weight. Physical activity burns kcal, increases the proportion of lean to fat body tissue, and raises the basal metabolic rate.

Persons with physically disabling conditions also benefit from moderate amounts of physical activity. Although this population tends not to perform regular exercise, it is still at risk for chronic diseases for which risk may be reduced by performing regular moderate exercise appropriate to the level of physical abilities. Other benefits include increased stamina and muscle strength and improvement of feelings of well-being by potential reduction of anxiety and depression.[2]

Currently, disparities in physical activity levels exist among American subgroups. More women than men report no leisure time physical activity, more African Americans and Hispanic Americans than whites, more older adults than younger, and less affluent Americans than more affluent Americans. This means that generally women, African Americans and Hispanic Americans, older adults, and the less affluent are not exercising sufficiently to gain the health benefits associated with physical activity.[3] Health care providers can reduce these disparities by teaching patients about the benefits of exercise and providing information or referrals for exercise programs.

Physical activity need not be strenuous to achieve healthful benefits. Even people who are usually inactive can improve their health by becoming moderately active on a regular basis. As we counsel clients and patients in community and acute care settings, we can incorporate suggestions for simple fitness activities into care plans. The *2008 Physical Activity Guidelines for Americans* makes the following recommendations regarding the quantity, intensity, and type of exercise to promote health and reduce risk for major chronic diseases, psychological well-being, and a healthy body weight:[2]

BOX 9-1   MYPLATE: PHYSICAL ACTIVITY

Why Is Physical Activity Important?*
Regular physical activity can produce long term health benefits. People of all ages, shapes, sizes, and abilities can benefit from being physically active. The more physical activity you do, the greater the health benefits.

Being physically active can help you:
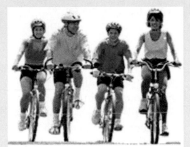
- Increase your chances of living longer
- Feel better about yourself
- Decrease your chances of becoming depressed
- Sleep well at night
- Move around more easily
- Have stronger muscles and bones
- Stay at or get to a healthy weight
- Be with friends or meet new people
- Enjoy yourself and have fun

When you are *not* physically active, you are more likely to:
- Get heart disease
- Get type 2 diabetes
- Have high blood pressure
- Have high blood cholesterol
- Have a stroke

Physical activity and nutrition work together for better health. Being active increases the amount of calories burned. As people age their metabolism slows, so maintaining energy balance requires moving more and eating less.

Some types of physical activity are especially beneficial:
- *Aerobic activities* make you breathe harder and make your heart beat faster. Aerobic activities can be moderate or vigorous in their intensity. Vigorous activities take more effort than moderate ones. For **moderate activities**, you can talk while you do them, but you can't sing. For **vigorous activities**, you can only say a few words without stopping to catch your breath.
- *Muscle-strengthening activities* make your muscles stronger. These include activities like push-ups and lifting weights. It is important to work all the different parts of the body - your legs, hips, back, chest, stomach, shoulders, and arms.
- *Bone-strengthening activities* make your bones stronger. Bone strengthening activities, like jumping, are especially important for children and adolescents. These activities produce a force on the bones that promotes bone growth and strength.
- *Balance and stretching activities* enhance physical stability and flexibility, which reduces risk of injuries. Examples are gentle stretching, dancing, yoga, martial arts, and t'ai chi.

*Accessed June 14, 2012, from http://www.choosemyplate.gov/physical_activity/why.html.

Adults (aged 18-64):
- *Moderate-intensity aerobic activity:* 2 hours and 30 minutes a week, **or** *vigorous-intensity (aerobic)* 1 hour and 15 minutes (75 minutes) a week **or** equivalent combination of moderate- and vigorous-intensity aerobic physical activity. Complete in intervals of at least 10 minutes, best distributed over the week.[2]
- *Additional health benefits:* moderate-intensity aerobic physical activity increased to 5 hours (300 minutes) a week **or** 2 hours and 30 minutes vigorous-intensity physical activity **or** equivalent combination of both.[2]
- *Muscle-strengthening activities:* 2 or more days a week using all major muscle groups.[2]

Older Adults (aged 65 and older):
- *Follow adult guidelines:* If movement is limited due to chronic conditions, adults can be as physically active as possible. Avoid inactivity. Focus on activities that sustain or increase balance.[2]

Sedentary Individuals
Generally, sedentary people can do little activity without the early onset of fatigue or discomfort. For these individuals, it is best that physical activity be included as part of their life-style. For example, taking a 10-minute walk three times a day plus stretching and strengthening activities provides adequate physical activity without the strain of fatigue or discomfort.

Moderately Active Individuals
Moderately active people are those who can participate in 30 minutes of physical activity with minimum fatigue. They are generally interested in improving cardiovascular health; however, many of these individuals may wish to decrease body fat or increase muscle mass. If the goal is to lose fat, the total kcal expended are more important than the intensity level of the activity. Moderately active individuals should also engage in resistance exercises that involve major muscle groups (Box 9-2).

Vigorously Active Individuals
This category generally includes recreational athletes, competitive athletes, and elite and Olympic-level athletes. These individuals not only want to develop cardiovascular fitness but also look to enhance their performance and move to the next level in their sport. In most cases, the training intensity should match the intensity of the sport. For example, a cyclist works primarily on aerobic training. The basketball player would perform some aerobic and anaerobic training.

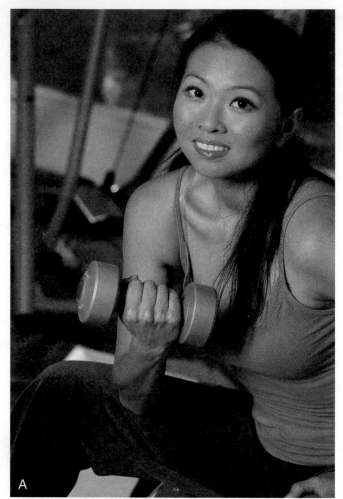

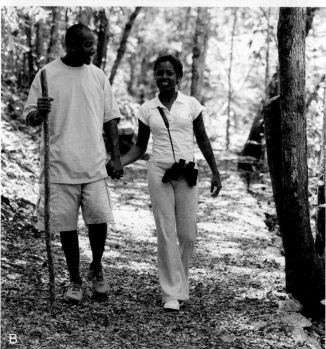

Weight-bearing exercises, including strength training **(A)** and brisk walking **(B)** are beneficial for bone health. (Photos.com.)

BOX 9-2 EXAMPLES OF MODERATE AMOUNTS OF ACTIVITY*

	Less Vigorous, More Time ↑
Washing and waxing a car for 45-60 minutes	
Washing windows or floors for 45-60 minutes	
Playing volleyball for 45 minutes	
Playing touch football for 30-45 minutes	
Gardening for 30-45 minutes	
Wheeling self in wheelchair for 30-40 minutes	
Walking 1¾ miles in 35 minutes (20 minutes/mile)	
Shooting basketballs for 30 minutes	
Bicycling 5 miles in 30 minutes	
Dancing fast (social) for 30 minutes	
Pushing a stroller 1½ miles in 30 minutes	
Raking leaves for 30 minutes	
Walking 2 miles in 30 minutes (15 minutes/mile)	
Water aerobicizing for 30 minutes	
Swimming laps for 20 minutes	
Playing wheelchair basketball for 20 minutes	
Playing basketball for 15-20 minutes	
Bicycling 4 miles in 15 minutes	
Jumping rope for 15 minutes	
Running 1½ miles in 15 minutes (10 minutes/mile)	
Shoveling snow for 15 minutes	↓ More Vigorous,
Walking stairs for 15 minutes	Less Time

*A moderate amount of physical activity is roughly equivalent to physical activity that uses approximately 150 kcal of energy per day, or 1000 kcal per week. Some activities can be performed at various intensities; the suggested durations correspond to expected intensity of effort.
Data from U.S. Department of Health and Human Services, Public Health Service, Centers for Disease Control and Prevention: *Report of the Surgeon General: Physical activity and health*, Washington, DC, 1996, U.S. Government Printing Office.

Special Populations

Adults with physical disabilities can follow the adult guidelines (Figure 9-5). If necessary, activity can be adapted to abilities. Inactivity should be avoided.[2]

Pregnant women and those individuals with physical disabilities (see Figure 9-5) or health problems such as diabetes, hypertension, or cardiovascular disease can follow the same principles of prescribing intensity with a few adaptations:[2]

- The more severe the condition, the lower the intensity of exercise.
- Women who are healthy during pregnancy and postpartum can do moderate-intensity aerobic activity for at least 2 hours and 30 minutes a week. Those with an established vigorous-intensity aerobic activity can continue as long as their condition remains consistent. Activity levels should be discussed with health care providers. Pregnant women should not participate in

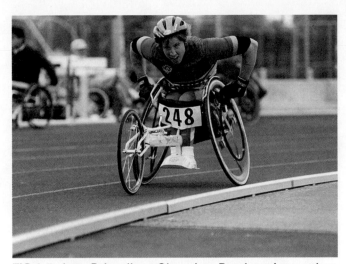

FIG 9-5 Jean Driscoll, an Olympian, Paralympian, author, and advocate for people with disabilities, was born with spina bifida. During her career as an elite wheelchair racer, Jean won 2 Olympic silver medals and 12 Paralympic medals. (Copyright 1995 Curt Beamer, PVA Publications, Sports 'n Spokes, Phoenix.)

high-intensity exercise after their first trimester because of the increase in body core temperature. (See Chapter 11 for exercise guidelines during pregnancy.)

- Individuals who have diabetes or hypertension need to be more aware of their conditions and carefully monitor their exercise intensity. Depending on the frequency and intensity of exercise, levels of medications may need adjustment.

Strength Training

Strength training has become a popular way to stay in shape. It is an integral part of an overall exercise program. Strength training involves lifting various types of weights to build muscle strength and endurance. It may differ from weight lifting. With strength training, improvement is gauged by increased muscle mass. In contrast, weight lifting may be a competitive sport in which individuals lift weights in specific body weight divisions.

Proper strength training exercise programs can reliably increase muscle size and strength in men and women of all ages. The stimulus for muscle growth is overload: resistance greater than that to which the muscle has been accustomed must be imposed. Beginners may start with 3-pound weights and progress to higher weights as strength increases. Research shows that moderately active people can achieve significant gains in strength by performing one set of 8 to 12 repetitions.

Most of us know that aerobic exercise, such as running and cycling, is good for the heart, making it stronger and more efficient. However, strength training has benefits for cardiovascular health, too. It can help improve blood cholesterol levels, burn fat, and contribute to our well-being. Strength training may also protect against back problems, osteoporosis, and minor injuries. Recent studies show that strength training builds muscle mass of adults in their 80s. Increased muscle mass improves strength and flexibility, both of which reduce the risk of injuries caused by poor muscle coordination and resulting falls.[4]

Bone responds to the force of gravity and to muscular contraction. Physical exercise forces bone to adapt to the stresses imposed on it. When stressed, bones become larger and stronger. Weight-bearing exercises (e.g., walking, jogging, weight [strength] training) are beneficial for bone health. The density and health of bone tissue are of particular concern for women. Being physically fit through aerobic and weight-bearing exercise is a good defense against osteoporosis, for which women are at greater risk. Fortunately, this can be accomplished through daily brisk walking or jogging. Other strategies for reducing the risk of osteoporosis are listed in Chapter 8.

For some clients, the development of a simple strength-training program with a certified exercise physiologist (or certified personal trainer) may be appropriate as a valuable addition to individual health care plans. Such a program may be beneficial for nursing professionals as well.

Bodybuilding

In recent years there has been increased interest and participation in bodybuilding. Bodybuilders work to develop muscle mass, strength, and muscle definition through a combination of diet, weight training, and aerobic exercise. Unlike weight lifting and other traditional sports that involve strength, bodybuilders exercise to improve their physique as a form of athletic performance.

To prepare for competition, bodybuilders diet and exercise to reduce their body fat. Unfortunately, many bodybuilders follow a number of dietary practices that may place them at risk for health problems. Bodybuilders are susceptible to misinformation about muscle growth and development because they want quick results and may not understand the dietary requirements of muscle gain. Instead, they may consume protein or amino acid powders and supplements in the belief they will provide extra energy and increase muscle mass and strength. These beliefs are reflected in endorsements for a variety of protein and amino acid supplements found in popular fitness and strength magazines. Claims for fast muscle development are made for everything from bee pollen to specific types of exercise equipment.

Suggested dietary intake composition for bodybuilders consists of 55% to 60% carbohydrate, 25% to 30% protein, and 15% to 20% fat for off-season (no competitive events) and precontest (6 to 12 weeks before event) phases.[5] Off-season dietary regimens should maintain positive energy balance at about 15% higher than usual energy intake. This provides sufficient energy for workouts and for muscle anabolism. For the precontest phase, bodybuilders can be in a slight negative energy balance, consuming about 15% less than the usual energy intake. The lower intake allows for the utilization of body fat for energy and better muscle definition, assuming protein and carbohydrate intakes are sufficient for adequate maintenance of muscle mass.[5]

The composition of muscle is approximately 70% to 75% water, 15% to 22% protein, and 5% to 7% other materials, including inorganic salt, lipids, glycogen, enzymes, and minerals. Exercise, though, is the single most important factor in increasing the size, strength, and endurance of muscles.

FOOD AND ATHLETIC PERFORMANCE

Physical activity and nutrition have been associated with health since the time of ancient Greece. Hippocrates said, "All parts of the body which have a function, if used in moderation and exercised in labors in which each is accustomed, become thereby healthy, well-developed, and age more slowly, but if unused and left idle they become liable to disease, defective in growth and age quickly."[6] More than 2000 years later, this advice is still consistent with our knowledge about nutrition, physical fitness, and health.

Physically active people of all ages and levels of competition are seeking information to enhance their training and achieve a competitive edge. They want to know what kinds of foods to eat and specific dietary regimens to follow. The nutritional needs of athletes are basically no different from nonathletes, with the exception of kcal and fluids. A diet that provides a variety of foods supplying 45% to 65% of kcal intake from carbohydrate; 20% to 35% of kcal intake from fat; and 10% to 35% of kcal intake from protein is recommended for health and performance.[7] However, some forms of heavy training increase the requirement for certain nutrients. For example, carbohydrates are an important source of energy during endurance exercise, and therefore runners, cyclists, and swimmers may need more carbohydrates (60% to 70% of their total kcal intake) than other individuals.

Nutrition can affect an athlete in many ways. At the most basic level, nutrition is essential for normal growth and development and for maintaining good health. By staying healthy, an athlete will feel better, train harder, and be in better condition. Among comparable athletes, good eating habits can be the factor that determines the winner. However, these good habits do not come from the pregame meal or even from what the athlete eats the week before competition. They are built daily over a long period.

A number of dietary patterns will provide good nutrition. MyPyramid can be a useful outline for athletes of what to eat every day. Each food group provides some—but not all—of the nutrients an athlete needs. Foods in each of the six food categories of MyPyramid provide kcal from different combinations of carbohydrate, protein, and fat (see www.mypyramid.gov). For example, fruits provide kcal from carbohydrates, and milk products contain carbohydrate, protein, and varying amounts of fat.

Athletes should eat at least the minimum number of servings for each group daily to meet energy needs. Depending on their body size and level of training, some athletes may need more than the larger number of servings (Box 9-3).

Nurses and other health professionals should have a basic understanding of the nutritional needs of athletes to provide fundamental information and to conduct a simple assessment or screening of nutritional status as influenced by athletic activities. Referrals to a registered dietitian with expertise in sports nutrition is appropriate for athletes and

---

BOX 9-3	BENEFITS OF SNACKING

Snacking provides the following benefits:
- Helps the athlete get enough kcal without having to eat large amounts of food at any one meal; this is especially important for staying awake in class and helping to curb hunger pains during practice. Snacking supports academic and physical performance.
- Helps to replace muscle glycogen stores and fluids lost during practice or competition.
- Supplies vitamins and minerals the athlete may not get in regular meals.

Whatever kind of snacker you are, ask yourself the following questions:
1. What nutrients do snacks provide?
2. Do I need the extra calories?
3. How can these snacks fit into the total day's diet?

---

coaches with more specific concerns, such as the creation of individualized eating plans to support training and competitive needs.[8]

Kilocalorie Requirements

As noted earlier, kcal requirements vary greatly from person to person and are affected by activity level, body size, age, and climate. Body size affects kcal requirements more than any other single factor. The smaller the athlete, the lower the kcal requirement.

Some sports demand high-energy expenditure, whereas others do not. A frequently asked question is "How many kcal should I consume?" Athletes are consuming enough kcal if they are maintaining their best competitive yet healthy weight. Ideally, kcal intake should balance energy expended. If intake is consistently more or less than an athlete's requirement, weight gain or weight loss will occur, both of which can affect performance.

Many athletes are concerned about their appearance and thus eat less to keep their body weight and percentage of body fat low. However, restricting kcal can have a negative impact on health and performance. As kcal intake decreases, so does nutrient intake. A minimum requirement for college athletes is 1800 to 2000 kcal a day. Eating less than this amount can leave the athlete feeling weak and listless and may lead to iron deficiency, stress fractures, and, for women, *amenorrhea* (lack of menstruation) and osteoporosis.

On the other hand, increasing kcal intake to gain weight may also be difficult for athletes. Too much food can cause discomfort, especially if a workout takes place soon after eating. Furthermore, when balancing school, work, and practice, little time is available to eat. Small meals and snacks become an important source of nutrients. How often to snack depends on body size and kcal needs.

Water: The Essential Ingredient

Water is the nutrient most critical to athletic performance. Without adequate water, performance can suffer in less than an hour. Water is necessary for the body's cooling system. It also transports nutrients throughout the tissues and maintains adequate blood volume.

During exercise there is always the risk of becoming dehydrated (fluid volume deficit), especially when the temperature is hot. When athletes sweat, they lose water. Although sweat rates vary among people, losing as little as 2% to 3% of weight via sweat can impair performance.[9] When the water lost via sweat is not replaced, blood volume falls and body temperature rises, causing confusion and loss of coordination. To replace the lost water, athletes must consume extra fluids.

The athlete's sense of thirst is not the best indicator that the body needs water; fluid needs may be greater than thirst can gauge. Adequate water intake before, during, and after an event or practice session is of utmost importance. The following guidelines by the American College of Sports Medicine ensure adequate fluid replacement, leading to optimal performance.[9]

- Eat a nutritionally balanced diet and drink adequate fluids during the 24-hour period before an event.
- Consume 2 cups (16 ounces) of fluid 2 hours before exercise, followed by another 2 cups 15 to 20 minutes before exercise and 4 to 6 ounces of fluid every 10 to 15 minutes during exercise.
- Drink cool beverages to reduce body core temperature. Cool beverages are best for activities lasting less than 1 hour.
- Consume sport drinks to enhance fluid intake and absorption and help delay fatigue in endurance events lasting longer than 1 hour.
- After exercise, consume sport drinks to enhance palatability and further promote fluid replacement.

Stress the importance of adequate fluid intake. Clients should weigh themselves nude before and after exercise to determine fluid replacement needs. Sweat loss of 1 pound (2.2 kg) of body weight is equal to 2 cups (480 mL) of water.

How can athletes be sure they are well hydrated? One criterion of hydration is that urine should be basically clear in color throughout most of the day. Athletes should also weigh themselves before and after workouts. For every pound lost, an athlete needs to drink 2 cups of fluid (see Chapter 8 for effects of a fluid volume deficit).

Athletes completing endurance events or slower runners in races who continually drink fluid without an equivalent loss of fluid through sweat or urination may so overhydrate as to experience *hyponatremia* (low blood sodium). Fluid volume deficit (dehydration) is much more common. Awareness of dehydration and hyponatremia is important because medical treatment differs even though the symptoms appear similar.

Sport Drinks

Athletes often wonder which is better for replacing fluids during exercise—water or sport drinks. The number one goal is to remain well hydrated. Whether the athlete drinks water or a sport drink is his or her choice. Cool water is what the body really needs during activities lasting less than 1 hour. However, athletes participating in endurance events requiring more than 90 minutes of continuous moderate to heavy exercise, such as distance running or cycling, may benefit from sport drinks that contain carbohydrate and electrolytes (sodium and potassium). Sports drinks provide fluids to keep the athlete well hydrated and provide extra carbohydrate for energy.

A major consideration in fluid replacement is how quickly the fluid empties from the stomach. To hydrate the total body, the fluid needs to leave the stomach quickly to be distributed throughout the body. Although larger volumes of fluid empty more rapidly from the stomach, many athletes cannot exercise with a full stomach. Cool fluids empty faster from the stomach than warm fluids. Kcal content is also important. The greater the kcal content of a beverage, the slower the emptying rate.

Carbohydrate: The Energy Food

Carbohydrate stores in the body (glycogen) are limited. Low levels of muscle glycogen can impair performance. Consuming carbohydrates before and during exercise will delay the onset of fatigue and allow the athlete to compete longer.

How much carbohydrate should an athlete eat each day to replace muscle glycogen? It depends mostly on body size. An athlete with more muscle mass will require more carbohydrate. Carbohydrate requirements also depend on intensity and level of training. Athletes participating in high-energy sports that require short bursts of energy (e.g., basketball, tennis, football, soccer) need about 5 g of carbohydrate per kilogram of body weight daily to maintain muscle glycogen stores. Endurance athletes who train aerobically for more than 90 minutes daily may need up to 10 g of carbohydrate per kilogram of body weight to replace glycogen.[9] Individuals who exercise regularly to maintain conditioning do well with general guidelines of high-complex carbohydrate diets, as represented by MyPyramid. The *Teaching Tool* box, How Much Carbohydrate Do You Need? shows how to calculate carbohydrate requirements.

Both types are effective in replenishing glycogen in the muscles. However, complex carbohydrates provide vitamins, minerals, and fiber as well. Examples of complex carbohydrates include whole grains, bread, potatoes, pasta, cereal, fruits, and fruit juices. Simple sugars include maple syrup, molasses, honey, and table sugar.

✳ TEACHING TOOL

How Much Carbohydrate Do You Need?

1. Divide body weight in pounds by 2.2 lb/kg to determine body weight in kilograms. For example:
   154 lb ÷ 2.2 lb/kg = 70 kilograms body weight
2. Multiply each kilogram of body weight by 5 grams to determine the number of grams of carbohydrate needed daily. For example:
   70 kg × 5 g = 350 g of carbohydrate daily

Carbohydrate Loading

Carbohydrate loading is the process of changing the type of foods eaten and adjusting the amount of training to increase glycogen stores in the muscle. This concept first became of interest around 1939 when scientists studied the effects of dietary manipulation on the ability to perform prolonged hard work. They found that men consuming a high-carbohydrate diet for 3 days could perform heavy work twice as long as men fed a high-fat diet for the same 3 days.[10] Since then, researchers have investigated several techniques for increasing glycogen levels in the muscles.

To achieve maximum muscle glycogen stores through carbohydrate loading, athletes should consume a high-carbohydrate diet as part of their regular training program. At least 60% (preferably 60% to 70%) of their total kcal should come from carbohydrate. For the athlete eating 3000 kcal a day, this represents a minimum of 450 g of carbohydrate daily. Three days before competition, exercise should taper off to allow muscles to rest. Dietary carbohydrates should be increased to 60% to 70% of total kcal. This technique of combining rest and increased carbohydrate intake encourages greater glycogen storage. Kcal intake may need to be reduced to compensate for less training.

Carbohydrate loading is usually recommended only for athletes engaged in continuous exercise lasting more than 90 minutes, although benefits may be gained for shorter events as well. It is not recommended for athletes participating in short-term events such as sprints or in sports such as football, baseball, and wrestling; nor should individuals with diabetes or hypoglycemia consider this dietary pattern that affects carbohydrate metabolism. Furthermore, the degree of benefit from carbohydrate loading varies among individuals. Therefore, athletes should determine before competition the value of this regimen for them and should refer to specific resources for detailed recommendations. The potential negative side effects of carbohydrate loading include increased water retention and weight gain, stiffness, cramping, and digestive problems.[11]

A more practical concern is whether athletes are eating enough carbohydrate on a daily basis to maintain adequate levels of muscle glycogen for training and workouts. See the Websites of Interest at the end of this chapter for sites that determine adequate carbohydrate intake to maximize muscle glycogen stores.

Protein

The importance of protein for athletes has been a subject of controversy for many years. Many athletes and coaches believe that a high-protein diet supplies extra energy, enhances athletic performance, and increases muscle mass. There is no evidence, however, that eating more protein than needed improves athletic ability.

Although carbohydrate and fat are the major fuels used for energy, studies indicate that protein use increases during exercise, and under certain conditions protein may contribute significantly to energy metabolism.[11] Two factors that influence the use of protein as an energy source are the length of exercise and the carbohydrate content of the diet. The body may depend on protein for an increased percentage of energy in prolonged exercise (greater than 90 minutes), particularly when carbohydrate intake is low.

The Dietary Reference Intake (DRI) for protein for sedentary adults is 0.8 g per kilogram of body weight per day.[7] Research suggests that athletes need between 1.5 and 2 g of

---

BOX 9-4   IS A SNACK BAR *JUST* A SNACK BAR?

Do you grab a snack bar before heading to the gym? Why? Is it high in protein? Is it high in energy?

Snack or energy bars tend to be either high in protein *or* high in energy. They are often expensive and may not be necessary. If the "snack" is to provide some quick energy before exercise, then the bar should be high in carbohydrate energy. Having a high-protein bar that may also be high in fat before exercise won't provide you with quick energy; it takes longer for the protein and fat to be digested and absorbed.

Protein bars are appropriate if one's protein intake is low or if the bar is a meal replacement. Popular among bodybuilders, protein bars are considered a way to maintain protein intake throughout the day. For some, the bar functions as a minimeal in addition to regularly planned meals, adding calories and protein to maintain lean body mass. Most bodybuilders consume an adequate protein intake even for muscle-building purposes.

Perhaps the bottom line is to determine which type of snack bar fulfills a particular need at an appropriate cost and whether it is edible (tastes good). And remember that a well-planned snack, such as a piece of fruit plus some raisins and nuts or a handful of almonds, may provide the same nutrients and satiety for a lot less cost.

Data from Antonio J: Sports supplements. Protein bars may enhance lean body mass, *Strength Condition J* 27(4):1524, 2005; and Zaveri S; Drummond S: The effect of including a conventional *snack* (cereal *bar*) and a nonconventional *snack* (almonds) on hunger, eating frequency, dietary intake and body weight, *J Hum Nutr Diet* 22(5): 461-468, 2009.

---

protein per kilogram of body weight per day.[9] For a 150-pound (68-kg) athlete (runner), this amounts to 102 to 136 g of protein per day. Factors such as kcal intake, protein quality, and type and intensity of the sport are important considerations. The lower the kcal intake, the higher the protein requirements. This is one reason why protein intake is often a concern among female athletes because many do not consume enough calories.

The type of protein eaten also affects the amount of protein needed. The 1.5 to 2 g of protein per kilogram of body weight recommendation is based on a diet containing animal foods. Athletes who eat meat, fish, poultry, eggs, milk, or cheese will have little problem meeting their protein needs. Strict vegetarian athletes, however, will need to plan their diets more carefully to ensure that their protein needs are met. Protein bars may be used to supplement protein and energy intakes for athletes. Products should be carefully chosen to avoid excess intake of protein and simple sugars masked as dietary supplement bars (Box 9-4).

Protein and Amino Acid Supplements

The use of protein and amino acid supplements is a common practice among athletes. Various combinations of individual amino acids are sold to athletes with the promise that the acids will stimulate the release of growth hormone and thus increase muscle mass. Promoters claim that amino acids can build muscle, aid fat loss, provide energy, speed up muscle repair, and improve endurance. Others claim that they are more readily digested and absorbed than the protein consumed in foods.

The question is: Do athletes need to take these supplements, or can they get the protein they need from food alone? Many athletes eat more than the recommended amount of protein (and thus amino acids) from food alone. Amino acids as building blocks of all proteins are found in a wide variety of foods, from pork chops to bread and from beans and peas to milk and tacos. Because the body cannot store extra protein, excess protein and amino acids are broken down and used for energy or stored as fat. If protein or amino acid supplements provide more nutrients than needed for protein functions, the body treats supplements the same as any excess source of protein.

It is safer and cheaper to take amino acids in a glass of milk, a turkey sandwich, or other protein-rich foods. Muscle size and strength increase only after weeks of work. If athletes want to gain muscle mass, they need to become involved in a resistive strength training program and consume a diet rich in carbohydrates.

Fat

In athletic performance, carbohydrate and fat are the major sources of energy. The amount of fat used during exercise depends on the duration and intensity of exercise, the degree of prior training, and the composition of the diet. Exercise performed under aerobic conditions will promote fat use as a source of energy. There is a good reason to increase your body's ability to burn fat as fuel; using fat as a source of energy will spare muscle glycogen.

Athletes need a certain amount of fat in their diets and on their bodies for optimal health and performance. The challenge is eating a diet that provides the right amount. The position of the American Dietetic Association, Dietitians of Canada, and the American College of Sports Medicine recommends moderate energy intake of 20% to 25% energy from fat.[8] Because each athlete is different, some may eat less and some slightly more than the recommended range of kcal from fat. Many athletes cannot get the kcal they need without eating a little extra fat. However, fat intakes greater than 35% of total kcal have been associated with increased risk of certain diet-related diseases (e.g., heart disease, obesity, cancer).

To lower fat intake, athletes should choose lean meats, fish, poultry, and low-fat dairy products. Fat and oils should be used sparingly in cooking, and fried foods and high-fat snacks should be eaten in moderation. (See Chapter 5 for strategies designed to lower dietary fat intake.)

Vitamins and Minerals

A balanced diet generally supplies enough vitamins and minerals to meet the needs of most athletes, and consuming more has not been shown to improve performance. Nevertheless, use of supplements by high school and college athletes is common. Use is even higher among elite athletes. Female athletes tend to use vitamin/mineral supplements more than

men, and patterns exist among sport groups; for example, bodybuilders, cyclists, and runners are bigger supplement users than wrestlers and basketball players.

There are reportedly many reasons why athletes take vitamin/mineral supplements, such as for extra energy, to make up for a poor diet, to recover quicker after exercise, and for general well-being. The problem is that athletes may view supplements as "good" and therefore harmless. Such beliefs can lead to excessive intakes. For many athletes, the level of nutrients consumed from food alone is greater than 200% of the DRI. With the addition of a supplement, combined food and nutrient intakes can exceed 1000% of the DRI. Toxicity and adverse health effects can occur from consuming high doses of vitamins and minerals over a long period.

On the other hand, athletes in "thin-build" sports (e.g., gymnastics, figure skating, wrestling, distance running) often consume low-calorie intakes and thus are at risk for vitamin and mineral deficiencies. For these athletes, supplementation with a multivitamin/mineral providing 100% of the DRI can be beneficial.

Ergogenic Aids

In athletics, the term **ergogenic aids** is used to describe drugs and dietary regimens believed by some to increase strength, power, and endurance (Table 9-4). Because winning is often a matter of a split second, it is easy to see why athletes are continuously looking for the competitive edge. The fact that more and more nutritional supplements are marketed to athletes presents a challenge to coaches, trainers, nutritionists, and health care providers to provide sound nutrition information.

The nutritional supplements used by athletes constantly change. Often, as athletes find that one doesn't work, they search for another. Today commonly used nutritional aids include creatine monohydrate (a protein), chromium picolinate, beta-hydroxy-beta-methylbutyrate (HMB), and dehydroepiandrosterone (DHEA). Although the use of DHEA is banned in some states, athletes still use it. With the exception of creatine, research has not shown these supplements to have a significant effect on performance. Despite a lack of scientific basis for the claims associated with these products, their widespread use continues.

Nutritional supplements are a multimillion-dollar business. Athletes are a prime target for the marketers of these products. Athletes make good consumers because, like many Americans, they believe that if a little is good, a lot is better. It is not uncommon for an athlete to consume five or six different supplements a day and not know what substances are in them. Many of the supplements athletes purchase from specialty nutrition stores and mail-order catalogs are not subject to the regulations established by the U.S. Food and Drug Administration (FDA), and this presents another concern. Athletes have no way of knowing whether these nutritional supplements are safe.

Taking several different supplements at one time, or one containing a large amount of one nutrient such as vitamin A, can be toxic. There is also the risk of nutrient-nutrient

TABLE 9-4	ERGOGENIC AIDS MARKETED TO ATHLETES		
SUBSTANCE	**DESCRIPTION**	**CLAIMS**	**ACTUAL EFFECT**
Arginine, lysine, ornithine	Amino acids	Stimulate release of human growth hormone	No proven effect
Antioxidant vitamins C, E, beta carotene	Compounds that may prevent free-radical damage	Prevent muscle damage from oxidation following high-intensity exercise	Some evidence of proven benefit
Caffeine*	Stimulant	Improves performance; increases fatty acid; oxidation; spares glycogen	Some evidence of proven benefit
Carnitine	Facilitates the transfer of long-chain fatty acids into the mitochondria	Enhances energy levels; decreases	No proven effect on body fat
Creatine	Protein/amino acids	Increases intramuscular creatine; increases power output; promotes increase in lean body mass	Some evidence of proven benefit
Dehydroepiandrosterone (DHEA)	Hormone	Increases energy, increases muscle mass, decreases body fat	More research is needed to confirm these observations
Ginseng	Extract of ginseng root	Reduces fatigue and improves endurance, strength, and recovery from exercise	No proven effect
Hydroxy beta methylbutyrate (HMB)	Metabolite of the amino acid leucine	Increases in lean body mass, decreased body fat, increased strength	More research is needed to confirm these observations

*The use of caffeine is considered a form of doping by the International Olympic Committee (IOC). The IOC has set an upper limit of 12 mcg/mL of caffeine in the urine.

interactions, in which an excess of one nutrient can interfere with the body's ability to use another nutrient. This may occur when excessive amounts of one amino acid are consumed; the body's use of other amino acids may be affected.

OVERCOMING BARRIERS

American "Couch Potatoes"

The term *couch potatoes* became part of our slang terminology several years ago. The term refers to people who just sit on the couch and vegetate (do nothing) while watching television, viewing movies, or playing video games. Those of us who do more sitting than doing often end up soft and fluffy like mashed potatoes. How did we fall into such habits?

More than likely, couch potatoes have always existed. Habits that develop during childhood and adolescence may predispose us to lead sedentary lifestyles (see the *Cultural Considerations* box, Field Trips to Fast-Food Restaurants). If as children our favorite activities involved watching television and sports events rather than playing sports or being physically active, we may end up as couch potato adults. If our parents were also sedentary, we did not have fitness role models.

What has changed is that more focus is being placed on the health benefits of physical fitness. We now know a sedentary lifestyle puts us more at risk for heart disease, some cancers, diabetes, hypertension, and obesity. Even if our body weight is low, we are still at risk for health problems if we are sedentary. These chronic diseases drain the productive and economic resources of our society. Now is a good time for couch potatoes to transform their ways and turn into roadrunners.

Psychosocial Dimensions of Fitness

When most people hear the word *fitness*, they visualize a young, "athletic" person. Our image of fitness needs to become synonymous with healthy. One way to get closer to this image is to encourage our clients (and ourselves) to initiate and maintain regular physical activity within our everyday lives. A way to open a dialog with clients about exercise is to discuss the concept of "fitness personality." Fitness personality takes into account our individual traits and relates those to different sports and exercise programs.

To allow for positive matches to take place, seven psychosocial dimensions of activities can be considered. These dimensions include sociality of sports and exercise; degree of control or spontaneity; intrinsic and extrinsic motivation; aggression or sport assertiveness; competitive, collaborative, or individualistic options; mental focus; and risk taking or risk avoiding. The degree to which the psychosocial challenges meet the expectations of the individual, the more likely an increase in self-esteem and compliance may occur.[12]

Using the Fitness Personality Profile (Figure 9-6), an individual can note a sport of interest and determine which

🌐 CULTURAL CONSIDERATIONS

Field Trips to Fast-Food Restaurants?

To initiate lifestyle behavior changes among high-risk, ethnically diverse, low-income adults, eight community nursing centers (CNCs) of the Midwest Nursing Centers Consortium, conducted a 16-week course titled Wellness for a Lifetime for clients of the center. The purpose of the course was to promote increased physical activity and to improve the quality of dietary intake of the participants.

Created by a multidisciplinary team, Wellness for a Lifetime was based on health behavior theory and included culturally appropriate content. Each CNC was provided with complete course content including themes for support group discussions. Course topics included foods and nutrition; stretching and exercising basics; relationship between chronic diseases and diet and activity; and stress reduction strategies. The course was interactive including trips to grocery stores and fast-food restaurants, and exploring walking routes.

All the CNCs have the same purpose: to deliver primary care that blends traditional medical management with primary prevention and community based health promotion approaches.

Sites differ in the delivery of the primary care. At each site the nurse educators customized the course to meet the needs of the population of that center including language, age, and ethnicity. The course was quite successful at all sites and participants requested it to continue past 16 weeks.

Application to nursing: CNCs provide services within neighborhood settings. By being "part of the neighborhood," the CNCs were able to recruit clients for the course who might not have otherwise participated. The physical activity levels of the ethnically diverse populations served increased. Describing the need for exercising may not be enough; actually leading clients through an exercise session or on a walking route models appropriate behaviors.

Although the Wellness for a Lifetime course was developed with culturally appropriate content, each site still needed to modify content to meet the specific needs of its population such as offering the sessions in various languages (Spanish, Chinese, or Russian). When using other health education tools, we may need to modify aspects of the programs to meet the needs of our own.

Data from Anderko L et al: Wellness for a lifetime: Improving lifestyle behaviors of low-income, ethnically diverse populations, *Ann Fam Med* 3(Suppl 2):S35-S36, 2005.

psychosocial traits are most required. Or one can assess for each trait where on the scale he or she ranks and determine if a sport or exercise program is best. The profile can also be used to develop a certain trait. Perhaps a person works alone in an office every day and wants to use physical activity as a way to be more social. He or she might choose martial arts as opposed to cardio conditioning.[12] The ultimate goal is to increase regular physical activity so that more Americans are healthy and fit.

Exercise Makes You Hungrier: Myth or Fact?

Does exercise make us hungrier? Do we have a greater physiologic need for food when using our bodies more? Or is the hunger psychologic?

During and immediately after exercise, our digestive system basically slows down. Blood flow through the main digestive organs slows; the blood concentrates on reaching the large muscles that need all the nutrients and oxygen possible to do their work. This means that any foodstuff in the digestive tract takes longer to be processed. When we complete and recover from exercising, the digestive process resumes.

However, we may experience low blood glucose levels, depending on how long ago we ate and the amount of exercise we completed. Until the body recovers from the exercise, a glass of juice or other light snack best serves the needs of the body to raise blood glucose to a comfortable level.

Sustained regular exercise does cause a physiologic need for more food. The work of exercise uses additional kcal. Although we may be hungrier and take in more kcal, we also use more kcal. The equation of kcal input and output can still

balance. The bonus is that we will have stronger bodies with more stamina.

TOWARD A POSITIVE NUTRITION LIFESTYLE: MODELING

Want to begin a fitness routine but don't know how to get started? Although motivation is essential, sometimes the basic steps of getting started are the hardest. Should exercise be done in the morning, at lunch, or at night? Must you exercise every day, or is three times a week sufficient? How is this done?

A technique to assist in changing behavior is called *modeling*; modeling can be used as an education strategy with patients or may be personally applied to our own lifestyles. Modeling is replicating or imitating the behavior of someone else.

For simplicity, let's apply this technique to you. You are molding your behavior to be similar to that person's behavior. Approaches to modeling include visualization by imagining you doing what the other person does or discussion with the person to discover how the desired behavior is performed.

Application to a fitness routine could use both approaches. Perhaps a friend has an established fitness routine, and you would like to begin to work out also. To use visualization, first imagine the friend preparing for the workout, exercising, and resting afterward. Then substitute yourself for the friend. Imagine getting your exercise clothes ready, setting the alarm clock, getting dressed to exercise, exercising, and then resting

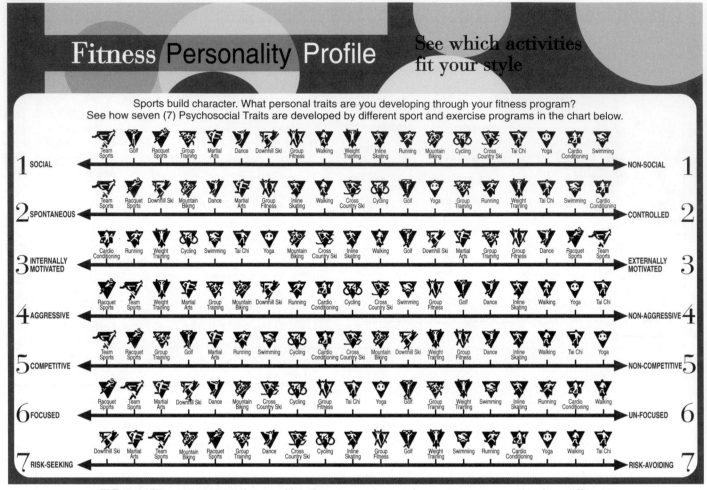

FIG 9-6 Fitness personality profile. Sports and exercise programs emphasize different psychosocial dimensions. Pairing personality traits with psychosocial dimension demands may allow for better adherence to an exercise program or to the development of new desired personality traits. (Courtesy James Gavin, PhD, Department of Applied Human Sciences, Concordia University, Montreal, Quebec, Canada.)

afterward. Do this for several days and then actually exercise.

The other approach is to talk with friends or family members who exercise regularly. Find out how they prepare for workouts. What motivation techniques to maintain a fitness program do they use? How many times per week do they exercise? How do they deal with everyday interruptions to their exercise program such as examinations, sick children, or work crises? After adjusting their techniques to your circumstances, do the exercises yourself.

SUMMARY

The ability to perform work, produce change, and maintain life all requires energy. ATP is the fuel for all energy-requiring processes in the body. We convert the energy from the food we eat into ATP energy.

There are two related energy pathways. The aerobic pathway depends on oxygen; the anaerobic pathway functions without oxygen. The physical demands of different sports require specific sources of energy. Carbohydrate in the form of glucose is the only fuel to be used anaerobically without oxygen to produce ATP. During low- to moderate-intensity exercise, muscle cells mainly use fat for fuel.

Our daily energy requirement depends on three major components: basal metabolism, physical activity, and the energy to metabolize food. Each of these components is affected directly or indirectly by many factors including our age, gender, and body size. Physical exercise is important to our long-term health and well-being because increased physical activity leads to improved fitness and other physiologic changes that may reduce the risk of chronic diseases such as heart disease, cancer, diabetes, and obesity. A combination of aerobic exercise and strength training is recommended for overall fitness.

The nutritional needs of athletes are generally no different from those of nonathletes, with the exception of kcal and fluids. Many different dietary patterns can meet the athlete's nutrition needs. Carbohydrate is an important nutrient for both health and athletic performance. Athletes should eat enough carbohydrate daily to maintain adequate levels of muscle glycogen for training and workouts. Protein require- ments of athletes may be slightly greater than that of seden- tary individuals. Most athletes, however, get enough protein in their diets. There is no need for them to take protein powders or amino acid supplements. For the most part, research has shown that nutritional supplements including vitamins and minerals have little effect on performance in athletes who consume a balanced diet.

THE NURSING APPROACH

Case Study: Nutrition for an Athlete

Tom, an 18-year-old freshman student on the university track team, was preparing for a marathon running event. He had been given instructions about diet from his coach but wanted to confirm the information with the nurse at the student health center. He had trained hard and was highly motivated to do his best in the race.

ASSESSMENT

Subjective (from patient statements)

- "I eat healthy, following MyPyramid guidelines."
- "I'm wondering how I should do carbohydrate loading before the marathon."
- "I would like to know what type of sports drinks I should drink, and how much and when I should drink them."
- "Please tell me about protein powders."

Objective (from physical examination)

- Height 5'9", weight 140 pounds.
- Blood pressure 120/80. Temperature 98.4° F, pulse 60, res- pirations 16
- Lean with well-defined muscles

DIAGNOSES (NURSING)

Readiness for enhanced nutrition as evidenced by desire to know about carbohydrate loading before a marathon race, sports drinks, and protein powders

PLANNING

Patient Outcomes

Short term (at the end of this visit):

- Tom will state specific plans for carbohydrate loading, hydra- tion, and protein supplements.
- He will discuss the rationale for each dietary plan.

Nursing Interventions

1. Assess Tom's knowledge of nutrition and teach him about nutrition for the athlete.
2. Caution Tom to avoid steroids.

IMPLEMENTATION

1. Assessed Tom's knowledge of nutrition.
   It is important to know the beliefs of an individual so that his knowledge can be confirmed or corrected. Teaching should proceed from the familiar to new information. Teaching should be centered on the learning needs.
2. Taught him the correct procedure for carbohydrate loading.
   During endurance training, at least 60% of calories should come from carbohydrates. A few days before the endurance event, exercise is tapered down to allow muscles to rest, and carbohydrates are increased to help build glycogen stores in the muscles and liver. On the day of the event, a light carbohydrate meal is consumed before the race.

3. Taught him that hydration is important before the event. About six ounces of sports drinks should be consumed every 15 to 20 minutes during an event lasting longer than 90 minutes.
   Water is needed to cool the body and prevent dehydration. Carbohydrate supplies energy, and sodium and potassium replace electrolytes lost through sweat.
4. Taught Tom that endurance athletes may have higher protein needs than the general population but probably do not need protein powders.
   Endurance and strength-trained athletes may need 1.5 to 2 g protein/kg body weight per day. These recommenda- tions are usually met through diet alone because most Amer- icans actually consume almost twice the recommended amount of protein. Female athletes, though, may need to be aware of their protein intake in relation to their overall caloric intake
5. Cautioned him to avoid steroids.
   Even when not asked about steroids, the nurse should address them for health promotion. Steroids are synthetic hormones that are anabolic and androgenic, taken by some athletes to increase muscle size and strength. Very danger- ous, they can cause premature closure of bone growth, liver injury, heart disease, high blood pressure, sterility and many other physical effects.
6. Referred Tom to a dietitian to discuss specific personal diet questions and concerns.
   Although a nurse is qualified to discuss general nutrition, spe- cific individualized diets should be planned by a dietitian.

EVALUATION

Short term (at the end of the visit):

- Tom was able to state correct plans for consuming carbohy- drates, sports drinks, and protein foods.
- He was able to explain valid rationales for his plans.
- He stated that he does not take steroids and will continue to avoid them.
- Goals met.

DISCUSSION QUESTIONS

Tom went to a dietitian to work out a personalized meal plan, and he reported to the dietitian after the race. He was able to finish his marathon running event but was not among the fastest runners. He planned to do more training.

1. Describe one prerace dinner meal that would provide high protein and about 60% carbohydrate.
2. Would the basic principles in this case study be the same for a young woman who planned to run a marathon? What might be different?

APPLYING CONTENT KNOWLEDGE

Darren, a college student, just started an aerobic exercise plan to lose some fat. Because he feels tired, he stops by the college health center and chats with a nurse practitioner about his exercise program. He asks, "If my muscles use simple carbohydrates for energy, why isn't it okay for me to have a soda and a candy bar rather than a regular meal? It's all kcal, isn't it?" How might the nurse practitioner respond?

WEBSITES OF INTEREST

The Physician and Sportsmedicine (Journal) Online

www.physsportsmed.com
Supplies clinical and personal health resources on nutrition, personal fitness, exercise, and physical rehabilitation.

American College of Sports Medicine (ACSM)

www.acsm.org
Promotes developing active lifestyles for people of all ages.

Healthier US Initiative

http://HealthierUS.gov
As part of the HealthierUS Initiative, supports and educates to improve people's lives, prevent and reduce the costs of disease, and promote community health and wellness.

REFERENCES

1. Merriam-Webster OnLine: *Dictionary: Definition of athlete*, Springfield, Mass, 2010, Author. Accessed February 16, 2010, from www.webster.com.
2. U.S. Department of Health and Human Services: *2008 Physical Activity Guidelines for Americans*, Washington, DC, 2008, U.S. Government Printing Office. Accessed February 16, 2010, from http://healthierus.gov.
3. U.S. Department of Health and Human Services, Public Health Service: *Healthy People 2010*, ed 2, Washington, DC, 2000, U.S. Government Printing Office, Accessed February 16, 2010, from http://healthypeople.gov.
4. Henwood TR, Taaffe DR: Strength versus muscle power-specific resistance training in community-dwelling older adults, *J Gerontol A Biol Sci Med Sci* 63(1):83-91, 2008.
5. Lambert CP, et al: Macronutrient considerations for the sport of bodybuilding, *Sports Med* 34(5):317-327, 2004.
6. Simopoulos AP: Opening address: nutrition and fitness from the first Olympiad in 776 BC to 393 AD and the concept of positive health, *Am J Clin Nutr* 49(5 Suppl):921-926, 1989.
7. Institute of Medicine, Food and Nutrition Board: *Dietary DRI References: The essential guide to nutrient requirements*, Washington, DC, 2006, The National Academies Press.
8. Nutrition and athletic performance—Position of the American Dietetic Association, Dietitians of Canada, and the American College of Sports Medicine, *J Am Diet Assoc* 109:509-527, 2009.
9. American College of Sports Medicine: *American College of Sports Medicine offers guidance to athletes on preventing hyponatremia and dehydration during upcoming races* (news release), Indianapolis, 2005 (July 26), Author. Accessed May 1, 2006, from www.acsm.org/publications/newsreleases2005/HyponatremiaDehydration.htm.
10. Christensen E, Hansen O: Arbeitsfahigkeit and Ernahrung, *Skand Arch Physiol* 81:160-171, 1939.
11. Williams MH: *Nutrition for fitness and sport*, ed 9, New York, 2009, McGraw-Hill.
12. Gavin J: Pairing personality with activity: New tools for inspiring active lifestyles, *Phys Sportsmed* 32(12):17-24, 2004.

Management of Body Composition

All people—the fat, the thin, and the in between—can benefit by adopting attitudes and behaviors that over time should promote the body composition appropriate to each individual's genetic makeup and contribute to true wellness.

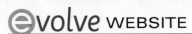 WEBSITE

http://evolve.elsevier.com/Grodner/foundations/

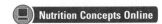 Nutrition Concepts Online

ROLE IN WELLNESS

What does weight or fatness mean to us as members of our contemporary culture? We step on the scale frequently, we read the numbers, and we often seem to get a message that extends beyond the simple mass of heaviness of our bodies. What message does the scale deliver? For some members of our culture, the figures on the scale convey something about their physical health. For others, the scale measures attractiveness. Sometimes it measures a sense of empowerment, of being in control of our lives. How can one simple assessment convey so many powerful interpretations? This chapter explores the meanings of weight or fatness in our contemporary culture and challenges these meanings and how they relate to wellness.

Because it is body fat that is really the issue, our focus is on fat rather than on weight. In addition, we use the approach of *management of body composition; specifically body fat levels,* rather than achievement of ideal body fatness. In this context, *management* is defined as the use of available resources to achieve a predetermined goal. This definition recognizes that individuals differ in the resources available to them and in the goals they set.

Consideration of the dimensions of health helps emphasize that managing body composition is more than just counting calories. Managing body composition levels by decreasing or increasing body fat or lean body mass is, if appropriate, an aspect of the *physical* dimension of health. Adequate levels of body fat allow the body to function most efficiently. The *intellectual* dimension of health provides the skills to understand and critique the role of society in molding our attitudes toward the shapes of our bodies. Regardless of body size, our *emotional* health depends on our developing positive self-esteem. The *social* dimension of health may not

be affected by body fat levels, although those at either extreme of body size may need to develop a circle of friends and family who accept their size differences. The *spiritual* dimension of health is sometimes tested as a belief in a higher being, providing support for some individuals struggling with behavior changes related to food consumption.

BODY COMPOSITION, BODY IMAGE, AND CULTURE

Body Image

The phrase *body image* refers to the perceptions we have of our bodies. Although body image can refer to the functioning of the body, most often it deals with our ideas, feelings, and experiences about the physical appearance or attractiveness of our bodies. Individuals have a distorted body image when their perceptions are inconsistent with reality. For example, most people with anorexia nervosa view their bodies as disgustingly fat when in fact they are emaciated. Body image is important because it may affect how we feel about ourselves and how we behave.

Body Perception

All of us have notions as to what makes a body attractive. Fortunately we all don't agree on some of the fine distinctions. In general, however, from where did our notions of attractiveness arise? Why do we think men should look strong and women soft? Many of our notions of attractiveness are so ingrained that we are unaware of them. Apparently, biology and culture interact to set the standards. It is probably this biologic influence that causes us to admire an appearance of strength in men and soft curves in women. Genetics also determines the potential for other characteristics of appearance, such as height, color of skin, shape of nose, and texture of hair.

However, within these biologically determined characteristics we make great distinctions as to what is attractive and desirable. At different times and places, humans have had widely differing notions of what constitutes an attractive man or woman. As far as fatness is concerned, a rotund figure has often been considered evidence of fertility and well-being. Prehistoric figures of women with massive breasts and hips have been unearthed all over Europe and are believed to have been symbols of good fortune and fertility. Over time, styles in attractiveness would come and go, sometimes favoring a full figure, other times favoring slenderness. Both fatness and thinness were viewed as unhealthy when carried to an extreme, but generally there was not a great deal of interest in weight.

As America entered the twentieth century, things changed. There developed a preference for slenderness that has not abated. Why this change in perception of attractiveness occurred and endured is not completely clear. Probably it was the coming together of several factors. These include concerns about the effects of an increasingly sedentary lifestyle, a heightened interest in fashion, the development of the medical profession, and increased knowledge of nutrition, as well as the self-interests of various promoters who saw profit to be gained by creating an anxiety about fatness.[1]

After World War II we entered an era of especially strong cultural influences. Mass media created a web of communication of a magnitude and efficiency that was never before possible. Now notions of attractiveness are shared quickly around the globe. Furthermore, sales promotion is a motive that underlies much of the communication. The outcome has been a view of beauty that homogenizes individual differences into a general sameness, decreeing the same size and shape for all.

Body Image: Illusions versus Reality

The effects of these conflicting cultural pressures are bewildering and, for some individuals, overwhelming. Physical attractiveness is narrowly defined as thinness and firmness and becomes, for some, the expression of personal worth. There follows an urgency to be sure one is thin enough. This concern is compelling for those fat and thin alike.

Most of us weigh ourselves regularly and have a good idea of our current weight. The figure on the scale, however, does not always agree with how fat we feel. Figure 10-1 shows an example of the type of instrument that investigators use to assess differences between actual, perceived, and preferred body size. The investigator instructs the subjects to mark the figure that is most like the way they feel at that time, as well as the figure that they consider ideal for themselves. When these figures are compared with an objective assessment, regardless of their actual size, the subjects usually have greatly overestimated their size.

Body Preferences: Gender Concerns

Investigators also use figure rating scales to determine how men and women differ in size preferences; they ask you which

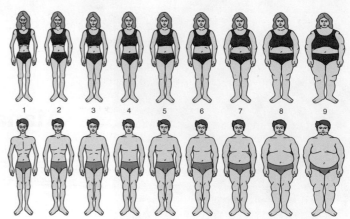

FIG 10-1 An example of a figure rating scale. (Modified from Stunkard AJ, Sorensen T, Schulsinger F: Use of the Danish adoption register for the study of obesity and thinness. In Kety SS: *Genetics of neurological and psychiatric disorders, ARNMD series,* vol 60, New York, 1983, Raven Press.)

figure is most like how you would like to be, which is most like how you currently are, and which you think is most attractive to the opposite sex. Ideally, the answers to these three questions would be closely clustered, indicating that you are fairly satisfied with your size. For men, that is usually the case. Women, however, on average consider themselves much fatter than they think is ideal. Originally it was assumed that the women's dissatisfaction represented a desire to appear more slender and, therefore, more attractive to men. Usually, however, women's personal ideal is thinner than the figure they think men would choose, challenging the assumption that women want to be thin to attract men. An alternative interpretation is that both men and women interpret a slender body as evidence of being in control of one's life.[2]

Body Acceptance: A Key to Wellness

Why is body image important? A negative body image may affect how we feel about ourselves generally: *body image* tends to become *self-image.* Furthermore, a negative body image may influence our health behaviors. We may feel defeated that because our bodies are so bad, it is not worth working hard to improve our health. At other times we may feel drawn to various kinds of risky behaviors in a frantic attempt to make our bodies more acceptable. We may strive mightily to meet the societal standards of attractiveness and thinness, but, given our individual genetic makeup, we cannot all succeed. Although humans have an awesome potential for growth and development, there are limits to the changes we can make and sustain in our body size and shape.[2]

If we have a healthy and positive body image, we evaluate various aspects of our bodies fairly realistically, finding some characteristics positive and others less so. Those we consider weak or unattractive, we accept in a dispassionate way, much the same way that we accept that we don't all have beautiful singing voices or the ability to throw a great curveball. We understand that our bodies have multiple aspects, that there is more to our bodies than their size and shape. Our healthy body image is influenced by our awareness of how our bodies

SOCIAL ISSUES
Dealing With Our Own Prejudices

We live in a world in which fat intolerance or fat phobia (fear of fat) is the last socially acceptable prejudice. "Fatism" even seems to have similarities with racism. As a society, we are committed to self-improvement. Consequently, it may feel wrong to question the directive that all those who deviate from the ideal size and shape should dedicate themselves to rectifying the situation. Our fat intolerance may be motivated by the best intentions to be helpful to ourselves and to others, but like all prejudices, it diminishes the people to whom it is applied.

This prejudice is especially problematic when it exists among health professionals. Obese people often report they feel degraded by their health care encounters and therefore avoid seeking medical help. The traditional medical model holds the patient responsible for the existence of a health problem; this moralistic philosophy tends to justify blaming the patient for choosing to be fat or thin. Although this prejudice could be expected to interfere with their effectiveness, health professionals seem to possess high levels of fat intolerance. Consider these facts from National Association to Advance Fat Acceptance (NAAFA):

Medical Professionals

In a study of 400 doctors, the following was found:
- One out of three listed obesity as a condition to which they respond negatively, ranked behind only *drug addiction, alcoholism, and mental illness.*
- Obesity was associated with *noncompliance, hostility, dishonesty, and poor hygiene.*
- Self-report studies show that doctors view obese patients as *lazy, lacking in self-control, noncompliant, unintelligent, weak-willed, and dishonest.*
- Psychologists ascribe more pathology, more negative and severe symptoms, and worse prognosis to obese patients

compared with thinner patients presenting identical psychological profiles.

In a survey of 2449 overweight and obese women, the following was found:
- 69% experienced bias from doctors.
- 52% experienced recurring incidents of bias.

In one survey of nurses, the following was found:
- 31% said they would prefer not to care for obese patients.
- 24% said that obese patients "repulsed them."
- 12% said they would prefer not to touch obese patients.

Consequences
- Avoidance of proper care
- Reluctant to seek medical care
- Cancellation or delay of medical appointments
- Delay important preventative health care
- Doctors seeing overweight patients:
  Spend less time with patient
  Engage in less discussion
  Show reluctance to perform preventive health screenings (i.e., pelvic exams, cancer screenings, mammograms)
  Do less intervention
- Appropriate-sized medical equipment not available:
  Stretchers
  MRIs
  Blood pressure cuffs
  Patient gowns
  Etc.

What about you? Have you been successful in questioning and replacing your own prejudices? Are you able to accept yourself and your body? As a future health professional, are you prepared to empower your patients to work toward total wellness, including the Health At Every Size (HAES) philosophy and habits?

Data from NAAFA: *Healthcare*, 2009. Accessed February 23, 2010, from www.naafaonline.com/dev2/the_issues/health.html.

function and how they look. This image affects and is affected by socio-demographic factors. Body image satisfaction may be related to the degree of overweight and to psychologic distress represented by depression and low self-esteem.[3] Understanding and accepting what we can and cannot expect to achieve in pursuit of the ideal body is a key to wellness. Only with this understanding can we establish goals to guide our behaviors toward health (see the *Social Issues* box, Dealing With Our Own Prejudices).

MANAGEMENT OF BODY FAT COMPOSITION

If we say that individuals must choose their own values and goals, it is impossible to state one goal for everyone. Nevertheless, we can identify some probable commonalities. Surely most of us would define a goal of maximizing the quality and length of our lives. We probably can go further and say that our goal is to achieve the best possible health, including emotional, social, intellectual, physical, and spiritual aspects. This chapter proceeds on the premise that we can agree on some version of this goal. Most of us would also agree that too little

and too much fat are likely to compromise physical health. In addition, we assume that the relationship between fatness and well-being is limited. That is, being slender does not guarantee happiness and health in all its aspects, nor is being heavy a sentence of unhappiness and illness.

Association of Body Fatness with Health
Physical Health

Most of our evidence of the association between fatness and physical health comes from epidemiologic studies. Epidemiologic research investigates the distribution of disease in a population and seeks to explain associations between causative factors and the disease. This type of research usually involves thousands of subjects and may be longitudinal (i.e., involving observations over a number of years). Because it is not practical to measure fatness in these large studies, weight is usually measured instead. Weight is most meaningful when considered in relationship to height. A convenient way to determine fatness is to calculate body mass index (BMI), a value derived by dividing one's weight in

TABLE 10-1   BODY MASS INDEX TABLE

	NORMAL						OVERWEIGHT					OBESE					
BMI	19	20	21	22	23	24	25	26	27	28	29	30	31	32	33	34	35
Height (Inches)	Body Weight (Pounds)																
58	91	96	100	105	110	115	119	124	129	134	138	143	148	153	158	162	167
59	94	99	104	109	114	119	124	128	133	138	143	148	153	158	163	168	173
60	97	102	107	112	118	123	128	133	138	143	148	153	158	163	168	174	179
61	100	106	111	116	122	127	132	137	143	148	153	158	164	169	174	180	185
62	104	109	115	120	126	131	136	142	147	153	158	164	169	175	180	186	191
63	107	113	118	124	130	135	141	146	152	158	163	169	175	180	186	191	197
64	110	116	122	128	134	140	145	151	157	163	169	174	180	186	192	197	204
65	114	120	126	132	138	144	150	156	162	168	174	180	186	192	198	204	210
66	118	124	130	136	142	148	155	161	167	173	179	186	192	198	204	210	216
67	121	127	134	140	146	153	159	166	172	178	185	191	198	204	211	217	223
68	125	131	138	144	151	158	164	171	177	184	190	197	203	210	216	223	230
69	128	135	142	149	155	162	169	176	182	189	196	203	209	216	223	230	236
70	132	139	146	153	160	167	174	181	188	195	202	209	216	222	229	236	243
71	135	143	150	157	165	172	179	186	193	200	208	215	222	229	236	243	250
72	140	147	154	162	169	177	184	191	199	206	213	221	228	235	242	250	258
73	144	151	159	166	174	182	189	197	204	212	219	227	235	242	250	257	265
74	148	155	163	171	179	186	194	202	210	218	225	233	241	249	256	264	272
75	152	160	168	176	184	192	200	208	216	224	232	240	248	256	264	272	279
76	156	164	172	180	189	197	205	213	221	230	238	246	254	263	271	279	287

Data from Clinical guidelines on the identification, evaluation, and treatment of overweight and obesity in adults: The evidence report. From National Institutes of Health: *Aim for a healthy weight*, NIH Pub. No. 05-5213, Bethesda, Md, 2005 (August), U.S. Department of Health and Human Services.

kilograms by the square of one's height in meters (Table 10-1). This formula for BMI results in a value that correlates well with body fatness.

If we were to plot the findings of epidemiologic studies of the association of BMI and the risk of certain diseases or mortality from all causes, we would usually produce a U-shaped curve such as that shown in Figure 10-2.[4] This curve means that individuals at both extremes of fatness—those very thin and those very fat—are at increased risk. Those at a more moderate fatness level have the lowest risk for the four leading causes of death in the United States: heart disease, some types of cancer, stroke, and diabetes. It is a surprise to many people that the low end of the fatness range, or underweight, shows an increased risk, which provides strong evidence that one can be too thin.

It is possible that the lowest BMI in these types of curves reflects low levels not of fat but of the lean body components.[4] The higher risks at the low BMI levels probably reflect some degree of body wasting, including lean body mass, possibly caused by smoking or the effects of disease. To understand the effect of fat on mortality, we need to measure body composition (fat and lean) and not rely on weight alone. Although the factors contributing to this increased risk of extremely low weight are not completely clear, they are thought to differ from the factors associated with increased risk of heavy individuals.

Physically disabled individuals are at greater risk for obesity because of physical inactivity, muscle atrophy, and

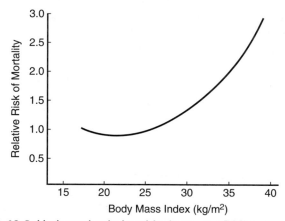

FIG 10-2 U-shaped relationship between BMI to excess mortality in adults. Relative risk was defined as 1 for adults with BMIs between 20 and 25. (From Stipanuk MH: *Biochemical, physiological, & molecular aspects of human nutrition*, Philadelphia, 2006, Saunders.)

metabolic energy alterations. Strategies implemented to prevent weight gain support all dimensions of health.

Obesity and Physical Health

Because we have far more fat people in this country than thin ones, let's consider first the impact of excess fat or obesity on physical health. Obesity can be defined as excessive fatness. More quantitative definitions traditionally used in medicine and the popular press are that weights greater than 110% of desirable weight equal overweight and weights greater than 120% of desirable weight equal obesity. These definitions assume a precision in interpreting risks of fatness that is simply not available. Use of BMI provides another tool for providing a quick assessment of weight in relationship to height. But, as will be discussed, BMI does not account for distribution of body fat, nor is it accurate for muscular individuals.

As research has extended beyond merely relating BMI to mortality risk, we have become aware that, between extreme emaciation and great obesity, just knowing how fat a person is doesn't tell us much about their health. If we consider how the body fat is distributed, we can improve our understanding. Without knowing the individual's total fatness or BMI, we can still make fat-mediated predictions about health risk. Higher levels of body fat around the waist seem to be more dangerous than fat in the buttocks and thighs. Fat located in the abdominal area is called visceral fat and seems to be especially related to risk. People with high levels of visceral fat are prone to a cluster of metabolic risk factors, including high blood pressure (hypertension of ≥130/85 mm Hg); low level high-density lipoproteins (men <40 mg/dL; women <50 mg/dL); elevated triglycerides (≥150 mg/dL); and impaired fasting glucose.[5] When three or more of these criteria are present, the condition is referred to as the *metabolic syndrome*.[5]

The metabolic syndrome, apparently the result of complex endocrine interactions, increases the risk of atherosclerosis, heart disease, stroke, and diabetes mellitus. Diabetes mellitus is characterized by inadequate insulin activity. In the metabolic syndrome, levels of insulin are usually normal or even elevated, but obese people have developed a resistance to their own insulin. Although they have high levels of this hormone in their blood, the insulin fails to control blood glucose levels. As a result, type 2 diabetes mellitus (DM) may develop. Type 2 DM is the most common type and is highly, but not exclusively, associated with obesity.

Obesity also increases the risk of health conditions that affect well-being but aren't usually life threatening. Examples include menstrual irregularities, infertility, gallbladder disease, and some types of arthritis. Table 10-2 lists health issues for which obesity increases risk.

Bear in mind that obesity does not increase all types of health risks (see the *Health Debate* box, Is Obesity a Chronic Disease?). In fact, risks of some types of cancer and of osteoporosis are lower, and risks of other conditions (e.g., infectious diseases, chronic lung disease, liver disease, injuries) are no higher among obese people than the general population.

Unanswered questions. Up to this point we have shown some convincing evidence that obesity compromises physical health. However, to get a balanced perspective, we must consider some important issues and unanswered questions. First, we must recognize that most studies show considerable variability in the effect of fatness on health. Three factors identified that may be involved in the variability are fat distribution, age, and sex. Even considering these factors, however, there

TABLE 10-2	POTENTIAL HEALTH CONCERNS ASSOCIATED WITH OR AT GREATER RISK FOR OBESE INDIVIDUALS

Cancer
Colon cancer
Endometrial cancer
Esophageal cancer
Gallbladder cancer
Kidney cancer
Postmenopausal breast cancer

Metabolic Disease
Cardiovascular disease
Hyperlipidemia
Hypertension
Nonalcoholic fatty liver
Stroke
Type 2 diabetes

Reproductive Disorders
Birth defects
Cesarean section
Fetal macrosomia
Infertility
Maternal death
Miscarriage
Preeclampsia
Stillbirth

Other
Asthma
Depression
Osteoarthritis
Sleep apnea

Adapted from Table 1.3, p. 35, Power ML, Schulkin J: *The evolution of obesity*, Baltimore, MD, 2009, The Johns Hopkins University Press.

is still a lot of variability in risk. For example, it is widely agreed that obesity increases the risk of developing type 2 DM, but little consideration is given to the fact that most obese adults do not develop diabetes.

What accounts for this variability? Why is obesity more of a risk to young adults than to older ones? How do risks differ between men and women? Most large-scale studies of risk have included whites living in the United States or Canada as subjects. What about risks of other ethnic groups? The limited information available indicates that racial and ethnic factors may be important. In addition, why is it that in recent decades Americans have gotten fatter, yet rates of mortality caused by heart disease have dropped significantly? As scientists sort out the various genetic influences on fatness and on vulnerability to various diseases, many of these questions will be answered (see the *Cultural Considerations* box, Globesity).

Does losing weight make health risks go away? And what about weight gain? We don't have strong evidence that weight

◑ HEALTH DEBATE
Is Obesity a Chronic Disease?

Is obesity a chronic disease? Or do some people simply weigh more than others? And if the latter is true, is health possible at any size? There are social and medical implications of both positions.

The basis of obesity as a chronic disease is its association with illness and death from other diseases such as hypertension, coronary artery disease, and diabetes. To qualify as a chronic disease, the disorder must be of slow onset, continue over a long period, may reoccur, and have symptoms affecting the whole body. If obesity becomes medicalized—recognized as a chronic disease—there can be reimbursement by health insurance companies for treatment and additional funds for research. At this time, obesity treatment, if prescribed by a primary health care provider, may be reimbursed. Treatment generally continues to be of the associative disorders rather than directly of the excessive body weight.

The flip side of the medicalization of obesity is whether it is possible to be "healthy" and "fit" at any size or body weight. If health determinants other than weight are used to assess health, then it is possible. Criteria of physical fitness, normal range blood lipid, blood cholesterol, blood glucose, and blood pressure readings and the absence of weight-associated diseases may provide more health than continual weight loss regimens. The physical and psychologic stress of attempting weight loss among individuals who are healthy based on the above criteria may be more harmful than remaining at a higher, though stable, weight. Over the course of time, attempts to lose weight often result in the cycle of weight loss/weight gain or yo-yo dieting, which increases body weight. The goal of weight management is good health achieved through stable weight. For many, it is more realistic to realize the benefits of good health at higher than average weights than to be unhealthy struggling with inadequate dietary intakes in addition to the other negative behaviors and effects associated with weight loss dieting.

What do you think? Should obesity be considered a chronic disease or can health be achieved at every size?

⊕ CULTURAL CONSIDERATIONS
Globesity

More than 300 million adults are obese, while another billion are overweight. Each year about 2.6 million people die from disorders related to being overweight or obese. Globesity, the spread of rising obesity levels throughout the world, seems to be centered on globalization and development tied to poverty. Hunger and malnutrition are no longer leading contributors to mortality; particularly in Latin America, obesity has joined the list. This may be partly due to "nutrition transition" in which traditional local foods and preparation styles are being replaced by highly processed foods that tend to be higher in calories, fat, and sodium and deficient in fiber, iron, and vitamin A—in essence "bad" nutrition or malnutrition.

Another potential factor of globesity is level of development and economy of regions. When incomes rise in poorer countries, people often gain weight and become fatter because more food can be purchased. In developed and transitional economies, greater income is associated with lower body weights. Why are poverty and overweight tied together? Studies show that short stature and growth stunting because of fetal and early life malnutrition are related to obesity in adulthood. It's as if the body is trying to catch up for early damages but cannot be satisfied. In addition, cultural views may represent excess body fat as prosperity to some minority and socioeconomic subgroups. The family has enough wealth to afford sufficient amounts of food to eat well enough to the point of fatness. Higher-educated socioeconomic subgroups, with knowledge of health risk factors, tend not to view overweight in this manner.

Regardless of the cultural and economic reasons that fuel globesity, the health costs of obesity-related disorders are the same, including type 2 diabetes mellitus (DM), coronary artery disease, hypertension, and certain cancers. Developing countries still struggling with the ravages of undernutrition will struggle even more attempting to deal with disorders of overnutrition.

Application to nursing: As we work with populations from varying cultural, economic, and global perspectives, we can be aware that values of excess body fat may have different meanings to others. We may need to initiate discussions about prosperity and the notion of healthy body weight management as being economically "very valuable."

Data from Eberwine D: Globesity: The crisis of growing proportions, *Perspect Health* 7(3):6-11, 2002; World Health Organization: *10 facts on obesity*, February 2010. Accessed on February 23, 2010, from http://www.who.int/features/factfiles/obesity/facts/en/index1.html.

---

loss reduces health risk. The literature is mixed about the long-term health effects of weight loss; some epidemiologic studies show increased risks following weight loss, whereas others show no effect or a diminished risk.[6] Important factors seem to be whether the weight was lost in response to a voluntary effort, the health condition of the person initially, and the pattern of weight changes (many gains and losses, one sustained loss, or other patterns).

Most epidemiologic studies include only initial weight, final weight, and mortality. This level of evidence is inadequate to illustrate the effect of sustained weight changes. One of the studies attempting to provide the needed information is the Nurses' Health Study, which has monitored for 20 years the health of more than 100,000 female nurses. This study shows that nurses who gained 22 pounds or more after the age of 18 had increased mortality risk in middle age.[7]

Chronic dieting and risk. One issue of contemporary concern is the effect of repeated or chronic dieting on risk. Given our cultural concern about fatness and the extremely limited success of most weight-loss attempts, there is a high likelihood that an overweight or obese adult will have tried to lose weight many times. Is it possible that some of the observed negative effects of obesity are really the outcomes of a lifetime of unsuccessful dieting? Although animal studies and some limited observations of humans support this hypothesis, reviews of the evidence conclude the risks were

A Work in Progress

Sometimes it seems as though I've been on a diet all my life, although I can trace my relationship with my weight back to one crucial day during the year I was 8. My father, having noticed that my 12-year-old brother and I were both approaching the top of our age-weight range, decided to take us to a nutritionist. I am sure that she was nice, but all I remember from the meeting was a deep sense of shame rising up from inside me and a chart that hung on our fridge listing the caloric content of common foods. The idea was that my brother and I were to monitor our eating and keep our daily intake between 1200 and 1800 calories. Although I'm sure he had only the best intentions, to this day I'm not sure what my father expected. Thus began my first diet.

During those awkward middle years, I developed a skewed image of myself. I chose to hear only the teasing and none of the praise and began to believe I would be chubby forever. The summer before my freshman year of high school, I discovered the world of sports, however. In order to try out for the field hockey team, I had to be able to run 3 miles. The coach passed out a training guide to those who signed up, and I followed it to the letter. On the first day of tryouts, I found myself keeping pace alongside the team captain, and my baby fat soon disappeared.

But although I was healthy and in shape, I still obsessed about my weight. Over the next 4 years, I became bulimic. When that didn't work, I would put myself on a regimen of 1000 calories a day, even during field hockey season. I developed irritable-bowel syndrome due to the stress I was placing on my body. When I graduated from high school, I weighed 125 pounds, right in the middle of the recommended weight range for my age, gender, and height. Yet I still saw myself as fat.

During college little changed. I was learning about other aspects of my identity, developing my skills and receiving praise for my talents. I exercised regularly and avoided the "freshman 15." Yet when I looked around at the tall, waiflike young women on my campus, I could not shake my insecurities.

During my junior year of college, I went abroad to Spain. I immersed myself in a culture of home-cooked meals, walking, and late nights. There I dropped below 120 pounds for the first time in my life. I wore a size 4 by the time I left, and I was happy with my body. When I returned home, the attention I received for my new figure boosted my confidence even more. Back in New York City my senior year, I spent thousands of dollars on new clothes. But deep down inside, nothing had changed. Those same anxieties were lying buried, waiting for the opportunity to emerge again. When I look at pictures of myself from that time, I am both scared and in awe of the person I see. Behind the shining surface there is nothing but darkness.

Immediately after college I entered a fast-track program for new teachers in the New York City public school system. My first year teaching was exhausting, both physically and emotionally. I was usually broke, and on my third day of teaching, the World Trade Center was attacked. I could see the smoke from the Twin Towers from my bedroom window in Brooklyn. I gained almost 20 pounds in 10 months.

Over the next 4 years my weight increased steadily until, a year before my wedding, I realized I weighed almost 160 pounds. It was then that I turned to a well-respected weight loss program. Since the thought alone of attending meetings embarrassed me, I signed up online. The first time around, it didn't work for me, but I returned. And through the program, I was forced to be aware of what I ate. More important, I learned portion control. I now consider myself a lifetime member.

I have come to see my body as a work in progress. I don't measure my self-worth based on the numbers on a scale, but I do place a great deal of importance on my health. My struggle with my weight is a part of who I am, but it does not define me. My goal is no longer to fit some idea of who I ought to be, but to feel like my true self: healthy and happy in my skin.

Judith Zaft Grodner
Montclair, New Jersey

not strong enough to justify discouraging people from making repeated attempts to lose weight[6] (see the *Personal Perspectives* box, A Work in Progress).

Obesity and Emotional/Social Health

For many years investigators have searched for a psychopathology that would fit most obese people and would help explain their fatness. Their efforts failed, for although a minority of overweight people suffer from a variety of mental health problems, no set of psychologic problems typical of obesity has been identified.[8] Our culture's extreme stigma against fatness extracts a tremendous toll on people who are obese. Social, economic, and other types of discrimination against obese people are widely practiced. This may lead to impaired self-image and feelings of inferiority, which in turn may contribute to social isolation and depression.

Some people feel so guilty about their fatness that they hide away and put their lives on hold until they can achieve slenderness.

Other people (both obese and slender) who are concerned about their weights develop a characteristic known as *restrained eating*. Restrained eaters try to use willpower to restrict their eating to a level below their natural **appetite** (desire for food). Their restraint is susceptible to disruption by various disinhibitors, especially stress. When experiencing disinhibition, restrained eaters usually binge. The binge may be a response to the **hunger** (physiological need for food) denied for days or weeks. It may be guided by black-and-white thinking such as "If I can't be perfect, I might as well give up." Thus restrained eating makes management of body composition harder.

As is the case with threats to physical health, the psychosocial risks are not uniform. Many people who are obese feel good about themselves and lead active, productive lives with a variety of positive relationships with other people.[9]

Underweight and Physical Health

Although the number of individuals struggling with being underweight is a fraction of those concerned with being overweight, we still need to consider issues related to physical health and underweight. Underweight is defined as 15% to 20% below weight standards. BMIs of 18.5 or lower are considered underweight and are associated with illness and greater risk for mortality as BMI decreases further. The causes of underweight may include genetics, malabsorption of nutrients, metabolic disorders caused by wasting diseases such as cancer, extreme psychologic or emotional stress, excessive expenditure of energy in athletics, and/or voluntarily restricting dietary intake as in anorexia nervosa.[9]

Health problems may be associated with underweight if they are caused by undernutrition or disease. A medical and nutritional assessment should be conducted. These health problems may include malfunctioning of the adrenals, pituitary, thyroid, and gonads. Disruption of the menstrual cycle may also occur in addition to decreased immune system functions.[9] Extreme underweight caused by illness is called the *wasting syndrome* and is most often associated with human immunodeficiency virus (HIV) and acquired immunodeficiency syndrome (AIDS). This syndrome is discussed in Chapter 22.

In contrast, healthy underweight individuals may find their level of underweight is problematic and want to gain weight. Nutrition therapy can be beneficial for both categories—healthy underweight and underweight caused by illness—by providing an analysis of dietary intake patterns and by assisting with eating strategies to ensure regular meals and planned snacks to increase the overall kcal and nutrient intake.[9]

Strategies may include simple changes such as choosing juices and milk beverages over water, exercising to build lean body mass for physical and psychologic benefits, and individualizing eating plans to accommodate the foods most enjoyed.[9]

HEALTHY BODY FAT

Functions of Fat

Although we tend to think of body fat as something to be avoided, it serves a number of vital functions. As discussed in Chapter 5, we could not live without some body fat. For most people, the major portion of body fat is storage fat. A layer of this fat under our skin provides protection from extremes of environmental temperatures, and cushions of fat defend many internal organs against physical trauma. Storing fat provides an efficient means of stockpiling energy so we can endure moderate fasts. In addition to this storage fat, there is a small amount of fat that serves vital functions such as membrane integrity; this minimal amount of fat is termed *essential*. Although we must always allow for

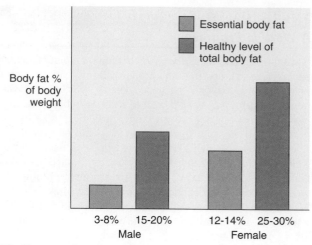

FIG 10-3 Male and female body fat levels. Essential body fat, minimum level of body fat for biologic functions; total body fat, range of level of body fat that provides for biologic functions but that does not have potential to negatively affect health. (From Rolin Graphics.)

individual differences, essential fat in men seems to be 3% to 8% of their body weight. When appropriate amounts of storage fat are added to essential fat for men, we derive a recommended range for total fat of 15% to 20% of body weight. In women the concept of essential fat must be expanded to include gender-specific fat in their breasts, pelvic region, and buttocks, which is apparently an evolutionary feature providing energy during childbearing and lactation. Thus for women the minimum levels of fatness compatible with health are based on the essential fat plus the gender-specific fat and are in the range of 12% to 14% of body weight; healthy levels of total fat range from 25% to 30% (Figure 10-3).

Sometimes athletes and dancers may strive for body fat levels below these ranges. There is concern that low body fat levels may be responsible for the menstrual irregularities experienced by many athletic women. Amenorrhea is associated with bone loss and increased risk of fractures. Early work indicated that most girls do not begin menstruation unless their bodies are at least 17% body fat and do not continue regular periods without 22% body fat. Modern methods of assessing body composition do not support these exact fatness levels as predictive of menstrual performance for all physically active women, but body fatness is considered an important factor. The fat level associated with the best athletic performance may not be the best level for all around long-term health. Working to achieve a lower percent body fat can be tempting; the desirability of doing this should be carefully assessed, considering the effect on strength, general health, menstruation, and other individual factors.

Body Fat Distribution

From both a health and an appearance perspective, it is not only the amount of fat but also its location that is important. Spend a few minutes at a popular swimming pool and notice the diverse patterns of fat distribution. Differences related to gender, age, and stage of development become apparent. Fat patterns may also vary among ethnic groups. These distinctions are genetically determined, and although the amount of exercise can affect the tone of the underlying muscle, it cannot change the pattern of distribution.

Imagine the various adult shapes seen at the swimming pool; try to classify them as either apples or pears. Apples (android body type) are biggest around the waist, and pears (gynoid type) are biggest in the hips, buttocks, and upper thighs. Although some evenly proportioned people will fit neither category, probably most of the pears are women and most of the apples are men and older women. Although this swimming pool visualization may seem frivolous, it focuses attention on the location of fat, which largely determines its effect on health. As discussed earlier, fat that is in the abdominal cavity seems to be much more dangerous than lower-body fat or fat under the skin in the abdominal area.

Although some sophisticated techniques accurately assess fat distribution patterns, a good estimate is possible by comparing waist circumference to that of hips (Figure 10-4).[10] For men it is healthier to have a waist-to-hip ratio of less than 0.95 to 1, whereas women should have a ratio of 0.8 or less. The diameter of your waist alone provides a good estimate of the fat in your abdominal area; waist measurements more than 40 inches for men and more than 35 inches for women are at greater risk for the various chronic diseases associated with obesity.[11]

The two types of fat distribution also differ in their rate of turnover, with visceral fat being much more easily lost and also more quickly regained than subcutaneous abdominal fat or lower-body fat. This is one of the factors contributing to men's apparent greater ease in losing and regaining fat. It is ironic that although the typical female fat pattern of lower-body obesity is more benign, women tend to be more concerned with their fatness than do men.

Body Fat Storage

Most of the fat in our bodies is stored in special cells called **adipocytes**. These cells have a nucleus, mitochondria, and other organelles just as other cells do, but as Figure 10-5 illustrates, these features are usually squeezed over to the side to make room for the droplet of stored fat.

The fat in this droplet is in the form of triglycerides, the same type of molecule making up most of the fat we eat. These triglycerides are synthesized from glucose, glycerol, fatty acids, and some amino acids that are carried to the adipocyte by the bloodstream. The stored fat is in a constant state of flux, with some triglycerides breaking down while others are built. The net effect of this flux—that is, how much fat is in storage—is the result of our energy balance at that time. If we need energy, the balance shifts to favor breakdown and release of fatty acids and glycerol to be transported to various cells, where they are oxidized or converted to other needed molecules. When we have a ready supply of energy, especially shortly after a meal, the balance tilts toward storage.

At birth most of us have relatively small numbers of adipocytes, but during the next few years, these cells increase in

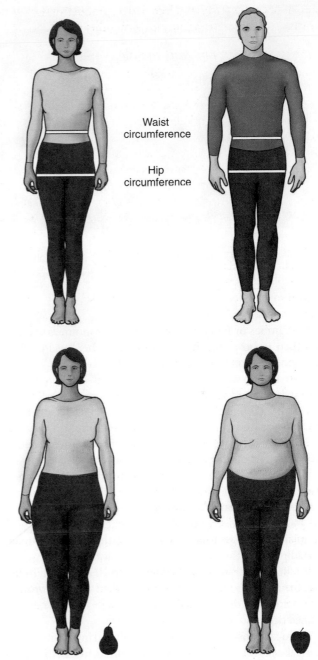

FIG 10-4 Apple (android) and pear (gynoid) body shapes. To estimate your fat distribution, measure the circumference of your waist and your hips. Divide your waist measurement by your hip measurement. You are an apple if you are a man and your waist-to-hip ratio is greater than 0.95 to 1 or if you are a woman and your waist-to-hip ratio is greater than 0.8. You are a pear if you are a woman and your waist-to-hip ratio is less than 0.8.

number (a type of growth known as **hyperplasia**) and in size (**hypertrophy**). Hypertrophy occurs whenever we continue in positive energy balance for any time. Hyperplasia, however, is more specialized, occurring during the growth spurts that accompany normal development. These growth-related times of hyperplasia occur during infancy, the preschool years, adolescence, and pregnancy. The adolescent increase

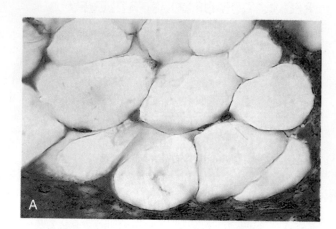
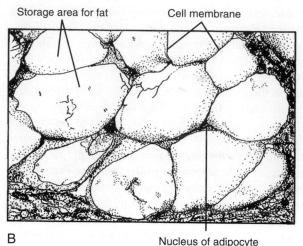

FIG 10-5 Filled adipocytes. **A,** Photomicrograph. **B,** Sketch of photomicrograph. Note the large storage spaces for fat inside the adipocytes. (A, From Ed Reschke; A and B In Thibodeau GA, Patton KT: *Anatomy & physiology,* ed 6, St Louis, 2007, Mosby.)

in the number of fat cells is much more pronounced among girls than in boys, and it results in the higher level of body fat normal for girls in comparison with boys.

Most evidence indicates that once these cells form the process of adipocyte hyperplasia, there is no natural means of reducing the number. Knowing there are predictable times of adipocyte hyperplasia, scientists once thought if we carefully controlled our energy balance during those critical periods, we would have lifetime insurance against becoming too fat. Unfortunately, we now know this is not true. If conditions are right, new adipocytes can form at any stage of life.

If more energy is consumed than expended, fat storage will go on until the fat droplet reaches its maximum size. If the positive energy balance continues, the body will make new adipocytes, thereby expanding the storage capacity. The stored fat is relatively equally divided, so all cells contain less than their maximum capacity. We are then able to continue to expand our storage capacity as long as the positive energy balance persists.

When fat is lost, whether through reduced intake, increased physical activity, or illness, fat is mobilized from adipocytes to meet energy needs. This reduces the size of the droplet of stored fat, producing a smaller adipocyte.

If we have been obese and then lose a lot of fat, our adipocytes may become quite tiny—smaller than the cells of people who were never fat. Our bodies seem to monitor the size of adipocytes, interpreting the shrunken cells as evidence of imminent starvation. We may then feel compelled to eat more. Although the response mechanisms are not fully understood, clearly the effects on metabolism and drive to eat developed as a means to reverse the threat of further loss. This set of responses is a major part of the theory of set point, discussed later in this chapter.

Measuring Body Fatness

Body weight is the most common way to estimate fatness. Weight is used even though our bodies are made up not only of fat but also bone, muscle, and other nonfat tissue known as *lean body mass.* Weighing works fairly well as a means to determine fatness because usually the lean body mass changes slowly. Therefore, we assume if the scale shows we are a pound heavier this week than we were last week, the change is caused by a gain of fat.

There are several situations in which weight is not a good measurement of fatness. One involves fluctuations in body fluid; fluid retention that occurs before menstruation or during hot weather may be interpreted as fat gain, and losses in a sauna may appear to be fat losses. In these circumstances, normalizing the fluid balance makes the apparent fat change promptly disappear. On the other hand, the scale is also misleading for anyone whose amount of lean body mass deviates from what is expected. A bodybuilder has a higher portion of lean body mass than the average person and thus will weigh more at the same height. Someone who suffers from a wasting disease has less lean tissue.

Because weighing is so convenient, it remains a useful assessment. However, if we really need to know how fat we are, we must resort to other means, which generally involve other measurements of the size of the body (anthropometric measurements) or assessments that distinguish between fat and other body components on the basis of their physical differences. Of the latter group, underwater weighing (**densitometry**) is the most widely accepted and is often used as a standard to assess the validity of other measures. Unfortunately, densitometry apparatus is bulky and expensive, and not everyone is willing or able to be submerged.

A practical alternative is **bioelectric impedance analysis (BIA)**, a method often offered at health fairs and health and fitness centers. This method uses electrodes placed at the wrists and ankles to monitor the ease of passage of a mild electrical current. Fat is a poor conductor of electricity; the conductivity occurs through the nonfat parts of the body. BIA actually estimates the amount of lean body mass, and then the amount of fat is calculated from the difference

BOX 10-1	BODY MASS INDEX CLASSIFICATIONS
<18.5	Underweight
18.5-24.9	Normal
25-29.9	Overweight
30-39.9	Obese
≥40	Extreme obesity

between the lean body mass and the total weight. BIA is safe, inexpensive, easily performed, and reasonably accurate, but it is not considered sensitive enough to detect day-to-day changes experienced by someone trying to gain or lose fat. Hydration levels, though, may affect accuracy of the BIA readings. Other methods of assessing fat level include triceps skinfold and mid–upper arm circumference (see Chapter 14), but likewise these are unable to detect day-to-day changes.

Interpreting Body Fatness Measures

To interpret fatness measures, we have to agree on some criteria. Because our focus is achieving wellness rather than current fashion standards, we direct our attention to health-related criteria. Before we consider various measurement systems, let us emphasize the importance of individual interpretations. All systems are based on averages; however, we're all aware that there is no average person. Consider these factors that affect our clients' and our own body configurations, our values, our personal and family health history, the fatness level at which we feel best, and what we find achievable. The systems we review should not be construed as iron-clad laws but merely guidelines (Box 10-1).

Interpreting Weight

A convenient way to interpret weight is to determine BMI. As mentioned earlier, BMI is calculated by dividing the weight in kilograms by the square of the height in meters. This yields a value that can be interpreted without further reference to height. BMI can be determined and related to the associated health risk by consulting Table 10-1. BMI levels apply equally well to men and women without adjustment. BMIs in the normal to lower overweight category are associated with the least health risks.[11] Although some controversy exists as to whether the standards should be increased with age, health risk evidence supports increasing the recommended range by one unit for each decade beyond 24 years.[4] Thus for people ages 25 to 34 years, the recommended range would be 20 to 25 BMI.

Bear in mind that although BMI is widely used and convenient, it is still a measure of weight and has all the shortcomings of using weight to estimate fat. When both weight and fat are measured on the same men and women, there are usually some individuals who have weight-to-height ratios considered normal but levels of body fat that are beyond what is recommended; they are normal weight to height but obese. On the other hand, there are other individuals who are overweight but not "overfat"; this group is most likely to include very physically active persons.

REGULATION OF BODY FAT LEVEL

Our bodies form fat as a way of storing energy between eating episodes. When excess energy is available, we synthesize triglycerides and store them in adipose cells. When we have a shortage of energy, those stored triglycerides break down and the energy stored in them is used. Thus the bottom line in adjustment of body fat levels is the status of the body's energy balance: when energy intake exceeds expenditure, we gain fat; when it is less than expenditure, we lose fat. Sounds simple, doesn't it? But in fact, it's not simple at all. Our bodies are much more complex than the teeter-totter that is often used to illustrate energy balance. Many factors affect the rate of energy intake and expenditure. We all are familiar with the concept that some cars get good gas mileage and others don't. Humans have many systems regulating the mileage we get from our food energy. The previous chapter explored some of these factors.

Changes in Body Fatness

Levels of body fatness change when a disequilibrium in energy balance is established and maintained for a period. A pound of body fat is roughly equivalent to 3500 kcal. Thus a cumulative positive balance of that magnitude should cause an estimated weight gain of 1 pound, whereas a negative balance of the same size should result in the loss of about a pound of fat. Recall that energy balance is determined by the relationship of the energy intake to the energy expenditure. The intake side of the equation is simple: it represents the kcal value of the food and drink consumed. The expenditure side is more complex, including the energy required just to keep the body going when at rest (resting energy expenditure, or REE), the energy cost of exercise, and the energy expenditures incurred by eating (called the *thermic effect of food* [TEF]). The levels of these expenditures are major factors in determining whether we will gain weight, lose weight, or stay the same weight on a given level of intake.

Chapter 9 considered how changes in one's physical activity change the energy balance, an important factor when trying to achieve healthy levels of fatness. In addition to the effect of physical activity, the rate of energy expenditure is affected by a number of factors that cause individuals to vary significantly in the efficiency of their energy use. Difference of REE may occur because of ethnicity. African Americans may have lower REE than whites. This may affect efforts to prevent childhood/adolescent obesity among this group.[12] Although factors affecting basal metabolic rate (BMR) and TEF are of interest, there is no safe and practical way to alter them. Nevertheless, understanding these influences helps us interpret what we see in the outcomes of the weight management efforts.

Genetic Influences on Body Size and Shape

Genetic effects on body weight are researched through family studies and investigations of specific genes and their mechanisms. The similarities of BMI among first-degree family members are best explained by genetic similarity. This

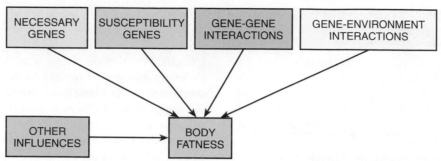

FIG 10-6 Genetic factors and causes affecting body fatness levels. (Modified from Bouchard C: Genetic factors and body weight regulation. In Dalton S, editor: *Overweight and weight management*, Gaithersburg, Md, 1997, Aspen.)

accounts for an increased risk of obesity for the first-degree relatives of obese individuals. Family studies reveal that obese children tend to be the offspring of obese parents. However, such studies cannot separate out the intermingled effects of natural genetic factors with those of the environment.[13] Adoptive studies, though, favor the effects of genetic over environment. The adult weight of adoptive children mostly resembles the BMI of their biologic parents rather than their adoptive parents. This tendency negates or lessens the effects of environment on weight.

Genetic influences related to obesity include the hormones leptin and ghrelin. Leptin, produced by adipocytes, has a role in the complex system of the regulation of body weight and fat regulation. Leptin inhibits food intake and regulates long-term appetite. The size of adipose stores is regulated through messages transmitted by leptin between the brain and leptin receptors. Mutations in functions of leptin and leptin receptors may have a role in the development of obesity. This association is more theoretical than diagnosable.[13] In addition, leptin has a role in supporting functions of the body requiring substantial amounts of energy such as reproduction and puberty. Leptin regulates these actions based on the adequacy of nutrient stores.[14]

Another hormone of interest is ghrelin, which is produced by the stomach and increases the appetite or food intake of humans (and rodents). When weight is lost, changes in appetite and energy use occur. Ghrelin, circulating in plasma, is part of the adaptive response of the body to weight loss by leading the body to regain lost weight. As such it acts as a long-term regulator of body weight. Consequently, depending on genetic predisposition, ghrelin may make maintaining weight loss harder—especially when the weight loss is through restrictive dieting. Its effect is less so when weight loss is through the severe gastric bypass surgical intervention (see p. 215), probably because the stomach, under that circumstance, produces less ghrelin.[15]

Studies of leptin and ghrelin are ongoing. Such studies significantly contribute to the understanding of the chemistry of appetite control and demonstrate that there are genetic factors associated with obesity. The work also serves to remind us that human fatness is complex, influenced by the interaction of many factors, both genetic and environmental.

The efforts of the scientists conducting these studies reveal that the role of genetics in fatness is complex. There is no single gene for human fatness or thinness. It is true that there are a couple of rare syndromes (e.g., Prader-Willi and Bardet-Biedl) in which obesity is clearly determined by a genetic factor that also produces mental retardation. In these rare cases, there is a gene necessary for the production of the syndrome. These genes are called *necessary genes;* the syndrome cannot occur in their absence. Otherwise, fatness must be considered a multifactorial phenotype; that is, the displayed characteristic (phenotype) is the product of numerous genetic and environmental factors. The main genetic influences come from susceptibility genes—genes that do not in themselves produce a certain characteristic but rather affect the susceptibility to other factors (Figure 10-6). Interactions between genes and gene-environmental influences as well as nongenetic influences complete the scheme of factors contributing to differences in fatness levels.

Regardless of one's genetic makeup, one's fatness is also influenced by nutritional, psychologic, economic, and social factors. In addition, there are many different types of obesity and thinness. When a family is characterized by a marked degree of fatness or thinness, casual observations are unable to distinguish between the effects of a shared environment, shared genetics, or both. By extensive study of large numbers of people, geneticists have learned that a significant amount of the influence on one's fatness (and characteristics such as metabolic efficiency contributing to fatness) is genetic. Somewhat more influence comes from cultural or environmental influences shared by a family, and the remaining influence is related to factors beyond the shared genes and shared environment within a family.

How would genes affect the amount and distribution of fat? Research suggests there is a strong genetic influence on certain components making up the energy balance equation: basal or resting metabolic rate, TEF, and the energy cost of light exercise (see Chapter 9). Investigators also found genetic influences on the ability to use ingested fat for energy, on taste preferences, and on the ability to achieve a high level of physical conditioning. These findings help explain why people differ in their ease of gaining or losing weight. Nevertheless, for almost every component studied, there were not only genetic but also environmental factors involved.

Although genetics plays a part in the level of body fatness, it is not the only factor. The extent of its influence probably varies from person to person.

Set Point and Body Fatness

Many of our body characteristics are regulated so they are maintained at a constant level or within a narrow range. This is true of body temperature, the level of glucose in our blood, blood pressure, the acidity of body fluids, and many other features. Departure from the usual levels of these variables is usually a clear indication that something is wrong. Usually when the problem is corrected, the characteristic returns to its usual level. This usual or natural level is called the set point. Actually, this term usually indicates not a single point but rather a narrow range defining the natural level for the characteristic. The adjustments our bodies make to return to the set point are called *defending the set point.* Thus we can define set point as a natural level (of some characteristic) that the body regulates or defends.

Because energy is a high priority for the body, the level of energy stores is not left to chance without regulation. Indeed, as described, the weight (and body fatness) of most adults is remarkably stable, returning to the usual level after minor gains and losses. In spite of minor gains over the years, this is true of fat and thin people alike.

For the most part, our adult weights are pretty constant. Something regulates them; there is evidence that we defend a set point. This regulation is skewed toward prevention of weight loss rather than avoidance of weight gain. Furthermore, it is clear that among adult humans there is quite a range of set points for body fatness.

Any theory describing set point mechanisms must be able to describe three components: (1) some characteristic that the body monitors, (2) some kind of messenger to carry the information to the central nervous system (CNS), and (3) some mechanism of response to exert the control. Evidence suggests that fatness, lean body mass, and body mass in general are all monitored.

Our major attention will be on the possible mechanisms of response, the actual regulation. The only options for exerting this control are (1) changing the amount of energy ingested, (2) changing the level of physical activity, or (3) changing the efficiency with which we use ingested and stored energy. These options are exercised through overlapping neural, endocrine, and metabolic mechanisms to exert both short- and long-term adjustments. Defending our bodies' fat stores is a matter of some complexity. Undoubtedly, this complex system with lots of checks and balances and backup schemes reflects the fact that energy is of prime importance to our survival.

The concept of a set point for body weight or composition is still controversial. Some of the controversy involves the question of set point versus set range. Other experts debate what characteristic (weight, fat, or lean body mass) is under regulation. Still others resist the concept because they feel it discourages individual responsibility for one's own health behaviors. The importance of these controversies is that they do not refute the basic concept.

Food Intake Adjustments

In discussing the regulation of food intake, one aspect of set point control was identified. When an individual's weight or fatness is below what the body perceives as appropriate, the drive to eat is activated. Although the person experiences short-term satiety, this long-term hunger drive apparently is maintained as long as the lower weight exists. Although an individual may learn to ignore this drive, there is no evidence it goes away. The individual is vulnerable to disinhibition, leading to potential excessive food intake or binge eating. It seems to take effort and attention to resist this hunger drive. People don't always have the psychologic energy to devote to this resistance.

Some people come back from a holiday or other situation during which they overate and gained weight, saying, "I ate so much then that I'm just not hungry now." Unfortunately, this type of hunger adjustment is rare. It is much more common for people to experience their usual degree of hunger and usual intake even after a period of overeating. The regulation system works poorly, if at all, in limiting food intake in this situation. Fortunately, the energy use efficiency part of regulation works somewhat better.

Adjustments in Energy Use

The body can adjust the efficiency of energy use in numerous ways; only a few are examined here. A fundamental mechanism of control is the rate of energy metabolism. This is implemented primarily in adjustments in the REE. The level of the TEF and the energy cost of a given amount of physical activity are probably affected as well. REE is a major component of total energy expenditure and usually accounts for at least half of total energy expenditure. Reducing food intake produces a prompt and significant depression in REE, which drops promptly and stays depressed throughout the period of lowered intake. If the reduction in intake is not too great, the drop in REE may be sufficient to prevent weight loss; this is a successful defense of set point. With greater dietary restriction, weight is lost, producing a departure from set point (at least temporarily). When weight is lost, there is less body to use energy; this also depresses REE. Thus these adjustments greatly slow the rate of weight loss. Most often the weight is then regained.

Figure 10-7 shows the total energy expenditure responses of obese and nonobese individuals who overate or dieted under carefully monitored conditions. When the individuals overate so they increased their body weight by 10%, their total energy expenditure was significantly increased. When they dieted so they lost the extra weight, their energy expenditure returned to the initial level. When the obese members of the group continued dieting until losses of 10% to 20% were achieved, their energy expenditure dropped well below the baseline level.

The energy effect occurs whenever food intake is reduced significantly—in dieters, in victims of disasters, in those

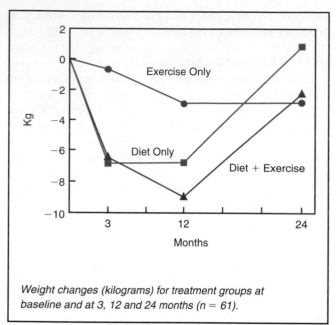

Weight changes (kilograms) for treatment groups at baseline and at 3, 12 and 24 months (n = 61).

FIG 10-7 Typical outcome of serious attempts to lose weight. (From Skender ML, et al: Comparison of 2-year weight loss trends in behavioral treatments of obesity: Diet, exercise, and combination interventions, *J Am Diet Assoc* 96:342-346, 1996, with permission from the American Dietetic Association.)

suffering from illness, in anyone whose food intake is reduced. There is some concern that yo-yo dieters, people who repeatedly diet and lose weight only to regain, may lose the ability to raise their REEs during the regain phase, making it harder to lose weight again and to maintain the loss. At this time there is not good evidence from research to demonstrate that this failure of REE recovery occurs.

Longer studies have shown that the REE and total energy expenditure stay depressed as long as the weight loss is maintained. This means that one's usual amount of food will go further than it did before. One will now gain weight on intakes that previously supported a steady weight. The body is fighting to preserve itself, defending its set point. Although the amount of the decrease in REE seems relatively small to have such an effect, the REE represents energy expenditure in every second of every day; it adds up fast.

Excursions into overeating trigger an increase in energy expenditure. In many people this increase is sufficient so they can overeat periodically without gaining weight. In that case the set point was successfully defended. On the other hand, there are limits to the ability to expand energy expenditure, and if overconsumption is sustained, weight gain usually occurs and the set point is reestablished at a higher level.

Total energy expenditure is also reduced when the level of physical activity is reduced. Restriction of food intake usually produces a reduction in the level of voluntary activity. This phenomenon was first observed in naturally occurring famines—the starved were seen to reduce their activity to the lowest possible level, moving only as absolutely necessary. This seems to be a natural way to conserve the limited energy

supply; it occurs whether the restriction is the product of a natural disaster or a self-imposed diet.

Determinants of Set Point Ranges

Are we born with our regulatory systems set for slenderness or fatness? Exactly what is it that determines set point? Definitive answers are not available yet, but here are some probable answers. Observations of weight histories suggest that set point ranges are mainly a matter of the body's adjustment to the maximum size or fatness achieved. The combination of each person's genetic makeup, cultural heritage, environmental experience, and voluntary behavior leads to the development of his or her adult body size and composition. The body seems to assess this size and composition and uses it to establish the set point.

This is easiest to understand in the case of adipocytes. Once formed, they are maintained for life. If their size becomes smaller than usual (because the person has lost fat), the body sets in motion the mechanisms previously described to refill the cells to their usual size. This means that set point can easily be adjusted upward. One's set point may be at a level of fatness that seems too high or too low. Clearly, set point weight or fatness is not synonymous with what we usually consider ideal or desirable levels.

Changing Set Point

The previous discussion shows that the set point regulatory mechanisms dampen the effects of conscious changes in eating and exercise. However, the set point effects also can be overridden by consistent changes in voluntary behaviors of eating and exercise. If these behaviors lead to a consistent positive energy balance, we gain fat and adjust our set points upward. Usually this seems to be a true change in set point; the new level of fatness becomes one that can be maintained without a great deal of effort.

Unfortunately, the situation related to a negative energy balance is not parallel. As shown, those rare enduring weight losses seem to be maintained only through continuing effort. A study illustrated the magnitude of the effort required by assessing the energy expenditures of women attempting to maintain weight they lost. Only those who had a high level of exercise were successful in sustaining their losses for 1 year; the amount of exercise these women performed was the equivalent of 80 minutes daily of moderate exercise, such as brisk walking, or 35 minutes daily of vigorous aerobic exercise.

Another investigation studied the food intake of people enrolled in the National Weight Control Registry.[11] To be included in this registry, a person must have maintained a weight loss of at least 30 pounds for a year or more. These successful maintainers report they continued to diet, with the women consuming an average of about 1300 kcal a day and the men slightly less than 1700 kcal. Both men and women ate very low levels of fat, approximately 24% of their kcal, and exercised on a regular basis, most daily. Achieving such low levels of fat intake requires constant attention to one's food choices. These studies are encouraging in that they show that some people are successful in altering their environment and in changing their habits so the effort required is manageable. On the other hand, the level of effort is significant and may explain why many people are unable to withstand the set point pressure.

Various pharmacologic substances that have been proposed to aid weight loss by reducing the appetite or increasing energy expenditure are sometimes described as having the ability to adjust the set point downward. These substances have only temporary effects. As soon as the medication is discontinued, the effect disappears and the set point forces are reestablished. Furthermore, some individuals find that the medication loses its effectiveness over time.

Scientists have looked for factors that would change set point by affecting the rate of breakdown or synthesis of storage fat in adipocytes. Many enzymes and other factors influence these processes, but the search for a factor that could be externally controlled without bodily harm has not been successful to date.

Set Point Is Not the Whole Story

This discussion of set point has focused on physiologic factors regulating fatness. As important as these factors are, we must not lose sight of the fact that one's level of fatness is influenced by environmental and psychosocial factors as well. In fact, because the physiologic influences are basically beyond our control, we usually focus on these other factors. Nevertheless, set point often helps us understand what is going on with our weights.

When Body Fatness Deviates from Usual

In spite of these various regulatory systems, our population includes many people whose fatness deviates from usual, resulting in obesity or emaciation. Obesity and emaciation have been tied to disordered eating, resulting in the development of clinically diagnosable eating disorders. Binge-eating disorder may result in obesity, whereas anorexia nervosa may lead to emaciation. Obesity and emaciation in these instances represent a continuum of disordered eating. The eating disorders of anorexia nervosa, bulimia nervosa, and binge-eating disorder are discussed in Chapter 12. This section considers deviation of body fatness not caused by eating disorders but from other determinants of health.

Incidence of Obesity

If someone asks, "What is the incidence of obesity or overweight in the United States?" the answer would depend on the definition of obesity and the age, gender, and ethnicity of those studied. If we use an obesity definition of BMI 27.3 for women or 27.8 for men (definitions that include not only those frankly obese but also those with mild obesity) and apply that definition to adult Americans in general, we find that roughly 33% of those older than 20 years of age meet the criterion.[16] This incidence of fatness represents a significant upturn in levels that had been relatively stable since 1960. Generally, more women than men are overweight, especially African American and Hispanic American

women. The incidence usually increases with age up to about age 50, and then levels off until age 60, then declines.[16] The higher incidence among ethnic minorities seems to reflect combined genetic and environmental influences. Generally, the incidence of obesity is inversely related to socioeconomic status.

Overweight among children is defined as BMI at or above the 95th percentile of the 2000 Centers for Disease Control and Prevention BMI-for-age growth charts.

It is especially alarming that the incidence of overweight among children and adolescents has increased sharply in recent decades. Within a 20-year period, overweight among American children aged 6 to 18 years increased from 6% to 16%. Significant racial and ethnic differences also developed. Larger percentages of African American and Mexican American children are overweight compared with white non-Hispanic children. At especially high risk of overweight are African American girls (23%) and Mexican American boys (27%).[17] A decade ago, there were no weight differences among adolescent boys aged 12 to 18 years; now there are significant differences. Presently, among American adolescents, overweight occurs among 15% of white non-Hispanic males, 20% of African American males, and 27% of Mexican American males.[17]

Compared with the prevalence of fatness among adults, these figures do not seem startling. However, these figures represent an increase of two- to threefold over the past 20 years. There is considerable ethnic influence of obesity among young people, roughly paralleling that found among adults in this country.[16] Significant portions of obese young people grow to be obese adults. Add to early-onset obese persons those who become obese as adults and it appears that the incidence will continue to increase. This increase of obesity is a worldwide phenomenon (refer to the *Cultural Considerations* box, Globesity).

Success of Attempts to Lose Weight

Ironically, during the time reflected in the statistics presented earlier, Americans were busily engaged in trying to lose weight, primarily through diet and exercise but also through surgery, jaw wiring, pills, hypnosis, acupuncture, sweating devices, and other systems. Actually, the number of people who describe themselves as being "on a diet" increased somewhat in the past 10 years or so. Since 180 million Americans regularly use low-calorie or sugar-free foods and beverages,[18] it becomes clear that restricting one's intake has become an accepted way of life. Unquestionably, a high level of weight loss activity occurs, yet the incidence of obesity continues at an all-time high.

Considering these facts, what is the success of weight loss attempts? Many of the commercial programs and products don't release data on the long-term effectiveness of their systems. None of those for which data are available produce significant weight losses that are sustained for more than a year in the majority of people who try them. If we ignore the downright fraudulent methods and consider only those systems designed to induce a negative calorie balance through reduced intake or increased activity, we find that although losing weight is not easy, maintenance is the real pitfall.[11]

The challenge to not only lose weight but to maintain the loss is even greater for those who are severely obese. Surgical intervention, specifically gastrointestinal surgery for obesity, also called bariatric surgery, is an alternative that continues to be an effective approach to providing long-term weight loss for those who are unable to lose weight through diet and exercise or have significant obesity-related disorders. Significant weight loss of 20% to 25% of body weight by 90% of patients occurs with successful surgery. Weight loss is maintained for more than 5 years by 50% to 80% of patients compared with only about 5% by other weight loss approaches.[11] All forms of bariatric surgery have disadvantages and risks;[19] the procedures are serious medical interventions.

Specific criteria to qualify for surgery include the following:[19]

- A body mass index (BMI) of 40 or more—about 100 pounds overweight for men and 80 pounds for women
- A BMI between 35 and 39.9 and a serious obesity-related health problem such as type 2 DM, heart disease, or severe sleep apnea (when breathing stops for short periods during sleep)
- An understanding of the operation and the lifestyle changes needed to be made

The procedures succeed by altering the digestive process, resulting in limiting food intake or combining limitation with malabsorption. Intake may be restricted by placing a band around the upper portion of the stomach (adjustable gastric banding) or a band with staples to form a small stomach pouch (vertical banded gastroplasty). To consume foods without nausea or discomfort, only $\frac{1}{2}$ to 1 cup of food can be eaten at one time, and even then the food needs to be of soft texture, moist, and chewed well. Combined procedures restricting intake and causing malabsorption include Roux-en-Y gastric bypass (RGB), which involves creating a small stomach pouch and attaching a section of the small intestine to the pouch, thereby reducing the amounts of calories and nutrients absorbed by the body.

Another more complicated procedure is the biliopancreatic diversion (BPD), which involves removing the lower portion of the stomach and connecting the remaining pouch directly to the final segment of the small intestine. Often a duodenal switch is formed that allows for additional nutrient absorption, reducing the nutrition deficiency risk that is common with BPD. The combined procedures ultimately lead to greater weight loss, providing quicker relief from obesity-related disorders such as type 2 DM, sleep apnea, and hypertension, but they have more risks during surgery and are more likely to cause nutritional deficiency from decreased nutrient absorption.

Patient acceptability for surgery should be based on an evaluation by a multidisciplinary team consisting of at least a physician, a psychiatrist, and a registered dietitian. The dietitian focuses on the assessment of weight history, food-related behaviors (such as binge-eating disorder), and efforts

related to weight loss. Lifestyle behaviors that may be barriers to acclimating to necessary changes after surgery need to be realistically discussed with the patient. Nutrition counseling support is important not only immediately following surgery but also for a substantial time afterward. Postoperative dietary intake for individuals with RGB is particularly important to prevent nutritional deficiencies that can lead to protein-calorie malnutrition and other nutrient deficiency related disorders. For all types of bariatric surgery, in order to maintain health, continue weight loss, and counter gaining weight back, appropriate food choices and portion sizes still need to be monitored, in addition to regular physical activity.

Surgical interventions are extreme and intended for the morbidly obese. The typical outcome of serious attempts to lose weight (without surgical intervention) is shown in Figure 10-7. In a group setting, these individuals followed a low-calorie diet, exercised, or did both for 3 months, and then did the same things on their own for another 9 months. Then they tried to maintain their losses more than a year, but at the end of this time their weights were not significantly different from when they started.

Repeat dieting. Do you know someone who diets repeatedly, never eats without feeling guilty, and yet remains fat? Dieting changes the act of eating from a simple, enjoyable process into something complicated and laden with guilt and other moral overtones. Hunger is interpreted as temptation, and responding to it becomes evidence of weakness or even sin. After repeatedly denying the call of hunger, most dieters lose touch with the sensations of hunger. Hunger becomes confused with being tired, bored, sad, or other feelings. Dieters rarely eat to satiety; they either force themselves to stop short of satisfaction or they become disinhibited and eat far beyond satiety. Their physiologic regulatory cues are completely tuned out. They usually develop two lists of foods: virtuous ones that they eat when they are being "good" and forbidden foods that are constant pitfalls. Rather than increasing the ability to regulate food intake to meet body needs, dieting makes this regulation more precarious.

Certainly one of the harmful aspects of repeat dieting is the sense of personal failure accompanying the almost inevitable weight gains. Dieters feel pressured not only by those with a commercial interest but also by health care professionals, friends, and family to try every new weight loss plan that comes along. Most plans do produce initial losses, and dieters are lured into thinking that significant and lasting losses are obtainable. Dieters ignore the powerful and automatic adjustments in metabolism and hunger driving weight loss triggers. Bodies naturally adjust to restore the lost fat. When the weight comes back, dieters may internalize the failure of their diets and suffer feelings of inadequacy spreading to other areas of their lives.

Gain/loss cycles are not benign. They may lead to nutritional inadequacies, confused food habits, loss of sensitivity to physiologic hunger cues, diminished self-confidence, and loss of self-esteem. Furthermore, as more data about the effect of weight changes become available, we may find that it exacerbates the health risks associated with obesity.

Time for Some New Approaches

This book takes a nontraditional stance regarding attempts to change body composition. Health care professionals who are convinced that diets (even the good ones) don't work have instead chosen to share an approach emphasizing acceptance of diversity in body size and shape and emphasizing not achieving an ideal body composition but instead promoting feelings of wellness, personal satisfaction, and well-being. It is our philosophy that except for acute medical conditions, it is inappropriate to give specific weight loss advice. This is an attitude shared by a number of health care professionals. Instead, all people—the fat, the thin, and the in-between—can benefit by adopting attitudes and behaviors that over time should promote the body composition appropriate to each individual's genetic makeup and contribute to true wellness. To emphasize the lifelong nature of this approach, we will refer to maintenance approaches rather than to efforts to change body composition.

DEVELOPING A PERSONAL APPROACH

Gain, Lose, or Maintain: A Wellness Approach

Although it is untrue that we can mold our bodies to any size or shape we desire, we do have the power to change our attitudes and behaviors if needed so that we can achieve satisfaction and wellness at the body composition most natural for each of us. This section describes some guidelines that are equally applicable to nurses and to their patients who are fat, thin, or just right. This concept is commonly referred to as a *nondiet approach.* All of the behaviors recommended focus on long-term changes. Those who adopt these attitudes and implement these behaviors can expect to feel more comfortable with their bodies and probably better about themselves in general. If we eat well and are physically active, we will look and feel good. Body fatness may or may not change. Although this approach may seem discouraging, the harmful and disheartening effects of diets and other programs that promise a lot but deliver only worse problems will be avoided. Appendix D, Kcal-Restricted Dietary Patterns, provides dietary procedures for those few people who have a serious health condition that justifies the risks of traditional weight-loss efforts (see also the *Health Debate* box, Can "Commercial" Diet Programs Teach Healthy Eating Habits?).

Establishing Realistic Goals

In setting goals, consider two almost opposing factors: (1) our unique and individual values, needs, and characteristics, and (2) the limits to the extent of control we have over our bodies and our level of fatness. It is fashionable to deny any limits to this control, but objective observation will reveal the fallacy in that thinking. Aspiring to total control is neither realistic nor healthy for most of us. In goal-setting we need to consider what is practically feasible.

Changing Behavior

The most important goals are those related to changes in behavior. By choosing appropriate behaviors for change, we can work toward establishing habits that will become almost self-sustaining. The behavioral goals should be related to each person's unique needs. For example, in examining his lifestyle, one person may discover that he is always out of food and running out to grab whatever he can find, usually pizza and convenience store items. He may try to establish a habit of planning and shopping for the next week every Sunday afternoon. For him, this behavior change automatically leads to better food choices. For a different person, this particular goal might be irrelevant.

The *Teaching Tool* box Principles of Behavior Change outlines basic principles of behavioral modification applicable to choosing appropriate changes. In recent decades it has become popular to make superficial use of the principles of behavioral change in weight loss programs. These techniques had limited success because they were presented as just a list of handy hints (e.g., eat on a smaller plate, put down the fork between bites) rather than the individualized system described in the box. Don't confuse these principles with those hints having little to do with the original concepts.

Normalizing Eating

The goal here is to reclaim eating as a comfortable and natural process. It involves being in tune with the needs of one's body and its signals about those needs.

Enjoying Eating

Normal eating should be enjoyable. Eating is a very sensual process and has the potential to be highly pleasant. Unfortunately, the ubiquitous dieting mentality dictates a love-hate relationship with food. We tend to label the foods we most love sinful and off-limits. Then we long for them and feel dissatisfied with the more ordinary foods we allow ourselves.

In normalizing eating we strive to retain the enjoyment of the process. This involves eating with awareness, relaxation, and without guilt, allowing ourselves to eat, in appropriate quantities, all the foods we enjoy. It may also involve expanding our pleasure by learning to enjoy a wider variety of foods.

Enjoyment can be enhanced by keeping meals and snacks simple enough that the true flavors of each item can be tasted. Not only do toppings, sauces, and the like usually involve the addition of extra sugars and fats, but they also obscure flavors.

In spite of all this emphasis on enjoyment, normal eating does not mean depending on food as a major source of pleasure. Just as drinking a tall, cold glass of water is a joy when we are thirsty (but is without appeal when we're not thirsty), eating should be a natural source of pleasure and not a preoccupation. We are not advocating that we all live to eat (Box 10-2).

Letting Hunger and Satiety Guide Eating

As discussed earlier, most of us guide our eating not only by physiologic cues to hunger and satiety but also by

HEALTH DEBATE

Can "Commercial" Diet Programs Teach Healthy Eating Habits?*

With the ever advancing epidemic of obesity in the United States, health professionals are constantly telling the American population, "Don't gain weight! Lose weight!" But at the same time the health professionals are also saying, "Don't go on a diet! Stay away from those dangerous fad diets advertised on television!" So what is the average person suppose to do? How do we expect nondietary experts to lose weight even while we health professionals struggle with our own weight control? Surely there must be some positive aspects of weight loss programs that we can use in our national "battle of the bulge."

This box presents discussion of healthy food aspects of programs like Weight Watchers—focusing on moderation and portion control; and intake of fruits, vegetables, and fiber—and the South Beach Diet—emphasizing whole grains and fruits and vegetables—as helping individuals to normalize eating patterns and food portions, *after* the first 2 weeks of deprivation! Perhaps we need to change our approach to using commercial diet programs. Let's consider how to customize a program whether online or through books. This applies to men and women.

Portion Sizes

Programs that either provide premeasured food *or* have no limit on portion sizes do us a disservice. After years of eating out of control or even just "eating" our usual servings, our portions may be just too large for our caloric needs. It is better to spend a few weeks with measuring cups learning that your favorite cereal bowl actually holds three servings of cereal, not just one.

Cooking Skills

Eating out may be convenient, but it is more nutritious and economical to cook simple meals. Some programs include easy-to-follow recipes that taste good to both dieters and nondieters. Because more families consist of busy two-career parents, and children have many extracurricular activities,

children may grow up without learning basic cooking skills. As young adults they can easily teach themselves by following simple directions. Better healthy eating programs provide recipes for novice cooks.

Personal and Time Management

Goal-oriented individuals succeed. They plan and follow through. These skills are woven into the higher-quality weight management programs. Planning ahead, shopping, and cooking for meals for the week involve time management skills. Consider if a week includes difficult social events involving food and how to cope with them; some programs are flexible enough to educate participants as to strategies for dealing with such situations.

Food Records

Food records or journaling has become an established means for keeping track of foods eaten. It is a diary of all that is consumed including portion sizes and time of day. Studies show more success occurs when written records are kept of food intake when attempting to normalize food consumption. There are now "blogs" or personal diaries online of individuals' food struggles that all can read. A person's food record may be part of an online program of a commercial weight loss program or may be a free program available on the Internet.

Food for Thought?

When a commercial weight loss program advertises that if we do exactly as the program states, we will lose weight, run the other way! A healthy eating plan to manage body weight should be customized to our individual needs. To achieve this, we must take personal responsibility for creating our own strategy for healthy eating.

What is your opinion? Is there a role for commercial weight loss programs? How would you advise your clients who need to manage their body weight?

*This discussion does not advocate the use of any named commercial diet program.

TEACHING TOOL

Principles of Behavior Change

Set a positive, specific, and achievable objective. It is helpful to frame a goal in terms of the exact behavior to be practiced. Objectives like "I want to eat better" or "I don't want to be so inactive" fail to give you any guidance about how to achieve them and what constitutes success. On the other hand, an objective such as eating vegetarian meals five times a week can orient you in a helpful direction right from the start. It is easier to replace a behavior with a new one than to just stop doing it. Break down major behaviors into smaller, less daunting parts, and try only a few changes at a time.

Establish a system for monitoring the behavior to be changed. This observation helps to assess success in changing the behavior and assists in determining what contributes to and detracts from mastery.

Modify the environment so that it supports the change. If you were trying to eat more vegetarian meals, for instance, it would be helpful if the environment included vegetarian cookbooks

and ingredients and opportunities to be with vegetarian friends.

Set up a plan for rewarding successes. Be sure to choose rewards that will be appreciated but are appropriate to the magnitude of the achievement. The reward should be as immediate as possible. Long-range rewards can seem immediate by awarding points toward the reward.

Recruit support from friends and family. These people may want to be helpful but may not be skilled at it. Tell them of your objectives and how they can help, but do not make them responsible for personal behaviors.

Allow enough time for a new behavior to become a habit. A simple new behavior like taking smaller bites practiced faithfully for 3 weeks, should be well on the way to becoming habit. More complex lifestyle behaviors take much longer to change, usually at least 4 months. Under stress, most of us revert to old habits, so have a plan for how to deal with this.

BOX 10-2 MYPLATE: WEIGHT MANAGEMENT

The MyPlate food guidance system can also be used for weight management. Several tools of MyPlate can be used to supervise our own energy in/out equation to maintain, lose, or gain weight depending on our individual health needs. These tools are available through www.MyPlate.gov.

Potential MyPlate Tools

- MyPlate Plan: a customized food guide providing recommended number of daily food group serving amounts based on an individual's age, gender, and activity level.
- Super Tracker: an online dietary and physical activity personal assessment tool providing information on diet quality, activity levels, nutrition information based on assessment, and links to related resources. The Food Calories/Energy Balance feature automatically determines energy balance by subtracting the energy expended from physical activity from food calories/energy consumed. Energy balance history can be saved for up to one year on the Super Tracker. The Tracker presents the components of the energy balance equation and allows the user to understand the relationship between good nutrition, regular physical activity, and weight management.

✴ TEACHING TOOL

Mindless Eating Revealed

Based on years of studying the psychology of our food choices and quantities consumed, Dr. Wansink, Cornell University professor of psychology, food marketing and nutrition, and director of the Cornell Food and Brand Lab, has revealed some of the cues and influences that govern our mindless consumption of calories. He notes that "The best diet is the one you don't know you are on." The mindful eating approach may be supportive when working with clients needing to improve their dietary intake. Dr. Wansink suggests that rather than trying to "eat right," try to "eat better."

Your Mindful Eating Plan

- **Your Mindless Margin.** By making 100- to 200-calorie changes in your daily intake, you feel deprived and backslide.
- **Mindless Better Eating.** Focus on reengineering small behaviors that will move you from mindless overeating to mindless better eating. Five common places to look (diet danger zones) include meals, snacks, parties, restaurants, and your desk or dashboard.
- **Mindful Reengineering.** To trim your mindless margin, you can use basic diet tips, but a more personalized approach is to use food trade-offs or food policies. Both give you a chance to eat some of what you want without making it a belabored decision.
- **The Power of Three.** Design three easy, doable changes that you can mindlessly make without much sacrifice.
- **Mindless Margin Checklist.** Use this daily checklist to help you move from mindless overeating to mindless better eating.

Data from Wansink B: *Mindless eating: Why we eat more than we think,* New York, 2006, Bantam Dell; www.MindlessEating.org.

environmental and cognitive factors. Of these three sets of stimuli, only the physiologic cues are triggered by the body's needs. Therefore, normalizing eating involves letting hunger and satiety guide eating. It means eating when hungry even if it is not a traditional mealtime, and it means stopping with the first signs of satiety even if there is still food on the plate.

Although it would seem that eating this way would be easy, trying to implement this advice is actually challenging. A person may fear that if the cognitive control tells us what we should be eating is relinquished, all control will be lost and huge amounts eaten. A few people actually do go through such a period—a pretty scary experience. Nevertheless, when they trust that they can eat again as soon as hunger dictates, most find they are no longer driven to continue eating such large quantities.

A great many people actually have a different problem: they have ignored their hunger/satiety cues for so long that they no longer sense them. Reversing this lack of awareness involves relearning how to feel and identify the body's signals for satiety. An individual can start this process by carefully noting feelings when several hours pass without eating. Then the person should interrupt a meal midway through it and examine body sensations for satiety cues. A few minutes will be needed to perceive the satiety. If there are no cues to satiety, eating should continue but be stopped again to assess satiety after a few more bites.

Most people are less aware of their satiety signals than of hunger cues. Eating slowly may enhance awareness of satiety. Keeping meals and snacks simple may help, too. Some research indicates there is a component of satiety tied to specific tastes: the greater the variety, the more food is required to reach satiety because each component is activated by the array of sensations. This may be responsible for eating behaviors at generous buffets. (See the *Teaching Tool* box Mindless Eating Revealed.)

Sensations of hunger are often confused with those of tiredness, anxiety, relief of anxiety, and other states. Distinguishing the difference may require work. It may be helpful to keep a journal of the various sensations observed.

Minimizing the Use of Food to Meet Emotional Needs

Probably all humans use food and eating to help them deal with emotions. We use food for expressing positive feelings, celebrating good fortune, rewarding hard work, and creating a sense of companionship. Eating as a means of handling negative emotions such as boredom, frustration, anger, or loneliness is especially problematic for many people. Compared with some other ways of responding to strong emotions, eating may be relatively benign, but when we rely on it as our main means of coping, our consumption patterns may have little or no relationship to our physiologic needs. This emotion-driven eating often is followed by feelings of guilt that may feed into the original negative feelings, creating a destructive cycle.

Minimizing emotional eating requires being aware of feelings and any associated eating. For personal understanding or as an adjunct to patient education, a journal or eating record can help achieve this awareness by monitoring feelings, hunger, and eating. Records kept for several weeks catch a range of moods. Examine the records from both the perspective of what triggered eating and of how the feelings were expressed or handled.

When we practice eating in response to hunger, we will probably use food less to meet emotional needs. However, if a pattern of eating in response to feelings rather than to hunger still occurs, or if we regularly use food to deal with certain emotions, we need to learn some alternative ways to respond to emotions. We can often be our own best resource for discovering alternative responses by using the records to identify coping behaviors that are already working and that can be used more often. Books are available that deal with making these kinds of changes. Counseling also can help.

Although we are probably never going to completely give up using food to meet emotional needs, it is worth considering how to do so effectively so that we may increase awareness of how food consumption and emotions are connected. The following guidelines may help:

- Be aware of the reasons behind food use. Verbalize the intended function of the food. Eat food slowly and with concentration.
- Eat without guilt. If this type of eating occurs only rarely, there is nothing about which to feel guilty.
- Arrange a safe circumstance for eating. If some rich, creamy chocolate is just the thing needed, that's fine. Have some, but make sure there is no danger of overdoing it. Buy just one piece, eat in public, or do whatever is necessary to ensure that a reasonable amount can be enjoyed without feeling at risk of bingeing.

Eating Regularly and Frequently

Our bodies have evolved so that we function best when we eat several times a day at times spaced throughout our waking hours. Unfortunately, our modern hurried lifestyle often makes eating balanced meals inconvenient. We tend to snack on what is handy early in the day and do most of our eating between 5 PM and bedtime. This pattern has several undesirable effects, as follows:

- It puts the greatest food intake at the least active time of day. This means that the energy ingested must be stored as fat to await use the next day. Because many individuals do not efficiently mobilize stored fat for energy, they probably feel sluggish and curtail their activity the next day.
- It may mean long stretches of time with little food. During these times we often find it too inconvenient to eat, and therefore we deny our hunger or stave it off with inadequate snacks. By late afternoon our hunger, now joined by tiredness and frustrations of school and work, overwhelms us, and we eat frantically, often far

more than we need. Thus this pattern runs counter to our goal of hunger-directed eating. Furthermore, with little or nothing to break the overnight fast, it's hard to get a good start in the morning.

- The quick meals or snacks we grab during the day usually are high in sodium and fat with little nutritive value.

There is nothing magical about three meals a day. Five may be better. Fewer than three results in long fasting times and may induce the problems described earlier. Whatever pattern works best, it should space food throughout active hours and should not produce overwhelming hunger or the drive to consume excessively. For most of us, how often we eat has to reflect the difficulties of providing ourselves with nourishing options throughout the day. Normalizing eating involves planning ahead to ensure that we don't get caught without any alternatives to chips and candy bars.

Adopting an Active Lifestyle

Does physical exercise help maintain a desirable body composition? The conclusions from research are contradictory and confusing. A lot of the confusion disappears when distinguishing between what is possible in a controlled laboratory experiment and what is probable in the reality of most people's lives. Although exercise is not a panacea, it is one of the few factors consistently associated with success in maintaining a healthy body composition.

Increase Energy Expenditure

Exercise is mechanical work that requires energy; it takes more energy to stand than to sit, to walk than to stand, and so on. Furthermore, vigorous exercise has the potential to increase the rate at which energy is used, even beyond the period of activity. However, for the level of exercise most people are able to accommodate in their lives, the daily effect on energy expenditure is in the range of a few hundred kcal. Most authorities believe that the beneficial health effects of exercise are far greater than can be accounted for by the direct effect on energy balance of these few hundred kcal.

Maintain Lean Body Mass

Many factors conspire to reduce our levels of lean body mass. These include aging, sedentary lifestyles, wasting caused by illness, and dieting. Exercise reduces the effect of these factors by increasing or maintaining the muscles of the body that directly affect lean body mass levels.

Improve Many Health Conditions

Exercise reduces a variety of risk factors for hypertension, coronary artery disease, and diabetes mellitus. These conditions are associated with increased obesity. Yet even without changes in body fat levels, exercise can decrease heart rate, reduce blood pressure, and improve the blood lipid profile.

Change Your Outlook

Practically every investigation studying people who are successful in long-term maintenance of a healthy body fatness level finds that exercise is an important factor. Its influence cannot be accounted for on the basis of a direct effect on energy balance because the amount of kcal used may not be high. Instead, exercise seems to help because it changes how people feel about themselves and about their ability to be in charge of their own lives. Regular, enjoyable exercise increases our awareness and level of comfort with our own body. It provides a good time for thinking and problem solving. It reinforces our commitment to wellness and increases the likelihood that other wellness behaviors will be maintained.

Differences in Responses to Exercise

When two friends exercise together regularly, but only one of them seems to be changing size, they probably have different responses to exercise. In a study of such differences, 31 obese women faithfully exercised for 90 minutes a day four or five times a week.[20] They didn't change their way of eating. After 6 months, two-thirds of the women had decreased levels of body fat, whereas the other women had increased levels. Both groups had improved cardiorespiratory fitness, carbohydrate metabolism, and blood lipid profiles. In addition, women in both groups deserved to feel proud of their accomplishments.

Differences in the response to exercise may be related to gender, fat distribution patterns, ability to exercise vigorously, and appetite response to exercise. Our bodies respond differently, and our level of fatness is a poor indicator of the beneficial effects of exercise.

Individualized Exercise

Most of the health benefits of exercise are maintained only as long as the exercise is continued regularly. Therefore, it is alarming that most people who start an exercise program drop out. Although many factors undoubtedly contribute to this picture, a major one involves attempting exercise that is too difficult for one's physical condition. This is especially true for older or heavier individuals. Driven by sayings such as "It doesn't count if it isn't aerobic," or "No pain, no gain," regimens may be attempted that are initially too demanding. The goal for health benefits is to do 30 minutes or so of aerobic exercise three or more times a week, preferably most days of the week. To develop fitness, at least 60 minutes a day tends to be needed. Time can be taken to work up to these levels. An exercise diary is a good way to monitor one's progress.

We are more likely to exercise if we have access to a variety of activities we enjoy, such as walking, swimming, biking, gardening, sports, or even housecleaning; there are many options.

OVERCOMING BARRIERS

Prospects for the Future

During our lifetime, will the day arrive when no one will have to worry about being too fat, too thin, or too displeasingly shaped? There are several avenues leading to such a future:

we could learn how to prevent deviations from healthy amounts and distributions of fat, we could learn how to effectively treat them, or we could become so accepting of individual differences that deviations were no longer defined as problems. All avenues will probably be important, but even when considered together, they will probably be insufficient to lead to such a future.

Alarming Trends

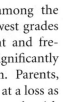

Surveys have revealed some alarming trends among the children of this country. Children in even the lowest grades of school are already obsessed with their weight and frequently place themselves on diets, yet there is a significantly increased incidence of obesity among children. Parents, teachers, and health care professionals usually feel at a loss as to how to deal with this combination, particularly as the risk of weight-associated disorders such as childhood type 2 DM increases. The instinctive response is to restrict the child's intake, but the evidence overwhelmingly indicates that this response only creates a terror of not getting enough to eat and contributes to a sense of being ugly and generally unacceptable.

It is not clear what has led to these trends among children, but many suspect that physical inactivity accompanied by a rather generalized passivity may be involved. Furthermore, children are not free of the cultural messages that equate slenderness with happiness—thus the practice of dieting early in life.

Americans want to be physically active, but they are working longer hours and spending more time getting to work or school. When the workday is over, concerns about the safety of our neighborhoods may keep us inside and inactive. It will be interesting to see how physical activity is affected by new communication technologies that make it possible for more people to work from home. As our country's demographics change, we will have more ethnic diversity. We know that there are major ethnic differences in the incidence of obesity and of eating disorders. However, what causes these differences is unclear, and we certainly are not prepared to deal with them at this time.

Multiple Etiologies Complicating Treatment and Prevention

"Coming Soon: A Drug to Cure Fatness." This title may appear in the tabloids, but the likelihood of a medication that could reverse all types of obesity (or emaciation) is unlikely because there are too many different causes. More than 40 different models of obesity have been demonstrated in laboratory animals.[21] Humans living in the real world are much more complex. Even within a single individual are numerous factors contributing to fatness level. At one time, doctors thought giving thyroid hormone would reverse all obesity, but experiences proved that only a small proportion of individuals were good candidates. Some people lost weight with thyroid treatments, only to regain in response to other factors. The administration of medications may be helpful in some situations, but a pharmaceutical cure-all is unlikely. Likewise, prevention efforts will have to be multifaceted to address all the factors involved.

Acceptance through Prevention Efforts

At this time, it seems prevention is our best hope for a better future concerning fatness. Effective prevention has to encourage behaviors that promote total wellness on a long-term basis. Experience is demonstrating that this requires people to view themselves as valuable and worthy of effort. The Vitality campaign mounted by the Canadian Ministry of National Health and Welfare is a good example of this approach.[22] Designed to promote healthy weights, the Vitality program urges Canadians to feel good about themselves, eat well, and be active (see Appendix B).

Although programs in the United States are generally more traditional in their pressure to lose weight, we have begun to see some changes. Some recommendations recognize that for the many people who are unable to achieve slenderness, a goal of a *healthier weight* is more realistic. A healthy weight may be viewed as a weight at which a person can physically move comfortably, maintain without undue restriction of food intake (but following healthy eating guidelines) or without excessive exercise, and live without experiencing any weight-related associative disorders such as diabetes, hypertension, coronary artery disease, or high blood lipid levels. If associative disorders do develop, lifestyle changes can be initiated to achieve a *healthier weight*. The definition of healthier weight involves a weight loss of 10 to 16 pounds accompanied by healthy lifestyle behaviors.

In response to increasing concerns about weight-related health disorders, similar concepts of healthier weight are being incorporated into many health promotion programs to change perspectives regarding healthy weight and management of body composition. These programs focus not on encouragement of dieting and weight loss but rather on prevention of obesity and promotion of healthy eating and exercise habits. Thus as more such programs are launched by government health departments, hospitals, and nonprofit health organizations, we may see that good prevention campaigns also lead toward greater acceptance of individual differences in body size, shape, and fatness (Box 10-3).

Role of Nurses

Approaches to weight and body composition management are being reformulated. Recognition that traditional weight loss approaches to eat less and exercise more are not successful and are often counterproductive is growing and is forcing health professionals to consider alternative and adjunct approaches. Some of these approaches were presented in this chapter. Acceptance of genetic limitations and redefining weight management goals provides health professionals and their clients with potentially achievable objectives to achieve and maintain health.

Within these changes it is important for nurses to understand that the role of the dietitian is evolving from a counselor/educator who gives only dietary advice to a therapist who practices advanced counseling skills using psycho-

---

BOX 10-3	HEALTH CARE BILL OF RIGHTS

1. To have a policy in the health care system against discriminating practices based on weight, size or health status.
2. To have access to affordable quality medical care, social services and adequate physical accommodations, equipment and testing facilities in the health care setting.
3. To have access to affordable and appropriate health insurance.
4. To have complete and accurate explanations of all treatments.
5. To have a full say in the modality of treatment; including the areas of analgesia and anesthesia.
6. To have the right to refuse treatment.
7. Access and treatment should not hinge on the acceptance or enrollment in any type of weight loss program.
8. To have or provide access to a patient advocate, either an individual or organizational representative of our choice, to play an active role in our medical care.
9. All caregivers are to act in a professional manner free of ridicule, coercion and harassment; and they should be informed about the latest research in the areas of bariatrics, nutrition, metabolism and genetics with regard to "obesity."
10. To privacy and confidentiality of all medical records, following federal and local laws.

Copyright 2008 NAAFA, P.O. Box 22510, Oakland CA 94609
Telephone: (916) 558-6880

www.naafaonline.com/dev2/education/brochures/Healthcare_Bill_of_Rights-EDITED.pdf

---

dynamic models of therapy to assist and coach clients. This new view expands nutrition therapy and involves a shift from a short-term to a long-term approach. Weight management is a lifelong process and so incorporates broader lifestyle skills to achieve healthy weight goals. Dietitians can coach clients about the process of food choice, shifting the responsibility of decision-making about food and portion control to the client who is then armed with skills and support from dietetic counseling. The goal is to ensure enjoyment of eating while still maintaining a healthy lifestyle. Everyone should be able to enjoy his or her favorite foods but make conscious choices about where, when, and how much of the food is eaten.

Dietitians are often part of multidisciplinary teams that incorporate primary health care providers, physicians, nurses, behavior therapists, exercise therapists, and psychologists. Nurses can provide support during the formal and informal interactions within the health care system. An important aspect of this support involves nurses considering their attitudes toward their own bodies and toward clients who struggle with their weight, body image, and possible associated health concerns. In addition, nurses need to be knowledgeable about the lifestyle changes and food choices to achieve long-term body composition management to further support client success. This may necessitate further specialization as a member of a multidiscipline health team.

TOWARD A POSITIVE NUTRITION LIFESTYLE: EXPLANATORY STYLE

In his book *Learned Optimism,* Dr. Martin Seligman, a psychologist and professor, explores applications of explanatory styles to everyday life situations.[23] As a component of personal control, *explanatory style* is the way in which a person regularly explains why events happen. An individual with a pessimistic explanatory style spreads learned helplessness by having a pervasive negative view that no matter what he or she does, nothing will change. In contrast, a person with an optimistic explanatory style feels able to stop the reaction of learned helplessness and understands events in a more positive way. An optimistic person feels competent that he or she can change the course of events.

Explanatory style has been studied in relation to health and wellness. A person's approach to dealing with issues of physical health can be helped or hindered by cognitions about personal control over health conditions and maintenance. Seligman notes the following:[23]

- The way we think, especially about health, changes our health.
- Optimists catch fewer infectious diseases than pessimists do.
- Optimists have better health habits than pessimists do.
- Our immune system may work better when we are optimistic.
- Evidence suggests that optimists live longer than pessimists.

How does this information apply to body fat management? Having an optimistic explanatory style may mean accepting one's body as it is and acting in ways to improve health by attempting to eat well and exercise regularly. A pessimistic explanatory style would judge one's body negatively and would not attempt behaviors to improve body composition because physical attributes would be understood to be permanent and thus unchangeable. Consider other ways that explanatory styles affect the approach of our patients toward their illnesses and the effect of our explanatory styles on strategies of nursing care.

SUMMARY

Lifelong management of body fat levels provides a more holistic health approach to body size than does body weight. Management is defined as the use of available resources to achieve a predetermined goal. This definition recognizes that individuals differ in the resources available to them and in the goals they set. Goals for body fat levels must take into account an individual's genetic and family factors as well as those of society and health.

Ways of measuring body fat composition include densitometry and bioelectric impedance analysis. In addition to simple body weight, BMI provides another way to interpret weight levels. Weight may be maintained by set point, through which the body regulates its most natural weight.

Body size, as an issue of health status, is still a concern among many health professionals. Individuals at both extremes of fatness—those very thin and those very fat—are at increased risk for certain health-related disorders. Obesity, however, does not increase all types of health risks, nor are all obese individuals ill. Risks of some types of cancer and of osteoporosis are lower for the obese than for others.

Body acceptance is a key to wellness. Biology and culture interact to set standards of body image, perceptions, and social models of attractiveness. Because of individual genetic makeup, different body types and sizes may not fit the cultural ideals. The goal is to reclaim eating as a comfortable and natural process. This means being in tune with one's body's needs and its signals about those needs. A part of body composition management is the incorporation of regular exercise. Exercise increases energy expenditure, promotes maintenance of lean body mass, improves many health conditions, and changes one's outlook. Differences in bodies' responses to exercise may be related to gender, fat distribution patterns, ability to exercise vigorously, and appetite response to exercise. Future considerations of body composition management include prevention of deviations from healthy levels and distributions of fat, development of effective treatments, and the cultivation of acceptance of individual differences.

THE NURSING APPROACH

Case Study: Weight Management

His mother brought 10-year-old Jake to the clinic for a physical exam before the start of Little League baseball. The mother said she hoped the sport would help control Jake's weight. Concerned about his rapid weight gain during the last year, she indicated that Jake was not very active, and he loved to eat.

ASSESSMENT

Subjective (from patient statements)

- "My friends tease me. They call me Fat Albert."
- "I get tired easily when I have to run, and I'm always the last one to finish a race."

- "I hope the team won't laugh at me if I run slower than the other boys."
- "I usually spend my time playing computer games or watching TV. I like to eat snacks when I watch TV."
- "We usually eat fast foods two or three times a week. Desserts and french fries are my favorites."

Objective (from physical examination)

- Height 55 inches, weight 102 pounds
- Weight at the 95th percentile, BMI 24 (>95th percentile for children his age)

THE NURSING APPROACH—cont'd

Case Study: Weight Management—cont'd

- Blood Pressure 120/80 (117/75 is 90th percentile for his age)

DIAGNOSIS (NURSING)

Imbalanced nutrition: more than body requirements related to overeating and inactive lifestyle as evidenced by weight at 95th percentile, frequently eats fast foods, usually sits for activities, friends tease him about his weight, and BP at 90th percentile

PLANNING

Patient Outcomes

Short term (at the end of this visit):
- Jake will identify healthy foods and state his intent to substitute them most of the time for foods high in fat and sugar.
- He will agree to watch less TV, play fewer computer games, and actively play every day.

Long term (phone follow-up after one month):
- No weight gain, weight stable

Nursing Interventions

1. Assess Jake's knowledge of healthy food choices.
2. Encourage healthy food choices and activities.
3. Inform Jake and his mother about potential serious health problems from obesity.

IMPLEMENTATION

1. Used a picture board to see if Jake could point to the healthier food choices.

   Assessment of knowledge and skills helps determine learning needs.

2. Showed Jake pictures of foods with equivalent calories—large serving sizes of healthy foods and small servings of high-fat, high-sugar foods. Said it was important to choose nutritious food and limit portion sizes when eating a treat.

   Many people are visual learners. Pictures can communicate comparisons without a lot of words. Portion sizes help determine calories consumed.

3. Gave him a list of the healthier choices at fast-food establishments.

   Information and choice can empower individuals. The child should be encouraged to take responsibility for his own choices when possible.

4. Encouraged Jake's mother to have healthy food on hand for after-school snacks.

   By providing nutritious food choices, parents can help control weight gain and promote good health.

5. Recommended avoiding more weight gain and praised Jake for playing baseball.

   Praise and encouragement can reinforce healthy choices. Weight maintenance rather than weight loss is usually recommended for a child who is overweight or obese. As the child grows taller, he will help even out weight proportionally.

6. Suggested to Jake that he spend less time at the TV and computer and spend more time playing—for example, riding a bike or swimming.

   Active sports will help burn calories and could improve his self-esteem and socialization with friends.

7. Showed Jake and his mother how his weight compared to standard growth charts for boys his age. Reported Jake's high blood pressure for his age group and discussed potential complications of obesity: hypertension, insulin resistance (precursor to type 2 diabetes), high cholesterol levels (precursor to coronary heart disease), joint problems, and sleep apnea.

   Knowledge of potential complications can motivate an individual to adopt a healthy lifestyle.

8. Ordered fasting lab tests, including lipid panel, insulin level, and blood glucose.

   Baseline lab results help determine predisposition to complications and could indicate need for treatment.

9. Referred Jake and his mother to a dietitian for a dietary consult. Asked them to record and bring a 2- or 3-day food journal.

   The dietitian can individualize food patterns and make compliance easier.

EVALUATION

Short term (at the end of the first visit):
- Jake was able to identify the healthier foods and fast-food choices.
- He stated the intention to try to eat smaller portions of food and food that is lower in fat and sugar.
- He stated willingness to watch less TV and practice baseball and running.
- Goals met.

Long term (in one month at a follow-up phone call):
- Jake's mother reported that Jake's weight was stable, and they had met with the dietitian.
- Goals met.

DISCUSSION QUESTIONS

1. Why do you think Jake was not asked to adopt a rigid weight loss plan?
2. List five snacks that you could recommend for the mother to have on hand for Jake.

❓ APPLYING CONTENT KNOWLEDGE

Carol eats a moderately low-fat diet, doesn't overeat, and exercises three or four times a week. Her body fat level is about 32%. Her friend, Barbara, also eats a moderately low-fat diet, doesn't overeat, and exercises three or four times a week. However, compared with Carol, Barbara's body fat level is in the low range of 22%. Explain how their body fat levels could differ.

WEBSITES OF INTEREST

The Obesity Prevention Small Step

www.Smallstep.gov

Encourages families to make small dietary and physical activity changes—in other words, "small steps" toward healthier lifestyles.

Shape Up America!

www.shapeup.org

Provides evidence-based information, educative tools, and strategies for achieving weight management.

National Association to Advance Fat Acceptance (NAAFA)

www.naafa.org

Works toward improving the quality of life for fat people and eliminating size discrimination through public education, advocacy, and member support.

REFERENCES

1. Stearns PN: *Fat history: bodies and beauty in the modern West*, New York, 1997, New York University Press.
2. Brownell KD: Personal responsibility and control over our bodies: When expectation exceeds reality, *Health Psychol* 10:303-310, 1991.
3. Friedman KE, et al: Body image partially mediates the relationship between obesity and psychological distress, *Obes Res* 10(1):33-41, 2002.
4. Stipanuk MH: *Biochemical, physiological, & molecular aspects of human nutrition*, Philadelphia, 2006, Saunders.
5. Reaven GM: Metabolic syndrome: Definition, relationship to insulin resistance, and clinical utility. In Shils ME, et al, editors: *Modern nutrition in health and disease*, ed 10, Philadelphia, 2006, Lippincott Williams & Wilkins.
6. Hu FB: *Obesity epidemiology*, New York, 2008, Oxford University Press.
7. Manson JE et al: Body weight and mortality among women, *N Engl J Med* 333:677-685, 1995.
8. Vaidya V: Psychosocial aspects of obesity, *Adv Psychosom Med* 27:73-85, 2006.
9. Mahan LK, Escott-Stump S: *Krause's food & nutrition therapy*, ed 12, St Louis, 2008, Elsevier.
10. Shape Up America! *Measurement tools*, Washington, DC, 2005-2006, Author. Accessed February 23, 2010, from www.shapeup.org.
11. American Dietetic Association: Position of the American Dietetic Association: Weight management, *J Am Diet Assoc* 109:330-346, 2009.
12. Tershakovec AM, et al: Age, sex, ethnicity, body composition, and resting energy expenditure of obese African American and white children and adolescents, *Am J Clin Nutr* 75(5):867-871, 2002.
13. Hill JO, et al: Obesity: Etiology. In Shils ME, et al, editors: *Modern nutrition in health and disease*, ed 10, Philadelphia, 2006, Lippincott Williams & Wilkins.
14. Brodsky I: Hormones and growth factors. In Shils ME, et al, editors: *Modern nutrition in health and disease*, ed 10, Philadelphia, 2006, Lippincott Williams & Wilkins.
15. Cummings DE, et al: Plasma ghrelin levels after diet-induced weight loss or gastric bypass surgery, *N Engl J Med* 346(21):1623-1630, 2002.
16. U.S. Department of Health and Human Services, Public Health Service: *Leading Health Indicators, Healthy people 2010*, ed 2, Washington, DC, 2000, U.S. Government Printing Office. Accessed August 19, 2010, from www.health.gov/healthypeople.
17. Federal Interagency Forum on Child and Family Statistics: *America's Children: Key National Indicators of Well-Being, 2009*, Federal Interagency Forum on Child and Family Statistics, Washington, DC, 2009, U.S. Government Printing Office. Accessed February 23, 2010, from http://childstats.gov/americaschildren/index.asp.
18. Calorie Control Council: *Trends and statistics: Dieting figures*, Atlanta, 2010, Author. Accessed February 23, 2010, from www.caloriecontrol.org/press-room/trends-and-statistics.
19. Weight-Control Information Network (WIN), National Institute of Diabetes & Digestive & Kidney Diseases, National Institutes of Health: *Bariatric surgery for severe obesity*, NIH Publication No. 08–4006, Bethesda, Md, 2009 (March), U.S. Department of Health and Human Services. Accessed February 23, 2010, from http://win.niddk.nih.gov/publications/gastric.htm.
20. Lamarche B, et al: Is body fat loss a determinant factor in the improvement of carbohydrate and lipid metabolism following aerobic exercise training in obese women? *Metabolism* 41:1249-1256, 1992.
21. Björntorp P, Brodoff BN, editors: *Obesity*, Philadelphia, 1992, Lippincott.
22. Health Canada: *Reflecting on VITALITY—Lessons learned from the development, implementation and evaluation of VITALITY*, Ottawa, Ontario, Canada, 2004 (April 24), Author. Accessed February 23, 2010, from www.hc-sc.gc.ca/fn-an/nutrition/weights-poids/reflecting-retour-vitality_e.html.
23. Seligman MEP: *Learned optimism*, New York, 2006, Alfred A. Knopf.

Life Span Health Promotion: Pregnancy, Lactation, and Infancy

Following conception and continuing until parturition (childbirth), many metabolic, anatomic, hormonal, psychologic, and physiologic changes take place in the mother.

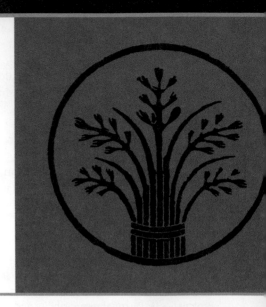

evolve WEBSITE

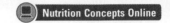

http://evolve.elsevier.com/Grodner/foundations/

Nutrition Concepts Online

Chapters 11, 12, and 13 cover the topics of life span health promotion. These chapters not only address the basic nutrition requirements of pregnancy, infancy, childhood, adolescence, and adulthood through older adulthood but also consider the factors that affect health promotion. As presented in Chapter 1, the goal of health promotion is to increase the level of health of individuals, families, and communities. Health promotion strategies often focus on lifestyle changes leading to new, positive health behaviors.

Development of these behaviors may depend on knowledge, techniques, and community supports. Knowledge is learning new information about the benefits or risks of health-related behaviors. Techniques are strategies used to apply new knowledge to everyday activities. By applying our knowledge, we modify lifestyle behaviors. Community supports are available (environmental or regulatory measures) that support new health-promoting behaviors within a social context.

ROLE IN WELLNESS

The prenatal period is characterized by numerous physiologic, psychologic, and social changes in the mother in preparation for birth and care of the infant. It is a time when a woman often expresses interest and motivation in improving her eating habits, realizing she is the sole source of nourishment for her developing baby. Following birth, lactation leads to changes for the mother. Although providing human milk for one's infant is exhilarating, the 24-hour demands of a newborn lead to a reorganization of everyday life and can sometimes be overwhelming. Societal and cultural influences also may affect the acceptability of breastfeeding.

The goal of health promotion is to prepare a woman for these changes by helping her become knowledgeable and responsible for her own health and the well-being of her infant. Few experience this alone. A spouse, significant other, and family members can be sources of support to further the goals of health promotion. A father-to-be often needs guidance as he grapples with his own expectations of his future responsibilities. Health professionals can use this opportunity to assist individuals to establish healthful habits, such as eating well, being physically active, and avoiding alcohol and drug use.

This chapter explores pregnancy, lactation, and infancy through the framework of nutritional requirements and health promotion. The five dimensions of health (physical, intellectual, social, emotional, and spiritual) provide insight into the issues associated with these topics. The *physical health* of the newborn depends on the nutrients consumed by the expectant mother and on the teratogens avoided. Preparation before conception to take on the responsibilities of pregnancy and future parenting requires application of knowledge exercising the *intellectual health* dimension. *Emotional health* may be strained as some women develop postpartum depression after delivery; recognition and treatment of this disorder is crucial to the well-being of both mother and child. The *social health* relationships of mothers and fathers may be altered as lifestyle changes occur because of their new social status as parents. *Spiritual* dimension of health is affected because the creation of new life is one of life's miracles regardless of one's religious or humanistic beliefs.

NUTRITION DURING PREGNANCY

Although the influence of nutrition on the course of pregnancy was assumed for some time, it was not until the twentieth century that research provided a scientific basis to substantiate such assumptions. Appropriate nutrition intake during pregnancy is integral to a successful pregnancy.

TABLE 11-1	NEW RECOMMENDATIONS FOR TOTAL AND RATE OF WEIGHT GAIN DURING PREGNANCY, BY PREPREGNANCY BMI			
GAIN	TOTAL WEIGHT		RATES OF WEIGHT GAIN*	
			SECOND AND THIRD TRIMESTER	
PREPREGNANCY BMI	RANGE IN KG	RANGE IN LBS	MEAN (RANGE) IN KG/WEEK	MEAN (RANGE) IN LBS/WEEK
Underweight (<18.5 kg/m²)	12.5-18	28-40	0.51 (0.44-0.58)	1 (1-1.3)
Normal weight (18.5-24.9 kg/m²)	11.5-16	25-35	0.42 (0.35-0.50)	1 (0.8-1)
Overweight (25.0-29.9 kg/m²)	7-11.5	15-25	0.28 (0.23-0.33)	0.6 (0.5-0.7)
Obese (≥30.0 kg/m²)	5-9	11-20	0.22 (0.17-0.27)	0.5 (0.4-0.6)

*Calculations assume a 0.5-2 kg (1.1-4.4 lbs) weight gin in the first trimester (based on Siega-Riz et al., 1994; Abrams et al., 1995; Carmichael et al., 1997).

From Institute of Medicine and National Research Council: *Weight gain during pregnancy: Reexamining the guidelines*, Washington, DC, 2009, The National Academies Press.

fetus and the placenta. Inadequate weight gain by the mother during pregnancy suggests she may not have received the proper nutrients during pregnancy. Poor weight gain may then lead to intrauterine growth retardation in the infant. Infants born small for gestational age (SGA) or low birth weight are more likely to require prolonged hospitalization after birth or be ill or die during the first year of life. SGA is when an infant is born at a lower birth weight than expected for the length of gestation, while low birth weight is a weight less than 5.5 pounds (2500 g) at birth. Additionally, infant mortality rate, which in part reflects maternal weight gain, is regarded as one measure of a country's health and well-being. Although the 2007 infant mortality rate for the United States (6.8 per 1000 live births) continued an all-time low first reached in 1996 (6.9 per 1000 live births),[2] it still remains far greater than other developed countries. Infant mortality rates are higher among non-Hispanic black infants than among non-Hispanic white and Hispanic infants.[2]

There is strong evidence that the pattern of weight gain is just as important as the absolute recommended weight gains, as shown in Table 11-1. Failure to gain adequately during the second trimester of pregnancy is associated with poor infant birth weight, even if the net gain falls with in the recommendations.

A balance must be struck regarding weight gain during pregnancy. Although women who are underweight or normal weight (as defined by body mass index [BMI]) are counseled to eat sufficiently to promote adequate gain, caution must be observed in counseling women who enter pregnancy overweight or obese. Overweight and obese women should gain enough weight to support the fetus and maternal support tissues but without increasing total body fat. There are increased risks for operative delivery, increased maternal postpartum weight, gestational diabetes, and other long-term health consequences when maternal weight goes beyond the guidelines, particularly among women who are obese before pregnancy.[1] In addition, there may be subpopulations such as minorities and low-income women who need special guidance regarding weight gain during pregnancy. Figure 11-1 summarizes possible determinants and effects on gestational weight gain.

Additional issues arise when women who have underdone gastric bypass surgery become pregnant. Because of smaller stomach size, less food is consumed, and intestinal absorption of nutrients may be compromised. Recommendations are to delay pregnancy until at least a year after bypass surgery and to seek nutrition therapy to support adequate nutrient absorption and energy intake.

Energy and Nutrient Needs during Pregnancy

The Dietary Reference Intakes (DRIs) recommend increases during pregnancy of all nutrients *except* vitamin D, vitamin E, vitamin K, phosphorus, fluoride, calcium, and biotin (Table 11-2). There are separate dietary recommendations for adolescents who are pregnant.

Energy

It is difficult to estimate the true energy cost of pregnancy, but the best estimates place the total energy cost somewhere between 68,000 kcal and 80,000 kcal. The increase accommodates the rise in maternal BMR during pregnancy, as well as the synthesis and support of the maternal and fetal tissues.[1] The current recommendation is for a woman to consume an extra 300 kcal per day during the second and third trimesters of pregnancy. Although she is eating for two, the expectant mother need not and should not double her food intake. An extra sandwich and a glass of milk can easily provide the additional 300 kcal per day, providing she was eating well before pregnancy. Personal preference may guide particular food choices to provide the extra kcal, as long as the foods are nutritious.

What happens if a pregnant woman fails to increase her energy intake during pregnancy? The best-known example in the twentieth century occurred in Holland during World War II. Infants born during the famine of 1944 and 1945 had smaller birth weights and birth lengths when compared with infants born either before or after the famine.[3] Recent research shows that when women who begin pregnancy in energy deficit (e.g., those who are chronically undernourished in developing countries) are provided with energy supplementation throughout the course of pregnancy, there is a positive effect on maternal weight gain and infant birth weight.[4] On

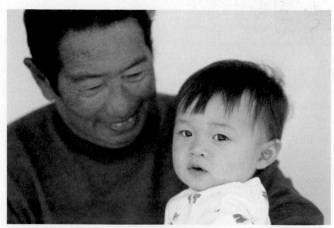

Grandparents can be a source of support to further the goals of health promotion.

Successful pregnancy outcomes include a viable infant of acceptable birth weight, an infant free of congenital defects, and a favorable long-term health outlook for both mother and infant.

Body Composition Changes during Pregnancy

Following conception and continuing until parturition (childbirth), many metabolic, anatomic, hormonal, psychologic, and physiologic changes take place in the mother. This chapter focuses on those most affected by or affecting nutrient intake.

Hormones of Pregnancy

There are numerous steroid hormones, peptide hormones, and prostaglandins influencing the course of pregnancy. Some of them, such as the placental hormones *human placental lactogen* and *human growth hormone,* are produced only during pregnancy. Others, including insulin, glucagon, and thyroxine, are present in altered amounts compared with the nonpregnant state and have profound influences on metabolism throughout gestation.

Progesterone and estrogen have a particularly strong influence on pregnancy. The action of progesterone promotes development of the endometrium (mucous membrane of the uterus) and relaxes the smooth muscle cells of the uterus. This relaxation serves to both help the uterus expand as the fetus grows and prevent any premature contractions of the uterus. The same effect also influences other smooth muscle cells, such as the gastrointestinal (GI) tract. The resulting slowing of the GI tract during pregnancy may increase the absorption of several nutrients, most notably iron and calcium. One perhaps annoying consequence of this decreased gut motility is the promotion of constipation. Progesterone causes increased renal sodium excretion during pregnancy. The body compensates for this sodium-losing mechanism by increasing aldosterone secretion from the adrenal gland and renin from the kidney. Sodium restriction during pregnancy, once thought to prevent hypertensive disorders of pregnancy, is actually harmful because it reduces plasma volume and cardiac output.

Estrogen promotes the growth of the uterus and breasts during pregnancy and renders the connective tissues in the pelvic region more flexible in preparation for birth.

Metabolic Changes

Profound changes in maternal metabolism occur during pregnancy, and successful adaptation to these changes is necessary for a favorable pregnancy outcome. The basal metabolic rate (BMR) rises during pregnancy by as much as 15% to 20% by term. This increase is caused by the increased oxygen needs of the fetus and the maternal support tissues. There are alterations in maternal metabolism of protein, carbohydrate, and fat. The fetus prefers to use glucose as its primary energy source. Changes occur in maternal metabolism to accommodate this need of the fetus. The adaptation allows the mother to use fat as the primary fuel source, thus permitting glucose to be available to the fetus.[1] Increased macronutrient and micronutrient intake by the mother during pregnancy ensures that these increased metabolic needs are met.

Anatomic and Physiologic Changes

Plasma volume doubles during pregnancy, beginning in the second trimester. Failure to achieve this plasma expansion may result in a spontaneous abortion, a stillbirth, or a low birth weight infant. One of the results of this increase in plasma volume is a hemodilution effect, or dilution of the blood. In other words, measured components in the plasma such as hemoglobin, serum proteins, and vitamins will appear to be at lower levels during pregnancy because there is a greater volume of solvent (the plasma) relative to concentrations of solute (the components). Cardiac hypertrophy occurs to accommodate this increased blood volume, accompanied by an increased ventilatory rate.

In the kidneys, the glomerular filtration rate (GFR) increases to accommodate the expanded maternal blood volume being filtered and to carry away fetal waste products. As a result of this increase in GFR, small quantities of glucose, amino acids, and water-soluble vitamins may appear in the urine. Although minor losses may be acceptable, a woman who excretes large amounts of protein may experience a more serious problem called *preeclampsia,* or pregnancy-induced hypertension, which needs strict medical monitoring. Preeclampsia is described in more detail later in the chapter.

As mentioned, progesterone may slow GI motility during pregnancy, leading to constipation, heartburn, and delayed gastric emptying. In late pregnancy, these problems may be exacerbated by the weight of the uterus and fetus as they compress the abdominal cavity.

Weight Gain in Pregnancy

There are three components to maternal weight gain: (1) maternal body composition changes, including increased blood and extracellular fluid volume; (2) the maternal support tissues, such as the increased size of the uterus and breasts; and (3) the products of conception, including the

WEIGHT GAIN DURING PREGNANCY

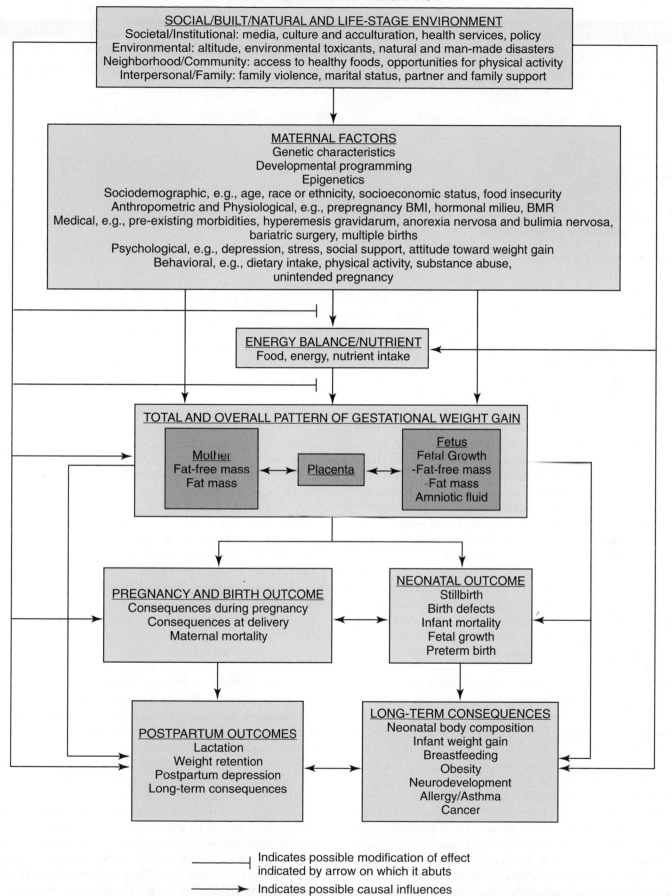

FIG 11-1 Summary of possible determinants and effects of gestational weight gain. (From the Institute of Medicine and the National Research Council: *Weight gain during pregnancy: Reexamining the guidelines,* Washington, DC, 2009, The National Academies Press.)

TABLE 11-2	DRIs TO MEET NEEDS OF PREGNANCY AND LACTATION		
	ADULT WOMEN (25-49 YEARS OF AGE)	**PREGNANT WOMEN (THIRD TRIMESTER)**	**LACTATING MOTHERS***
Energy (kcal)	2200	2500	2700
Protein (g)	46	71	71
Vitamin A (RE)	800	800	1300
Vitamin D (mcg)†	5	5	5
Vitamin E (mg α-TE) mg	15	15	19
Vitamin C (mg)	60	70	95
Thiamine (mg)	1.1	1.4	1.5
Riboflavin (mg)	1.1	1.4	1.6
Niacin (NE mg)	14	18	17
Vitamin B_6 (mg)	1.3	1.9	2
Folate (mcg)	400	600	500
Vitamin B_{12} (mcg)	2.4	2.6	2.8
Calcium (mg)†	1000	1000	1000
Phosphorus (mg)	700	700	700
Iron (mg)‡	15	30	15
Zinc (mg)	12	15	19
Iodine (mcg)	150	175	200
Selenium (mcg)	55	65	75

*During the first 6 months of lactation.
†Adequate Intake.
‡The increased iron requirement for pregnancy cannot be met by the usual American diet or from body stores; thus a supplement of 30 to 60 mg of elemental iron is recommended.
DRIs, Dietary Reference Intakes; *NE,* niacin equivalent; *RE,* retinol equivalent; *α-TE,* alpha tocopherol equivalent.
From Institute of Medicine, Food and Nutrition Board: *Dietary DRI References: The essential guide to nutrient requirements,* Washington, DC, 2006, The National Academies Press.

the other hand, some research suggests that women in the United States who are well nourished do not increase their total energy intake by a full 300 kcal per day and still have a positive pregnancy outcome. Most likely, in the third trimester, many women decrease their energy expenditure in pregnancy by decreasing activity, thereby giving a net increase in energy intake.[5]

Pregnancy is not a time to restrict kcal or to lose weight, even if the mother begins the pregnancy as overweight. This may be particularly important to emphasize to the adolescent population. The mother should be encouraged to eat at least the minimum number of servings recommended during pregnancy from MyPyramid (Box 11-1). The interactive MyPyramid Plan for Moms creates a personalized dietary food pattern based on height, weight, age, and other characteristics. Sample menus can be helpful in showing the pregnant woman how MyPyramid can be used (Box 11-2).

Protein

The Recommended Dietary Allowance (RDA) for protein during pregnancy is 71 g per day for adolescent and adult women. Women can easily obtain this in the American diet; the use of special protein powder supplements is not recommended. Pregnant patients may be counseled to include appropriate sources of protein providing vitamins, minerals, and moderate amounts of fat. Clients from low-income populations may need counseling or other assistance to ensure protein intake is sufficient; these clients may qualify for

food vouchers through the Special Supplemental Nutrition Program for Women, Infants, and Children (WIC) of the U.S. Department of Agriculture (see the *Social Issues* box, Providing the Essentials).

The increase in protein intake over the nonpregnant state is necessary to build and maintain the variety of new tissues of pregnancy. A woman experiencing nausea and vomiting in the first trimester of pregnancy may find it difficult to increase sources of protein in her diet, particularly if meats (which have a strong cooking odor) aggravate the nausea. If this is the case, she should consume small amounts of high-quality protein as tolerated.

Vitamin and Mineral Supplementation

The DRIs are increased during pregnancy for most vitamins and minerals. Vitamins of concern are vitamins A and D. While the RDA for vitamin A is 750 to 770 mcgRAE (Retinol Activity Equivalents) preformed vitamin A, the Tolerable Upper Intake Level (UL) is set at 2800 to 3000 mcgRAE preformed vitamin A per day because of the potential for birth defects from excessive intake.[6] Similarly, excessive vitamin D during pregnancy may cause birth defects so that the Adequate Intake (AI) (5 mcg per day) and UL (50 mcg per day) are the same for women regardless of physiological state.[6] Micronutrient needs may be met with a balanced diet, with a few notable exceptions including folate and iron. All supplementation during pregnancy should be in the form of prenatal type multivitamin-mineral supplements as recommended by primary health care providers or dietitians.

BOX 11-1 **Myplate Pregnancy and Breastfeeding**

Health & Nutrition Information for Pregnant & Breastfeeding Women

When you are pregnant or breastfeeding, you have special nutritional needs. This site is designed just for you. It has advice you need to help you and your baby stay healthy.

First – visit your doctor or health care provider if you haven't already. Every pregnant woman needs to visit a doctor regularly. Only he or she can make sure both you and your baby are healthy. Your doctor can also prescribe a safe vitamin and mineral supplement, and anything else you may need.

Next – get you own Daily Food Plan for Moms. Your Plan will show you the foods and amounts that are right for you. Enter your information for a quick estimate of what and how much you need to eat. Or, enter the foods you eat into the Super-tracker to see how your food choices compare to what you need.

Then – learn more by choosing a topic from the menu below. "Sources of information" will take you straight to the government's best advice on pregnancy and breastfeeding.

Making Healthy Choices in Each Food Group

Follow your Daily Food Plan for Moms and eat the amount recommended for each food group. Include the foods listed below—they are the best sources of some nutrients you need when you are pregnant or breastfeeding.*

Vegetable Group

(choose fresh, frozen, canned, or dried)
- Carrots
- Sweet potatoes
- Pumpkin
- Spinach
- Cooked greens (such as kale, collards, turnip greens, and beet greens)
- Winter squash
- Tomatoes and tomato sauces
- Red sweet peppers

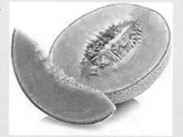

These vegetables all have both vitamin A and potassium. When choosing canned vegetables, look for "low-sodium" or "no-salt-added" on the label.

Fruit Group

(choose fresh, frozen, canned, or dried)
- Cantaloupe
- Honeydew melon
- Mangoes
- Prunes
- Bananas
- Apricots
- Oranges

- Red or pink grapefruit
- 100% prune juice or orange juice

These fruits all provide potassium, and many also provide vitamin A. When choosing canned fruit, look for those canned in 100% fruit juice or water instead of syrup.

Dairy Group

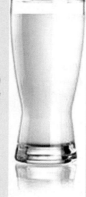

- Fat-free or low-fat yogurt
- Fat-free milk (skim milk)
- Low-fat milk (1% milk)
- Calcium-fortified soymilk (soy beverage)

These all provide the calcium and potassium you need. Make sure that your choices are fortified with vitamins A and D.

Grain Group

- Fortified ready-to-eat cereals
- Fortified cooked cereals

When buying ready-to-eat and cooked cereals, choose those made from whole grains most often. Look for cereals that are fortified with iron and folic acid.

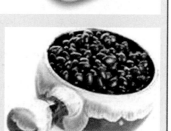

Protein Foods Group

- Beans and peas (such as pinto beans, soybeans, white beans, lentils, kidney beans, chickpeas)
- Nuts and seeds (such as sunflower seeds, almonds, hazelnuts, pine nuts, peanuts, and peanut butter)
- Lean beef, lamb, and pork
- Oysters, mussels, crab
- Salmon, trout, herring, sardines, and pollock

NOTE: Do not eat shark, swordfish, king mackerel, or tilefish when you are pregnant or breastfeeding. They contain high levels of mercury. Limit white (albacore) tuna to no more than 6 ounces per week. Learn more about the safety of eating seafood during pregnancy. (Go to Food Safety at www.choosemyplate.gov for more information about safety of eating fish during pregnancy.)

All of these foods provide protein. In addition, beans and peas provide iron, potassium, and fiber. Meats provide heme-iron -which is the most readily absorbed type of iron. Nut and seeds also contain vitamin E. Seafood provides omega-3 fatty acids.

Accessed June 14, 2012 from http://www.choosemyplate.gov/pregnancy-breastfeeding.html

*The foods on this list are the best sources of one or more of the following nutrients: vitamin A, vitamin E, potassium, and iron. Food sources of these nutrients are included because when choosing a typical mix of food choices in each food group, the intake patterns may not meet dietary standards for pregnant and/or breastfeeding women for these nutrients. Accessed June 14, 2012, from http://www.choosemyplate.gov/pregnancy-breastfeeding/making-healthy-food-choices.html.

BOX 11-2   SAMPLE MENU FOR PREGNANT WOMEN

Breakfast

Orange juice	½ cup
Whole grain toast	1 slice
Banana	½ medium
Oatmeal	1 cup
Skim milk	1 cup

Midmorning Snack*

Lunch

Roast beef (2 oz lean) sandwich on whole grain bread with lettuce and tomato

Green salad	1-1½ cups leafy greens, 1 tbsp balsamic vinegar dressing
Orange wedges	1 cup
Skim milk†	1 cup

Midafternoon Snack*

Dinner

Sesame chicken (or fish)	4 oz
Broccoli	1½ cup
Sweet potato	1 medium
Mixed salad (carrots, tomato, 1½ cups spinach, romaine lettuce)	
Olive oil	2 tsp
Fresh lime juice or vinegar	2 tsp
Whole grain bread	1 slice
Butter	1 tsp
Fresh fruit salad	½ cup
Skim milk	1 cup

Snack* (Evening if Needed)

Some examples are:

Cereal (ready to eat) ¾ cup with skim milk (½ cup)

Fresh or frozen berries (½ cup) with nonfat yogurt (½ cup)

Apple/pear with cheese (1 oz) or peanut butter (1 tbsp)

Fruit and yogurt shake

Open-face peanut butter and apple sandwich

*Snacks are all interchangeable

†Assumes water consumed throughout the day as a beverage in addition to skim milk.

Folate. Substantial research has demonstrated that folate is important for the prevention of neural tube defects (NTDs) such as spina bifida and anencephaly, one of the most common congenital malformations in the United States. Approximately 2500 to 3000 infants are born with NTDs each year in the United States, with an equal number likely lost to pregnancy termination and additional unknown numbers of spontaneous abortions. The U.S. Public Health Service and the American Academy of Pediatrics now recommend all women of childbearing age who are capable of becoming pregnant receive a daily intake of 400 mcg of synthetic folic acid (from vitamin supplements, fortified grains, and other foods). Although fortification has been implemented, education continues to be needed to encourage awareness of folic acid intake by women of childbearing age. During pregnancy the DRI increases to 600 mcg dietary folate equivalents (DFE) per day.[6]

SOCIAL ISSUES
Providing the Essentials

Nutrient-dense foods are the foundations for healthy expectant mothers and their offspring. Women at low socioeconomic levels may have difficulty affording these essentials. One way to ensure adequate nutrition is through a federal government program, such as the USDA's Special Supplemental Nutrition Program for Women, Infants, and Children (WIC). Over 9.2 million women, infants and children receive the benefits of WIC.

The WIC program began in 1974 and currently operates through approved clinics in all 50 states. Eligible participants must live in an area served by WIC, meet federal income guidelines (income no greater than 185% of U.S. poverty level), and have a nutritional risk factor such as anemia, poor weight gain during pregnancy, previous low birth weight infant, or inadequate diet. Pregnant and postpartum women (up to 12 months' postpartum if breastfeeding, 6 months if not) are eligible to participate, as well as infants and children up to 5 years of age.

WIC provides vouchers for foods including fresh fruits and vegetables high in protein, vitamin C, vitamin A, iron and calcium—nutrients having shown to be lacking in this population. Participants are offered nutrition education or nutrition counseling, receive testing for anemia, receive routine anthropometric monitoring, and obtain referrals to other health care resources.

Community health care nurses can refer clients to local WIC programs for assistance. Contacting the city, county, or state health departments can identify the closest WIC clinic.

Iron. The RDA for iron during pregnancy is 27 mg per day. This level may be difficult to achieve with a normal diet, which maintains recommended fat and kcal guidelines. Therefore, all women should take a supplement with 30 mg ferrous iron daily beginning in the second trimester to prevent iron deficiency anemia in pregnancy.[1]

Iron deficiency anemia is one of the most common complications of pregnancy. The iron requirement increases secondary to the expansion of the maternal red cell volume. Iron deficiency anemia can mean impaired oxygen delivery to the fetus, which may have severe consequences. In addition, during the last trimester, the fetus stores iron in its liver to use during the first 4 months of life.

As discussed in Chapter 8, an unusual behavior associated with iron deficiency is pica. *Pica* is characterized by a hunger and appetite for nonfood substances including ice, cornstarch, clay, and even dirt. These substances contain no iron and may lead to loss of additional minerals, particularly when clay and dirt are consumed. Intestinal blockages caused by consumption of these substances may be life-threatening. Of particular concern is the practice of pica during pregnancy when the risk and implications of iron deficiency anemia are most severe. Although more common among African American women, pica has been diagnosed among all ethnic groups within all socioeconomic levels. A challenge to obstetric

BOX 11-3	SPECIAL NEEDS POPULATIONS

Special considerations are needed during pregnancy for the following:
- Adolescents
- Vegetarians
- Women older than 35 years of age
- Women who are underweight
- Women who are overweight
- Women with phenylketonuria
- Women with multiple pregnancies
- Women who smoke or use drugs or alcohol
- Women with concurrent medical problems

nurses is to elicit information about this type of dietary behavior when assessing clients.

Calcium. The AI for calcium is 1000 mg per day for women and 1300 mg per day for adolescents, neither of which is an increase over the nonpregnant state.[6] Although calcium needs are great during pregnancy, particularly for mineralization of the fetal skeleton, changes occur in maternal calcium homeostasis, which results in an increase in intestinal calcium absorption. Many women, particularly adolescents, may not consume the AI for calcium before pregnancy. Women who are unable to consume rich sources of calcium may need to seek advice from a dietitian/nutrition specialist to determine whether supplements are necessary.

Nutrition-Related Concerns

Some pregnant women require particular attention through the course of pregnancy because of exposure to potential teratogens, problematic lifestyle behaviors, or development of medical conditions unique to pregnancy. Box 11-3 lists special needs populations of pregnant women.

A number of nonnutritive substances that women may be exposed to during pregnancy may have the capability to act as teratogens. A teratogen is an agent that is capable of producing a malformation or a defect in the unborn fetus. Some anomalies are apparent at birth or shortly after, such as NTDs or a cleft lip or palate. Other defects such as delayed growth or learning deficits may not be noticeable for several months or even years. Potential teratogens include caffeine, drugs, alcohol, and tobacco. Other concerns affecting the course and outcome of pregnancy include strenuous exercise, maternal age, and medical conditions requiring nutrition intervention such as hypertension, diabetes, phenylketonuria, and human immunodeficiency virus (HIV) infection. Although not nutritional in nature, the effect of teratogens on the course of pregnancy may be so serious as to warrant at least a brief review.

Caffeine

Whether a woman should refrain from caffeine consumption during pregnancy has been a matter of debate. Caffeine (1-, 3-, 7-trimethyxanthine) may alter deoxyribonucleic acid (DNA) and, in some individuals, may alter circulating levels of neurotransmitters and increase blood pressure.[7] It has been argued that any or all of these effects may have direct adverse consequences on the developing fetus. However, there is enough evidence suggesting that caffeine is not a human teratogen, and even at modest doses (<300 mg/day or about 2 cups or less of coffee), there is no increased risk of spontaneous abortion or preterm labor. It doesn't affect birth weight, gestational age, or fetal growth.[7] There may be small reductions in birth weight at very high levels of consumption. The important issue may be that heavy use of nonnutritive substances such as coffee, tea, and cola may displace needed nutrients in the diet and thus interfere with prenatal development. Moderation of caffeine use during pregnancy as opposed to complete elimination is reasonable advice.

Drugs

A pregnant woman should not consume any over-the-counter or prescription medications unless prescribed by her primary health care provider. The growing fetus, particularly during the period of organogenesis in the first trimester, is highly susceptible to insult.

Although not a direct nutrient concern, the acne medication isotretinoin (Accutane) contains high levels of retinoic acid in the form of a vitamin A analog. This medication causes fetal malformations such as craniofacial abnormalities and microcephaly (abnormal smallness of head with brain underdevelopment) when ingested in the periconceptional period. The current recommendation is that women of childbearing age not use isotretinoin for the treatment of acne.

This recommendation is consistent with a large body of animal data that show that consumption of large quantities of preformed vitamin A during pregnancy results in an excess of malformations such as anencephaly (defective brain development), cleft palate, spina bifida, webbed fingers or toes, and facial malformations. Vitamin A crosses the placenta by simple diffusion. Because it is fat soluble, the excess vitamin A can accumulate in the fetal tissues and may cause damage by interfering with cellular growth and differentiation during critical periods of development.[8]

Alcohol

The use of alcohol during pregnancy may produce fetal alcohol syndrome (FAS) or fetal alcohol spectrum disorder (FASD) in the infant. Symptoms include central nervous systems defects and specific anatomic defects such as a low nasal bridge, short nose, flat midface, and short palpebral fissures (separation between the upper and lower eyelids) (Figure 11-2).

There is no safe level of alcohol intake during pregnancy. FAS is not confined to heavy drinkers; anyone who uses alcohol during pregnancy places the infant at risk of this preventable syndrome. Therefore, *all* pregnant women should be urged to cease consumption of *all* alcoholic beverages. Because alcohol use by pregnant women has been increasing, health care providers should screen women for alcohol use and counsel clients appropriately.

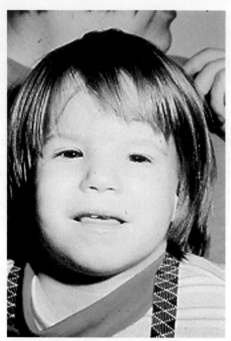

FIG 11-2 A young child with fetal alcohol syndrome features. (From Streissguth AP, et al: Teratogenic effects of alcohol in humans and laboratory animals, *Science* 209[4454]:353-361, 1980.)

Tobacco

Considerable research has been conducted on the effects of cigarette smoking during pregnancy. Women who smoke during pregnancy are at greater risk for several adverse outcomes including prematurity, low birth weight, SGA, stillbirth, placenta previa (location in lower uterine area), abruptio placentae (separation from uterine wall), and, postnatally, sudden infant death syndrome (SIDS). Smoking during pregnancy may cause prolonged effects of impaired intellectual performance and decreased attention span in the offspring. Poor nutrition during pregnancy will compound the risks associated with smoking.[9]

Foodborne Illness

Foodborne illness is a concern during pregnancy. Pathogens such as *Listeria monocytogenes*, *Salmonella* species, and *Toxoplasma gondii* are high risk for a pregnant woman and her fetus. In addition, commonly consumed foods may contain pathogens, not usually viewed as high risk, which can be problematic during pregnancy. Food safety strategies take on greater importance as a woman's body has reduced immunity or protections against pathogen. Box 11-4 highlights these concerns.

Exercise

Women with normal pregnancies should stay active during pregnancy, but the intensity of exercise is a matter of debate. Strenuous exercise was thought to divert blood to the exercising muscles and thus reduce the blood supply to the fetus. There was also speculation that intense exercise would place

---

| BOX 11-4 | FOOD SAFETY RISKS FOR PREGNANT WOMEN AND NEWBORNS |

During pregnancy, women and their unborn children are more likely to become very ill from food poisoning. Newborns and infants also are at risk because their immune systems are not fully developed. Infections from foodborne illness can be difficult to treat and can recur in these groups.

In addition to keeping good food safety habits, there are certain foods that pregnant women should not eat:

- Rare, raw or undercooked meats and poultry (rare hamburgers, carpaccio and beef or steak tartare)
- Raw fish (including sushi, sashimi, ceviche and carpaccio)
- Undercooked and raw shellfish (clams, oysters, mussels and scallops)
- Fish containing high levels of mercury (swordfish, tilefish, king mackerel and shark)
- Refrigerated smoked seafood
- Unpasteurized dairy products ("raw" milk and cheeses)
- Some fresh soft cheeses (Brie, Camembert, blue-veined varieties and Mexican-style queso fresco) unless made with pasteurized milk
- Raw or undercooked eggs (soft-cooked, runny or poached)
- Food items that contain undercooked eggs (unpasteurized eggnog, Monte Cristo sandwiches, French toast, homemade Caesar salad dressing, Hollandaise sauce, some puddings and custards, chocolate mousse, tiramisu and raw cookie dough or cake batter)
- Raw sprouts (alfalfa, clover and radish)
- Deli salads
- Unpasteurized fruit and vegetable juices
- Refrigerated pate or meat spreads

Some ready-to-eat foods require reheating before use. These foods include hot dogs, luncheon and deli meats and fermented and dry sausages. Throw away packaged items once the "use-by" date has passed. If you think you have contracted a foodborne illness, contact your health-care provider immediately.

From the American Dietetic Association: *Food safety risks for pregnant women and newborns.* Author. Accessed on February 28, 2010, from www.eatright.org/Public/content.aspx?id=5984&terms =foodborne+illness+pregnancy.

---

the mother at risk for premature labor. More recent research shows the short-term metabolic changes associated with exercise pose no problem for the fetus. On the other hand, strenuous work conditions may pose risks for adverse pregnancy outcome. Heavy lifting and a heavy work pace may increase the risk of low birth weight infants[10]

Based on these studies, there is no reason for women to discontinue established exercise programs during pregnancy. However, if beginning a new exercise program, a woman should keep a pulse rate below 140 beats per minute and work toward 1 hour of physical activity 3 days a week. The level of intensity should result in a heart rate between 120 and 130 beats per minute. Walking, swimming, and stationary cycling are appropriate to achieve the benefits of reducing risk of gestational diabetes, maintaining or improving fitness, and easing the stress of labor.[11]

Maternal Age

Adolescents and women older than 35 years of age are at higher risk for poor pregnancy outcome. In any assessment of the nutritional status of the pregnant teen, there are several important factors to consider. These include the growth pattern of the mother, the psychologic maturity of the mother, the lack of economic resources to provide for the infant, and delay in seeking medical care. Dietary factors to assess are the poor dietary habits typical of many teens, frequency with which meals are eaten away from home each day, and the possible preoccupation with weight gain during pregnancy. This is still a major public health problem in the United States affecting medical and nutritional status. Nutritional counseling targeted specifically for this age group is beneficial at reducing the risk of adverse outcomes commonly seen among this group[11] (Figure 11-3).

Women who become pregnant after the age of 35 years have distinct nutritional needs, reflecting their longer medical history, potential long-term use of oral contraceptives (which may affect folate levels), and the possibility of a longer history of poor eating habits. In addition, older women are at risk for nutrition-related complications such as gestational diabetes. Careful nutritional evaluation of these patients can be useful in providing guidance to reduce the risk of nutritional imbalances that cause pregnancy complications.

Preeclampsia

Preeclampsia, also known as pregnancy-induced hypertension, is considered hypertension with proteinuria (excess protein in urine) after 20 weeks' gestation.[1] Clinically, the mother experiences a sudden and severe rise in arterial blood pressure, rapid weight gain, and marked edema, often necessitating immediate delivery of the fetus to save the life of both mother and infant.

Preeclampsia may occur in as many as 3% to 5% of pregnancies and is one of the leading causes of prematurity and maternal and fetal death. Risk factors for preeclampsia are listed in Box 11-5.

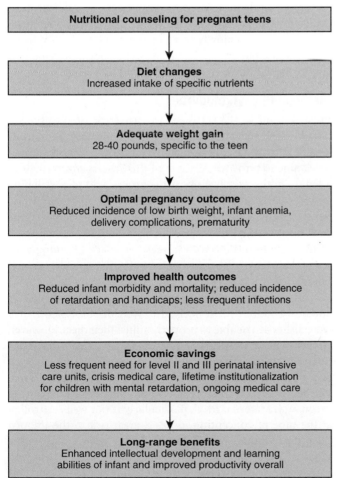

FIG 11-3 Nutrition counseling during teen pregnancy. (From Mahan KL, Escott-Stump S: *Krause's food & nutrition therapy,* ed 12, Philadelphia, 2008, Saunders.)

Flowchart contents:
- Nutritional counseling for pregnant teens
- **Diet changes** — Increased intake of specific nutrients
- **Adequate weight gain** — 28-40 pounds, specific to the teen
- **Optimal pregnancy outcome** — Reduced incidence of low birth weight, infant anemia, delivery complications, prematurity
- **Improved health outcomes** — Reduced infant morbidity and mortality; reduced incidence of retardation and handicaps; less frequent infections
- **Economic savings** — Less frequent need for level II and III perinatal intensive care units, crisis medical care, lifetime institutionalization for children with mental retardation, ongoing medical care
- **Long-range benefits** — Enhanced intellectual development and learning abilities of infant and improved productivity overall

BOX 11-5   RISK FACTORS AND SYMPTOMS OF PREECLAMPSIA

Risk Factors
First pregnancies
Diabetes mellitus (type 1; type 2)
Hypertension (for at least 4 years)
Advanced maternal age
African American heritage
Multiple pregnancies
Renal disease
Age at conception:
- 19 years or younger
- 40 years or older
Preeclampsia in earlier pregnancies:
- Family history of mothers or sister having preeclampsia
- Family history: hypertension, vascular disease
- Being researched: Inflammatory response, insulin resistance, and oxidative stress
Symptoms
- Headaches (continuous and severe)
- Hypertension (change compared with usual level)
- Edema of hands and face
- Sudden weight gain
- Excessive nausea and vomiting
- Vomiting blood
- Smaller amounts of urine or no urine
- Blood in urine
- Rapid heartbeat
- Dizziness and blurred or double vision
- Sudden blindness
- Ringing or buzzing sound in ears
- Drowsiness
- Fever
- Pain in the abdomen
- Slowed fetal growth
- Protein in urine (proteinuria)

Preeclampsia may progress to eclampsia. Eclampsia may result in seizures that can be fatal to the mother and the infant. The cause of eclampsia is unknown, and there is no screening test available.[1]

Nutrition support during preeclampsia includes provision of a well-balanced diet with generous sources of protein to replace losses in proteinuria and with adequate vitamins and minerals. It should supply a sufficient amount of energy. Energy intake should not be limited in an attempt to restrict maternal weight gain.

Currently low vitamin D status is being studied as an associative factor of preeclampsia. Lower levels have been reported in women with preeclampsia, particularly dark-skinned women from northern latitudes whose levels are lower than white women in the same area. Nonetheless, any women with preeclampsia may be experiencing hypovitaminosis D, and testing should be conducted. For those with low levels, dietary changes and/or supplementation may be appropriate.[12]

Diabetes Mellitus

Women with preexisting diabetes mellitus (DM) (type 1 and type 2) require specialized care during pregnancy. Pregnancy significantly affects insulin requirements. Control of glucose levels and avoidance of ketosis by adjusting nutrient intake and insulin dosage lend support for health birth outcomes. There is an increase risk of birth defects, especially of the heart and central nervous system.[1] Other complications include macrosomia (larger body size), hypoglycemia, erythremia (abnormal increase of red blood cells), and hyperbilirubinemia. Hyperbilirubinemia is a neonatal condition of excessively high levels of bilirubin (red bile pigment) leading to jaundice, in which bile is deposited in tissues throughout the body.

These infants may experience hypoglycemia after birth. The maternal source of glucose is no longer available, and because glucose readily crosses the placenta, levels of glucose in utero tend to be high, especially if the diabetes has been poorly controlled. Infants born to mothers with diabetes require immediate monitoring in the neonatal intensive care unit (NICU).

Fortunately there may be a decreased prevalence of many of the maternal and fetal complications associated with DM when normal blood glucose level (normoglycemia) is achieved before conception and maintained throughout pregnancy. The current recommendation is for women to achieve tight glucose control *before* conception to maximize the likelihood of a healthy mother and infant while avoiding perinatal risks. Control includes prudent blood glucose monitoring, adherence to diet, moderate exercise, and strict adherence to the prescribed insulin regimen. Total energy intake and energy distribution will likely need modification during pregnancy because of the increased energy needs of pregnancy. Insulin dosages will require adjustment because many of the hormones of pregnancy, such as estrogen, progesterone, human chorionic, somatotropin, and maternal cortisol, act in an antagonistic fashion with insulin. All women with diabetes

should discuss drug treatment options with their physician before conception.

Gestational diabetes mellitus (GDM) is a form of diabetes occurring during pregnancy, most commonly after the twentieth week of gestation. Pregnancy affects glucose control and insulin needs. For nondiabetic women, insulin sensitivity is decreased by placental and ovarian hormones. In response, more insulin is secreted to ensure appropriate glucose levels. The pancreatic reserves of approximately 5% to 10% of women are unable to compensate and do not secrete adequate insulin, and gestational diabetes develops. Patients experience abnormal carbohydrate metabolism in a manner similar to other persons with diabetes. Of all forms of diabetes during pregnancy, GDM is the most common, affecting 4% of all pregnancies.[13] All women should undergo screening for GDM during the second trimester, with repeat testing for women who may be borderline.

Treatment of GDM consists primarily of dietary control combined with moderate exercise leading to an appropriate weight gain. Insulin may be required if glycemic control is not achieved through dietary control and exercise. Risk factors for GDM include delivery of a previous large infant, prepregnancy weight, family history of diabetes, ethnicity (see the *Cultural Considerations* box, Gestational Diabetes: Screening Guidelines Based on Ethnicity?), a prior perinatal death, glycosuria, and maternal age greater than 30 years (Box 11-6). The majority of women with GDM have normal glucose tolerance following delivery, but they may remain at risk for type 2 diabetes mellitus later in life.

Maternal Phenylketonuria

Phenylketonuria (PKU) is an inborn error of metabolism characterized by extremely low levels of the enzyme phenylalanine hydroxylase, which catalyzes the conversion of phenylalanine to tyrosine. Absence of this crucial enzyme causes a failure in the metabolism of the amino acid phenylalanine and low levels of tyrosine. Successful treatment of this disorder occurs by adhering to a strict diet low in phenylalanine and supplemented with tyrosine beginning in the first week of life. Failure to detect the disease or a lack of compliance with the dietary therapy results in irreversible mental retardation.

Thirty years ago most patients with PKU did not conceive and bear children. Most likely, they were disabled before they were diagnosed or able to properly adjust their diets. However, with the advent of neonatal PKU testing in all 50 states, diagnosis and treatment of the disorder allow many young women to lead normal, productive lives, including having children. Women with PKU require specialized nutrition care during pregnancy. Maternal PKU, particularly if not well controlled at the time of conception, poses a great risk to the unborn offspring. Mothers with untreated PKU have a high likelihood of experiencing spontaneous abortion or having an infant born with microcephaly, mental retardation, congenital heart defects, or intrauterine growth retardation, even if the infant does not have the genetic defect. Conscientious adherence to a low-phenylalanine diet may lessen, but not

⊕ CULTURAL CONSIDERATIONS

Gestational Diabetes: Screening Guidelines Based on Ethnicity?

African Americans, Latinas, and Asians are more at risk for the development of gestational diabetes (GDM) than are Caucasians. Regardless of the type of screening tests used, the highest prevalence of GDM is among Asians, Latinas, African Americans, and then Caucasians. There are sensitivity and specificity variation responses of each ethnic group, so a single screening threshold such as 140 mg/dL may not be the most efficacious level to use for all groups to determine the presence of GDM. Perhaps race/ethnicity specific glucose-screening test thresholds should be used.

A retrospective cohort study of 14,058 pregnant women meeting study criteria were screened for gestational diabetes between January 1988 and December 2001 in San Francisco, Calif. Based on the ethnicities self-reported, there were four ethnic groups of Caucasian, African American, Hispanic or Latina, and Asian. The results suggest that it may be prudent to adjust threshold values based on ethnicity in order to strengthen sensitivity and decrease false-positive rates of the glucose-loading test. Additional research, though, is needed to assess if this will result in improved outcomes.

Application to nursing

This study considers that race and ethnicity may affect the threshold values of screening tools that in turn influence treatment decisions. Criteria for diagnosis may reflect this difference formally in the future. The need for quality prenatal care is once again emphasized. In nursing practice, clients can be made aware early in prenatal education of risk factors of gestational diabetes, particularly if of a higher risk racial/ethnic group.

From Esakoff TF, et al.: Screening for gestational diabetes: Different cut-offs for different ethnicities? *Am J Obs Gyn* 193(3 S1):1040-1044, 2005.

---

completely eliminate, the risk of an adverse pregnancy outcome.[14] Total nutrient intake and maternal weight gain should be monitored throughout pregnancy.

All young women with PKU should continue their low-phenylalanine diets throughout the childbearing years. Family planning is strongly encouraged to establish safe phenylalanine levels before conception and to educate women regarding the high risk of poor pregnancy outcome, even with good dietary control.

Human Immunodeficiency Virus Infection

In the United States most of the female cases of HIV infection are among women of childbearing age. Pregnancy may put an additional strain on the already fragile immune system because the hormones and proteins of pregnancy (including estrogen, progesterone, human chorionic gonadotropin (HGC), alpha fetoprotein, corticosteroids, prolactin, and alpha globulin) have immunosuppressive effects.

The HIV-infected woman experiencing an opportunistic infection during pregnancy has increased needs for kcal, protein, vitamins, and minerals. Weight gain must be strictly

---

BOX 11-6	RISK FACTORS AND SYMPTOMS OF GESTATIONAL DIABETES MELLITUS

Risk Factors
- Obesity
- Advanced maternal age
- African or Hispanic heritage
- Recurrent infections
- Gestational diabetes in previous pregnancy
- In a previous child having a congenital malformation or birth defect and/or unexplained death of fetus or newborn
- Previous newborn weighing more than 9 pounds

Symptoms
Often there are no symptoms, but the following may occur:
- Increased thirst
- Increased urination
- Weight loss with increased appetite
- Fatigue
- Blurred vision
- Frequent infections including those of the bladder, vagina, and skin
- Nausea and vomiting

---

monitored, although there are no specialized weight gain recommendations for this population.

Overcoming Barriers: Relief from Common Discomforts during Pregnancy

The following information discusses the common discomforts during pregnancy and methods of relief.

Nausea and Vomiting

Nausea and vomiting during the first trimester of pregnancy can be annoying, but they generally begin to subside by the beginning of the second trimester. Symptoms of morning sickness may actually occur at any time throughout the day, although vomiting tends to be more common between 6 AM and noon. Although the etiology of nausea and vomiting during pregnancy is unknown, it may be caused by hormonal factors such as a rise in estrogen or the placental hormone HCG. Stress or fatigue may exacerbate the condition. There is no cause for alarm unless the mother begins to lose weight or becomes severely dehydrated. If she cannot retain either foods or fluid for 6 hours or longer, a physician should be contacted.

If nausea or vomiting persists into the second trimester or severely interferes with the mother's life, it may be a more serious condition. Hyperemesis gravidarum is severe and unrelenting vomiting and usually requires intravenous replacement of nutrients and fluids. If the mother receives total parenteral nutrition or nasogastric tube feedings for the treatment of hyperemesis gravidarum, appropriate levels of vitamins and minerals should be included, with careful monitoring and follow-up.

There are no specific foods to avoid, but many women find it is helpful to eat small, frequent meals; drink liquids between rather than with meals; and avoid fried and greasy foods. Some women find it helpful to reduce coffee intake and to prepare meals near an open window to avoid cooking odors. If nausea on getting out of bed in the morning is a problem, dry toast or crackers eaten before getting out of bed may provide relief. Snacks to keep handy while working or traveling might include dried fruit, crackers, and small cans of juice.

Heartburn

In late pregnancy, when the fetus rapidly grows in size, the uterus pushes up against the stomach, which may cause a feeling of fullness in the mother. Additionally, because of the action of progesterone (which can cause relaxation of smooth muscles), a relaxation of the gastroesophageal sphincter may occur, resulting in some reflux of gastric contents into the lower esophagus. This is the cause of the heartburn so common during the final weeks of pregnancy. The best dietary remedies include eating small, frequent meals; avoiding foods high in fat; drinking fluids between rather than with meals; limiting spicy foods; and avoiding lying down for 1 to 2 hours after eating. Many women find relief by wearing loose-fitting clothing around the abdomen. Expectant mothers should not take antacids without approval of a primary care provider. Heartburn generally disappears after delivery of the infant.

Constipation

Constipation is common during the first and third trimesters of pregnancy. During the first trimester, progesterone (which slows GI motility) may be responsible. In the third trimester, the growing fetus crowds the other internal organs, again possibly slowing GI motility. Although bothersome, constipation responds well to dietary treatment. A generous intake of fiber, such as whole grain cereals, fresh fruit, and raw vegetables, as well as inclusion of plenty of fluids should alleviate constipation. Moderate exercise such as a daily walk also may help. The recommendations for alleviating constipation also help prevent hemorrhoids. Over-the-counter laxatives or enemas should not be used unless prescribed by a physician.

NUTRITION DURING LACTATION

All sexually mature female mammals possess milk-producing mammary glands and are able to produce milk specifically formulated to provide optimum growth and development for their offspring. Although there are historical accounts of wet nurses and even artificial feeding implements dating back to Greek and Roman times, breastfeeding (lactation) was the primary mode of infant feeding until this century in the United States and around the world.

Since World War II, however, there has been a dramatic decline in the incidence and duration of breastfeeding worldwide. Currently close to 60% of mothers in the United States initiate breastfeeding at hospital discharge, but by 5 to 6 months after birth, only about 20% of American infants are

---

BOX 11-7 BENEFITS OF BREASTFEEDING

- Provides immunologic protection to the infant against many infections and diseases (especially respiratory and gastrointestinal)
- Offers uniquely suited nutrient composition with high bioavailability
- Reduces risk of food allergy in the infant
- Promotes infant oral motor development
- Offers convenience: always fresh, available, and at the right temperature
- Is generally less expensive than formula feeding
- May protect infant against some chronic diseases such as type 1 diabetes and childhood leukemia
- Promotes mother-infant bonding
- Facilitates uterine contractions and controls postpartum bleeding
- Promotes return to prepregnancy weight

---

breastfed.[15,16] In many developed countries, such as Sweden, all women initiate breastfeeding and continue for most of the infant's first year of life. Although there is not one isolated cause for poor breastfeeding rates in the United States, it can be attributed to a multitude of causes. These include the advertising of breast milk substitutes, lack of support for the breastfeeding mother, lack of knowledge of lactation by health care professionals, short postpartum hospital stays, and the rise in maternal employment without appropriate facilities to nurse infants or pump and store breast milk.[17]

The American Dietetic Association and the American Academy of Pediatrics have policy statements advocating exclusive use of human milk as the preferred feeding choice for infants for at least the first 6 months of life.[15,17] Ideally, breastfeeding should occur for the entire first 12 months accompanied by appropriate weaning foods. Although primary nourishment is provided by breast milk for the first 6 months, introduction of complementary foods may range from 4 to 8 months, depending on individual feeding behaviors and needs. Breastfeeding offers advantages for both infant and mother (Box 11-7).

Anatomy and Physiology of Lactation

The human breast begins development in utero and goes through two further stages of change after birth: at puberty and during pregnancy. The mature human breast consists of a system of alveoli and ducts. Myoepithelial cells surround the milk-producing glands, located in the alveoli. The ductules emerge from the alveoli to carry the milk to the lactiferous ducts, which eventually empty into the lactiferous sinuses. The lactiferous sinuses are located behind the areola, or the darkened area of the nipple where the infant latches on during nursing (Figure 11-4).

Throughout the course of pregnancy, the breast tissue undergoes considerable development. Under the influence of progesterone, the lobules or alveoli increase in size and number, and estrogen stimulates proliferation of the ductal

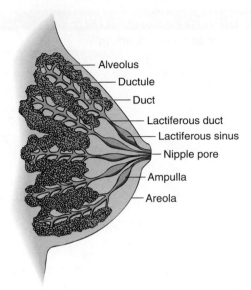

FIG 11-4 Detailed structural features of the human mammary gland. (From Rolin Graphics.)

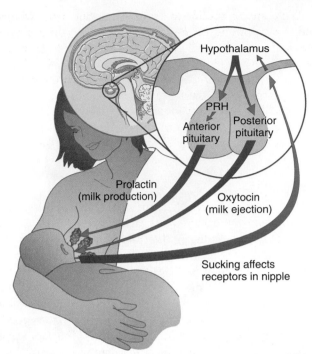

FIG 11-5 Maternal breastfeeding reflexes. (From Mahan KL, Escott-Stump S: *Krause's food & nutrition therapy,* ed 12, Philadelphia, 2008, Saunders.)

system. Together, these changes render the breast completely capable of milk production after delivery. An uncommon occurrence is a failure of the breasts to undergo development during pregnancy. A woman who does not notice any changes in her breasts during pregnancy, particularly if she is pregnant for the first time, should receive postnatal assistance to determine her ability to fully lactate. Most women are able to fully lactate with no problems. Actual size of breast has no bearing on the ability to breastfeed.

Lactation is a normal process beginning when various hormones interact following delivery of the infant. Before the onset of labor, there is a rise in serum levels of oxytocin. This hormone is instrumental in initiating the uterine contractions of labor that bring about birth. Oxytocin and another hormone, prolactin, set off the lactation process. Prolactin is primarily responsible for milk synthesis; oxytocin is involved with milk ejection from the breast.

When an infant is allowed to suckle after birth, a nerve impulse is sent to the mother's hypothalamus. This stimulates the anterior pituitary to secrete prolactin, which then stimulates milk production in the alveolar cells (Figure 11-5). The infant sucking stimulus initiates the release of oxytocin from the posterior pituitary. The flood of oxytocin into the breast tissue causes the myoepithelial cells around the glands to contract, thereby ejecting the milk into the infant's mouth. This is called the *let-down reflex,* or the *milk-ejection reflex.* Many women report feeling a tingling sensation in their breasts when the let-down occurs. Additionally, if a mother hears her infant's cry or sees another infant, she may experience a let-down accompanied by a rush of milk ejecting from her breasts. Deterrents to the let-down reflex may include fatigue, stress, alcohol, smoking, and some prescription medications.

An important point to note is that milk production is a supply-and-demand mechanism. The more an infant is allowed to nurse, the more nerve stimulation there will be,

resulting in a rise in prolactin levels followed by increased milk production. There should be no restrictions placed on the number of times an infant, particularly a newborn, nurses per day.[17]

Of particular value is colostrum which is the fluid secreted from the breast during late pregnancy and the first few days postpartum. When consumed by a newborn, colostrum provides immunologic active substances (maternal antibodies) and essential nutrients.

Promoting Breastfeeding

To increase the incidence and duration of breastfeeding in the United States and around the world, health care professionals can take measures ensuring that appropriate breastfeeding policies are adopted and practiced in hospitals providing maternity care. In 1991 the World Health Organization and UNICEF launched the Baby Friendly Hospital Initiative. The initiative includes "Ten Steps to Successful Breastfeeding" that the hospital must be willing to take to become infant friendly. Among the steps is breastfeeding education for all mothers, no separation of mother and infant following birth except for medical reasons, and no supplemental feedings unless medically indicated.[18] Nurses play a key role in prenatal counseling and in postpartum support to help mothers successfully establish and maintain lactation. Obstetric nurses should consult a lactation specialist if an infant or mother has difficulties initiating breastfeeding.

Another influence on successful lactation is acceptability of lactation within the cultural and ethnic communities of which the mother is a part. Cultures in which breastfeeding is common include Chinese, Finnish, Indian, Saudi Arabian,

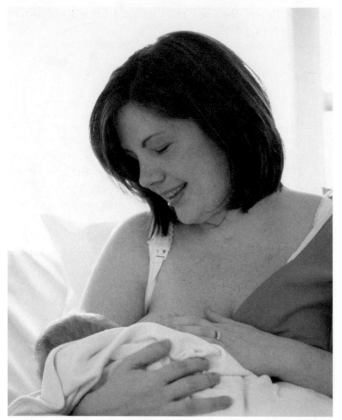

Successful breastfeeding depends on the health and nutritional status of the mother, her attitude toward breastfeeding, and support from health care providers and family. (Photos.com.)

Muslim, South African, and Swedish. In the following cultures, breastfeeding is common, but infants are not given colostrum because it is considered bad or unclean: Cambodian, Filipino, Haitian, Japanese, Korean, Laotian, Mexican, and Vietnamese.[19] Socioeconomic and education levels are influences that help or hinder a mother's attempt at successful lactation. Organizations such as La Leche League or community-based mothers' groups may provide invaluable support to nursing mothers, particularly those nursing for the first time (see the *Personal Perspectives* box, Testament to Breastfeeding).

Energy and Nutrient Needs during Lactation

A large proportion of the energy stores laid down as adipose tissue during pregnancy are mobilized in lactation. Both BMR and maternal activity return to their prepregnant levels. The energy cost of milk production is approximately 500 to 800 kcal per day, depending on the volume of milk production. The RDA recommends increases for protein (71 g per day) and for most of the vitamins and minerals over the normal adult levels. The mother can meet most of these increases by consuming a well-balanced diet (see Table 11-2).

A woman need not avoid certain foods while breastfeeding unless a problem occurs. For example, some infants are fussy following the mother's consumption of gas-producing vegetables such as cabbage, onions, and broccoli.

Adequate fluid intake is important during lactation. The average woman produces 750 to 1000 mL of milk per day. She can replace this fluid through consumption of water or juice. Coffee or cola drinks should be avoided or used on a minimal basis. They act as diuretics in the mother's body, and caffeine, a stimulant, passes into breast milk in small amounts. The old myth stating that alcohol helps a mother relax and enhances milk production should not be followed. Alcohol not only passes into milk, thus becoming available to the infant, but it also may inhibit oxytocin, consequently reducing the let-down reflex.

Despite the desire of most women to return to their prepregnancy weight quickly, rapid weight loss should not be encouraged while breastfeeding; milk reduction may result. Research shows that women may achieve weight loss without compromising their nutritional intake or the infant's when breastfeeding without the use of supplementary formula continues for at least 6 months. Sufficient milk may be provided with a modest caloric reduction for healthy lactating women with a 1 lb per week loss. An energy intake of at least 1800 kcal per day should be maintained for adequate lactation regardless of maternal fat stores.[12]

Contraindications to Breastfeeding

Common colds, the flu, and even most illnesses requiring short-term antibiotic therapy do not require cessation of breastfeeding. A number of maternal illnesses or conditions, however, are contraindications to breastfeeding:

- Active tuberculosis
- Human immunodeficiency virus/acquired immunodeficiency syndrome (HIV/AIDS)
- Herpes simplex lesions on the maternal breast
- Maternal alcoholism
- Maternal drug addiction
- Malaria
- Maternal chicken pox (first 3 weeks postpartum only)
- Maternal breast cancer requiring treatment

Most medications for mild illnesses are safe for the mother to take while breastfeeding. Mothers should always remind their health care providers that they are nursing an infant should the need for a medication arise. The American Academy of Pediatrics has classified medications into five categories based on safety considerations. For mild illnesses, as well as for chronic diseases, a medication compatible with breastfeeding can usually be found and substituted for one that is contraindicated.[20] The amount of the maternal dose of drug actually secreted into the milk depends on the route of administration, the size of the molecule, ionization, the pH of the medication, solubility, and protein binding.[21] Health care providers might keep this information in mind as they consider prescription medications for nursing mothers.

The Centers for Disease Control and Prevention (CDC) recommend that all women in the United States infected with HIV not breastfeed their infants.[22] In developing countries where the risk of death from diarrhea caused by inappropriate bottle feeding is far greater than the risk of transmission of HIV via human milk, the World Health Organization recommends that breastfeeding continue in these situations.[23] The woman with active AIDS and opportunistic infections is unlikely to have the physical strength to successfully lactate.

Because of the advent of hepatitis B vaccinations given at birth, hepatitis B is no longer a contraindication to breastfeeding. However, there is mother-to-infant transmission of hepatitis C, and therefore mothers with hepatitis C should not breastfeed.

NUTRITION DURING INFANCY

Energy and Nutrient Needs during Infancy

Dramatic changes in growth and development occur during the first 12 months of life. In the first year, a human infant is expected to triple its birth weight and increase its length by 50%. In addition, after birth, organs such as the kidney and brain continue to develop and mature. In no other period of life do growth and development occur so rapidly. To support this rapid growth and development, the appropriate balance of all nutrients is essential. At the same time, parents, caregivers, and health care professionals must realize that infants have specialized nutrient needs. Advice that is appropriate for adults, and even older children, is inappropriate for infants, particularly with regard to fat and fiber intake and weight gain patterns.

Energy

Adequate energy intake will be reflected in satisfactory gains in length and weight as plotted on a National Center for Health Statistics (NCHS) growth chart (www.cdc.gov/growthcharts/clinical_charts.htm). Infants should not have a restricted fat intake. Well-meaning parents should not place their infants on low-fat diets. Human milk, in fact, is high in cholesterol and fat content. Omega-3 fatty acids are plentiful in human milk, particularly if the mother includes fish in her diet on a regular basis. These fatty acids have been found to be essential for proper brain and nervous system development.[24,25]

Protein

Protein needs of infants have been hard to determine because of the difficulty of performing nitrogen balance studies on this population. Requirements are estimated based on the intake and growth rates of normal, healthy breastfed infants. Protein requirement is highest during the first 4 months of life when growth is the most rapid. It is suggested infants receive 2.2 g/kg/day from birth to 6 months of age and 1.6 g/kg/day for the second half of the first year.[25] An excess of protein in an infant's diet can be problematic. Protein has a significant influence on renal solute load. The infant kidney is immature and unable to handle the large renal solute loads of an adult. Therefore, increasing a normal infant's protein intake above the recommended amount should be avoided.

Vitamins and Mineral Supplementation

The DRIs may be consulted for appropriate levels of vitamins and minerals for infants. Breast milk or commercial formula should provide infants with all the vitamins and minerals needed for proper growth and development (Table 11-3).

During the third trimester of pregnancy, the fetus stores iron in its liver to be used during the postnatal period. By 4 months of age, this supply of iron is usually depleted. The

TABLE 11-3	RECOMMENDED SUPPLEMENTATION OF INFANT DIETS			
TYPE OF FEEDING	IRON	VITAMIN D	FLUORIDE	VITAMIN K
Human milk	1 mg/kg/day*	10 mcg/day	0.25 mg/day	Single intramuscular dose of 0.5 to 1 mg or oral dose of 1 to 2 mg
Formula	Iron-fortified formula		0.25 mg/day†	Single intramuscular dose of 0.5 to 1 mg or oral dose of 1 to 2 mg

*May be provided through iron-containing foods after 6 months of age.
†If fluoride content of water is less than 0.3 part per million.
Adapted from Committee on Nutrition, American Academy of Pediatrics, *Handbook of pediatric nutrition,* ed 6, Elk Grove Village, Ill, 2009, American Academy of Pediatrics.

iron in breast milk, although lower in absolute amounts, is more bioavailable than iron from commercial formula. Many breastfed infants do not need to be supplemented with iron. However, their iron levels should be assessed periodically. Infants who consume commercial formula should use the iron-fortified variety to prevent iron deficiency anemia.

Humans are able to manufacture vitamin D through exposure to the sun; many young infants may not receive enough sun exposure for adequate synthesis. Breast milk contains vitamin D, but it may not be present in levels sufficient to prevent vitamin D–related rickets. There are several documented cases of vitamin D–related rickets, particularly among fully breastfed infants who receive little or no sunlight exposure.[26] Therefore, it is recommended that all breastfed infants receive a daily oral supplement of vitamin D, unless they receive substantial sunlight exposure. Vitamin D can be toxic, so the recommended dosage should not be exceeded. Because vitamin D is present in commercial infant formula, formula-fed infants need not receive a supplement. Use of milk alternatives such as rice beverage ("rice milk") and soy health food beverage also has resulted in rickets. These alternatives, which are low in protein, calcium, and vitamin D, are not nutrient dense in comparison with breast milk, formula, or cow's milk. Health care providers need to emphasize to caregivers that although the term "milk" is used in reference to these beverages, they are not nutritionally equal to milk produced by humans or by animals.

The water supply of most major cities in the United States contains fluoride as a preventive measure against tooth decay. The availability of fluoride may be particularly important for infants and young children whose teeth are developing. Routine fluoride supplementation is not recommended for infants younger than 6 months of age. Older infants may need to receive fluoride if their local water supply is not fluoridated, but an assessment of total exposure to fluoride (via water, or juice prepared from local water source) should be made before systemic fluoride is prescribed. For example, many rural families who rely on well water should have water supplies assessed for fluoride content. Excess fluoride can result in fluorosis, or mottling of tooth enamel, so precise dosing is critical.

Newborns are vulnerable to vitamin K deficiency (and thus hemorrhaging) in part because they lack intestinal bacteria to synthesize the vitamin. As a preventive measure, U.S. hospitals routinely give infants 0.5 to 1 mg of vitamin K by injection or 1 to 2 mg orally, once shortly after birth.

Food for Infants

The ideal food for the first 4 to 6 months of life is exclusive use of breast milk, which has the correct balance of all the essential nutrients as well as immunologic factors that protect the infant from acute and chronic diseases. The breast should be offered at least 10 to 12 times per 24 hours in the first several weeks. As the infant develops a stronger suck, more milk will be extracted with each nursing session, and the frequency of feeding may decline. Although there is no specified time the infant should stay on the breast, between 10 and 15 minutes per breast (offering both breasts per session) is a good recommendation. It is important to realize this is a *general* guideline because all infants have different nursing styles. It may in fact be more appropriate to watch the *infant*—not the *clock*—in an effort to allow the infant to dictate when satiety is reached. The *Teaching Tool* box, Guidelines for Successful Breastfeeding, offers some suggestions to facilitate breastfeeding.

If a mother chooses not to breastfeed or if she has a medical condition contraindicating breastfeeding, a variety of formulas made from either cow's milk or soy are available. In addition, a number of specialty formulas, such as protein hydrolysate formulas, are available for infants with medical problems. The parents should consult their primary health care provider or nutrition care specialist to identify the most appropriate formula for their infant.

Formulas are either ready-to-feed, with no mixing required, or are a powder or liquid concentrate to be mixed with water (Box 11-8). To reduce the chance of lead leaching into water, tap water should be run for 2 minutes after it has been standing in the pipes, and only cold water should be used for formula preparation. The formula should be mixed exactly as stated on the package, unless otherwise directed by a primary health care provider. Adding insufficient water can result in a high renal solute load, placing strain on the immature infant kidneys; overdiluting will precipitate undernutrition.

For parents or caregivers who may be non–English speaking or have low literacy skills, pictorial mixing instructions may be useful. Alternatively, asking the caregiver to demonstrate appropriate formula mixing may be suitable. Formula

Guidelines for Successful Breastfeeding

Although breastfeeding is the most natural and easiest way to feed infants, mothers who decide to breastfeed will welcome the following suggestions:

- Offer both breasts at each nursing session.
- Open infant's mouth wide to latch on correctly.
- Place at least 1/2 to 3/4 inch of the areola in the infant's mouth, not just the nipple.
- Check that the infant's lips make a tight seal around the breast.
- Sore nipples are usually caused by incorrect positioning; position the infant correctly in a tummy-to-tummy fashion or in a "football hold." Support newborn's head and back with extra pillows on the mother's lap or with the mother's arm cradling infant.
- Do not limit nursing time in the first several days. This does not prevent sore nipples and may hinder milk production.
- Remember: milk is produced by supply and demand—the more often the infant nurses, the more milk produced.
- Expect growth spurts at approximately 10 days, 2 weeks, 6 weeks, and 3 months. At these times, expect a fussy infant who wants to nurse frequently.
- Offer no bottles of formula or water while the milk supply is being established. The artificial nipple may confuse the infant, and substitute feedings that replace breast stimulation may diminish milk production.
- Once milk supply is established, breast milk may be expressed manually or by a pump and saved in a bottle in the refrigerator (up to 48 hours) or in the freezer (several months).
- Learn your infant's cues for satiety.

BOX 11-8   FORMULA PREPARATION

1. Clean all necessary equipment and wash hands before preparing formula.
2. Read formula label and dilute formula exactly as recommended by the manufacturer.
3. Use cold tap water for preparation of concentrated or powdered formula, unless directed otherwise by physician or nurse.
4. Never heat formula in a microwave oven.
5. Discard unused formula after 2 hours.

---

should never be heated in a microwave oven because microwaves heat food unevenly. Contents of a bottle appearing to be cool on testing may actually have portions that could scald an infant. All unused formula at the end of a feeding should be discarded if not used within 2 hours because of contamination by saliva enzymes and bacteria. Home-prepared formulas made from evaporated milk, popular in some cultures, are likely to be low in iron, vitamin C, and other essential nutrients and should be avoided.

Before 1 year of age, cow's milk, regardless of fat content or form (evaporated, liquid, or dried), should not be fed to infants. The fat in cow's milk is less digestible than the fat in breast milk or formula and contains less iron and more sodium and protein. These higher levels of solutes may lead to dehydration caused by increased urine volume to reduce solute levels in the body. Deficiencies of other nutrients, such as vitamin C, essential fatty acids, zinc, and possibly other trace minerals, develop because cow's milk is a poor source of these nutrients.

Cow's milk may be introduced after 1 year of age when at least two-thirds of energy needs are fulfilled by foods other than milk. The delay in cow's milk consumption reduces the risk of developing a milk allergy. Reduced fat and nonfat milk is not recommended until age 2.

Introduction of solid foods. Solid foods may be added to the infant's diet between the ages of 4 and 6 months. Infants who are introduced to solid foods before this time may be prone to excessive kcal intake, food allergies, and GI upset. Many parents and even some health care professionals believe offering an infant cereal in the evening will promote sleeping through the night. This belief, however, is not supported by research.

Two basic issues when considering the introduction of solid foods to the infant's diet are how to introduce them and what foods to introduce.

How to introduce solid foods. Parents and other caregivers may be anxious to introduce foods other than breast milk or formula to their infant's diet. Health professionals can assure them that it's best for the infant to be developmentally ready for solid foods. The infant should be able to sit with some support; move the jaw, lips, and tongue independently; be able to roll the tongue to the back of the mouth to facilitate a food bolus entering the esophagus; and show interest in what the rest of the family is eating. For example, the infant may try to reach and grab an item off of a family member's plate at mealtime. Likewise, parents should become familiar with satiety cues so as not to overfeed the infant. To indicate fullness the infant may turn the head to the side, refuse to open the mouth, or grimace when the spoon comes close to the mouth. The caregiver should respect these cues. The infant should never be force-fed. If the infant is overtired or is not interested in food, he or she ought to be removed from the high chair and the foods offered again later.

At the age of 9 to 12 months, an infant may enjoy self-feeding. Although this may be a messy process, caregivers should encourage the development of these skills through food exploration (Figure 11-6).

Appropriate solid foods during the first year of life. The second half of the first year of life should be thought of as a transitional period; breast milk or formula is still the primary food, and the solid foods are complementary. Solid foods should be introduced gradually and one at a time with a 4- to 5-day interval between new foods. This timing is suggested because if the infant has any type of allergic reaction such as GI upset, upper respiratory distress, or skin reactions (e.g., eczema, hives), the offending food can be easily identified. Families with a documented history of allergies should delay introduction of solid foods until the infant is about 6 months

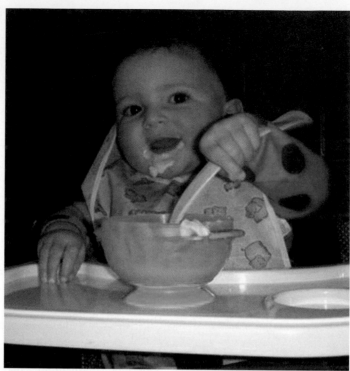

FIG 11-6 A messy experience as an 11-month-old infant strives to feed herself with a spoon.

old. If solid foods are introduced too early, the large protein molecules of the offending food may cross the intestinal barrier and elicit an immunologic response in the infant. As the gut matures, it is less likely to allow large unhydrolyzed proteins to cross the mucosa.

Solid foods offered to the infant need not be commercial. Home-prepared foods are a good, practical alternative. There should be strict attention to sanitary food preparation procedures. Although infants should not be offered excessive sweets, naturally sweet fruits such as peaches offer them a taste satisfaction. Although salt should not be added to an infant's food, complete elimination of sodium from foods in the diet is neither practical nor recommended.

A variety of textures, colors, and tastes is important for infants, whether they receive home-prepared or commercial infant foods. The *Personal Perspectives* box, Developing "Nutrition Intelligence," provides strategies introducing infants and older children to a diverse selection of foods. General guidelines for infant feeding are listed in Table 11-4.

Beverages during the first year of life. Fruit juice, particularly apple juice, is offered to many infants. Fruit juice can make an important contribution to the diet as a source of vitamin C, water, and possibly calcium (if fortified). Its use, though, needs to be monitored. From age 6 to 12 months, no more than 4 to 6 fluid ounces per day should be offered. Excess fruit juice (more than 12 fluid ounces per day) may lead to diarrhea from carbohydrate malabsorption, growth failure, or, in some children, obesity caused by excess calories.[27,28] Juices can be diluted with water, providing a beverage with less sweetness. All fruit juices given to infants (and children) should be pasteurized.

TABLE 11-4	SOLID FOODS DURING THE FIRST YEAR OF LIFE	
AGE	**FOOD**	**FOODS TO AVOID IN THE FIRST YEAR OF LIFE**
4-5 months	Iron-fortified infant cereal	Honey (may cause infantile *Clostridium botulinum* poisoning); hot dogs, grapes, hard candies, raw carrots, popcorn, nuts, peanut butter (choking hazards); skim milk (insufficient calories); cow's milk (potential allergen, may replace breast milk or formula); egg whites (potential allergen)
5-6 months	Strained fruits and vegetables	
6-8 months	Mashed or chopped fruits and vegetables Juice from a cup	
9-12 months	Crackers, toast, cottage cheese, plain meats, egg yolk, finger foods	

Baby Bottle Tooth Decay

Baby bottle tooth decay (BBTD), also known as *nursing bottle caries, nursing bottle mouth,* and *nursing bottle syndrome,* is a distinctive pattern of tooth decay in infants and young children. It most commonly affects the maxillary incisors, although other teeth may be affected as well. From 5% to 15% of all children may be affected, but precise prevalence figures are difficult to obtain.[29] For BBTD to develop, the

PERSONAL PERSPECTIVES

Developing "Nutrition Intelligence"

Alan Greene, MD, is a practicing physician who also teaches at Stanford University School of Medicine, but he is most known for advocating the green baby movement. The movement entails raising our young in a natural manner that is most supportive of their well-being and sustaining for our communities and world. He has coined the phrase "nutrition intelligence" to represent having a full understanding and experience of eating and enjoying great wholesome food. This excerpt is from his book Feeding Baby Green: The Earth-Friendly Program for Healthy, Safe Nutrition.

The Eight Essential Steps for Teaching Nutritional Intelligence

These eight simple steps to teaching nutritional intelligence will help you lay a strong foundation for building a healthy and delicious future for your child.

1. *Take Charge!* You are your child's first teacher and the primary agent of change in the way she approaches what she eats. It's not an overstatement to say that unless you take steps to prevent it, your child's food style will likely become a blend of the way you eat and the predominant American kids' food culture—weighted strongly toward the latter. The prevailing current is strong, but by making conscious choices now, you can make a lasting difference in your child's health and his enjoyment of food.

2. *Use Windows of Opportunity.* Every child has his or her own unique developmental process. Yet the stages of early development—from birth through about the end of the second year—provide special opportunities for you to make a deeper impact on future choices more easily than it will be later on. Learn to advance your child's food development in coordination with other unique stages of development that you see happening in your baby. Being out of sync often leads to food battles or refusing healthy food. Working together is one of life's joys.

3. *Engage All the Senses.* Use your baby's senses, even before birth, to help teach her to love great food, to create a deep sense of familiarity and joy about these healthy foods, and to help forge the comfort foods of her future. Enlist food's many flavors, aromas, and textures, and even its appearance and the language you use to talk about food....

4. *Choose the Right Amount.* The amount of food your child eats—before birth and after—not only affects growth now but can change hunger, metabolism, and health far into the future. Learn how to tell how much and what to feed your child at every age, and how to help her learn how much is just right for her.

5. *Choose the Right Variety.* Repetition is critical to acquiring tastes for new flavors, but so is novelty. A balanced diet is just that: a wide variety of colors and types of foods that meet all of your child's nutritional needs....

6. *Customize Needs for Every Body.* Learn to use foods to help address your family's specific health issues, including ADHD, allergies, asthma, cancer, diabetes, ear infections, and eczema. Learn to adapt the Feeding Baby Green program if you or your child has the "bitter taste" gene, and to fit your food preferences, schedule, beliefs, or culture.

7. *Exercise!* Exercise really is good for every body—yours and your child's. It's closely linked to how a body desires and uses food every day. Working in tandem with good nutrition, it's the best start you can give your baby. ...

8. *Reap the Benefits of Green.* Making connections—with where food comes from, with how it is prepared, and with others who share the food—is a powerful way to instill love for real food. The basics are simple: Eat seasonally. Eat locally. Grow something together. And choose organic. Avoiding extra hormones and toxic synthetic chemicals in our food and food containers is good for the environment and great for your baby.

From Greene A: *Feeding baby green: The earth-friendly program for healthy, safe nutrition*, San Francisco, Calif, 2009, Jossey-Bass.

mouth requires the presence of fermentable carbohydrate and a pathogenic organism.

BBTD commonly occurs in infants who are allowed to sleep with a bottle of milk, juice, or other sweetened liquid. As the infant falls asleep, the vigorous suck-swallow pattern that normally occurs during feeding diminishes. Moreover, saliva production decreases, resulting in a loss of saliva's buffering action in the mouth. Liquid pools in the infant's mouth, particularly behind the central incisors, becoming a ready source of fermentable carbohydrate for the bacteria colonizing the oral cavity. The acid produced by bacterial metabolism then destroys tooth enamel and initiates caries.

Prevention of BBTD is important for long-term dental health. Infants should never be put to bed with a bottle of milk, formula, juice, or other sweetened liquid. If a bottle is needed at bedtime, it should be plain water only. Oral hygiene may begin as soon as teeth erupt by a daily gentle cleaning of the tooth surfaces with gauze or a washcloth. Finally, sharing of food and utensils between adults and infants should be

discouraged because of transmission of bacteria from the adult to the infant. Weaning from the bottle should occur as soon as the child can drink from a cup.

Special Nutritional Needs

The nutrition requirements of children with congenital or acquired health problems deserve special attention. These infants often have increased nutrient requirements, increased losses, or malabsorption. Significant drug-nutrient interaction often takes place as well. Although it is beyond the scope of this chapter to describe all of the children's special needs one might encounter in practice, a few of the major disorders are outlined. In all of these cases, a registered dietitian should be a part of the medical team.

The Premature and Low Birth Weight Infant

An infant is considered premature if born before 37 weeks' gestation. Low birth weight infants may be full term or premature but weigh 2500 g or less at birth. As medical technology becomes increasingly sophisticated, infants are surviving at younger ages and lower weights. However, their developmental outlook may still be tenuous. Nutrition support of these infants plays a crucial role in successful long-term outcome. The major issues of concern in the premature infant are low birth weight, immature lung development, poor immune function, immature GI and neurologic function, insufficient production of digestive enzymes, inadequate bone mineralization, and minimal energy and mineral reserves.

Because the coordinated suck-swallow reflex is not fully developed until an infant reaches 34 weeks' gestation, initial feeding of the premature infant may need to be via total parenteral nutrition, tube feeding, or gavage feeding. Many criteria influence the route of nutrient delivery, and thus each infant should receive an individualized nutrition assessment by a registered dietitian who specializes in high-risk pediatrics.

Premature infants have increased needs for protein, kcal, calcium, phosphorus, sodium, iron, zinc, vitamin E, and fluids. The best feeding choice for a premature infant is mother's milk with the addition of "human milk fortifier," which adds additional minerals and protein needed by the premature infant. Although the infant may not suckle well or may tire easily at the breast, the nurse can play a key role in helping the mother pump and store her milk in the neonatal nursery. The milk may then be given by gavage even when the mother is not present. If the mother chooses not to breastfeed, a variety of specialized infant formulas are available to meet the special nutritional requirements of the infant.

Research suggests these formulas should be fortified with long-chain fatty acids to mimic what would be delivered via the placenta. Long-chain fatty acids are essential for proper retinal and neurologic development. Premature and low birth weight infants require continual nutrition follow-up after discharge for at least the first year of life because they are at risk for feeding problems, developmental delays, and growth retardation.

Cystic Fibrosis

Cystic fibrosis (CF) is an autosomal recessive disorder and is the most common genetic disorder among white populations, affecting roughly 1 in 2000 live births. Clinical features of the disease include chronic pulmonary disease, pancreatic exocrine insufficiency, and increased sweat chloride. The nutrition considerations facing children with CF include growth failure and energy and protein malnutrition. The chronic pulmonary dysfunction leads to malnutrition caused by an increased metabolic rate, increased energy requirement, and frequent use of antibiotics, which can cause anorexia. Steatorrhea, maldigestion, and malabsorption are common because of the lack of lipase secretion in the pancreas. Because of these increased needs as well as greater losses, patients are not always able to meet nutrition needs.

To prevent frank protein and energy malnutrition and resulting growth failure, the Consensus Committee of the Cystic Fibrosis Foundation recommends that all CF patients receive a comprehensive nutrition assessment every 3 to 4 months. Care of the CF patient should be multidisciplinary, and each nutrition assessment plan should be individualized to promote optimal growth and development.[30] Further nutrition interventions are discussed in Chapter 18.

Failure to Thrive

Failure to thrive (FTT) is defined as a fall of two standard deviations in weight gain over an interval of 2 months or longer for infants younger than 6 months of age or over an interval of 3 months or longer for infants older than 6 months of age.[31] An alternative definition is a weight-for-length measurement less than the fifth percentile or weight for age below the third percentile.[32]

FTT may have organic causes, such as an underlying metabolic disorder. Congenital heart disease or HIV infection may cause such an increased energy requirement that oral intake is not able to keep up with metabolic need.

Nonorganic FTT may be diagnosed when no medical reason for poor growth can be recognized. There may be psychosocial causes of the FTT such as either extreme of parental attention (neglect or excessive attentiveness).[33] Neglect may include inadequate maternal-infant bonding, poverty, child abuse, or neglect. Treatment for nonorganic FTT must include nutrition intervention to promote weight gain and therapy to correct developmental delays and any psychosocial problems in the home environment.[33]

Inborn Errors of Metabolism

Phenylketonuria. All 50 states have newborn screening programs to detect PKU. When discovered early, dietary therapy can begin immediately, and long-term prognosis is good. Without treatment, phenylalanine and its metabolites reach toxic levels in the blood, resulting in damage to the central nervous system, including mental retardation. Likewise, because phenylalanine cannot be converted to tyrosine, low or absent tyrosine may contribute to the mental retardation.

Treatment consists of a low-phenylalanine diet to be followed throughout the individual's life. In infancy the use of a special formula such as Lofenalac is recommended. Partial breastfeeding is permitted, but phenylalanine levels in the infant's blood must be monitored carefully.[14] As PKU children are introduced to solid foods and make the transition to table foods, meals require careful planning. The use of low-protein breads and pastas is advised. This condition requires close monitoring of dietary intake by specialized dietitians.

Galactosemia. Galactosemia is another rare, autosomal recessive disorder caused by an enzyme deficiency and is part of the newborn screening panel. Absence of the enzyme galactose-1-phosphate uridylyltransferase results in an inability to metabolize galactose. Because the milk sugar lactose is a disaccharide of glucose and galactose, these infants are unable to tolerate any milk products containing lactose. Manifestations include diarrhea, growth retardation, and mental retardation. Treatment is dietary therapy excluding all milk products, including human milk. Soy formulas and casein hydrolysate formulas are acceptable. Even with lifelong diet therapy, there may be long-term health consequences such as nervous system or ovarian dysfunction.[14] Specialized pediatric dietitians closely monitor the diet of infants and children who have this disorder.

Other inborn errors of metabolism that require nutrition therapy include urea cycle disorders, maple syrup urine disease, and homocystinuria.

TOWARD A POSITIVE NUTRITION LIFESTYLE: REFRAMING

Reframing means to change the way a situation or concept is understood to a different frame that equally suits and explains the situation. Pregnancy and all of the recommendations in this chapter could be viewed as a worrisome burden to the expectant mother. Her body will swell in size, and others may tease her for the weight she gains. Based on what she hears about pregnancy, it sounds as if every action and every morsel of food consumed will affect the health of her unborn child. Anxiety replaces excitement over the beginning of a new life.

Reframing pregnancy can improve the well-being of the expectant mother physically and emotionally. Nurses can encourage mothers to view the weight gain of pregnancy as a natural feminine process enhancing fetal growth and development. Dietary and lifestyle suggestions can be presented as proactive behaviors to support the nutrient needs of the expectant mother and those of the fetus. A more positive frame of pregnancy provides a reassuring gestational period full of anticipatory excitement.

SUMMARY

From before conception and through infancy, health promotion concepts are intricate components of wellness. Good nutrition habits form a foundation for proper growth and development. The importance of nutrition during pregnancy, the benefits of breastfeeding, and the establishment and maintenance of positive eating styles during infancy are crucial to overall health goals. Nutrition services should play a role in all health care delivery systems, not only as a vehicle to prevent chronic disease but also as an important part of comprehensive health care for chronic disease such as DM, inborn errors of metabolism, and CF.

Women need to be knowledgeable of dietary patterns providing for nutritional requirements of pregnancy. They should understand the impact of smoking, drugs, and alcohol on the course of fetal development. Health professionals need to review risk factors and never assume the public is knowledgeable of these dangers. Women whose pregnancies are at high risk, such as those complicated by DM, should have early and regular nutrition services provided during routine prenatal care; specific education may be needed to sensitize them to their special medical and nutritional needs.

Lactation is a natural, physiologic process beginning shortly after delivery. It completes the cycle of the female body from pregnancy through motherhood. Human milk is the best health promoter for the neonate. The majority of women can successfully breastfeed when given proper instruction, support, and follow-up. The nursing professional is in a good position to provide such care. Breastfeeding should begin immediately after birth and continue every 2 to 3 hours during the initial weeks postpartum.

Lactating women should continue to consume a diet with adequate sources of protein, energy, vitamins, and minerals. Despite the desire of most women to return to their prepregnancy weight quickly, rapid weight loss should not be encouraged while breastfeeding.

Health promotion, attending to the needs of the total person, begins as soon as an infant is born. Sound nutrition practices during the first year of life lay the foundation for good health. The ideal food for the first 4 to 6 months of life is breast milk. Supplemental foods may be introduced one at a time at 4 to 6 months of age. Breast milk (or formula) should continue until the infant reaches 1 year of age. Children with medical problems may require specialized nutrition support.

THE NURSING APPROACH

Case Study: Breastfeeding

Rebecca, age 24, delivered her first child two days before meeting with the nurse practitioner. She said she and the baby boy, Bobby, were doing well, but she had some questions about breastfeeding.

ASSESSMENT
Subjective (from patient statements)
- "He nurses OK and seems happy, though he wants to eat every two hours."
- "My nipples are not sore, but I feel really tired."
- "I plan to keep breastfeeding until Bobby is about six months old. I like the closeness I feel to him."
- "I'm wondering what to do about feeding when I need to leave the baby with my husband for a few hours."
- "How do I know if Bobby is getting enough to eat?"

Objective (from physical examination)
- Birth weight 7 pounds 10 ounces and length 19.7 inches

Continued

THE NURSING APPROACH—cont'd

Case Study: Breastfeeding—cont'd

- Newborn at 50th percentile for weight and length
- Loose yellow stool and light yellow urine in diaper

DIAGNOSIS (NURSING)

1. Effective breastfeeding as evidenced by the newborn infant "nurses OK and seems happy," the mother likes the closeness, newborn at 50th percentile for weight and height, and loose yellow stool and light yellow urine in infant's diaper
2. Readiness for enhanced knowledge as evidenced by questions about saving milk and evaluating adequacy of milk intake

PLANNING

Patient Outcomes

Short term (at the end of this visit):
- Rebecca will state how she can determine if the infant is eating enough.
- She will state how she can save milk for the infant for times when she cannot breastfeed.
- She will identify resources for continued success with breastfeeding.

Long term (follow-up visit after four weeks):
- Weight gain of infant as expected
- Rebecca will say she is satisfied with breastfeeding.

Nursing Interventions

1. Assess Rebecca's feelings about breastfeeding.
2. Encourage good nutrition and answer questions about breastfeeding.
3. Provide resources for Rebecca.

IMPLEMENTATION

1. Assessed Rebecca's feelings and attitudes about breastfeeding.

   The nurse can accept and support a woman's decision to breastfeed or bottle feed. If the mother is not successful with breastfeeding, the nurse can try to help her. If the mother is not happy with breastfeeding, the nurse should present her with an alternate choice of using formula in bottles.
2. Encouraged drinking at least 3000 ml of water, milk, and juices per day, and eating a well-balanced diet per recommendations from MyPyramid.gov.

   Adequate hydration, adequate nutrients, and extra kcal (about 500 kcal more than usual) are needed to support lactation and the health of the mother. Alcohol and caffeine should be avoided because they can be secreted in the breast milk.
3. Reviewed benefits of breastfeeding.

   It is rewarding for the mother to know that the infant may have fewer infections, fewer allergies, and easier digestion with breast milk. It is usually more convenient and economical to breastfeed rather than bottle feed.
4. Discussed how to express breast milk and save it in a bottle.

   Milk may be expressed manually or by a pump. It needs to be saved in a bottle in the refrigerator (up to 48 hours) or in the freezer (several months). Cleanliness and good hand washing are essential.
5. Discussed how to determine if the infant is getting enough milk.

   Breastfeeding should be done on a demand schedule, and the infant should generally be content after eating. At least six wet diapers and one bowel movement per day indicate adequate hydration and milk. Weight gain should follow a standard growth chart.
6. Provided literature about breastfeeding and La Leche League support groups and wrote down a contact number for the clinic.

   Written materials reinforce learning. Contacts and support personnel are helpful when questions arise about breastfeeding.

EVALUATION

Short term (at the end of the first visit):
- Rebecca identified how to determine if the infant is getting enough milk.
- She demonstrated how to express milk and stated how she can save milk.
- She said she might contact someone from La Leche support group.
- Goals met

Long term (in one month):
- Infant gained weight and remained in 50th percentile for height and weight.
- Rebecca reported her satisfaction and infant's contentment after breastfeeding
- She reported infant has a bowel movement with each feeding and urinates several times a day.
- Rebecca said she rented a breast pump and was able to save enough milk to go on a date with her husband while the grandmother cared for the infant.
- Goals met.

DISCUSSION QUESTIONS

At the follow-up visit, Rebecca said she was drinking a lot of diet cola to increase her fluid intake and production of breast milk. She was restricting her calorie intake so that she could quickly lose the 25 pounds she needed to lose to get back to prepregnancy weight.

1. Role-play a conversation the nurse could have with Rebecca about her fluid intake and her restriction of calories.
2. How soon should Rebecca add solid food to the infant's diet? What food may be tolerated best?

APPLYING CONTENT KNOWLEDGE

Elena, age 18, is a client at the city Special Supplemental Nutrition Program for Women, Infants, and Children (WIC); she is beginning her third trimester of pregnancy. She attended nutrition education classes taught by the WIC nutritionist. The nutritionist, though, is concerned because Elena has not been gaining sufficient weight to support her pregnancy but is otherwise healthy. The nutritionist suspects that Elena does not understand the relationship between her dietary intake and the health of her fetus. The nutritionist asks you as a WIC nurse to reinforce these concepts when Elena comes in for her monthly checkups. What will you discuss with Elena?

WEBSITES OF INTEREST

BabyCenter

www.BabyCenter.com

Covers a full range of topics ranging from preconception through infancy.

March of Dimes

www.modimes.org

Supplies information and resources on all aspects of pregnancy and genetic disorders to prevent birth defects.

La Leche League

www.lalecheleague.org

Advocates breastfeeding through education, information, and support through publications, conferences, and local chapter meetings.

REFERENCES

1. Turner RE: Nutrition during pregnancy. In Shils ME, et al, editors: *Modern nutrition in health and disease*, ed 10, Philadelphia, 2006, Lippincott Williams & Wilkins.
2. Heron M, et al: Annual summary of vital statistics: 2007, *Pediatrics* 125(1):4-15, 2010.
3. Smith C: The effect of wartime starvation in Holland upon pregnancy and its product, *Am J Obstet Gynecol* 53:599-608, 1947.
4. Bitler PM, Currie J: Does WIC work? The effects of WIC on pregnancy and birth outcomes, *J Policy Anal Manage* 24(1): 73-91, 2005.
5. Butte NF, King JC: Energy requirements during pregnancy and lactation, *Public Health Nutr* 8(7a):1010-1027, 2005.
6. Institute of Medicine, Food and Nutrition Board: *Dietary DRI References: The essential guide to nutrient requirements*, Washington, DC, 2006, The National Academies Press.
7. Clausson B, et al: Effect of caffeine exposure during pregnancy on birth weight and gestational age, *Am J Epidemiol* 155(5):429-436, 2002.
8. Rothman KJ, et al: Teratogenicity of high vitamins A intake, *N Engl J Med* 333:1369-1373, 1995.
9. Muscati SK, Koski KG, Gray-Donald K: Increased energy intake in pregnant smokers does not prevent human fetal growth retardation, *J Nutr* 126:2984-2989, 1996.
10. Vrijkotte TG, et al: First-trimester working conditions and birth weight: a prospective cohort study, *Am J Public Health* 99(8):1409-1416, 2009.
11. American College of Obstetics and Gynecology (ACOG): Exercise during pregnancy and the postpartum period, *ACOG Committee Opinion* 267:171-173, 2002.
12. Erick M: Nutrition during pregnancy and lactation. In Mahan LK, Escott-Stump S, editors: *Krause's food & nutrition therapy*, ed 12, Philadelphia, 2008, Saunders.
13. Anderson JW: Diabetes mellitus: Medical nutrition therapy. In Shils ME, et al, editors: *Modern nutrition in health and disease*, ed 10, Philadelphia, 2006, Lippincott Williams & Wilkins.
14. Elsas II LJ, Acosta PB: Inherited metabolic diseases: Amino acids, organic acids, and galactose. In Shils ME, et al, editors: *Modern nutrition in health and disease*, ed 10, Philadelphia, 2006, Lippincott Williams & Wilkins.
15. American Academy of Pediatrics: Policy statement on breastfeeding and the use of human milk, *Pediatrics* 115(2):496-506, 2005.
16. Tully MR: Working & breastfeeding: Helping moms and employees figure it out, *AWHONN Lifelines* 9(3):198-203, 2005.
17. American Dietetic Association: Position of the American Dietetic Association: Promoting and supporting breastfeeding, *J Am Diet Assoc* 109:1926-1942, 2009.
18. Hofvander Y: Breastfeeding and the Baby Friendly Hospitals Initiative (BFHI): Organization, response and outcome in Sweden and other countries, *Acta Paediatrica* 94(8):1012-1016, 2005.
19. Blaumslag N: Breast-feeding: cultural practices and variations. In Hamosh M, Goldman AS, editors: *Human lactation 2: Maternal and environmental factors*, ed 9, New York, 1986, Plenum Press.
20. Bailey B, Ito S: Breast-feeding and maternal drug use, *Pediatr Clin North Am* 44:41-54, 1997.
21. American Academy of Pediatrics: Breastfeeding and the use of human milk, *Pediatrics* 115:496-506, 2005.
22. Centers for Disease Control and Prevention (CDC): Achievements in public health. Reduction in perinatal transmission of *HIV* infection—United States, 1985-2005, MMWR. *MMWR Morb Mortal Wkly Rep*, 55(21):592-597, 2006.

23. Coutsoudis A, et al: HIV, infant feeding and more perils for poor people: new WHO guidelines encourage review of formula milk policies, *Bull World Health Organ*, 86(3):210-214, 2008.

24. Gibson RA, Makrides M: Long-chain polyunsaturated fatty acids in breast milk: Are they essential? *Adv Exp Med Biol* 501:375-383, 2001.

25. Avestad N, et al: Growth and development in term infants fed long-chain polyunsaturated fatty acids: A double-masked, randomized, parallel, prospective, multivariate study, *Pediatrics* 108(2):372-381, 2001.

26. Wagner CL, Greer FR, Section on Breastfeeding and Committee on Nutrition: Prevention of Rickets and Vitamin D Deficiency in Infants, Children, and Adolescents, *Pediatrics*, 122:1142-1152, 2008.

27. American Academy of Pediatrics: The use and misuse of fruit juice in pediatrics, *Pediatrics* 107(5):1210-1213, 2001.

28. Stephens, Mark B, et al: Clinical inquiries. When is it OK for children to start drinking fruit juice? *J Fam Pract* 58(9):E3, 2009.

29. Mohan A, et al: The relationship between bottle usage/content, age and number of teeth with mutans streptococci colonization in 6-24 month old children, *Community Dent Oral Epidemiol* 26:12-20, 1998.

30. Michel SH, et al: Nutrition management of pediatric patients who have cystic fibrosis, *Pediatr Clin North Am* 56(5):1123-1141, 2009.

31. Wright C, et al: New chart to evaluate weight faltering, *Arch Dis Child* 78:40-43, 1998.

32. Batchelor JA: Has recognition of failure to thrive changed? *Child Care, Health and Dev* 22:235-240, 1996.

33. Krugman SD, Dubowitz H: Failure to thrive, *Am Fam Physician* 68(5):879-884, 2003.

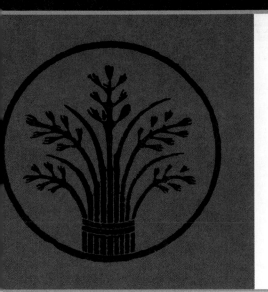

Life Span Health Promotion: Childhood and Adolescence

Once we pass the specific nutrition and health necessities of pregnancy and infancy, the rest of the life span categories share more similarities than differences regarding nutrient intake and dietary patterns.

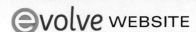 **WEBSITE**

http://evolve.elsevier.com/Grodner/foundations/

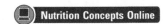 Nutrition Concepts Online

This chapter continues the exploration of the life span categories of childhood and adolescence. Once we pass the specific nutrition and health necessities of pregnancy and infancy, the rest of the life span categories share more similarities than differences regarding nutrient intake and dietary patterns. In striving to increase the level of health of individuals, families, and communities, the degree of knowledge appropriate at each stage varies and the techniques reflect these limitations. Community supports reveal the commitment of the society regarding health issues.

ROLE IN WELLNESS

The nutrient requirements of humans are basically the same throughout the life span. What differs, depending on age, is the amount of nutrients required and frequency of food consumption (dietary patterns) recommended; these differences are caused by physiologic and psychosocial needs. For example, consider the amount of food individuals are able to consume at one time. Toddlers can eat only small amounts at one time. They depend on planned snacks to provide their full assortment of nutrients. Adolescents, however, can eat large quantities but also need time throughout the day to eat. In contrast, older adults still have high nutrient needs but require less energy and therefore need more nutrient-dense foods.

The five dimensions of health also apply to the nutrition needs of children and adolescents. Knowledge of the relationship between adequate nutrient intake and good health empowers children to practice health-promoting behaviors that enhance *physical health*. *Intellectual health* skills are used by children to make decisions about food choices; considering our public health concerns about childhood overweight, these skills can be quite valuable. *Emotional health* is sup-

ported when caregivers provide guidance for children to use food for nourishment and enjoyment, not as a means of emotional comfort. The *social* dimension of health is strengthened by including children in the preparation of food, which teaches them the social skills of cooperation. The *spiritual* dimension is developed by sharing meals with family members as a form of communication and bonding.

LIFE SPAN HEALTH PROMOTION

Stages of Development

The life span stages reflect psychologic and physiologic maturation. Approaches to health promotion take into account these stages and their impact on nutrient requirements, eating styles, and food choices.

Childhood (1 to 12 Years)

The accelerated growth of infancy slows down by about age 1, marking the transition to childhood. Growth then occurs unevenly until puberty heralds the onset of adolescence. This growth deceleration during childhood results in varying hunger levels, reflecting physiologic need. Awareness of these fluctuations by parents and caregivers allows children to stay in tune with their internal hunger cues.

Nurses sensitive to normal growth patterns as affected by genetics and environmental influences can help families to understand the growth curves of their children. Height, weight, and head circumferences are used with the standard growth charts from the National Center for Health Statistics to monitor growth (available at www.cdc.gov/growthcharts). See Chapter 14 for a detailed description of clinical nutrition assessment procedures.

Childhood categories are based on a combination of psychosocial and physiologic developmental stages. Physiologic requirements are the basis of the age and gender divisions of the Dietary Reference Intakes (DRIs). This discussion highlights the nutrients of concern—protein, iron, calcium, and zinc. For other specific age-related nutrient recommendations, refer to the DRI tables inside the front cover.

Children depend on adults for the provision of food. A discussion of the nutrient needs of the growing body is not complete without a discussion of the role of adults in nourishing children. Children are influenced by adults and model the behaviors of adults. Adults control all the quantity and quality of foods prepared and the environment within which foods are presented for consumption. The children themselves, however, control the actual amount consumed.

Ellen Satter, a registered dietitian and therapist, describes the feeding relationship as the interactions or patterns of behaviors that surround food preparation and consumption within a family. This description reveals the contextual nature of food preparation and consumption. Her advice to parents and caregivers is about "the division of responsibility. You are responsible for what your child is offered to eat, but he is responsible for how much of it he eats and even whether he eats."[1]

Adults are responsible for not only what meals are offered but also *when* meals are offered. Regularity of mealtimes at home—breakfast and dinner—helps support success at school. Breakfast supplies energy in the morning for school learning (see the *Teaching Tool* box, What's the Best Breakfast?); dinner supports the ability to complete homework, study, and relax before bedtime. Most children eat lunch away from home and either bring a prepared lunch from home or purchase meals through a school lunch program. (School lunches are discussed later in this chapter under the heading "Community Supports.")

Snacks boost daily nutrient intake; for children whose energy and general dietary intake are adequate, snacks may sometimes include sweets such as cookies and even an occasional candy bar. A common myth is that sugar makes children hyperactive, yet studies have shown no convincing evidence that consumption of sugar causes attention-deficit/hyperactivity disorder. High-sugar-containing foods, however, can displace more nutritious foods and contribute to nutrient deficiencies (such as of calcium and dietary fiber) or excessive caloric and dietary fat intake. Of significant concern is childhood excess adiposity or overweight.[2] (See "Overcoming Barriers" later in this chapter.) No food should be forbidden; frequency and quantity should be the guides.

Children too young for school may attend day care programs if their parents work. The impact on their nutrition may be positive or negative depending on the quality and attitude of the programs toward nutrition and mealtimes. Most young children, regardless of parental employment, attend some form of preschool; for many, the food and social experiences broaden acceptance of a variety of foods and eating styles.

Although adults may have predominant influence over the eating behaviors of children, another primary influence for some children is television. The influence of TV commercials has been studied extensively and is most often condemned as

TEACHING TOOL

What's the Best Breakfast?

Foods considered best for breakfast have changed. Although traditional breakfasts consist of eggs, bacon, white toast, and whole milk, this combination is now recognized as being too high in fat and protein. In addition, in the rush of morning preparation, few of us have the time to prepare this type of meal. Nonetheless, breakfast, which breaks our fast, is an important contributor of nutrients and energy.

As we teach clients and their families about nutrition and optimum dietary intake patterns, we can assure them that breakfast can be simple yet still provide appropriate levels of nutrients. Following are some ideas for parents to use to ignite their children's breakfast appetites:

- For children (and adults) who eat and run, have quick foods available such as fruit, granola bars (low fat/low sugar), muffins (low fat/low sugar), and raisins/nuts.
- For older children, offer to prepare a simple breakfast. Although they are able to prepare their own meal, the extra nurturing—and time saved—will be appreciated.
- For creating appetites, toast bread while family members are dressing. The enticing scent will spark their taste buds.
- For picky eaters, create small smorgasbord plates with several choices such as a small container of yogurt, crackers with cheese, and some pear slices.
- Many of the healthy snacks listed in Box 12-1 can alternate as breakfast foods for everyone.
- Be a role model by also eating breakfast yourself.

negatively influencing children's food choices. In addition, watching television when eating family meals appears to affect the types of foods served, which results in consumption of foods higher in fat and lower in fiber. This possibly reflects the categories of foods most often advertised on television.[3] Parents and caregivers can watch television with their children to assess the type of products advertised and then discuss their nutritional value. As more healthful products are marketed, even if targeted at adults, acceptance by children may increase. Occasional treats of advertised products may lessen their appeal if children are accustomed to high-quality snacks and meals.

The Acceptable Macronutrient Distribution Range (AMDR) for daily dietary fat intake recommends about 30% kcal intake. This level of dietary fat intake may also assist with obesity prevention and emphasizes fruits, vegetables, and complex carbohydrates. It is easier to enjoy whole foods that are naturally low in fat throughout childhood than to convert one's eating style as an adult. Other AMDR include for carbohydrates 45% to 65% kcal; for protein 5% to 20% kcal for young children and 10% to 30% kcal for older children; added sugars should not exceed 25% of total calories; and adequate intake dietary fiber of 19 g/day for children 1 to 3 years, 25 g/day for 4 to 8 years, 31 g/day boys 9 to 13 years, and 26 g/day girls 9 to 13 years.[2]

Despite national dietary recommendations, trends in children's total energy intake are increasing. Although calories

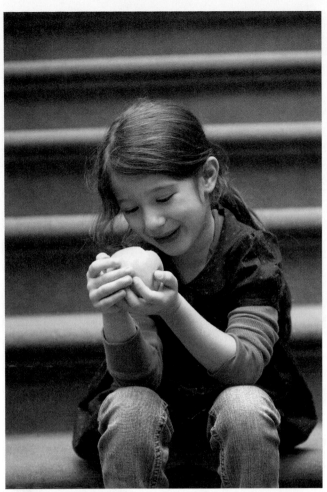

Making low-fat foods a habit throughout childhood is easier than trying to change one's eating style as an adult. (Photos.com.)

Child Health Education for Foreign-Born Parents

Providing child health education for foreign-born parents presents special concerns related to language and culture. An innovative, culturally relevant approach should be used to present basic child health information in English, with translators present as facilitators. Foreign-born parents who need a partial or complete language interpretation then have readily available access to translation support. Parents can ask questions, provide comments and suggestions, and evaluate the presentation through the translator. Because participants can be grouped with an appropriate translator, each presentation can accommodate more than one language.

The presentation, conducted in English, is paced to allow for discussions. Child care is provided in a nearby setting. This allows parents to focus on the presentation without the concern of child care. Vocabulary relative to health care is developed from English into the parents' primary language with the support of the translator.

Application to nursing

This is an example of one cultural-specific strategy used to meet minority and ethnic health needs. Nurses are also encouraged to provide translated health education materials for the populations with whom they teach.

Data from Baker R: Child health education for the foreign-born parent, *Issues Compr Pediatr Nurs* 24:45-55, 2001.

increased, total intake of milk, vegetable, soups, breads, grains, and eggs decreased, and intake of fruits, fruit juices, sweetened beverages, poultry, and cheese increased. When food groups are considered, about 16% of U.S. children did not meet any food group recommendations, whereas only 1% consumed recommended amounts for all food groups. Approximately two-thirds of U.S. children do not consume suggested servings of fruits and vegetables. Consumption of whole grains is extremely low, with consumption of two or more servings of whole grains daily by less than 13% of children. Those who did meet dietary recommendations had intakes that were high in fat. Consider that for some children, their principal vegetable is french fries. These findings indicate that nutrition education is still needed for parents and their children. (The *Cultural Considerations* box, Child Health Education for Foreign-Born Parents, offers suggestions for educating foreign-born parents about their child's health.)

Health professionals need to use careful wording when discussing nutrient restriction or reduction for children. Several infants have developed failure to thrive, not because of neglect or lack of food but because of parental over vigilance about fat, both dietary and body.[4]

Stage I: Children 1 to 3 Years Old

Usually referred to as "toddlerhood," the age span of 1 to 3 years old is a busy time for young children. They are dealing with issues of autonomy. Often food and eating create an arena for asserting newly discovered independence. The eating relationship between parent (or caregiver) and child is forming, and adult reaction to autonomy sets the stage for future encounters.[1] Consistency of mealtimes is important. Meals are best accepted when hunger, tiredness, and emotions are still controllable; an overly tired child just cannot eat. Equally important is fostering self-reliance by allowing young children to feed themselves in a manner most appropriate for their psychomotor abilities. Regardless of the messy results, attempts to self-feed provide the roots of self-empowerment crucial to overall physical and psychologic development (Figure 12-1).

Hunger, rather than adult meal schedules, guides the child's perception of time to eat. Meals for toddlers are based on the same design and food selections as adults, only in smaller portions. (Of course, overly spicy foods may not be acceptable to young taste buds.) Snacks are a necessity in addition to meals. Toddlers are able to eat only small amounts at each meal or food encounter. Planned snacks provide required additional nourishment between meals to ensure an adequate dietary intake.

Nutrition requirements. Growth, basal metabolic rate (BMR), and endless activity require an energy supply of 1300 kcal/day for ages 1 to 3. Protein needs increase to 16 g

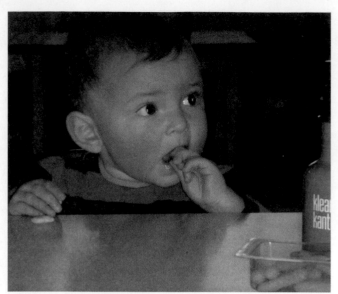

FIG 12-1 Allowing toddlers to feed themselves promotes physical and psychologic development.

to meet the demands of growing muscles. For children aged 1 through 6 years, a general guideline is one fruit or vegetable serving equals one level-measuring tablespoon of fruit or vegetable per year of age. A serving of bread or cereal is equal to about one-fourth of an adult's serving. Up to age 3, children should consume two or three 8-ounce cups of milk per day or about 16 to 24 ounces per day, and meats or meat substitutes can be offered at least twice per day.[5] Caregivers should be advised that alternative milk products such as rice milk and soymilk, unless sufficiently fortified, may not provide the same quality of nutrients as animal-derived foods.

When children are between 1 and 3 years old, introduce lower-fat versions of commonly eaten foods. Fat-containing foods should not be obsessively restricted; however, high-fat foods are often filling and may displace other nutrient-containing foods.

This is also a prime time to introduce toddlers to a variety of foods. (See Chapter 11, Personal Perspectives *Developing "Nutrition Intelligence."*) Toddlers imitate the adults around them; therefore, adults can model behavior by eating a variety of foods themselves. Clever introductions to foods are always helpful to catch the attention and appetite of toddlers. Broccoli is more than just a vegetable; cut up, it looks like little trees. Peas steamed in their pods are not just peas but green pearls waiting to be discovered.

Although breast milk or formula is the milk of choice until age 1, toddlers should drink breast milk, whole milk, or formula until age 2, after which low-fat or skim milk is best. Sometimes toddlers consume too much milk or juice, particularly if they are given an unlimited number of servings. Perhaps drinking from feeding bottles throughout the day simply becomes a habit. Unfortunately, the child fills up on milk or juice, both low sources of iron, and then does not have an appetite for iron-containing foods such as meat, fish, poultry, eggs, or legumes. Iron deficiency anemia may

develop. Additionally, apple juice is sweet tasting and has few nutrients beyond carbohydrate kcal. Frequent consumption may habituate young children to sweet drinks. Later, apple juice may be replaced with sugar-laden sodas or beverages, which displace more nutrient-dense beverages. One possible solution is to dilute juices with water. Milk can be served with meals and diluted juices drunk between meals. Parents and caregivers can view bottles as cups or glassware. Few of us drink from a cup continually while watching television, reading, or playing games. Similarly, once past infancy, young children's use of feeding bottles and/or lidded cups or "sippy" cups should be viewed as beverages as part of a meal or snack.

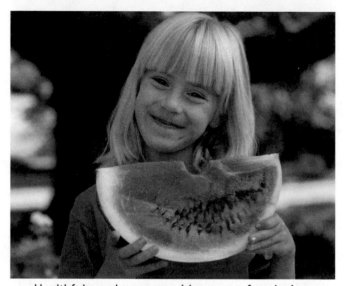

Healthful snacks can provide energy for playing.

Stage II: Children 4 to 6 Years Old

The stage of 4 to 6 years old is characterized by independent eating styles, although modeling of adults still occurs. Children of this age clearly understand the time frame of meals and can save their appetite for meals. Snacks are still an integral part of the child's nutrient intake. Far from the messy eating styles of toddlers, these children accept foods more easily if presented separately, not mixed in a casserole style. Variations of hunger and appetite levels may confuse parents and caregivers. The most practical approach is to be respectful of these variations of hunger; this diffuses power plays over food consumption.

New foods can continue to be introduced. Children may require repeated exposures, as many as 8 to 10 attempts, before acceptance occurs. For some families, backup meal plans can encourage trying new foods. For instance, if a child does not accept a new dish after a reasonable attempt, the child may be allowed to prepare a meal of a peanut butter sandwich or cereal and fruit. By establishing backup meals in advance, parents avoid becoming short-order cooks preparing three or more individualized meals for dinner.

Another approach is to have at least one meal (eaten at home) include new foods along with favorite foods. In addition to the new foods, the child will recognize some familiar foods on his or her plate. A meal can consist of a sampling of food items; several will probably be acceptable.

At this stage children can develop a sense of responsibility for healthful food selections. They can understand that although all foods are okay, some foods such as fruits, vegetables, and low-fat foods can be eaten more often than others. After participating in a 3-month nutrition education demonstration project to decrease cholesterol and cardiovascular risk, some of the children ages 4 to 10 reduced their kcal intake of fat by about 9% by replacing higher-fat food with lower-fat foods within the same food group. These same children also increased their overall intake of fruits, vegetables, and very-low-fat desserts. Their total calorie and nutrient intake remained appropriate.[6]

Sometimes children develop food jags, wanting to eat only a narrow range of foods. Parents and teachers can educate the child that each food contains a different assortment of nutrients and offer substitute choices that contain additional nutrients, with the child making the final selections. Eventually food jags diminish and the child consumes a broader selection of foods.

Nutrition requirements. Energy requirements jump to 1800 kcal/day at 4 to 6 years of age, reflecting continued growth and activity levels. Protein needs increase to 24 g.

Stage III: Children 7 to 12 Years Old

The years from 7 to 12 are tumultuous. Although actual growth may slow down, the body is preparing and seemingly storing up for the puberty growth spurt. Puberty may begin for girls from around age 9; boys may reach puberty in the early teen years. This prepuberty time may be reflected by weight buildup; an increase in chubbiness is not alarming if moderate eating and physical activities are maintained. Adults must be careful not to overreact, or they may plant the seeds of eating disorders. To rule out overeating, children can be asked if they are really hungry for food or whether they are only tired or thirsty. These are different sensations. A child can be reminded to "stop eating when you are full" (Figure 12-2). If hunger returns, a snack can be provided. By taking time to consider these sensations, children can stay in touch with internal cues of true hunger.

Exposure to other dietary patterns takes place as children spend more time away from home at school and socializing with friends. Peer influence at school lunchtime increases; having the right kind of lunch may be as important as wearing the right kind of clothes. Adults need to be sensitive to these issues. As long as a basic lunch of some protein, complex carbohydrates, and a beverage (preferably milk, juice, or water) is consumed, missing nutrients can be adjusted for later in the day, especially through after-school snacks.

It is at this age—when midmorning school snacks disappear and school lunch scheduling has more to do with numbers of students than with actual lunchtime appetites—that after-school hunger may intensify. This is the time to provide healthful snacks or at least stock the kitchen shelves with an assortment of nutrient-dense treats (see Box 12-1).

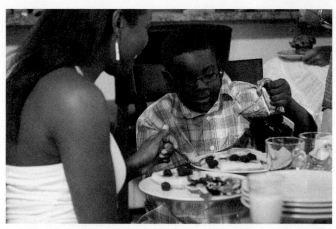

FIG 12-2 Young children should not be pushed to "clean their plates" at mealtime if they seem to be finished eating so as not to override natural feelings of satiety. (Photos.com.)

BOX 12-1   HEALTHY SNACKS

Snacks are a way to bridge energy levels between meals. They are not meant to be so energy dense that intakes during meals are compromised or that daily total caloric intakes are significantly increased. Frequent snacking (or nonstop eating) throughout the day has been associated with increased body weight in children (and adults!).

Here are some suggestions:

- Ready-to-eat cereals: reserve presweetened cereals as special snack treats or mix a sweet cereal with a less sweet cereal—the best of both worlds
- Snack smorgasbord: cut-up apples and oranges, popcorn, cheese, crackers, and cookies
- Fruit juice packs
- Low-fat chocolate milk packs
- Open-face peanut butter sandwich (child-made) with cut fruit, jelly, coconut, and raisins
- Sliced apple or pear with thin spread of nut butter (peanut, almond, or cashew)
- Fresh or canned fruit (in fruit juice) with cottage cheese (in 4-ounce sizes)
- English muffins (oat bran, raisin, and sourdough) with a small amount of fruit spread
- Healthier Danish: a slice of toasted bread with low-fat ricotta cheese and preserves
- Bagels with a spread of whipped cream cheese, margarine/butter, or nut butter (peanut, almond, or cashew); freeze a variety of bagels
- Smoothies or fruit shakes made with skim milk or fruit juice, plain or fruit-flavored yogurt, fresh or frozen fruit—just mix in a blender
- Leftovers from lunch or dinner; a bowl of soup with bread for dipping instead of a prepackaged snack

---

If children purchase snacks away from home, adults can develop guidelines with children this age to maintain positive eating styles.

The intent is to supplement the nutrients received during meals with nutrient-dense snacks so the total caloric and nutrient intake is adequate to meet the needs of growth at each childhood stage. Snacking, though, seems to have changed in definition and frequency. A recent study of 31,337 children and adolescents assessed snacking and meal intake trends from 1977 to 2006. On average the number of calories and eating events (a total of snacks and meals) increased substantially over time. Compared to the 1970s, about half of American children average 4 snacks a day, while others consume snacks and meals as many as 10 times a day or basically nonstop eating. This means that an excessive number of calories, most likely less-nutrient-dense snack foods, are being consumed and the consumption of nutrient-dense meal time foods are decreasing. While the increase of snack calories is only 168 kcal, this number represents an average, signaling that for many children the excess intake is higher. With increased eating episodes, there can be a concern that eating is not due to physiological hunger but to a habit from needing a constant state of satiation.[7]

Nutrition requirements. Energy needs for 7- to 12-year-olds increase to 2000 to 2200 kcal/day. Protein requirements rise to between 28 and 46 g depending on sexual maturity. Sexual maturity leads to an increase of lean body mass, particularly for boys. Lean body mass requires more dietary protein for growth and maintenance.

Mineral needs increase as well. Because of increased bone growth and mineralization, calcium Adequate Intake (AI) recommendations jump from 800 mg/day at age 8 to 1300 mg/day throughout adolescence. Iron and zinc allowances increase as well. Well-chosen dietary intakes will provide sufficient amounts of these nutrients. Marginal intakes of zinc have been noted among schoolchildren that are finicky eaters; low zinc intakes can affect growth rates.[8]

Childhood Health Promotion (1 to 12 Years)
Knowledge

The growth cycle of this age span is important for both parents and children to understand. Attention to issues related to weight, appropriate appetite, and meal patterning is crucial for positive eating relationships and may prevent the development of eating disorders. By understanding the relationship of nutrients and kcal to their growth needs, children possess sufficient information to take responsibility for certain aspects of their food choices and dietary patterns. Children with special needs who are challenged by physical and/or mental limitations may require additional support to achieve nutritional adequacy (Box 12-2). Ultimately, however, adults must provide nourishment for children and guidance as to positive health behaviors.

Techniques

Several techniques can be used with children this age. MyPyramid for Kids is similar to the adult version but presents games and other creative approaches for children to visualize and understand the serving sizes and types of foods that result in a balanced nutrient intake. These can be found at www.mypyramid.gov (Figure 12-3). Another source for appropriate techniques is the "Fruits & Veggies, More

---

BOX 12-2   NUTRITION NEEDS OF CHILDREN WITH SPECIAL NEEDS

Although the basic nutrition needs of all children are the same, some children may be challenged by the limitations of physical and mental differences and the physical and pharmacologic consequences of chronic disease treatment. The ability to self-feed may be highly related to life expectancy. Enhancing feeding skills to the greatest extent possible is an involved procedure. Nutrition education has valuable skills and experiences to offer. Keep the following issues in mind:

- All children can enjoy working together to prepare foods. The process of measuring, mixing, arranging, and *eating* food that they helped to prepare enhances self-esteem and provides the acquisition of other skill competencies such as math, science, and interpersonal skills of cooperation.
- Positioning of children with physical handicaps may require adaptive equipment and alternative eating strategies for special conditions. Oral stimulation before eating may be required for children with low muscle tone, and certain textures of foods may be better received than others. If chewing and swallowing are problematic, textures of foods may need adjustment. Low muscle tone may also affect functioning of the large intestine and require adequate fiber and water to reduce the risk of constipation.
- Medications may increase or decrease appetite. Caregivers and teachers should be aware of these effects and time meals and snacks to be offered when hunger is the strongest.
- Children with sensory integration difficulties may be sensitive to textures, temperature, and even colors of foods. Accommodate preferences when possible to ensure adequate nutrition and to provide the children a sense of control over food choices.
- Children experiencing growth retardation or malnutrition should be reassessed by a registered dietitian to determine if alternative feeding strategies can improve the child's nutritional status. Parents should regularly receive assessments of nutritional status to fully understand their children's conditions.
- Periodic nutritional assessments of children with special needs should be conducted by registered dietitians who have the expertise to evaluate nutritional status and offer practical strategies for everyday eating situations.

Data from Fung EB, et al: Feeding dysfunction is associated with poor growth and health status in children with cerebral palsy, *J Am Diet Assoc* 102(3):361, 373, 2002; and correspondence on Society for Nutrition Education (SNE) list/serv February 19, 1998, from Susan Piscopo, associate professor, University of Malta; Sharon Davis, education director, Home Baking Association; Collette Janson-Sand, associate professor, University of New Hampshire, and others.

Matters" site. Resources for parents and children are available at www.fruitsandveggiesmorematters.org.

Community Supports

Community supports for children are currently divided into two categories based on location and services or education

10 tips

Nutrition Education Series

choose MyPlate

10 **tips** to a great plate

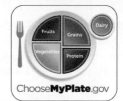

ChooseMyPlate.gov

Making food choices for a healthy lifestyle can be as simple as using these 10 Tips.
Use the ideas in this list to *balance your calories*, to choose foods to *eat more often*, and to cut back on foods to *eat less often*.

1 balance calories
Find out how many calories YOU need for a day as a first step in managing your weight. Go to www.ChooseMyPlate.gov to find your calorie level. Being physically active also helps you balance calories.

2 enjoy your food, but eat less
Take the time to fully enjoy your food as you eat it. Eating too fast or when your attention is elsewhere may lead to eating too many calories. Pay attention to hunger and fullness cues before, during, and after meals. Use them to recognize when to eat and when you've had enough.

3 avoid oversized portions
Use a smaller plate, bowl, and glass. Portion out foods before you eat. When eating out, choose a smaller size option, share a dish, or take home part of your meal.

4 foods to eat more often
Eat more vegetables, fruits, whole grains, and fat-free or 1% milk and dairy products. These foods have the nutrients you need for health—including potassium, calcium, vitamin D, and fiber. Make them the basis for meals and snacks.

5 make half your plate fruits and vegetables
Choose red, orange, and dark-green vegetables like tomatoes, sweet potatoes, and broccoli, along with other vegetables for your meals. Add fruit to meals as part of main or side dishes or as dessert.

6 switch to fat-free or low-fat (1%) milk
They have the same amount of calcium and other essential nutrients as whole milk, but fewer calories and less saturated fat.

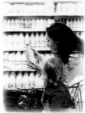

7 make half your grains whole grains
To eat more whole grains, substitute a whole-grain product for a refined product—such as eating whole-wheat bread instead of white bread or brown rice instead of white rice.

8 foods to eat less often
Cut back on foods high in solid fats, added sugars, and salt. They include cakes, cookies, ice cream, candies, sweetened drinks, pizza, and fatty meats like ribs, sausages, bacon, and hot dogs. Use these foods as occasional treats, not everyday foods.

9 compare sodium in foods
Use the Nutrition Facts label to choose lower sodium versions of foods like soup, bread, and frozen meals. Select canned foods labeled "low sodium," "reduced sodium," or "no salt added."

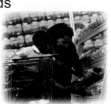

10 drink water instead of sugary drinks
Cut calories by drinking water or unsweetened beverages. Soda, energy drinks, and sports drinks are a major source of added sugar, and calories, in American diets.

USDA
United States
Department of Agriculture
Center for Nutrition
Policy and Promotion

Go to www.ChooseMyPlate.gov for more information.

DG TipSheet No. 1
June 2011
USDA is an equal opportunity provider and employer.

FIG 12-3 Be a heathy rote model for children. (Accessed June 14, 2012, from http://www.choosemyplate.gov/food-groups/downloads/TenTips/DGTipsheet1ChooseMyPlate.pdf.)

offered: (1) school food service and (2) classroom nutrition education.

School food service. The National School Lunch Program (NSLP) was established to protect the health and wellness of American children. Formalized in 1946, the program provides lunches at varying costs, depending on family income, to all schoolchildren at public and nonprofit private schools and residential child care institutions. At the federal level the program is administered by the Food and Nutrition Service (FNS) of the U.S. Department of Agriculture (USDA), at the state level by various agencies, and locally by school boards. As an entitlement program, the NSLP provides funds to all schools that apply and meet the criteria of eligibility. Currently, about 95% of all school districts participate in this program. Every school district is required to implement a local school wellness policy to focus on obesity prevention and through modification of school environments support healthy eating habits and physical activity.[9]

At participating schools, there are two types of eligibility to qualify for free or reduced price meals; both usually require family to complete and return application forms. Categorical eligibility is based on the child's household receiving food stamps from the Supplemental Nutrition Assistance Program (SNAP) or Temporary Assistance for Needy Families (TANF) or participating in the Food District Program on Indian Reservations (FDPIR), and free meals for the homeless, runaways, and children of migrant workers. Income-based eligibility offers reduced-price meals to children whose household income is below 185% of the federal poverty level; free meals are available to those falling below 130% of the poverty level. Through the process of direct certification, school districts qualify children without requiring submission of family applications. School districts work with state or local SNAP, TANF, and FDPIR agencies to certify children in households. During the 2008-2009 school year, NSLP served meals daily to 31.2 million children. About 60% of these children received free or reduced-price lunches.[9]

Specific nutrient guidelines regulate the meals served through this program. At times the definition of these guidelines has been controversial because of their nutritional impact on children and their economic impact on the farmers and food producers supplying the food. Some foods are available at reduced cost because of federal surplus commodities programs. Although wholesome, these may have higher fat contents than would otherwise be used in the preparation of school lunches. Fresh fruits and vegetables may be passed over for canned fruits and vegetables that are not as acceptable to children and at times not as nutritious. Whole milk, cheeses, and high-fat meats may be served more often because of economics, despite the health objectives of consuming lower-fat foods. Meals served may not meet the lower-fat and higher fruits and vegetable consumption of current dietary recommendations.

Basically, lunch must provide approximately one-third or more of the recommended levels for key nutrients, providing no more than 30% kcal from fat and less than 10% of kcal from saturated fat. For low-income children participating in the program, this provides one-third to one-half of their daily intake.[9]

The School Breakfast Program was created in 1966 to support schools by providing morning meals in areas where children ride buses to school and/or most mothers are in the work force, particularly in economically disadvantaged areas. The program has reduced tardiness and decreased absenteeism. It is administered through the same governmental offices as the School Lunch Program and is also an entitlement program. During the 2008-2009 school year, more than 86,000 schools and institutions participated in the School Breakfast Program, serving 10.8 million children. More than 81% of the participants qualify for free or reduced-priced meals. More than 47% of the children from low-income families receive both school lunch and school breakfast.[9]

An assortment of foods can comprise breakfast, but the program requires milk (either as a beverage or with cereal), a serving of fruit (either whole or as juice), and two servings of a bread/cereal product or meat/meat alternative or a combination of bread and meat servings. The breakfast is designed to provide one fourth or more of the daily recommended level for key nutrients and limits fat to no more than 30% kcal with less than 10% kcal of saturated fat.

During summer, the Summer Food Service Program for Children (SFSP) functions through a range of eligible organizations including schools, summer camps, and community agencies, as well as various federal, state, and local government departments. The purpose is to serve meals to school-age children when schools are not in session in communities where children depend on school meals as an essential component of their daily nourishment.[9]

School nurses and community health nurses should be aware of these programs as a valuable source of nutrition. Sometimes children do not participate because school payment policies create a stigma associated with participation. Intervention by a health professional may be required to ensure that children's health needs are met in a socially sensitive manner. As health advocates, nurses may be able to highlight the importance of school lunch and breakfast programs to educational administrators and the community at large.

Classroom nutrition education. Health has been taught for many years in most school systems. What vary are the depth of school health curricula and the qualifications of the instructors. Both may affect the quality of the nutrition education. Although basic nutrition facts can be taught within a short-term health course, lifestyle changes that affect dietary patterns take longer to achieve. Unless they have special preparation, instructors may not feel comfortable teaching the intricate and ever-changing discipline of nutrition. This may lead to either poor-quality teaching or the imparting of negative attitudes toward nutrition and food selections.

Adolescence (13 to 19 Years)

The adolescent years are marked by change. Not only does puberty initiate growth acceleration, but emotional and social developmental struggles also occur as academic and

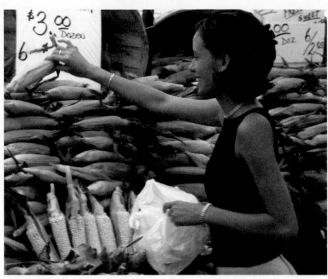

Teens can help shop for and plan meals that meet the family's nutritional needs while incorporating alternative food styles.

personal responsibilities escalate. Adults often assume that teenagers can take care of themselves. Although teens need to take responsibility for their behavior and overall health status, they still need the guidance and nurturing of caring adults. There is a fine line between allowing adolescents to be responsible and neglecting their needs. Adult involvement is still necessary to provide physical and emotional support during the stressful years of adolescence.

Part of the physical and emotional support includes creating guidelines for dietary patterns and providing food for consumption. Creating guidelines means maintaining a household in which meals are available, even if family members may not be able to eat together. Knowing that dinner just needs to be reheated means someone was thinking of the welfare of all family members. Of course, shared responsibility for meal preparation may be an appropriate component of family duties. A kitchen stocked with nourishing snack foods and ingredients for simple meals helps to make stressful, chaotic teenage schedules more manageable.

Older teens may be adjusting to the new demands of the college environment, including adapting to dining hall meals. Some campuses provide flexible meal plans with several locations for meal acquisition around campus. Others offer salad bars and food "stations" to provide a variety of selections. Individuals requiring special dietary requirements such as kosher meals or lactose-reduced meals should discuss these issues with food service staff or with student service personnel.

As their sense of social awareness develops, some teens may adopt a vegetarian dietary pattern. Creative planning on the part of the teen and the family meal planner results in meals meeting everyone's nutritional needs without compromising personal convictions.

Discussions of the eating habits of teens tend to be critical of their fast-food consumption. Fortunately, most teens can

✳ TEACHING TOOL

Fast-Food Choices

We might as well accept it: Fast-food restaurants are part of our everyday lives. Because they provide quickly prepared foods that are usually reasonably priced and in convenient locations, fast-food chains are here to stay. Although many health professionals complain about the high-fat, high-sodium, and calorie-laden foods provided, consumers continue to flock to these locales. Rather than fight a losing battle, we serve the needs of our clients best by providing guidelines for making healthier selections when time is short and hunger great.

Choose plainer food items such as a plain hamburger instead of a specialty burger that has more fat-laden toppings, or select a grilled chicken sandwich rather than a fried chicken sandwich. A request for "no sauce" can lower the fat content significantly.

INSTEAD OF:	SOMETIMES CHOOSE:
Specialty burger* 570-660 kcal; 280-360 kcal fat (32-40 g fat)	Quarter-pound burger 430 kcal; 190 kcal fat (21 g fat)
	Bacon cheeseburger (regular size) 400 kcal; 200 kcal fat (22 g fat)
	Grilled chicken sandwich[†] 450-530 kcal; 160-230 kcal fat (18-26 g fat)
Fried chicken sandwich* 710 kcal; 390 kcal fat (43 g fat)	Grilled chicken sandwich[†] 450-530 kcal; 160-230 kcal fat (18-26 g fat)
	Fried chicken sandwich without mayonnaise 500 kcal; 180 kcal fat (20 g fat)

*There are also other specialty sandwiches that are much higher in kcal and fat content.
[†]Order without mayonnaise sauce to save 110 kcal.
Data from Kuhl KM: *Fast food facts,* Fort Worth, Texas, Author. Accessed April 10, 2010, from www.fastfoodfacts.info.

afford the extra kcal that typically higher-fat foods such as hamburgers, fries, and pizza may contain. If teens have grown up accustomed to well-balanced meals, they will more than likely still prefer those meals to high-fat delights. Eating in fast-food restaurants, where prices tend to be inexpensive, may have more to do with socializing among peers than with nutrient values.

When fast foods become the mainstay of an individual's diet, regardless of age, some nutrients such as vitamin A and C may be lacking and overconsumption of dietary fats and kcal may occur. Although teens may be seen at such restaurants, most other customers consist of families with young children as well as older adults. Fast foods affect the nutrient intake of all ages (see the *Teaching Tool* box, Fast-Food Choices).

Nutrition Requirements

Because of the natural physiologic differences between adolescent males and females, nutrient requirements from age 9 and older are divided by gender. Females need about 2200 kcal and 45 g of protein daily. Recommendations for males are 2500 to 2900 kcal and 45 to 59 g of protein daily. These values for kcal and protein reflect the increased lean body mass developing in males. They do, however, only represent suggested amounts; physical activity, either work or athletic endeavors, affects the actual nutrient needs for both males and females.

Calcium AI recommendations are the same for both genders, 1300 mg per day, to allow for skeletal growth (particularly for boys) and for bone mineralization, a prime physiologic function during adolescence. Bone mineralization for girls is a concern because teenage girls often don't consume enough calcium-rich foods.

Teenage girls and sometimes teenage boys are at risk for dieting-related disorders and eating disorders. By regularly underconsuming nutrients during a time when the human body is completing maturation, girls are at risk for various deficiencies as they progress to adulthood and the nutrient requirements of potential pregnancies. In addition to calcium, iron allowances are important to fulfill, particularly for girls who begin menstruation; iron is also needed by boys, whose accelerated growth necessitates an increased blood volume and lean body mass.

Adolescence Health Promotion (13 to 19 Years)
Knowledge

The adolescent body benefits from a dietary intake most similar to an adult's; however, some nutrient needs are greater. Energy requirements are higher than at any other time of life, especially for adolescents involved in competitive athletics. Calcium recommendations increase to ensure adequate mineralization of bones. Tolerance for alternative food styles enhances overall dietary intake and allows for the acceptance of dietary suggestions to maintain appropriate nutrient consumption.

Teenagers can comprehend the body's physiology and nutrient needs. Ideally this information should be taught within family life, health, or science curricula in schools. This knowledge provides a rationale for consumption of nutrient-dense foods, especially as preparation for sports activities. Although adults may supply provisions for meals and snacks, especially those that can be reheated, ultimately most adolescents take responsibility for their own nutrient intake.

Awareness of the risk factors and symptoms of disordered eating and drug/alcohol abuse can be provided through health classes or interactions with health and educational professionals and parents. Even mild substance abuse in the face of the increased nutritional needs of adolescence can compromise nutritional status. For example, alcohol adversely affects absorption of folate and zinc, two nutrients required for normal growth. Nurses need to be aware of the indicators of substance abuse so they can guide adolescents into treatment. Nutrition assessment, intervention, and support are part of comprehensive physical and psychologic rehabilitation of all substance abusers.

Techniques

Similar to techniques for children, the concepts of MyPyramid and "Fruits & Veggies, More Matters" provide a basis for adolescent food choices (adolescents use MyPyramid for adults). Often the forces overriding good food choices are lack of time and scheduling demands. One strategy accommodating both is to ensure the availability of simple meals that are easily eaten and reheatable. Scheduling of meals in a home or institutional setting (e.g., school cafeterias, dining halls) can take into account school, sports, work, and recreational agendas. To improve the quality of food choices, adolescents should be included in meal planning and food preparation.

Community Supports

Except for federal government programs serving children and adults, no food programs are specifically targeted at adolescents.[9,10] At a time when teens are developmentally ready to be empowered to take care of themselves, society provides few supports. In fact, school, sports, and work schedules often hinder adolescents from taking responsibility for their health behaviors. Television, radio, the Internet, and print messages rarely promote healthy behaviors. Although the increased interest in physical pursuits of basketball, soccer, biking, skateboarding, weight lifting, and other recreational sports enhance fitness, the nutrition component is often overlooked or cloaked in misinformation. This is an area to which all health professionals should be sensitive.

One of the few community supports is a comprehensive school health program. The depth of health issues covered varies and may not include sufficient nutrition guidance, but at the least, these programs highlight basic concerns of nutrition and health.

OVERCOMING BARRIERS

Food Asphyxiation

Asphyxiation from food is possible at any point along the life span, but toddlers and older adults tend to be more at risk. (Older adults are discussed in Chapter 13.) As toddlers first become accustomed to a variety of food textures and substances, they sometimes misjudge the size of food being chewed or may be too active when eating and accidentally swallow before sufficiently chewing. Some foods that are potential problems are peanut butter (large clumps can stick in the throat), peanuts, popcorn, hot dogs, potato chips, hard candies, gum, grapes, and foods containing bones (e.g., beef, poultry, fish). Efforts by parents and caregivers to serve appropriate foods to young children can prevent choking incidents; adults with responsibility for caring for children should know how to perform the Heimlich maneuver.

Children can be reminded to chew food well and sit quietly while eating (Box 12-3).

Lead Poisoning

Lead poisoning can be an invisible health hazard. Found in old paint dust or chips, enameled porcelain fixtures (bathtubs), and soil or air from industrial and transportation pollution, excessive amounts of lead can be absorbed into the body. Children are most at risk; they naturally absorb greater amounts of minerals than adults. Nutritional deficiencies of iron, calcium, and zinc tend to increase the absorption of lead. Lead poisoning and iron deficiency anemia are sometimes diagnosed concurrently. Excessive exposure to lead can permanently affect cognitive and perceptual abilities. These reduced functions affect learning ability.[11]

Role of Nurses

School and community nurses in higher-risk areas should be sensitive to this risk to both physical and intellectual health. Higher-risk areas for children include lower socioeconomic areas with poor housing conditions. Once lead poisoning is determined through blood testing, local health departments work with families to ascertain the sources of contamination in the home or school environment, while physicians implement lead-reduction therapy.

Overall levels of lead in the environment are lower than in the past because of standards established and enforced by the Environmental Protection Agency. Levels of lead in some communities, however, are still high enough by Centers for Disease Control and Prevention standards that primary prevention activities to further reduce lead poisoning should remain a community-wide goal.

Obesity

During childhood and adolescence, weight and height continually change. This affects the standard measurements used to assess body composition of fat and lean mass. Therefore, standards used to evaluate obesity in adults are inappropriate to apply directly to children. Gender and age also affect body composition during growth. For example, during adolescence, fat redistributes differently for males and females. Males gather body fat centrally around the waist, whereas females tend to collect body fat gluteally on the lower body. Overweight may be determined by a body mass index (BMI) of 30 or greater and/or by skinfold measurements.[12]

The prevalence of obesity or excessive body fat composition among American children and adolescents increased substantially over the past 30 years. Among children aged 6 to 18 years the proportions that were overweight increased from 6% in 1980 to 16% by 2002. Racial, ethnic, and gender differences reveal that black non-Hispanic girls and Mexican American boys were at greater risk of being overweight than other American children (23% and 27%, respectively). Severe overweight or obesity has increased more quickly than even the increases of moderate overweight.[12]

The etiology of these changes is not obvious but may be considered multifactorial. Eating more food as snacks and meals away from home may be a subtle factor for children and adults. These food portions are larger and higher in calories and dietary fat than those eaten at home. Another factor may be the increase of sedentary lifestyles. Physical activity has decreased with a related decline of fitness. Although TV watching has not increased substantially over the years, children may be more sedentary than in the past because they play video and computer games and "surf" the Internet. Physical and behavioral environmental influences also affect the level of physical activity. If facilities are not available or not safe to use, activity is limited. Concerns over increasing numbers of latchkey children (grade-school children arriving home without adult supervision until the evening) focus on the use of food for emotional comfort and security. All of these factors affect the influence of genetics, which may predispose children toward heavier weights and should be considered as interventions are considered.

Clinical assessment of childhood overweight consists of completing a health history, including the pattern of weight gain, emotional health status, and physical activity patterns. If BMI is greater than 30, a further discussion of weight issues may be appropriate, but first a consultation with parents or guardians may be appropriate to determine if intervention is warranted.

As with adults, intervention regarding weight should be initiated only when the patient is motivated or is experiencing weight associative disorders. Conducting a 24-hour recall provides an opportunity to engage in a discussion of dietary intake patterns such as excessive or imbalanced intake of non-nutrient-dense foods such as sodas, sweets, and fast foods. (This type of discussion may be appropriate regardless of the child's weight.) Physical examinations need to be sensitive to the child regarding his or her weight and body issues. If weight is excessive, the assessment can determine if weight causes physical symptoms such as sleep apnea. Morbidly obese adolescents may require a more comprehensive physical examination and intervention approaches.

Type 2 Diabetes Mellitus

Obesity during childhood when combined with lack of physical activity is of significant concern as risk factors for type 2 diabetes mellitus (type 2 DM). Until recently, type 2 DM was just a concern of older adults, but with the significant increase in childhood overweight combined with lack of physical activity and poor-quality dietary intakes, the age of risk has gotten progressively younger. Risk is multidimensional because genetics and race also predispose individuals. Asians develop diabetes at lower body weights than people of other races; Hispanics and African Americans appear to develop diabetes in greater numbers than other ethnic groups. Increased risk is also tied to the everyday lifestyle habits often set in childhood; such habits as sedentary activities (video games/TV) and fat/sweet excessive snacking have a lasting impact on diabetes risk. As the incidence of type 2 DM increases among the American adult population, the behaviors that put these adults at risk are being adopted by their children.[13]

BOX 12-3   CHOKING RISK PREVENTION

Choking risk prevention for young children can be approached through the following measures:

1. Appropriate selection of foods based on size, shape, and texture
2. Application of prevention strategies, and just in case:
3. Knowledge of the Heimlich maneuver procedures for use with children

Food Selection for Choking Risk Prevention

Size

Both small and large pieces of food can cause choking. Small, hard pieces of food may get caught in the airway if they are swallowed before being chewed well. Larger pieces, those that are more difficult to chew, are more likely to complete block the throat. Examples include the following:

- Nuts
- Raw carrots, broccoli, or cauliflower
- Hard fruit, especially with peels, such as crisp apples

Shape

Food items shaped like a tube may cause choking because they are more likely than other shapes to completely block the throat. Examples include the following:

- Hot dogs
- Link sausage
- Whole carrots
- Grapes
- Frozen banana pieces

Texture

Foods that are firm, smooth, or slick may slide down the throat into the airway. Examples include the following:

- Hard candy
- Whole-kernel corn
- Peanuts, especially Spanish peanuts

Dry, hard foods may be hard to chew but easy to swallow whole. Examples include the following:

- Hard pretzels
- Tortilla chips
- Popcorn

Sticky foods can stick to the back or roof of the mouth and block the throat and are difficult to remove. Examples include the following:

- Nut butters alone
- Processed cheese chunks or slices
- Gummy bears
- Marshmallows
- Fruit roll-ups

Hard-to-chew foods that are fibrous and tough can present hazards. Examples include the following:

- Bagels
- Steak, roast, or other fibrous meats
- Meat jerky
- Toddler biter biscuits

Applying Prevention Strategies

- **Always supervise eating:** Children do best when sitting to eat. It lets them concentrate on chewing and swallowing. Join the children at the table. Eating or drinking while running or playing is a distraction and can cause choking problems.
- **Decrease outside distractions:** Such as television, games, pets, and so on, during meals and at snack times.
- **Cut food into bite-size pieces or thin slices:** Grind or mash tough food.
- **Cook food until soft, especially beans, pasta, and rice:** These foods are favorites but need to be soft enough to chew easily.
- **Steam vegetables, such as carrots and broccoli.**
- **Eating in cars/buses may also cause problems:** It is hard for the driver to safely pull over fast enough if a child is choking.
- **Serve small amounts of food at a time:** Keep portion size small. With babies be sure the mouth is clear before giving the child another spoonful of food.

Heimlich Maneuver

Choking is fairly common. Choking deaths occur most commonly in children younger than 3 years old and in senior citizens, but they can occur at any age. The Heimlich maneuver has been valuable in saving lives and can be administered by anyone who has learned the technique.

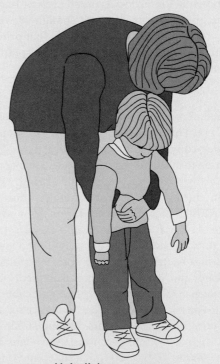

Heimlich maneuver.

From Child Care Health Program, Public Health—Seattle & King County: *Preventing choking on food by children: Safe practice guidelines for child care facilities,* Seattle, 2005, updated October 2008, Author. Accessed September 20, 2010 from www.kingcounty.gov/healthservices/health/child/childcare/education/choking.aspx.

TABLE 12-1	RECENT SOCIETAL CHANGES THAT AFFECT CHILDREN'S DIET AND ACTIVITY PATTERNS
CHANGE	**CONSEQUENCES**
More families with working parents	Parents unable to supervise children's meals and active play
Neighborhoods and parks perceived as increasingly unsafe	Children unable to play outside without supervision
Reduced tax revenues for schools	Introduction of soft drink contracts, vending machines, fast food, and food advertising in schools
Limits on school physical education	Less play during and after school
Increased agricultural production	Increased competition for market share; promotion of more junk food directly to children
Increased demands for convenience foods	More eating occasions; more calories consumed
Greater consumption of food prepared outside the home	Larger portions; more calories consumed
Business deregulation	Unrestricted marketing to children
Television deregulation	More commercials for junk foods during children's programming
Increased use of computers	Food marketing on the Internet; more sedentary behavior
Increased media consolidation	Alliances with food companies to market to children
Increased Wall Street expectations for corporate growth	Expansion of fast-food chains, food products, and marketing to children

From Nestle M: Preventing childhood diabetes: The need for public health intervention, *Am J Public Health* 95(9):1497-1499, 2005.

Type 2 DM is almost completely preventable by balancing energy intake with energy output. This may sound like a simple solution, but as the rates of obesity and type 2 DM increase among children, particularly Hispanic and African American children, societal changes seem to fuel the risk factors, creating much more complex situations. Societal changes affect family structures, educational system, communities, consumer demands, food production and business practices, all of which affect behaviors associated with overweight and diabetes risk for all ages.[13] Table 12-1 lists the consequences of these changes.[13]

Present prevention efforts focus on the responsibility of the individual to reduce one's risk factors for overweight and diabetes. Instead, a public health approach would be more effective.[13] A public health approach provides community supports to ease the transition to positive health-promoting behaviors. For example, local governments can create and provide funds for after-school programs for different types of physical activities suitable for children of varying ages.

Treatment

Treatment, if warranted, must include the family. The goal is to maintain the current weight of the child while growth continues. Children should not be "dieting," but guidance can be provided to the child and caregivers as to healthier eating patterns. Education about dietary patterns such as MyPyramid and food choices to restructure dietary intake patterns may be sufficient and should be conducted by a dietitian who has the expertise to work with children and their families. The goal of treatment should not be to reach an "ideal weight" but to develop and maintain a healthy lifestyle that includes acceptance of diverse body sizes.

Successful treatment programs include the Stop Light Diet[12] and CATCH study.[14] The Stop Light Diet has been an effective weight reduction program for children and young adolescents. Foods are categorized as green, yellow, and red, based on whether the food can be eaten freely, with caution, or only on rare occasions. By focusing on increasing fruit and vegetable intake, decreases in fat and carbohydrate intake may occur. Programs with specific recommendations such as emphasizing foods that families are encouraged to eat, rather than foods to restrict, tend to be more effective.[12] The Children's Activity Trial (CATCH), an intervention study, was successful in changing physical activity and dietary behaviors of children. The effects were maintained through adolescence.[15] By emphasizing physical activity in addition to dietary concerns, long-term results may be sustained (see also the *Teaching Tool* box, Strategies for Healthy Weights).

Role of Nurses

Nurses support the goals of health promotion of overweight children by being sensitive to the emotional, social, and physical dimensions associated with weight and body composition. As allies, nurses create an affirming medical environment for large children by awareness of their own behavior when conducting physical examinations, such as quietly recording weight rather than announcing weight aloud in a medical office or school setting. Pediatric offices should also have examining gowns large enough to adequately be used by larger pediatric patients.

Iron Deficiency Anemia

For children, poverty is a significant risk factor for iron deficiency anemia. Economically deprived children of inner cities are most at risk because of the dual risk of lead poisoning, which reduces the amount of iron absorbed by the body, and chronic hunger that limits the intake of adequate nutrients. Lead poisoning and iron deficiency each contribute to learning failure. Ability to learn is decreased because cognitive and motor abilities are altered, and this limits the ability

TEACHING TOOL

Strategies for Healthy Weights

What's a family to do? How do we support the efforts of our clients to raise their children with healthy weight habits? Following are some strategies from the American Heart Association for families and children:

1. Be a positive role model. If parents are practicing healthy habits, it's a lot easier to convince children to do the same.
2. Set specific goals and limits, such as 1 hour of physical activity a day or two desserts per week other than fruit. When goals are too abstract or limits too restrictive, the chance for success decreases.
3. Don't reward children with food. Candy and snacks as a reward encourage bad habits. Find other ways to celebrate good behavior.
4. Make a game of reading food labels. The whole family will learn what's good for their health and be more conscious of what they eat. It's a habit that helps change behavior for a lifetime.
5. Make dinnertime a family time. When everyone sits down together to eat, children are less likely to eat the wrong foods or snack too much. Get the kids involved in cooking and planning meals. Everyone develops good eating habits together, and the quality time with the family will be an added bonus.

From the American Heart Association, *Top ten ways to help children develop healthy habits,* Dallas, undated, Author. Accessed March 20, 2010, from http://www.americanheart.org/presenter.jhtml?identifier=3033747.

to explore, focus, and benefit from the education environment. Although poor Americans of any group are at risk, African American, Hispanic American, and Native American children are most likely to have inadequate intakes of iron.

Malnourished children may be developmentally delayed and unable to benefit from educational experiences. The effects of iron deficiency anemia may begin in childhood and carry through adolescence and into adulthood, limiting the productivity and potential accomplishments of individuals.

Although iron deficiency has been recognized as a public health issue for many years, it is still a concern. It is possible that federal government programs to increase nutrition status among poor Americans may actually work against decreasing iron deficiency. For example, the U.S. Federal Commodity Food Program releases cheese and butter to the poor. Not only are these foods high in fat but they also are particularly poor sources of iron and may contribute to the continuing prevalence of iron deficiencies.[11] Another contributing factor may be that in 1997, the USDA began to allow the School Lunch Program to substitute yogurt for meat/protein requirements.[12] For the general population, the effect on iron intake may be minimal, but for economically disadvantaged children, the amount of iron consumed through school lunch servings of meat, poultry, fish, and beans is significant. The effects of chronic poverty and malnutrition are so intertwined that simple nutritional intervention will not overcome the deficits of social deprivation.[15]

Role of Nurses

Nurses, particularly school nurses, can educate teaching staff about the relationship between iron deficiency and learning ability. Children may be labeled as slow learners and "behavior problems" when iron deficiency may be the true cause of learning difficulties.

Food Allergies and Food Intolerances

Food allergies and food intolerances pose nutritional and social challenges for children, their families, and caregivers. Although adults may also experience adverse responses to foods, infants and children are most commonly affected. About 6% to 8% of children and 0.5% to 2% of adults have documented food allergies.[16] Commonly affected individuals are those with asthma and hay fever.

Food Allergy

A food allergy is the overreaction of the immune system to a food protein or other large molecule that has been absorbed and interacts with the immune system, which produces a response. The body produces antibodies to protect itself from the foreign substance, the protein allergen. The reaction causes a variety of physical symptoms that occur immediately (less than 2 hours), intermediately (2 to 24 hours), or delayed (more than 24 hours).[17] The most common food allergies experienced by children are peanuts, milk, eggs, and wheat. Seafood and peanuts are more common among older children and adults. Cross-reactivity also occurs. For example, if a person is affected by a ragweed allergy, reaction to melons and bananas may occur.[17]

Symptoms may include skin, respiratory, and gastrointestinal reactions (Box 12-4). Reactions may affect breathing ability if the upper airway becomes obstructed because of swelling. If the symptoms are treated as asthma instead of a true food allergy, the misdiagnosis may trigger more serious physical responses and a continuation of symptoms because the offending food may continue to be consumed.

Reactions for a small number of individuals may be so severe as to be life threatening. This type of reaction is called anaphylaxis and may occur immediately after eating the food substance. Peanuts, eggs, shellfish, and nuts may cause anaphylaxis in sensitive individuals. Symptoms may include hives, breathing difficulties, and unconsciousness. It requires immediate medical care or a plan of action in case inadvertent consumption of the offending food occurs. Caregivers, whether parents, school officials, family, or friends, must be aware of the potential reaction and the appropriate and immediate treatment for the anaphylaxis response.[18]

Risk factors. Risk factors include heredity, gastrointestinal permeability, and environmental factors. Heredity is a risk factor because if parents have allergies, their children are most at risk. Gastrointestinal permeability affects the amount of the antigen inappropriately absorbed. Environmental factors can increase food allergic responses. Environmental factors include increased exposure to inhalant seasonal allergies such as pollen and cold weather and other

BOX 12-4 POTENTIAL SYMPTOMS OF FOOD ALLERGIES

Gastrointestinal System
Nausea
Abdominal cramping
Vomiting
Gastroesophageal reflux
Gastrointestinal bleeding
Oral and pharyngeal pruritus (itchiness)

Respiratory System
Rhinitis (inflamed nasal membranes and discharge)
Cough
Hoarseness
Asthma
Stridor (high-pitched sound from trachea/larynx obstruction)
Chest tightness
Dyspnea (shortness of breath)

Neurologic System
Headache (migraine)
"Feeling of impending doom"

Dermatologic System
Itching
Contact dermatitis
Flushing
"Goose bumps"
Eczema (itchy, crusty rash)
Erythema (redness of skin/mucous membranes)
Urticaria (itchy skin eruptions)

Cardiovascular System
Syncope (brief lapse of consciousness)
Hypotension (abnormally low blood pressure)
Dizziness
Loss of consciousness

Genitourinary System
Uterine bleeding
Uterine cramping

Data from Hubbard SK: Medical nutrition therapy for food allergy and food intolerance. In Mahan LK, Escott-Stumps S, editors: *Krause's food & nutrition therapy*, ed 12, Philadelphia, 2008, Saunders; Smith LJ, Munoz-Furlong A: Management of food allergy. In Metcalfe DD, Sampson HA, Simon RA, editors: *Food allergy: Adverse reactions to food and food additives*, ed 2, Cambridge, Mass, 1997, Blackwell Science.

environmental allergens of dust, mold, dust mites, smoke, and stress.

Food Intolerance

In contrast to a food allergy, **food intolerance** is an adverse reaction to a food that does not involve the immune system. The symptoms are triggered by a reaction of the body to a food. Pharmacologic properties of foods (e.g., tyramine in aged cheese, theobromine in chocolate), metabolic disorders (e.g., lactose intolerance), or idiosyncratic responses may cause the reaction.[19] Lactose intolerance is an example of a food intolerance (see Chapter 4). The lack of the enzyme lactase limits the digestion of lactose, leading to physical symptoms of bloating, flatulence, diarrhea, and nausea. The resulting symptoms can be similar to and mistaken as a food allergy. Treatment, though, is different than for a true allergy. For lactose intolerance, products are available that contain reduced lactose, or there are pills (e.g., Lactaid) that break down lactose, thus easing digestion. In contrast, if the symptoms are caused by a food allergy, the offending substance in milk—the milk proteins—is not affected by the reduction of lactose (a carbohydrate) and the immune system response and symptoms would still occur.

Diagnosis

Determination of whether a reaction is caused by a food allergy or by intolerance requires consultation with a health care provider specializing in allergies. Diagnosis involves a health history and physical examination, food and symptom diary, biochemical and immunologic testing, and a food elimination procedure.[16] The health history records symptoms, including the reaction time from ingestion to symptoms and a family allergy history, in addition to traditional information of health histories. The physical examination assesses weight and height patterns to determine whether potential malnutrition may be present because of the effects of the food allergies. Related allergenic symptoms such as eczema are noted. A food and symptom diary keeps track of amounts of food consumed, time and day of consumption, and any resulting symptoms. This information is valuable to begin to isolate potential food allergens. Biochemical testing such as a complete blood count rules out symptoms caused by conditions unrelated to food allergies. Immunologic testing through skin pricking of individual foods assists in identifying potential food allergens based on reactive immunologic adverse reactions, such as swelling and welts at the site of the skin prick.

A food elimination process consists of not eating foods suspected of being allergenic for 2 weeks to allow the person to become symptom-free. Guidance during this phase is crucial to ensure complete compliance. Adequate nutrition can be sustained by substitution of other foods to provide nutrients lost by the elimination of allergenic foods. A registered dietitian should be consulted for appropriate elimination diets. To ensure the accuracy of the diagnosis, a food challenge is implemented. This consists of consuming the allergenic food and assessing the responsive symptoms. Severe reactions are possible. Consequently, food challenges should be conducted in an appropriate health care setting. Another protocol is to conduct a double-blind, placebo-controlled food challenge. Rechallenges may be conducted after several years to assess if the food allergy is still present.[16]

Treatment

The only way to treat a food allergy is to avoid consumption of the food. Referral to a registered dietitian for nutrition counseling is important, and family and caregivers should be included in the nutrition counseling process. Nutrition

BOX 12-5 LABEL TERMINOLOGY FOR MILK, WHEAT, AND SOY INGREDIENTS

Milk, wheat, and soy may be contained in a variety of ingredients, as indicated in the following lists:

Milk

Buttermilk solids	Lactalbumin
Caramel color/flavoring	Milk
Casein	Milk solids
Caseinate	Natural flavoring
Cream	Sodium caseinate
Curds	Whey

Wheat

Enriched flour	Modified starch
Flour	Modified food starch
Gluten	Vegetable starch
Graham flour	Vegetable gum
Hydrolyzed vegetable protein	Wheat
Malted cereal syrup	Wheat bran
Seminola	Wheat germ
Starch	Wheat starch
Gelatinized starch	

Soy

Hydrogenated oils	Soybean oil
Natural flavoring	Vegetable broth
Soy	Vegetable shortening
Soy flour	Vegetable starch
Soy protein	Vegetable gum

Data from Hubbard SK: Medical nutrition therapy for food allergy and food intolerance. In Mahan LK, Escott-Stumps S, editors: *Krause's food & nutrition therapy,* ed 12, Philadelphia, 2008, Saunders; Smith LJ, Munoz-Furlong A: Management of food allergy. In Metcalfe DD, Sampson HA, Simon RA, editors: *Food allergy: adverse reactions to food and food additives,* ed 2, Cambridge, Mass, 1997, Blackwell Science.

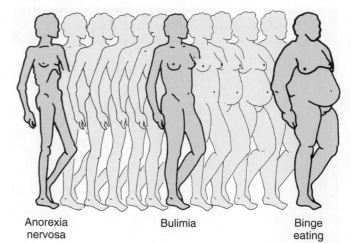

FIG 12-4 **Continuum of eating disorders.** Although physical conditions vary, underlying psychologic characteristics are held in common across the continuum. (From Worthington-Roberts BS, Williams SR: *Nutrition throughout the life cycle,* ed 4, New York, 2000, McGraw-Hill.)

Anorexia nervosa   Bulimia   Binge eating

counseling identifies alternative sources of nutrients to ensure appropriate substitutions for the foods eliminated. Nutrition counseling also assists in teaching how to use food labels to recognize the different terms of allergenic items (Box 12-5). Valuable assistance is provided by organizations such as the Food Allergy Network, which provides a newsletter, informational website, and other educational supports. Planned nutrition counseling follow-up sessions should be considered to assess progress in complying with dietary recommendations.

Role of nurses. Awareness of food allergies and the nutrition adequacy issues associated with specific food elimination supports the health promotion goal of clients. Appropriate referrals to nutrition counseling can assist in avoiding nutrient deficiencies and frustrations with compliance.

Eating Disorders

Eating disorders are a group of behaviors fueled by unresolved emotional conflicts, symptomized by altered food consumption. Disorders include anorexia nervosa, bulimia nervosa, and binge eating. These represent a continuum from the starvation of anorexia nervosa to the uncontrollable excessive food intake of binge eating (Figure 12-4). Mostly women are affected, but men are also susceptible.

Although disordered food consumption is the overt symptom of eating disorders, changed nutrient intake is not the cause. Nourishment becomes a symbolic issue when individuals experiencing eating disorders are not able to deal directly with their emotions and instead nourish their psyches by either excessively restricting food or consuming extremely large quantities of foods that may then be purged. Eating properly cannot cure eating disorders. Underlying psychologic concerns must first be addressed. Nurse-client relationships often provide informal opportunities to discuss dietary patterns; detection of early signs allows for further assessment or treatment (Figure 12-5).

Etiology

The etiology of eating disorders tends to be assigned to our Western obsession with thinness. For many American women, dieting (restrictive food intake) is a way of life from early adolescence on. Most who are caught in the web of the culture of thinness experience chronic dieting syndrome. Chronic dieting syndrome can be described as a lifestyle inhibited or controlled by a constant concern about food intake, body shape, or weight that affects an individual's physical and mental health status. Only a small percentage of these chronic dieters manifest eating disorders. Additional risk factors must be present for eating disorders to evolve. Common risk factors include low self-esteem, depression, participation in appearance or endurance sports, history of sexual abuse, or self-regulatory difficulties. The influence of risk factors is cumulatively mediated by the context of the individual in relation to societal and familial variables (see the *Teaching Tool* box, Resources for Eating Disorders).

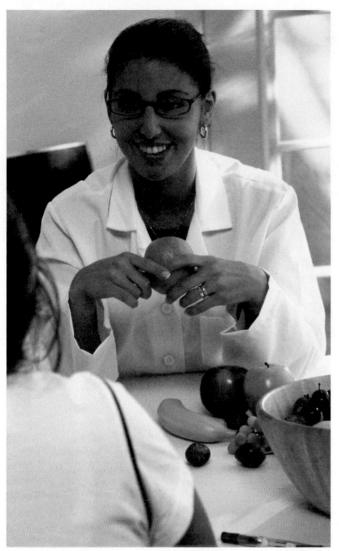

FIG 12-5 Nurse-client relationships often provide informal opportunities to discuss dietary patterns. If early signs of disordered eating are detected, further assessment or treatment can be initiated. (Photos.com.)

Anorexia Nervosa and Related Eating Disorders, Inc. (ANRED) is an organization dedicated to the education, prevention, and dissemination of treatment resources on many disordered eating conditions.

Diagnosis

Uniform criteria for these psychiatric disorders are established by the American Psychiatric Association and published in the *Diagnostic and Statistical Manual of Mental Disorders*, fourth edition (DSM-IV).[20] Periodic revisions allow for updating disorder criteria and for adding newly recognized conditions. The DSM-IV criteria for clinical diagnosis of anorexia nervosa (AN), bulimia nervosa (BN), eating disorder not otherwise specified (EDNOS), and binge-eating disorder (BED) are listed in Box 12-6 (see also the *Personal Perspectives* box, Growing Up with an Anorexic Mother).

Anorexia nervosa. Anorexia nervosa is characterized as the refusal to maintain normal body weight through self-imposed starvation. Because of distorted body images, individuals who experience this disorder do not see themselves as underweight and continue to restrict their food intake, often in a ritualistic manner. Some experience binge-eating episodes that are also associated with bulimic behaviors. Psychologic characteristics include obsession with body shape and weight and an intense phobia of obesity. Chronic restrictive dieting is coupled with self-imposed limitation of food selection, hoarding, or hiding of food. Although their personal food intake is restricted, anorexics often prepare food for others; otherwise they avoid food-related events. When questioned about their food intake, they deny the disorder and weight loss. Anorexics tend to be overly perfectionist *model children* who are introverted, reserved, or possibly socially insecure. A profile of low self-esteem or a family history of anorexia or depression often exists, as well as compulsive behaviors in areas other than food intake. Other areas of compulsion may include excessive exercise, ritualized personal hygiene habits, and intensive study and work behaviors. Bingeing behaviors, if present, are similar to those of bulimia nervosa.

Physical dimensions may include amenorrhea; fatigue yet appearance of hyperactivity; dehydration; electrolyte imbalances including abnormally low levels of magnesium, zinc, phosphorus, and calcium in circulating blood; and metabolic alkalosis or metabolic acidosis caused by laxative abuse. Cardiovascular problems may develop such as hypotension (abnormally low blood pressure), dysrhythmias, and sinus bradycardia (unusually slow heartbeat). Also present may be hormonal imbalances of reduced levels of estrogen or testosterone, hypothermia, and hypertension. Lanugo (soft white hair covering the body) is a late-stage effect, as is edema not caused by premenstrual conditions or other medical

BOX 12-6 EATING DISORDERS: AMERICAN PSYCHIATRIC ASSOCIATION DIAGNOSTIC CRITERIA

Anorexia Nervosa (AN)

A. Refusal to maintain body weight at or above a minimally normal weight for age and height (e.g., weight loss leading to maintenance of body weight less than 85% of that expected; or failure to make expected weight gain during period of growth, leading to body weight less than 85% of that expected)

B. Intense fear of gaining weight or becoming fat, even though underweight

C. Disturbance in the way in which one's body weight or shape is experienced, undue influence of body weight or shape on self-evaluation, or denial of the seriousness of the current low body weight

D. In postmenarcheal females, amenorrhea (i.e., the absence of at least three consecutive menstrual cycles)

1. *Restricting type*: During the current episode of AN, the person has not regularly engaged in binge eating or purging behavior.

2. *Binge eating/purging type*: During the current episode of AN, the person has regularly engaged in binge eating and purging behavior.

Bulimia Nervosa (BN)

A. Recurrent episodes of binge eating. An episode of binge eating is characterized by both of the following:

1. Eating, in a discrete period of time (e.g., within any 2-hour period), an amount of food that is definitely larger than most people would eat during a similar period of time and under similar circumstances

2. A sense of lack of control over eating during the episode (e.g., a feeling that one cannot stop eating or control what or how much one is eating)

B. Recurrent inappropriate compensatory behavior to prevent weight gain, such as self-induced vomiting; misuse of laxatives, diuretics, enemas, or other medications; fasting; or excessive exercise

C. The binge eating and inappropriate compensatory behaviors both occur, on average, at least twice a week for 3 months

D. Self-evaluation is unduly influenced by body shape and weight.

E. The disturbance does not occur exclusively during episodes of AN.

1. *Purging type:* During the current episode of BN, the person has regularly engaged in self-induced vomiting or the misuse of laxatives, diuretics, or enemas.

2. *Nonpurging type:* During the current episode of BN, the person has used other inappropriate compensatory behaviors such as fasting or excessive exercise but has not regularly engaged in self-induced vomiting or the misuse of laxatives, diuretics, or enemas.

Eating Disorder Not Otherwise Specified (EDNOS)

This category is for disorders of eating that do not meet criteria for any specific eating disorder. For example:

1. For females, all of the criteria for AN are met except that the individual has regular menses.

2. All of the criteria for AN are met except that, despite significant weight loss, the individual's current weight is in the normal range.

3. All of the criteria for BN are met except that the binge eating and inappropriate compensatory mechanisms occur at a frequency of less than twice a week or for a duration of less than 3 months.

4. The regular use of inappropriate compensatory behavior by an individual of normal body weight after eating small amounts of food.

5. Repeatedly chewing and spitting out, but not swallowing, large amounts of food.

Binge Eating Disorder (BED)

A. Recurrent episodes of binge eating in the absence of the regular use of inappropriate compensatory behaviors characteristic of BN

B. Binge episodes must occur at least 2 days per week for a period of 6 months.

From American Psychiatric Association: *Diagnostic and statistical manual of mental disorders, DSM-IV-TR*, ed 4, (text revision) Washington, DC, 2000, American Psychiatric Association.

conditions. Other physical conditions may include metabolic changes, constipation, and symptoms associated with starvation, including loss of muscular strength, endurance, aerobic capacity, speed, and coordination. Vitamin, mineral, and protein deficiencies may also develop, leading to loss of bone mass and permanent damage to body organs. Approximately 0.2% to 1.3% of the general population is affected. Mortality for anorexia nervosa is between 5% and 10%.[21]

Bulimia nervosa. Bulimia nervosa is called the *binge and purge syndrome;* bulimic behaviors include experiencing repetitive food binges accompanied by purging or compensatory behaviors. Bingeing is defined as feeling out of control when eating, resulting in the consumption of excessive amounts of food. In response to bingeing, the individual with bulimia purges using laxatives, diuretics, or self-induced vomiting or uses inappropriate compensatory behaviors of fasting, diet pills, or excessive exercise. Bingeing is one of the primary characteristics of bulimia. A *binge* consists of the consumption of excessively large quantities of food in a short period of time with a feeling of being unable to control the amount consumed. An average of two binges per week for 3 months accompanied by several other psychologic and physical dimensions constitutes a diagnosis of BN. Binge foods tend to be of high-kcal value and require minimal preparation. Sleep, abdominal pain, or self-induced or drug-induced vomiting terminates the binge.

Purging and other compensatory behaviors to counteract binges are other characteristics of bulimia. Compensatory behaviors include self-induced vomiting and the use of emetics (substances that cause vomiting), diuretics, and laxatives as purging agents. Fasting or restrictive dieting, appetite suppressants, and excessive exercise may serve as

Growing Up with an Anorexic Mother

Although most individuals with eating disorders are in their teens and early 20s, these disorders can strike at most any age. Particularly difficult is anorexia nervosa, for which the struggle to recover may be lifelong. Family members may be affected psychologically and physically as their loved ones experience this disorder. Consider the following excerpt from an article by Mark Stuart Ellison.

"A hamburger on whole wheat toast and don't cut it." Those words are indelibly etched in my mind. That's how my mother would order whenever she ate out. Although the hamburger was never to her liking and she would never eat the toast, the order was always the same. I recall the extraordinary patience and compassion of waiters and waitresses trying to please someone who was unpleasant. My mother had anorexia nervosa.

My mother died of anorexia at age 49; I was 17. As an attractive young woman, my mother, at 5'4" weighed a voluptuous 135 lbs. During the course of her illness, she weighed as little as 60 lbs, while exercising to exhaustion. The circumstances surrounding her illness had caused me to become socially withdrawn years earlier. I am now 34 years old and have only recently begun to emerge from that isolation.

When I was 9, I witnessed a horrifying scene. The bathroom door in our apartment was slightly ajar. My mother was in the bathroom, squirming on the toilet seat, my father struggling to hold her on the bowl. I was terrified. I didn't know what was happening.

A few minutes later, paramedics took her to the hospital on a stretcher. Mom had had one too many enemas and suffered the consequences on that day. From then on, my mother was in and out of hospitals for the rest of her life and never lived with me again.

As an anorexic she was ever-present; as a mother, she was absent. I have only begun to fill in the blanks in my own life.

From Ellison MS: Growing up with an anorexic mother, *AABA Newsletter*, Summer 1995.

compensatory behaviors. The use of emetics in particular to induce vomiting may have serious medical consequences; fatal incidences associated with bulimia have been reported.[21]

Psychologic dimensions of bulimia encompass obsessions with body shape and weight associated with chronic restrictive dieting. Binge eating and purging are *triggered* by stressful events or initiated as a group activity as part of a social event. Episodes of bingeing are accompanied by a loss of self-control and low self-esteem. Individuals tend to lack the ability to apply appropriate coping skills. Addictive disorders, depression, and family history of obesity, bulimia nervosa, or sexual abuse may be present.

Physical characteristics may include weight fluctuation, amenorrhea, and fatigue. Dental health is affected because dental caries (from excessive simple-sugar consumption) develops and dental enamel erosion (from acidic vomitus) occurs. Purging may lead to dehydration and electrolyte imbalances, particularly with abnormally low levels of chloride, sodium, and calcium in circulating blood; laxative abuse may result in metabolic acidosis. Recurrent episodes of vomiting may cause metabolic alkalosis, bruising of the dorsal surface of the hands (from inducing vomiting), sore throat, swollen salivary glands (especially parotid glands), hormonal imbalances, bloodshot eyes (particularly after vomiting), and broken blood vessels on the face. Rare complications may include gastric rupture, esophageal tears, and cardiac dysrhythmias. Chronic use of emetics may lead to cardiac and skeletal abnormalities.

Eating disorders not otherwise specified (EDNOS). This category covers disordered eating behaviors that do not meet the full criteria of AN or BN but still impact physical and mental health. The occurrence of symptoms and their severity vary compared to those of anorexia and bulimia. Binge-eating disorder (BED) is an EDNOS that often occurs with obesity.[21] It is commonly called *compulsive overeating*. Individuals with this disorder frequently engage in binge-eating behavior not accompanied by purging or compensatory behaviors.

Psychologic dimensions are reflected by binges *triggered* by stressful events or dysphoric moods, including anxiety and depression. The binge eating may occur in secret or private settings and be accompanied by a sense of loss of control. Individuals appear to lack appropriate coping skills. After bingeing episodes, they experience low self-esteem, shame, remorse, or depression. Other addictive disorders may be present in addition to obsessive behaviors in nonfood areas. A family history of obesity, depression, or addictive disorders is likely.

Physical characteristics may include obesity with increased risk of joint pains, breathing difficulties, coronary artery disease, elevated blood cholesterol levels, hypertension, and gastrointestinal tract disturbances. BED, however, is not the only etiologic factor of obesity. Obesity may also be caused by excessive kcal consumption not associated with emotional turmoil, poor eating habits, sedentary lifestyle, or genetic factors. Conversely, BED may be present in the absence of obesity if the criteria of recurrent binges associated with emotional upset and a sense of loss of control occur.

Nutritional Therapy

Dietary patterns in eating disorders may be fractured to a point at which meals are nonexistent or so redefined as to lose all meaning. A challenge in treatment is the relearning of meal patterns.

Medical nutrition is the use of specific nutrition services to treat an illness, injury, or condition. It involves assessment and treatment including diet therapy, counseling, and the use of specialized nutrition supplements. Because medical nutrition is an integral component of eating disorder recovery, knowledge of the process of nutritional care is beneficial for all health care professionals who interact with patients who have eating disorders. As the medical, nursing, and psychologic staffs implement their therapeutic approaches, they will be aware of the medical nutrition objectives. Although underlying psychologic issues are worked on through psychologic therapy, the registered dietitian works with the patient to bring about changes in the patient's food- and weight-related behaviors. This collaborative effort occurs in various phases of outpatient or inpatient therapy and constitutes nutrition intervention.

Objectives of nutrition intervention include (1) separate food- and weight-related behaviors from feelings and psychologic issues; (2) change food behaviors in an incremental fashion until food intake patterns are normalized; (3) slowly increase or decrease weight; (4) learn to maintain a weight that is healthful for the individual without using abnormal food- and weight-related behaviors; and (5) learn to be comfortable in social eating situations.

The effectiveness of the multidiscipline approach to treatment is caused by the recognition that the complex etiology of eating disorders requires the expertise of various health professionals. With the dietitian addressing the food- and weight-related behaviors, the psychologic team members can focus on the psychologic issues while the medical and nursing personnel rectify the physical ramifications of the disorder.

Role of nurses. Nurses are members of the therapeutic multidisciplinary team along with physicians, psychiatrists, psychologists, and dietitians. The therapeutic orientation of nursing care depends on the philosophy and clinical modalities of individual treatment programs. Although nurses are central to the staffing of inpatient programs, their participation in outpatient programs may be marginal. If outpatient treatment is within a holistic clinic attending to medical and psychologic concerns, the role of nurses is integral. Most outpatient treatment tends to be direct care between the client and a health specialist such as a psychologist or dietitian.

Nurses have an educational role in the prevention of eating disorders. By providing information about nutrition and normal eating patterns to parents, caregivers, and children, healthier feeding relationships can evolve. This can help diffuse the behavior of using food as an emotional outlet. Additionally, nurses can be accepting of all body types, taking care to be sensitive to issues of weight and size when providing basic health care. Nurse-client relationships often provide informal opportunities to discuss dietary patterns; if early signs of disordered eating are detected, further assessment or treatment can be initiated before a clinically diagnosable disorder develops (see the *Social Issues* box, When an Eating Disorder Is Suspected, Who Is Responsible for Intervention?). Referral to a dietitian with special training in eating disorders should be considered.

TOWARD A POSITIVE NUTRITION LIFESTYLE: PSYCHOSOCIAL DEVELOPMENT

Psychosocial development occurs during childhood through adolescence. This continual process is most often assessed through the work of Erik Erikson. Erikson's stages of ego development consider the emotional, cultural, and social forces that mold an individual's personality. Divided into

SOCIAL ISSUES

When an Eating Disorder Is Suspected, Who Is Responsible for Intervention?

Perhaps it is a daughter, son, sibling, friend, or roommate. An eating disorder is suspected; too much weight is lost, little is eaten or too much is eaten, and vomiting and other purging is observed. What should you do?

Too often, denial occurs, not only by the person with disordered eating but by her family and friends as well. It's easier to ignore what is happening than to risk becoming involved. On the other hand, sometimes overinvolvement happens when family and friends become so embroiled in the battle to eat or not eat that the disorder becomes the center of relationships. Few relationships can survive well based on struggling with eating issues.

When an eating disorder is suspected, the first action is to talk directly to the person about it. She may be waiting for someone to confront her and tell her these behaviors are not okay; such an encounter may be a trigger for her to seek professional help. If that is not sufficient, friends may choose to contact family members who may have more influence and responsibility for the health of the individual. In a college dormitory setting, resident life personnel should be contacted. They are often specially trained to assist students with eating disorders. It is unfair for the eating disorder of a roommate to negatively affect the lives of the others. Roommates can best help the person by intervening, however risky such actions may be to the friendship.

Once intervention begins, new rules often have to be negotiated. Food and related eating behaviors can no longer be the focus of relationships. Each person becomes responsible for her own intake of nourishment. Although meals may be shared, food policing needs to be curtailed. Parents will need to refrain from pushing food to their child who is anorexic; friends may need to ignore second helpings of a friend who is bulimic. Other rules may evolve; if an individual still binges, she must replace the food she consumes. If the binge is followed by purging, she must completely clean the bathroom after vomiting. The goal is that the person must be responsible for her or his own actions without interfering with the rights of others. Though friends and family may analyze how their behaviors might have supported this illness, ultimately the struggle to heal is the individual's alone.

Data from Siegel M, Brisman J, Weinshel M: *Surviving an eating disorder: Strategies for family and friends,* New York, 1997, Harper Perennial.

stages, this process involves the resolution of psycho-social conflicts. The resolution for children from ages 2 to 3 years is self-confidence and self-control; 4 to 5 years is independence; 6 to 11 years is competence; and 12 to 18 years is sense of self and loyalty.

Each resolution skill has applicability to food preparation and consumption. Children 2 to 3 years of age attain self-confidence and self-control by using acceptable social skills when eating with others and only taking appropriate portions to allow enough for everyone. Allowing children to choose and prepare safe and appropriate snacks can encourage independence for 4- to 5-year-olds. Competence is exhibited by 6- to 11-year-olds by preparing simple meals and assisting in the meal preparation for the family. A sense of self among teens occurs as they successfully negotiate com-

plicated school schedules, extracurricular activities, or work schedules while still allowing time and energy for adequate nutrition because they value the importance of health promotion behaviors.

SUMMARY

The nutrient requirements of humans are basically the same throughout the life span. Overall, the issues of health promotion and disease prevention apply regardless of age. This chapter focuses on those issues most tied to nutrition-related concerns such as prevention of diet-related disorders (e.g., coronary artery disease, some cancers, type 2 diabetes mellitus, and obesity) and emphasizes dietary patterns rather than specific nutrients.

The life span stages reflect psychologic and physiologic maturation. They include childhood (ages 1 through 12),

adolescence (ages 13 through 19), and adulthood. Approaches to health promotion take into account these stages and their effect on nutrient requirements, eating styles, and food choices. Health promotion depends on knowledge, techniques, and community supports. Each stage of development requires different approaches and is supported in various ways by the larger community. Barriers to health promotion during childhood and adolescence may include food asphyxiation, lead poisoning, overweight/diabetes, iron deficiency anemia, food allergies and intolerances, and eating disorders.

THE NURSING APPROACH

Case Studies: Toddler and Adolescent

CASE STUDY #1: TODDLER

Tracy, age 18 months, and her mother Judy are visiting the family nurse practitioner (FNP) for Tracy's annual checkup. After the physical examination, the FNP asks Judy how Tracy is eating. Judy responded, "I'm concerned; Tracy doesn't seem to be eating very well." The nurse interviewed Judy further.

ASSESSMENT

Subjective (from the mother's statements)

- "Tracy used to eat a lot before she started walking."
- "How will I know she is getting enough food?"
- "What should I be primarily concerned with at this age?"
- "Are the jars of prepared foods healthy?"
- "Tracy doesn't seem interested in eating."
- "What can I do to get her to eat?"

Objective (from physical examination of Tracy)

- Weight 24 pounds, height 31.5 inches (50th percentile for 18-month-old girl)
- Tested for growth and development using the Denver II screening toolkit: result 50th percentile in all categories (personal social, fine motor adaptive, language and gross motor)
- Healthy appearance

DIAGNOSIS (NURSING)

Readiness for enhanced knowledge as evidenced by mother's questions and concerns about her toddler's nutrition and growth and development

PLANNING

Patient Outcomes

Short term (at the end of this visit):
- Judy will verbalize ways she can improve Tracy's nutrition.
- Judy will state her intent to seek further nutrition information at MyPyramid.gov.

- Judy will express relief that Tracy's growth and development are normal.

Long term (at the next visit in six months):
- Tracy will remain at or near the 50th percentile for growth and development.
- Tracy will remain healthy.
- Judy will state that she is more at ease regarding Tracy's eating behaviors.

Nursing Interventions
- Answer the mother's questions and concerns.
- Refer Judy to MyPyramid.gov.
- Reassure the mother that Tracy's growth and development are normal.

IMPLEMENTATION

1. Answered the following questions, based upon knowledge of growth and development:

a. "She used to eat a lot before she started walking."
Because growth slows abruptly after the first year of life, the toddler's appetite is smaller than the infant's.

b. "How will I know she is getting enough food?"
The actual amount of food eaten daily will vary from one child to another. It is recommended that parents place small amounts of food on a plate and allow the child to eat it and then ask for more rather than serve a large portion that he or she cannot finish. One level tablespoon of each food served is a good start.

c. "What should I be primarily concerned with at this age?"
The primary dietary concern is the prevention of iron deficiency anemia. Sources of iron such as meat may be rejected. Cooked eggs, specifically the yolk, offer a valuable source of iron that can be incorporated easily.

d. "Are the jars of prepared foods healthy?"
The use of prepared toddler foods during the transition from infancy to early childhood presents special concerns. These products may not provide the nutrient or food range needed

THE NURSING APPROACH—cont'd

Case Studies: Toddler and Adolescent—cont'd

by the child. It is important to read the information label of all prepared foods.

e. "Tracy doesn't seem interested in eating."

The eating behavior and habits of the young child present one of the major barriers in providing adequate nutrition. The toddler often begins to use the meal event as an occasion to assert individuality, control of the environment, and simple exploration of food textures and qualities. Definite food preferences and food fads emerge.

f. "What can I do to get her to eat?"

- Offer simple, single foods. Toddlers often reject mixtures of foods.
- Offer a variety of foods but repeat the same foods often enough so that the toddler recognizes them.
- Do not use food as a reward or punishment for behavior.
- Schedule meals and sleep periods so that the child is awake and alert during mealtime.
- Serve small portions and offer seconds after the first portion is eaten.
- Do not offer raw carrots, celery, peanuts, or other such foods that could be easily aspirated.
- Allow the toddler to self-feed; this is a major way to strengthen independence.
- Offer finger foods and allow a choice between two types of food to help promote independence.
- Serve nutritious finger foods such as pieces of chicken, slices of bananas, and pieces of cheese and crackers.

2. Referred Judy to MyPyramid.com for further nutrition information.

The MyPyramid site says the information is for toddlers at least 2 years old. However, much of the information is pertinent to an 18-month-old child. Becoming familiar with this resource can help the mother anticipate what she can do for Tracy as she grows.

3. Reassured Judy that Tracy's growth and development was normal.

Parents appreciate the assurance that a child is growing and performing within a normal range.

EVALUATION

Short term (at the end of the visit):

- Judy verbalized ways that she could improve Tracy's nutrition.
- Judy stated that she would go to MyPyramid.gov to seek more nutrition information.
- Judy expressed relief that Tracy was growing and developing at a normal rate.
- Goal met.

DISCUSSION QUESTIONS

1. Tracy is beginning to establish some eating patterns. Besides providing adequate nutrition for the toddler, how could this mother be a role model for healthy eating?
2. Which of these nurse's instructions would be applicable to a preschooler?

CASE STUDY #2: ADOLESCENT

Brenda, a 16-year-old junior student in high school, came to see the school nurse with complaints of abdominal discomfort. As the nurse interviewed and examined Brenda, the nurse learned that Brenda was concerned about her friend who had anorexia nervosa. The nurse suspected that Brenda also had some anorexic behaviors. Brenda's school record indicated she weighed 129 pounds six months earlier, but current weight was only 109 pounds.

ASSESSMENT

Subjective (from patient's statements)

- "My stomach hurts. I don't have any energy today."
- "I don't remember when my last period was. It probably was a few months ago. I am not sexually active."
- "I have not had any diarrhea or vomiting. I tend more to be constipated. No one in my family has been sick."
- "I haven't eaten anything unusual. I frequently skip lunch at school. I would rather spend the time running. I exercise every day."
- "I always feel so fat."
- "I am worried about my friend Sonya, who is in the hospital with anorexia nervosa. Her mother said Sonya just about died two days ago. That scares me."

Objective (from physical examination)

- Blood pressure: 108/60; temperature: 97.4° F; pulse: 68; respirations: 14
- Height 5 feet 6 inches, weight 109 pounds
- Abdomen tender, bowel sounds hypoactive
- Appears thin, pale; skin dry, hair dull

DIAGNOSES (NURSING)

1. Imbalanced nutrition: less than body requirements related to regular exercise and insufficient intake of food (possible anorexia nervosa) as evidenced by 84% ideal body weight, 16% weight loss in six months, feels fat, skips meals, abdominal discomfort, loss of menstruation, constipation, fatigue, dull hair and BP 108/60
2. Fear related to severe consequences of anorexia nervosa as evidenced by concern for anorexic friend and "that scares me."

PLANNING

Patient Outcomes

Short term (at the end of this visit):

- Brenda will agree to see a physician for a physical examination and lab tests.
- Brenda will agree to eat small meals frequently throughout the day and to return to the school nurse once a week to report eating and activity and to check weight.

Long term (in four months):

- Gradual weight gain, preferably about one pound per week
- Regular pattern of eating
- Return of menstrual periods, energy, shiny hair
- No abdominal pain and no constipation

THE NURSING APPROACH—cont'd

Case Studies: Toddler and Adolescent—cont'd

Nursing Interventions

1. Express concern for Brenda's friend and state observations that Brenda has some danger signs of poor nutrition.
2. Contact parents regarding the need for Brenda to get follow-up medical care and professional care.

IMPLEMENTATION

1. Expressed concern for Brenda and her friend. Conveyed a nonjudgmental attitude and praised Brenda for seeking help from the school nurse.
   Establishing trust facilitates open discussion about health concerns.
2. Assessed Brenda's knowledge of possible consequences of anorexia nervosa and its treatment, and then corrected misunderstandings.
   Fear may be a motivating factor for behavioral changes. Full information may lead to wiser choices.
3. Told Brenda that she needs to see a physician to determine the cause of her discomfort and evaluate her general health.
   A medical doctor can assess her health, determine a diagnosis, and prescribe care.
4. Related the nurse's observations of Brenda's health to poor nutrition and emphasized benefits of healthy eating.
   It is common for people with anorexia nervosa to deny eating problems and to not associate health difficulties with poor nutrition. Striving for desirable physical characteristics (e.g., shiny hair) and comfort (e.g., lack of constipation) may motivate behavior changes.
5. Gave her a chart indicating normal weights for adolescents her height and showed her how her weight was much lower than expected.
   An individual who has distorted body image may see a more accurate picture of personal weight when comparing own weight to the expected weight on the chart.
6. Helped Brenda set goals to avoid further weight loss and helped her identify possible changes she could make in her lifestyle.
   Involving the individual in planning contributes to empowerment and a sense of control. Small steps may be needed to reach desired changes.
7. Suggested eating small portions of nutrient dense foods more frequently, including whole grains, milk, fruits, and vegetables.

Low calories may initially be necessary to prevent refeeding syndrome. Because of early satiety, food intake should be spread throughout the day. These foods will provide nutrients needed for normal metabolism and function, and fiber and adequate water will help reduce constipation. Quantities may be increased gradually.

8. Asked Brenda to visit the nurse once a week for several weeks. Asked her to keep a food and activity record for the next week, and bring it to the school nurse.
   Frequent monitoring of weight helps track improvement (or lack of improvement) and helps an individual to be accountable. Food records can be used for praise of positive eating when accompanied by stable weight or weight gain. Imbalance of activity versus food may aid discussion and further planning.
9. Telephoned Brenda's parents to invite them to come for a discussion of possible health problems of Brenda and to advise them of the need for medical follow-up and counseling.
   Parents have the responsibility to protect the health of their children and seek medical care as needed. They may not be aware of eating problems. Should the physician diagnose anorexia nervosa, a referral can be made for counseling.

EVALUATION

Short term (at the end of the visit):
- Brenda said she would see a doctor.
- She reluctantly agreed to record her food intake and activity for one week and return to see the school nurse each week for a few weeks.
- Short-term goals met.

DISCUSSION QUESTIONS

1. What foods might be acceptable to Brenda for frequent small meals?
2. How can the nurse know if Brenda's food diary is an honest recording of food and fluids actually consumed by her?
3. What would be a reasonable weight gain for Brenda at the end of one month?

Nursing Diagnoses-Definitions and Classification 2009-2011. Copyright © 2009, 1994-2009 by NANDA International. Used by arrangement with Blackwell Publishing Limited, a company of John Wiley & Sons, Inc.

APPLYING CONTENT KNOWLEDGE

Daphne is upset about the way her young children eat. "Although I have the nanny prepare meals for them, they just don't sit still to eat. They seem to want to just grab foods from the time they get home from school until they go to sleep." When Daphne was asked about her eating style and that of her husband, she responded, "Oh, we both work crazy hours, so we don't have time to eat regular meals. We just grab a bowl of cereal or have leftovers from takeout orders." What strategies would you share with Daphne to change the eating styles of her young children?

WEBSITES OF INTEREST

The Food Allergy & Anaphylaxis Network (FAAN)

www.foodallergy.org

Educates about food allergies and anaphylaxis responses by providing support, research, and publications such as special product alert notices.

GirlsHealth

www.girlshealth.gov

Focuses on health topics for girls (ages 10 to 16) and motivates behaviors with positive, supportive, and non-threatening messages.

KidsHealth

www.kidshealth.org

Provides information for children, teens, and parents on health, food, and fitness including games and colorful animations.

REFERENCES

1. Satter E: *How to get your kid to eat ... but not too much*, Palo Alto, Calif, 1987, Bull Publishing.
2. American Dietetic Association: Nutrition Guidance for healthy children ages 2-11 years, *J Am Diet Assoc* 108(6):1038-1047, 2008.
3. Coon K, et al: Relationship between use of television during meals and children's food consumption patterns, *Pediatrics* 107:e7, 2001.
4. Krugman SD, Dubowitz H: Failure to thrive, *Am Fam Physician* 68(5):879-884, 2003.
5. Heird WC, Cooper A: Infancy and childhood. In Shils ME, et al, editors: *Modern nutrition in health and disease*, ed 10, Philadelphia, 2006, Lippincott Williams & Wilkins.
6. Dixon LB, et al: The effect of changes in dietary fat on the food group and nutrient intake of 4- to 10-year-old children, *Pediatrics* 100(5):863-872, 1997.
7. Piernas C, Popkin BM: Trends in snacking among U.S. children, *Health Affairs*, 29(3):398-404, 2010.
8. Cole CR, Lifshitz F: Zinc nutrition and growth retardation, *Pediatr Endocrinol Rev* 5(4):889-896, 2008.
9. Food Research & Action Center: *National School Lunch Program* (December 2009); *School Breakfast Program* (December 2009); *Summer Food Service Program for Children*, Washington, D.C., Author. Accessed March 19, 2010, from www.frac.org.
10. Food and Nutrition Service, U.S. Department of Agriculture: *Food distribution programs* (Jan 2006), www.fns.usda.gov/fdd.
11. Wood RJ, Ronnenberg AG: Iron. In Shils ME, et al, editors: *Modern nutrition in health and disease*, ed 10, Philadelphia, 2006, Lippincott Williams & Wilkins.
12. Dietz WH: Childhood obesity. In Shils ME, et al, editors: *Modern nutrition in health and disease*, ed 10, Philadelphia, 2006, Lippincott Williams & Wilkins.
13. Nestle M: Preventing childhood diabetes: The need for public health intervention, *Am J Public Health* 95(9):1497-1499, 2005.
14. Treuth MS, Griffin IJ: Adolescence. In Shils ME, et al, editors: *Modern nutrition in health and disease*, ed 10, Philadelphia, 2006, Lippincott Williams & Wilkins.
15. Karp R: Malnutrition among children in the United States: The impact of poverty. In Shils ME, et al, editors: *Modern nutrition in health and disease*, ed 10, Philadelphia, 2006, Lippincott Williams & Wilkins.
16. Kim JS: Food allergy: diagnosis, treatment, prognosis, and prevention, *Pediatr Ann*, 37(8):546-551, 2008.
17. Hubbard SK: Medical nutrition therapy for food allergy and food intolerance. In Mahan LK, Escott-Stumps S, editors: *Krause's food & nutrition therapy*, ed 12, Philadelphia, 2008, Saunders.
18. Smith LJ, Munoz-Furlong A: Management of food allergy. In Metcalfe DD, Sampson HA, Simon RA, editors: *Food allergy: Adverse reactions to food and food additives*, ed 2, Cambridge, Mass, 1997, Blackwell Science.
19. Sampson HA: Diagnosis and management of food allergies. In Shils ME, et al, editors: *Modern nutrition in health and disease*, ed 9, Philadelphia, 1999, Williams & Wilkins.
20. American Psychiatric Association: *Diagnostic and statistical manual of mental disorders (DSM-IV TR 2000)*, ed 4, text revision, Washington, DC, 2000, American Psychiatric Publishing, Inc.
21. American Dietetic Association, Position of the American Dietetic Association: Nutrition intervention in the treatment of anorexia nervosa, bulimia nervosa, and other eating disorders, *J Am Diet Assoc* 106(12):2073-2082, 2006.

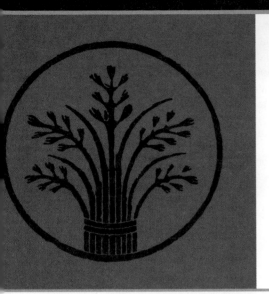

Life Span Health Promotion: Adulthood

Aging is a gradual process that reflects the influence of genetics, lifestyle, and environment over the course of the life span.

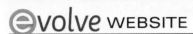 WEBSITE
http://evolve.elsevier.com/Grodner/foundations/

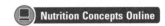 **Nutrition Concepts Online**

ROLE IN WELLNESS

By the time young adults reach their early 20s, growth levels off and the body achieves a state of homeostasis. Mental capacity is fully developed as young people begin to assume their roles in adult society. How this transition is experienced depends on cultural views of growing older. Does growing older confer social privileges of respect and authority? Or does it mean the loss of youth and good times? How we accept new responsibilities within family and intimate relationships may affect our overall health status and level of wellness.

Layered on cultural perceptions of aging is the complexity of today's world. Through telecommunications we are exposed to and influenced by numerous world and local events in ways unimaginable to previous generations. Similarly, educational and employment opportunities seem endless; yet some adults are caught in cycles of underemployment and unemployment as the marketplace evolves, and others, through economic misfortune, are homeless. Additionally, each stage of adulthood presents particular life stressors. How we cope with these stressors and those of society affects adult nutritional status.

The five dimensions of health affect the health promotion of adulthood. Beginning health-promoting habits early in life and continuing them through older adulthood maintains *physical health*. Our *intellectual health* provides the ability to change and adapt as circumstances vary according to age and related responsibilities for our health. The symbolic representation and occasions defined by certain foods are often tied to our *emotional* well-being. Food provides a means of communication; customs surrounding eating behaviors vary among cultures and ethnic groups; exposure to these differences is rewarding and enhances *social health*. The support of our religious and charitable communities provides an added

dimension to *spiritual health* promotion and to recovery from disease and illness.

Although previous chapters have addressed nutrition for adults, this section addresses the different influences on nutritional lifestyles through the adulthood stages of the early years (20s and 30s); the middle years (40s and 50s); the older years (60s, 70s, and 80s); and the oldest years (80s and 90s).

AGING AND NUTRITION

Aging is a gradual process that reflects the influence of genetics, lifestyle, and environment over the course of the life span. The purpose of cell creation begins changing around age 30. No longer supplying new cells for growth and development, cell metabolism slows down and instead creates new cells to replace old cells. At older ages, this process of cell replication slows even more, and the effects of aging on body organs begin to appear. Some body systems are more affected than others, and the changes may begin to affect nutritional status. Other organ functions that may be altered include taste and smell, saliva secretions, swallowing difficulties, liver function, and intestinal function. For example, the gastrointestinal tract functions are diminished by reduced production of gastric juices such as hydrochloric acid, which results in decreased absorption of nutrients. The systems and the effects of aging are listed in Table 13-1.

How an individual body responds to these changes reflects health status across the life span. Consequently, everyone ages differently. The role of nutrition during the life span categories of adolescence through the middle years (40s and 50s) provides a foundation to adequately support body processes to effectively deal with the effects of lifestyle and environmental factors. Nutrient intake and dietary patterns directly influence the risk of developing the chronic

TABLE 13-1	EFFECTS OF AGING	
EFFECT ON NUTRITIONAL STATUS	CAUSED BY	ORGAN INVOLVED
↓Ability to taste salt and sweets	↓Taste buds	Tongue and nose
↓Palatability of food	↓Taste and olfactory nerve endings	
↓Food intake		
↓Taste and smell		
Reduced sense of thirst/dry mouth	↓Saliva production	Salivary glands
Difficulty chewing		
Minor effects on swallowing (but may progress to dysphagia)	Muscle contractions may malfunction	Esophagus (and swallowing process)
↓Bioavailability of vitamins, minerals, proteins	↓Hydrochloric acid (HCl) secretion and intrinsic factor	Stomach
↓Absorption of vitamin B$_{12}$ and folate	↓Pepsin	Stomach
↓Drug doses (adjustments possible to prevent overdosing)	↓Production of drug-metabolizing enzymes	Liver

Data from Rosenberg IH, Russell RM, Bowman BB: Aging and the digestive system. In Munro HN, Danford E, editors: *Nutrition, aging, and the elderly*, New York, 1989, Plenum Press.

BOX 13-1	15 WAYS TO PROMOTE SUCCESSFUL AGING: SUGGESTIONS FROM OLDER ADULTS

1. Simplify your life; identify priorities and set limits.
2. Pay attention to yourself: your body, your mind, and your spirit.
3. Continue to teach, continue to learn; teach a class, take a class.
4. Plan some serious leisure activities (painting, woodwork) and do them.
5. Let yourself laugh and let yourself cry—both are important.
6. Be flexible; learn to navigate change.
7. Be charitable; make it a practice to give (wisdom, experience, money, time, yourself).
8. Be financially astute; invest early for retirement.
9. Get a life; you'll live better in retirement if you do.
10. Practice good nutrition and exercise; discover your internal and external motivators.
11. Think about your past and future; write your autobiography.
12. Be involved; discover what has meaning for you.
13. Be positive; have hope and believe there is a tomorrow.
14. Link with others—relationships are important.
15. Become mortal and deal with your mortality.

From Kershner H, Pegues JM: Productive aging: A quality of life agenda, *J Am Diet Assoc* 98(12):1445-1448, 1998.

disorders of osteoporosis, coronary artery disease, diabetes, hypertension, and obesity. The effect of nutrient intake, though, is mediated by lifestyle behaviors, including physical activity, stress, smoking, alcohol consumption, and exposure to environmental factors. For example, how a young woman eats and the amount of exercise she performs affect the density of her bones and the level of lean body mass of her body. If her nutrient intake is adequate and the exercise is weight bearing, she may reduce her risk of osteoporosis (as well as the risk of the other chronic disorders) decades later when she is in her 60s or 70s.

Productive Aging

The concept of productive aging considers the many psychosocial influences on successful aging. *Productive aging* refers to an overall process of aging that is dependent on attitudes and skills developed over the course of one's life. These attitudes and skills prepare an individual to adapt to the transitions of life and maintain a personal sense of experiencing a productive, meaningful life.[1] Successful aging considers that different criteria of success apply during the older years compared with those of the earlier life span categories. Box 13-1 is a list of 15 ways to promote successful aging that was developed from suggestions by older adults.[1]

STAGES OF ADULTHOOD

The Early Years (20s and 30s)

Students tend to imagine that once they finish high school or college and enter the working world, they will then be able to eat better, sleep more, and generally take better care of themselves than they do during their hectic school years. Unfortunately, that is rarely the experience of young adults. Many find that their lifestyles may be even more time restricted, and positive health behaviors such as regular meal patterns and exercise may fall by the wayside.

These years mark a transition from one stage of the life span to another; young adults separate from their family of origin, focus on personal and career goals, and often face reproductive decisions (Figure 13-1). As such, it is a prime time to either refine or establish an eating style that promotes health, possibly preventing future development of diet-related diseases. National surveys, though, continue to report that few adults consume the health-promoting recommended intakes of fruits and vegetables. As of 2007, 76% of American adults reported consuming fewer than 5 servings of fruits and vegetables a day.[2] A self-review or assessment by a nutrition professional can assist in creating a personal schedule that allows time for planning and preparation of simple yet high-quality meals.

Many women bear children during these years. The nutrition and health requirements of pregnancy are detailed in Chapter 11. Layered on these needs during this life span stage

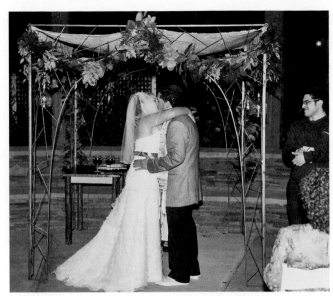

FIG 13-1 The early years of adulthood often include the forming of long-term relationships. (Copyright Jean Kallina, 2005.)

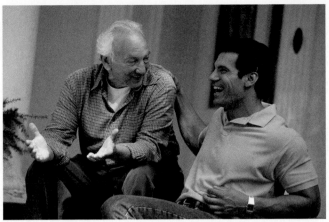

FIG 13-2 The parenting roles often shift during the middle years of adulthood. (Photos.com.)

are often employment and other family commitments, all of which affect nutritional and health behaviors. Physically caring for young children, although eminently rewarding, may be exhausting. Throughout the mother's pregnancy and during childbearing, the father's role in terms of health issues is often ignored. Although the woman's body is nourishing fetal development, the father is under stress as he prepares to support additional responsibilities. Fathers also need to be at optimum health, especially during the first few years of child-rearing when physical stamina is put to the test.

Nutrition Requirements

Growth tends to be completed by the late teens for women and early 20s for men, as reflected by the Dietary Reference Intake (DRI) (see the inside front cover). For women, the Recommended Dietary Allowance (RDA) for energy is 2200 kcal daily; for men, it is 2900 kcal. This reflects the typical differences in body weight and lean body mass of men and women. When this stage includes a departure from high school or college sports training, energy intake should be reduced to meet actual need, or weight gain could occur. A teenage boy's serious athletic training may require as much as 5000 to 6000 kcal a day to maintain weight. Switching to a desk job and exercising for 1 hour per day does not equal previous energy requirements.

The RDA for protein increases for women from 46 to 50 g and for men from 58 to 63 g daily; these ranges reflect lean body mass growth that may occur in both men and women through about age 24. Vitamin and mineral needs do not significantly change. Calcium and phosphorus needs for men and women decline after age 18 because skeletal growth is almost complete. Daily Adequate Intake (AI) recommended calcium levels up to age 18 are 1300 mg, dropping to 1000 mg from 19 years on. For phosphorus, RDA levels up to age 18

are 1250 mg a day, dropping to 700 mg from 19 years on. Maintaining calcium and iron intake continues to be a concern for women because of their often-restricted intake of food during dieting. (See also Box 7-1 or Box 8-3 regarding nutrients and their functions.)

The Middle Years (40s and 50s)

The years from 40 to 50 are marked by a continuation of family demands and career involvement. Some middle-year adults may be faced with caring for aging parents (Figure 13-2); this increased stress and responsibility may be offset by the seemingly reduced parenting of their own children. As older children leave for college or move into their own residences, the resultant "empty nest" necessitates rediscovering preparation of dinners for two or, for single parents, dinners for one. With family meals no longer a requirement, many middle-year adults often have the finances and time for restaurant dining. However, making the transition to food preparation styles and dietary patterns that maintain healthful dietary patterns is crucial.

The impact of continued positive dietary patterns coupled with regular exercise provides continued prevention or delay of diet-related diseases such as type 2 diabetes mellitus (type 2 DM) and coronary artery disease. Increased stamina is an additional benefit from such behaviors.

Nutrition Requirements

During the middle years, cell loss rather than replication occurs. Kcal needs decline as lean body mass is lost and replaced by body fat that is less metabolically active. Women in particular experience an increase in body fat composition. Body fat increases can be slowed by exercise and strength training to continue maintenance of lean body mass. After age 50, daily energy needs drop from 2200 to 1920 kcal for women and from 2900 to 2300 kcal for men. It is a challenge to meet the same nutrient needs with reduced kcal intake. Protein needs remain constant for both genders. Iron requirements for women drop from 18 to 8 mg, which reflects reduced iron loss because of menopause. (See also Box 7-1 or Box 8-3 regarding nutrients and their functions.)

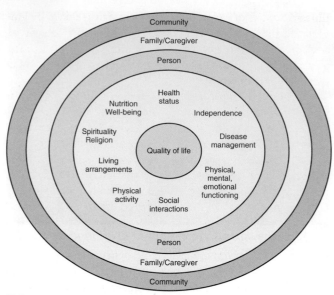

FIG 13-3 Factors that influence of the quality of life of adults 60 years and older. (From American Dietetic Association: Position of the American Dietetic Association: Nutrition across the spectrum of aging, *J Am Diet Assoc* 105(4):616-633, 2005, with permission from the American Dietetic Association.)

Overall, dietary patterns that are nutrient dense and feature lower-fat protein foods coupled with fiber-containing fruits, vegetables, and grains best meet the nutrient needs of middle-year adults.

The Older Years (60s, 70s, and 80s)

The United States has never had a population with as high a percentage of older adults as it will have soon. As our life span increases in years, senescence (older adulthood) is for many a time of life for continued professional or career advancement and recreational enjoyment. Others are in transition, adjusting to retirement and settling into new patterns of activities. Gerontology, the study of aging, has provided insights into the emotional, physical, and social aspects of the later years of life. Preparation for the social and physical transitions of aging actually begins many years earlier, as individual approaches to lifestyle health behaviors, career fulfillment, and leisurely pursuits evolve.

Overall, quality of life for older adults depends on factors that influence daily experiences. These factors include health status; nutrition well-being; spirituality; living arrangements; physical activity; social interactions; physical, mental, and emotional functioning; disease management; and level of independence (Figure 13-3). The level of wellness experienced during this stage of life often reflects the quality of life resulting from health behaviors through the several life span stages.

Physical Activity

A lifetime of physical fitness and good nutrition allows an individual to enter these years with more stamina, cardiovascular conditioning, and solid health-promoting habits that

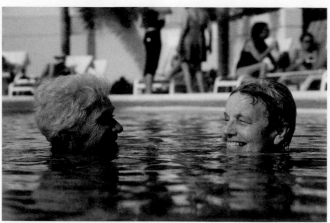

FIG 13-4 Socializing assists with the adjustments of the older years. (Photos.com.)

enable him or her to overcome the inevitable slowing down or physical limitation of the later years (Figure 13-4). Even those who were not always active have been shown to benefit from regular exercise. Strength training has improved the muscle tone and stamina of older men and women.[3]

Physical, Mental, and Emotional Functioning

During these later years, individuals may struggle with the deaths of family members and friends and adjustment to retirement. Although some delight in retirement, others view retirement as a loss of social status. This combination of death and loss of status may lead to isolation and depression, leading to loss of appetite (anorexia) or other forms of malnutrition. The economic realities of retirement without a solid financial base may thrust some older adults into unexpected poverty, because Social Security and Medicare payments may not be sufficient to adequately cover living and medical expenses. Resources for food purchases may be limited and negatively affect nutritional status. Unless social networking and family supports are strong, these conditions may persist. Older adults may abuse alcohol as a way to deal with these perceived difficult events.

Disorientation or senility often associated with aging may be caused by improper use of medications, marginal nutrient deficiencies (e.g., vitamin B_{12}), or simple dehydration. Older clients may intentionally restrict fluids because of incontinence, nocturia (excessive urination at night), or the inability to get to the toilet on their own. Some older adults lose their sense of thirst and forget to consume enough fluids. Fluid requirements in older adults remain the same as in younger adults (about 8 cups daily is sufficient) unless a medical condition or medication prescribes otherwise. The signs of dehydration are listed in Box 13-2. Medical diagnosis should be sought to determine the specific etiology of these signs.

Nutrition Well-Being

Nutrition status may be affected by restricted access to food and ability to prepare meals. Shopping may be difficult without transportation, and mobility to walk through stores

BOX 13-2	SIGNS OF DEHYDRATION IN OLDER ADULTS

Confusion
Weakness
A hot, dry body
Furrowed tongue
Decreased skin turgor (may not be valid finding in older adults)
Rapid pulse
Elevated urinary sodium

BOX 13-3	RISK FACTORS FOR MALNUTRITION OF OLDER ADULTS

Alcoholism
Anorexia
Chewing and swallowing problems (dysphagia)
Consuming only one meal a day
Dental difficulties
Depression or dementia
Diabetes
Diminished physical functioning
Feeding problems
Food purchasing/preparation difficulties
Impaired acuity of taste and smell
Living in long-term care institution
Loss of spouse
Taking multiple medications
Nerve disorders
Poverty
Pulmonary disease
Surgery

Data from Chernoff R: Nutrition and health promotion in older adults, *J Gerontol A Biol Sci Med Sci* 56 Spec 2(2):47-53, 2001; copyright the Gerontological Society of America.

may be limited. Funds for food may be constrained, and often food quantities available are beyond the amounts that can be used by individuals living alone. Once foods are purchased, preparation may be affected by physical limitations caused by progressive chronic illnesses such as arthritis. Some older adults may no longer have an interest in cooking. Others have become so frightened about foods containing too much fat or cholesterol that they become malnourished. For individuals in this age bracket, there is not sufficient evidence to warrant restrictive dietary intake; in actuality, malnutrition and underweight are more detrimental than excess dietary fat and cholesterol intake. Box 13-3 lists risks factors for malnutrition of older adults.

Dietary management for older adults may be more complicated than for other stages of adulthood. For example, obesity is viewed as a form of malnutrition of an older adult.[4] For younger adults, reducing body mass index (BMI) decreases health risks. For older adults, decreased BMI may be associated with increased risk of strokes. Having an average BMI provides healthful weight reserves during times of

illness.[4] Studies of weight reduction strategies seldom include older participants, so their complex physiologic, behavioral, and social needs are not considered. Additionally such strategies may overly limit intake of essential nutrients, further increasing malnutrition.[4]

Another aspect of older adult dietary management is protein adequacy. Total body protein decreases as aging progresses. Although the loss of skeletal muscle is the most noticeable body protein lost, organ tissue, blood components, and immune bodies are also affected, including compromised wound healing, loss of skin elasticity, reduced ability to battle infection, and longer recuperation from illness and surgeries.[5] Dietary intake may be further altered when these physical factors combine with social factors, leading to reduced protein intake. Consumption of micronutrients found in protein foods also may be limited, leading to deficiencies of B_{12}, A, C, D, calcium, iron, zinc, and others.[6] This need, combined with the greater turnover of whole-body protein of aging bodies, results in older adults needing greater dietary protein intake (1 g/kg body weight) compared with younger adults (0.8 g/kg body weight).[5] Frail elderly women are most at risk for these micronutrient deficiencies.

Living Arrangements

Living arrangements also affect nutritional status. A variety of living arrangements exists for older adults. Although many continue to live in their own homes or with family members, some opt for retirement communities, and others, because of health conditions, may reside in long-term care facilities or nursing homes. Living in one's own home provides the freedom to prepare and eat foods whenever desired; illness, however, may make shopping for food and preparing it difficult. Retirement communities may provide transportation to food stores and more social events involving meals (Figure 13-5), although residents still are responsible for their own food preparation. Long-term care facilities usually provide prepared meals, but the style of cooking may not be as appealing or comforting as home-prepared meals.

A challenge for meeting the nutritional needs of institutionalized older adults is that the DRIs used to guide nutrient levels are intended to meet the needs of healthy older adults. Adjustments are necessary for individual circumstances of acute or chronic illness to achieve rehabilitation, recuperation, or maintenance to reduce the risk of further complications.[7] Consequently, it is now recommended that diets in long-term care facilities be liberalized to improve dietary intake of this age group.[8]

Dietary patterns and preferences of older adults are the result of long-established habits. When they are ill, lonely, or under stress, older adults may strongly prefer foods they associate with pleasant memories. Ethnic favorites may provide security and comfort. The psychologic and social meanings of foods can play an important part in helping an older client recover from illness or adjust to changed circumstances.

Demographic and lifestyle characteristics may, as noted, put older adults at nutritional risk. Factors may include gender, smoking, alcohol abuse, dietary patterns, educational

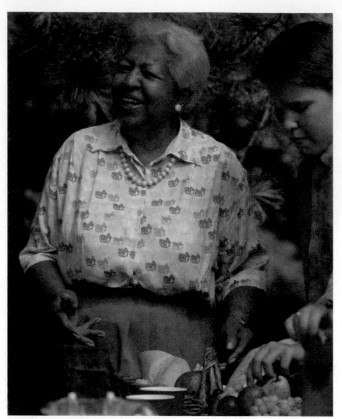

FIG 13-5 Companionship makes mealtimes more enjoyable for older adults. (Photos.com.)

the use of vitamin B_{12} supplements or consumption of foods fortified with vitamin B_{12} to meet the RDA of 2.4 mcg/day (see also Box 7-1 or Box 8-3 regarding functions of nutrients).

Other factors may affect nutritional status. A marginal deficiency of zinc can alter the sensitivity of taste receptors. This deficiency heightens the ability to taste bitter and sour flavors and reduces sweet and salty sensations; excessive use of sugars and salt to make foods taste appealing may result.

Overconsumption of simple sugars and sodium may exacerbate other diet-related disorders such as diabetes and hypertension. As the muscularity of the digestive system weakens, constipation may be a problem, especially after a lifetime of low-fiber foods. Constipation may be alleviated by slowly increasing consumption of whole-wheat products, fruits, vegetables, and fluids, as well as increasing exercise. The Modified MyPyramid for Older Adults, developed by Tufts University, highlights nutrient-dense foods and fluid intake while also suggesting different forms of foods that may be more easily available (Figure 13-6).

Dental health may also affect the ability of older adults to be well nourished. Loss of teeth caused by periodontal disease limits the ability to chew foods such as meats, a prime source of zinc. Chewing ability for some may still be compromised even after dentures have been fitted to replace missing teeth. Dentures may need to be periodically refitted. When dentures do not fit properly, some people do not use them. Instead, they tend to eat foods that can be gummed rather than chewed.

The Oldest Years (80s and 90s)

As life expectancy increases in years, the number of those in the most golden years rises. Although nutrient needs remain basically stable, the effects of aging may continue to reduce the ability of the body to absorb and synthesize nutrients. Optimum nutrition continues to be critical. The healthiest of the oldest develop individual patterns of dietary intake that most meet their physical and social needs.

The *Personal Perspectives* box, Settling into a New Home, provides some first-person insight into the transition one 80-year-old woman experienced on moving from her home to an adult independent living community.

Nutrition Requirements

Malnutrition and underweight become a concern during this stage (see Box 13-3). As food preparation becomes more physically difficult to accomplish, kcal intake may diminish. Illness and accompanying medications may reduce appetite; malnutrition is associated with increased complications. Relatives, friends, and health care professionals can assist in ensuring that adequate meals are available and consumed (Box 13-4). Those in the oldest years may be most at risk for dehydration. Particularly at risk are African Americans and men. Risk increases because of decreased ability of the kidneys to concentrate urine, limited movement, drug interactions, and malfunctioning thirst sensation. Limited ability to move

level, dental health, chronic illnesses, and living situations. Interventions to assist older adults need to account for these influences and should view support services through a continuum of care. Continuum of care provides continuity of care while the older individual moves through different living situations and services as health, medical, and supportive services are provided in suitable care environments. Care settings may range from acute medical settings to community and daycare, from assisted-living retirement housing to traditional nursing home facilities and hospices.

Nutrition Requirements

The DRIs remain constant from age 51 years and older for men and women, except for vitamin D. What does change is the ability of the body to either process or synthesizes certain nutrients. Synthesis of vitamin D is reduced; the AI for vitamin D for individuals older than age 70 increases to 15 mcg a day compared with 10 mcg a day for ages 51 to 70 years. Older adults either need more exposure to sunlight to produce required amounts of vitamin D or require a supplement if so diagnosed by a physician, qualified nutritionist, or dietitian. Because of decreased production of gastric juices and intestinal enzymes, digestion and absorption may be reduced, further highlighting the need for optimum nutrient intake. The production of the intrinsic factor required for vitamin B_{12} absorption also may be reduced, increasing the risk of pernicious anemia. New recommendations suggest

Modified MyPyramid for Older Adults

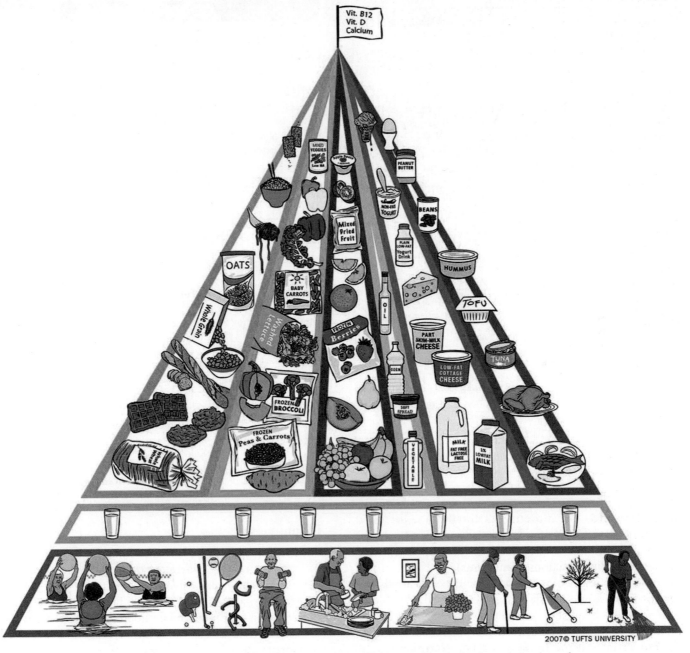

FIG 13-6 Modified MyPyramid for Older Adults. The pyramid emphasizes the value of consuming adequate fluids by the use of glasses as the base of the pyramid and suggests forms of food such as precut frozen vegetables or canned fruit in single-serve packaging, which may be more convenient for older adults. (From Lichtenstein AH, et al: Modified MyPyramid for Older Adults. *J Nutr,* 138:78-82, 2008.)

Settling into a New Home

When 80-year-old Yetta Kaemmer moved to an adult independent living community after living in her own home, she made some adjustments, including eating meals with others every day in the congregate dining room, no longer needing to even cook for herself.

It's like living in a hotel. I don't have to cook, and I always have someone to eat with. Every morning I go to the dining room for breakfast. It's good to be dressed and have a schedule to follow. By the time breakfast is over, you forget about the aches and pains you woke up with. For lunch I have something in my refrigerator to eat, or I may go out. Before dinner I relax by watching television. Then I always freshen my makeup and go to the dining room to eat at my assigned table with three others. When new people arrive, they sometimes feel awkward until they get to know others, especially when entering the dining room for dinner, since everyone seems to know each other. After dinner, there is often a program to attend.

Although we are served balanced meals, we actually eat more food than before, since we have full dinners every night. There are always choices of appetizers, main dishes, and desserts. You get to choose. And so most of us have put on a few pounds!

I don't really miss cooking. Sometimes, though, I will feel a twinge in the supermarket when I see the ingredients of favorite meals I used to prepare. I made a real good meatloaf and, for company, Cornish hens each with a pineapple ring and cherry. Oh they would look so nice!

Yetta Kaemmer
Teaneck, N.J.

BOX 13-4 **STRATEGIES FOR OVERCOMING BARRIERS TO GOOD NUTRITION**

Counteract Decreased Senses of Taste and Smell
Recommend smokers refrain from smoking at least 1 hour before meals.
Suggest sipping water before and during the meal to moisten a dry mouth.
Amplify flavors with the use of seasonings other than salt.
Recommend chewing food thoroughly to fully release flavor and aroma.
Vary food textures and flavors.

Encourage Social Interaction
Find others who are willing to share food preparation and mealtimes.
Investigate congregate meal programs available through senior citizen centers, religious organizations, and hospital community outreach programs.
Avoid noisy dining areas if hearing aids are used.

Present Food Attractively
Use colorful foods and table settings.
Provide enough lighting to see food clearly.

Provide Outside Support
Arrange for Meals-on-Wheels for homebound adults.
Refer eligible clients to the Food Stamp Program, Emergency Food Assistance Program, Child and Adult Care Program, or community food banks or soup kitchens.
Locate grocery stores with delivery service.
Refer to the Expanded Food and Nutrition Education Program (EFNEP) of the Cooperative Extension Service for recipes, meal suggestions, and budgeting assistance.
Refer to home health nurse for routine nutrition screening and appropriate interventions.

may increase fears of incontinence that lead to decreased fluid intake. Nearly half of older adults hospitalized as Medicare patients experience dehydration[8] (see also Box 7-1 or Box 8-3 regarding functions of nutrients).

Although assessment is the responsibility of all health care professionals, home health nurses are particularly able to conduct routine nutrition screening and implement appropriate interventions to prevent or halt malnutrition among this population (see the *Teaching Tool* box, Nutrition Screening Initiative).[9] Government and community meal programs help fill this need and are discussed later in "Community Supports."

ADULT HEALTH PROMOTION

Knowledge

Health promotion integrates nutrition education and focuses on three areas of knowledge: (1) adequate intake of nutrients found in foods (rather than supplements), (2) the relationship between diet and disease, and (3) moderate kcal intake coupled with regular exercise for physical fitness and obesity prevention.

Techniques

Many strategies can be used for adult health promotion:
1. *To reduce risk of diet-related disorders such as coronary heart disease, some cancers, type 2 DM and obesity, consider:*
   - Scheduling routine food shopping so staples such as fruits, vegetables, and grains are available for meal preparation.
   - When shopping, occasionally compare fat content of commonly purchased foods with similar products; purchase the lower-fat product.
   - Aiming to limit visible fat-containing foods.
   - Reorganizing work and personal priorities if necessary to allow time for meal preparation and consumption; for example, get up earlier for breakfast, pack a lunch or afternoon snack, preplan easy-to-prepare dinner menus.
   - Keeping track of dietary intake using MyPyramid or the Fruits & Veggies—More Matters plan. Review Chapter 5 for other dietary fat-lowering techniques and Chapter 4 for approaches that increase the use of complex carbohydrates and fiber-containing foods.

Nutrition Screening Initiative

As the risk of malnutrition among older adults becomes recognized, the American Dietetic Association, the American Academy of Family Physicians, and the National Council on Aging developed the Nutrition Screening Initiative (NSI) project to identify individuals older than 65 who are at nutritional risk. A simple-to-use screening tool is based on key risk factors that may represent determinants of undernutrition or malnutrition. Individuals or caregivers who can consult with a health professional for further guidance can use the tool.

Determine Your Nutritional Health

The warning signs of poor nutritional health are often overlooked. Use this checklist to find out if you or someone you know is at nutritional risk. Read the statements below. Circle the number in the *yes* column for those that apply to you or someone you know. For each *yes* answer, score the number in the box. Total your nutritional score.

	YES
• I have an illness or condition that made me change the kind or amount of food I eat.	2
• I eat fewer than two meals per day.	3
• I eat few fruits, vegetables, or milk products.	2
• I have three or more drinks of beer, liquor, or wine almost every day.	2
• I have tooth or mouth problems that make it hard for me to eat.	2
• I don't always have enough money to buy the food I need.	4
• I eat alone most of the time.	1
• I take three or more different prescribed or over-the-counter drugs a day.	1
• Without wanting to, I have lost or gained 10 pounds in the past 6 months.	2
• I am not always physically able to shop, cook, and feed myself.	2
TOTAL	

Total Your Nutritional Score

0-2 *Good!* Recheck your nutritional score in 6 months.

3-5 *You are at moderate nutritional risk.* See what can be done to improve your eating habits and lifestyle. Your office on aging, senior nutrition program, senior citizens center, or health department can help. Recheck your nutritional score in 3 months.

6 or more *You are at high nutritional risk.* Take this checklist the next time you see your doctor, dietitian, or other qualified health or social service professional and mention any problems you may have. Ask for help to improve your nutritional health.

From the Nutrition Screening Initiative, a project of American Academy of Family Physicians, American Dietetic Association, and National Council on the Aging; funded in part by a grant from Ross Laboratories, a division of Abbott Laboratories.

2. *To reduce osteoporosis risk and strengthen bone health, consider:*
   • Focusing on routine dietary habits—for example, drink a glass of milk at lunch each day. A food pattern assessment can assist in creating a practical calcium consumption plan.
   • Reviewing Chapter 8 for other approaches to increasing calcium consumption.

3. *To decrease the risk of sodium-sensitive hypertension and coronary artery disease, consider:*
   • Adopting the DASH (Dietary Approach to Stop Hypertension) eating plan, which focuses on increasing intake of fruits and vegetables. See Chapter 8 for more details.
   • Learning food categories that are generally salty, and either consume them only occasionally or, if available, purchase low-sodium versions of products. See Chapter 8 for other sodium-reducing strategies.
   • Reducing overall fat intake, particularly saturated fat.

4. *To achieve a healthy body weight and decrease the possibility of diet- and lifestyle-related obesity, consider:*
   • Responding to actual hunger with low-fat, high-fiber foods (with occasional splurges), rather than focusing on dietary restrictions.
   • Exercising regularly to increase stamina, strength, and a sense of wellness. Depending on conditioning, incorporate exercise gradually. A 10-minute walk may be comfortable for some, but others can begin with more strenuous endeavors.
   • Consulting Chapters 9 and 10 for related strategies (see also the *Cultural Considerations* box, Live Long and Prosper … the Okinawa Way!).

Community Supports

Government, corporate, and social institutions create the environments and structures that can support lifestyle health promotion behaviors. Although the actions of these institutions affect particular groups of the public, employees, or communities, it is the individual who can choose to reap the rewards.

Government agencies such as the U.S. Food and Drug Administration (FDA) create regulations that either provide consumer information for decision making (e.g., nutrition labeling) or control the quality of foods, which in turn affects the nutrient viability of manufactured products.

Food manufacturers as an institution were challenged by an earlier *Healthy People* goal to increase to at least 5000 the number of processed food products that are reduced in fat and saturated fat. This objective was achieved.[10] The intent of this goal was to make it easier for consumers to reduce their intake of fat and saturated fat through manufactured products. Not all health professionals are in favor of this approach. Some suggest that it is better to choose foods that are naturally low in fat than to consume prefabricated foods that may lose other nutritious properties during the manufacturing process.

Another objective of the earlier *Healthy People* objectives concerns eating outside the home. The purpose of this

⊕ CULTURAL CONSIDERATIONS

Live Long and Prosper ... the Okinawa Way!

Ageism, discrimination against the elderly, would cease to exist if we followed the lifestyles of the "successful-aging" elders of the Japanese island of Okinawa. According to the ongoing Okinawa Centenarian Study that began in 1976, the elders who follow Okinawa traditional ways experience lower levels of heart disease, stroke, and cancer; are generally healthier; and more physically active for a greater number of years compared with other worldwide populations.

Because most of the present Okinawa centenarians are disabled, frail, and physically and/or cognitively impaired, the researchers decided to study the small number of successful-aging centenarians who are able to care for themselves by accomplishing activities of daily living (ADLs) and live independently in their villages. Although findings show genetic factors to be significant for their longevity and wellness, environmental factors may be even more important. The blend of these environmental factors of culture, attitude, and habits as an aspect of wellness may be understood through the definition of health as the blending of the five dimensions of health.

Okinawan Longevity and Wellness through the Five Dimensions of Health

- *Physical health* (efficient body functioning): *Nuchi gusui* and *hara hachi bu* address efficient body functioning through nourishing the body. *Nuchi gusui* means "let food be your medicine" by consuming a plant-based diet of fruits, vegetables, whole grains, sweet potatoes, legumes, fish, tofu, and other soy products. About 15 different foods, in small portions, are eaten every day. *Hara hachi bu* translates as eating in moderation until just about almost full. This approach allows the hypothalamus time to signal the brain that hunger has been satisfied, preventing overconsumption. The healthiest elders tend to be the most physically active who work, garden, and pursue interests.
- *Intellectual health* (use of intellectual abilities): Rural Okinawan society views aging as a valuable achievement. Intellectual ability allows for acceptance of the aging process while maintaining one's active role in the community. Birthdays from ages 73 to 100 are observed with symbolic gestures such as elders patting family and friends to impart their good health and good fortunes.

- *Emotional health* (ability to control emotions): *Taygay* represents a calm and relaxed approach to life. Traditional Okinawan society encourages being able to deal with stressors while maintaining appropriate control of one's emotions.
- *Social health* (interactions and relationships with others): *Yuimaru* is the principle of mutual assistance upon which Okinawan society is based. This concept applies to all ages as *moais* (groups of individuals who may be friends or work together) provide support for each other over many years. For the elders, their *moais* are important social links, providing daily interaction over shared pots of tea to discuss the news of the day.
- *Spiritual health* (cultural beliefs about the purpose of life): "*Isha-hanbun, yuta-hanbun*" is a proverb meaning "To best understand your problem, see both a doctor and a shaman." This addresses the balance of life to be aware of spiritual as well as physical well-being. Okinawan pursuits such as T'ai chi and karate provide both physical and spiritual benefits.

Application to nursing: Although we may not find ourselves in the semirural environment of the Okinawan villages in which these elders live, we can draw some strategies from their lifestyles to apply to our nursing practice.

For elderly clients from diverse cultural backgrounds, we need to be mindful that they may have lost touch with their *moais*. Perhaps they have recently moved to live with their adult children or have lost a spouse, or both. In addition to medical care, suggestions for seeking out a new *moai* may be most helpful. Art classes, card games, or discussion groups at a local senior center may be helpful in addition to medication for hypertension.

As we advocate for behavior change by our clients, particularly around food choices, consideration of the meaning of food is valuable. Asking an elder to make sweeping food changes is very unsettling. Perhaps introducing the traditional Okinawan concepts of *nuchi gusui* ("let food be your medicine") and *hara hachi bu* (eating in moderation until about almost full) may initiate a lively discussion about food choices and quantities consumed. Your client will remember "that interesting discussion I had with the friendly nurse."

Data from Buettner D: The secrets of long life, *Nat Geogr* 208(5):2-27, 2005; Weil A: Longevity lessons from the Okinawans, *Dr. Andrew Weil's self-healing,* November 2005, p. 8; Suzuki M, et al: Successful aging: Secrets of Okinawan longevity, *Geri Gero Int* 4:S180, 2004; *Okinawa Centenarian Study,* http://okinawaprogram.com.

objective is to increase to at least 90% the proportion of restaurants and institutional food service operations that offer identifiable low-fat, low-kcal food choices, consistent with the Dietary Guidelines.[10] It has been difficult to assess progress toward this objective because the operational definition of *food choices* is so broad.

Recently, in New York City, an ordinance was passed that requires restaurants and food chains with 10 or more locations in Manhattan to post the nutrient content of foods served. This information may be posted on signs as in fast-food restaurants or on menus in traditional restaurants.

Whether this will influence consumer choices is yet to be determined, but at least the possibility of informed decision making is available. Ordinances banning the use of trans fats when preparing foods for direct consumption by consumers in restaurants and other food outlets have been implemented and instituted in other cities in the United States.

Corporations can support health promotion activities by offering comprehensive employee health promotion programs to their employees. This can be accomplished through wellness centers providing programs about healthy lifestyles.

Although most corporations may not be able to provide on-site gyms or similar facilities, some have arranged for corporate discounts at local gym facilities.

Government agencies and community groups provide socioeconomic support within the community. Government programs include the SNAP/Food Stamp Program, Emergency Food Assistance Program, and community food banks and meals. The new recommended name for the Food Stamp Program is Supplemental Nutrition Assistance Program (SNAP), which provides coupons toward the purchase of foods for people with low incomes. By boosting food purchasing power, overall nutrient intake is improved. This program is administered nationally by the U.S. Department of Agriculture (USDA) and on the state and local levels by welfare or human services agencies. The federal government pays the actual food assistance costs; administration costs are divided among the other agencies.

As an entitlement program, SNAP is available to all who are eligible without restriction of age or family size. Financial and nonfinancial factors of households are considered to determine eligibility. Financial factors include income and economic resources such as savings or vehicles; nonfinancial considerations consist of a variety of factors such as social security eligibility, citizenship, and work requirements. Gross incomes must meet certain percentages of the poverty level based on overall factors; the level of support varies based on family membership and net income.[11]

The Food and Nutrition Service of the USDA administers The Emergency Food Assistance Program (TEFAP). Various local agencies may administer the program. State agencies determine their own criteria for eligibility based on household income. The program serves two functions: to reduce government-held surplus dairy commodities and to supplement the dietary intake of low-income households through the distribution of basic commodities. The types of foods distributed vary between actual surplus foods and foods purchased especially for this program. In addition to dairy products of nonfat dry milk and cheese, TEFAP has distributed canned meat, peanut butter, citrus juices, legumes, dried potatoes, and canned and dried fruit. Some of this program's funds are used by states to fund emergency feeding programs such as soup kitchens or food banks.[11]

Community food banks and emergency feeding programs may be partially funded by TEFAP in addition to support by foundations and other charitable organizations (Figure 13-7). Some programs also collect food from the surrounding community and surplus donations from supermarkets and restaurants. Personnel at these facilities are usually volunteers from youth groups, religious organizations, and civic associations. Food banks often provide a bag of food staples to help bridge the gap that may occur when food stamps and monthly welfare support are exhausted before the beginning of the next month. Emergency feeding programs such as soup kitchens may provide hot meals as a safety net to assist individuals among lower socioeconomic populations to avoid malnutrition.[11]

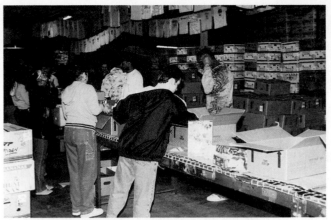

FIG 13-7 FoodBank volunteers sorting foods. (Courtesy Community FoodBank of New Jersey, Hillside, N.J.)

Supports specifically for older adults include the Child and Adult Care Food Program and the Senior Nutrition Program. Community groups may sponsor some of the government programs or may develop their own local programs.[11]

The Child and Adult Care Food Program provides meals and snacks for children up to age 12 and to senior citizens and specific categories of handicapped people participating in daycare programs that are nonprofit, licensed, or receive agency approval. Reimbursement rates differ for programs that serve children and adults. Family income of the participants may be considered. Similar to other programs, it is administered on the federal level by the Food and Nutrition Service of the USDA and on the state level by human services or education departments. Adult daycare programs may be administered locally by a variety of community sponsors. For children, eligible programs include Head Start, after-school programs, family daycare, and other approved sites.[11]

The Senior Nutrition Program serves only older adults and was created to offer inexpensive meals, education, and socialization. The Congregate Meals Program and Home-Delivered Meals Program are both part of the Senior Nutrition Program. This program provides for those in financial need as well as for those in social need. Eligibility is open to everyone aged 60 years or older; spouses of participants may also be served regardless of their age. To participate in the Home-Delivered Meals Program, individuals must reside in the program service area and be unable to prepare their own meals. Meals are generally provided Monday through Friday. Those receiving meals at home may also be given frozen meals for weekend consumption.[11] Distribution of meals varies among programs.

OVERCOMING BARRIERS

Food Asphyxiation

Older adults may be at risk for asphyxiation of food because of reduced chewing ability from loss of teeth or poorly fitting dentures. Neurologic conditions such as Parkinson's disease and effects of stroke may result in chewing and swallowing difficulties (dysphagia) that may cause asphyxiation. Counseling older adults about problematic foods may avert asphyxiation. Referrals to a registered dietitian with expertise in these disorders should be considered.

Stress

Stress can affect all aspects of well-being. Although the actual cause of stress may not be related to dietary intake and meal patterns, nutrient intake may be altered. The *normal* stressors of contemporary life may lead individuals to be so busy that they forget to eat or do not make appropriate food selections, particularly for breakfast and lunch. Some may overeat to soothe their nerves, and others may lose their appetite entirely. If these actions become habitual, inappropriate eating patterns reduce the ability to cope with stressors.

Other impediments may occur. Stress may lead the gastrointestinal tract to produce excessive gastric juices. The resulting indigestion may lead to the development of peptic ulcers. The anxiety of stress could also cause loss of appetite, which further reduces nutrient intake and can affect the absorption of nutrients, including minerals, protein, and vitamin C. Emotional stress increases the release of some hormones such as adrenaline, which has a role in the breakdown of bone tissue during bone remodeling. Excess production of adrenaline in response to repetitive stressors affects bone health and is a risk factor for osteoporosis. The stressors of everyday life may occasionally cause an increase of urinary nitrogen output; however, the amount is not significant. Extreme levels of stress caused by environmental or physiologic factors can substantially increase nitrogen loss, requiring therapeutic intervention; these interventions are detailed in Chapter 15.

Women's Health Issues

Adult women must take responsibility for their own nutritional intake, but most often they are also the caregivers and food and nutrition gatekeepers who influence the nutritional status of multiple generations within their families. Consequently, health promotion activities, services, and other medical/educational efforts should support women to adopt appropriate nutritional approaches to achieve health and wellness. The diseases for which women are most at risk include osteoporosis, coronary artery disease, hypertension, cerebrovascular disease, certain cancers, diabetes, and weight-related disorders.[12] These health problems are more common among minority women, who are more at risk for these chronic diseases. Their access to preventive and medical care may be limited by greater incidence of poverty and other socioeconomic factors that further impair their health status.[12]Although these disorders are discussed in detail throughout this book, specific concerns for women regarding breast cancer and related issues are presented here.

Cancer

About one third of cancer mortality may be due to dietary or nutritional influences such as energy intake or body weight.

Risk factors are different among the varied forms of cancer. The three top cancers among North American females are cancers of the breast, lung and bronchus, and colon and rectum. Because cancer is the second leading cause of death in North America, guiding clients to follow dietary recommendations to reduce cancer risk is important.[12]

The role of diet in the development of cancer has not been uncovered to the extent that the relationship between diet and other diseases such as coronary artery disease (CAD) has. It is expected that diet-gene interactions and other discoveries will result in biomarkers for cancer as presently exist for CAD with cholesterol. Studies exploring areas of nutrient and cancer associations are ongoing and will influence the dietary guidelines of the American Cancer Society and the World Cancer Research Fund/American Institute for Cancer. Presently these dietary recommendations promote plant-based diets that emphasize minimally processed foods. Recommended corollary lifestyle behaviors include maintaining healthy weight and leading physically active lifestyles. Table 13-2 shows risk and dietary factors related to cancers of the breast, lung, colon and rectum, endometrium, cervix, and ovary.[12]

Menopause

Recommendations to increase fruits, vegetables, and grains address not only a possible reduced risk of cancer but also the increased risk for coronary artery disease for which women are more at risk after menopause. Menopause is characterized by the decreased production of estrogen and progesterone, which results in the termination of menses. For about 3 to 7 years before menopause, a range of symptoms may be experienced, including changes in menstruation, night sweats, hot flashes, insomnia, loss of bone density, and mood swings. This cluster of symptoms is called perimenopause.

Controversy continues regarding whether such symptoms should be treated with hormone replacement therapy (HRT), which often reduces the effects of perimenopause and menopause, or whether to proceed with the natural course of female physiology without the use of HRT. Decisions regarding HRT need to take into account a woman's genetic and medical history and the extent to which menopausal symptoms are affecting her quality of life because of the possible increased risk of stroke and endometrial and breast cancer from HRT.

An alternative approach to menopausal symptoms is to consume foods containing phytoestrogens, particularly soy in the form of foods or isoflavone extracts, which appear to replicate some of the functions of estrogen. This function, though, is not nutritional but actually pharmacologic. Other supplements used to decrease menopausal symptoms are *Ginkgo biloba,* black cohosh, and flaxseed. Overall, the potential benefits, risks, and combination of supplements with food and/or medications remain uncertain.[12] Nutrition approaches to reduce symptoms continue to focus on quality of dietary choices and healthy weight maintenance.

An increased intake of fruits, vegetables, and whole grains—including calcium-containing foods—accompanied

TABLE 13-2	GENERAL RISK AND DIETARY FACTORS ASSOCIATED WITH CANCERS OF THE BREAST, LUNG, COLON, RECTUM, ENDOMETRIUM, CERVIX, AND OVARY

FACTORS AFFECTING ENERGY AND/OR NUTRITIONAL STATUS	CANCER					
	BREAST	LUNG	COLON/RECTUM	ENDOMETRIUM	CERVIX	OVARY
Avoidance of obesity	+ + (postmenopausal) − (premenopausal)	?	+ +	+ +	0	?
Physical activity	+ +	?	+ +	+	?	?
Dietary fat						
Total	?	?	?	?	?	−
Saturates	?	?	−	?	?	−
Monounsaturates	?	?	?	?	?	
Polyunsaturates	?	?	?	?	?	?
Trans fatty acids	?	?	−	?	?	?
n-3s	?	?	?	?	?	?
Meat/protein	?	?	− − For processed & red meats	?	?	?
Fruits and vegetables	+	+ +	+	?	+	+
Refined carbohydrate	?	?	−	?	?	?
Dietary fiber	?	?	+	?	?	?
Minerals			Calcium (+) Selenium (?)			
Vitamins			Folate (+ +)			
Alcohol	− −	?	−	?	?	?
Caffeine	0	?	?	?	?	?
Other	Breastfeeding (+ +) Soy (?)					Galactose (?)

− = Probable/possible evidence of harm (studies showing associations either are not so consistent or the number or type of studies is not extensive enough to make a definitive judgment).
? = Insufficient evidence to conclude benefit or risk.
0 = No association.
+ = Probable/possible evidence of benefit (studies showing associations are either not so consistent or the number or type of studies is not extensive enough to make a definitive judgment).
+ + Probable evidence of benefit
− − Probably evidence of harm
Modified from American Dietetic Association: Position of the American Dietetic Association and Dietitians of Canada: Nutrition and women's health, *J Am Diet Assoc* 104(6):984-1001, 2004, with permission from the American Dietetic Association.

by decreased consumption of dietary fat—especially animal-derived fat—is appropriate to provide a solid nutritional basis as women progress through the life span. This dietary pattern provides possible protection for all diet-related chronic disorders.

Men's Health Issues

Although most major health research studies have used men, particularly white men, as research subjects, the emphasis on male-only health issues is not as great as it is for female health issues, such as menopause and breast cancer. With the exception of testicular cancer and prostate cancer, other health obstacles also affect women as well as men. Consequently, the discussion on alcohol abuse has significance for women, although it has a higher incidence among men.

Alcohol

Moderate alcohol consumption is recognized as beneficial for lower risk of coronary artery disease. Although moderate is

defined as 14 drinks per week, the National Institute on Alcohol Abuse and Alcoholism guidelines recommend that older adults limit consumption to one alcohol drink per day.[13] Alcohol is the most commonly used and abused drug in the United States. Although both men and women use it, the death rate from alcohol abuse is more than twice as high for men as for women. Native Americans are most at risk for chronic alcohol ingestion problems. Alcohol abuse is severe among this group and affects the physical, mental, social, and economic well-being of many Native Americans. Excessive alcohol consumption is associated with poverty, violent crimes, birth defects, suicide, and sexual and domestic abuse. The pattern of excessive intake often begins during adolescence and continues through the adult years.[14]

Chronic consumption of large amounts of alcohol affects nutritional status. Appetite is diminished and is associated with limited nutrient absorption, metabolism, and excretion, and it further increases the effects of aging. Other medical and social problems emerge. Medical conditions include cirrhosis of the liver and cancer of the liver and gastrointestinal tract, including the mouth, pharynx, larynx, and esophagus. Social problems include impaired driving while intoxicated, which has resulted in significant mortality and morbidity. Family functioning may also be altered when excessive consumption of alcohol begins to affect an individual's ability to parent and to function in the work setting. Community resources are available to help individuals reduce their consumption of alcohol.

Prostate Cancer

Although diet-related cancers such as colon cancer are discussed under "Women's Health Issues," men are also at risk for such cancers. Prostate cancer, of course, affects men only and is most likely a result of multifactor causes including genetics, hormones, environment, virus, and diet. Prostate cancer is noted for an association with fat intake, particularly saturated fat. It appears that consumption of animal fat is most closely associated with the aggressive prostate cancer that is most lethal. As with breast and colon cancer, increased consumption of fruits, vegetables, and whole grains, which lowers intake of animal-derived saturated fat, may not only reduce risk of these cancers but also is heart healthy and may help reduce blood pressure and decrease risk of type 2 DM. Men older than age 40 should be encouraged to undergo an annual digital rectal examination or other form of prostate cancer screening because overt symptoms may not occur until the cancer is advanced. Prostate cancer is the most common cancer among American men.[15] African American men have a higher incidence rate than other Americans and should be screened regularly.[15]

Dietary approaches to prevent prostate cancer are being explored. Some studies imply that lycopene, an antioxidant naturally occurring in tomatoes and other fruits and vegetables, may reduce the risk of prostate cancer. Intervention studies in which human subjects alter their diets are needed to assess the efficacy of lycopene. Other studies report inconsistent findings as to the prevention of prostate cancer through the consumption of fruits and vegetables. Consequently, the consumption of a low-fat, plant-based diet has not been shown, as yet, to decrease the risk of prostate cancer. Nonetheless, such a diet affords other potential benefits such as decreased risk of hyperlipidemia, hypertension, and cardiovascular disease.[15]

TOWARD A POSITIVE NUTRITION LIFESTYLE: RATIONALIZING

Rationalization is one of the psychologic defense mechanisms used to protect our sense of self when we are under stress. When our behaviors, feelings, or perceptions are irrational or unreasonable, we may use rationalization to assign reasonable explanations to ourselves as to why we behaved as we did.

For example, from adolescence on through the older years, some individuals rationalize their poor eating habits. The list of reasonable explanations may include not enough time to prepare better meals, lack of knowledge of nutrition, or lack of cooking skills. Although these may be reasonable explanations, they do not help improve nutritional status. Often these types of rationalizations make it harder to change unproductive behaviors.

Consider the same explanations in a more positive way:
- Not enough time to prepare better meals but can reorganize schedule to create time.
- Lack of knowledge of nutrition or of cooking skills but can take a nutrition or cooking course or read books on nutrition and use simple cookbooks to learn basic skills.
- Instead of continuing negative rationalization, positive rationalization may provide the means to change.

SUMMARY

Aging is a gradual process that is different for each individual depending on the influence of genetics, lifestyle, and environment across the life span. Productive aging takes into account the many psychosocial influences of successful aging. Many of these factors may affect nutrient intake.

The role of nutrition in each of the adult life span categories reflects the value of adequate nutrient intake to reduce the risk of chronic disorders of osteoporosis, CAD, DM, hypertension, and obesity. During the early years (20s and 30s), establishment of positive health behaviors is desirable. These years are the childbearing and child rearing years, with health implications for both women and men. The middle years (40s and 50s) are years of career and family demands. Chronic diet-related diseases, such as type 2 DM and CAD, may occur during these years. Positive dietary and exercise behaviors may provide protection. Nutrient needs for women change as menopause occurs. In particular, adequate calcium consumption is recommended to offset loss of bone density. The older years (60s, 70s, and 80s) are most reflective of lifestyle behaviors practiced over many years. Psychosocial issues of dealing with the deaths of loved ones, adjustment to retirement, and changes in living arrangements and economic status may affect the adequacy of nutrient intake. During the older years, nutrients remain the same as in earlier years, except for vitamin D, for which the AI is increased. During the oldest years (80s and 90s) malnutrition and underweight are of concern.

A variety of techniques and community supports are available to implement health promoting objectives of these life span categories. Other barriers to health promotion during the adult years include food asphyxiation, stress, and health issues particular to women and men.

THE NURSING APPROACH

Case Studies

PART 1: YOUNG ADULT VEGAN

Julie, age 25, came to the nurse practitioner's office for an annual physical required by her employer. She stated that her health is good. She is single and has no children. Results from lab tests obtained the day before the visit included low hematocrit, low hemoglobin, and microcytic hypochromic (small pale) red blood cells.

ASSESSMENT

Subjective (from patient statements)

- "I have been a vegan for 1 year."
- "I don't use any animal products because I value animal rights."
- "My menstrual periods are regular, but the bleeding tends to be somewhat heavy."
- "I have been a little tired lately, but I have been very busy, and I exercise hard."
- "I haven't been taking vitamins. I don't think they are necessary."

Objective (from physical examination and lab results)

- 5 feet 6 inches tall, weighs 120 pounds
- Skin and conjunctivae appear pale.
- Low hemoglobin, microcytic hypochromic red blood cells

DIAGNOSIS (NURSING)

Imbalanced nutrition: less than body requirements related to vegan diet and "somewhat heavy" menstruation as evidenced by low hemoglobin and microcytic hypochromic red blood cells, "I have been a little tired lately," pale skin and conjunctivae, 92% ideal body weight.

PLANNING

Patient Outcomes

Short term (at the end of this visit):

- Julie will identify food sources to correct common problems in a vegan diet.
- She will state her intention to take a vitamin/mineral supplement daily.

Long term (follow-up visit after one month):

- Lab results for hematocrit, hemoglobin, and red blood cells will be closer to normal.
- Julie's weight will be stable, and she will state that she has more energy.

Nursing Interventions

1. Assess Julie's usual dietary intake and knowledge of healthy balance in a vegan diet.
2. Discuss possible nutritional problems with a vegan diet and how to correct them.
3. Prescribe multiple vitamins with iron and other minerals.

IMPLEMENTATION (Also see Chapter 6.)

1. Asked Julie to recall everything she ate or drank yesterday and then to compare those foods to her usual eating.
   A diet recall is an effective tool for assessing a patient's diet.
2. Notified Julie that lab tests showed anemia, and explained possible causes.
   Loss of blood from menstruation can reduce hematocrit and hemoglobin and iron. Vegan diets may lack iron, vitamin B_{12}, and folate, all necessary for production of red blood cells.

3. Conducted a physical exam and ordered a transferrin lab test. Informed Julie that she would receive a follow-up phone call and possibly a prescription for iron tablets.
   Red blood cells that are microcytic and microchromic usually indicate iron deficiency anemia. Transferrin levels will be low when a deficiency of iron results from blood loss and/or inadequate dietary intake of iron. The nurse practitioner can prescribe ferrous sulfate to restore adequate iron reserves.
4. Discussed food sources of iron.
   Nonheme iron (from plants) is found in vegetables, legumes, dried fruits, whole grain cereals, and fortified dry cereals. Nonheme iron is not absorbed as readily as heme iron (from animals), but absorption of iron may be increased by eating foods containing ascorbic acid (vitamin C) in the same meal. Tea and coffee contain tannins that bind the iron and thus reduce absorption.
5. Discussed food sources of vitamin B_{12} and folate, adding that folate is important for all women of childbearing age to prevent spinal bifida in early stages of fetal development.
   Vitamin B_{12} is found in nature only in animal sources. Fortified foods (some soy drinks and cereals) and vitamin supplements may contain vitamin B_{12}. Folate is widely available in foods, especially leafy green vegetables, legumes, breakfast cereals, and some fruits and juices.
6. Prescribed multivitamin tablets with iron and other minerals, and recommended taking one each day with orange juice.
   Daily supplements may provide missing or insufficient nutrients in the diet, such as iron and vitamin B_{12}. Orange juice contains ascorbic acid (vitamin C), which increases absorption of iron.
7. Encouraged Julie to get sufficient vitamin D and calcium.
   Adequate vitamin D and calcium (and exercise) are needed to prevent osteoporosis. The most common source of vitamin D and calcium is milk, but dairy products are not included in a vegan diet. Some synthesis of vitamin D occurs in the presence of sunshine. Some foods (breads, cereals, orange juice, and soy milk) may be fortified with calcium. Tofu, lentils, and broccoli are good sources of calcium. Spinach and tea contain binders of calcium (oxalic acid in both, and also tannins in tea), reducing absorption of calcium.
8. Discussed the importance of getting sufficient calories and quality protein from foods.
   Sufficient calories are needed to prevent protein catabolism. Animal sources of protein contain all essential amino acids and thus are complete proteins. Only one plant source (soy milk) contains all essential amino acids. When used alone, individual grains, beans, and nuts are incomplete in essential amino acids. However, when a variety of beans, nuts, and grains are eaten, amino acids become complete and balanced.
9. Asked Julie to set up a return appointment for a one-month follow-up visit.
   Follow-up is important to evaluate success of treatments and to further explore causes for blood loss if indicated.

Continued

THE NURSING APPROACH—cont'd

Case Studies—cont'd

EVALUATION

Short term (at the end of the first visit):

- Julie identified several sources of iron, folate, calcium, and vitamins B$_{12}$, and D.
- She stated the importance of getting a variety of plant proteins and sufficient calories.
- She stated her intention to take a multivitamin tablet (with minerals) with orange juice on a daily basis.
- She set up an appointment for follow-up in one month.
- Goals met.

DISCUSSION QUESTIONS

1. At the follow-up visit, the nurse may decide to encourage Julie to add eggs and dairy products to her diet. What additional nutrients would be obtained from these foods?
2. If Julie had children, she might ask them to be vegans. Would this be a good diet for the whole family?

PART 2: A GERIATRIC ASSESSMENT PROGRAM

Health care professionals advocate keeping older adults in their homes as long as possible. Avoiding institutionalization is often the best way to maintain quality of life for older adults and to minimize expense associated with nursing homes or other institutional settings. However, older adults who live alone or with their spouses or children may still not have the highest possible quality of life if they suffer from undiagnosed mental or physical problems or if they do not receive the supportive services they need. They may benefit from an assessment of their health, functional abilities, and need for health-related or home maintenance services. Such an assessment is usually done through a local geriatric assessment program sponsored by a hospital or community agency.

A family member or primary care provider acting on behalf of older adults usually makes the contact with a geriatric assessment team individual. The assessment team is composed, in most instances, of a physician or primary health care provider who is a geriatrician, a nurse practitioner, a registered dietitian, and a social worker. The team members visit the person in the place of residence and do a complete health assessment, including nutritional assessment, an assessment of ADLs, and an evaluation of the physical surroundings and the social support available to the individual.

An example of how this system works is as follows. An older woman lives alone and her family is concerned that she does not adequately care for herself and that there might be safety hazards. Maybe the woman needs to see a medical specialist or needs physical therapy, or she may be depressed and need medication. The team may discover that this client does not eat a balanced diet or does not take in a sufficient quantity of food. She may have significant functional limitations in ADLs, making it impossible for her to cook or to shop for groceries often enough to get fresh vegetables, fruit, and milk.

After this thorough assessment is completed, which may take several hours; a written plan is developed for the client and perhaps for the family. In relation to nutrition, the plan may include teaching the client about the need to change her diet or may involve contacting the Home-Delivered Meals Program or providing a community volunteers who can shop for groceries for this older adult. An alternative recommendation might be to hire a home health aide who would cook at least one meal per day for the client.

This type of assessment and planning service is invaluable to many older adults in the community. They and their families know they need help, but they often don't know what they need until they consult health professionals. A geriatric assessment program provides an integrated approach to meeting all of the identified unmet needs in this population and may result in a healthier and happier aging process.

🔍 APPLYING CONTENT KNOWLEDGE

Jennifer and Peter are in their late 40s. Recently Peter was diagnosed with high blood cholesterol levels. His doctor told him to cut down on fats and cholesterol, but he is confused about what to order at the daily business lunches he must attend. Jennifer has noticed that she is starting to put on weight and wonders if it has to do with perimenopause or if she is just eating more than usual. In addition, Jennifer's mother has just moved in with them because she could no longer afford her own home. Jennifer is concerned because her mother seems to eat little during the day. Her mother is alone all day because Jennifer and Peter work. What advice might you give to this family?

WEBSITES OF INTEREST

American Optometric Association

http://www.aoa.org/nutrition.xml

Explores the relationship of diet and nutrition to eye health through the life span.

Office of Minority Health and Health Disparities (OMHD)

http://www.cdc.gov/omhd

Aims to eradicate health disparities for vulnerable and at-risk populations and to maximize the health impact of the Centers for Disease Control and Prevention (CDC) on the U.S. population.

National Women's Health Information Center

http://www.womenshealth.gov/

Functions as a single point-of-entry for federal and private sector sources on women's health issues; created by the Office on Women's Health, Department of Health and Human Services.

REFERENCES

1. Kerschner H, Pegues JM: Productive aging: A quality of life agenda, *J Am Diet Assoc* 98(12):1445-1448, 1998.
2. Centers for Disease Control and Prevention (CDC): *Prevalence and trends data, behavioral risk factor surveillance system survey data*, Atlanta, 2007, U.S. Department of Health and Human Services. Accessed April 4, 2010, from http://apps.nccd.cdc.gov/BRFSS.
3. Liu CJ, Latham NK: Progressive resistance strength training for improving physical function in older adults, *Cochrane Database Syst Rev*, 2009 (3). *Cochrane AN*: CD002759 *Date of Electronic Publication*: 2009 Jul 18.
4. Chernoff R: Dietary management for older subjects with obesity, *Clin Geriatr Med* 21(4):725-733, 2005.
5. Chernoff R: Protein and older adults, *J Am Coll Nutr* 23(6 Suppl):627S-630S, 2004.
6. Chernoff R: Micronutrient requirements in older women, *Am J Clin Nutr* 81(5):1240S-1245S, 2005.
7. Position of the American Dietetic Association: Liberalization of the diet prescription improves quality of life for older adults in longer term care, *J Am Diet Assoc* 105:1955-1965, 2005.
8. Position of the American Dietetic Association: Nutrition across the spectrum of aging, *J Am Diet Assoc* 105(4):616-633, 2005.
9. Millen BE, et al: The elderly nutrition program: An effective national framework for preventive nutrition interventions, *J Am Diet Assoc* 102(2):234-240, 2002.
10. U.S. Department of Health and Human Services: *Healthy People 2010: Understanding and improving health*, ed 2, Washington, DC, 2000, U.S. Government Printing Office. Accessed April 6, 2010, from www.health.gov/healthypeople.
11. Food Research and Action Center: *Federal food programs*, Washington, DC, [undated], Author. Accessed April 6, 2010, from www.frac.org/federal-foodnutrition-programs/.
12. Position of the American Dietetic Association and Dietitians of Canada: Nutrition and women's health, *J Am Diet Assoc* 104(6):984-1001, 2004.
13. Mukamal KJ, et al: Alcohol consumption and risk of coronary heart disease in older adults: The Cardiovascular Health Study, *J Am Geriatr Soc* 54(1):30-37, 2006.
14. Galvan FH, Caetano R: *Alcohol use and related problems among ethnic minorities in the United States*, December 2003, National Institute on Alcohol Abuse and Alcoholism (NIAAA), Accessed April 6, 2010, from http://pubs.niaaa.nih.gov/publications/arh27-1/87-94.htm.
15. National Cancer Institute: *Prostate cancer prevention*, Author. Accessed April 6, 2010, from www.cancer.gov/cancertopics/pdq/prevention/prostate/healthprofessional.

PART 4

Overview of Nutrition Therapy

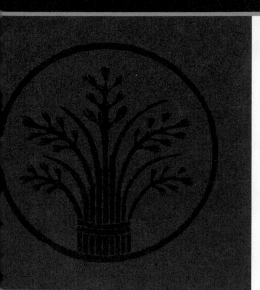

Nutrition in Patient Care

During these trying times for patients and staff alike, food becomes very important, both physiologically and psychologically, to patients because it is often one of the few familiar experiences patients encounter in a hospital.

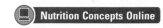

Nutrition Concepts Online

evolve WEBSITE
http://evolve.elsevier.com/Grodner/foundations/

ROLE IN WELLNESS

The first three parts of this text discuss basic nutrition as it relates to wellness. Part 4, "Overview of Medical Nutrition Therapy," provides information for nursing professionals on how nutrition pertains to the physiologic stresses of disease states.

Although Hippocrates made the link between nutrition and disease almost 3000 years ago, the modern medical community has just recently made the same discovery. The tremendous advances of medical technology are fundamentally important if the recipient is malnourished or is at nutritional risk. Nutritional risk is the potential to become malnourished because of primary (inadequate intake of nutrients) or secondary (caused by disease or iatrogenic affects) factors. Capacity for recovery from illness or disease depends on nutritional status. Poor nutritional status delays or prevents recovery, whereas good nutritional status promotes healing and recovery. It is therefore important to determine the nutritional status of those undergoing medical treatment or cure.

Sometimes dietary modifications are required to allow the body to heal, adjust to physical disability, prepare for diagnostic tests, or prepare for surgical procedures. Nutrition therapy may involve changes in dietary intake to liquefied or pureed foods, tube feeding, or intravenous (IV) nourishment. This chapter discusses promotion of wellness through typical progressive hospital diets, enteral formulas, and parenteral nutrition.

Because wellness is the goal of caring for patients, the physical, intellectual, social, emotional, and spiritual dimensions of health are applicable to the issues of this chapter. The *physical health* dimension is affected because dietary alterations may affect overall nutritional status; careful nursing supervision can ensure adequate nutrient intake. The *intellectual*

dimension is tested because nurses and caregivers are in the tricky position of observing patient eating patterns and then assessing whether problems are caused by illness or food availability. Nurses need the intellectual skills to determine when to alert the clinical dietitian. The *emotional health* dimension can be challenged if the loss of symbolic foods, particularly if modifications are long term or permanent, stresses emotional health. Nurses can be sensitive to this aspect of dietary modification and help patients to create new symbols to replace the old. The *social health* dimension may be altered when patients are served meals in their rooms. Feelings of isolation may deprive mealtimes of their function of social relatedness. The *spiritual health* dimension is affected because some foods have spiritual or religious significance to individuals, such as bread and wine used for Communion or matzoh used during the Jewish holiday of Passover. When such foods are not permitted because of enteral problems, individuals should consult their spiritual or religious advisors.

NUTRITION AND ILLNESS

Nurses are usually the first health care workers with whom the hospitalized patient comes into contact. By using information from nursing assessments, they are in a good position to identify patients in need of nutritional services. Furthermore, hospital size or staffing may necessitate nursing staff to perform some basic nutrition screening, nutrition assessment, and nutrition education.

When more in-depth knowledge of aspects of nutritional care beyond basic nutrition interventions are needed; this care is provided by registered dietitians (RDs). They conduct nutritional assessments, provide nutrition therapy, and serve as a valuable resource for the nursing staff. Nutrition therapy (also called *medical nutrition therapy*) is the provision of

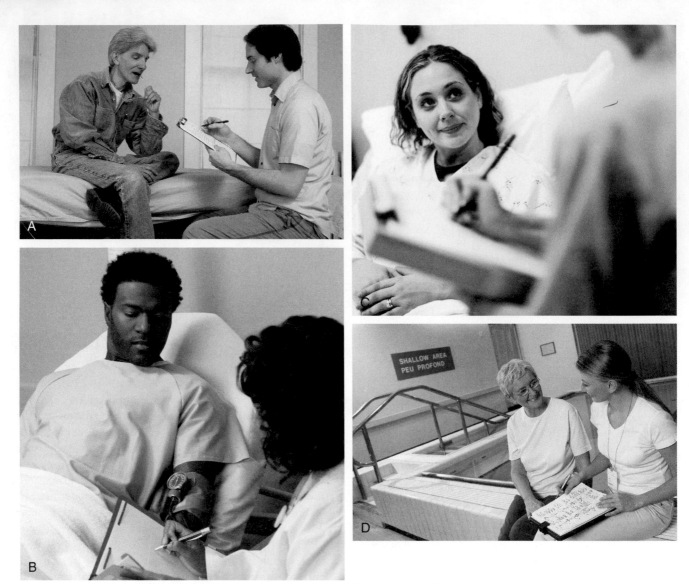

FIG 14-1 A-D, Patients are interviewed by many health care professionals.

nutrient, dietary, and nutrition education needs based on a comprehensive nutritional assessment to treat an illness, injury or condition. Occasionally, RDs may be assisted by dietetic technicians when taking diet histories, collecting information for nutritional screenings and assessments, and working directly with patients who are having problems with foods.

Modern health care settings—acute care hospitals—can play havoc with patients' nutritional status. During their hospitalization, patients admitted in good nutritional status encounter several elements—psychologic and physiologic—that can potentially put them at nutritional risk. If patients are admitted in compromised nutrition status, as many are, risks are even greater and of more consequence.

Hospital Setting

Imagine you have been taken to a place where, after answering a multitude of questions about your insurance, financial status, and **durable power of attorney** (a legal document in which a competent adult authorizes another competent adult

to make decisions for him/her in the event of incapacitation), you are whisked off to a sterile-looking room that you must share with a stranger. In this room your clothes are replaced with a thin, flimsy gown that won't close in the back. You answer more questions about your medical history from the nurse who admits you. Once he or she finishes, a resident/intern comes into your room to ask many of the same questions and conduct a physical examination (Figure 14-1).

During a stay in the hospital, your eating habits are open to scrutiny, possibly provoking guilty feelings. You're away from your own refrigerator, and meals are served on a schedule that may or may not coincide with your personal meal schedule. Although the food is prepared with the utmost care, it will be different from home cooking (just like any food eaten away from home). Depending on your diagnosis, the food is likely to be modified in texture, consistency, nutrients, or energy. When you're waiting for meals to be served (you still haven't gotten used to eating in bed), different hospital staff routinely enter your room to ask more questions, draw

Sharing an Orange

Machines were whirling as I entered the cardiac intensive care unit to visit my husband Lenny's grandmother. I didn't know what to expect. Grandma Ethel was the most energetic older adult I ever knew. Eighty-six years old, still running her own gift shop, and always ready to go out with Lenny and me, until she had this heart attack.

Grandma Ethel was sitting upright in a chair with all kinds of wires attached to her body. She was pale but immediately her radiant smile spread across her face. She said, "Come and sit, have lunch with me," as she invited me to share the hospital lunch that was on a tray in front of her. Now I certainly wasn't going to eat any of her lunch, especially hospital food. But I was definitely needed. She wanted the soup, but with the wires and being somewhat weak, couldn't get the lid off the Styrofoam cup. So I came to the rescue. Uncover the lid from the plate of soft chicken and mashed potatoes? Again I was handy. Open the juice container and decaffeinated coffee cup? Who knew I was so competent?

"Michele, here have the orange." The orange was in a bowl surrounded by plastic wrap. I gently suggested she should have it because it was good for her. "No, I'm too full. Take it home . . . take it home for the boys [my sons; her great-grandsons] and take the brownie too!" I then realized that the real issue was not to feed Grandma Ethel's body, but to let her soul feed us. Her soul needed to nourish us with her gift of a sweet orange and a rich brownie. And we were nourished.

Michele Grodner
Montclair, N.J.

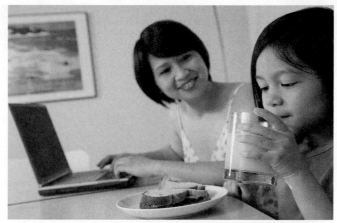

FIG 14-2 Food provides emotional comfort as well as nutrition, especially for children. (Photo.com.)

blood, take you elsewhere in the hospital for tests that may or may not be invasive, and ask you about your elimination habits and what you have eliminated, if anything.

Many patients who enter hospitals are miles away from their homes, family, and friends. Although no malfeasance is intended, little privacy is afforded hospital patients while they undergo tests and examinations that may provide them with critical information regarding their prognosis or life expectancy. During these trying times for patients and staff alike, food becomes very important, physiologically and psychologically, to patients because it is often one of the few familiar experiences encountered in a hospital setting (see the *Personal Perspectives* box, Sharing an Orange).

Particularly with hospitalized toddlers and adolescents, food can become a battleground because of its emotional connotations (Figure 14-2). As you will see in this chapter and those following, food or alternative nourishment can mean the difference between a good or poor prognosis for many patients' morbidity or mortality (see the *Cultural Considerations* box, Asking the Right Questions for Cultural Competence).

Bed Rest

Occasionally, complete bed rest is prescribed as part of patients' medical care, or patients may be unable to ambulate

because of the severity of their illness or because they are "hooked up" to a multitude of necessary life-saving equipment at bedside. Although it is often necessary or unavoidable, complete bed rest can cause injurious effects on a patient's body.[1] Skin integrity may be compromised after just 24 hours of immobilization, and after 3 days of lying supine in bed, muscle tone, bone calcium, plasma volume, and gastric secretions diminish. In addition, glucose intolerance and shifts in body fluids and electrolytes may also occur. Nursing personnel can provide care that may help prevent or delay injurious effects of bed rest by frequently turning patients and stimulating the skin and underlying muscles by providing skin care (e.g., applying skin lotion) and passive exercises for the extremities, respectively.

Malnutrition

Many patients admitted to hospitals are at nutritional risk, whereas other may develop malnutrition during their hospitalization.[2] These patients may be experiencing hypermetabolism or have physiologic stress from injury or illness that increases nutritional needs, further increasing nutritional risk. Additionally, nutritional needs may be further compromised because of, for example, periodic need for an empty gut for laboratory testing or diagnostic procedures. Likely problems may develop from hospital routine causing inadequate nourishment in some cases, including the following:[3]

- Highly restricted (nutritionally incomplete) diets remaining on order or unsupplemented too long
- Unserved meals due to interference of medical procedures and clinical tests
- Unmonitored patient appetite

Each ill or injured patient is a unique person and needs individual treatment and care.[3] Nursing personnel can be a fundamental factor in prevention of malnutrition by paying particular attention to patients' diet orders, recognizing potential risk when patients have had nothing but clear or full-liquid diets for more than 24 hours, and contacting the RD to evaluate patients' nutritional risk.

🌐 CULTURAL CONSIDERATIONS
Asking the Right Questions for Cultural Competence

Health care professionals strive for cultural competence when providing care to patients in a variety of health care settings. By doing so, they provide truly comprehensive health care. Cultural competence involves understanding the attitudes and knowledge of each cultural group in relation to how foods protect health and maintain wellness.

It is difficult to know all of the specific cultural food practices of diverse groups in North America. The use of the Cultural Nutritional Assessment Guide, presented here, is essential as part of a patient's health history. The information obtained from the patient or family member by health care professionals ensures cultural competent practice.

Cultural Nutritional Assessment Guide
- What nutritional factors are influenced by the client's cultural background? What is the meaning of food and eating to the client?
- With whom does the client usually eat? What types of foods are eaten? What is the timing and sequencing of meals?
- What does the client define as food? What does the client believe comprises a "healthy" versus an "unhealthy" diet?

- Who shops for food? Where are groceries purchased (e.g., special markets or ethnic grocery stores)? Who prepares the client's meals?
- How are foods prepared at home—type of food preparation, cooking oils used, length of time foods are cooked (especially vegetables), amount and type of seasonings added to various foods during preparation?
- Has the client chosen a particular nutritional practice such as vegetarianism or abstinence from alcohol or fermented beverages?
- Do religious beliefs and practices influence the client's diet (e.g., type, amount, preparation, or delineation of acceptable food combinations [e.g., kosher diets])? Does the client abstain from certain foods at regular intervals, on specific dates determined by the religious calendar, or at other times?

If the client's religion mandates or encourages fasting, what does the term *fast* mean (e.g., refraining from certain types or quantities of foods, eating only during certain times of the day)? For what period of time is the client expected to fast?
- During fasting, does the client refrain from liquids/beverages? Does the religion allow exemption from fasting during illness? If so, does the client believe that an exemption applies to him or her?

Cultural Nutritional Assessment Guide from Andrews M, Boyle J: *Transcultural concepts in nursing care,* ed 4, Philadelphia, 2002, Lippincott Williams & Wilkins.

NUTRITION INTERVENTION

The tremendous advances of medical technology are fundamentally unimportant if the recipient is malnourished or is at nutritional risk. Most patients entering the health care system are prone to have nutrition problems and will have special nutritional needs depending on their injury or illness. Patients at nutritional risk need to be identified so high-quality nutrition care can be provided.[4] Poor nutritional status may lead to complications that may lead to increased morbidity and mortality, length of stay, and cost of care.[5] For nutrition intervention to be efficacious and successful, a systematic, logical strategy is necessary. The nutritional care process provides such an approach (Box 14-1).

Screening

In long-term care, assessments must be completed on all residents within 14 days of admission. The Joint Commission (TJC) requires all patients admitted to a hospital to be screened within 48 hours of admission.[6] "Nutrition screening is the process of identifying characteristics known to be associated with nutrition problems."[7] It is not possible, or necessary, to complete a full nutrition assessment on every patient. It is necessary, however, to have a system in place to quickly identify patients at risk for nutritional problems, such as malnutrition.[7]

Nutrition screening can be executed by registered dietitians, dietetic technicians, dietary managers, nurses, physicians, or other trained personnel. Whether or not RDs are engaged in performing nutrition screening, they are responsible for providing input into development of suitable screening parameters to make certain the screening process addresses the correct parameters.[7] The nutrition screening process has the following characteristics:[8]
- It may be completed in any setting.
- It facilitates completion of early intervention goals.
- It includes collection of relevant data on risk factors and interpretation of data for intervention/treatment.
- It helps determine the need for a nutrition assessment.
- It is cost effective.

A referral process may be necessary to ensure a patient is referred to an RD, who will conduct the nutrition assessment, make nutritional diagnoses, and provide nutrition care.

Nutritional Assessment

The nutritional care process is often performed during a comprehensive nutritional assessment conducted by dietetic professionals, who work synergistically with nursing personnel to provide this essential component in medical care. A comprehensive nutritional assessment is a procedure conducted by dietetic professionals to determine appropriate medical nutrition therapy based on identified needs of the patient. This process uses data collected from several

BOX 14-1 AMERICAN DIETETIC ASSOCIATION'S NUTRITION CARE PROCESS

Definition of the American Dietetic Association's Nutrition Care Process (NCP)

Providing nutrition care employing the American Dietetic Associations's (ADA's) NCP starts when a patient is recognized as being at nutritional risk and requiring additional support to attain or maintain positive nutritional status. The NCP is defined "as a systematic problem-solving method that dietetics professionals use to critically think and make decisions to address nutrition-related problems and provide safe and effective quality nutrition care." It is composed of the following four separate but interrelated and associated steps:

1. Nutrition assessment
2. Nutrition diagnosis
3. Nutrition intervention
4. Nutrition monitoring and evaluation

Each stage builds upon the preceding one, but the process is not necessarily linear. Figure 14-3 provides a visual illustration of the model.

Step 1: Nutrition Assessment

Techniques such as those outlined previously in the chapter are used to systematically obtain information necessary to deter-

mine or reassess whether a nutrition problem (or diagnosis) exists. If so, the problem is diagnosed using a PES (problem, etiology, signs/symptoms) statement in Step 2 of the NCP.

Step 2: Nutrition Diagnosis

Before nutrition intervention can take place, the nutrition problem(s) must be identified. This is accomplished with the nutrition diagnosis. Standardized language has been developed to make the nutrition diagnosis clear to other nutrition and health care professionals. When the nutrition problem has been identified, it is labeled with a specific, standardized diagnostic term. The nutrition diagnosis statement or PES statement is organized in three distinct parts: the problem (P), etiology of the problem (E), and signs and symptoms associated with the problem (S). Typically nutrition diagnoses fall into three categories or domains: intake, clinical, and behavioral-environmental.

Here is an example of how a nutrition diagnosis is written:

Disordered eating pattern related to harmful belief about food and nutrition as evidenced by reported use of laxatives after meals and statements that calories are not absorbed when laxatives are used.

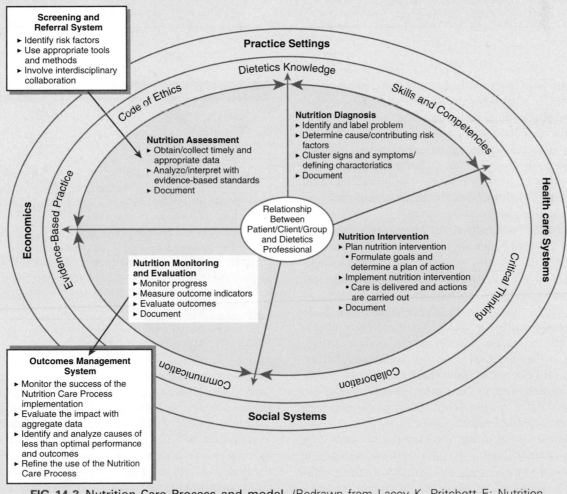

FIG 14-3 Nutrition Care Process and model. (Redrawn from Lacey K, Pritchett E: Nutrition Care Process and model: ADA adopts road map to quality care and outcomes management, *J Am Diet Assoc* 103(8):1062, 2003, with permission from the American Dietetic Association.)

Continued

| BOX 14-1 | AMERICAN DIETETIC ASSOCIATION'S NUTRITION CARE PROCESS—cont'd |

Step 3: Nutrition Intervention

Intervention begins once the nutritional diagnosis is identified. It is generally aimed at the etiology (E) of the nutrition diagnosis and is directed at reducing or eradicating effects of the signs and symptoms (S). Nutrition interventions are intended to modify a nutrition-related problem, and are comprised of two interconnected components: planning and implementation. Nutrition diagnoses are prioritized in the planning component, whereby implementation is the "action phase." The plan is communicated and carried out, data continued to be collected, and the nutrition intervention is revised as necessary. Four categories or domains of nutrition intervention have been identified:

- Food and/or nutrient delivery
- Nutrition education
- Nutrition counseling
- Coordination of care

Step 4: Nutrition Monitoring and Evaluation

The point of the nutrition monitoring and evaluation step in the NCP is to measure improvement made by the patient in meeting nutrition care goals. Patients' progress is examined by determining if the nutrition intervention is being executed and by providing evidence that the intervention is/is not altering the patients' nutritional status. Nutrition monitoring and evaluation terms are organized into four categories or domains:

- Food/nutrition-related history
- Biochemical data, medical tests, and procedures
- Anthropometric measurements
- Nutrition-focused physical findings

In summary, the Nutrition Care Process allows for continuous monitoring and evaluation of the patient. As the condition of the patient changes, plans or interventions change, and diagnoses and/or interventions change. Or if the patient does not respond to interventions, new interventions can be developed. Additionally, any/all nutrition interventions should be planned along with patients and/or their caregivers or significant others. For more detailed information regarding the Nutrition Care Process, please refer to the following references.

References

American Dietetic Association: *International dietetics and nutrition terminology (IDNT) reference manual. Standardized language for the nutrition care process*, ed 2, Chicago, 2009, American Dietetic Association.

Lacey K, Pritchitt E: Nutrition Care Process and model: ADA adopts road map to quality care and outcomes management, J Am Diet Assoc 103(8):1061-1072, 2003.

---

different sources to assess patients' nutritional needs, often using the ABCD approach: **A**nthropometrics, **B**iochemical tests, **C**linical observations, and **D**iet evaluation. Each part of this process is important because there is no one parameter that directly measures nutritional status or determines nutritional problems or needs. Thus a combination of these parameters must be used to interpret the overall nutrition picture presented by patients within the context of their personal, social, and economic backgrounds.*

Anthropometric assessment. Anthropometric measurements are determined by simple, noninvasive techniques that measure height and weight, the head, and skinfold thicknesses. Effectiveness of single anthropometric measurements is limited, but certain serial measurements can be useful to assess body composition changes or growth over time. Standardized techniques must be used to obtain valid and reliable measurements. Evaluation of anthropometric data involves comparison of data collected with predetermined reference limits or cutoff points that allow classification into one or more risk categories and, in some cases, identification of the type and severity of malnutrition.[9] Discussion of various anthropometric measurements follows.

Height. Stature (height/length) is important in evaluating growth and nutritional status in children. In adults, height is needed for assessment of weight and body size. Height should

---

| BOX 14-2 | MEASURING HEIGHT |

1. Have patient stand erect with weight equally distributed on both feet.
   a. If the legs are of unequal length, place boards under the short limb to make the pelvis level.
   b. When possible, make sure the head, shoulder blades, buttocks, and heels all touch the vertical surface.
   c. Instruct patient to let arms hang free at the sides with palms facing the thighs.
2. Have patient look straight ahead (so the line of vision is perpendicular to the body), take a deep breath, and hold that position while the horizontal headboard is brought down firmly on top of the head. (Measurer's eyes should be level with the headboard to read the measurement.)
3. Read the measurement to the nearest 0.1 cm or ⅛ inch.

From Lee RD, Nieman DC: *Nutritional assessment*, ed 4, New York, 2007, McGraw-Hill.

be measured using a fixed measuring stick or tape on a true vertical, flat surface with no carpeting. If this is not available, the movable measuring arm on platform clinic scales may be used with reasonable accuracy, although it tends to produce lower measures.[10] The patient should be measured standing as straight as possible, without shoes or head coverings, with the heels together, and looking straight ahead (Box 14-2).

Accurate heights are important in nutritional assessment. Many calculations used to determine energy requirements and needs are based on height and weight. Heights are not always available in the medical records of hospitalized patients. When heights are documented, it is often unclear

---

*Note that information described in the anthropometric, biochemical, clinical, and dietary assessment data is not all-encompassing. Only parameters of particular interest to nursing are discussed.

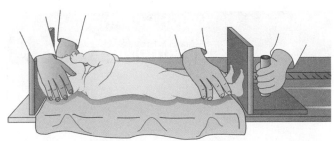

FIG 14-4 A recumbent length board used to take height measurements horizontally. (From Mahan LK, Escott-Stump S: *Krause's food & nutrition therapy*, ed 12, St. Louis, 2009, Saunders.)

BOX 14-3	MEASURING RECUMBENT BED HEIGHT

1. Remove pillows and make bed level.
2. Straighten the patient out in bed but with the feet flexed.
3. With a clipboard or ruler, extend perpendicular lines from the top of the head and the bottom of the feet out to the side of the bed.
4. Mark the two positions on the bed sheet and measure the distance between them to the nearest 0.5 cm.

Data from Gray D: Accuracy of recumbent height measurement, *JPEN J Parenter Enteral Nutr* 9:712-715, 1985.

---

whether they are reported by the patient or measured. Asking patients about their height does not always produce accurate information. On average when asked, people report being slightly taller than they actually are.[11] Men overstate height more often than women (men—0.46 in. [1.22 cm]; women—0.68 in. [0.68 cm]), and the extent of overstating height increases as people age.[11] If the height of a patient recorded in the medical record is not a measured height, it should be documented as a stated height.

When measuring infants and children (younger than 2 to 3 years) who cannot stand or others unable to stand erect without assistance, recumbent measures can be taken while the subject is lying down or reclining. A recumbent length table can be used. A recumbent length table or board has a fixed headboard, a movable footboard, and a permanent measuring tape along the side (Figure 14-4). To measure a patient, he or she should be placed supine on the board or table with shoulders and legs flat against the measuring board (table) and arms at the sides. The head should firmly touch the headboard while the line of vision is perpendicular to the board or table. Soles of the feet should be vertical, and the footboard should touch the bottom of the feet so that the soft tissue is compressed. Length can be recorded from the measure at the footboard. Two people are often needed to take an accurate measurement.[10]

When the patient is comatose, critically ill, or unable to be moved for other reasons, taking a recumbent bed height may be possible (Box 14-3).[12] Note that when compared with standing height, bed height is significantly greater by at least 2%.[12]

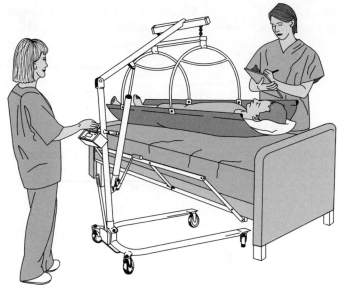

FIG 14-5 If a patient is nonambulatory, a bed scale can be used to measure patient weight.

A more accurate measurement for patients who cannot stand is knee height. Knee height is more accurate when measured in a recumbent rather than a sitting position.[13,14] This measurement is minimally affected by aging. In older adults, knee height can be measured to estimate height by using the following formulas[15]:

$$\text{Male height (cm)} = 64.19 - (0.04 \times \text{age}) \cdot [2.02 \times \text{Knee height (cm)}]$$

$$\text{Female height (cm)} = 84.88 - (0.24 \times \text{age}) \cdot [1.83 \times \text{Knee height (cm)}]$$

The special calipers necessary for measuring knee height are available from Ross Laboratories in Columbus, Ohio.

Weight. When accurately measured, body weight is a simple, gross estimate of body composition. In fact, body weight is one of the most important measurements in assessing nutritional status and is used to predict energy expenditure.[16] Beam scales with movable but nondetachable weights or accurate electronic scales are recommended to obtain accurate results. Spring scales are not recommended. If the patient is nonambulatory, wheelchair or bed scales should be used (Figure 14-5).[10] Scales should be checked for accuracy periodically and recalibrated when necessary. Like heights, actual measured weights are more accurate than patients' estimated weights because men slightly overreport their weight (men—0.66 lbs [0.30 kg]), and women report slightly less than it actually is (–3.06 lbs [–1.39 kg]).[11]

For accurate weights, patients should be clothed in their underwear or hospital gown. Weights should be measured at the same time of day and after voiding. The patient should stand still with the weight evenly distributed on both feet while weight is recorded to the nearest 0.1 kg, or 0.25 pound.[10]

As a nutritional screening tool, weights can be used to recognize changes that may be representative or suggestive of serious health problems. Magnitude and direction of weight change are more meaningful when dealing with sick or debilitated patients than standardized desirable weight references (see Table 14-1). Percent weight change is a useful nutrition index and may be computed as follows:

% Weight change = (Usual weight − Actual weight)
÷ Usual weight × 100

For example, Mrs. Welch is admitted to your unit. Her weight on admission is 120 pounds. During the admissions interview, she indicates that 3 months ago she weighed 135 pounds. Her percent weight change from usual weight is

$$(135-120) \div 135 \times 100 = 15 \div 135 \times 100$$
$$= 0.11 \times 100$$
$$= 11\% \text{ Weight change}$$

Mrs. Welch's (actual) weight is 11% less than her usual weight.

% Weight change from admission weight
= (Usual weight − Actual weight)
÷ Admission weight × 100

For example, Mr. Tucker is a patient in the long-term care facility where you work. When he was admitted more than a year ago, he weighed 180 pounds. He has weighed 170 pounds for the past 6 months, but today you weigh Mr. Tucker and he weighs 165 pounds. His percent weight change from admission weight is

$$(170-165) \div 180 \times 100 = 5 \div 180 \times 100$$
$$= 0.0278 \times 100$$
$$= 2.78\%, \text{ or } 3\% \text{ Weight change}$$

Mr. Tucker's (actual) weight is 3% less than his admission weight.

% Weight change since nutrition intervention
= (Usual weight − Actual weight)
÷ Preintervention weight × 100

For example, Mrs. Bussard was placed on a feeding tube because her weight has decreased from her usual weight of 130 pounds to 115 pounds. She has been on the feeding tube for 1 week, and when you weigh her today, she weighs 122 pounds. Her percent weight change since nutrition intervention is

$$(130-122) \div 115 \times 100 = 8 \div 115 \times 100$$
$$= 0.067 \times 100$$
$$= 6.96\%, \text{ or } 7\% \text{ Weight change}$$

Mrs. Bussard's weight has increased 7% since the tube feedings were initiated.

Care should be taken to identify patients with ascites, edema, or dehydration because their weight changes may be more a reflection of their fluid status than actual changes in body composition. If more than 1 pound is gained in a day's time, it may be indicative of excess fluid. It is also important to examine any unplanned weight loss the patient might experience, as indicated in Table 14-1. Reported or

TABLE 14-1	WEIGHT CHANGE AS AN INDICATOR OF NUTRITIONAL STATUS	
% WEIGHT CHANGE	**TIME PERIOD**	**NUTRITIONAL STATUS**
1%-2%	1 week	Moderate weight loss
>2%	1 week	Severe weight loss
5%	1 month	Moderate weight loss
>5%	1 month	Severe weight loss

measured percent weight losses of these magnitudes could be cause for alarm.

For older adult patients who cannot be weighed because of the severity of their medical condition, or if bed or chair scales are not available, Chumlea and colleagues[17] have developed gender-specific equations used to predict body weight in people 60 to 90 years of age. The estimated weights are based on recumbent measures of arm circumference (AC), calf circumference (CC), subscapular skinfold (SSF), and knee height (KH).

Women: Weight (cm) = [0.98 × AC (in cm)] + [1.27 × CC (in cm)] + [0.4 × SSF (in mm)] + [0.87 × KH (in cm)] 62.35

Men: Weight (cm) = [1.73 × AC (in cm)] + [0.98 × CC (in cm)] + [0.37 × SSF (in mm)] + [1.16 × KH (in cm)] 81.69

Another challenge in obtaining weights occurs in patients who have missing body parts because of accidents or amputation. Figure 14-6 shows the approximate percent of body weight contributed by individual body segments so desirable weight can be calculated.

Body mass index. Body mass index (BMI) is a ratio of weight to height and has been associated with overall mortality and nutritional risk.[18,19] BMI does not determine body composition (lean body mass or adipose) but is a dependable gauge of total body fat, which is interrelated with risk of disease.[20] While measurements are valid for men and women, BMI measurements do have limits:[19,20]

- BMI has not been validated in acutely ill patients
- BMI may underestimate body fat in the elderly and others who have lost muscle mass
- BMI may overestimate body fat in individuals who have a muscular build

You can determine BMI by referring to Table 10-1 or by dividing weight in kilograms by height in squared meters using the following three steps:

1. Divide weight in pounds by 2.2 to convert it into kilograms.
2. Multiply height in inches by 2.54 and divide the result by 100 to convert height to meters; then multiply height in meters by itself (that is, square it).
3. Divide weight in kilograms (result of step 1) by the square of height in meters (result of step 2). The result is BMI.

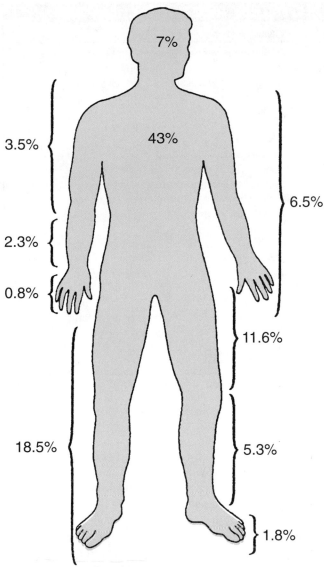

FIG 14-6 Approximate body weight percentages. (Modified from Brunnstrom S: *Clinical kinesiology,* Philadelphia, 1962, FA Davis.)

$$BMI = Weight \ (kg) \div Height \ (m)^2$$

The desired BMI range for healthy adults is 18.5 to 24.9 kg/m², which reflects a healthy weight for height. Although at low risk for health problems, people with BMIs of 25 to 29.9 kg/m² are approximately 20% above desirable levels. A BMI of less than 18.5 kg/m² is classified as underweight (Table 14-2) and is associated with risk factors such as respiratory disease, tuberculosis, digestive disease, and some cancers.[21]

Waist circumference. Waist circumference is an economical and straightforward measure that can be used to assess abdominal fat content. BMI and waist circumference highly associate obesity with risk for disease, and both should be used to classify overweight/obesity and estimate disease risk.[19,22,23] A circumference greater than 40 inches in men and 35 inches in women indicates risk for disease. It should be noted that visceral adiposity may vary among racial and ethnic groups.[22]

TABLE 14-2	CLASSIFICATIONS OF OVERWEIGHT AND OBESITY BY BODY MASS INDEX (BMI)
	BMI (kg/m²)
Underweight	<18.5
Normal	18.5-24.9
Overweight	25.0-29.9
Obesity	≥30

Biochemical assessment. Many routine blood and urine laboratory tests recorded in patients' charts are useful in providing an objective assessment of nutritional status. However, care should be taken in interpreting test results for a number of reasons. First, there is no single test available for evaluating short-term response to medical nutritional therapy. Laboratory tests should be used in conjunction with anthropometric data, clinical data, and dietary intake assessments. Second, some tests may be inappropriate for certain patients; for example, serum albumin might not be useful in the evaluation of protein status in those patients with liver failure because this test assumes normal liver function. Third, laboratory tests conducted serially will give more accurate information than a single test. Although, serial measures can be obtained in long-term care settings, patients in acute care facilities are rarely hospitalized long enough to obtain serial measures. Therefore, it might be more appropriate to compare test results with known standards.

The most important biochemical parameters are visceral protein status and immune function. Visceral protein status is assessed through tests of serum albumin and prealbumin. (**Visceral proteins** include proteins other than muscle tissue, such as internal organs and blood.) Immune function is evaluated based on total lymphocyte count (TLC). The test results of these biochemical assessments provide useful information to determine the effects of nutritional factors or of medical conditions on the health status of patients (Table 14-3).

Serum albumin. Serum albumin provides an assessment of visceral protein status. Normal values are within 3.5 to 5 g/dL. For nutritional analysis, values between 2.8 and 3.5 g/dL indicate compromised protein status; values less than 2.4 g/dL suggest possible kwashiorkor. This test is most useful when used to monitor long-term nutrition changes because normal values may still be found among patients who are recently malnourished. In addition, if patients are experiencing dehydration (hemoconcentration) or have received infusions of albumin, fresh frozen plasma, or whole-blood serum albumin, levels may appear normal. However, as a tool to assess long-term changes, the effects of dehydration and infusions would dissipate. Alternate causes of abnormally low values may be infection and other stressors (especially with poor protein intake), burns, trauma, congestive heart failure, fluid overload, and severe hepatic insufficiency.[24,25]

TABLE 14-3 BIOCHEMICAL PARAMETERS AND HOW THEY ARE TESTED

SERUM PROTEIN	FUNCTION	COMMENTS
Albumin Normal: 3.5-5.0 g/dL Depletion: 　Mild: 3.0-3.4 g/dL 　Moderate: 2.4-2.9 g/dL 　Severe: <2.4 g/dL Half-life ~ 14-20 days	Maintains plasma oncotic pressure; carrier for small molecules	Not sensitive or specific for acute protein malnutrition or response to nutrition therapy; affected by hydration status, disease state, clinical condition Can be used as prognostic indicator of morbidity, mortality, and severity of illness
Transferrin Normal: 200-400 mg/dL Depletion: 　Mild: 150-200 mg/dL 　Moderate: 100-149 mg/dL 　Severe: <100 mg/dL Half-life ~ 8-10 days	Binds iron in plasma and transports to bone marrow	Inversely correlated with body's iron stores; elevated concentration often indicates early iron deficiency Will decrease during acute illness Verify with laboratory whether lab is direct measurement or calculated
Prealbumin (transthyretin, thyroxin-binding prealbumin) Normal: 16-40 mg/dL Depletion: 　Mild: 10-15 mg/dL 　Moderate: 5-9 mg/dL 　Severe: <5 mg/dL Half-life ~ 2-3 days	Carrier protein for thyroxin Combined with retinol-binding protein, transports vitamin A	Influenced less by intravascular fluid volume Not affected as early or as significantly with liver disease (compared with albumin) More likely to be a reflection of recent dietary intake than accurate indicator of nutritional status

Adapted from (compiled from components in tables and text) Moore MC: *Pocket Guide to Nutrition Assessment and Care*, ed 6, St. Louis, 2009, Mosby Elsevier; Thompson CW: Laboratory assessment. In Charney P, Malone AM, editors: *ADA Pocket Guide to Nutrition Assessment*, ed 2, Chicago, 2009, American Dietetic Association; Lee RD, Nieman DC: *Nutritional Assessment*, ed 4, Boston, 2007, McGraw Hill.

Prealbumin. Prealbumin (thyroxine-binding prealbumin) also can provide a measure of visceral protein status assessment. Normal values range from 16 to 40 mg/dL. This test is useful in monitoring short-term changes in visceral protein status because of its short half-life of 2 days. Compromised protein status is indicated when levels are between 10 and 15 g/dL. Possible kwashiorkor is a potential diagnosis when levels are less than 10 mg/dL. A nonnutritional cause of normal values despite patient malnutrition is chronic renal failure. Other factors that result in abnormally low levels of prealbumin include surgical trauma, stress, inflammation, infection, and liver dysfunction.[24,25]

Clinical assessment. Clinical assessment incorporates data from several sources: medical history, social history, and physical examination. Many environmental factors can affect nutritional status. This information can be found by reviewing the patient's medical record or through direct interview. Social or family factors may also affect nutrient intake or past or present medical conditions that influence nutrient use. Many physical signs and symptoms associated with malnutrition are also an integral part of assessing nutritional status.

Features associated with nutritional deficiency may be considered through historical and clinical categories.[24,25] Historical findings may include alcohol abuse, poverty, avoidance of specific food groups (e.g., fruits or vegetables), weight loss, drug use (or abuse), family history of inborn errors, and cigarette smoking. Clinical features are extensive, including surgery or wounds; blood loss; dull, dry, pluckable hair; fever; and bleeding gums. Findings may be organized by symptoms

of the eyes, face, skin, muscles, tongue, and central nervous system. Table 14-4 provides additional data about historical and clinical features in relation to nutritional status.

Dietary intake assessment. There are several methods for collecting information regarding actual and habitual dietary intake. Most commonly, data are collected using diet/food recall (retrospective) or diet/food records (prospective). Each method has its pros and cons, so it is important to choose a method best suited to the type of information needed. These data provide information regarding intake of kcal, protein, carbohydrate, fat, vitamins, minerals, and fluid, which can be calculated manually using food composition tables or analyzed by computer software. More than 100 programs are available to analyze dietary intake. Evaluation of software needs and systems suitable to meet those needs is important when selecting an appropriate software package.[10]

24-Hour diet recall. In this method, the patient is asked by a trained interviewer to report all foods and beverages consumed during the past 24 hours. Detailed description of all foods, beverages, cooking methods, brand names, condiments, and supplements, along with portion sizes in common household measures, is included. Food models, measuring cups, life-size pictures, or abstract shapes (squares, circles, rectangles) are used to assist the patient in estimating correct portion sizes of foods consumed. This method is useful in screening or during follow-up to evaluate adaptation of or compliance with dietary recommendations. The advantages of this method are that it is quick (only 15 to 20 minutes are needed) and it can be used with most age groups. Because it is retrospective, the patient does not modify his or her actual intake. The information can be obtained by face-to-face interview, telephone, or patient self-reporting. Some of the drawbacks for this method are that it relies on the memory, motivation, and awareness of the patient. Because this is only a single day's intake, it may not be representative of the patient's actual diet.

Food records. Estimated or measured food records can provide a more realistic picture of a patient's usual intake. All foods, beverages, snacks, and supplements are recorded by the patient, usually over 1 to 7 days using household measures. The patient must be trained with food models, measuring cups, or other measuring devices that will help ensure recording of proper or actual portion sizes. Cooking methods, recipe ingredients, and descriptions need to be recorded as completely and accurately as possible. Often, record keeping like this influences the recorder's standard food choices but only in some cases. In some instances, the recorder is also asked to record locations, times, events, and feelings in addition to foods eaten if information is needed to identify behavioral as well as nutritional patterns. A 7-day food record is considered optimal for gathering this kind of information,

but it does tend to be tedious. Shorter periods are less representative of usual intake, but a 3-day record (including 2 weekdays and 1 weekend day) can be acceptable. Obviously for this method of dietary data collection, the patient must be literate, numerate, and well motivated.[10]

Kcalorie counts. In an acute or a long-term care setting, one of the most common forms of food records is a kcal count. This term is a little misleading because in actual practice, all nutrients can be assessed, but kcal and protein intakes are parameters usually quantified. Information gathered in this manner is often used to determine the adequacy of patients' daily oral intake or to document need for nutritional support (any nutrition intervention used to minimize patient morbidity, mortality, and complications). Nursing observations are essential for early identification of malnutrition and prevention of iatrogenic weight loss during the hospital stay. Staff responsible for recording intake must be accurate in their recordings. It is important to record foods and beverages consumed in measurable amounts (e.g., cups, ounces, teaspoons, tablespoons, mL) or in percentage of amount eaten (50% baked chicken, 75% bread, 25% green beans). Subjective terms such as *two bites, ate well,* or *three*

TABLE 14-4 SIGNS THAT SUGGEST NUTRIENT IMBALANCE

AREA OF CONCERN	POSSIBLE DEFICIENCY	POSSIBLE EXCESS
Hair		
Dull, dry, brittle	Pro	
Easily plucked (with no pain)	Pro	
Hair loss	Pro, Zn, biotin	Vit A
Flag sign (loss of hair pigment in strips around head)	Pro, Cu	
Head and Neck		
Bulging fontanel (infants)		Vit A
Headache		Vit A, D
Epistaxis (nosebleed)	Vit K	
Thyroid enlargement	Iodine	
Eyes		
Conjunctival and corneal xerosis (dryness)	Vit A	
Pale conjunctiva	Fe	
Blue sclerae	Fe	
Corneal vascularization	Vit B_2	
Mouth		
Cheilosis or angular stomatitis (lesions at corners of mouth)	Vit B_2	
Glossitis (red, sore tongue)	Niacin, folate, vit B_{12}, and other B vit	
Gingivitis (inflamed gums)	Vit C	
Hypogeusia, dysgeusia (poor sense of taste, distorted taste)	Zn	
Dental caries	Fluoride	
Mottling of teeth		Fluoride
Atrophy of papillae on tongue	Fe, B vit	
Skin		
Dry, scaly	Vit A, Zn, EFAs	Vit A
Follicular hyperkeratosis (resembles gooseflesh)	Vit A, EFAs, B vit	
Eczematous lesions	Zn	

Continued

TABLE 14-4 SIGNS THAT SUGGEST NUTRIENT IMBALANCE—cont'd

AREA OF CONCERN	POSSIBLE DEFICIENCY	POSSIBLE EXCESS
Petechiae, ecchymoses	Vit C, K	
Nasolabial seborrhea (greasy, scaly areas between nose and lip)	Niacin, vit B_{12}, B_6	
Darkening and peeling of skin in areas exposed to sun	Niacin	
Poor wound healing	Pro, Zn, vit C	
Nails		
Spoon-shaped nails	Fe	
Brittle, fragile	Pro	
Heart		
Enlargement, tachycardia, failure	Vit B_1	
Small heart	Energy	
Sudden failure, death	Se	
Arrhythmia	Mg, K, Se	
Hypertension	Ca, K	
Abdomen		
Hepatomegaly	Pro	Vit A
Ascites	Pro	
Musculoskeletal Extremities		
Muscle wasting (especially temporal area)	Energy	
Edema	Pro, vit B_1	
Calf tenderness	Vit B_1 or C, biotin, Se	
Beading of ribs, or "rachitic rosary" (child)	Vit C, D	
Bone and joint tenderness	Vit C, D, Ca, P	
Knock-knee, bowed legs, fragile bones	Vit D, Ca, P, Cu	
Neurologic		
Paresthesias (pain and tingling or altered sensation in the extremities)	Vit B_1, B_6, B_{12}, biotin	
Weakness	Vit C, B_1, B_6, B_{12}, energy	
Ataxia, decreased position and vibratory senses	Vit B_1, B_{12}	
Tremor	Mg	
Decreased tendon reflexes	Vit B_1	
Confabulation, disorientation	Vit B_1, B_{12}	
Drowsiness, lethargy	Vit B_1	Vit A, D
Depression	Vit B_1, biotin, B_{12}	

Ca, Calcium; *Cu*, copper; *EFAs*, essential fatty acids; *Fe*, iron; *K*, potassium; *Mg*, magnesium; *Na*, sodium; *P*, phosphorus; *Pro*, protein; *Se*, selenium; *Vit*, vitamin(s); *Zn*, zinc.

swallows are not useful and cannot provide objective information needed to calculate protein and kcal intake.

Nutritional Risk

The nutritional care process involves assessing patients' nutritional status, estimating nutritional needs, and planning for nutritional intervention. If done appropriately, it allows for early intervention in both treatment of established malnutrition and prevention of malnutrition among those at high nutritional risk. Areas to consider regarding nutritional risk are age, weight, laboratory test results, (body) systems, and feeding modalities[24] (Table 14-5), each of which is detailed as follows:

- *Age:* Age-related high risk is possible for patients aged 75 years or older; for children, high risk most often occurs for those younger than the age of 5. Moderate nutritional risk occurs among adults between ages 65 and 75, and for children older than 5 years of age.
- *Weight:* Weight loss is a potential nutritional risk factor depending on its cause. The percentage of body weight lost combined with the evaluation or cause of the loss determines the possible level of risk (see Table 14-1).
- *Laboratory test results:* As noted previously, biochemical tests of albumin, TLC, and prealbumin levels provide an assessment of nutritional risk.
- *Systems:* Systems account for conditions of various body systems that present either moderate or high nutritional risk. Moderate nutritional risk may be experienced when a patient undergoes chemotherapy because of its effects on dietary intake. High risk is

TABLE 14-5 AREAS OF NUTRITIONAL RISK

DATA SOURCE	MODERATE RISK	HIGH RISK
Age	65-75 years of age Children more than 5 years of age	75 years of age or older Children less than 5 years of age
Weight	Evaluation of loss (i.e., self-induced)	5% weight loss in 1 month 10% loss in 6 months Length/height for age <5th percentile Weight/height <5th percentile or <80th percentile of standard
Laboratory	Albumin 3-3.5 g/dL	Albumin ≤3 g/dL TLC ≤1200 cells/mm^3
Systems*	Heart, antepartum, pain, orthopedics, selected oncology, short stay, chemotherapy	Renal, pancreas, gastrointestinal, liver, diabetes with pregnancy, eating disorders, oncology, transplants, any condition in children associated with development of protein calorie malnutrition
Feeding modalities	Transitional (stable) Some selected modified diets with education component	Parenteral nutrition, tube feeding, nothing per mouth (NPO), or clear liquids >3 days

*Systems for risk depend on the individual patient population at risk.
Data from Grant A, DeHoog S: *Nutritional assessment and support*, ed 5, Seattle, 1999, Anne Grant/Susan DeHoog.

incurred among individuals with eating disorders or diabetes when pregnant. (Other conditions are listed in Table 14-5.)

Feeding modalities: Moderate nutritional risk is associated with transition from restrictive therapeutic intervention to a regular dietary intake. Risk may also occur when patients are on modified diets that have potential to cause nutrient deficiencies. Patients may be at high risk when they are on parenteral feeding or tube feeding, are NPO (i.e., nothing by mouth), or on clear liquids for more than 3 days.

Nutritional assessment involves examination of anthropometric data, biochemical data, clinical data, and dietary data. It is important to remember that there is no one absolute index for measuring nutritional status. Accurate and meaningful assessment can be made only by incorporating data from several sources.

NUTRITIONAL THEORY

As will be discussed in the chapters to follow, specific diseases or conditions require modifications of nutritional components of a normal diet. Each modified diet has a purpose and rationale, and its use is usually determined by the physician or dietitian. To appreciate modified diets described in the following chapters, it will be helpful to have an understanding of the basis for these diets: the regular, general, or house diet.

The regular/general diet is designed to attain or maintain optimal nutritional status in people who do not require modified or therapeutic diets. Individual requirements for specific nutrients vary and are adjusted depending on gender, age, height, weight, and activity level. This diet is used to promote health and reduce risks for developing chronic diet-related diseases such as cardiovascular diseases or certain cancers. Depending on individual food choices, a regular diet can be adequate in all nutrients.

Dietary modifications of the regular diet may be made in two ways: quantitative or qualitative. Qualitative diets include modifications in consistency, texture, or nutrients, such as clear-liquid or full-liquid diets. Quantitative diets include modifications in number or size of meals served or amounts of specific nutrients, such as six small feedings or kcal-controlled diets used in the treatment of diabetes mellitus.

Whatever kind of meals or modified diets patients receive, much of patients' acceptance of the food is influenced by nursing personnel. For example, if a patient's primary caregiver expresses criticism about the food service, the patient is likely to do the same. It is also possible acceptance of modified diets may also be influenced by whether patients perceive nutrition to be an important part of their medical care and recovery. Patient education can make a difference in patient acceptance of meals. By explaining the rationale of why some foods are allowed and others are to be reduced or avoided, the nurse or dietitian may affect patient compliance with modified dietary intake. It is important to remember that food provides the energy and nutrients that aid in the healing process. Food left on the tray does not help the patient heal.

Food Service Delivery Systems

Because nursing personnel are often on the front line when food is delivered to patients, it is important to understand how meals are prepared and delivered to patients in hospitals and long-term care facilities. Food service in a health care setting is the responsibility of the director of the food and nutrition services department. This person may be either a management dietitian or a specially trained food service manager. He or she is responsible for hiring, terminating, and supervising staff; ordering and purchasing food and supplies; delivering food to patients and staff; and overseeing quality assurance issues. Clinical dietitians may work under the supervision of or alongside the food service director to assess patients' nutritional status, plan appropriate diets and nutrition intervention, and provide nutrition education. Other personnel from the food and nutrition service area include cooks, clerks, dishwashers, aides, and dietetic technicians. Clinical dietitians may also be members of a food service department. Their jobs involve direct patient care. Typically, only RDs (management and clinical) and dietetic technicians have the appropriate education and training in clinical nutrition and all of its applications, whether that is the delivery of food or the assessment of nutritional status.

Patients are often able to choose (from a menu) foods they will be served at mealtimes. Some institutions provide this service for patients who receive regular as well as modified diets. A menu for a modified diet lists only foods that are appropriate for a given type of patient. This practice allows patients to select foods they like and will eat. Although a dietitian can plan the most nutritious meals, if patients do not eat the food, they may be at risk in the long term. A selective menu system also affords patients the feeling of some control over their lives while hospitalized. (See the *Teaching Tool* box, Assisting Patients with Menu Selections, for more suggestions.)

Some institutions do not offer selective menus. In their place, a standard house diet that is adjusted (or modified) according to special nutritional needs is used. Although a selective menu may not be available, efforts can be made to ensure that patient food preferences are met. Simple changes or substitutions are common. Nursing personnel, on behalf of their patients, often interact with the staff of the food service system at their facility. It may be beneficial for nurses to familiarize themselves with the organization and food service system staff. Beneficial information includes the following:

- Telephone number of the clinical dietitian to request nutrition assessment or education
- Time schedule of meal service so requests or changes can be made *before* meals are delivered to patients

Location of the diet manual on the nursing unit, which is required in each unit by the Medicare Conditions of Participation for Hospitals and TJC; the diet manual is the reference (usually in a three-ring binder or online) that describes the rationale and indications for using a specific diet, lists allowed and restricted foods, and provides sample menus

Most of this information also applies to long-term care facilities, but there are a few additional concerns. Food service supplied to residents in long-term care facilities frequently relies exclusively on the food service department for nutritious foods and meals. Repetition and monotony also influence patient acceptance of foods and meals served. Therefore, it is of meticulous significance that these patients be given food they can and will eat because they are often at high nutritional risk.

Basic Hospital Diets

Clear liquid diets. Clear liquid diets may be used postoperatively or if a patient is scheduled for diagnostic tests (Box 14-4). A clear liquid diet consists of foods that are clear and liquid at room or body temperature, factors that help prevent dehydration and keep colon contents to a minimum.

Assisting Patients with Menu Selections

When we select food items from a restaurant menu while socializing with friends and family, the process is fun. However, choosing foods from the restricted hospital selections, often with little descriptive information, can be a difficult and sometimes intimidating chore when we are ill in a hospital. Some hospitals are going to paperless menus, instead using palmtop computers to read menus to patients for selections. As nurses, we are familiar with hospital forms and computer entries that require us to choose selections quickly; we cannot assume our patients also share that ability. Patients may need our help. Below are potential menu selection problems and possible solutions.

PROBLEM	SOLUTION
Patient has a low literacy level, is illiterate, has reduced visual abilities, or is too ill to read or write.	Read menu items to patient and mark his or her selections.
Patient does not understand the vocabulary used on menu (we cannot assume dietary terms are common knowledge).	Clarify for patient or ask for clarification from dietetic technician, dietitian, or food service personnel.
Patient often must select foods from menu a day in advance, often resulting in choosing too much or too little food (particularly a concern when appetite may be diminished from drug-nutrient interactions or from the effects of the illness).	Remind patients they are selecting food for the next day. If they have not selected enough food, offer them foods kept on the nursing unit for snacks or order additional foods from food service. If they have selected too much food, cover, date, and store appropriate foods for use later in the day.
Patient does not understand why some of his or her favorite foods are not included on the menu or why smaller amounts are served (when ill, familiar foods are most desired and comforting).	Menus are a great teaching tool for modified diets. Discuss dietary concerns of the patient's illness, explaining why specific foods are not included or only limited amounts allowed. Contact the registered dietitian (RD) to provide education for patient.

Although a good source of fluids and water, this modified diet is desolate when it comes to adequate amounts of protein, fat, and energy. In addition, the clear liquid diet is almost devoid of dietary fiber, which is one of the reasons it is used. Whereas this diet can provide adequate amounts of ascorbic acid (if an adequate amount of juice is consumed), it is nutritionally inadequate for almost all other required nutrients except water. Because of its limited choices, this diet is boring and does not meet patients' expectations for a meal. Because

BOX 14-4   TYPES OF DIETS

Liquid Diets

Indications for Clear Liquid Diet
Provide oral fluids; before/after surgery; prepare bowel for diagnostic tests (colonoscopic examination, barium enema, and other procedures); minimize stimulation of gastrointestinal (GI) tract; promote recovery from partial paralytic ileus (early refeeding); minimize residue in the GI tract; transition feeding from IV feeding to solid foods; acute GI disturbances; diarrhea

Contraindications for Clear Liquid Diet
Should not be used more than 24 hours; inadequate GI function; nutrient needs requiring parenteral nutrition

Indications for Full Liquid Diet
Provide oral fluids; after surgery; transition between clear liquids and solid food; oral or plastic surgery to the face and neck; mandibular fractures; patients who have chewing or swallowing difficulties; esophageal or GI strictures; diarrhea

Contraindications for Full Liquid Diet
Dysphagia

Pureed, Mechanical, or Soft Diets

Indications for Pureed Diet
Neurologic changes; inflammation or ulcerations of the oral cavity and/or esophagus; edentulous patients; fractured jaw; head and neck abnormalities; cerebrovascular accident

Contraindications for Pureed Diet
Situations in which ground or chopped foods are appropriate

Indications for Mechanical Soft Diet
Poorly fitting dentures; edentulous patients; limited chewing or swallowing ability; dysphagia; strictures of intestinal tract; radiation treatment to oral cavity; progression from enteral tube feedings or parenteral nutrition to solid foods

Contraindications for Mechanical Soft Diet
Situations in which regular foods are appropriate

Indications for Soft Diet
Debilitated patients unable to consume a regular diet; mild GI problems

Contraindications for Soft Diet
Situations in which regular foods are appropriate

a clear liquid diet is nutritionally inadequate, long-term use is discouraged.[26] Use of a clear liquid diet for more than 1 day can lead to compromised nutritional status and possible nutrient deficiencies. If the patient is already nutritionally depleted, insult is added to the injury.

Caution is also necessary in regard to the amount of caffeine patients might receive on clear liquid diets. Because food choices are so limited, patients might easily receive and consume excessive amounts of caffeine in the form of coffee, strong tea, or soft drinks containing caffeine. Excess caffeine consumption could lead to increased hydrochloric acid pro-

duction in the stomach, leading to an upset stomach, and contribute to sleeplessness.

Although few conditions contraindicate a clear liquid diet, it is important to reiterate that this diet should not be used as the sole means of nutrition for more than 24 hours in any condition. This diet should also not be used if the patient does not possess adequate gastrointestinal (GI) function. Clear liquid diets can be adjusted to accommodate other dietary modifications, such as sodium restriction, if necessary.

There is some thought that unsupplemented clear liquid diets are one of the causative factors in the incidence of hospital malnutrition.[27] One way to prevent this is quality assurance monitoring by the RD. This helps identify patients who have been on clear liquid diets too long, as well as those patients with any nutritional problems that result from use of the diet. Another way to monitor use of clear liquid diets would be to establish a policy that diet orders for clear liquid diets are valid for only 24 hours (similar to the time-restricted orders for antibiotics), thus allowing physicians to reevaluate the patient and the need for this nutritionally deficient diet. Each day the physician can reorder the diet with documented justification or choose a more appropriate source of nutrition. Along with this method, a mechanism to identify patients who have had clear liquid diets ordered more than three times would be necessary.

Full liquid diets. A full liquid diet is one that consists of foods that are liquid at room or body temperature. It is used to provide oral nourishment for patients who have difficulty chewing or swallowing solid foods. Unlike the clear liquid diet, the full liquid diet offers more variety, and commercial nutritional supplements can be used to supply adequate amounts of energy and nutrients to make it nutritionally complete.

There are a few potential hazards associated with full liquid diets that have caused this diet to be excluded in widely used diet manuals,[28] but it may still be found in most hospitals. Because all liquids are allowed, lactose-containing (milk-based) foods are included. This is usually not a problem, except for patients who are lactose intolerant. Most patients do not tolerate fat or lactose well after surgery, albeit temporarily. They may experience symptoms of GI distress such as nausea, vomiting, distention, or diarrhea when given lactose-rich liquids. This, plus evidence that supports rapid postoperative progression of the diet, has led to the elimination of the full liquid diet from many hospital settings.[28]

If a patient is to receive a nutritionally complete full liquid diet for an extended period, care should be given to reduce the high saturated fat and cholesterol content of the diet. One approach is to avoid excessive use of whole-milk products, ice cream, milk shakes, and eggs as protein sources (e.g., in custards). Another special concern is for patients with dysphagia who cannot swallow thin liquids. Chapter 17 discusses special adaptations that can be used.

Full liquid diets can be nutritionally complete if they are well planned and include between-meal snacks or nourishment from commercially prepared supplements. Amounts of the diet consumed by patients should be monitored daily to ensure adequate energy and nutrient consumption. One word of caution about possible problems with foodborne illness: raw eggs should never be used in the preparation of any food served to patients, and patients and their families should be educated about possible dangers of foodborne illness.

Mechanically altered diets. When a patient has problems chewing or swallowing, foods can be chopped, ground, mashed, and pureed. Consistency of food can be varied according to the patient's ability to chew and swallow. The nurse, dietitian, and patient should work together to evaluate the patient's needs for modifying consistency according to the food preferences.

Some foods, such as mashed potatoes and ice cream, are already a smooth consistency. For other foods, small amounts of liquids (e.g., broth, milk, gravies) can be added to reach the appropriate consistency needed. Any liquid added to pureed foods should complement the food and not conceal the food's original flavor. Care should be taken to add only enough liquid to achieve desired consistency yet allow nutritional quality of the food to be retained. Butter, margarine, gravies, sugar, or honey may be added to foods to increase kcal density. To make pureed foods more attractive, component pureeing may be used. For example, a cake-decorating tool (icing bag and tips) can be used to make pureed peas look like regular peas. Molds are also used to shape foods. For example, a pork chop can be pureed and then put into a pork chop–shaped mold and reheated in a microwave oven.

As mentioned previously, exact composition and consistency of a mechanically altered diet will vary depending on the patient's needs. These diets can be modified for additional needs such as low sodium, kcal control, or low fat. Care should be taken in evaluating the patient's needs for consistency. Food consistency should be altered only to the degree it is needed. If a patient needs only meats pureed, then only the meats should be pureed. If a patient needs only the foods or meats ground, then they shouldn't be pureed. Sometimes, foods just need to be chopped coarsely or finely. Edentulous patients can often chew solid or soft foods.

Soft diets. Soft diets are often used during transition from liquid diets to regular or general diets. Whole foods, low in fiber and only lightly seasoned, are used. This diet has traditionally been used for patients with mild GI problems. Food supplements or between-meals snacks may be used if needed to add kcal. Soft diets can contain "hard to chew" foods such as white toast. This diet is not appropriate for patients requiring mechanical soft diets.

Regular or general diets. A regular diet is used for patients who do not need dietary restrictions or modifications. Most hospitals offer self-select menus for regular diets and often for many modified diets. The regular diet serves as the basis for almost all modified diets.

Appendix E lists information about each of the basic hospital diets, which progress from a clear liquid to an unrestricted regular diet. Each step or diet of the progression provides appropriate texture and consistency as GI function increases. As healing proceeds, dietary restrictions decrease toward a regular diet.

"Diet as tolerated." Occasionally when patients are admitted, the physician writes an order for "diet as tolerated." It is also common for this diet to be ordered postoperatively. This permits patients' preferences and situations to be taken into consideration and also allows for postoperative diet progression at the patient's tolerance. "Diet as tolerated" helps to alleviate prolonged use of clear and full liquid diets. Furthermore, this diet order provides an excellent opportunity for collaboration by the nurse, dietitian, and patient to plan and provide food that is eaten, tolerated, and nourishing.

Enteral Nutrition

Any time the GI tract is used to provide nourishment, the feeding can be referred to as enteral nutrition. This includes liquid diets, soft and solid food diets, and special nutritionally complete formulas administered orally or via tubes. The consistency of the diet may be modified in progressive steps as in the following discussion and summarized in Appendix E, "Foods Recommended for Hospital Diet Progressions." However, when medical personnel talk about enteral nutrition, most often they are referring to specialized formula feedings.

Enteral Feeding by Tube

Frequently, patients are unable or unwilling to orally consume adequate nutrients and kcal. When this is the case and the GI tract is functioning, nutrients can be provided via feeding tubes placed into the alimentary tract (see the *Teaching Tool* box, Tube Feeding the Infant or Child). In fact, when the GI tract is functional, accessible, and safe to use, enteral feedings are preferred over parenteral nutrition because they are physiologically beneficial in maintaining the integrity and function of the gut.[26] In addition, enteral tube feedings are much less costly than parenteral nutrition for both the patient and the health care institution.

Enteral tube feeding can be part of routine care when a patient experiences protein-calorie malnutrition with 5 days of inadequate oral intake or with a reduced oral intake over the previous 7 to 10 days. Other conditions warranting tube feeding are severe dysphagia, major burns, a short gut from small bowel resection, or when intestinal fistulas (abnormal passages between the intestines) are present. Conditions under which enteral tube feedings are helpful, but not routine, include major trauma, radiation therapy, chemotherapeutic regimens, acute or chronic liver failure, or severe renal dysfunction. Enteral feeding is of limited or undetermined value if intensive chemotherapy results in GI tract dysfunction or if adequate postoperative oral intake is expected to resume within 5 to 7 days. Other conditions for which benefit is unclear are acute enteritis secondary to radiation, acute infection, active inflammatory bowel disease, and if less than 10% of the small intestine is intact after surgery.[29]

Types of formulas. Enteral nutrition by tube has been used since the late 1800s.[30] For years, enteral formulas were

✳ TEACHING TOOL

Tube Feeding the Infant or Child

Parents and caregivers need special support when their infants and children are tube fed. Assure them that the children can still be cuddled and can play without interfering with the tube nourishment. Teach the adults how the process works; they can be allies in helping young children accept and understand these procedures. Be sure to explain the procedures to the children as well. Dolls or stuffed animals can be used to explain how tube feeding helps speed the healing process.

Every infant and child has individual nutritional requirements based on growth needs and medical conditions. Check with the nurse or dietitian for appropriate rate, concentration, and volume of feedings. The following are some specific techniques to ensure adequate nutrient intake:

- Wash your hands with soap and water for at least 20 seconds (the time it takes to sing the "Happy Birthday" song twice).
- Flush feeding tube with 1-5 mL of water before and after each feeding, and before and after giving medications to prevent the feeding tube from clogging.
- Never add new formula to formula in the feeding container.
- Change the entire feeding setup every 24 hours.
- Place only 8 hrs of formula or 4 hrs of breast milk in feeding container at any given time.
- Make sure your infant or child has pleasant sensations during feedings: hold during feedings, suck on a pacifier, sit in a high chair, be a part of family meals.
- Give medications only in liquid form.
- Elevate the head of the bed 30 to 45 degrees.

Data from Cincinnati Children's Hospital Medical Center, *Nasojejunal tube feeding with enteral pump.* Accessed January 31, 2010, from www.cincinnatichildrens.org/health/info/abdomen/home/nasojejunal-kangaroo.htm.

prepared using foodstuffs, vitamin/mineral preparations, and a blender. Today an extensive variety of commercially prepared formulas are used. Some formulas are nutritionally complete, some are formulated for specific diseases or conditions, and others (modular) provide specific nutrients to supplement a diet or other formula. Commercial products are usually preferred over hospital or home-blended concoctions because they provide a known nutrient composition, controlled osmolality and consistency, and bacteriologic safety. They are also much easier to prepare and store. Many are nutritionally complete if consumed in the volumes recommended by the manufacturers.

Standard–intact formulas. Standard–intact formulas (or polymeric formulas) are composed of intact nutrients that require a functioning GI tract for digestion and absorption of nutrients. There are several categories of polymeric formulas that provide 1 to 2 kcal/mL. Standard–intact formulas can be categorized into blenderized food products, milk-based products, high-kcal lactose-free products, and normocaloric lactose-free products.

Normocaloric lactose-free products can be categorized into those that are isotonic, hypertonic, high nitrogen, and fiber containing. Blenderized formulas (1 kcal/mL) are a blenderized mixture of ordinary foods that usually contain milk products (lactose). They have a high viscosity and moderate osmolality. Blenderized formulas can be made by the dietary staff or in the patient's own home; they are also available commercially. Noncommercial formulas are low in cost but run the risk of bacterial contamination and variation in nutrient composition. Commercial formulas provide a sterile product with a fixed nutrient composition. Extreme caution should be exercised when using noncommercial (homemade) formulas because of the risk of foodborne illness. For patient safety, commercial formulas should be used.

Normocaloric (1 kcal/mL) lactose-free formulas have low osmolality, which generally makes them well tolerated. Hypercaloric (1.5 to 2 kcal/mL) formulas are designed to meet kcal and protein demands in a reduced volume and have moderate to high osmolality. High-nitrogen lactose-free formulas (1 to 2 kcal/mL) are designed to meet increased protein demands at usual or increased energy needs. They have low to moderate osmolality. Fiber-containing products are low osmolality and are used for patients with abnormal bowel regulation. These formulas contain fiber from natural food sources or soy polysaccharide.

Special formulas

Elemental formulas. Elemental formulas (predigested or hydrolyzed formulas) (1 to 1.3 kcal/mL) are composed of partially or fully hydrolyzed nutrients that can be used for patients with a partially functioning GI tract or those who have impaired capacity to digest foods or absorb nutrients, pancreatic insufficiency, or bile salt deficiency. These products are lactose-free and are usually hyperosmolar. They are not palatable and are best suited for administration by tube.

Modular formulas. Modular formulas (3.8 to 4 kcal/mL) are not nutritionally complete by themselves because they are single macronutrients such as glucose polymers, protein, or lipids. They are added to foods or other enteral products to change composition when nutritional needs cannot otherwise be met.

Specialty formulas. These products (1 to 2 kcal/mL) are designed to meet specialized nutrient demands for specific disease states such as diabetes, renal failure, liver failure, pulmonary disease, or human immunodeficiency virus/acquired immunodeficiency syndrome (HIV/AIDS). Some formulas may require supplementation with vitamins, minerals, or trace elements. Some are unpalatable, and most formulas are expensive.

Formula selection. The numerous types and brands of enteral feeding products on the market can make product selection a complex process. Choosing an enteral feeding formula includes the following considerations:

- What are the patient's digestive and absorptive capabilities?
- Do the patient's fluids need to be restricted?
- Does the patient have high metabolic requirements?

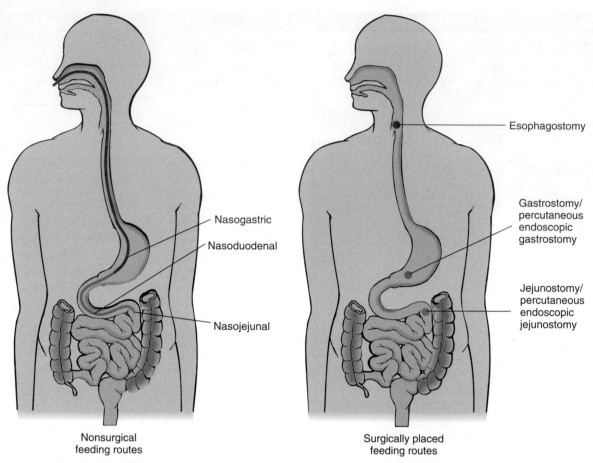

Nasogastric

Nasoduodenal

Nasojejunal

Esophagostomy

Gastrostomy/
percutaneous
endoscopic
gastrostomy

Jejunostomy/
percutaneous
endoscopic
jejunostomy

Nonsurgical
feeding routes

Surgically placed
feeding routes

FIG 14-7 Types of enteral feeding routes. (From Rolin Graphics.)

Whether a patient can digest and absorb nutrients indicates whether an elemental or polymeric formula should be used. Individual nutrient requirements determine the type and amount of tube-feeding formula. As with previous components of medical nutritional therapy, ongoing assessment of nutritional status and patients' tolerance of the formula is necessary.

Successful use of enteral feeding depends on the patient's condition, availability of access for feeding, and the patient's tolerance of the chosen enteral formula. Enteral feeding is the feeding route of choice because of benefits provided. Some of these benefits include improved use of nutrients, maintenance of gut mucosa and immunocompetence, decreased catabolic response to injury, administration safety, and lower cost.[31]

Feeding routes. In addition to choosing an appropriate tube-feeding formula, selecting the appropriate feeding tube and feeding route involves consideration of various factors. Patients' medical status and nutritional status often govern the length of the feeding tube (i.e., the portion of the GI tract into which the formula is delivered). Anticipated length of time that tube feeding will be required dictates whether the feeding tube should be surgically placed. If the tube feeding will be used for short duration, a nonsurgical placement can be made. If the feeding tube will be long term or permanent, surgical placement is necessary. Routes for tube feeding include the following (Figure 14-7):

Nasogastric: Tube is passed through nose to stomach.
Nasoduodenal: Tube is passed from nose to duodenum (small intestine).
Nasojejunal: Tube is passed through nose to jejunum (small intestine).
Esophagostomy: Tube is surgically inserted into the neck and extends to stomach.
Gastrostomy: Tube is surgically inserted into stomach.
Jejunostomy: Tube is surgically inserted into small intestine.

Placing the feeding tube into the stomach, duodenum, or jejunum through the nose is the simplest and most commonly used tube-feeding technique. This technique is preferred for patients who will resume oral feedings in the near future. Placement into the stomach simulates normal GI function but should be reserved for patients who are alert with intact gag and cough reflexes. Tube placement into the small intestine has less risk of aspiration, but elemental formulas are often required for easier absorption and continuous feedings are better tolerated. Surgical placement of the feeding tube is preferred when long-term use is anticipated or when obstruction makes insertion through the nose impossible. These procedures require surgery with general anesthesia. **Percutaneous endoscopic placement (PEG)** of a gastrostomy can be performed with minimal sedation and has fewer complications than surgical placement. PEG involves placing a feeding tube into stomach via the

TABLE 14-6   ADVANTAGES AND DISADVANTAGES OF ENTERAL FEEDING ROUTES

FEEDING ROUTE	CHARACTERISTICS	ADVANTAGES	DISADVANTAGES
Nasogastric	Tube extends from nose into stomach	Easy placement/easy to remove No surgery necessary Less expensive Medications can be administered	Greater risk of aspiration (compared with nasointestinal feeding) Gastric emptying must be monitored
Nasoduodenal or nasojejunal	*Nasoduodenal:* Tube extends from nose through pylorus into duodenum; tube must be advanced by peristalsis or videofluoroscopy *Nasojejunal:* Tube extends from nose through pylorus into jejunum and is usually placed by videofluoroscopy or endoscopy	Lessened risk of aspiration (compared with nasogastric feedings) Helpful in patients with gastroparesis	Requires placement via endoscopy Unable to monitor gastric motility
Gastrostomy or percutaneous endoscopic gastrostomy (PEG)	*Gastrostomy:* Tube placed through incision in abdominal wall into stomach *PEG:* Tube percutaneously placed in stomach under endoscopic guidance, secured by rubber "bumpers" or inflated balloon catheter	Intermediate/bolus feedings possible Patient comfort Size of tube allows medication administration and/or gastric decompression	Increased risk of aspiration in some individuals Stoma care required Potential for dislodgment of tube
Jejunostomy or percutaneous endoscopic jejunostomy (PEJ)	Jejunostomy: Types include needle catheter placement, direct tube placement, and creation of jejunal stoma that is catheterized intermittently PEJ: Weighted feeding tube (from PEG insertion) into duodenum; peristaltic action advances tube into jejunum	Early postoperative feeding possible Decreased aspiration risk	Smaller tube used, tube may clog easily Stoma care required Intraperitoneal leakage possible Volvulus possible

Data from American Dietetic Association: *Handbook of clinical dietetics*, ed 2, New Haven, Conn, 1992, Yale University Press; American Dietetic Association: *Manual of clinical dietetics*, ed 6, Chicago, 2000, American Dietetic Association.

esophagus and then drawing it through the abdominal skin using a stab incision. Table 14-6 describes the classifications, advantages, and disadvantages of feeding routes.

Method of administration. How enteral tube feedings are administered or given to patients is just as important as formula selection and feeding site. Proper administration safeguards delivery of the desired nutrients, enhances tolerance by the patient, and provides optimal nutrition support. Factors affecting decisions about appropriate methods of formula infusion include the patient's medical status, GI function, and feeding route. Tube feedings can be administered by three methods: continuous, intermittent, or bolus infusion.

Continuous infusion is generally the preferred method of feeding. This method provides controlled delivery of a prescribed volume of formula at a constant rate over a continuous period using an infusion pump. Although this method requires use of special equipment, it is preferred, especially when feeding into the small intestine, because it is similar to typical gastric emptying.[32,33]

Intermittent infusion involves delivering the total quantity of formulas needed for a 24-hour period in three to six equal feedings. Each feeding is usually delivered by gravity during a 30- to 60-minute period. This method represents a more normal feeding pattern, but patients often do not tolerate this method of feeding if the rate is too rapid. Although equipment needs are minimal, this method is time consuming because feedings must be closely monitored to ensure proper delivery rate.[32,33]

Bolus feedings involve infusing volumes of formula (250-500 mL) by gravity or syringe over a short period of time. This method requires minimal equipment and time but is associated with increased potential for aspiration, regurgitation, and GI side effects. This method should not be used for intestinal feedings.[32,33] Table 14-7 summarizes indications for and pros and cons of each feeding method.

Starting the tube feeding. Before initiating enteral tube feedings, placement of the feeding tube must be confirmed and documented. This can be done several ways. Radiologic confirmation of placement is often used to confirm

TABLE 14-7	ADMINISTRATION OF ENTERAL TUBE FEEDINGS		
METHOD	**INDICATIONS**	**ADVANTAGES**	**DISADVANTAGES**
Continuous	Patients who have not eaten for a significant period, debilitated patients, those with impaired GI function, patients with uncontrolled type 1 diabetes mellitus, intestinal feedings	Feedings can be administered at constant rate over 24-hr period, feedings can be cycled (allows formula to be delivered over shorter period, allowing patients freedom of movement and to promote oral intake if appropriate), gastric pooling minimized and fewer GI side effects experienced, continuous feeding into jejunum is similar to normal gastric emptying	Requires feeding pump if accuracy of volume delivered is required; continuous drip by gravity is possible, but less accurate
Intermittent	Feedings that are infused at specific intervals throughout the day (total volume of feeding divided and given 4-6 times/day)	Requires only simple equipment, can be used in home settings, may be more physiologic than continuous infusion, feedings can be administered by gravity over 30-90 minutes	In absence of pumps, feedings must be monitored vigilantly, may become time consuming depending on number of scheduled feedings per day, rate of intermittent infusion (rather than volume) seems to be a major reason for intolerance of tube feedings
Bolus	Appropriate *only* for feeding into the stomach, involves feeding large volumes of formula intermittently over short periods, usually by syringe	More manageable for the patient, rate of 30 mL/min or volume of 500-700 mL per feeding seems to be cutoff of physical tolerance limits	Associated with increased risk of aspiration, regurgitation, and GI side effects; not appropriate for postpyloric feedings

Data from Moore MC: *Pocket guide to nutrition assessment and care*, ed 6, St. Louis, 2009, Mosby/Elsevier.

placement after initial insertion. Thereafter, aspiration of gastric contents with a large syringe (60-mL) is used to reconfirm tube placement. The high osmolality of a hypertonic formula can lead to GI distress such as intestinal distention and osmotic diarrhea. Diluting tube feedings will lengthen the amount of time necessary before nutritional requirements can be met by the formula and feeding regimen. Rate of the feedings can be advanced to desired volume, and then concentration can be gradually increased until kcal and protein needs are met. Rate and concentration should never be advanced at the same time. If the feeding is not tolerated, rate or concentration can be reduced to the last level of tolerance, then gradually increased again. Other criteria to be considered to ensure optimal tolerance of the formula and safety of the feedings include solution temperature, prevention of bacterial contamination, prevention of aspiration, patency of tubing, administration of medications, and patient monitoring (Table 14-8).

Possible tube-feeding complications. Although tube feedings use the GI tract to nourish the patient, they are not without problems. Most are preventable, and all are correctable. Most problems can be prevented simply through the use of good hand washing techniques by nursing staff administering the feeding.

Tube-feeding complications can be categorized three ways according to the type of problem: GI, mechanical, or metabolic. GI problems include diarrhea, nausea and vomiting, cramping, distention, and constipation. Mechanical complications consist of tube displacement or obstruction, pulmonary aspiration, and mucosal damage. Metabolic difficulties involve hyperosmolar dehydration or overhydration; abnormal blood concentration levels of sodium, potassium, phosphorus, and magnesium (too high or too low); hyperglycemia; respiratory insufficiency; and rapid weight gain. Table 14-9 summarizes possible complications, probable causes, and suggested corrective actions.

Diarrhea, a common complication of enteral feedings, was once thought to be caused by hyperosmolar feeding solutions. More recently it has been determined that other factors may contribute to this problem. Patients receiving tube feedings are frequently placed on liquid forms of medications, and many of these medications contain sorbitol, which can cause diarrhea. Bacterial dysentery caused by *Clostridium difficile* is also a common cause of diarrhea. Diarrhea should not be attributed to tube-feeding formulas until other causes have been ruled out.[33]

Home enteral nutrition. Because of changing health care reimbursement patterns, demand for home tube feeding has been growing steadily. Although it provides opportunity and convenience for patients, home enteral nutrition (HEN) imparts responsibility that nurses and dietitians must assume and risks that must be anticipated. In addition to criteria already discussed regarding selection of appropriate candidates for tube feedings, other criteria that should be consid-

TABLE 14-8	CRITERIA FOR SAFE ADMINISTRATION OF ENTERAL TUBE FEEDINGS
CRITERIA	**CONSIDERATIONS**
Temperature	Administer solutions infused by continuous drip chilled
	Administer intermittent and bolus feedings at room temperature to decrease incidence of GI side effects
Prevention of bacterial contamination	Use closed feeding containers
	Prefilled, ready-to-feed closed systems are available for some products (less chance of contamination)
	Change extension tubing administration set and bag *daily*
	Never add new formula to old formula
	Do *not* hang feedings for longer than 4-8 hours
	Maintain ice in pouch of bag at all times while formula is running
Prevention of aspiration	Check tube placement before administration
	Tubes placed into small bowel are associated with decreased risk for aspiration
	Head of bed (HOB) should be elevated 30-45 degrees
	Consider adding vegetable food coloring to formula to allow for detection of aspirated tube feeding from pulmonary secretions (remember, this does not protect against aspiration)
Patency of tubing	Irrigate tubes every 6-8 hours with 40-50 mL of warm water (continuous feeds)
	For intermittent or bolus feedings, irrigate tubes after each feeding with 40-50 mL of warm water
	Flush tube with 40-50 mL of water each time feeding is stopped
	If tubing clogs, flush with 30-50 mL of warm water
	Systems are available that allow for self-flushing of the feeding tube (e.g., Ross Laboratories)
Medications	Medications administered through the feeding tube should be in *liquid form*
	Flush tubing before and after giving the medication with 20 mL of water to prevent clogging
	If medication is not available in liquid form, consult the pharmacist *before* crushing or diluting the medication (some medications are pharmacologically altered by mechanical manipulation)
	Never crush time-released, liquid-filled capsules or enteric coated medications
	Do *not* give sublingual medications through the tubing
	Because hyperosmolar liquid medications (KCl) may cause gastric irritation or diarrhea, dilute with water before administration
	Supplemental electrolyte preparations (KCl, NaCl, $NaPO_4$) increase the osmolality of the formula and may cause feeding tubes to clog
	Do not mix together multiple medications and deliver simultaneously unless the compatibility of the medications is known
	If feeding into the duodenum or jejunum instead of the stomach, check the effect of medication absorption
	Monitor patient response to medications given through the feeding tube and make changes needed
Monitoring	Confirm tube placement before initiating feeding and before each intermittent feeding
	Record urine glucose every shift until final feeding rate and concentration are established
	Record gastric residuals every 4 hours (gastric feedings only)
	Record bowel movements and consistency
	Record tolerance to feedings
	Record daily:
	Weight
	Intake and output
	Record weekly:
	Serum electrolytes and blood counts
	Chemistry profile (including liver function tests, phosphorous, calcium, magnesium, total protein, and albumin)
	Nitrogen balance, if appropriate
	Reassess nutrition indexes weekly, adjusting energy and protein as needed

Data from Moore MC: *Pocket guide to nutrition assessment and care*, ed 6, St. Louis, 2009, Mosby/Elsevier.

ered when sending a patient home on enteral nutritional therapy include the following:[33]

- Patient's nutritional needs cannot be met orally
- Appropriate enteral access is in place and functioning, and patient is tolerating tube-feeding regimen
- Patient and/or significant other is (are) able and willing to perform HEN techniques safely and effectively
- Underlying disease state is stable, and patient is ready for discharge and can be monitored in the home setting
- Affordable HEN supplies are available

TABLE 14-9	**TUBE-FEEDING COMPLICATIONS, CAUSES, AND CORRECTIVE ACTIONS**	
PROBLEM	**POSSIBLE CAUSE**	**CORRECTIVE ACTION**
Gastrointestinal		
Diarrhea (defined as more than four bowel movements per day or liquid stools greater than 200 g)	Protein-energy malnutrition (PEM)	Switch to isotonic formula and feed at slow rate (will allow intestine to adapt to refeeding)
	Infection, microbial contamination of formula	Confirm with stool, blood, or formula cultures; limit hang time of formula 8-12 hr, maintain ice in bag's pouch, change bag and tubing every 24 hr, and rinse after each bolus feeding or before filling bag for continuous feedings; use good handwashing technique
	Malabsorption	Check for pancreatic insufficiency; pancreatic enzymes replacement may be necessary; change to low-fat, lactose-free, or elemental formula; change to continuous feeding
	Bolus feeding, volume overload, rapid administration, dumping syndrome	If infusion rate or concentration was advanced recently, return to previously tolerated rate/concentration; change to continuous feeding; decrease bolus volume and increase frequency of feedings
	Hyperosmolar formula	If started, reduce rate and increase gradually; dilute formula or change to isotonic product; if starting, rate should begin at 25 mL/hr, increasing every 12-24 hr
	Medications	Evaluate types of medications as primary cause (diarrhea has been related to administration of antibiotics and antacids, potassium supplements, cimetidine, and sorbitol-containing drops) and the possibility for change; stool samples should be taken for *Clostridium difficile* culture and toxin; change to fiber-containing formula
	Hypoalbuminemia	Albumin levels <2.5 g/dL result in decreased colloidal osmotic pressure* with accompanying peripheral edema (which may involve GI tract); try peptide-based, low-fat formula with MCT†
	Decreased bulk transit time and providing bulk	Fiber-containing formulas may help control diarrhea by normalizing GI
Nausea and vomiting, cramping, distention	High osmolality	Dilute formula to isotonic concentration if gastric residuals are consistently high; consider changing to isotonic formula
	Patient position	Reposition patient on right side to facilitate passage of gastric contents through pylorus
	Rapid increase in rate, volume, or concentration	Return to slower rate, and advance by smaller increments; advance only when tolerating current rate
	Delayed gastric emptying	Stop feedings for 2 hr and check residuals; check residuals every 2-4 hr (continuous feedings) and before administration (bolus feedings); reduce fat content in tube feeding; consider transpyloric feeding; monitor for drugs or disease that may influence gastric or intestinal motility; ambulation may help
	Lactose intolerance	Change to lactose-free formula
	Cold formula	Warm formula to room temperature
	Gastrointestinal (GI) tract obstruction	Stop feeding immediately
	Excessive fat in formula	Change to low-fat formula

TABLE 14-9	TUBE-FEEDING COMPLICATIONS, CAUSES, AND CORRECTIVE ACTIONS—cont'd	
PROBLEM	**POSSIBLE CAUSE**	**CORRECTIVE ACTION**
Constipation	Dehydration	Monitor intake and output; add free water if intake not greater than output by 500-1000 mL/day
	Decreased fiber	Use formula with fiber; make sure patient gets adequate water
	Medications	Evaluate medication side effects; suggest stool softener or bulk-forming laxative
	Inactivity	Increase patient activity if possible
	GI tract obstruction	Stop feedings
Mechanical		
Tube displacement	Coughing, vomiting	Replace tube, confirm placement before restarting feeding
	Dislodgment by patient	Replace tube; restrain patient if necessary; consider alternate feeding route
	Inadequate taping of tube	Position tube; tape securely
Tube obstruction	Improperly crushed medication	Use liquid form of medication, medications should not be crushed without first checking with pharmacy; rinse tube with 20 mL warm water before and after giving medications
	Medications mixed with incompatible formula	Review drug/nutrient interaction guidelines; flush tubing before and after adding medications
	Insufficient tube irrigation; failure to irrigate	Flush tubing with 20-50 mL warm water before and after bolus feeding, every 4-8 hr during continuous feedings, and whenever tube is disconnected or feeding is stopped
Pulmonary aspiration	Patient lying flat	Elevate head of bed 30-45 degrees during continuous feedings and for at least 30-60 minutes after bolus feedings
	Absent or weak gag reflexes	Feed into duodenum or jejunum
	Gastric reflux	May be caused by feeding tube, change to smaller bore tube; feed into duodenum or jejunum
	Delayed gastric emptying	Monitor gastric residual; residual >200 mL in patients with gastrostomy tubes and 100 mL in patients with gastrostomy tubes may indicate intolerance; hold feedings, recheck residual in 1-2 hr
	Improper tube placement	Confirm tube placement with radiology; reconfirm placement before each feeding and periodically during continuous feeding by injecting air into stomach and listening with a stethoscope
Mucosal damage	Extended use of large-bore tubes	Conscientious mouth and nose care; consider changing to small-bore tubing or permanent gastrostomy or jejunostomy feeding tubes
	Decreased salivary secretions caused by lack of chewing; mouth breathing	Moisten lips and mouth; let patient chew sugarless gum, gargle, or suck on anesthetic lozenges if appropriate
Metabolic		
Hyperosmolar dehydration	Hypertonic formula used without adequate water	Begin hypertonic feedings at slower rate; dilute with free water; or consider isotonic formula
Overhydration (fluid overload)	Refeeding patients with PEM; fluid overload	Restrict fluids; use concentrated formula
Hyponatremia	Congestive heart failure (CHF), cirrhosis, hypoalbuminemia, edema, ascites	Restrict fluids, administer diuretics, use concentrated formulas
	Excess GI losses	Monitor serum Na levels and hydration status, replace Na as needed

Continued

TABLE 14-9	TUBE-FEEDING COMPLICATIONS, CAUSES, AND CORRECTIVE ACTIONS—cont'd	
PROBLEM	**POSSIBLE CAUSE**	**CORRECTIVE ACTION**
Hypernatremia	Dehydration	Calculate patient's fluid needs: 35 mL/kg can be used unless patient's condition alters fluid needs, <30 mL/kg for the elderly
Hypokalemia	Refeeding syndrome, insulin administration, diuretics, diarrhea	Monitor electrolytes daily, replete with parenteral potassium
Hyperkalemia	Renal insufficiency, metabolic acidosis, anabolic metabolism	Reduce potassium intake, consider changing to a lower potassium tube-feeding formula, assess renal function
Hyperphosphatemia	Renal insufficiency	Use phosphate binder, consider changing formula
Hypophosphatemia	Refeeding syndrome, insulin administration	Replace phosphorus with parenteral supplement; monitor serum levels daily; once patient is repleted, monitor weekly
Hypomagnesemia	Refeeding syndrome, alcoholism	Replete with parenteral magnesium sulfate; monitor serum levels daily; once patient is repleted, monitor weekly
Hyperglycemia	Diabetes mellitus; temporary insulin resistance or insulin deficiency	Monitor blood sugars frequently, adjust insulin dose; reduce rate of tube feeding until blood sugar controlled; avoid formulas high in simple carbohydrates
Increased respiratory quotient; excess CO_2 production; respiratory insufficiency	Overfeeding (kcal), especially in form of carbohydrates	Balance kcal provided from fat, protein, and carbohydrates; consider using a higher-fat formula or adding modular fat
Rapid, excessive weight gain	Excess kcal, excess fluids, electrolyte balance	Decrease concentration or amount of formula; evaluate electrolyte status

*Pressure difference between the osmotic pressure of blood and that of tissue fluid or lymph; it is an important force in maintaining balance between blood and surrounding tissue and is usually caused by large particles such as protein molecules that will not pass through a membrane. Also called oncotic pressure.

†Medium chain triglycerides (MCTs), distinguished from other triglycerides by having 8 to 10 carbon atoms. MCTs are easily digested.

Data from Moore MC: *Pocket guide to nutrition assessment and care*, ed 6, St. Louis, 2009, Mosby/Elsevier; Mueller C, Bloch AS: Intervention: Enteral and parenteral nutrition support. In Mahan LK, Escott-Stump S, editors: *Krause's food & nutrition therapy*, ed 12, St. Louis, 2008, Saunders.

Once a patient is considered an appropriate candidate for HEN, the nutrition care plan must be modified to an appropriate home plan that includes tailoring the enteral formula, route and method of administration, and feeding schedule. Amount or type of formula may need to be adjusted to meet the patient's long-term nutritional requirements. Blenderized formulas are strongly discouraged because of reasons previously discussed. Route of HEN administration should also be examined for its ability to meet the patient's long-term needs and adequacy. If at all possible, the patient should be included in this decision. Keeping the functional level of the GI tract and risk of aspiration in mind, method of administration (continuous, intermittent, or bolus) should be altered if necessary according to patient preference, convenience, and cost.[34] Feeding schedules may need to be arranged around family members' schedules or other daily routines. They should be planned to augment patient comfort and convenience and to maximize nutritional benefit.

The patient should be stabilized on the home feeding regimen while still hospitalized before patient education is initiated. Education should include oral instructions, written guidelines, staff demonstration, return demonstration by the patient and caregiver, and their assumption of full responsibility for tube feeding before discharge from the hospital.[34] Figure 14-8 is an example of a HEN training checklist.

Patients should also be referred to a source for obtaining supplies such as formula and administration equipment before discharge. Some patients may need help in obtaining financial assistance. Most often, referral to home health agencies provides the necessary supplies, equipment, and staff for home follow-up visits, as well as assistance with third-party payers.

Parenteral Nutrition

Fortunately, there are alternatives for providing nutrients to patients when they can't or won't eat and tube feedings are contraindicated. Parenteral nutrition (PN) affords the provision of energy and nutrients intravenously. When infused into a large-diameter vein, such as the superior vena cava or subclavian vein (Figure 14-9), parenteral nutrition is often called central parenteral nutrition (CPN) or total parenteral nutrition (TPN). When a smaller, peripheral vein is used (usually in the forearm), parenteral nutrition is called peripheral parenteral nutrition (PPN). Other terms also are used to characterize parenteral nutrition: central venous nutrition

PURPOSE AND INSTRUCTIONS: This checklist will assist in identifying instructional responsibilities and aid in training patients in the skills needed for performing home enteral nutrition (HEN).

The nurse and dietitian will jointly instruct the patient on tube feeding administration and cares.

Date and initial section when instruction/demonstration is completed

RNs: Document training in Nursing Notes.

RDs: Document training in Progress Notes.

STAGE I: INITIATION OF HEN PROGRAM

———— Patient assessment   (Dietitian-Nurse)
          Medical-social-nutritional history
——— Plan of care outlined   (Dietitian-Nurse)
——— Identification of dismissal date _____ (Nurse)
——— Home enteral coordinator notified   (Dietitian)

STAGE II: IMPLEMENTATION OF HEN TRAINING   (Dietitian)

INTRODUCTION TO HEN PROGRAM   (Dietitian)

——— Discuss purpose
——— Introduce manual *Instructions for Tube Feeding at Home*

EQUIPMENT   (Dietitian-Nurse)
Discuss purpose, assembly, use, care, and cleaning of equipment.

	Discuss	Demonstrate	Patient Demonstrate
Feeding tube	———	———	———
Feeding bag	———	———	———
Gavage syringe	———	———	———
Enteral pump (if needed)	———	———	———

FORMULA—FLUIDS   (Dietitian)
———Show formula.
———Discuss purpose, type, amount, formula concentrations, fluid needs.
———Discuss preparation.
———Discuss administration schedule.
———Discuss weight expectations.

FIG 14-8 Home enteral training checklist. (From Nelson JK, Weckwerth JA: Home enteral nutrition. In Skipper A, editor: *Dietitian's handbook of enteral and parenteral nutrition*, Rockville, Md, 1989, Aspen.)

(CVN), peripheral venous nutrition (PVN), and hyperalimentation (hyperal).

TPN may mean the difference between life and death for patients who cannot be adequately nourished via the GI tract. But because of serious complications that may occur from TPN, it should be preserved for severely malnourished patients undergoing chemotherapy and major surgery.[35] Factors that should be considered before initiating TPN are the nature of the patient's GI dysfunction, severity of malnutrition, degree of hypercatabolism, medical prognosis, and the patient's wishes.[35]

Components of Parenteral Nutrition Solutions

PN solutions contain the same nutrients and components found in any enteral nutrition source: water, amino acids, dextrose, electrolytes, vitamins, and trace elements. Fat is also included, often by means of piggyback administration or by adding it directly to the PN solution (usually called a three-in-one solution, which is discussed later).

Carbohydrates. The most common carbohydrate used in PN is dextrose monohydrate. Used as an energy source, it yields 3.4 kcal/g because of its hydrated form. Dextrose solutions are available in initial concentrations of 5% through 70%. Higher-glucose concentrations are useful when a patient's fluids need to be restricted; lower concentrations are often used to help control hyperglycemia. Concentrations greater than 10% (final concentration) are hypertonic and must be delivered via CPN because the larger central vein can dilute the solution rapidly without damaging the blood vessel. Dextrose solutions are mixed with amino acids and

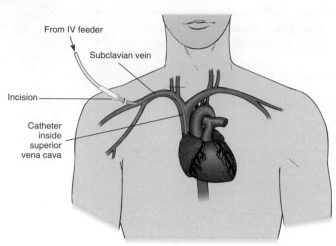

FIG 14-9 Placement of catheter for central parenteral nutrition, via the subclavian vein to the superior vena cava. (From Rolin Graphics.)

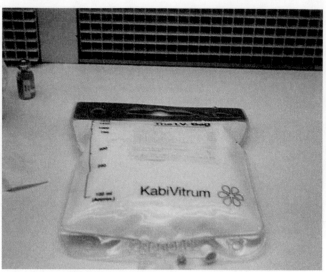

FIG 14-10 A three-in-one solution includes dextrose, amino acids, and lipids. (From Morgan SL, Weinsier RL: *Fundamentals of clinical nutrition*, ed 2, St. Louis, 1998, Mosby.)

other nutrients to form the final solution. Glucose needs and tolerances are important guidelines.[33]

Amino acids. Protein is provided in PN solutions as a mixture of essential and nonessential crystalline amino acids that are available with or without added electrolytes. It is important that the amino acids be used for protein synthesis and not be considered part of the solution's kcal source. Some facilities will not include protein kcal when calculating kcal content of PN solutions. Amino acid solutions are available in different concentrations as well as in different compositions of amino acids. Amino acid solutions are available for specialized protein needs such as renal failure, liver failure, stress, and trauma, but their efficacy is controversial.[33]

Fats. IV lipid emulsions are used as a concentrated energy source and to prevent the development of essential fatty acid deficiency. Commercial lipid emulsions are formulations of safflower oil, soybean oil, or a combination of the two, with glycerol added for isotonicity and egg phospholipid added as an emulsifying agent. The kcal density of lipid solutions is useful when volume restriction is necessary. A 10% fat emulsion yields 1.1 kcal/mL or 550 kcal per 500-mL bottle, and a 20% solution yields 2 kcal/mL or 1000 kcal per 500-mL bottle. Another plus for lipid emulsions is that kcal can be increased without increasing osmolality of PN solutions.[33]

Traditionally, lipid emulsions have been delivered peripherally using a piggyback system. Although IV lipids are useful in supplying most of the nonprotein kcal, care should be taken to not exceed 1 g of lipid/kg (adults).[33] Baseline serum triglyceride levels should be confirmed before administrating IV lipid emulsions and should be monitored according to institutional policy. If a lipid profile is ordered on a patient receiving lipids, the patient should not have received lipid emulsion for the 12 hours before blood is drawn.

Total nutrient admixtures. When lipid emulsions are added to dextrose and amino acid mixtures, the resulting solution is called a three-in-one mixture, or a TNA (Figure 14-10).[33] The advantage to this system is that it allows lipid

infusion over 24 hours, decreasing carbon dioxide production and reducing hepatic accumulation of fat induced by long-term glucose use.[33]

Electrolytes. Electrolytes and minerals can be provided by the general amino acid solution, as a combined electrolyte concentrate, or added separately as individual salts. Electrolytes and minerals are essential for normal body function and to accommodate excesses and deficiencies of minerals resulting from underlying disease processes. Commercial electrolyte solutions are available. Magnesium, phosphate, and potassium requirements increase in severely malnourished patients during refeeding or when higher levels of dextrose concentrations are used.[33]

Vitamins. Adult and pediatric multivitamin formulations for IV use are available commercially. In the event of frank vitamin deficiency, multiples of daily doses can be given in accordance with clinical status. Vitamin K is not included in adult preparations and must be given either intramuscularly or as an IV injectable added to the PN solution.

Trace elements. Trace elements are another essential component of PN solutions. Formulations that include zinc, copper, manganese, chromium, and selenium are available from commercial sources already combined, or institutional pharmacies may develop their own IV injectable formula.

Peripheral Parenteral Nutrition

PN solutions composed of less than 10% (final concentration) dextrose and/or less than 5% (final concentration) amino acids are hypertonic and can be administered only into central veins. PN solutions administered via peripheral veins must be isotonic to prevent damage to the vein. Isotonic PN solutions usually contain 5% to 10% dextrose (final concentration) and 3% to 5% amino acids, plus electrolytes, vitamins, minerals, and fat as needed. These nutrient components can provide only a limited amount of kcal and protein. PPN is most often used in situations in which only short-term nutrition support is needed in nonhypermetabolic conditions.

Monitoring Guidelines

Monitoring needs and protocols will vary among institutions and patient populations. Frequency of baseline parameter readings range from every 6 hours to a one-time baseline reading. Routine frequencies range from every 6 hours to biweekly or as needed. Specific parameters and recommendations for monitoring patients receiving TPN are listed in Box 14-5.

Complications

As with enteral tube feedings, complications can occur with PN. Most can be averted by following the recommendations for monitoring in Box 14-5. Others can be circumvented by adhering to stringent technique. Box 14-6 summarizes possible complications.

Technical complications are related to catheter placement and are not unique to parenteral nutrition. The most common technical complication results in pneumothorax, which can be prevented by careful insertion of the central line using proper technique. Septic complications, like technical complications, are not unique to parenteral nutrition. Infections can be local or systemic, and they usually occur because of poor technique in aseptic catheter care. Metabolic complications are the most common because metabolic requirements (electrolytes and energy) differ from patient to patient. The most common metabolic complication is hyperglycemia, which can be treated by administering insulin or by adding it to the solution, reducing the dextrose load, or ensuring total kcal load is not excessive.

Home Parenteral Nutrition

Home parenteral nutrition (HPN) enables selected patients who depend on PN to return to a reasonably normal lifestyle. A specialized catheter is used to reduce possibility of infection (Figure 14-11). The catheter is placed through a tunnel under the skin and exits the chest at a place where the patient or caretaker can care for it conveniently. As with HEN, HPN requires that both patient and caregiver are willing and able to perform daily procedures involved in administering the PN, which include monitoring laboratory values, temperature, weights, glucose measurements, and fluids. Home health care agencies may be used to provide equipment, supplies, and services.

Patients may be scheduled to receive HPN at night during sleep (cyclic TPN) to allow freedom to leave home or even work during the day. If the GI tract is functional, sometimes HPN is administered only selected nights per week to supplement oral intake. Although expensive, HPN costs less than hospitalization, allows the patient to leave the hospital sooner, and in many cases allows the patient to resume a productive lifestyle.

BOX 14-5   RECOMMENDATIONS FOR MONITORING PATIENTS RECEIVING TOTAL PARENTERAL NUTRITION (TPN)

Every 8 Hours
Vital signs
Temperature
Urine fractionals

Daily
Weight
Fluid intake and output
Serum electrolytes, glucose, creatinine, blood urea nitrogen (BUN) until stable; then twice weekly

Weekly
Serum magnesium, calcium, phosphorus, albumin
Liver function tests
Complete blood count
Review of actual oral, enteral, and TPN intake

Fluid Disorders
Urine sodium or fractional sodium excretion
Serum osmolality
Urine specific gravity

Protein Status
Nitrogen balance, serum prealbumin

Lipid Disorders
Serum triglycerides or lipid clearance test
Respiratory quotient
Essential fatty acids (if fat-free TPN is necessary)

Hepatic Encephalopathy
Plasma amino acids

Gastrointestinal Losses
Serum trace elements
Stool electrolytes

Respiratory Compromise
$Paco_2$
Indirect calorimetry, respiratory quotient

Acid-Base Disorders
Blood pH
Anion gap

Long-Term TPN
Body composition measures
Serum trace elements, vitamins

From Lenssen P: Management of total parenteral nutrition. In Skipper A, editor: *Dietitian's handbook of enteral and parenteral nutrition*, ed 2, Rockville, Md, 1998, Aspen.

BOX 14-6 COMPLICATIONS OF PARENTERAL NUTRITION

Technical Complications
Pneumothorax
Malposition of catheter
Subclavian artery puncture
Carotid artery puncture
Catheter embolism
Air embolism
Catheter obstruction
Thrombosis

Septic Complications
Catheter-related sepsis
Septic thrombosis

Metabolic Complications
Hyperglycemia
Hyperglycemic hyperosmolar nonketotic dehydration
Hypoglycemia
Hyperkalemia
Hypophosphatemia
Hypocalcemia

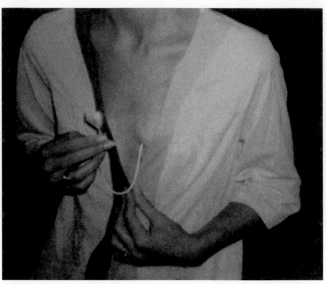

FIG 14-11 Catheter used for home central venous alimentation. (From Morgan SL, Weinsier RL: *Fundamentals of clinical nutrition*, ed 2, St. Louis, 1998, Mosby.)

Transitional Feedings

A period of adjustment, or weaning, is necessary before discontinuing nutritional support or when converting from one form of nutritional support to another. Transition to an adequate oral intake to maintain nutritional status will differ from patient to patient. Although the GI tract responds quickly to enteral feeding, patients who have been receiving TPN usually have decreased appetites and may take 1 to 2 weeks after complete cessation of TPN before they feel hungry; they may experience early satiety.[33] This necessitates gradual weaning from PN as enteral feeding (oral or tube) progresses to ensure continued adequate intake. Moreover, stopping TPN too quickly can result in hypoglycemia.

Parenteral to Oral or Tube Feeding

Long periods of PN without enteral feedings result in atrophy of the GI tract. If not contraindicated, minimal enteral intake (sips of dilute fruit juice) is encouraged to help maintain normal GI tract physiology and gut mucosal immunity. Before weaning from PN, judicious assessment of GI function is recommended to prevent problems with delayed gastric emptying, nausea, vomiting, or diarrhea.[33] As PN is tapered and oral or tube-feeding intake increases, it is important to document actual enteral intake, including fluids. This will facilitate maintenance of nutrient requirements. If oral feedings or isotonic formulas are not well tolerated, an elemental formula may be needed.

Tube to Oral Feeding

In addition to documentation of intake per tube and orally, it will be important to assess the patient's swallowing ability before offering oral feedings. Full liquids are usually offered first, followed by pureed or soft foods. Tube feedings should be stopped at least 1 hour before and after mealtime to promote appetite. As oral intake increases, tube-feeding volume should be decreased. When oral intake consistently exceeds two-thirds of energy requirements, the tube feedings can be discontinued.

SUMMARY

Although hospital nurses may perform some basic nutrition assessment and nutrition counseling, RDs can provide more in-depth knowledge of nutritional care, consult individually with patients, and participate in team meetings. Nurses, however, need to recognize that nutritional status of patients may be compromised by their stay in acute care hospitals, and be responsible for seeing that patients actually receive the nutrients they are served. Psychologic and physiologic aspects of illness, combined with effects of bed rest and the potential of iatrogenic malnutrition, emphasize the need for nutritional screening or monitoring to identify patients at nutritional risk.

Capacity for recovery from illness or disease depends in part on nutritional status. A comprehensive nutritional assessment is a procedure conducted by dietitians to determine appropriate medical nutrition therapy based on identified needs of the patient. Data are collected from several sources to assess patients' nutritional needs, often using the ABCD approach: **A**nthropometrics, **B**iochemical tests, **C**linical observations, and **D**iet evaluation. The nutritional care process provides for the unique nutritional needs of each patient. This can be accomplished through nutrition intervention to reduce nutritional risk. The nutritional care process, similar to the nursing process, uses a five-step procedure to identify and solve nutrition-related problems. The five steps are assessment, analysis, planning, implementation, and evaluation.

All patient nutrition is provided through food service delivery systems of acute care hospitals and long-term care facilities. Staff includes a director of the food and nutrition services department, clinical dietitians, as well as cooks, clerks, dishwashers, aides, and dietetic technicians.

To provide nutritional therapy, modified diets are developed to meet specific needs of patients as determined by the physician or dietitian. Dietary modifications of the regular diet may be made in two ways: qualitative or quantitative. Qualitative diet changes include modifications in consistency, texture, or nutrients. Quantitative diet changes include modifications in size and number of meals served or amounts of specific nutrients. By working together, nurses and dietetic professionals can most efficiently meet the nutritional and medical needs of patients.

Every patient deserves one of the most basic of all needs: nourishment. For obvious reasons, enteral nutrition (oral or tube feedings) is the preferred method of nutrition support. Feeding patients via the GI tract is safer, easier to administer, aids in maintaining GI tract integrity, and is as much as five times less expensive than PN. An array of commercial tube-feeding products that supply intact nutrients is available. When administered in the appropriate volume, 100% of the Dietary Reference Intakes (DRIs) for vitamins and minerals can be provided, as well as adequate amounts of energy and protein.

In those instances when patients are unable to obtain nutrition enterally, use of PN can literally be a lifesaving therapy. Peripheral or central infusions of amino acids, dextrose, fat emulsions, vitamins, and minerals can provide the ordinary or extraordinary nutrient needs of patients. Although not without risk, when managed through a team approach and routine monitoring, PN can provide a safe vehicle for meeting patients' nutritional goals.

THE NURSING APPROACH

Empathy and Dietary Teaching: Experiencing Modified Diets

An effective way for nursing students to learn about medical nutrition is to research modified dietary pattern guidelines and resources for specific disorders and conditions and then experience these diets personally. Following a modified diet even for 1 day provides students empathy with patients who need to change their regular eating habits and adhere to special dietary intakes. This dietary experience also supplies nursing students with strategies to reinforce teaching by dietitians.

PURPOSES OF THE EXPERIENCE

- Experience a modified diet (for health promotion or nutrition therapy) for 1 day (24 hours).
- Identify components or principles of the diet and specific foods allowed or restricted.
- Gain empathy for patients who are beginning nutrition therapy for disorders or conditions and need to adhere to modified dietary patterns.
- Reflect on teaching ideas for use with patients based on this experience.

CHOOSE ONE DIET AND FOLLOW IT FOR A 24-HOUR PERIOD OR LONGER

- High fiber and adequate liquid (for diverticulosis)
- Gluten-free (for celiac disease)
- Carbohydrate counting (for diabetes)
- Therapeutic Lifestyle Changes (TLC) diet (for coronary heart disease)
- Dietary Approaches to Stop Hypertension (DASH) diet (for hypertension)

ANSWER THESE QUESTIONS

1. List three health problems that may make this diet modification necessary or desirable.
2. What general guidelines were followed?
   a. What types of food were consumed?

   (1) Characteristics (e.g., food groups; temperature of foods; texture such as solid, pureed, or liquid)
   (2) Example foods
   (3) Rationale (scientific)
   b. What amounts of food were consumed?
   (1) Number of calories or specific measurements
   (2) Rationale
   c. At what time of day were foods consumed? (Create a food diary.)
   (1) Times and types of meals (e.g., breakfast)
   (2) Rationale
   d. What foods/beverages were avoided or restricted?
   (1) Specific foods/beverages
   (2) Rationale
3. What resources besides this textbook were used to learn about the diet?
4. What was your experience?
   a. How did you feel physically and/or emotionally?
   b. What did you learn by paying attention to food labels?
   c. What surprised you (e.g., foods you needed to include or foods you needed to eliminate)?
   d. What foods were challenging to include or eliminate (e.g., drinking eight glasses of water, consuming at least five fruits and vegetables a day, or eliminating soda)?
   e. What were other personal barriers that made following this diet difficult?
5. Are there special dietary products that may help people with this?
   a. Are special products needed? Why?
   b. What products (helpful or not) are available?
   c. Which of these products would you buy if on this diet for a month?
6. What are the pros and cons of this diet?
   a. Benefits
   b. Disadvantages and/or risks

Continued

THE NURSING APPROACH—cont'd

Empathy and Dietary Teaching: Experiencing Modified Diets—cont'd

7. What aspect of this experience gave you empathy for a patient who is following this diet?
   a. What dietary guidelines would be especially difficult if you followed this diet for 1 month? Why (e.g., cost, not wanting to be different from peers)?
   b. Was it necessary to learn a large amount of new information? Explain the steps taken to gain this information.
   c. Would it be difficult to follow this diet indefinitely? Discuss.

8. How would you teach a patient about this diet?
   a. What would you do to promote understanding of this diet (which foods and why)?
   b. What patient education materials would assist a patient to make wise food choices?
   c. What would be a reasonable goal that a patient could successfully achieve by the end of the first week?
   d. What would you recommend as the first step a patient should take when beginning this dietary pattern?

Nursing Diagnoses-Definitions and Classification 2009-2011. Copyright © 2009, 1994-2009 by NANDA International. Used by arrangement with Blackwell Publishing Limited, a company of John Wiley & Sons, Inc.

CRITICAL THINKING

Clinical Applications

Advances in medical technology have provided mechanisms to feed or nourish patients who once could not be fed or nourished. However, like most medical advances, it also provides dilemmas and difficult decisions about patient care. Nutrition care dilemmas occur when this technology will keep the patient alive, although the patient has no hope of ever living a normal life. What happens if a person loses decision-making capacity? Who should decide? What should be decided? Who should the surrogate be? What should that person do?

In a perfect world, the person should be a person designated by the patient while the patient still has decision-making capacity (durable power of attorney for health care). In the world we actually live in, when a patient does not have the capacity to make decisions or has not made an advanced directive, some family member without legal authority has to make decisions about life and death matters, often in a time of crisis. And what happens if family members of the patient do not agree on what should be done? Often, the dilemma involves legal action for resolution.

Such was the situation in the case of 41-year-old Terri Schiavo. Schiavo collapsed at home and experienced several minutes of oxygen deprivation to the brain in 1990, leaving her in a persistent vegetative state (PVS). In 1993, her husband decided to withdraw artificial nutrition, hydration, and life support on the grounds that she would not want to be kept alive this way. Her mother and father, the Schindlers, disagreed, and a controversy began in 1993 that lasted more than 12 years, going back and forth to court. What made the Schiavo case different from its predecessors (Karen Ann Quinlan of New Jersey and Nancy Cruzan of Missouri) was the involvement of Jeb Bush, then governor of Florida; the Florida state legislature; U.S. Congress; and 19 judges in six courts, including the Florida Supreme Court and federal courts. The courts continually sided with Terri's husband, whereas Bush and the Florida legislature sided with the Schindlers. Her feeding tube was removed on March 18, 2005, and Terri Schiavo died 13 days later. What are your thoughts about the following circumstances?

- An 85-year-old man who suffers from many physical problems, but is not terminally ill, refuses to be tube fed.
- A 57-year-old woman is hospitalized as a result of a severe psychiatric disorder that prohibits her from speaking or eating. She is bedridden in a fetal position and has a gastrostomy tube. She repeatedly dislodges the feeding tube and is combative when it is replaced.
- A 75-year-old woman's husband has requested termination of her nasogastric feedings. She is brain dead and has no living will.

WEBSITES OF INTEREST

Think Cultural Health

www.thinkculturalhealth.hhs.gov/
Supported by Office of Minority Affairs, site supplies resources and tools to promote cultural competency in health care.

National Center for Health Statistics
Centers for Disease Prevention and Control

www.cdc.gov/nchs/
Collects statistical data on every aspect of health status and use of health services by socioeconomic status, region, race or ethnicity, and other population attributes.

American Society of Parenteral and Enteral Nutrition (ASPEN)

www.nutritioncare.org
This association is dedicated to patients receiving the most appropriate nutritional therapy. Interactive features on the site allow users to post questions, register for conferences, and view links to other related organizations.

Data from Edelstein S: *Ethical dilemmas and decisions*, San Marcos, Calif, 1993, Nutrition Dimension; Jennings B: *Garrison Colloquium: The long dying of Terri Schiavo—private tragedy, public danger*, Garrison, NY, 2005 (May 20), The Hastings Center.

REFERENCES

1. Kortebein P, et al: Functional impact of 10 days of bed rest in healthy older adults, *J Gerontol A Biol Sci Med Sci* 63(10): 1076-1081, 2008.
2. Fessler TA: Malnutrition: a serious concern for hospitalized patients, *Today's Dietitian* 10(7):44-48, 2008.
3. Schlenkler E, Roth SL: *Williams' essentials of nutrition & diet therapy*, ed 10, St. Louis, 2010, Mosby.
4. Lacey K, Pritchitt E: Nutrition Care Process and model: ADA adopts road map to quality care and outcomes management, *J Am Diet Assoc* 103(8):1061-1072, 2003.
5. Lee RD, Nieman DC: *Nutritional Assessment*, ed 4, Boston, 2007, McGraw Hill.
6. The Joint Commission: *2009 Comprehensive accreditation manual for hospitals: the official handbook for Hospitals (CAMH)*, Oakbrook Terrace, Ill, 2009, Author.
7. Nelms MN, et al: *Understanding nutrition therapy and pathophysiology*, ed 2, Belmont, Calif, 2010, Wadsworth/ Thomson Learning.
8. Identifying patients at risk: ADA's definitions for nutrition screening and nutrition assessment, *J Am Diet Assoc* 94(8):838-839, 1994.
9. World Health Organization: *Physical status: The use and interpretation of anthropometry*, Technical Report Series 854, Geneva, 1995, Author.
10. Lee RD, Nieman DC: *Nutritional assessment*, ed 4, Boston, 2007, McGraw Hill.
11. Merrill RM, Richardson JS: Validity of self-reported height, weight, and body mass index: findings from the National Health and Nutrition Examination Survey, 2001-2006, *Prev Chronic Dis* 6(4):A121, 2009. Accessed January 24, 2010, from www.cdc.gov/PCD/issues/2009/oct/pdf/08_0229.pdf .
12. Gray D: Accuracy of recumbent height measurement, *JPEN J Parenter Enteral Nutr* 9:712-715, 1985.
13. Chumlea WC, et al: 1994. Prediction of stature from knee height for black and white adults and children with application to mobility-impaired or handicapped persons, *J Am Diet Assoc* 94:1385-1388, 1994.
14. Cockram DB, Baumgartner RN: Evaluation of accuracy and reliability of calipers for measuring recumbent knee height in elderly people, *Am J Clin Nutr* 52:397-400, 1990.
15. Chumlea WC, et al: *Nutritional assessment of the elderly through anthropometry*, Columbus, Ohio, 1984, Ross Laboratories.
16. Blackburn GL, Thornton PA: Nutritional and metabolic assessment of the hospitalized patient, *JPEN J Parenter Enteral Nutr* 1:11-22, 1977.
17. Chumlea WC, et al: Prediction of body weight for the nonambulatory elderly from anthropometry, *J Am Diet Assoc* 88:564-568, 1988.
18. Nelms M: Assessment of nutrition status and risk. In Nelms MN, et al, editors: *Understanding nutrition therapy and pathophysiology*, ed 2, Belmont, Calif, 2010, Wadsworth.
19. Lefton J, Malone AM: Anthropometric assessment. In Charney P, Malone AM, editors: *ADA Pocket Guide to Nutrition Assessment*, ed 2, Chicago, 2009, American Dietetic Association.
20. National Heart Lung and Blood Institute: *Obesity education initiative*. Accessed March 12, 2009, from www.nhlbi.nih.gov/ health/public/heart/obesity/lose_wt/risk.htm.
21. National Institutes of Health, National Heart, Lung, and Blood Institute: *Clinical guidelines of the identification, evaluation, and treatment of overweight and obesity in adults: the evidence report*, Pub No 98-4083, Bethesda, Md, 1998 (September), Author.
22. Moore MC: *Pocket Guide to Nutrition Assessment and Care*, ed 6, St. Louis, 2009, Mosby Elsevier.
23. American Dietetic Association Evidence Analysis Library: *Adult weight management guidelines*. Accessed January 24, 2010, from www.adaevidencelibrary.com.
24. Heimburger DC, Weinsier RL: *Handbook of clinical nutrition*, ed 3, St. Louis, 1997, Mosby.
25. Morgan SL, Weinsier RL: *Fundamentals of clinical nutrition*, ed 2, St. Louis, 1998, Mosby.
26. American Dietetic Association Nutrition Care Manual: *Clear liquid diet*. Accessed January 24, 2010, from www.nutritioncaremanual.org.
27. Murray DP, et al: Survey: use of clear and full liquid diets with or without commercially produced formulas, *JPEN J Parenter Enteral Nutr* 9:732-734, 1985.
28. American Dietetic Association Nutrition Care Manual: *Full liquid diet*. Accessed January 24, 2010, from www.nutritioncaremanual.org.
29. American Dietetic Association Evidence Analysis Library: *Critical illness nutrition practice recommendations*. Accessed January 31, 2010, from www.adaevidencelibrary.com.
30. Rombeau JL, Barot LR: Enteral nutrition therapy, *Surg Clin North Am* 61:605-620, 1981.
31. McClave S, et al: Guidelines for the provision and assessment of nutrition support therapy in the adult critically ill patient: Society of Critical Care Medicine (SCCM) and American Society for Parenteral and Enteral Nutrition (A.S.P.E.N.), *JPEN J Parenter Enteral Nutr* 33(3):277-316, 2009.
32. American Dietetic Association Nutrition Care Manual: *Tube feeding guidelines*. Accessed January 31, 2010, from www.nutritioncaremanual.org.
33. Mueller C, Bloch AS: Intervention: enteral & parenteral nutrition support. In Mahan LK, Escott-Stump S, editors: *Krause's food & nutrition therapy*, ed 12, St. Louis, 2008, Saunders.
34. Nelson JK, Weckwerth JA: Home enteral nutrition. In Skipper A, editor: *Dietitian's handbook of enteral and parenteral nutrition*, Rockville, Md, 1989, Aspen.
35. American Dietetic Association Nutrition Care Manual: *Parenteral/TPN guidelines*. Accessed January 31, 2010, from www.nutritioncaremanual.org.

Nutrition and Metabolic Stress

One of the first body functions affected by impaired nutritional status is the immune system.

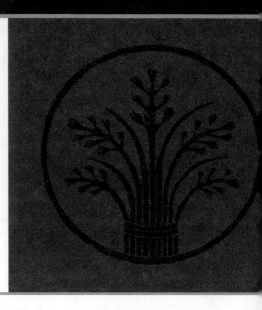

evolve WEBSITE

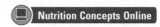

http://evolve.elsevier.com/Grodner/foundations/

ROLE IN WELLNESS

In its never-ending quest to maintain homeostasis, the human body responds to stress, physiologic or psychologic, with a chain reaction that involves the central nervous system and hormones that affect the entire body. Magnitude and duration of the stress determine just how the body will react. It is important for nurses to understand metabolic changes that take place in reaction to stress, both in uncomplicated stress that is present when patients are at nutritional risk and in more multifarious variations that result from severe stress brought about by trauma or disease.

IMMUNE SYSTEM

One of the first body functions affected by impaired nutritional status is the immune system. When metabolic stress develops, hormonal and metabolic changes subdue the immune system's ability to protect the body. This activity is further depressed if impaired nutritional status accompanies the metabolic stress. A deadly cycle often develops: impaired immunity leads to increased risk of disease, disease impairs nutritional status, and compromised nutritional status further impairs immunity. Recovery requires that this cycle be broken.

Role of Nutrition

For the immune system to function optimally, adequate nutrients must be available. A well-nourished body will not be ravaged by infections the way a poorly nourished body will be. (See the *Cultural Considerations* box, The Process of Balance, for a multicultural perspective on balanced eating for good health.) To prove this point, think of the leading causes of death in industrialized countries such as the United States. The majority are chronic diseases associated with lifestyle. In developing countries, however, infections lead to high morbidity and mortality rates, especially in children, largely because of the high rate of protein-energy malnutrition (PEM). The majority of people in the United States who have serious problems with malnutrition and infections are (1) those with severe medical problems, (2) those who suffer from major metabolic stress, (3) those who suffer from a diseased state that causes metabolic stress and/or decreased nutrient intake and/or nutrient malabsorption, and (4) those who have poor nutritional intakes as a result of socioeconomic conditions (e.g., poverty, homelessness).

Compromised nutritional status creates a vulnerable immune system by making it difficult to mount both a stress response and an immune response when confronted with a metabolic stress. A number of nutrients are known to affect immune system functioning. It is difficult to determine which specific nutrient factor results in symptoms when a patient is malnourished because of overlapping nutrient deficiencies combined with illness and accompanied by weakness, anorexia, and infection.[1]

Immune system components affected by malnutrition include mucous membrane, skin, gastrointestinal tract, T-lymphocytes, macrophages, granulocytes, and antibodies. The effects on the mucous membrane are that the microvilli become flat, which reduces nutrient absorption and decreases antibody secretions. Integrity of the skin may be compromised as it loses density, and wound healing is slowed. Injury to the gastrointestinal tract because of malnutrition may increase risk of infection-causing bacteria spreading from inside the tract to outside the intestinal system. T-lymphocytes are affected as the distribution of T cells is depressed. The effect on macrophages and granulocytes requires that more time is needed for phagocytosis kill time and lymphocyte

CULTURAL CONSIDERATIONS

The Process of Balance

What is a balanced way of eating for good health? To most Americans, the response is to eat foods from each of the food groups, with particular emphasis on fruits and vegetables. Among other cultures, foods consumed to achieve balance and good health do not follow the American food categories. The Chinese system of *yin-yang* sorts foods into *yin* (bean curd or tofu, bean sprouts, bland and boiled foods, broccoli, carrots, duck, milk, potatoes, spinach, and water) and *yang* (bamboo, beef, broiled meat, chicken, eggs, fried foods, garlic, ginger-root, green peppers, and tomatoes). Foods should be selected from each group to achieve balance. Which foods belong in each group may vary by region, but some foods such as rice and noodles are considered neutral. The overall goal is to maintain the harmony of the body with adjustments for climate variations and physiologic factors.

Balance is also the focus of the *hot-cold classification* of foods practiced in the Middle East, Latin American, India, and the Philippines. This concept is derived from the Greek humoral medicine based on the four natural world characteristics of air-cold, fire-hot, water-moist, and earth-dry related to the body humors of hot and moist (blood), cold and moist (phlegm), hot and dry (yellow/green bile), and cold and dry (black bile).

Although this concept is related to the development of disease and their remedies, it also applies to foods. The hot and cold aspects of specific foods are emphasized. This does not relate to the actual temperature of the foods but to their innate characteristics. To achieve balance, eating cold foods offsets hot foods. The list of foods in each category varies among subgroups within each culture. Often, younger generations follow this concept but without knowing that it is based on the hot-cold theory of balance.

Application to nursing: Each of the cultures, subscribing to the yin-yang concept and the hot-cold theory, has sizable populations in the United States. When treating Americans of Chinese, Indian, Latino, Middle Eastern, and Filipino descent, these concepts of food selection to achieve health and harmony may affect client food choices. Although healthy selections are often selected, subtle effects may occur. For example, within the hot-cold theory, pregnancy may be considered "hot" as are vitamins. Consequently, vitamins are not taken during pregnancy because to do so would not restore balance. If a client seems unwilling to follow dietary and supplement recommendations, discussion of these classifications and ways to remedy the situation can be created.

Data from Kittler PG, Sucher KP: *Food and culture in America: A nutrition handbook,* ed 5, Belmont, Calif, 2007, Wardsworth.

TABLE 15-1	ROLE OF NUTRIENTS AND NUTRITIONAL STATUS ON IMMUNE SYSTEM COMPONENTS	
IMMUNE SYSTEM COMPONENT	**EFFECTS OF MALNUTRITION**	**VITAL NUTRIENTS**
Mucus	Decreased antibody secretions	Vitamin B_{12}, biotin, vitamins B_6 and C
Gastrointestinal tract	Flat microvilli, increased risk of bacterial spread to outside GI tract	Arginine, omega-3 fatty acids
Skin	Integrity compromised, density reduced, wound healing slowed	Protein, vitamins A and C, niacin, zinc, copper, linoleic acid, vitamin B_{12}
T-lymphocytes	Depressed T-cell distribution	Protein, arginine, omega-3 fatty acids, vitamins A, B_{12}, B_6, folic acid, thiamine, riboflavin, niacin, pantothenic acid, zinc, iron
Macrophages and granulocytes	Longer time for phagocytosis kill time and lymphocyte activation	Protein, vitamins A, C, B_{12}, B_6, folic acid, thiamine, riboflavin, niacin, zinc, iron
Antibodies	Reduced antibody response	Protein, vitamins A, C, B_{12}, B_6, folic acid, thiamine, biotin, riboflavin, niacin

activation to occur. Antibodies may be less available because of damage to the antibody response[1]. Table 15-1 outlines how specific nutrient deficiencies affect immune system functions; note that fat and water-soluble vitamins, fatty acids, minerals, and protein are important for adequate functioning of most immune system components.

THE STRESS RESPONSE

The body's response to metabolic stress depends on the magnitude and duration of the stress. Stress sets up a chain reaction that involves hormones and the central nervous system that affects the entire body. Whether stress is uncomplicated (altered food intake or activity level) or multifarious

(trauma or disease), metabolic changes take place throughout the body.

According to Gould,[2] the body's constant response to minor changes brought about by needs or environment was first noted in 1946 by Hans Selye when he described the "fight or flight" response, or general adaptation syndrome (GAS). The body constantly responds to minor changes to maintain homeostasis. Research following Selye's work has identified that the stress response involves an integrated series of actions that include the hypothalamus and hypophysis, sympathetic nervous system, adrenal medulla, and adrenal cortex.[2] Significant effects of this response to stress are outlined in Table 15-2. These responses to stress produce multiple changes in metabolic processes throughout the body. The effect of

TABLE 15-2   EFFECTS OF THE STRESS RESPONSE*

TARGET ORGAN	HORMONAL RESPONSE	PHYSIOLOGIC RESPONSE	SIGNS/SYMPTOMS
Sympathetic nervous system and adrenal medulla	Norepinephrine	Vasoconstriction	Pallor, decreased glomerular filtration rate, nausea, elevated blood pressure
Adrenal medulla	Epinephrine	Vasoconstriction	See above
		Increased heart rate	Elevated blood pressure
		Vasodilation	Increased skeletal muscle function
		Central nervous system (CNS) stimulation	More alert, increased muscle tone
		Bronchodilation	Increased O_2
		Glycogenolysis, lipolysis, gluconeogenesis	Increased blood glucose
Adrenal pituitary and cortex	Cortisol (glucocorticoids)	CNS stimulation	Increased blood glucose, increased serum amino acids, delayed wound healing
		Protein catabolism, gluconeogenesis	
		Stabilize cardiovascular system	Enhance catecholamine action
		Gastric secretion	Ulcers
		Inflammatory response decreased	Decreased white blood cells (WBCs)
		Allergic response decreased	
		Immune response decreased	
	Aldosterone (mineralocorticoid)		Retain sodium and water, increased blood volume, increased blood pressure
Posterior pituitary	Antidiuretic hormone	Water reabsorbed, increased blood volume, increased blood pressure	
Other feedback mechanisms	Aldosterone and antidiuretic hormone	See above	See above

*Possible complications include hypertension, tension headaches, insomnia, diabetes mellitus, infection, heart failure, peptic ulcer, and fatigue.
Data from Gould BE: *Pathophysiology for the health-related professions*, ed 3, Philadelphia, 2006, Saunders.

different levels of stress on metabolic rate is illustrated in Figure 15-1.

Starvation

If someone must involuntarily go without food, that can be defined as *starvation*. If we withhold food from ourselves, such as when we try to lose weight, that act can be defined as *dieting* or *fasting*. Whatever the cause of inadequate food intake and nourishment, results are the same. After a brief period of going without food (fasting) or an interval of nutrient intake below metabolic needs, the body is able to extract stored carbohydrate, fat, and protein (from muscles and organs) to meet energy demands.

Liver glycogen is used to maintain normal blood glucose levels to provide energy for cells. Although readily available, this source of energy is limited, and glycogen stores are usually depleted after 8 to 12 hours of fasting. Unlike glycogen stores, lipid (triglyceride) stores may be substantial, and the body also begins to mobilize this energy source. As the amount of liver glycogen decreases, mobilization of free fatty acids from adipose tissue increases to provide energy needed by the nervous system. After approximately 24 hours without energy intake (especially carbohydrates), the prime source of glucose is from gluconeogenesis.[3]

Some body cells, brain cells in particular, use mainly glucose for energy. During early starvation (about 2 to 3 days of starvation), the brain uses glucose produced from muscle protein. As muscle protein is broken down for energy, the level of branched-chain amino acids (BCAA) consisting of leucine, isoleucine, and valine increases in circulation, although they are primarily metabolized directly inside muscle.[3] The body does not store any amino acids as it does glucose and triglycerides; therefore, the only sources of amino acids are lean body mass (muscle tissue), vital organs including heart muscle, or other protein-based body constituents such as enzymes, hormones, immune system components, or blood proteins. By the second or third day of starvation, approximately 75 g of muscle protein can be catabolized daily, a level inadequate to supply full energy needs of the brain.[3] At this point, other sources of energy become more available. Fatty acids are hydrolyzed from the glycerol backbone, and both free fatty acids and glycerol are released into the bloodstream. Free fatty acids are used as indicated earlier, and glycerol can be used by the liver to generate glucose via the process of gluconeogenesis.

As starvation is prolonged, the body preserves proteins by mobilizing more and more fat for energy (Figure 15-2). Ketone body production from fatty acids is accelerated, and

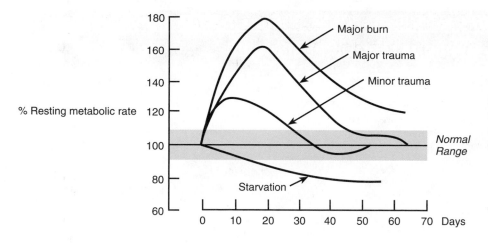

FIG 15-1 Percent resting metabolic rate. (From Kinney JM, et al: *Nutrition and metabolism in patient care*, Philadelphia, 1988, Saunders.)

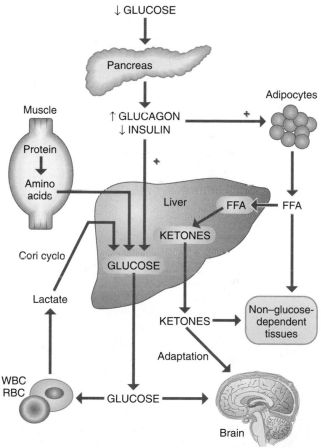

Fig 15-2 Metabolic changes in starvation. *FFA,* Free fatty acids; *RBC,* red blood cells; *WBC,* white blood cells. (From Simmons RL, Steed DL: *Basic science review for surgeons,* Philadelphia, 1992, Saunders.)

the body's requirement for glucose decreases. Although some glucose is still vital for brain cells and red blood corpuscles, these and other body tissues obtain the major proportion of their energy from ketone bodies. Muscle protein is still being catabolized but at a much lower rate, which prolongs survival.

An additional defense mechanism of the body to conserve energy is to slow its metabolic rate, thereby decreasing energy needs. As a result of declining metabolic rate, body temperature drops; activity level decreases, and sleep periods increase—all to allow the body to preserve energy sources. If starvation continues, intercostal muscles necessary for respiration are lost, which may lead to pneumonia and respiratory failure. Starvation will continue until adipose stores are exhausted.

Severe Stress

Whether stress is accidental (e.g., from broken bones or burns) or necessary (e.g., from surgery), the body reacts to these stresses much as it does to the stress of starvation—with a *major* difference. During starvation, the body's metabolic rate slows, becoming hypometabolic. During severe stress, the body's metabolic rate rises profoundly, thus becoming hypermetabolic.

The body's response to stress can be summarized by two phases: ebb phase and flow phase (Figure 15-3). The *ebb phase,* or *early phase* (Table 15-3), begins immediately after the injury and is identified by decreased oxygen consumption, hypothermia (lowered body temperature), and lethargy. The major medical concern during this time is to maintain cardiovascular effectiveness and tissue perfusion. As the body responds to injury, the ebb phase evolves into the flow phase, usually about 36 to 48 hours after injury.[4] The *flow phase* is characterized by increased oxygen consumption, hyperthermia (increased body temperature), and increased nitrogen excretion, as well as expedited catabolism of carbohydrate, protein, and triglycerides to meet the increased metabolic demands.[4] The flow stage will last for days, weeks, or months until the injury is healed.

Multiple stresses result in increased catabolism and even greater loss of body proteins. Unfortunately, some stresses that patients are obliged to endure are iatrogenic. Think, for example, of the series of stresses a patient admitted for elective surgery might experience. Preoperatively, most surgical patients receive only clear liquids or nothing by mouth (NPO). After surgery, they may remain NPO until the return

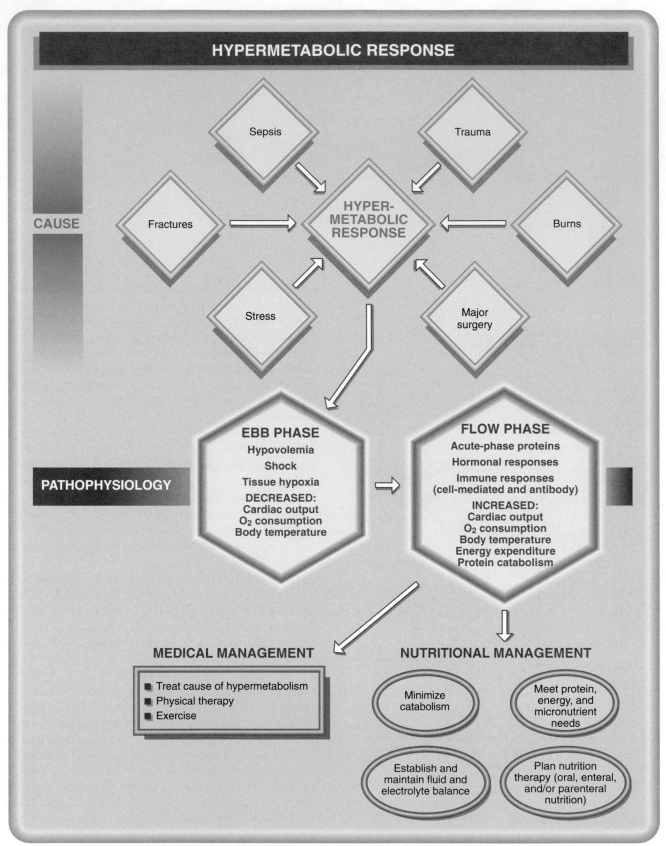

FIG 15-3 Hypermetabolic response to stress pathophysiology algorithm. (From Mahan LK, Escott-Stump S: *Krause's food & nutrition therapy,* ed 12, Philadelphia, 2008, Saunders. Algorithm content developed by John Anderson, and Sanford C. Garner, 2000. Updated by Marion F. Winkler and Ainsley Malone, 2002.).

TABLE 15-3	METABOLIC RESPONSES TO SEVERE STRESS	
EBB PHASE	**FLOW PHASE**
↓ Oxygen consumption	↑ Oxygen consumption
↓ Cardiac output	↑ Cardiac output
↓ Plasma volume	↑ Plasma volume
Hypothermia	Hyperthermia
	↑ Nitrogen excretion
↓ Insulin levels	Normal or elevated insulin levels
Hyperglycemia	Hyperglycemia
Hypovolemia	
Hypotension	
↑ Lactate	Normal lactate
↑ Free fatty acids	↑ Free fatty acids
↑Catecholamines, glucagon, cortisol	↑ Catecholamines, glucagon, cortisol
Insulin resistance	↑ Insulin resistance

of bowel sounds, and then progress through clear liquid and full-liquid diets until they can tolerate food.

If the patient is in poor nutritional status before the stress of surgery, he or she is at greater risk for developing pneumonia or a wound infection accompanied by fever as a result of decreased protein synthesis. As in starvation, energy requirements will be met from endogenous sources (within the body) if exogenous sources (outside the body) are not available or adequate. Thus intercostal muscles may be depleted, leading to pneumonia, or inadequate amino acids may be available to synthesize antibodies, leading to impaired immune response to infection. Either complication has a negative impact on metabolic demands.

Nutrients affected by hypermetabolic stress include protein, vitamins, and minerals, as well as related nutritional concerns for total energy and fluid intake. During moderate metabolic stress, protein requirements have been reported to increase from 0.8 g/kg body weight (amount recommended for an average healthy adult) to 1 to 1.5 g/kg body weight and for severe stress (e.g., thermal injuries exceeding 20% total body surface area) can rise to 1.5 to 2 g/kg body weight.[1] These levels are based on sufficient energy consumption to allow for protein synthesis. Requirements of vitamins and minerals all increase during stress. Tissue repair especially depends on adequate intakes of vitamin C, zinc, calcium, magnesium, manganese, and copper. At the least, Dietary Reference Intake (DRI) levels of nutrients should be consumed, preferably from foods rather than from vitamin or mineral supplements. Achieving requirements through food intake also supports provision of sufficient kcal to meet increased energy demands during critical illness.

Several formulas have been used to determine the energy needs of patients experiencing hypermetabolic stress. The Mifflin-St. Jeor equation best predicts resting metabolic rate (RMR).[5] Total energy expenditure can be determined by multiplying RMR by activity level and an injury factor.[6] Activity level considers energy required if the patient is confined to bed or is ambulatory. Severity of injury is a factor based on whether the injury is caused by major or minor surgery, mild to severe infection, skeletal or blunt trauma, or burns (based on percentage of body surface area affected) (Box 15-1).

Registered dietitians, in collaboration with the medical team, use these formulas to determine energy requirements. As factor assessments change, nurses can alert either the registered dietitian or other members of the medical team to ensure adequate energy provision.

Fluid requirements during hypermetabolic stress are based on age, reflecting age-related modifications of body composition. For adults younger than 55 years, fluid needs are calculated at 35 to 40 mL/kg body weight. Adults between the ages of 55 and 65 years require a lower amount, 30 mL/kg body weight; and for adults older than age 65, 25 mL/kg body weight is recommended.[7]

Effects of Stress on Nutrient Metabolism

Protein Metabolism

Even if adequate carbohydrate and fat are available, protein (skeletal muscle) is mobilized for energy (amino acids are converted to glucose in the liver). There is decreased uptake of amino acids by muscle tissue, and increased urinary excretion of nitrogen[8] (Figure 15-4). Some nonessential amino acids may become conditionally essential during episodes of metabolic stress. During stress, glutamine is mobilized in large quantities from skeletal muscle and lung to be used directly as a fuel source by intestinal cells (Figure 15-5).[9] Glutamine also plays a significant role in maintaining intestinal immune function and enhancing wound repair by supporting lymphocyte and macrophage proliferation, hepatic gluconeogenesis, and fibroblast function.[9]

Carbohydrate Metabolism

Hepatic glucose production is increased and disseminated to peripheral tissues, although proteins and fats are being used for energy. Insulin levels and glucose use are in fact increased, but hyperglycemia that is not necessarily resolved by the use of exogenous insulin[8,9] is present. This appears, to some extent, to be driven by an elevated glucagon-to-insulin ratio.[9]

Fat Metabolism

To support hypermetabolism and increased gluconeogenesis, fat is mobilized from adipose stores to provide energy (lipolysis) as the result of elevated levels of catecholamines along with concurrent decrease in insulin production.[8] If hypermetabolic patients are not fed during this period, fat stores and proteins are rapidly depleted. This malnutrition increases susceptibility to infection and may contribute to multiple organ dysfunction syndrome (MODS), sepsis, and death.[9]

Hydration/Fluid Status

Increased fluid losses can result from fever (increased perspiration), increased urine output, diarrhea, draining wounds, or diuretic therapy.[8]

Energy requirements are highly individual and may vary widely from person to person. Total kcal requirements are dependent on the basal energy expenditure (BEE) plus the presence of trauma, surgery, infection, sepsis, and other factors. The most accurate method to determine energy needs is indirect calorimetry. When indirect calorimetry cannot be performed, use of predictive formulas is necessary.

Predictive Formulas

Formulas with the best prediction accuracy for critically ill patients are Penn State (2003a version), Swinamer, and Ireton-Jones (1992), while inaccuracy of predicted and actual energy needs result in under- or overfeeding.

Penn State

$RMR = BMR (0.85) + V_E (33) + T_{max} (175) - 6433$

Basal metabolic rate (BMR) is calculated using the Harris-Benedict equation, minute ventilation (V_E) in liters per min (L/min), and maximum temperature (T_{max}) in degrees Celsius.

Swinamer

Energy Expenditure = 945 (BSA) − 6.4 (age) + 108 (T) + 24.2 (breaths/min) + 81.7 (VT) − 4349

Body surface area (BSA) in squared meters (m²), temperature (T) in degrees Celsius, and tidal volume (VT) in liters per minute (L/min).

Ireton-Jones

Spontaneously breathing Ireton-Jones Energy Equations (IJEE) (s) = 629 − 11 (A) + 25 (W) − 609 (O); *Ventilator dependent IJEE (v)* = 1925 − 10 (A) + 5 (W) + 281 (S) + 292 (T) + 851 (B)

Age (A) in years, body weight (W) in kilograms (kg), sex (S, male = 1, female = 0), diagnosis of trauma (T, present = 1, absent = 0), diagnosis of burn (B, present = 1, absent = 0), obesity >30% above initial body weight from body mass index >27 (present = 1, absent = 0).

Other formulas, particularly the Harris-Benedict formula (with or without adjustments for activity/stress), Ireton-Jones (1997), and the Fick equation are not appropriate to use for RMR determination in this population. These equations do not have adequate prediction accuracy because they were developed for the healthy population.

Protein Requirements

Additional protein is required to synthesize the proteins necessary for defense and recovery, to spare lean body mass, and to reduce the amount of endogenous protein catabolism for gluconeogenesis.

Vitamin/Mineral Needs

Needs for most vitamins and minerals increase in metabolic stress; however, no specific guidelines exist for provision of vitamins, minerals, and trace elements. It is usually believed that if the increased kcal requirements are met, adequate amounts of most vitamins and minerals are usually provided. In spite of this, vitamin C, vitamin A or beta carotene, and zinc may need special attention.

Fluid Needs

Fluid status can affect interpretation of biochemical measurements as well as anthropometry and physical examination. Fluid requirements can be estimated using several different methods.

Micronutrient Supplementation

Vitamin C: 500 to 1000 mg/day in divided dose
Vitamin A: one multivitamin tablet containing vitamin A, one to four times daily
Zinc sulfate: 220 mg, one to three times daily

ACTIVITY	ACTIVITY FACTOR	CLINICAL STATUS	ENERGY STRESS FACTOR	G PROTEIN/ KG BODY WT/DAY
Bed rest	1.2	Elective surgery	1-1.2	1-1.5
Ambulatory	1.3	Multiple trauma	1.2-1.6	1.3-1.7
		Severe infection	1.2-1.6	
		Peritonitis	1.05-1.25	
		Multiple/ long bone fractures	1.1-1.3	
		Infection with trauma	1.3-1.5	
		Sepsis	1.2-1.4	1.2-1.5
		Closed head injury	1.3	
		Cancer	1.1-1.45	
		Burns (% BSA)	1.8-2.5	
		0%-20%	1-1.5	
		20%-40%	1.5-1.85	
		40%-100%	1.85-2.05	
		Fever	1.2 per 1° C >37° C	

BSA, Body surface area.

FLUID REQUIREMENTS BASED ON:		WATER (ML)
Weight		100 mL/kg for first 10 kg
		50 mL/kg for next 10 kg
		20 mL/kg for each kg above 20 kg
Age and weight	16-30 yr (active)	40 mL/kg/day
	20-55 yr	35 mL/kg/day
	55-75 yr	30 mL/kg/day
	>75 yr	25 mL/kg/day
Energy	1 mL/kcal	
Fluid balance	Urine output + 500 mL/day	

Data from American Dietetic Association Evidence Analysis Library: *Determination of resting metabolic rate in critical illness.* Accessed February 14, 2010, from www.adaevidencelibrary.com; Heimburger DC, Ard J: *Handbook of clinical nutrition,* ed 4, St. Louis, 2006, Mosby; Moore MC: *Mosby's pocket guide to nutritional care,* ed 5, St. Louis, 2005, Mosby; Winkler MF, Malone AM: Medical nutrition therapy for metabolic stress: sepsis, trauma, burns and surgery. In Mahan LK, Escott-Stump S, editors: *Krause's food & nutrition therapy,* ed 12, Philadelphia, 2008, Saunders.

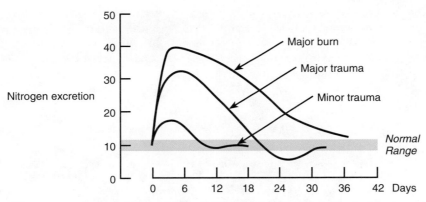

FIG 15-4 Nitrogen excretion. (From Kinney JM, et al: *Nutrition and metabolism in patient care*, Philadelphia, 1988, Saunders.)

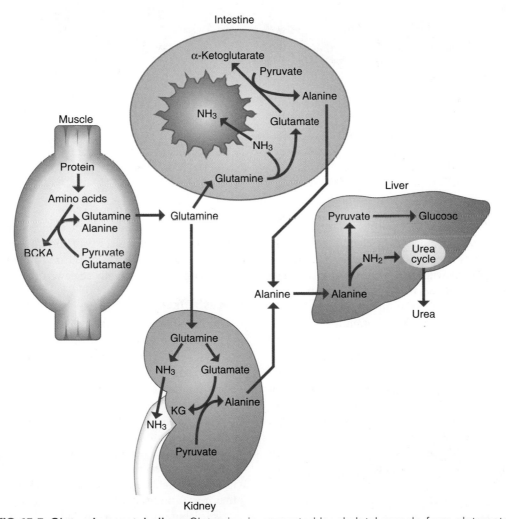

FIG 15-5 Glutamine metabolism. Glutamine is generated by skeletal muscle from glutamate by transamination. Glutamine is taken up by the intestine and kidney, where deamination and ammonia elimination occur. The glutamate formed is transaminated with pyruvate to form alanine, which goes to the liver for gluconeogenesis, and alpha-ketoglutarate (KG), which can be used for energy production by the muscle or kidney. *NH₂,* amine; *NH₃,* ammonia. (From Simmons RL, Steed DL: *Basic science review for surgeons,* Philadelphia, 1992, Saunders.)

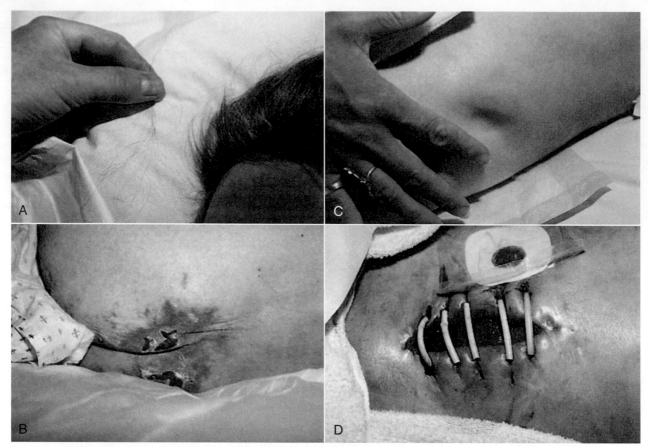

FIG 15-6 Clinical findings in kwashiorkor. **(A),** Easy, painless hair pluckability; **(B),** pitting edema; **(C),** skin breakdown; and **(D),** delayed wound healing. (From Morgan S, Weinsier R: *Fundamentals of clinical nutrition,* ed 2, St. Louis, 1998, Mosby.)

Vitamins and Minerals

Just as kcal needs increase during hypermetabolic conditions, so, too, do needs for most vitamins and minerals. And if kcal needs are met, the patient will most likely receive adequate amounts of most vitamins and minerals. Special attention, however, should be given to vitamin C (ascorbic acid), vitamin A or beta-carotene, and zinc.[6] Vitamin C is crucial for the collagen formation necessary for optimal wound healing. Supplements of 500 to 1000 mg/day are recommended.[6] Vitamin A and beta-carotene (vitamin A's precursor) play an important role in the healing process in addition to their role as antioxidants. Zinc increases the tensile strength (force required to separate the edges) of a healing wound. Supplements of 220 mg/day zinc sulfate (orally) when stable are commonly used.[6] Additional zinc may be necessary if there are unusually large intestinal losses (small bowel drainage or ileostomy drainage).[6]

Protein-Energy Malnutrition

Inadequate intake of energy, particularly from protein, can result in acute or chronic protein deficiency, or PEM. PEM can be primary or secondary. Primary PEM is the result of inadequate intake of nutrients. Secondary PEM results from inadequate nutrient consumption caused by some disease state that impairs food consumption, interferes with nutrient absorption, or increases nutritional requirements. PEM, kwashiorkor, and marasmus are presented in detail in Chapter 6 and only briefly reviewed here.

Kwashiorkor

The clinical syndrome kwashiorkor is diagnosed largely on the basis of results of laboratory tests on patients in the acute state of poor protein intake and stress. Although etiologic mechanisms are not understood, it appears that normal adaptive response of protein sparing seen in fasting fails. Kwashiorkor may develop in as little as 2 weeks.

Patients with kwashiorkor appear to be adequately nourished, tending to have normal fat reserves and muscle mass (or even above normal). However, findings such as easily plucked hair, edema, skin breakdown, and delayed wound healing are telltale signs of kwashiorkor (Figure 15-6) and that it is a condition of impaired protein synthesis.[6] Characteristic laboratory changes include reduced levels of albumin, prealbumin (transthyretin), and retinol binding protein.[6]

Marasmus

Another form of PEM—marasmus—is manifested by severe loss of fat and muscle tissue as a result of chronic energy deficiency. Unlike kwashiorkor, an individual with

BOX 15-2   REFEEDING SYNDROME

Refeeding a patient with protein-energy malnutrition can result in many complications if not initiated correctly. In fact, refeeding can be fatal if done too rapidly. Introduction of excess protein and kcal can overload various enzymatic and physiologic functions that may have adapted during malnutrition. As refeeding is initiated, rapid changes occur in thyroid and endocrine function, causing increased oxygen consumption, cardiac output, insulin secretion, and energy expenditure. Refeeding syndromes are associated more with parenteral (feeding via circulatory system; see Chapter 14) nutrition than enteral (feeding via GI tract; see Chapter 14), but discretion and common sense are of key importance in refeeding semistarved and chronically ill patients. The pathogenesis of refeeding syndrome is described in the following sections.

Phosphorus

During starvation, total phosphorus is greatly reduced. During refeeding there is an increase in cellular influx of phosphorus, leading to severe extracellular **hypophosphatemia**. This will occur in enteral and parenteral feeding but can be prevented by a slower rate of nutrient infusion. Hypophosphatemia can also cause **cardiac decompensation**. (Sodium shifts are thought to play a separate, additional role in cardiac overload.) In addition, hypophosphatemia can lead to tissue **hypoxia** and subsequent altered tissue function.

Potassium

Because potassium is greatly reduced from tissue, and under anabolic conditions, extracellular fluid levels fall (hypomagnesemia), which in turn can lead to cardiac depression, arrhythmias, neuromuscular weakness, irritability, and **hyporeflexia**.

Magnesium

Magnesium is also greatly reduced from tissue, and under anabolic conditions, extracellular fluid levels fall (hypomagnesemia), which in turn can lead to cardiac depression, arrhythmias, neuromuscular weakness, irritability, and hyporeflexia.

Glucose Metabolism

When glucose is reintroduced via high-glucose or high-volume enteral or parenteral feedings, the starved patient loses the stimulus for gluconeogenesis (an important adaptive mechanism during nutritionally depletion). Suppression of gluconeogenic glucose production leads to a corresponding decrease in amino acid use and negative nitrogen balance. Additionally, hyperglycemia can precipitate osmotic diuresis, dehydration, hypotension, hyperosmolar nonketotic coma, ketoacidosis, and metabolic acidosis. Hyperosmolar nonketotic coma and ketoacidosis are discussed in Chapter 19.

Fluid Intolerance

Refeeding with carbohydrate results in sodium and water excretion. With concurrent sodium ingestion, this can lead to a rapid expansion of extracellular fluid volume, which will result in fluid retention and subsequent weight gain. This enhanced fluid retention seen with carbohydrate refeeding may in turn be exacerbated because of the loss of tissue mass resulting from starvation.

Preventing Refeeding Syndrome

Nutrients should be reintroduced slowly to the malnourished patient while medical and metabolic status is closely monitored. Careful estimation of energy requirements should be made through a complete nutritional assessment (see Chapter 14). Care should also be taken to minimize fluid retention (weight gain >1 kg/wk can be assumed to be fluid retention and should be avoided) and provide adequate repletion of phosphorus, potassium, and magnesium on a daily basis. Weight and fluid balance should be monitored daily to assess the rate of weight regain. Refeeding formulas (whether enteral or parenteral) must also contain adequate amounts of other essential nutrients such as vitamins and minerals. Greater than routine amounts are not necessary, but their absence may be lethal. After 1 week, intake of kcal, fluid, and sodium can be liberalized without fear of consequences because the various metabolic equilibrations should have taken place.

Data from Marinella MA: The refeeding syndrome and hypophosphatemia, *Nutr Rev* 61(9):320-323, 2003; and Parrish CR: Much ado about refeeding, *Pract Gastroenterol* 29(1):26-44, 2005.

---

marasmus will appear thin and is weak and listless. Visceral protein (other than muscle proteins) stores are preserved at the expense of somatic proteins (skeletal muscle proteins): skeletal muscle is severely reduced, but laboratory values are relatively unremarkable (serum albumin is usually within normal range). Immunocompetence and wound healing are fairly well preserved in patients with marasmus. Marasmus is a chronic rather than acute condition. Treatment is directed toward gradual reversal of the downward trend. And although medical nutrition therapy or support is necessary, overly aggressive repletion of nutrients can lead to a life-threatening condition called refeeding syndrome.

Refeeding syndrome consists of the physiologic and metabolic complications associated with reintroducing nutrition (refeeding) too rapidly to a person with PEM. These complications can include malabsorption, cardiac insufficiency, congestive heart failure, respiratory distress, convulsions, coma, and perhaps death (Box 15-2).

Marasmus-Kwashiorkor Mix

This combined form of PEM develops when acute stress (surgery or trauma) is experienced by someone who has been chronically malnourished.[10] The condition becomes life threatening because of the high risk of infection and other complications. It is important to determine whether marasmus or kwashiorkor is predominant so appropriate medical nutrition therapy can be initiated. The undernourished, unstressed (hypometabolic) patient is at risk of complications such as those observed in refeeding syndrome, and the stressed patient at risk for kwashiorkor is more likely to suffer from underfeeding.[6]

TABLE 15-4 NUTRITIONAL CONCERNS IN MULTIPLE ORGAN DYSFUNCTION SYNDROME

SYSTEM	EFFECTS	SYSTEM	EFFECTS
Pulmonary	Acute respiratory distress syndrome (ARDS): patients requiring ventilator support may need higher lipid content in their diets (even with cardiac failure)	Central nervous system	Lethargy Altered level of consciousness Fever: increased energy needs Hepatic encephalopathy
Gastrointestinal	Abdominal distention and ascites Intolerance to internal feedings Paralytic ileus Diarrhea Ischemic colitis Mucosal ulceration Bacterial overgrowth in stool	Immune	Infection: increased energy needs Decreased lymphocyte count Anergy
Liver	Increased serum ammonia level		
Hypermetabolism	Decreased lean body mass Muscle wasting Severe weight loss Negative nitrogen balance Hyperglycemia	Gallbladder	Abdominal distention Unexplained fever: increased kcal needs Decreased bowel sounds

Data from Baldwin KM, Cheek DJ, Morris SE: Shock, multiple organ dysfunction syndrome, and burns in adults. In McCance KL, Huether SE, editors: *Pathophysiology: The biologic basis of disease in adults and children,* ed 5, St. Louis, 2006, Mosby; Escott-Stump S: *Nutrition and diagnosis-related care,* ed 6, Baltimore, 2007, Lippincott Williams & Wilkins.

Nurses can be key players in the recognition and prevention of any of the different forms of PEM. By being alert to clinical signs and laboratory values seen in kwashiorkor and marasmus, further deterioration of the patient's nutritional status can be prevented.

MULTIPLE ORGAN DYSFUNCTION SYNDROME

Multiple organ dysfunction syndrome (MODS) involves the progressive failure of two or more organ systems at the same time (e.g., the renal, hepatic, cardiac, or respiratory systems).[11,12] It may occur following trauma, severe burns, infection, or shock; it usually results from an uncontrolled inflammatory response and can progress to organ failure and death.[11,13] MODS commonly begins with lung failure followed by failure of the liver, intestine, and kidney.[13] Myocardial failure generally manifests later, but central nervous system changes can occur at any time.[13] The pathogenesis of MODS is complex but usually results in the initiation of the stress response and release of catecholamines,[11] producing a hypermetabolic state in the patient.[13] Higher levels of kcal and protein are necessary to meet increased metabolic demands. How patients are fed is also important. Early enteral feedings (see Chapter 14) appear to maintain gut mucosal mass and barrier function and promote normal enterocytic growth in the gut. This is not possible with parenteral feedings (Table 15-4).

SURGERY

In a perfect world, all patients undergoing surgery would be at optimal nutritional status to help them tolerate the physiologic stress of the surgery and temporary starvation that follows. But all too often, surgical patients may be malnourished secondary to the medical condition causing the need for surgery. Additionally, they may experience anorexia, nausea, or vomiting, which decrease their ability to eat. Fever may increase their metabolic rate. Or nutritional needs may not be met because of malabsorption. For surgery to be successful, patients who are malnourished or in danger of malnutrition must be identified so corrective action may be arranged. Before surgery, patients are typically limited to NPO to prevent aspiration. Oral intake is generally resumed when bowel sounds return, usually 24 to 48 hours after surgery. The postoperative diet usually progresses from clear liquid to solid foods as tolerated.

BURNS (THERMAL INJURY)

Burns are customarily defined as electrical, thermal, chemical, or radioactive. They produce tissue destruction that results in circulatory and metabolic alterations that require the compensatory response to injury (Table 15-5). Actual cause of burns may be thermal or nonthermal, such as chemical, electrical, or radioactive sources. Thermal burns are usually characterized as contact (hot solid object), flame (direct contact with flames), or scald injuries (heated liquid).[11] These events have significant effects on nutritional status.

Burns are generally classified by physical appearance and symptoms associated with the affected skin and are often described in terms of percent of body surface burned (Figure 15-7). First-degree burns (or partial-thickness injury) involve only the epidermis, resulting in simple reddening of the area with no injury to underlying dermal or subcutaneous tissue.[11,12] Sunburns are an example of first-degree burns caused by ultraviolet radiation damage to skin. First-degree burns heal within 3 to 5 days without scarring.[11] Second-degree burns (superficial partial-thickness injury and deep partial-thickness injury) involve two categories of burn depth

with distinctly different characteristics.[11] Superficial partial-thickness burns are characterized by redness and blistering that affect the epidermis and some dermis.[11,12] Deep partial-thickness burns are characterized by destruction of epidermis and dermis (resulting in a waxy, white, mottled appearance), leaving only skin appendages such as hair follicles and sweat glands.[11] Second-degree burns take weeks to months to heal. Third-degree burns (full-thickness injury) are characterized by destruction of the entire epidermis, dermis, and frequently the underlying subcutaneous tissue. Occasionally, muscle or bone tissue may be destroyed.[11] Third-degree burns do not heal and require skin grafts[11] (see the *Personal Perspectives* box, Love, Greg & Lauren, for one couple's struggle with the aftermath of severe burns).

In addition to pain management, wound care, and infection control, nutrition support is recognized as one of the most significant considerations of patient care.[11,13] The first 24 to 48 hours of treatment for burn patients are dedicated to replacement of fluid and electrolytes. Fluid needs are based on the patient's age, weight, and extent of the burn.[14] Total body surface area (TBSA), used to estimate the extent of the burn, can be estimated using the "rule of nines" (Figure 15-8). Thermal injury wounds will heal only if the patient is in an anabolic state. Therefore, feeding should be initiated as soon as the patient has been hydrated.[14] Very early enteral feeding (within 4 to 12 hours of hospitalization) has been

TABLE 15-5	NUTRITIONAL GOALS FOR BURNED PATIENTS	
GOAL	**ACTION**
Minimize metabolic response	Control environmental temperature
	Monitor fluid and electrolyte balance
	Control pain and anxiety
	Cover wounds early
Meet nutritional needs	Provide adequate kcal to prevent weight loss >10% of usual body weight
	Provide adequate protein for positive nitrogen balance and maintenance or repletion of visceral protein stores
Prevent Curling's ulcer	Provide antacids or continuous enteral feedings

Modified from Winkler MF, Malone AM: Medical nutrition therapy for metabolic stress: Sepsis, trauma, burns and surgery. In Mahan LK, Escott-Stump S, editors: *Krause's food & nutrition therapy,* ed 12, Philadelphia, 2008, Saunders.

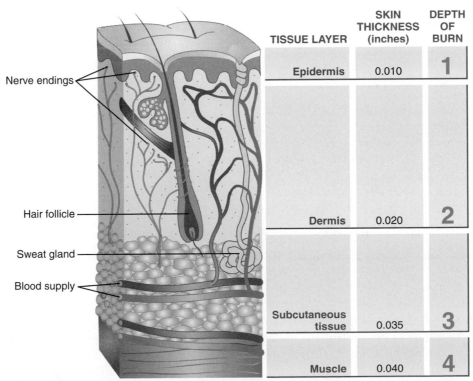

TISSUE LAYER	SKIN THICKNESS (inches)	DEPTH OF BURN
Epidermis	0.010	1
Dermis	0.020	2
Subcutaneous tissue	0.035	3
Muscle	0.040	4

Nerve endings
Hair follicle
Sweat gland
Blood supply

FIG 15-7 Interpretation of burn classification based on damage to the integument. (From Mahan LK, Escott-Stump S: *Krause's food & nutrition therapy,* ed 12, Philadelphia, 2008, Saunders.)

PERSONAL PERSPECTIVES

Love, Greg & Lauren

On September 11, 2001, at 8:48 AM, Lauren Manning, a senior vice president, partner, and director of global data sales for Cantor Fitzgerald, was entering the lobby of One World Trade Center in New York City. As the first of two planes dove into the World Trade Center buildings, an explosive fireball ran through the lobby. Lauren was burned on more than 82.5% of her body. The following is an excerpt from her husband's day-by-day e-mail account in the months following the tragedy of Lauren's struggle to heal and survive for her son, Tyler, and her husband. Consider the effect of serious injuries on patients, their families, and the medical personnel who assist in the healing process.

From: Greg

To: Everyone

Date: Saturday, September 29, 2001, 12:40 AM

Subject: Lauren Update for September 28 (Friday)

Today was a stable day. Lauren still has the septic infection, which they are fighting with antibiotics, but her lungs are functioning well, as is her stomach, two very important factors. The oxygen and the protein intake she is receiving through a feeding tube are needed to build new tissue and for her skin to heal.

I have a better understanding now of something the doctor told me about doing Lauren's grafts. He said he would "mesh 3-1" when doing autografts. Basically, a special machine is used to create a mesh pattern in the donor skin—her own skin—that permits it to cover an area three times as large as the site from which it was taken. The homograft, or skin-bank skin, is then placed over this mesh, creating a layer that enables the autograft beneath to heal better. The goal is for the mesh to take and for healing to occur in the open spots. More than one graft is often necessary to finish each site.

The grafts already done look good, which means the majority have probably taken. Unfortunately, the infection does have an adverse effect on the healing process, both of the grafts and of the donor sites. That is why Lauren's time in the burn ICU is such a balancing act. Negative factors have to be controlled so that positive factors can win out. The good aspect for Lauren is that she was strong and healthy going in, so she has managed to keep herself mostly stable, a word that has become very important for the families of all the burn patients.

Her nurse explained to me tonight how Lauren's various systems were adjusting on their own to maintain stability. For example, her heart was pumping faster to maintain her blood pressure despite a slight dilation of blood vessels due to infection. A glass-half-full type of sign.

I put two pictures—of Lauren and of Lauren, Tyler, and my dad—up on her wall. The pictures are an important way for the nursing staff to make a connection to her. They are all looking forward to meeting her when she is more awake, later in her treatment course.

That alone should tell you how difficult the work is that these nurses do; the patients arrive gravely injured, frequently unable to communicate, and highly critical. The medical and nursing staffs often fight for weeks to keep the patient improving; this is well before they have a chance to encounter the patient's personality. The staff first gets to know the patient through the family visitors, and the photographs help the staff connect with the life they are trying to help the patient return to.

The WTC disaster families have been there for 17 days now, and we know each other well. This bonding between families is due to the utter stress of the situation; we have all spent days, now weeks, and hopefully will spend months, worrying minute to minute about a loved one's condition. It is the same as if a surgical procedure were to last for weeks on end. We learn to read the facial expressions and voices of doctors and nurses.

So we, the waiting, speak to each other, and to the staff psychologists and chaplain and the Red Cross volunteers who wander through, and we are visited by Good Samaritans of all types, who provide food. ... And in the end, we alone understand what we are going through: we are the loved ones of critically injured patients from a massive tragedy in which most victims either died or walked out under their own power.

We, the waiting, are therefore at somewhat of a disconnect from the world at large, which is pursuing closure (not my favorite word), whether coping with loss of a family member; coming to terms with having one's life saved by something so trivial as arriving late for work; or honoring the heroism of lost firefighters and police.

Most of the world is already viewing the attacks from a distance, but we are pretty much still there at Time Zero, with the outcome unknown. However, we are all making it through, with the help of the huge support networks that have sprung up all around us. Including y'all. ... It really does help us, me and Lauren, to know how many people care.

Love,

Greg & Lauren

Update: Lauren Manning left home for work on September 11, 2001, and returned home on March 15, 2002. She continues to regain the life she had, including running, biking, getting back to work, and just being there with and for her son as he grows up.

From Manning G: *Love, Greg & Lauren,* New York, 2002, Bantam Books.

shown to be successful in decreasing the hypercatabolic response, decreasing the release of catecholamines and glucagon, reducing weight loss, and shortening the length of the hospital stay.[15]

Nutritional goals for patients with burns are outlined in Table 15-5. Several methods may be used to estimate energy and protein needs in burn patients when indirect calorimetry is not available. Energy needs vary according to the size of the burn.[13] One of the simplest and easiest to use is the Curreri formula (adults), as follows:[16]

- (25 kcal × kg of body weight) + (40 kcal × %TBSA)
- 15 to 18 kcal × kg body weight if patient >125% regular body weight
- Burns >50%, use a maximum value of 50%.

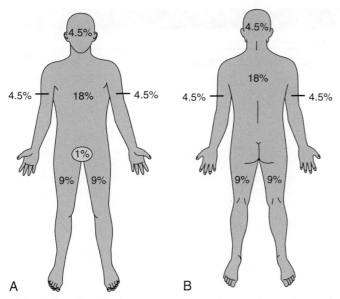

FIG 15-8 Rule of nines—a commonly used assessment tool with estimates of the percentages (in multiples of nine) of the total body surface area burned. **A,** Adults (anterior view). **B,** Adults (posterior view). (From Thompson JM, et al: *Mosby's clinical nursing*, ed 5, St. Louis, 2002, Mosby.)

Estimates using the Curreri formula may exceed actual energy needs,[12,16] but it is not uncommon for a patient to need 4000 to 5000 kcal.[12]

Protein lost through urine and wounds, increased protein use for gluconeogenesis, and wound healing increase protein needs in burned patients.[13] It is therefore important that kcal from protein are not calculated into total energy needs. Carbohydrates and fats are good for protein sparing (nonprotein energy sources).[13] Whether a patient receives adequate amounts of energy or protein is best evaluated by wound healing, graft take, and basic nutritional assessment parameters.[13]

In conjunction with increased energy demands, vitamin and mineral needs are generally increased in burn patients, but exact requirements are not known.[13] Most patients will receive vitamins in excess of the recommended intake because of their high kcal intakes, but special consideration should be given to vitamin C (collagen synthesis, immune function) and vitamin A (immune function and epithelialization). Supplements are commonly recommended.[13]

SUMMARY

The stress response of the body also affects nutritional status. Whether the stress response is caused by physiologic or psychologic determinants, the entire body is affected. Metabolic changes take place in reaction to stress. This includes changes caused by uncomplicated stress that is present when patients are at nutritional risk and severe stress caused by trauma or disease. The functioning of the immune system is also affected by the hormonal and metabolic changes that occur when metabolic stress develops. The immune system's ability to protect the body is further depressed if impaired nutritional status accompanies the metabolic stress.

THE NURSING APPROACH

Case Study: Nutritional Needs during Physical Stress

Daniel, age 65, developed pneumonia two days after his left hip replacement. He is receiving physical therapy, IV antibiotics, supplemental oxygen, and a high-kcal, high-protein diet. The hospital dietitian met with Daniel to individualize his diet, based on his Orthodox Jewish religion.

ASSESSMENT
Subjective (From Patient Statements)

- "The muscles in my chest ache from coughing, and my hip hurts."
- Pain rating: 3 of 10
- "I don't feel like eating, but if I have to eat, I want to observe dietary laws for an Orthodox Jew."
- "I feel tired and sometimes short of breath."

Objective (From Physical Examination)

- Eats small amounts of food, then pushes the food tray away
- Drinks about 1200 mL of fluid per day (mostly water)
- Tympanic temperature 101.2° F

- Crackles in lungs bilaterally
- O₂ saturation 90% with oxygen at 6 liters via cannula
- White blood count 12,000/mm³
- Productive cough, with thick yellow sputum
- Surgical wound on left hip intact without redness or drainage

DIAGNOSIS (NURSING)

Imbalanced nutrition: less than body requirements related to inadequate food intake (secondary to shortness of breath and discomfort) and increased metabolic stresses (surgery, infection, and fever) as evidenced by "I don't feel like eating," eats small amounts then pushes meal tray away, drinks about 1200 mL of fluid per day

PLANNING
Patient Outcomes

Short term (by discharge to a rehabilitation center in five days):
- Eating moderate amounts of food, especially protein-rich and nutrient-dense foods

Continued

THE NURSING APPROACH—cont'd

Case Study: Nutritional Needs during Physical Stress—cont'd

- Drinking at least 2000 mL per day
- No weight loss
- No shortness of breath, O_2 saturation 95% without supplemental oxygen
- Afebrile (no fever)
- White blood cell (WBC) count below 10,000/mm³
- Decreased or absent crackles in lungs
- No signs of infection of surgical wound on left hip

Nursing Interventions

1. Provide high-kcal, high-protein diet.
2. Maintain dietary intake according to Orthodox Jewish kosher dietary laws.

IMPLEMENTATION (Also see Chapter 6 and Appendix H.)

1. Asked Daniel's family to bring in kosher ground meat and special serving dishes.
   Ground meat provides high protein and requires little energy for chewing. If the hospital does not have a kosher kitchen, kosher meals may be ordered from special suppliers. Family members may be able to obtain kosher food and reassure the patient that it is truly kosher. Meat (no pork or shellfish) must be properly slaughtered, blessed by a rabbi, and cooked in a kosher kitchen. Dishes reserved for meat must be separated from dishes for milk, and meat cannot be served in the same meal as milk.

2. Asked Daniel and his family to inform nursing or dietary staff about special dietary needs, particularly for upcoming holidays and the Sabbath.
   Culturally sensitive staff will ask individuals and families how they can meet special dietary needs.

3. Provided rest periods and oral care before meals, and gave pain medicine as needed.
   Rest helps increase patient energy, and a fresh mouth promotes appetite. Patients eat more food when comfortable.

4. Pointed out the high-protein and nutrient-dense foods on meal trays and encouraged Daniel to eat them first.
   When patients can eat only small amounts of food, nourishment is better if they choose nutrient-dense foods.

5. Conferred with the dietitian and physician concerning high-kcal, high-protein snacks between meals.
   Increased kcal are needed to compensate for metabolic stresses, and additional protein is needed for healing and building up immunity. Frequent small meals are easier to consume than large meals when the patient is short of breath. Some doctors prefer to limit milk products for patients

with respiratory problems because of potential phlegm. Milk-based supplements must be served several hours before or after meats, according to Jewish dietary laws.

6. Provided a vitamin/mineral supplement, as prescribed by the physician.
   Bone healing requires adequate calcium and vitamin D. Vitamins A and C help promote wound healing. B vitamins are needed in stressful conditions.

7. Offered water frequently between meals and encouraged drinking 2000 mL of fluid per day.
   Fluid intake is needed to replace fluids lost during fever. Additional fluids help thin sputum, making it easier for the patient to cough up the sputum. Liquids during meals should be minimized if patient feels full after eating little food.

8. Recorded intake and output and weighed the patient daily.
   Records can help show balance or imbalance of fluid intake (by mouth and by intravenous fluid) and fluid output (urine). Adequate nutrition is needed to prevent weight loss.

9. Encouraged Daniel to get a pneumonia shot this year and a flu shot every year.
   Serious respiratory infections may be prevented by immunizations. Generally only one pneumonia shot is given, preferably when an adult becomes 65 years old. Influenza shots must be received by the patient annually, usually in the fall. Health promotion is an important nursing responsibility.

EVALUATION

Short term (at discharge to the rehabilitation center on the fifth day):

- Daniel was eating moderate amounts of food.
- He was drinking 2000 mL of fluids per day.
- No weight loss
- No shortness of breath, O_2 saturation 95% without supplemental oxygen
- Tympanic temperature 99° F
- WBC 9500/mm³
- Decreased crackles in lungs
- No signs of infection of surgical wound on left hip
- Goals met

DISCUSSION QUESTIONS

1. How would Daniel's diet plan be different if he did not request a Kosher diet?
2. Compare and contrast a diet for a patient with pneumonia versus a patient with severe burns.

CRITICAL THINKING

Clinical Applications

Kristin, age 19, is a member of her college's cheerleading team and was involved in a serious motor vehicle accident when the team was returning from a game. She was admitted through the emergency department of your hospital suffering from multiple fractures and contusions. Kristin is 5 feet 5 inches tall and weighed 120 pounds before the accident. Because she is young, looked healthy, and is somewhat muscular from being a cheerleader, the physician did not request a consult for the dietitian to evaluate Kristin's nutritional status. After 2 weeks in intensive care, she developed pneumonia. The nurse learned that before the automobile accident, Kristin had been using a commercial weight loss product and was consuming approximately 400 kcal/day for 3 months before the accident in an attempt to "make weight" so that she could remain on the cheerleading team.

1. How did the very-low-calorie diet (VLCD) affect Kristin's nutritional status?
2. Why did Kristin develop pneumonia?
3. Describe the variety of stresses Kristin experienced.
4. Could the pneumonia have been prevented? How?

WEBSITES OF INTEREST

Burnsurgery.org

www.burnsurgery.org
Offers up-to-date educational tools on burn care and treatment for health professionals.

KidSource OnLine!

www.kidsource.com/kidsource/content2/ecoli/anna.1.html
Presents support and resources on parenting resources including a parent's personal account of her daughter's experience with MODS caused by an *Escherichia coli* infection.

REFERENCES

1. Nelms MN, Fraizier C: Immunology. In Nelms MN, et al: *Nutrition therapy and pathophysiology*, ed 2, Belmont, Calif, 2010, Cengage/Thomson.
2. Gould BE: *Pathophysiology for the health-related professions*, ed 3, Philadelphia, 2006, Saunders.
3. Cahill GF: Starvation: Some biological aspects. In Kinney JM et al, editors: *Nutrition and metabolism in patient care*, Philadelphia, 1988, Saunders.
4. Bessey PQ, Wilmore DW: The burned patient. In Kinney JM et al, editors: *Nutrition and metabolism in patient care*, Philadelphia, 1988, Saunders.
5. American Dietetic Association Evidence Analysis Library: *Estimating RMR with prediction equations: what does the evidence tell us?* Accessed February 6, 2010, from www.adaevidencelibrary.com.
6. Moore MC: *Pocket guide to nutrition assessment and care*, St. Louis, 2009, Mosby/Elsevier.
7. Nelms MN: Fluid and electrolyte balance. In Nelms MN, et al: *Nutrition therapy and pathophysiology*, ed 2, Belmont, Calif, 2010, Cengage/Thomson.
8. Gottschlich MM: The burn patient. In Lysen LK, editor: *Quick reference to clinical dietetics*, Boston, 2006, Jones and Bartlett.
9. Heimburger DC, Ard J: *Handbook of clinical nutrition*, ed 4, St. Louis, 2006, Mosby.
10. Winkler MF, Malone AM: Medical nutrition therapy for metabolic stress: Sepsis, trauma, burns and surgery. In Mahan LK, Escott-Stump S, editors: *Krause's food & nutrition therapy*, ed 12, Philadelphia, 2008, Saunders.
11. Baldwin KM, et al: Shock, multiple organ dysfunction syndrome, and burns in adults. In McCance KL, Huether SE, editors: *Pathophysiology: The biologic basis for diseases in adults and children*, ed 6, St. Louis, 2008, Mosby.
12. Escott-Stump S: *Nutrition and diagnosis-related care*, ed 6, Baltimore, 2007, Lippincott Williams & Wilkins.
13. Winkler MF, Malone AM: Medical nutrition therapy for metabolic stress: Sepsis, trauma, burns and surgery. In Mahan LK, Escott-Stump S, editors: *Krause's food & nutrition therapy*, ed 12, Philadelphia, 2008, Saunders.
14. Saffle JR, Larson CM, Sullivan J: A randomized trial of indirect calorimetry-based feedings in thermal injury, *J Trauma* 30:776-782, 1990.
15. Chiarelli A, et al: Very early nutrition supplementation in burned patients, *Am J Clin Nutr* 51:1035-1039, 1990.
16. American Dietetic Association Nutrition Care Manual: *Burns: calculations for nutrition assessment*. Accessed February 14, 2010, from www.nutritioncaremanual.org.

16

Interactions: Complementary and Alternative Medicine, Dietary Supplements, and Medications

Herbs are not innocuous but can have significant effects on the bioavailability of foods, nutrients, and drugs.

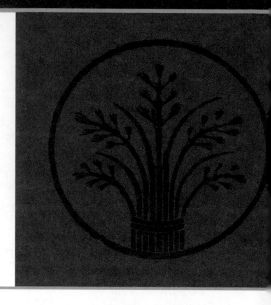

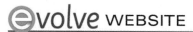 **WEBSITE**

http://evolve.elsevier.com/Grodner/foundations/

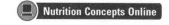 **Nutrition Concepts Online**

ROLE IN WELLNESS

This chapter first discusses the roles of complementary and alternative medicine (CAM) as they interact with conventional medicine. Dietary supplements, a component of CAM, have become an everyday part of life for many Americans. Because supplement use has substantially grown, part of this chapter discusses supplements as an influence that interacts with health status. This chapter closes with consideration of the interactions occurring among medications, food, nutrients, and herbs. These interactions can limit the bioavailability of medications or nutrients and can even cause serious symptoms that affect blood clotting and blood pressure.

The five dimensions of health provide additional perspectives as CAM, dietary supplements, and medications interact with health. The *physical health* dimension can be affected when dietary supplements interact with medications and inadvertently alter the effects of medications. *Intellectual health* becomes valuable because critical thinking skills are required to assess the efficacy and appropriateness of incorporating alternative medicine therapies. *Emotional health* may be enhanced as complementary approaches address stress and anxiety that sometimes occur when dealing with chronic disorders. *Social health* can be supported by several alternative modalities, such as yoga and T'ai chi, which often involve classes that provide a social support group (Figure 16-1). The last dimension, *spiritual health*, can evolve by adopting modalities such as meditation and biofeedback, which provide physical and spiritual benefits by using the body to heal itself.

COMPLEMENTARY AND ALTERNATIVE MEDICINE

CAM has become a significant component of health care in the United States. Consider that more than a third of Ameri-

cans use CAM therapies, and others take herbal and dietary supplements that total a combined out-of-pocket cost of $27 billion per year.[1] To address this increased interest in CAM, the National Institutes of Health created the National Center for Complementary and Alternative Medicine (NCCAM). For this discussion, the categories of CAM as outlined by NCCAM will be used. The CAM categories simplify the distinctions between the systems of healing and the related modalities but provide an adequate overview of the methods of application.

According to NCCAM, **complementary and alternative medicine** consists of a cluster of medical and health care approaches, methods, and items not associated with conventional medicine.[2] Medical doctors and doctors of osteopathy practice conventional medicine, which is also called *allopathy,* and Western medicine, as do other allied health professionals such as registered nurses, nurse practitioners, registered dietitians, and physician assistants. Some conventional physicians may also incorporate CAM in their practices. Studies of CAM therapies are being conducted; previously the efficacy of these therapies tended to be anecdotal based on the self-reported experiences of individuals. Some CAM systems such as Ayurveda, which includes the modality of yoga, and Traditional Chinese Medicine, which encompasses acupuncture, have been used for healing for thousands of years, thereby precluding the immediate need for "proof." Nonetheless, well-designed studies are needed to continue to identify the efficacy of particular modalities for specific disorders (see the *Cultural Considerations* box, Global Strategies on Traditional and Alternative Medicine). Providing support for such studies is part of the mission of NCCAM.

To continue with definitions, **complementary medicine** refers to non-Western healing approaches used at the same time as conventional medicine.[2] For instance, a patient

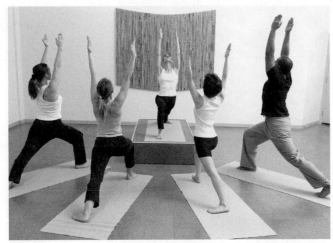

FIG 16-1 Participating in yoga class may help support social, physical, and spiritual health. (Photos.com.)

CULTURAL CONSIDERATIONS

Global Strategies on Traditional and Alternative Medicine

The global plan of the World Health Organization (WHO) provides guidelines for countries to develop national policies to evaluate and regulate traditional or complementary/alternative medicine (TM/CAM) to ensure its availability to populations throughout the world.

The global plan supports strategies to expand the availability and uniformity of traditional medicine. Supporting this goal has led to a sharing of successful endeavors that adapt traditional practice to self-help approaches. Some innovative strategies include the creation of "medikits" for use in isolated areas of Mongolia and the distribution of "your medicine in your garden" booklets to medically underserved regions south Asia. These efforts enhance the accessibility of health care and provide role models for other countries.

Traditional practice has not been formalized as part of the health care systems of African nations. China, North and South Korea, and Vietnam have integrated TM/CAM into their health systems. In developing countries, TM/CAM can provide health care availability, whereas a third of the populations currently do not have access to medical personnel or facilities.

Application to nursing: An additional concern is that TM/CAM may be inappropriately used as its benefits are translated from one culture to another. Nurses working with diverse cultural groups can be aware of the TM/CAM practices of patients' culture of origin. A prime example is the herb *ma huang* (ephedra). In China, ma huang is used for a short period to reduce respiratory congestion. In the United States ma huang was marketed as a dietary aid to reduce weight and to increase energy potential. When used long term, the herb caused strokes, heart attacks, and more than 10 deaths among young, otherwise healthy adults. Consequently, encouraging the creation of policies to regulate TM/CAM will lead to positive use of traditional knowledge by all.

Data from World Health Organization: *Report of the WHO Interregional Workshop on the use of traditional medicine in primary health care, Ulaanbaatar, Mongolia, 23-26 August 2007,* Geneva, 2009, Author. Accessed February 23, 2010, from http://apps.who.int/medicinedocs/en/m/abstract/Js16202e/.

who attempts to lower hypertension takes prescription medications (conventional) but also attends yoga classes (complementary) for physical and psychologic benefits. In contrast, **alternative medicine** replaces conventional medical treatment.[2] An example is the use of herbal supplements to treat cancer instead of surgical intervention or chemotherapy. **Integrative medicine** merges conventional medical therapies with CAM modalities for which safety and efficacy, based on scientific data, have been demonstrated.[2]

Integrative medical centers are available that are hospital based and under the direction of physicians and other conventional health professionals. Advanced practice nurses with master of science degrees in holistic health are often at the forefront of the integrative care provided. For example, a patient recovering from heart bypass surgery can be referred to a center for integrative medicine. Once there, a board-certified nurse practitioner or physician evaluates the patient and may recommend complementary approaches of therapeutic massage for stress reduction and yoga for exercise to assist recovery. All services are provided within the same health care facility. Insurance companies have slowly but steadily increased coverage for such treatments.

According to NCCAM, CAM therapies can be divided into five categories: alternative medical systems; mind-body interventions; biologically based therapies; manipulative and body-based methods; and energy therapies.[2]

Alternative Medical Systems

Alternative medical systems develop outside mainstream Western medical approaches. These systems are based on holistic structures that incorporate distinctive philosophies and applications. Alternative medical systems evolving from Eastern cultures include *Traditional Chinese Medicine (TCM)* and *Ayurveda* (Asian Indian derivation). Western cultures have produced *naturopathic medicine* and *homeopathic medicine.*[2]

The Eastern practice of TCM is a system based on the forces of nature understood through the fundamental concept of *yin* and *yang.* Illness is viewed as an imbalance of these two

forces that are opposites of each other. Yin is dark, night, feminine, and contracting; yang is light, day, masculine, and expanding. The imbalance of these two forces affects *Qi,* the life force. Therapeutic modalities, such as acupuncture, massage, meditation, incense, diet, herbs, and T'ai chi (exercise of slow movements), aim to reduce symptoms and restore energy balance. For example, **acupuncture** is the use of fine needles placed in the 2000 specific acupuncture points on the body to open blockages of the flow of Qi or life force and thus restore balance (Figure 16-2).

The Eastern practice of Ayurveda is 5000 years old, evolving from the Indian subcontinent. As an alternative medical system, **Ayurveda** focuses on diet and herbal remedies that emphasize the use of body, mind, and spirit to prevent and treat disorders.[2]

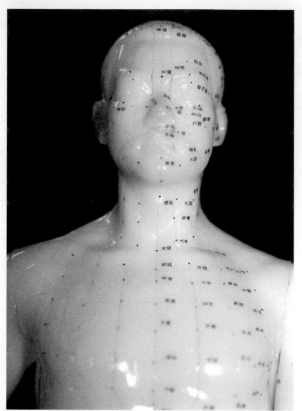

FIG 16-2 Acupuncture points are marked on the upper torso of this model. This practice uses fine needles placed in some of the 2000 specific points on the body to ultimately restore balance. (Copyright 2006 by JupiterImages Corporation.)

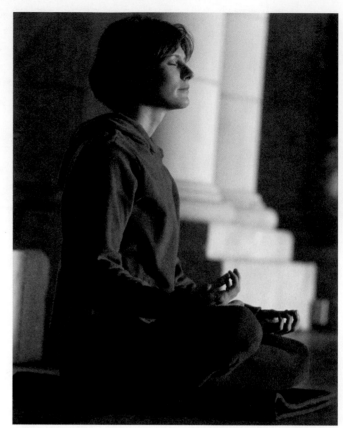

FIG 16-3 One advantage of meditation is that it can be practiced anywhere. (Photos.com.)

The Western approach of naturopathic medicine is based on the use of the body's natural healing forces to recover from disease and to achieve wellness.[2] This system incorporates techniques from Eastern and Western traditions. Techniques may include acupuncture, exercise, massage, and dietary alterations.

Homeopathic medicine is an alternative medical system through which a small amount of a diluted substance is prescribed to relieve symptoms for which the same substance, given in larger amounts, will cause the same symptoms. This theory is called *"like cures like."*[2]

Training in homeopathic medicine is necessary for practitioners to be able to diagnose and treat disorders appropriately. Individuals with the same illness may each receive different treatments because homeopathic practitioners focus on the needs of the specific individual, not on the disorder. Although the amounts of medications prescribed will usually not interfere with conventional medications, patients should reveal the use of homeopathic treatments to their health care providers.

Mind-Body Interventions

The focus of mind-body intervention is to expand the mind's ability to influence physical functions. These modalities include meditation, faith healing or prayer, biofeedback, and such therapies that influence behavior through creative approaches of music, dance, and art therapy.[2]

Several of these modalities are commonly recommended and are used not only for physical healing but also for stress reduction and other concerns related to contemporary life. Meditation is a self-directed technique of relaxing the body and calming the mind. Based in Eastern religions, meditation evolved from religious practice. Meditation calms the mind and body through guided imagery and rhythmic breathing (Figure 16-3). Faith healing is healing by invoking divine intervention without the use of conventional or surgical therapy. Faith healing is a form of prayer that is either practiced individually or as a group; the practice is often associated with religious institutions or communities. Biofeedback involves the use of special devices to convey information about heart rate, blood pressure, skin temperature, and muscle relaxation to enable a person to learn how to consciously control these medically important functions. Patients need several training sessions to become able to produce the desired responses on their own.

Biologically Based Therapies

Biologically based therapies encompass materials found in nature. These materials include nutrients, food, and herbs. This category incorporates dietary supplements, alternative dietary patterns, aromatherapy, and other alternative natural treatments such as shark cartilage for cancer treatment.[2]

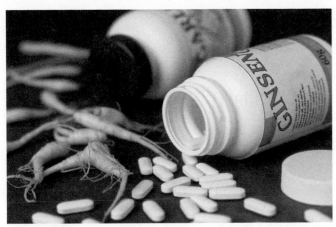

FIG 16-4 Dietary supplements are processed into various forms, including tablets, liquids, capsules, extracts, powders, concentrates, gel caps, liquids, and powders. (Photos.com.)

Dietary supplements are substances consumed orally as an addition to dietary intake (Figure 16-4). The ingredients of dietary supplements may include one or more of the following: minerals, vitamins, amino acids, herbs, plant extracts, enzymes, metabolites, and organ tissues.[3] Dietary supplements are processed into various forms, including tablets, liquids, capsules, extracts, powders, concentrates, gel caps, liquids, and powders. There are special requirements for supplement labeling. Under the Dietary Supplement Act of 1994, dietary supplements are considered foods, not drugs.[3] Because of the popularity of use, extensive range of supplements available, and connections to nutrition, the next section of this chapter explores supplements.

An alternative dietary pattern is the macrobiotic diet. The macrobiotic dietary pattern evolves from the yin-yang philosophy of opposing forces. By consuming a balance of foods that contain yin and yang characteristics, some believe that health may be maintained, disease possibly prevented, and treatment achieved. Although the macrobiotic diet was originally intended for general good health, it has recently become most associated with treatment for cancer even though the traditional medical community does not advocate its benefit. This occurred because the Japanese philosopher who originated this concept views cancer as an imbalance caused by dietary, environmental, and social and personal factors affecting an individual. Locations of cancer are even tied to yin-yang with yin cancers in the upper parts of the body and in hollow organs and yang cancers in the lower body and in more dense organs.

Because all foods are categorized as yin or yang, dietary recommendations would, for example, support consumption of yang foods to offset a yin cancer. Also considered are the person's age, sex, activity levels, and climate. Although the original macrobiotic diet consisted of a rigid 10-step program, the current version is not as restrictive and is health promoting. The core diet focuses on consumption of whole cereals and grains as 50% to 60% of intake with 40% to 50% from other foods, preferably organically grown, with minimal intake of animal foods except for small amounts of white fish. Consequently, intake of fatty foods, milk products, processed foods, and eggs are to be avoided because the belief is that such foods contain toxins that cause illness. Because this diet is low in fat and high in fiber and plant foods, it appears to support the health and recovery of individuals with cancer when used in conjunction with conventional treatments for cancer. The safety of the macrobiotic diet depends on the implementation to support sufficient intake of calories and nutrients. This requires substantial commitment to food preparation with planning to ensure nutrient adequacy.[4]

Aromatherapy is using extracts or essences of herbs, flowers, and trees in the form of essential oils to support health and well-being.[2] The essential oils are added to candles, oils, and lotions through which the aroma is dispersed and inhaled with subsequent physiologic responses. Often, the essential oils are an integral part of massage therapy. Applications of aromatherapy continue to increase. Pillows can be purchased that have a special pocket in which to place essential oils to provide aromatherapy while one sleeps. A dental practice in New York City now offers aromatherapy along with foot massages to decrease stress while dental procedures are conducted.[5] In a number of breast cancer treatment centers, nurses use essential oils and massage to reduce anxiety and discomfort of patients during chemotherapy treatments.

Manipulative and Body-Based Methods

Manipulative and body-based methods involve manipulation or movements of body parts. These methods include osteopathic or chiropractic manipulation, massage, and bodywork.

Osteopathic manipulation is a part of osteopathic medicine. Although osteopathic medicine is considered part of conventional medicine, it differs in its view of disease as stemming from the musculoskeletal system.[2] This approach is based on the assumption that the systems of the body function together. Therefore, disturbances in one system may affect other systems. Some osteopathic physicians conduct osteopathic manipulation, which is a method of hands-on actions to reduce pain, reinstate function, and promote health and well-being.[2]

Chiropractic manipulation addresses the ties between body structure (particularly of the spine) and function and how those ties affect the maintenance and return to health.[2] Manipulative therapy is the foundation of treatment.[2]

Massage therapy is the manipulation of muscle and connective tissue to improve function and to enhance relaxation and well-being; trained massage therapists conduct manipulation. Massage therapists do not diagnose and treat disorders, as do practitioners of osteopathy or chiropractic. Instead, their treatment is adjunct to other medical interventions or may be used to generally enhance physical and psychologic health.

Health benefits occur because massage strengthens and loosens the muscles and connective tissue. This is turn, allows better blood flow through the body, increases the removal of metabolic waste products, and stimulates the release of endorphins and serotonins in the brain and nervous system.

Several types of massage therapy exist; each form addresses different aspects of body muscularity. These massage therapies may include Swedish massage that focuses deeply on muscles; sports massage that kneads deeply into muscles most affected by athletic pursuits, and Trager massage that through gentle massage along with rhythmic rocking of body parts creates physical and psychologic relaxation. Massage therapy continues to emerge as it gains popularity as a health-promoting technique.

Energy Therapies

Energy therapies manipulate energy fields. Two kinds of energy therapies are biofield therapies and bioelectromagnetic-based therapies. Biofield therapies influence energy fields that encircle and go through the body. Whether these energy fields exist has not been determined based on Western scientific research. Nonetheless, these therapies manipulate body biofields by placing hands around or on the body, thereby changing the movement of energy.

Biofield therapies include Qi gong, reiki, and therapeutic touch. Qi gong is a modality of TCM that merges breathing regulation, movement, and meditation to increase the flow of Qi or life force in the body. This practice of Qi gong enhances circulatory and immune function.[2] Reiki means "universal life energy" in Japanese. The energy therapy bearing the name "reiki" is based on the belief that by healing the patient's spirit, the physical body will also heal. Spirits are healed when a reiki practitioner channels spiritual energy, or universal life force, through to the patient.[2] Therapeutic touch is a version of the ancient technique called *laying-on of hands*. Therapeutic touch is based on facilitating the flow of energy in and around the body. The therapist proceeds to identify and undo blockages to promote healing. Therapists, while in a meditative state, move their hands above patients to determine blockages in energy fields and then clear blockages by the downward motions of their hands around, but not actually touching, the patients' bodies. The healing energy powers of therapists are transferred to patients to restore energy balance within their bodies.[2]

Bioelectromagnetic-based therapies consist of the unusual use of electromagnetic fields. These fields include magnetic fields, pulsed fields, and direct or alternating current fields.[2] Although magnets have been used for a long time as healing tools, the efficacy of their use has not, as yet, been validated.

Application to Nursing

Familiarity with these CAM modalities is valuable. Although some do not directly affect nutrition status, many indirectly do by increasing awareness of the holistic nature of healing of which nourishing the body is fundamental. Acceptance without judgment of alternative healing approaches provides a more secure environment for patients to feel supported in their quest for health (see the *Personal Perspectives* box,

Everyday Experiences in Complementary and Alternative Medicine). Referrals can be made to nutritionists who have special training in integrating CAM therapies with dietary recommendations.

DIETARY SUPPLEMENTS

Knowledge of nutrients began to be discovered at the beginning of the twentieth century. First, the role of vitamins in preventing deficiency diseases was revealed. More recently, other nutrient-related substances such as concentrated garlic, fish oils, and psyllium came into use for believed health benefits. The concept of dietary supplements evolved because of the growing body of knowledge resulting in the availability of substances in the form of pills, powder, and liquid to enhance the quality of dietary intakes.[6] As the effects of nutrients on health continued to be learned, knowledge of the inappropriate eating habits of Americans increased. Consequently, the value of dietary supplements to rectify poor eating habits caught the attention of the American public as an easier way to improve health than by changing eating behavior.

Throughout this time, physicians tended to discount the value of dietary supplements, including vitamin supplementation. Instead, physicians and dietitians strongly recommended that all nutrients be consumed through food rather than supplements.[6] The view of supplementation of essential nutrients has changed somewhat during the past few years. Supplements may be recommended as a safety net for poor dietary intake. As a safety net, vitamin/mineral supplements at 100% or less of the Dietary Reference Intake (DRI) are appropriate. Additional vitamin/mineral supplements are also recommended for some specific nutrients for certain subgroups within the population. For example, calcium and vitamin D supplementation is suggested for adults older than 70 years because the new DRI for calcium and vitamin D for this age group is higher than what most individuals can generally consume.

Regulation and Labeling

The range of dietary supplements, though, has expanded from vitamins and minerals to a diverse selection of substances including herbs, protein powders, fatty acid capsules, natural and synthetic energy, and growth enhancers. Regulation to control the identity, potency, contents, and labeling of these substances is currently under the Dietary Supplement Health and Education Act (DSHEA) of 1994.

DSHEA establishes a definition of dietary supplements as products that supplement dietary intake and contain one or more of the following:[3]

- A vitamin or a mineral
- An herb or other botanical
- An amino acid
- A dietary substance for use by man to supplement the diet by increasing the total dietary intake
- A concentrate, metabolite, constituent, extract, or a combination of the preceding ingredients

PERSONAL PERSPECTIVES
Everyday Experiences in Complementary and Alternative Medicine

CAM therapies may seem unfamiliar, but we need not look hard to find individuals who praise CAM therapies for improving their health and sense of well-being. Access to CAM therapies is becoming more accessible to everyone and may be covered by health insurance programs. Following is a compilation of comments about CAM experiences from individuals of varying ages.

"I was having problems with incontinence because of a neurogenic bladder, and the usual drugs weren't helping or I couldn't tolerate them. My physician of integrative medicine suggested trying acupuncture. After about two months of weekly treatments, the incontinence was no longer a problem. I continued with sessions for a total of six months to possibly address other health concerns. Now two years later, I am still doing well."

"Acupuncture helped reduce my irritable bowel symptoms."

"Hot flashes were driving me crazy! I refused to go on hormone replacement therapy but had to do something because the hot flashes were disturbing my sleep and my husband's. I started taking yam extract but then stopped. At first it worked but then didn't. The soy seemed to help much more."

"I have a neuropathy problem with my feet that causes them to get extremely cold or really numb or very painful. Since I am very sensitive to many medications, it was suggested that I try capsaicin—the hot pepper stuff—on my feet. This works really well on my feet, but I couldn't continue to use it because I wear contact lenses. The active ingredient is the same stuff that's used in pepper spray. You can't get it off your hands, it goes through latex and other gloves, so you get it in your eye when putting in or taking out contacts. And it burns!"

"Meditation is wonderful to calm you down and bring focus to your inner self. It is not easy to do, because you have to completely clear your mind."

"Perhaps the best thing about meditation and yogic breathing is that it forces me to stop and take time out of the day to just be. One of the yogic breaths I learned helped me through two childbirth labors and I still use it during dental procedures to stay centered and ignore other body sensations."

"Reiki requires training. When doing it on yourself, I found it to be similar to meditation because you are directing all of your energy on one particular area/part of your body or problem."

"My father, who is very traditional and conservative, is practically a spokesperson now for glucosamine and chondroitin sulfate supplements to help his joints. He's 69 and says they allow him to still play 6 sets of tennis every Tuesday night."

"Varicose veins in my legs were really bothering me, so I tried an herbal preparation with horse chestnut extract in it … that plus exercise really made a difference."

Michele Grodner
Montclair, N.J.

NOTE: Health care providers should be consulted before using alternative and complementary approaches because some may interact with medications and/or affect other body processes.

Based on this definition, dietary supplements are to be considered foods; they are not drugs or food additives. This distinction affects the way they are regulated and actually eases the approval process. Drugs require more strident testing for safety and efficacy and food additives must also meet more stringent criteria. Consequently, dietary supplements can enter the marketplace much quicker with fewer data confirming their function.

If a manufacturer distributes a product containing a new dietary ingredient, the manufacturer must notify the U.S. Food and Drug Administration (FDA) 75 days before the product is to be released. In addition, the manufacturer must also provide data regarding the safety and efficacy of the product. Supplements already on the market or supplement ingredients previously used are considered generally safe and do not need reapproval.[3]

Labeling of dietary supplements must follow the format used for nutrition labels (see Chapter 2). This means that the label needs to identify the product as a dietary supplement and must include the name and amount of each item contained in the product. Labels may also include approved statements of health claims such as are allowable on food product labels. For example, a claim may be made that a diet containing soluble fiber from whole oats and psyllium may reduce the risk of coronary heart disease. Other health-related claims may also be made about the effect of the supplement on the "structure or function" of the body as well as on "general well-being." Claims related to reducing the risk of nutrition deficiency diseases are also acceptable. In addition, if claims are made, the label must include the statement "This statement has not been evaluated by the Food and Drug Administration. This product is not intended to diagnose, treat, cure, or prevent any disease."[3]

Supplement Use

In the past, use of supplements was limited to a small group of individuals, and supplements were available in an equally small number of locations such as health food stores and specialty shops. Currently, supplements are available through numerous outlets including supermarkets, drugstores, mail-order companies, and Internet websites. Sales of dietary supplements have increased tremendously from about $8 billion in 1994 to an estimated $24 billion in 2010.[7]

Consider that the reason for the increased use of dietary supplements is that consumers have self-care goals for which dietary supplements provide perceived value. Concurrently, such self-care goals may reflect consumers experiencing alienation from conventional health care systems.[3] This alienation may be why patients do not reveal their use of dietary supplements to their health care providers.

About 22.8 million consumers use herbal supplements rather than prescription drugs, and 19.6 million use herbs with prescription medications.[3] These consumers may either view the dietary supplements as not really "medicine" or fear that their health care providers might not approve of their self-care goals. Not revealing supplement use may result in misuse of substances or interaction with prescription and over-the-counter (OTC) drugs (Table 16-1). Consequently, it is most important to question patients in detail to ascertain use of supplements beyond prescription medications.

Looking to the Future

The consumption of dietary supplements as part of American dietary patterns will continue to evolve. Physiologically active substances have been added to food products, resulting in a category of foods called *functional foods*. Functional foods are generally regarded as foods that provide good health by containing physiologically active food components. This may include foods that have been modified to increase nutrient density including fortified, enriched, or enhanced foods.

Some functional food components are marketed as dietary supplements, such as herb-enriched beverages. Care must be taken, though, because the amounts and sources of herb and other phytochemical ingredients are not sufficiently regulated.[8] A fruit juice beverage may contain the herb St. John's wort, which may be effective for the treatment of mild depression, but it must be taken regularly for several months for a response to occur. Consuming a small amount in a juice beverage is ineffective for depression treatment and pointless for any other purpose.

Health professionals can be aware of the range of products available and advise patients accordingly based on basic principles of good health. As the public becomes more educated about phytochemicals as a natural component of whole foods, perhaps the perception of dietary supplements will change. For example, tomatoes naturally contain lycopene, a phytochemical. Instead of taking a supplement containing lycopene, consumption of tomatoes would provide the same benefit. Nonetheless, the development of functional foods will continue because of several factors. These factors include (1) an aging population concerned about health; (2) increased cost of health care; (3) growth of self-care regarding health; (4) continued evidence of the affect of dietary intake on disease prevention and treatment; and (5) changes in food regulation that appear to support the expanded growth of dietary supplements and functional foods.[8]

Application to Nursing

Nurses can understand the appeal of dietary supplements as an aspect of self-care. Compliance with conventional medications and recommended dietary and lifestyle changes can also be suggested as an aspect of self-care to decrease risk or to alleviate a disorder. It is also possible that patients may use supplements instead of conventional medications because of high prescription costs. If this is the case, patients can be referred to social services or pharmaceutical company programs that may be able to assist financially. Information on dietary supplements when appropriate can be offered to patients, which they can then discuss with their primary health care providers. An example would be to provide information on a dietary supplement such as the herb chamomile (*Matricaria recutita* or *Matricaria chamomilla*), which seems to stimulate digestion and may decrease inflammation and spasms of the gastrointestinal (GI) tract. Chamomile may also be calming. However, if an individual has ragweed allergy, allergic reactions can occur. Consequently, a patient can discuss dietary supplement use with a primary health care provider.

Referral to registered dietitians for nutrition therapy involving dietary supplements or for general nutrition counseling is always an option. Health professionals and the public can consult the American Dietetic Association's website (www.eatright.org) for guidance on meeting specific health promotion or nutrition therapy goals. Registered dietitians are trained to consider several factors when advising on nutrient and other dietary supplements. Factors considered include the level of scientific evidence available on the substance, demographics (i.e., age, gender), disease states, clinical parameters (e.g., blood pressure and weight), medications (prescribed and OTC) currently used, and risks or benefits of the substance. Dietary supplements should always be complementary to a sound diet. Dietary intake should first be adjusted to fulfill nutrient gaps before dietary supplements are used.[9]

MEDICATIONS

Drug-Nutrient Interactions

Drug-nutrient interactions become more of a concern as the use of dietary supplements increases along with continued use of OTC medication and the plethora of prescription drugs. In essence, dietary supplements may act as drugs, particularly when patients take many medications. The rule of eights may apply, which is that if a patient takes eight or more medications and/or supplements, there are bound to be some drug-drug or nutrient-drug interactions.

All drugs produce physiologic effects; some of these effects are unintended (side effects) and constitute the risks of medication use. The amount and rate of drug absorption can be affected by the composition and timing of food intake. Conversely, food intake, absorption, and metabolism can be altered by medication. Drug-nutrient interactions have the potential to reduce drug efficacy, interfere with disease control, foster nutritional deficiencies, influence food intake, or provoke a toxic reaction.[10] The Joint Commission (TJC) strongly recommends evaluation of drug and diet combinations. Documentation of these interactions, which may be done by the registered dietitian or nurse, is essential in complying with TJC standards. In addition to medications, use of alcohol and street drugs also affect nutritional status and nutrient requirements.

TABLE 16-1   AT LEAST IT'S NATURAL!

Herbal remedies and dietary supplements are not regulated by the FDA, so the purity, potency, and safety of these products can and do vary. Manufacturers' claims of efficacy and safety are not subject to the same rigorous testing that is mandatory for medications. It is likely for herbs and dietary supplements to be contaminated with other herbs, pesticides, herbicides, and other products during growth, harvesting, preparation, and storage. Moreover, active chemical components in the herb may not be standardized. This leads to dissimilar potencies from lot to lot, or even from capsule to capsule within the same lot. Safety, toxicity, and the likelihood of adverse interactions with other medications or treatments frequently have not been tested, particularly in children. Patients contemplating use of herbs and dietary supplements should proceed with caution and seek out products only from reliable manufacturers.

The reason many people give for using herbal remedies and food supplements is based in tradition ("The Chinese have been using this for thousands of years!") and extensive and aggressive marketing as "miracle cures" for what might ail a person rather than scientific data. Many turn to herbal remedies because they are "natural" and therefore seen as harmless. Well, hemlock, nightshade, mistletoe berries, belladonna, and poison ivy are all "natural" plants. What many do not realize is that "natural" is not synonymous with "safe"—especially when they combine herbs with medications.

HERB	TRADITIONAL USE*	DRUG(S) THAT INTERACT WITH THE HERB	ADVERSE EFFECTS/DRUG INTERACTIONS
Chamomile (English) (*Chamaemelum nobile, Matricaria recutita*)	Indigestion, reduce tension and induce sleep, eczema, irritation of mucous membranes following chemotherapy or radiation (for cancer)	Anticoagulants: heparin, warfarin (Coumadin)	May increase bleeding time
		Benzodiazepines: alprazolam (Xanax), chlordiazepoxide (Librium), diazepam (Valium), flurazepam (Dalmane), lorazepam (Ativan), temazepam (Restoril), triazolam (Halcion)	Binds to benzodiazepine receptors, which may alter effect of drug
		Central nervous system (CNS) depressants: alcohol, anticonvulsants, antiemetics, antihistamines, antipsychotics, antivertigo drugs, barbiturates, hypnotics, opioids, tricyclic antidepressants, paraldehyde (Paral)	May add to sedative effect
Chasteberry (*Vitex agnus-castus*)	Premenstrual syndrome (PMS), menopausal symptoms, amenorrhea, and other menstrual irregularities, fibrocystic breasts	Hormone replacement therapy, oral contraceptives	Herb binds to estrogen receptor, may counteract oral contraceptives
Dong quai (*Angelica sinensis*)	Menstrual irregularities and menopausal complaints	Anticoagulants	May increase bleeding time; if using concurrently, obtain prothrombin time and International Normalized Ratio (INR) to rule out interactions
Echinacea (*Echinacea angustifolia, E. pallida, E. purpurea*)	Decrease duration of colds	Immunosuppressants: azathioprine, basiliximab, cyclosporine, daclizumab, interferon, muromaonab-CD3, mycophenolate, sirolimus, tacrolimus, corticosteroids	May decrease immunosuppressant effect
Ma Huang, Ephedra (*Ephedra sinica, E. equisetina, E. intermedia*)	Bronchodilator, decongestant, CNS stimulant, diuretic	Amitriptyline (Elavil)	Drug may decrease hypertensive effect of ephedrine

Continued

TABLE 16-1	AT LEAST IT'S NATURAL!—cont'd		
HERB	**TRADITIONAL USE***	**DRUG(S) THAT INTERACT WITH THE HERB**	**ADVERSE EFFECTS/DRUG INTERACTIONS**
		Anticonvulsants	Sympathomimetic effects, which may interfere with drug
		General anesthetics	Concurrent use may result in arrhythmias
		Caffeine and other xanthine alkaloids	Increased effects and potential toxicity
		Monoamine oxidase inhibitors (MAOIs)	Increased sympathomimetic effects
		Antihypertensives: angiotensin-converting enzyme (ACE) inhibitors, alpha blockers, angiotensin II receptor blockers, beta blockers, calcium channel blockers, diuretics	May decrease effectiveness of drug due to stimulant effect
		Insulin/oral hypoglycemic agents	Possible hyperglycemia with concurrent use
		Methylphenidate (Ritalin)	May displace drug from adrenergic neurons, which may decrease effectiveness of drug
		Morphine	Increases analgesic effect
		Oxytocin (Pitocin)	Possible hypertension
Evening primrose oil (*Oenothera biennis L*)	PMS, eczema, diabetic neuropathy, fibrocystic breasts, rheumatoid arthritis	Phenothiazines: chlorpromazine (Thorazine), fluphenazine (Prolixin), prochlorperazine (Compazine), promethazine hydrochloride (Phenergan)	May increase risk of seizures
		Anticoagulants	May increase risk of bleeding
Ginkgo (*Ginkgo biloba*)	Improved blood flow, protection against free-radical damage, attention-deficit/hyperactivity disorder (ADHD), dementia, macular degeneration, mental performance	Aspirin or Coumadin	May increase risk of bleeding
Ginseng American (*Panax quinquefolius*)	ADHD, stress reduction, chronic fatigue syndrome, fibromyalgia, age-related memory loss, menopausal cloudy thinking	Insulin/oral hypoglycemic agents	May enhance hypoglycemic effect
Panax or Asian (*Panax ginseng*)		Oral contraceptives/hormone replacement therapy	May alter effectiveness of exogenous hormones
		General anesthetics	Should be discontinued 7 days before surgery, herb increases risk of hypoglycemia and bleeding
		Caffeine and other stimulants	Red ginseng (steamed) may be additive to stimulant effect
		Immunosuppressants	Ginseng has immunostimulant activity and should not be used concurrently
		MAOIs	Potentiates phenelzine, causing manic symptoms
Kava (or kava kava) (*Piper methysticum*)	Sleep disorders, antianxiety, tension headaches, menopausal anxiety, fibromyalgia	Alprazolam (Xanax)	Synergistic CNS activity of alprazolam

TABLE 16-1	AT LEAST IT'S NATURAL!—cont'd		
HERB	**TRADITIONAL USE***	**DRUG(S) THAT INTERACT WITH THE HERB**	**ADVERSE EFFECTS/DRUG INTERACTIONS**
		Alcohol, tranquilizers (barbiturates), and antidepressants	May potentiate action
		Antiparkinsonian drugs	May increase tremors and make medications less effective
Senna (*Cassia senna*)	Laxative, weight loss,	Any drug	May reduce intestinal absorption
		Antiarrhythmics	May potentiate drug
		Corticosteroids	May cause hypokalemia
		Digoxin/cardiac glycosides	May increase effects
		Diuretics	May interfere with potassium-sparing effect
St. John's wort	Depression, seasonal affective disorder	Theophylline and beta-2 agonists	Possibility of increased anxiety
		Selective serotonin reuptake inhibitors (SSRIs)	Serotonin syndrome (sweating, agitation, tremor)
Valerian (*Valeriana officinalis*)	Sleep disorders, ADHD, menstrual cramps	Sedatives, barbiturates, CNS depressants, general anesthetics, thiopental	May intensify effects

*Not an exhaustive listing.
From Long S: Drug-nutrient interactions. In Schlenker ED, Long S, editors: *Williams' essentials of nutrition & diet therapy,* ed 10, St. Louis, 2010, Mosby.
Data from Kuhn MA, Winston D: *Herbal therapy and supplements. a scientific and traditional approach,* ed 2, Philadelphia, 2007, Lippincott; Kemper K, Gardiner P, Chan E: "At least it's natural." Herbs and dietary supplements in ADHD, *Contemp Pediatr* 9:116-130, 2000. Accessed April 11, 2009, from *www.contemporarypediatrics.com*; Kemper K, Gardiner P, Conboy LA: Herbs and adolescent girls: avoiding the hazards of self-treatment, *Contemp Pediatr* 3:133-154, 2000. Accessed April 11, 2009, from *www.contemporarypediatrics.com*.

Risk Factors of Drug-Nutrient Interactions

Determination of risk for drug-nutrient reactions depends on characteristics of the individual, including age, physiologic status, multiple drug intake, hepatic and renal function, and typical dietary intake.

Age

Older adults are more at risk for drug-nutrient reactions because of the greater variety of medications used and reduced physiologic functioning affecting drug use. Older patients often experience several different disorders simultaneously, each with complications and medications that may interact. Nutritional status may be compromised because of physical and social dimensions that affect their ability to procure and prepare nutritious meals. The high rate of drug reactions noted among older adults also may be caused by a combination of these factors, including drug misuse or overuse.

Young children also can be affected by drug-nutrient interactions. Use of vitamins/minerals, dietary supplements, and OTC medications intended for adults can result in drug-nutrient reactions because the substances will be metabolized differently by the developing body systems of children.

Physiologic Status

Impaired ability to absorb, metabolize, or excrete nutrients and medications because of disorders of the GI tract and reduced hepatic and renal functioning increases the risk of drug-nutrient reactions. Postoperative trauma or injury may also trigger atypical physiologic responses to drug-nutrient interactions. Age alters physiologic status as the body matures. Drug doses can vary depending on a person's weight and metabolic function as an aspect of age-related physiologic status. Use of medications during pregnancy requires caution because of the multiple effects on the fetus and on the nutritional status of the mother.

Polypharmacy (Multiple Drug Intake)

Certain types of illness or disease groups tend to require combinations of therapeutic drugs plus other medications, including OTC drugs, for relief of symptoms. The resulting drug-nutrient reactions may be related to the disease itself or be a reaction to medications. For example, intestinal bleeding often causes iron deficiency anemia among patients with arthritis. This intestinal bleeding is a common side effect of long-term use of nonsteroidal anti-inflammatory drugs (NSAIDs), either prescribed or OTC, taken to reduce the symptoms of arthritis. Other chronic conditions such as hypertension and diabetes may result in similar drug-nutrient interactions. If other acute disorders develop, the combination of medications may affect nutrient availability or function.

Influence of Typical Dietary Intake

The basis of a person's nutritional status depends on foods regularly consumed; the nutritional content of these foods affects body functions. A well-nourished individual is better able to withstand a medical regimen that may affect nutrient functioning. In contrast, individuals who are malnourished or marginally deficient in nutrient intake are more at risk for complications of drug-nutrient reactions as the body's stores of nutrients are diminished. For example, individuals who excessively consume alcohol tend to be marginally deficient in a number of nutrients either because of inadequate food intake (alcohol is an appetite depressant) or because of drug (alcohol)-nutrient interactions. If illness necessitates therapeutic drug intervention, nutritional status may be further compromised, increasing the likelihood of drug-nutrient interactions.

Prescription and Over-the-Counter Medications

We receive an avalanche of messages to use medications to cure every ailment we experience. Knowledge of medications is not confined to health care providers because television, radio, and print media present advertisements about prescription drugs. Often, the descriptions of the disorders seem to apply to most of the audience, so much so that patients now approach primary health care providers requesting prescriptions for conditions for which they have not yet been diagnosed.

Although the public has become more educated about prescription drugs, OTC medications may be viewed as harmless because prescriptions are not required. Harmless they are not. A number of OTC medications that were originally prescription medications are now available without prescriptions. Although the directions for use tend to be lower doses than when used as a prescription drug, interactions with other medications, foods, nutrients, and supplements such as herbs may occur (Table 16-2). For example, antiulcer agents or histamine blockers such as ranitidine (Zantac) and famotidine (Pepcid) are available OTC.

TABLE 16-2	MEDICATIONS THAT AFFECT FOOD AND/OR NUTRIENTS			
DRUG CLASS	**EXAMPLES**	**ACTION**	**NUTRIENTS AFFECTED**	**HOW TO AVOID**
Alcohol, particularly excessive use	Beer, wine, spirits	Increases turnover of some vitamins; substitution of alcohol for food	Vitamin B_{12}, folate, and magnesium	Limit alcohol consumption to <2 drinks per day for men, <1 drink per day for women
Analgesics, NSAIDs, and anti-inflammatory agents	Salicylates (aspirin), ibuprofen (Motrin, Advil), naproxen (Anaprox, Aleve, Naprosyn), acetaminophen (Tylenol)	Increases loss of vitamin C and competes with folate and vitamin K	Vitamin C, folate, vitamin K	Increase intake of foods high in vitamin C, folate, and vitamin K; take with 8 oz water
Antacids	Aluminum antacids, H_2 blockers	Inactivates thiamin; decreased absorption of some nutrients	Thiamin B_1	Foods containing thiamin (B_1) should be consumed at a different time; depending on antacid, possibly magnesium, phosphorus, iron, vitamin A, and folate Take antacid after meals; take iron, magnesium, or folate supplements separately by 2 hours; take separately from citrus fruit or juices or calcium citrate by 3 hours
Antiulcer agents (histamine blockers)	Ranitidine (Zantac), Cimetidine (Tagamet), famotidine (Pepcid)	Decreases vitamin absorption	Vitamin B_{12}	Consult physician or registered dietitian regarding vitamin B_{12} supplementation

TABLE 16-2	**MEDICATIONS THAT AFFECT FOOD AND/OR NUTRIENTS—cont'd**			
DRUG CLASS	**EXAMPLES**	**ACTION**	**NUTRIENTS AFFECTED**	**HOW TO AVOID**
Antibiotics	Tetracycline, Ciprofloxacin (Cipro)	Chelation of minerals; ingestion with caffeine may increase excitability and nervousness	Calcium, magnesium, iron, and zinc; caffeine	Take tetracycline at least 1 hr before or 2 hr after a meal; do not take with caffeine-containing products
Antineoplastic drugs	Methotrexate	Causes mucosal damage, which may cause decreased nutrient absorption	Folate and vitamin B_{12}, also see *Antibiotics*	Consult physician or registered dietitian regarding supplementation
Anticholinergics	Amitriptyline (Elavil), chlorpromazine (Thorazine)	Saliva thickens and loses ability to prevent tooth decay	Fluids	Increase intake of fluids
Anticonvulsants	Phenobarbital, Phenytoin (Dilantin)	Increases metabolism of folate (possibly leading to megaloblastic anemia), vitamin D (especially in children), and vitamin K	Folate, vitamin D, and vitamin K	Increase folate, vitamins D and K intake
Antidepressants	Lithium carbonate, Lithane, Lithobid, Lithonate, Lithotabs, Eskalith	May cause metallic taste, nausea, vomiting, dry mouth, anorexia, weight gain, and increased thirst	Fluids	Drink 2-3 L of water per day and take with food, consistent sodium intake
Antihyperlipidemics	Cholestyramine (Questran), colestipol (Colestid)	Binds bile salts and nutrients	Fat-soluble vitamins (A, D, E, K), folate, vitamin B_{12}, and iron	Include rich sources of these vitamins and minerals in diet
Antituberculosis	Isoniazid (INH)	Inhibits conversion of vitamin B_6 to active form	Vitamin B_6	Vitamin B_6 supplementation is necessary to prevent deficiency and peripheral neuropathy
Corticosteroids	Prednisone, Solu-Medrol, hydrocortisone	Increases excretion	Protein, potassium, calcium, magnesium, zinc, vitamin C, and vitamin B_6	Increase intake of foods high in protein, potassium, calcium, magnesium, zinc, vitamin C, and vitamin B_6
Loop diuretics	Furosemide (Lasix)	Increases mineral excretion in urine	Potassium, calcium, magnesium, zinc, sodium, and chloride	Include fresh fruits and vegetables in diet
Thiazide diuretics	Hydrochlorothiazide (HCTZ)	Increases excretion of most electrolytes, but enhances reabsorption of calcium	Potassium, calcium, magnesium, zinc, sodium, chloride, and calcium	Increase intake of foods high in potassium, calcium, magnesium, zinc, sodium, chloride, and calcium
Potassium-sparing diuretics	Triamterene (Dyrenium)	Hyperkalemia	Potassium	Avoid potassium-based salt substitutes
Laxatives	Fibercon, Mitrolan	Decreases nutrient absorption	Vitamins and minerals	Consult physician or registered dietitian regarding supplementation

Continued

TABLE 16-2. MEDICATIONS THAT AFFECT FOOD AND/OR NUTRIENTS—cont'd

DRUG CLASS	EXAMPLES	ACTION	NUTRIENTS AFFECTED	HOW TO AVOID
Sedatives	Barbiturates	Increases metabolism of vitamins	Folate, vitamin D, vitamin B_{12}, thiamin, and vitamin C	Increase intake of foods high in folate, vitamin D, vitamin B_{12}, thiamin, and vitamin C
Mineral oil	Agoral Plain	Decreases absorption	Fat-soluble vitamins (A, D, E, K), beta carotene, calcium, phosphorus, and potassium	Take 2 hr apart from food and fat-soluble vitamins
Oral contraceptives	Estrogen/progestin	May cause selective malabsorption or increased metabolism and turnover	Vitamin B_6 and folate	Increase foods high in B_6 and folate

NSAIDs, nonsteroidal anti-inflammatory drugs.
From Long S: Drug-nutrient interactions. In Schlenker ED, Long S, editors: *Williams' essentials of nutrition & diet therapy,* ed 10, St. Louis, 2010, Mosby.
Data from Anderson J, Bland SE: Drug-food interactions, *J Pharm Soc Wisc,* Nov/Dec:28-35, 1998; Bobroff LB, Lentz A, Turner RE: *Food/ drug and drug/nutrient interactions: what you should know about your medications,* Gainesville, 1994, University of Florida Cooperative Extension Service, Institute of Food and Agricultural Science. Available at http://edis.ifas.ufl.edu/topic_food_and_drugs; Food and Drug Administration/National Consumers League: *Food & drug interactions* [brochure], Washington, DC, Authors.

Although they were originally prescription drugs for ulcer treatment, ads suggest their use for ordinary indigestion caused by overeating or eating spicy, high-fat foods. Both are dietary distress situations that can be remedied by dietary behavior change rather than medication. Regular use of these histamine blockers can decrease absorption of vitamin B_{12}, which is a problem for older adults who are often the target audience for these medications.

Effects of Drugs on Food and Nutrients

Most drug absorption occurs through the GI mucosa, predominantly in the small intestine. Before drugs can be absorbed, they must first be metabolized and dissolved in gastric juices of the stomach. The speed with which the drug leaves the stomach depends on the gastric emptying time, which affects the rate of drug absorption. The rate of drug absorption may either increase or decrease based on the amount of food in the GI tract. In the fasting state, the medication leaves the empty stomach quickly and is absorbed from the small intestine. For some drugs that is too quick because time is needed for disintegration into absorbable particles. For those drugs, it is better to take the medication in the fed state in which the stomach, containing food, empties more slowly, especially after consuming large meals, heated food, and meals with fat, all of which slow emptying time.

Drugs can alter food intake, nutrient absorption, metabolism, and excretion. These drugs include prescription medications, OTC drugs, and even alcohol. If a nutrient binds with a medication, decreased solubility of both the nutrient and drug can result. Drugs used to lower serum cholesterol levels bind with fat-soluble vitamins and bile salts. As a result, both the bile salts and vitamins are excreted. Some drugs can decrease the amount of digestive enzymes available and thereby decrease nutrient absorption. Drugs that decrease transit time in the GI tract will also decrease nutrient absorption. The tables in this chapter provide information on selected drug-nutrient interactions.

Mineral status can be affected by drugs, resulting in either depletion or overload. Depletion may occur from the simultaneous use of several medications that each has the side effect of mineral depletion. A common source of mineral depletion is the use of potassium-depleting diuretics in addition to the use of laxatives that also may cause potassium loss. Older adults often use these products; their dietary intake may be marginal in mineral content as well. Overload may occur in instances in which renal function is compromised and potassium-sparing diuretics (e.g., spironolactone) and potassium supplements are used. Patient education is vital regarding the use of potassium supplements. Clear information is essential; patients should be taught about the kind of diuretic they are taking and potential side effects to reduce inappropriate supplementation.

Medications can also alter food intake by acting as appetite depressants or stimulants (Box 16-1), altering taste sensations (Box 16-2), or producing nausea and vomiting, which further decrease appetite. The *Teaching Tool* box, Minimizing Drug Side Effects, provides a number of specific suggestions.

Drugs may cause additional nutrition problems by affecting GI tract motility (which can change nutrient absorption) or GI tract pH. Drugs also may cause injury of GI mucosa,

BOX 16-1 SELECTED DRUGS THAT AFFECT APPETITE

Appetite Stimulants

Antidepressants
Amitriptyline (Elavil, Endep)
Clomipramine HCl (Anafranil)
Monoamine Oxidase Inhibitor (MAOI)
Tranylcypromine Sulfate (Parnate)

Antihistamines
Astemizole (Hismanal)
Cyproheptadine HCl (Periactin)

Bronchodilator
Albuterol Sulfate (Proventil, Ventolin)

Steroids
Anabolic Steroids
Oxandrolone (Anavar)
Corticosteroids
Hydrocortisone (Cortef)
Glucocorticoids
Dexamethasone (Decadron)
Methylprednisolone (Medrol)

Tranquilizers
Lithium Carbonate (Lithane)
Benzodiazepines
Chlordiazepoxide HCl (Librium)
Diazepam (Valium)
Prazepam (Centrax)
Phenothiazines
Chlorpromazine HCl (Thorazine)
Promethazine HCl (Phenergan)

Appetite Depressants

Amphetamines
Benzphetamine HCl (Didrex)
Fenfluramine HCl (Pondimin)
Phenylpropanolamine (Dexatrim, Dimetapp, Triaminic)

Antidysrhythmics
Digitalis
Digitoxin (Crystodigin, Digitoxin)
Digoxin (Digoxin, Lanoxin)

Antibiotics
Amphotericin B (Fungizone)
Gentamicin (Garamycin)
Metronidazole (Flagyl)
Zidovudine (AZT)

Antidepressant
Fluoxetine HCl (Prozac)

Antihistamine
Azatadine Maleate (Optimine)

Antihypertensive
Amiloride and Hydrochlorothiazide (Moduretic)
Captopril (Capoten)
Chlorthalidone (Hygroton)

Muscle Relaxant
Dantrolene Sodium (Dantrium)

Stimulant/Anti-ADD
Methylphenidate HCl (Ritalin)

Data from Pronsky ZM. *Food-medication Interactions,* ed 15, Birchrunville, Pa, 2008, Food-Medication Interactions.

BOX 16-2 SELECTED DRUGS THAT ALTER TASTE

Antidysrhythmic
Amiodarone (Cordarone)

Antiarthritic/Chelating Agent
Penicillamine (Cuprimine, Depen)

Antibiotics
Ampicillin
Clarithromycin (Biaxin)

Anticonvulsant
Phenytoin (Dilantin)

Antidepressants
Clomipramine HCl (Anafranil)
Fluoxetine HCl (Prozac)

Antifungal
Griseofulvin (Fulvicin, Grifulvin V, Grisacrin)

Antigout
Allopurinol (Zyloprim)

Antihypertensives
Captopril (Capoten)
Labetalol HCl (Normodyne, Trandate)

Antimanics
Lithium Carbonate (Eskalith, Lithane, Lithobid)
Lithium Citrate (Cibalith-S)

Antiparkinsonian
Levodopa (Dopar, Larodopa)

Antiviral/Anti-HIV
Didanosine (Videx)

Muscle Relaxant
Dantrolene Sodium (Dantrium)

Muscle Relaxant/Antispasmodic
Baclofen (Lioresal)

Stimulant/Amphetamine
Dextroamphetamine Sulfate (Dexedrine)

Data from Pronsky ZM: *Food-medication interactions,* ed 15, Birchrunville, Pa, 2008, Food-Medication Interactions.

✳ TEACHING TOOL
Minimizing Drug Side Effects

A number of drugs have side effects—symptoms not caused by the illness for which the drugs have been prescribed but as physiologic responses of the body to the drug itself. The side effects may be mild or quite bothersome. Some may be serious enough to warrant a change in medication. Before using these strategies as education tools, consult the client's primary health care provider to ascertain if additional medical intervention is required.

Side Effect: Diminished Appetite
- Consider eating several small meals or snacks throughout the day.
- Describe a setting and atmosphere for mealtimes that enhances appetite. Assist the client in exploring approaches to encourage an optimum eating environment.
- Discuss client's favorite foods. Brainstorm about how recipes can be adapted to comply with dietary therapeutic plans.

Side Effect: Modified Taste Sensations
- Visit a dentist regularly to maintain oral hygiene.
- Mask the taste of medications, if needed, with fruit sauces such as applesauce, crushed pineapple, or milk products. First determine if combinations are acceptable and not contraindicated.

Side Effect: Increased Appetite
- Alert client to the appetite (and craving sweets) stimulant effect of certain medications.

- Evaluate client's typical dietary intake. Suggest high-fiber foods to provide a quick sense of feeling full.
- Advise limiting availability to high kcal foods and drinks to minimize excess kcal intake.
- Increase activity.

Side Effect: GI Tract Irritation and Discomfort
- Advise client to sit up or stand after taking medications that have the potential to cause heartburn or indigestion.
- Reduce intake of fat, greasy, and/or highly acidic foods, including citrus juices and tomato products.
- Limit food intake in the evening to prevent reflux.
- Control consumption of spicy foods, peppermint, colas, chocolate, alcohol, pepper, decaffeinated coffee, and caffeine if these produce gastric discomfort.

Side Effect: Nausea
- Control liquid intake by serving after meals or drink only small quantities with meals.
- Sustain adequate fluid volume; cold, carbonated, or clear liquids are easier to tolerate.

Side Effect: Dry or Sore Mouth
- Consume softer, moist foods such as applesauce, puddings, pureed foods, and mashed potatoes.
- Include iced and cold foods throughout the day; consider ice pops, frozen yogurt, ice cream, sorbets, and cooled melons.
- Encourage oral hygiene before and after eating.
- Avoid mouthwashes, which can further dry the oral mucosa.

Data from Pronsky ZM: *Food-medication interactions,* ed 15, Birchrunville, Pa, 2008, Food-Medication Interactions.

---

development of drug-nutrient compounds, decreased bile acid function, and depressed nutrient transport mechanisms (Table 16-3). Nutrient metabolism and excretion may be modified by drug therapy in a mechanism similar to that of nutrient absorption, with the addition of effects caused by physical characteristics of solubility and stability of the drug.

The metabolic and excretion rate of the drug itself may also interfere with nutrient metabolism and excretion. Nutrient metabolism can be affected by vitamin analogs that compete metabolically with the vitamin. Certain medications act as vitamin antagonists, preventing vitamins from completing metabolic functions. Warfarin (Coumadin), the anticoagulant, is a vitamin K antagonist that prevents the activation of the storage form of vitamin K; blood clotting, for which vitamin K is a factor, is then reduced. The converse, the effect of vitamin K on warfarin, is explored in *The Nursing Approach* box near the end of this chapter. Other drugs, such as oral contraceptives, may cause marginal deficiencies of B vitamins and vitamin C by causing increased use of these vitamins. Excretion of nutrients may be altered if a medication results in retention of a drug normally excreted. As described in relation to mineral depletion, some diuretics

are potassium sparing, causing the body to conserve more potassium than usual; other diuretics are potassium depleting. Depending on the type of diuretic, dietary support of additional food sources of potassium may be warranted. Table 16-2 presents information on how various drug classes affect food intake, nutrient absorption, metabolism, and excretion.

Conversely, foods and nutrients may affect drug action, producing uncomfortable side effects. Most noteworthy are the adverse side effects associated with monoamine oxidase inhibitors (MAOIs). MAOIs, such as phenelzine (Nardil) and tranylcypromine (Parnate), may be prescribed to treat depression. These drugs inhibit the enzyme monoamine oxidase. The function of monoamine oxidase is to inactivate tyramine, a compound found in some foods. Without monoamine oxidase, the level of tyramine increases the release of norepinephrine. Elevated levels of norepinephrine may cause increased blood pressure, headache, pallor, and heart palpitations. Life-threatening severe hypertension can develop. Patients who take MAOIs should avoid foods and drugs that contain tyramine. OTC medications list warnings when appropriate, but foods are not so labeled. An important

TABLE 16-3	DRUGS THAT MAY CAUSE NUTRITIONAL PROBLEMS	
NUTRITIONAL PROBLEM	DRUGS	USE
May cause depression that results in weight fluctuation	Carbidopa/levodopa	Antiparkinsonian
	Beta blockers	Antihypertensive
	Clonidine	Antihypertensive
	Benzodiazepines	Antianxiety
	Barbiturates	Antianxiety
	Anticonvulsants	Epilepsy
	Histamine H_2 blockers	Peptic ulcer disease
	Calcium channel blockers	Antihypertensive
	Thiazide diuretics	Antihypertensive
	Digoxin	Antidysrhythmic
May delay gastric emptying time	Anesthetic agents	Anesthesia
	Opiates	Narcotic
	Tricyclic antidepressant	Antidepressant
	Clonidine	Antihypertensive
	Calcium channel blockers	Antihypertensive
	Nitrates	Antianginal
	Meperidine	Analgesic
	Theophylline	Bronchodilator
	Caffeine	Stimulant
May increase gastric emptying time	Metoclopramide	Antiemetic
	Cisapride	Cholinergic enhancer
	Bethanechol	Cholinergic
	Erythromycin	Antibacterial
Can cause folate deficiency	Phenytoin	Seizures
	Methotrexate	Antimetabolite
	Trimethoprim	Antibacterial
Can cause drowsiness, may cause missed meals	Antihistamines	Allergies
	Beta blockers	Antihypertensive
	Skeletal muscle relaxants	Relieve stiffness, pain, discomfort
	Antiemetics	Nausea and vomiting
	Benzodiazepines	Antianxiety
	Antipsychotics	Psychotic disorders
	Antidepressants	Depression
May cause nausea and vomiting	Selective serotonin reuptake inhibitors (SSRIs)	Antidepressant
	Antibiotics	Antibacterial
	Antineoplastic agents	Chemotherapy
	Digitalis	Antidysrhythmic
	General anesthetics	Anesthesia
	Theophylline	Bronchodilator
	Opioid derivatives	Narcotic

Data from Losben N: Dietitians and consultant pharmacists: A team approach to improved quality care (in *The Consultant Pharmacist*), Alexandria, Va, 1997, American Society of Consultant Pharmacists. Accessed February 21, 2010, from www.ascp.com/public/pubs/tcp/1997/dec/dietitians.html; MedlinePlus: *Drugs & supplements,* Bethesda, Md (updated January 2006), U.S. National Library of Medicine and National Institutes of Health. Accessed February 21, 2010, from http://medlineplus.gov.

component of patient education is for patients who take MAOIs to know which foods contain significant levels of tyramine (Box 16-3).

Effects of Food and Nutrients on Drugs

Medications must be absorbed to have a therapeutic effect. Food intake, or lack thereof, in addition to composition of the food may affect drug absorption. The timing of drug administration and meals also has clinical significance. If absorption is increased by the presence of food, medication should be taken with a meal or a snack. If drug absorption is depressed by the presence of food in the stomach, optimum absorption occurs if medication is taken at least 1 hour before or 2 hours after eating or tube feeding. Table 16-4 lists some common drug classes whose absorption is affected by food. A specific food example is grapefruit juice. Grapefruit juice, sometimes used to take medications, can affect the bioavailability of certain drugs (Box 16-4).

The established drug administration schedules in health care facilities often conflict with the optimal bioavailability

BOX 16-3   TYRAMINE-CONTAINING FOODS

Avoid: Contain High Tyramine Levels

Aged Foods

Hard (aged) cheeses and meats, salami or mortadella, air-dried sausage

Pickled/Smoked Foods

Smoked or pickled fish, herring in brine, sauerkraut, kimchi

Fermented

Fermented bean curd, miso, broad beans, fava beans

Extracts

Hydrolyzed protein extracts (in many processed foods), concentrated yeast extracts, brewer's yeast

Use with Caution in Small Servings
(¼ to ½ cup; 2 to 4 oz)

Aged Foods

Bologna, pepperoni, aged kielbasa sausage, liverwurst

Pickled/Smoked Foods

Smoked meats and fish, Schmaltz herring in oil, pate, lumpfish roe

Beverages

Red and white wines, port wines, distilled spirits, coffee,* cola*

Fermented Foods

Soy sauce, yogurt, and cream from unpasteurized milk

Fresh Foods

Fresh liver, avocado, figs, bananas, raspberries, chocolate,* peanuts

*Caffeine in amounts greater than 500 mg may intensify reactions.
Data from McCabe BJ: Dietary tyramine and other pressor amines in MAOI regimens: A review, *J Am Diet Assoc* 86:1059-1064, 1986; and Pronsky ZM, *Food-medication interactions*, ed 15, Birchrunville, Pa, 2008, Food-Medication Interactions.

of the drug. Absorption response can be altered in 77% to 93% of drugs by the presence of food in the digestive tract.[11] Concomitant food intake with drug administration usually delays absorption of the drug, but this may or may not decrease the amount of drug absorbed. As a general guideline, drugs should be given at least 1 hour before or 2 hours after a meal unless the medication causes GI distress when taken on an empty stomach. Such timing should enhance drug absorption and decrease hindrance of nutrient absorption. Tube feedings present other issues of drug-nutrient interactions (Box 16-5).

Effects of Herbs on Food, Nutrients, and Drugs

As discussed earlier, herbs are not innocuous but can have significant effects on the bioavailability of foods, nutrients, and drugs. Rather than support health, the interactions may cause additional health problems. Table 16-1 lists numerous herbs and potential drug interactions that may result. For example, taking the herb feverfew for migraines may interfere with warfarin by further inhibiting blood platelet formation. Even taken alone, feverfew decreases blood clotting and should be discontinued 2 weeks before surgery.

Of particular concern are the effects of certain commonly used herbs on surgery. Ginkgo, feverfew, garlic, ginger, ginseng, dong quai, and danshen affect blood clotting. Other herbs, such as valerian, kava kava (which may also cause liver damage), and St. John's wort, can prolong narcotic and anesthesia drug effects.

Application to Nursing

Table 16-5 stresses the importance of herb regulation and the need for education both for the public and for health care professionals. This table describes herbal products patients may use to treat selected conditions. When used medicinally, herbs should be prescribed by health care professionals who have knowledge of the herbal actions so that the desired benefits are produced without the negative side effects. Because herbs are easily available, many individuals self-diagnose and treat themselves without consultation with trained health care professionals.

Because herbs are not considered medications, patients often do not volunteer information regarding their use when they are asked, "What medications do you regularly take?" Consequently, nurses can assist this process by asking more detailed questions about supplement intake, such as the following.

- Do you use any dietary supplements? (Direct patient to include in the answer vitamins, minerals, botanicals, amino acids, concentrates, and extracts.)
  - If so, what dosage do you take? What other directions do you follow, such as taking with meals or at bedtime?
- What is the purpose of taking the dietary supplement? (Avoid questions like "What is that supposed to do?" because such implied skepticism can embarrass the patient and discourage honest reporting of supplement use.)
- Have you experienced any side effects?
- Do you take an herbal product, herbal supplement, or other "natural remedy"?
  - If so, do you take any prescription or nonprescription medications for the same purpose as the herbal product?
- Have you used this herbal product before?
- Are you allergic to any plant products?
- Are you pregnant or breastfeeding?
- Are you seeing an herbalist, acupuncturist, naturopathic practitioner, nutritionist, or natural healer?
- Is your physician or primary health care provider aware that you take these supplements (in addition to any prescribed medications)?

Keep an open mind about alternative supplements and medications, and remain current with new findings in this quickly changing area.

Text continued on page 368.

TABLE 16-4	FOODS AND/OR NUTRIENTS THAT AFFECT MEDICATIONS				
DRUG CLASS	**EXAMPLES**	**USE**	**ACTION**	**FOOD/ NUTRIENTS**	**HOW TO AVOID**
Alcohol, particularly excessive use	Beer, wine, spirits	Lower inhibitions, CNS depressant	Slows absorption	Food	Consume alcohol with food or meals
Analgesics and NSAIDs	Salicylates (aspirin), Ibuprofen (Motrin, Advil), naproxen (Anaprox, Aleve, Naprosyn), Acetaminophen (Tylenol)	Pain and fever	Alcohol ingestion increases hepatotoxicity, liver damage, or stomach bleeding	Alcohol	Limit alcohol intake to <2 drinks per day for men, <1 drink per day for women
Antiulcer agents (histamine blockers)	Cimetidine (Tagamet)	Ulcers	Increased blood alcohol levels; reduced caffeine clearance	Alcohol; caffeine-containing foods and beverages	Limit caffeine intake; limit alcohol intake to <2 drinks per day for men, <1 drink per day for women
Antibiotics	Ciprofloxacin (Cipro)	Infection	Decreases absorption	Dairy products	Avoid dairy products
Anticoagulant	Warfarin (Coumadin)	Blood clots	Reduced efficacy; increased anticoagulation	Vitamins K and E (supplements) may reduce efficacy; alcohol and garlic may increase anticoagulation	Limit foods high in vitamin K: broccoli, spinach, kale, turnip greens, cauliflower, Brussels sprouts; avoid high dose of vitamin E (400 IU or more)
Antineoplastic drugs	Methotrexate	Cancer	Increased hepatotoxicity with chronic alcohol use	Alcohol	Avoid alcohol
Antiemetic	Amitriptyline HCl (Elavil), chlorpromazine HCl (Thorazine)	Antidepressant; antipsychotic/ antiemetic	Increased sedation	Alcohol	Avoid alcohol
Anticonvulsants Antidepressants: MAOIs	Phenobarbital Phenelzine (Nardil), tranylcypromine (Parnate)	Seizures, epilepsy Depression, anxiety	Increased sedation Rapid, potentially fatal increase in blood pressure	Alcohol Foods or alcoholic beverages containing tyramine	Avoid alcohol Avoid beer; red wine; American processed, cheddar, bleu, Brie, mozzarella, and Parmesan cheeses; yogurt; sour cream; beef or chicken liver; cured meats such as sausage and salami; game meats; caviar; dried fish; avocados; bananas; yeast extracts; raisins; sauerkraut; soy sauce; miso soup; broad (fava) beans; ginseng; caffeine-containing products (colas, chocolate, coffee, tea)

Continued

TABLE 16-4   FOODS AND/OR NUTRIENTS THAT AFFECT MEDICATIONS—cont'd

DRUG CLASS	EXAMPLES	USE	ACTION	FOOD/ NUTRIENTS	HOW TO AVOID
Antihistamine	Fexofenadine (Allegra), loratadine (Claritin), cetirizine (Zyrtec), astemizole (Hismanal)	Allergies	Increases drowsiness and slows mental and motor performance	Alcohol	Use caution when operating machinery or driving
Antihypertensives	ACE-inhibitors, angiotensin II receptor antagonists, beta blockers, verapamil HCl	Hypertension	Reduced effectiveness	Natural licorice (glycyrrhiza glabra) and tyramine-rich foods	Avoid these foods
Antihyperlipidemics (HMG-CoA reductase inhibitors) or statins	Atorvastatin (Lipitor), lovastatin (Mevacor), pravastatin (Pravachol), simvastatin (Zocor)	High serum LDL cholesterol	Enhances absorption; increases risk of liver damage	Food/meals; alcohol	Lovastatin should be taken with evening meal to enhance absorption; avoid large amounts of alcohol
Antiparkinson	Levodopa (Dopar, Larodopa)	Parkinson's disease	Decreased absorption	High-protein foods (eggs, meat, protein supplements); B_6	Spread protein intake equally in 3-6 meals per day to minimize reaction; avoid B_6 supplements or multivitamin supplement in doses <10 mg
Antituberculosis	Isoniazid (INH)	Tuberculosis	Reduced absorption with foods; increased hepatotoxicity and reduced INH levels with alcohol	Alcohol	Take on empty stomach; avoid alcohol
Bronchodilators	Theophylline (Slo-bid, Theo-Dur)	Asthma, chronic bronchitis, and emphysema	Increased stimulation of CNS; alcohol can increase nausea, vomiting, headache, and irritability	Caffeine, alcohol	Avoid caffeine-containing foods/ beverages (chocolate, colas, teas, coffee); avoid alcohol if taking theophylline medications
Corticosteroids	Prednisolone (Pediapred, Prelone), methyl prednisolone (Solu-Medrol); hydrocortisone	Inflammation and itching	Stomach irritation	Food	Take with food or milk to decrease stomach upset
Hypoglycemic agents	Chlorpropamide (Diabinese), metformin (Glucophage)	Diabetes	Severe nausea and vomiting	Alcohol	Avoid alcohol

ACE, Angiotensin-converting enzyme; CNS, central nervous system; INH, isoniazid; LDL, low-density lipoprotein; NSAIDs, nonsteroidal anti-inflammatory drugs.

From Long S: Drug-nutrient interactions. In Schlenker ED, Long S, editors: Williams' essentials of nutrition & diet therapy, ed 10, St. Louis, 2010, Mosby.

Data from Bland SE: Drug-food interactions, J Pharm Soc Wisc Nov/Dec:28-35, 1998; Bobroff LB, Lentz A, Turner RE: Food/drug and drug/ nutrient interactions: what you should know about your medications, Gainesville, 1994, University of Florida Cooperative Extension Service, Institute of Food and Agricultural Science. Available at http://edis.ifas.ufl.edu/topic_food_and_drugs; Brown CH: Overview of drug interactions, US Pharm 25(5), 2000. Accessed April 11, 2009, from www.uspharmacist.com; U.S. Food and Drug Administration/National Consumers League: Food & drug interactions [brochure], Washington, DC, Authors.

BOX 16-4 GRAPEFRUIT "JUICES UP" CERTAIN MEDICATIONS

Almost all oral drugs are subject to first-pass metabolism. That is, any substance the body views as a toxin (e.g., drugs, alcohol) goes through the liver via hepatic portal circulation, thus removing some of the active substance from blood before it enters general circulation. This means a fraction of the original dose of the drug will not be "available" to systemic circulation because it has undergone biotransformation. In other words, bioavailability of the drug has been altered, or lowered. One mechanism responsible for this is an enzyme system found in the intestinal wall and liver. The cytochrome P450 3A4 system (specifically CYP3A4-mediated drug metabolism) is responsible for first-pass metabolism of many medications. Most medications are lipid soluble and readily absorbed. To eliminate toxins (i.e., drugs) from the body, however, the cytochrome P450 system either breaks them down in the gut or changes the drug into a more water-soluble version in the liver, allowing it to be eliminated via urine.

Where does grapefruit juice come into play? Grapefruit juice blocks the CYP3A4 enzyme in the wall of the small intestine, thus increasing bioavailability of the drug. This means a higher serum drug level, which may cause unpleasant consequences, including side effects and/or toxicity.

What is it in grapefruit juice that does this? The precise chemical nature of the substance responsible for inhibiting gut wall CYP3A4 enzyme is unknown, but it is believed that more than one component present in grapefruit juice may contribute to the inhibitory effect on CYP3A4.

A single glass (8 oz) of grapefruit juice has the potential to increase bioavailability and enhance beneficial or adverse effects of a broad range of medications. These effects can persist up to 72 hours after grapefruit consumption, until more CYP3A4 has been metabolized. Interactions have been found between grapefruit juice and drugs, as outlined in the following table:

Interactions between Grapefruit Juice and Medications

CATEGORY	GENERIC NAME	BRAND NAME	EFFECT
Antihypertensive (calcium channel blockers)	Felodipine	Plendil	Flushing, headache, tachycardia, decreased blood pressure
	Nifedipine	Procardia, Adalat	
	Nimodipine	Nimotop	
	Nisoldipine	Sular	
	Nicardipine	Cardene	
	Isradipine	DynaCirc	
	Verapamil	Calan, Isoptin	Same as above plus bradycardia and atrioventricular (AV) block
Immunosuppressant	Cyclosporine	Neoral, Sandimmune, SangCya	Kidney toxicity, increased susceptibility to infections
	Tacrolimus	Prograf	
Statin (HMG-CoA reductase inhibitors)	Atorvastatin	Lipitor	Headache, gastrointestinal complaints, muscle pain, increased risk of myopathy
	Lovastatin	Mevacor	
Caffeine	Simvastatin	Zocor	Nervousness, overstimulation
Antianxiety, insomnia, or depression	Buspirone	BuSpar	Increased sedation
	Diazepam	Valium	
	Alprazolam	Xanax	
	Midazolam	Versed	
	Triazolam	Halcion	
	Zaleplon	Sonata	
	Carbamazepine	Tegretol	
	Clomipramine	Anafranil	
	Trazodone	Desyrel	
Protease inhibitors	Saquinavir	Fortovase, Invirase	Doubles bioavailability, resulting in increased efficacy or toxicity depending on dose and patient variability
Sexual dysfunction	Sildenafil	Viagra	Delayed absorption (takes longer to become effective)

Continued

BOX 16-4   GRAPEFRUIT "JUICES UP" CERTAIN MEDICATIONS—cont'd

MEDICATIONS CONSIDERED SAFE FOR USE WITH GRAPEFRUIT

Cetirizine	Zyrtec, Reactine
Fexofenadine	Allegra
Fluvastatin	Lescol
Loratadine	Claritin
Pravastatin	Pravachol

From Long S: Drug-nutrient interactions. In Schlenker ED, Long S, editors: *Williams' essentials of nutrition & diet therapy,* ed 10, St. Louis, 2010, Mosby.

Data from Bailey DG, et al: Grapefruit juice-drug interactions, *Br J Clin Pharmacol* 46(2):101-110, 1998; Guo L, et al: Role of furanocoumarin derivatives on grapefruit juice–mediated inhibition of human CYP3A activity, *Drug Metab Dispos* 28:766-771, 2000; Ho P, et al: Inhibition of human CYP3A4 activity by grapefruit flavonoids, furanocoumarins and related compounds, *J Pharm Pharm Sci* 4(3):217-227, 2001; Hyland R, et al: Identification of the cytochrome P450 enzymes involved in the N-demethylation of sildenafil, *Br J Clin Pharmacol* 51:239-248, 2000; Jetter A, et al: Effects of grapefruit juice on the pharmacokinetics of sildenafil, *Clin Pharmacol Ther* 71(1):21-29, 2002; Kane GC, Lipsky JJ: Drug-grapefruit juice interactions, *Mayo Clin Proc* 75:933-942, 2000; Pronsky ZM: *Food medication interactions,* ed 15, Birchrunville, Pa, 2008, Food Medication Interactions; Schmiedlin-Ren P, et al: Mechanisms of enhanced oral availability of CYP3A4 substrates by grapefruit constituents, *Drug Metab Dispos* 25(1):1228-1233, 1997; University of Illinois Chicago College of Pharmacy Drug Information Center: *Grapefruit juice interactions,* Chicago, 2005, Author. Accessed April 11, 2009, from www.uic.edu/pharmacy/services/di/grapefru.htm.

BOX 16-5   TUBE FEEDINGS AND DRUG-NUTRIENT INTERACTIONS

Drug-nutrient interactions can compromise pharmacologic and nutritional therapeutic objectives of safety, efficacy, and quality of care. Moreover, these interactions can affect cost effectiveness of health care. Before administering an oral drug through a gastric or nasogastric feeding tube, ask yourself the following questions:

1. Is the feeding tube placed correctly?
2. Can the medication be crushed and delivered through a feeding tube?
3. Will there be an interaction between the medication and the feeding solution?
    - If so, will the interaction degrade the nutritional components of the feeding solution?
    - Or alter the medication's availability?
    - Or clog the tube?
4. Will the medication change the osmolality or pH in the feeding system?
    - Or cause nausea, vomiting, cramping, or diarrhea?

Pharmacists have valuable expertise in optimizing prescriptions. The number of potential drug-feeding formula interactions is nearly endless, and new medications and feeding formulas are becoming available almost daily. Consultation with pharmacy services is recommended to detect possible incompatibilities and recommendations for appropriate alternative forms of medications if necessary. Questions regarding specific feeding formulas and adverse drug reactions can be directed to the dietitian.

These general guidelines will help nurses avoid common problems when administering oral drugs through a feeding tube.

POTENTIAL PROBLEM	SOLUTION
Should I administer the tablet or liquid form of the medication?	Whenever possible, use the liquid form of a drug because it bypasses the dissolution process. But be aware that many liquid medications are formulated for pediatric patients; therefore, large volumes must be dispensed to meet the required dose for adults. This often results in diarrhea as a result of excessive amounts of sorbitol in the adjusted dose.
Okay, I checked and the only form of the medication available is a tablet. What should I do?	If a tablet is the only preparation available, consultation with the pharmacist is mandatory. Some tablets can be crushed if they are simple, compressed tablets designed to dissolve immediately in the GI tract. Keep in mind that crushing the tablet allows it to enter the bloodstream faster. The difference may or may not be clinically significant. Always confirm the type of coating on the tablet with the pharmacy.
I've checked with the pharmacy and was told the tablet could be crushed. How do I do that?	Ideally, medication(s) should be crushed in the pharmacy. But if you must do it yourself, the best technique is to position a unit-dose tablet in a mortar without removing it from the package. Then crush the tablet by tapping it through the package with a pestle (to avoid tearing the package, don't grind). If the medication isn't packaged as a unit-dose, place it between two paper medicine cups and pulverize the tablet with the mortar and pestle. Mix the crushed tablet thoroughly with 15-30 mL water (5-10 mL for children), and administer through the feeding tube. Tubing must be flushed with a minimum of 30 mL of room temperature sterile water before and after administration of each medication.

BOX 16-5	TUBE FEEDINGS AND DRUG-NUTRIENT INTERACTIONS—cont'd
POTENTIAL PROBLEM	**SOLUTION**
It seems like it would be easier to add the medication to the feeding formula.	Never add medications directly to the feeding formula. This can alter the medication's therapeutic effect and disrupt the integrity of the feeding formula, causing it to resemble curdled milk.
The pharmacy has the prescribed medications in liquid form. Is there anything special I need to do?	Check whether dilution of the medication formulation before administration is required. Hypertonic, irritating, or viscous medications should be diluted in at least 30 mL of water immediately before infusion to avoid gastric irritation and diarrhea. In some cases, 90 mL of water may be necessary for dilution. Adjust water amounts appropriately for pediatric patients and patients on fluid restrictions. Document amount of water used on patient's intake and output records.
If sugar-coated tablets can be crushed, are there tablets that cannot be crushed?	Some types of tablets must not be crushed. These include: *Buccal or sublingual tablets* (e.g., nitroglycerin or isosorbide) are intended to be absorbed by veins under the tongue or in the cheek, thus bypassing the liver (avoiding first-pass effect) and protecting the medication from contact with other drugs, foods, and GI secretions that could affect the medication's potency or bioavailability. *Enteric coated tablets* (e.g., bisacodyl [Dulcolax] and ferrous sulfate [Feosol]) are formulated to inhibit release of the active drug until after the tablet has passed from the stomach into the small intestine. Moreover, the tablet's coating protects the stomach from irritation from the medication. Crushing the tablet would put an end to the protective coating. *Uncoated gastric irritants* (including aspirin) remain effective following crushing, but they are more apt to trigger undesirable GI reactions such as cramping or bleeding. Ask for an alternative form or different medication. *Sustained-release or effervescent tablets* (e.g., Slow-L, Procan SR, Theolair-SR, Inderal LA) were designed to dissolve and release medication gradually (they contain 2 or 3 doses of the medication). As a result, if crushed, the patient would get an overdose of the medication. In addition, the planned beneficial effects would not be maintained throughout the dosing interval.
The prescribed medication is in the form of a capsule. Can't I just place it in the tube and flush it down with some water?	Capsules should not be crushed, but you can open some and mix the contents with water: *Hard gelatin capsules* (e.g., ampicillin and doxycycline) contain a medication in a powdered form. The capsule can be opened (it's designed to separate in the middle) and the powder mixed thoroughly with water. *Sustained-release capsules* (e.g., Slo-bid and Feosol Spansules) release the active medication slowly, over time, through coated beads or pellets inside the capsules. They are designed to dissolve in the GI tract at different rates, lengthening the medication's duration of action. Obviously, crushing capsules or their contents would damage the timed-release coatings. A better alternative would be a liquid form or a simple compressed tablet that can be crushed (ascertain dosage frequency is increased appropriately). *Soft gel capsules* (e.g., chloral hydrate, some vitamin preparations) can be dispensed through a feeding tube by poking a pinhole in one end and squeezing out the liquid contents. The liquid contents can also be drawn up in a syringe. Neither method should be used if delivering an exact dose is important. Some of the drug will always remain inside the capsule. Dissolve the capsule in 15-30 mL of warm water (5-10 mL for pediatric patients), then administer. The drug-water mixture will also work if you plan ahead—dissolving the capsule can take as long as 1 hour.

Data from Lehmann S, Barber JR: Giving medications by feeding tube, *Nursing* 91:58-61, 1991; Lourenco R: Enteral feedings: Drug/nutrient interaction, *Clin Nutr* 20(2):187-193, 2001; and Belknap DC, et al: Administration of medications through enteral feeding catheters, *Am J Crit Care* 6(5):382-392, 1997.

TABLE 16-5	COMMONLY USED HERBAL PRODUCTS AND NUTRACEUTICALS THAT MAY BE USED TO TREAT SELECTED CONDITIONS*		
CONDITION/HERB	**USE**	**ASSOCIATED ADVERSE EFFECTS**
Asthma		
Tylophora indica, T. asthmatica	Inhibits histamine release	Sore mouth, loss of taste for salt, morning nausea and vomiting
Adhatoda vasica	Bronchodilator	Vomiting and diarrhea; lack of conclusive efficacy data
Picrorhiza kurroa	Bronchodilator	Vomiting, cutaneous rash, anorexia, diarrhea, itching, giddiness, headache, abdominal pain, increased dyspnea
Khellin	Bronchodilator	
Onion extract *(Allium cepa)*	May inhibit leukotriene and thromboxane	Delirium, tachycardia, nausea, high incidence of GI side effects
Ginkgo *(Ginkgo biloba)*	Smooth muscle relaxant	Clinical efficacy unproven
Anxiety and Depression		
Chamomile *(Chamaemelum nobile, Matricaria chamomilla, M. recutita)*	GI spasm or irritation, sedative	Therapeutic amounts may vary depending on effect chamomile has on an individual; side effects infrequent
Valerian *(Valeriana officinalis)*	Insomnia, mild to moderate anxiety, stress and tension, premenstrual tension, hyperactivity, depression, insomnia, migraine headaches	Side effects not reported, but if used in too large a dose initially, it may cause excitability
Passion flower *(Passiflora incarnate)*	Relaxation and sleep	Not recommended for children <2 years; use of decreased initial dose recommended for those >65 years
Kava *(Piper methysticum)*	Sedation, anticonvulsive, antispasmodic, central muscular relaxant	Prolonged use causes a temporary yellow coloring of skin, hair, and nails; may cause liver damage; not recommended for use with other CNS depressants, including alcohol
Hops *(Humulus lupulus)*	Insomnia, digestive aid, treatment of intestinal ailments	
Ginseng *(Panax quinquefolius, P. ginseng, Eleutherococcus senticosus)*	Increase energy, improve stamina, enhance memory	Typically mild and dose related; most commonly observed are nervousness, sleeplessness, nausea, and occasionally headache
St. John's wort *(Hypericum perforatum)*	Depression	Fatigue, pruritus, weight gain, emotional vulnerability; photosensitivity; decreased effectiveness of oral contraceptive therapy possible
Black cohosh *(Cimicifuga racemosa)*	Sedative, relaxant	Not for use in pregnancy
California poppy *(Eschscholzia californica)*	Hypnotic, tranquilizer	
Damask rose *(Rosa damascene)*	Antidepressant	Use only good quality of damask rose
Lemon balm *(Melissa officinalis)*		
Neroli oil *(Citrus aurantium)*		
Jamaican dogwood *(Piscidia erythrina)*	Insomnia, migraine	
Linden *(Tifia europaea)*	Reduces nervous tension	
Gotu kola *(Centella asiatica)*	Relaxant	Gotu kola may cause rash; avoid while pregnant or breastfeeding
Mugwort *(Artemisia vulgaris)*		
Skullcap *(Scutellaria lateriflora)*		
Vervain *(Verbena officinalis)*		
Pasque flower *(Anemone pulsatilla)*	Sedative action	Use only dried plant
Lavender *(Lavandula species)*	Sedative	Avoid high doses of lavender in pregnancy
Wild lettuce *(Lactuca virosa)*		Excess amounts of wild lettuce can lead to insomnia.

TABLE 16-5	COMMONLY USED HERBAL PRODUCTS AND NUTRACEUTICALS THAT MAY BE USED TO TREAT SELECTED CONDITIONS*—cont'd	
CONDITION/HERB	**USE**	**ASSOCIATED ADVERSE EFFECTS**
Wood betony (Stachys officinalis)		Large doses of wood betony can cause vomiting; avoid high doses in pregnancy
Cancer Prevention and Treatment		
Shark cartilage	Antiangiogenic effect	Doubtful oral bioavailability of biologically active components
Aloe vera	May stimulate macrophage function (antitumor activity)	May have deleterious effects in patients with AIDS
Echinacea (Echinacea angustifolia, E. pallida)	Immunostimulatory activity	Unknown whether effective orally
Mistletoe (Phoradendron species and Viscum species)	Potent inducer of cytokines stimulating release of TNF-α and interleukin-1	
Antioxidant vitamins A and E	May reduce risk of lung cancer by reducing formation of free radicals	Vitamin A can be toxic
Garlic and onion (Allium sativum and A. cepa)	May decrease nitrosamine formation	
Green tea	Antioxidant properties, inhibits nucleoside transport	Contradictory epidemiologic studies regarding efficacy in cancer
Chaparral (Larrea tridentate, L. divaricata, L. mexicana)	Antioxidant properties	Hepatoxic; unproven and dangerous
Ginseng (Panax quinquefolius, P. ginseng, Eleutherococcus senticosus)	Antiestrogen properties	More data needed
Laetrile	May have tumor static activity	Unproven
Goldenseal (Hydrastis canadensis)	May prevent carcinogenesis	Use may be limited by toxicity
Oregon grape root (Mahonia aquifolium, M. nervosa)		
Barberry root (Berberis vulgaris)		
Pineapple	May cause tumor regression	More study needed
Sweet and red clover (Trifolium pratense)	Stimulates macrophage activity	
Cloud fungus	Immunostimulatory activity	
Colds and Flu		
Anise (Pimpinella anisum)	Expectorant action	May cause contact dermatitis; avoid use while pregnant or breastfeeding
Boneset (Eupatorium perfoliatum)	Antipyretic; influenza	Individuals with hypersensitivity to the Asteraceae family (e.g., chamomile, feverfew) should avoid use
Coltsfoot (Tussilago farfara)	Antitussive	Possible hepatotoxicity; has abortifacient effects, should not be taken while pregnant or breastfeeding
Echinacea (Echinacea angustifolia, E. pallida)	Prophylaxis and treatment of cold and flu symptoms	Continuous use (>6-8 weeks) may lead to immunosuppression; contraindicated in autoimmune diseases
Purple coneflower (E. purpurea) is a different species with similar properties		
Horehound (Marrubium vulgare)	Controversial use as expectorant, antitussive, cough suppressant, digestive aid, appetite stimulant	Large doses have produced cardiac irregularities
Slippery elm (Ulmus rubra)	Demulcent and emollient to treat sore throats	Pollen can be an allergen; may cause contact dermatitis
Zinc lozenges	Reduces duration and severity of cold symptoms	Possible nausea, unpleasant taste

Continued

TABLE 16-5 **COMMONLY USED HERBAL PRODUCTS AND NUTRACEUTICALS THAT MAY BE USED TO TREAT SELECTED CONDITIONS*—cont'd**

CONDITION/HERB	USE	ASSOCIATED ADVERSE EFFECTS
Diabetes		
Karela *(Momordica charantia)*	Hypoglycemic	May sufficiently lower blood glucose to merit decrease in insulin or oral medications to avoid or minimize incidence of hypoglycemia; karela juice will cause greater decrease in blood glucose than when slices of karela are fried
Ginseng *(Panax quinquefolius, P. ginseng, Eleutherococcus senticosus)*	Hypoglycemic	Korean or Chinese ginseng may exert greater hypoglycemic effect than Japanese ginseng
Brewer's yeast	Hypoglycemic	May cause unfavorable variability in blood glucose control if medical staff is unaware of concomitant use with chromium
GS$_4$ *(Gymnema sylvestre)*	Hypoglycemic	May decrease insulin and glyburide requirements but should not be relied on for blood glucose control
Devil's claw *(Harpagophytum procumbens)*		May cause hyperglycemia
Hydrocotyle *(Centella asiatica)*		
Licorice *(Glycyrrhiza glabra; G. uralensis)*		
Ephedra or ma huang *(Ephedra sinica)*		
Dyslipidemia and Atherosclerosis		
Nicotine acid (niacin)	Reduces total serum cholesterol, LDL cholesterol, and triglycerides; increases HDL cholesterol	Should be used only under physician's supervision; may elevate blood glucose levels; severe hepatotoxicity may occur, especially with SR nicotinic acid products
Soluble fiber products (oat bran, guar gum, psyllium, and other dietary sources)	Can lower total serum cholesterol and LDL cholesterol depending on product and amount consumed	Flatulence, cramping, bloating, nausea, diarrhea, indigestion, heartburn
Fish oils (omega-3 fatty acids)	Inhibit platelet aggregation, lower triglyceride levels when consumed in high doses (20-30 g/day)	Triglyceride-lowering effect may diminish with continued use; produces variable effects (decreases and increases) on blood cholesterol levels; may increase bleeding risk
Vitamin E	200 International Units or more per day *may* reduce risk of CHD	
Garlic *(Allium sativum)*	Standardized powdered garlic products may produce modest reduction in total cholesterol	
Nuts	Lower plasma lipoprotein levels	
Beta-sitosterol	May produce modest reductions in total and LDL cholesterol	
Alfalfa seed *(Medicago sativa)*	May produce modest reduction in cholesterol	Potential toxic effects outweigh any advantages that might be obtained
Chromium	May produce modest cholesterol reductions; administration as picolinate salt seems to increase bioavailability	

TABLE 16-5 COMMONLY USED HERBAL PRODUCTS AND NUTRACEUTICALS THAT MAY BE USED TO TREAT SELECTED CONDITIONS*—cont'd

CONDITION/HERB	USE	ASSOCIATED ADVERSE EFFECTS
GI Problems		
Aloes (*Aloe barbadensis, A. ferox, A. africana, A. spicata*)	Orally a powerful cathartic and not generally recommended	A harsh purgative; less toxic laxatives are available. Contraindicated with hemorrhoids, kidney disease, intestinal obstruction, abdominal pain, nausea, or vomiting
Bilberry fruit (*Vaccinium myrtillus*)	Treatment of diarrhea	No known side effects or interactions
Cascara (*Rhamnus purshiana*)	Stimulant laxative	Do not take while pregnant or breastfeeding. Fresh bark may cause severe vomiting. Electrolyte imbalance with misuse; potentiates toxicities of cardiac glycosides and thiazide diuretics
Ginger (*Zingiber officinale*)	Treatment of motion sickness and nausea	May cause prolonged bleeding times; caution in patients on anticoagulant therapy. Reported to be an abortifacient, so avoid while pregnant or breastfeeding
Licorice (*Glycyrrhiza glabra; G. uralensis*)	Treatment of peptic ulcer, expectorant	Considered unsafe. Contraindicated in patients taking cardiac glycosides or thiazide diuretics
Peppermint (*Mentha piperita*)	Decreases muscle spasms of the GI tract. Treatment of abdominal pain. Enteric-coated capsules used to treat irritable bowel syndrome	Should not be used by infants or small children; tea from leaves can cause laryngeal and bronchial spasms. Overuse can lead to heartburn and relaxation of LES
Psyllium (*Plantago arenaria, P. psyllium, P. indica, P. ovata*)	Bulk-forming laxative for constipation, irritable bowel syndrome	Possibly interfere with absorption of other drugs. Bezoars (fibrous masses in GI tract) may occur if liquid intake is inadequate
Senna (*Cassia acutifolia; C. angustifolia, Senna alexandrina*)	Cathartic; used to treat constipation	Chronic use can result in electrolyte imbalance and potassium loss. May increase toxicity of cardiac glycosides and thiazide diuretics
Hypertension		
Garlic (*Allium sativum*)	Antihypertensive	Routine use not recommended. Avoid use of garlic with NSAIDs, anticoagulants, and drugs that inhibit liver metabolism (e.g., cimetidine) and drugs that may be affected by liver inhibition (e.g., propranolol, diazepam)
Grapefruit juice		May cause significant decrease in blood pressure if taken with nifedipine
Licorice (*Glycyrrhiza glabra; G. uralensis*)		May induce hypertension accompanied by hypokalemia. Patients taking oral contraceptives or thiazide diuretics may be predisposed to licorice toxicity if taken concomitantly
Yohimbine (*Pausinystalia yohimbe*)	May be used to treat impotence secondary to antihypertensive medications	May increase blood pressure. Should not be co-administered with tricyclic antidepressants or clonidine

*This table does not provide information on how to use herbs, nor is it an exhaustive look at every herbal product that may be used. Rather, the intent is to provide information regarding herbal products that patients may use.

AIDS, Acquired immunodeficiency syndrome; *CHD,* coronary heart disease; *CNS,* central nervous system; *GI,* gastrointestinal; *HDL,* high-density lipoprotein; *LDL,* low-density lipoprotein; *LES,* lower esophageal sphincter; *NSAIDs,* nonsteroidal anti-inflammatory drugs; *SR,* slow release; *TNF,* tumor necrosis factor.

Data from Miller LG, Miller WJ, editors: *Herbal medicinals: A clinician's guide,* New York, 1998, Pharmaceutical Products Press; Tyler VE: *The honest herbal,* ed 3, New York, 1993, Pharmaceutical Products Press.

SUMMARY

CAM is becoming a significant component of health care in the United States. CAM consists of a cluster of medical and health care approaches, methods, and items not associated with conventional medicine. Complementary medicine refers to non-Western healing approaches used at the same time as conventional medicine. In contrast, alternative medicine replaces conventional medical treatment. Integrative medicine merges conventional medical therapies with CAM modalities for which safety and efficacy, based on scientific data, have been demonstrated. CAM therapies can be divided into five categories: alternative medical systems; mind-body interventions; biologically based therapies; manipulative and body-based methods; and energy therapies. Familiarity with CAM modalities will promote a secure environment for patients.

Dietary supplements are substances consumed orally as an addition to dietary intake. The DSHEA of 1994 regulates supplement identity, potency, contents, and labeling under the supervision of the FDA. Supplement use has grown substantially and may interact with other medications and treatments.

Drug-nutrient interactions may occur. Nutrients and foods may interact with drug function; drugs may affect use of food and nutrients. Use of herbs as dietary supplements or as natural medications can interact with bioavailability of foods, nutrients, and drugs. Knowledge of potential interactions assists nurses to provide more comprehensive patient care.

THE NURSING APPROACH

Case Study: Food-Drug Interactions

Priscilla, age 56, talked with the nurse at the end of an office visit for follow-up related to anticoagulant medicine she was taking for atrial fibrillation (an abnormal rhythm of the heart). Priscilla's time with the doctor was very limited because he was called away on an emergency.

ASSESSMENT
Subjective (from patient statements)

- "My doctor says I am at risk for developing blood clots that could lead to a stroke. He has prescribed a medicine to thin my blood. I certainly don't want a stroke, but I'm concerned that I could have trouble bleeding."
- "The dietitian told me to limit foods high in vitamin K, but I don't remember what kinds of foods have large amounts of vitamin K."
- "I don't want anything to happen before my dental surgery next month. What precautions do I need to take?"
- "I told the doctor about the prescription drugs I take. Do I need to tell the doctor about the multiple vitamins and ginkgo that I take?"
- "I ordered the ginkgo from a website selling natural products after reading a lot of testimonials about how ginkgo has helped people improve their memory. I even read that you get a money-back guarantee."

Objective (from physical examination and health records)

- The patient's chart indicates a diagnosis of atrial fibrillation and a prescription for Coumadin (an anticoagulant).
- Prothrombin lab tests have been within therapeutic ranges, and the patient is scheduled for another prothrombin test today.
- Apical pulse 88, slightly irregular

DIAGNOSES (NURSING)
1. Deficient knowledge: interactions of foods, herbs, and medications related to incomplete information as evidenced by not remembering what foods should be limited with

Coumadin and wondering if the doctor should be informed about all supplements
2. Deficient knowledge: how to recognize authoritative health information on the Internet related to use of questionable website(s) as evidenced by "a lot of testimonials," "money-back guarantee," etc.

PLANNING
Patient Outcomes

Short term (at the end of this visit):
- Priscilla will recognize possible drug interactions and will share information about all of her over-the-counter medicines with the doctor.
- She will state plans to confer with the doctor about possible adjustments of Coumadin before her dental surgery.
- She will identify signs of possible bleeding.
- Priscilla will identify foods high in vitamin K.
- She will identify two authoritative sites on the Internet concerning herbs.

Long term (at next visit in six months):
- Priscilla will continue to get prothrombin lab tests monthly as prescribed.
- Her prothrombin tests will remain in a therapeutic range.

Nursing Interventions

1. Educate Priscilla about possible food-drug interactions and the need to keep doctors informed about all medicines.
2. Provide information about how to select authoritative Internet sites regarding health.

IMPLEMENTATION

1. Listed on the chart all medications Priscilla was taking. Informed Priscilla that *Ginkgo biloba* (in addition to Coumadin) could thin her blood and that vitamin K could work against the thinning effect.
The doctor must be informed about the patient taking ginkgo because it may interfere with platelet formation, thus potentiating the anticoagulant effect of Coumadin. Vitamin K sup-

THE NURSING APPROACH—cont'd

Case Study: Food-Drug Interactions—cont'd

plements could counteract the anticoagulant effect of Coumadin.

2. Informed Priscilla that she should contact her oral surgeon to see if she needed to adjust any medicines or supplements before her dental surgery.

The oral surgeon may want Coumadin and ginkgo discontinued for three days before surgery to reduce risk of bleeding. The surgeon may also discontinue her multiple vitamins because vitamin K could predispose to clot formation.

3. Encouraged her to continue to come to the lab monthly for prothrombin tests.

Follow-up lab tests must be done frequently to determine the correct dose of Coumadin.

4. Provided a list of signs of bleeding that she should report right away to the doctor if observed.

Hemorrhage is a dangerous effect of too much anticoagulation. The patient should watch for bleeding from small cuts, easy bruising, nosebleeds, and signs of blood in the urine or bowel movements. Premenopause women should also monitor their menstruation for heavy bleeding.

5. Gave a list of foods high in vitamin K and recommended that she minimize intake of those foods and be consistent in foods eaten.

If foods containing high amounts of vitamin K are increased, this could antagonize the anticoagulant effect of Coumadin. Foods high in vitamin K include dark leafy vegetables (and to a lesser extent dairy products, cereals, meats, and fruits). When a handout is given to a patient, the patient is more likely to remember the information discussed.

6. Pointed out to Priscilla that she may have used a questionable website regarding ginkgo. Explained reasons for questioning the site:
   • No professional credentials of authors and no contact information besides how to order products
   • No date for any of the information

• A commercial website, with a purpose to sell
• Message—too good to be true: a quick fix, cure-all for a variety of conditions, natural without any side effects, testimonials rather than research studies and references to support effectiveness and safety of the product, promise of money-back guarantee

7. Suggested that Priscilla go to sites ending in .gov (government), or .edu (university or college) for authoritative nutrition information. Some .org (organization) sites and some .com (commercial) sites give excellent information, but others just sell products. The nurse recommended three good websites for information about herbs and supplements:
   • National Center for Complementary and Alternative Medicine, National Institutes of Health, www.nccam.nih.gov
   • Office of Dietary Supplements, National Institutes of Health, www.ods.od.nih.gov
   • Mayo Clinic, www.mayoclinic.com

EVALUATION

Short term (at the end of the visit):
• Priscilla was able to state possible interactions of Coumadin with vitamin K and ginkgo and shared information about all medicines taken.
• She verbalized major sources of vitamin K.
• She stated her intention to confer with her oral surgeon about medicines and to get regular follow-up blood testing.
• She identified signs of bleeding.
• She identified two websites to check for authoritative information about gingko.
• Short-term goals met

DISCUSSION QUESTIONS

1. Identify specific foods that are high in Vitamin K and thus should be avoided or limited while taking Coumadin.
2. What other high doses of vitamins could increase the anticoagulation effect of Coumadin?

Nursing Diagnoses-Definitions and Classification 2009-2011. Copyright © 2009, 1994-2009 by NANDA International. Used by arrangement with Blackwell Publishing Limited, a company of John Wiley & Sons, Inc.

■ CRITICAL THINKING

Clinical Applications

Faye, a 20-year-old student from Germany, seeks medical attention at the urging of her roommates, who report that her mood has become increasingly depressed during the past two semesters. She has become withdrawn and moody—a significant change from her affect since first coming to the United States to attend college. She is otherwise healthy. Faye reports a 5-pound weight loss during the past 3 months. She takes oral contraceptives for regulation of menses. Her mother has been treated for depression with *Hypericum perforatum* (St. John's wort) by the family physician for the past 10 years. Faye reports smoking a pack of cigarettes per day. Plans are to treat her with 50 mg sertraline (Zoloft) per day and to provide counseling therapy. During the diet history, the dietitian asks Faye if she uses any over-the-counter vitamins, minerals, or herbal supplements. She tells the dietitian

that her mother suggested she try St. John's wort because in Germany it is prescribed to treat depression. Faye did as her mother suggested because it is available without prescription in the United States.

1. Faye's depression will be treated with sertraline, a selective serotonin reuptake inhibitor (SSRI). How do SSRIs work?
2. What is St. John's wort?
3. How is St. John's wort used in the United States? How is it regulated?
4. How does St. John's wort work as an antidepressant?
5. Does St. John's wort have any side effects?
6. How is St. John's wort used in Europe?
7. Why do you think people are interested in alternative medicine and herbal treatments?
8. What is your immediate concern regarding Faye's use of St. John's wort?

Modified from Nelms MN, Long S, Lacey K: *Medical nutrition therapy: A case study approach*, ed 3, Belmont, Calif, 2009, Cengage/Wadsworth.

WEBSITES OF INTEREST

American Botanical Council

www.herbalgram.org

Disperses information and research findings to encourage appropriate use of phytomedicines and medicinal plants.

National Center for Complementary and Alternative Medicine (NCCAM)

www.nccam.nih.gov

Promotes scientific research on CAM and distributes information to the public and health professionals on the efficacy of CAM modalities.

Office of Dietary Supplements (ODS)

http://dietary-supplements.info.nih.gov

Supports research and distributes findings about dietary supplements to the public and a resource to other federal agencies.

REFERENCES

1. Committee on Use of Complementary and Alternative Medicine by the American Public, Board on Health Promotion and Disease Promotion, Institute of Medicine: *Complementary and alternative medicine in United States*, Washington, D.C., 2005, National Academies Press.

2. National Center for Complementary and Alternative Medicine (NCCAM), National Institutes of Health: *What is CAM?* Bethesda, Md, 2002 (May) Updated February 2007, NCCAM Publication No. D347. Accessed February 22, 2010, from http://nccam.nih.gov/health/whatiscam/overview.htm.

3. Center for Food Safety and Applied Nutrition, Office of Nutritional Products, Labeling, and Dietary Supplements, Food and Drug Administration: *Dietary Supplement Labeling*, College Park, Md, 2005 (April) Updated May 2009, Author. Accessed February 22, 2010, from www.fda.gov/Food/DietarySupplements/default.htm.

4. Barrett S: Alternative nutrition therapies. In Shils ME, et al, editors: *Modern nutrition in health and disease*, ed 10, Philadelphia, 2006, Lippincott Williams & Wilkins.

5. Rapp E: Massage, aromatherapy, oils and a root canal, *New York Times*, July 21, 2002, NJ Section 10, page 1.

6. Thomas P: The regulation of dietary supplements, part 1: The 20th century through 1994, *The Dietary Suppl*, Jan/Mar 2000.

7. *National Business Journal*: Supplements 2010. Accessed February 22, 2010, from http://nutritionbusinessjournal.com/supplements/.

8. Position of the American Dietetic Association: Functional foods, *J Am Diet Assoc* 109:735-746, 2009.

9. Thomson C, et al: Guidelines regarding the recommendation and sale of dietary supplements, *J Am Diet Assoc* 102(8):1158, 2002.

10. Baldwin KM, et al: Shock, multiple organ dysfunction syndrome, and burns in adults. In McCance KL, Huether SE, editors: *Pathophysiology: The biologic basis for diseases in adults and children*, ed 5, St. Louis, 2006, Mosby.

11. National Center for Complementary and Alternative Medicine, National Institutes of Health: *NCCAM clearinghouse*, Bethesda, Md (updated February 2006), Author. Accessed February 21, 2010, from http://nccam.nih.gov/health/clearinghouse.

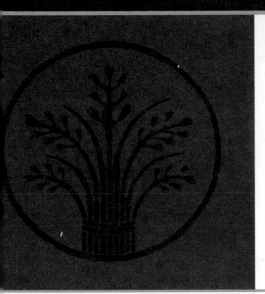

Nutrition for Disorders of the Gastrointestinal Tract

The ability to chew, swallow, digest, and absorb nutrients, while passing fiber and other substances on for elimination, may be compromised by disorders of the gastrointestinal tract.

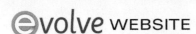 **evolve** WEBSITE

http://evolve.elsevier.com/Grodner/foundations/

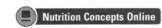 **Nutrition Concepts Online**

ROLE IN WELLNESS

Almost everyone experiences intermittent gastrointestinal (GI) complaints from time to time. Indigestion, gas, bloating, nausea, abdominal pain or cramping, diarrhea, and esophageal reflux are some of the symptoms occasionally experienced by healthy people. Many GI disorders produce significant nutritional implications, and in many situations diet is the cornerstone of therapy for GI complaints. Evaluation of a patient's GI symptoms requires a team effort to separate GI symptoms associated with dietary practices from those associated with GI disease or dysfunction. The registered dietitian's role is to help identify unusual dietary practices, nutritional inadequacies, or food intolerances through the use of an in-depth diet history.[1]

The simple act of eating an apple may no longer be easy for individuals with disorders of the GI tract. The ability to chew, swallow, digest, and absorb nutrients, while passing fiber and other substances on for elimination, may be compromised by disorders of the GI tract (Figure 17-1). These disorders affect provision of nutrients to all other organs and systems of the body, thereby influencing overall health.

Consider disorders of the GI tract through the five dimensions of health. The *physical health* dimension is most affected if the disorder is chronic and intensifies over time; eventually weight loss and nutrient deficiencies pose other health risks in addition to the primary GI tract disorder. *Intellectual health* is tested as the patient, caregivers, and dietetic and nursing staff work together to devise food combinations and textures that are physically and anesthetically acceptable to the patient; other disorders require constant vigilance to restrict inadvertent consumption of problematic foods (e.g., gluten for patients with celiac disease). *Emotional health* may be taxed when patients struggle with acceptance of dietary or

physical limitations; nurses can refer patients to disorder support groups as an additional therapeutic strategy. Some disorders may affect *social health* functioning. Nurses can provide patients with social strategies to deal with the physical ramifications of colostomies, dumping syndrome, and other disorders. *Spiritual health* and physical health of the GI tract may be enhanced by the practices of yoga and meditation, which are tied to teachings related to both mind and body.

DYSPHAGIA

The main focus of medical nutrition therapy for dysphagia is to provide nutrition in a form that fits specific anatomic and functional needs of the patient while maintaining or improving nutritional status and avoiding aspiration.[2] For patients with chewing or swallowing difficulties, diets must be devised to meet nutritional needs and prevent aspiration. Patients may also experience changes in consistency tolerance. Thickening agents provide varying levels of consistency to accommodate individual needs because thin liquids are usually more difficult to swallow.

We rarely think about swallowing, just as we don't think about breathing or our heart beating. Swallowing takes place in three stages, as outlined in Figure 17-2: oral preparation and transit, pharyngeal transit, and esophageal transit. A disorder affecting any of these stages may require medical nutrition therapy.

Patients sometimes give warning signs, including the following that they are at risk for swallowing problems:[2]

- Collecting food under the tongue, in the cheeks, or on the hard palate
- Spitting food out of the mouth, or tongue thrusting
- Inability to control tongue

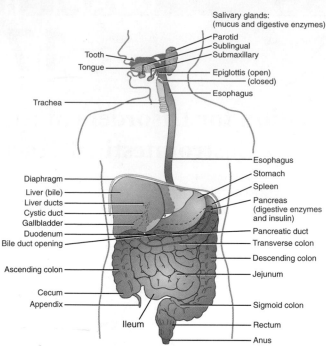

Salivary glands:
(mucus and digestive enzymes)
Parotid
Sublingual
Submaxillary
Tooth
Tongue
Epiglottis (open)
(closed)
Esophagus
Trachea

Esophagus
Diaphragm
Stomach
Liver (bile)
Spleen
Liver ducts
Pancreas
Cystic duct
(digestive enzymes
and insulin)
Gallbladder
Duodenum
Pancreatic duct
Bile duct opening
Transverse colon
Descending colon
Ascending colon
Jejunum
Cecum
Appendix
Sigmoid colon
Ileum
Rectum
Anus

FIG 17-1 The gastrointestinal tract. (From Mahan LK, Escott-Stump S: *Krause's food & nutrition therapy*, ed 12, Philadelphia, 2008, Saunders.)

- Excessively moving tongue
- Decreasing oral transit time
- Experiencing delay or absence of elevation of larynx while swallowing
- Coughing before or after swallowing
- Choking
- Drooling
- Experiencing gargled voice after eating or drinking
- Regurgitating food or liquid through nose, mouth, or tracheostomy tube
- Not taking in adequate amounts of food or fluids, resulting in weight loss
- Increasing time required to eat
- Resisting food, such as clenching teeth, pushing food away, clutching throat

Box 17-1 presents conditions that may cause dysphagia.

Nutrition Therapy

No two patients with dysphagia are alike. Therefore, diet must be individualized based on the swallowing ability of the patient and, of course, the patient's personal food preferences. Solid foods and liquids should be evaluated separately and modified based on texture, cohesiveness, density, viscosity, consistency, temperature, and taste. A nutritionally adequate diet for dysphagia involves considering these characteristics, along with careful planning to ensure nutritional adequacy. A three-stage dysphagia diet is outlined in Table 17-1.

When caring for patients with dysphagia, several aspects are of concern: bolus consistency, patient positioning, feeding rate, and specific swallowing techniques. Video-fluoroscopy swallow study (VFSS) determines the level of bolus consis-

tency the patient can tolerate. Different physiologic problems dictate the necessity for different consistencies of food. For example, the most common swallowing disorder in older adults who have experienced stroke is a delayed or absent pharyngeal swallow.[3]

Patients with this type of disorder need puréed foods to provide stimulation that provokes the reflex to swallow. If the pharyngeal swallow is reduced (but not delayed or absent), liquids tend to be the most difficult consistency for patients. Thickening agents can be used to acquire the appropriate consistency. For patients who have lost coordination of the upper esophageal sphincter (cricopharyngeal dysfunction), thin liquids are the most appropriate (see the *Personal Perspectives* box, The Pain of Parkinson's Disease).[4]

PERSONAL PERSPECTIVES
The Pain of Parkinson's Disease

When Don Kaemmer met his soon-to-be second wife, Yetta, he was a physically active 70-year-old widower. A few years after they wed, he developed a quickly advancing condition of Parkinson's disease that significantly affected his ability to speak and swallow. Here are some of Mrs. Kaemmer's reflections on dealing with her husband's dysphagia.

The doctor approached me and said, "I know what your husband had for dinner tonight." I just stared at him and thought how does he know? Hours after dinner that night, an ambulance brought Don to the hospital because of a kidney infection. While examining my husband, the doctor found partially chewed chicken in Don's mouth and throat. I thought Don swallowed his dinner but apparently not. An example of Parkinson's effect on daily activity became clear.

As the effects of the disorder progressed, my husband had trouble chewing and swallowing food and medications. I don't know if he was just too tired, too depressed, or didn't have an appetite to eat. He frequently looked as if he was wearing a mask with no emotion and said little. I often felt like a cheerleader trying to boost his spirits to get him to eat. How could he stay well if he didn't eat? I made soft foods like chicken soup with pieces of cut-up chicken and vegetables, split pea soup, puddings, and ice cream. During one hospital stay he had a supplement drink that he was willing to drink at home. It was expensive, so we would get a supply of it from the Veterans Administration because Don was entitled to benefits, having served in WWII. But toward the end, only small spoonfuls of ice cream or sherbet felt good. It took too much energy to drink. Instead of feeding with food, I nourished him by being there.

Yetta Kaemmer
Tamarac, Florida

One of the safest eating positions for patients who have trouble swallowing is upright. If patients cannot sit up by themselves, the head of the bed should be raised to provide support, and pillows and wedges should be used to support arms, head, neck, or trunk when necessary. The upright position allows gravity to assist with the passage of food along the esophagus and helps prevent choking and aspiration.[2]

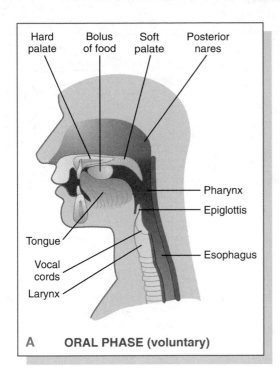

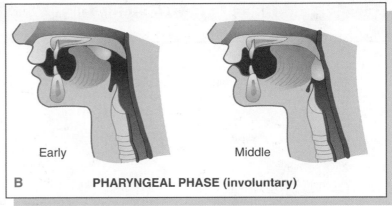

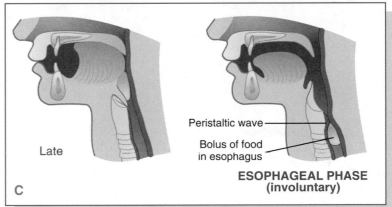

FIG 17-2 Swallowing occurs in three phases: **A**, Voluntary or oral phase. The tongue presses food against the hard palate, forcing it toward the pharynx. **B**, Involuntary, pharyngeal phase. Early: wave of peristalsis forces a bolus between the tonsillar pillars. Middle: soft palate draws upward to close posterior nares and respirations cease momentarily. Late: vocal cords approximate and the larynx pulls upward, covering the airway and stretching the esophagus open. **C**, Involuntary, esophageal phase. Relaxation of the upper esophageal (hypopharyngeal) sphincter allows the peristaltic wave to move the bolus down the esophagus. (From Mahan LK, Escott-Stump S: *Krause's food & nutrition therapy,* ed 12, Philadelphia, 2008, Saunders.)

BOX 17-1   CONDITIONS THAT CAUSE DYSPHAGIA

Achalasia
Acute cervical spinal cord injury
Alzheimer's disease/dementia
Amyloidosis
Amyotrophic lateral sclerosis (ALS, aka Lou Gehrig's disease)
Anoxia
Botulism
Cerebrovascular accident (CVA)/stroke
Chagas disease
Diabetes, type 1 (long-term)
Esophageal cancer
Esophageal varices
Gastroesophageal reflux (GERD)
Gastroparesis
Goiter
Guillain-Barré syndrome
Head and/or neck cancer, including brain stem tumors
Head injury

Human immunodeficiency virus (HIV) infection
Huntington's disease
Inflammatory masses
Intrinsic and extrinsic structural lesions
Lung inflammation, including Chronic obstructive pulmonary disease (COPD), with excessive secretions
Multiple sclerosis (MS)
Multiple system atrophy (MSA)
Muscular dystrophies (MD)
Myasthenia gravis
Parkinson's disease
Poliomyelitis
Postintubation trauma
Presbyphagia (swallowing difficulty of old age)
Scleroderma
Stricture or inflammation of pharynx or esophagus
Tumor or obstruction of throat

Data from American Dietetic Association: *Nutrition care manual,* Chicago, Author. Accessed February 28, 2010, from www.nutritioncaremanual.org.

Nutrition therapy for dysphagia

TABLE 17-1	THREE-LEVEL DYSPHAGIA DIET	
LEVEL	**RATIONALE**	**DESCRIPTION**
Level 1: Puréed	Suitable for people with severely reduced oral preparatory stage abilities, impaired lip and tongue control, delayed swallow reflex triggering, oral hypersensitivity, reduced pharyngeal peristalsis, and/or cricopharyngeal dysfunction.	Thick homogeneous textures are emphasized. Puréed foods should be "spoon-thick" or "pudding-like" consistency. No coarse textures, nuts, raw fruits, or raw vegetables allowed. Liquid or crushed medications (refer to physician or pharmacist for pharmoefficacy of medications) are required and may be mixed with puréed fruits. Liquids and water are thickened with commercial thickening agent as needed to recommended consistency.
Level 2: Mechanically altered	Intended for patients who can tolerate a minimum amount of easily chewed foods. May be suitable for people with moderately impaired oral preparatory stage abilities, edentulous oral cavity, decreased pharyngeal peristalsis, and/or cricopharyngeal muscle dysfunction.	No coarse textures, nuts, raw fruits (except ripe or mashed bananas), or vegetables, except as noted. Puréed or slurried bread, if necessary. Liquid or crushed medications may still be required (refer to physician or pharmacist for pharmo-efficacy of medications). Liquids and water thickened as needed with commercial thickening agent to recommended consistency.
Level 3: Advanced	Designed for patients who chew soft textures. Based on a soft diet; may be appropriate for individuals with mild oral preparatory–stage deficits.	Textures are soft with no tough skins, no nuts or dry, crispy, raw, or stringy foods. Meats should be moist and tender or casseroles with small chunks of meat allowed. Fluid consistency ordered separately: may be thin, nectar-thick, honey-like, or spoon-thick. Moist potatoes, rice, and dressing allowed. All soups except those with tough meat or vegetables. Soft, peeled fruit without seeds. Moist breads and cereals allowed. All fats except those with chunky additives.

Data from American Dietetic Association: *Nutrition care manual*, Chicago, 2009, Author. Accessed February 28, 2010, from www.nutritioncaremanual.org.

Sometimes patients eat too quickly or stuff their mouths too full of food and then choke when trying to swallow. Staff can observe and supervise patients while they eat to remind them to complete the swallowing sequence before taking their next bite of food.

Enlisting the aid of a speech therapist is usually necessary to teach the patient various techniques to compensate for swallowing problems. Techniques include the supra glottic swallow and the Mendelson maneuver. The supraglottic swallow is appropriate for patients with reduced laryngeal function. This method requires teaching the patient to take a breath before swallowing, consciously hold the breath during the swallow, exhale forcefully or cough gently after the swallow, and swallow again to clear the mouth. The Mendelson maneuver is helpful for individuals with cricopharyngeal dysfunction. The patient is taught to elevate the larynx voluntarily to the maximum level during a swallow to allow food to pass. When lubrication is a problem, nursing personnel can also use several techniques to assist the patient. Encouraging the patient to think or talk about food before mealtime can help stimulate the flow of saliva, which aids in the formation of a bolus and the chewing and swallowing process. Tart or sour foods can stimulate saliva production. Having the patient lick jelly from the lips, pucker them, hum, or whistle helps strengthen mouth muscles, which may help the patient, learn to close the lips around a fork or spoon.[5]

Feeding patients with swallowing difficulty is usually the responsibility of nursing personnel. The following safe procedures are recommended:[2,6]

1. Position patient upright, bent slightly forward, with the chin tucked and head tilted forward.
2. Eliminate distractions so the patient can focus all attention on the meal.
3. The person feeding should sit at or below patient's eye level while feeding.
4. Avoid asking patient to talk while eating.
5. Instruct the patient not to use liquids to clear the mouth of foods; in fact, they should be used only after the patient has cleared the food from the mouth. Encourage frequent dry swallows or coughing to help clear food from the mouth between bites.
6. Encourage small bites ($\frac{1}{2}$ to 1 teaspoon solid food or about 10 to 15 mL liquid), especially if patient's ability to manage food is impaired.
7. Allow adequate time to feed.
8. Use spoons rather than cups because patients have less difficulty taking food and liquid this way.
9. While patient eats, check for voice quality. A wet or gurgled voice indicates food may be resting on the vocal cords.

During the early stages of feeding, nursing supervision is necessary at meals to prevent or minimize swallowing problems. Patients should be reevaluated regularly to determine

- Increased levels of progesterone caused by pregnancy, oral contraceptives containing progesterone, late stages of the menstrual cycle
- Hiatal hernia (see Figure 17-3)
- Foods: chocolate, alcohol, mint, carbonated beverages, citrus fruits and juices, tomato-based products, caffeinated products, peppermint
- High-fat diets
- Smoking

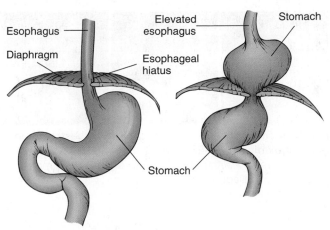

FIG 17-3 A, Normal stomach placement, compared with **B**, hiatal hernia. (From Rolin Graphics.)

whether any changes need to be made in the consistency of fluids or food. Evaluating and documenting the patient's food intake are also prudent to ensure adequate nutritional intake and status. If the patient's nutritional needs are not or cannot be met orally, alternative methods should be considered.[7]

For patients with dysphagia, mealtime can be made safe and nutritious, but it may be difficult to make eating the pleasure it once was. The one thing nursing personnel can do to make sure meals are as relaxing as possible is to let patients eat at their own pace. Patience on the part of nursing staff may be rewarded with patients who eat with minimal difficulty while maintaining their nutritional status.

Gastroesophageal Reflux Disease, Hiatal Hernia, and Esophagitis

More commonly known as *heartburn*, gastroesophageal reflux disease (GERD) is a frequent experience for some people. In fact, some consider it a normal state of being and never report the symptoms to their physicians. The reflux usually takes place within 1 to 4 hours after a meal.

Normally, the lower esophageal sphincter (LES) prevents stomach contents from entering the esophagus, but various factors often decrease sphincter pressure (Box 17-2 and Figure 17-3). Unlike gastric mucosa, esophageal mucosa can be damaged when exposed to gastric contents. If not treated, GERD can result in esophagitis (inflammation of the lower esophagus). The reflux is thought to be aggravated by reclining after eating, stress, and increased intraabdominal pressure. Increased intraabdominal pressure can occur with coughing, straining, bending, vomiting, obesity, pregnancy, trauma, ascites, tightly fitting clothing around the waist, lifting heavy objects, and exercising strenuously.[2] Older patients often experience respiratory symptoms of GERD, such as pneumonitis, chronic bronchitis, or asthma.

GERD is treated medically by reducing intraabdominal pressure and gastric acid production. Medical management can be divided into six stages (Box 17-3 and Figure 17-4). Stages 1 to 4 entail medical management, and stage 5 involves surgical intervention.[8] Table 17-2 summarizes medications that may be used to treat GERD, as well as their actions.

Lifestyle Modifications
- Head of bed elevated 6 inches
- Decreased fat intake
- Smoking cessation
- Weight reduction for obese patients
- Avoid recumbent positions for 3 hours postprandially
- Small, frequent meals
- Avoidance of certain foods (see Box 17-2)
- Avoidance of tight, waist-constricting clothing

As-Needed Pharmacologic Therapy
- Antacid or antacid product containing alginic acid
- Over-the-counter histamine H_2-receptor blocker
- Stool softeners

Scheduled Pharmacologic Therapy
- H_2-receptor blocker or prokinetic agent for 8 to 12 weeks
- For persistent symptoms, high-dose H_2-receptor blocker or proton pump inhibitor for another 8 to 12 weeks (or reconsider diagnosis)
- With documented erosive esophagitis, may use a proton pump inhibitor as first-line therapy

Maintenance Therapy
- Appropriate for patient with symptomatic relapse or complicated disease
- Lowest effective dosage of H_2-receptor blocker or proton pump inhibitor

Surgery
- May be appropriate in patient with severe symptoms, erosive esophagitis, or disease complications
- Laparoscopic fundoplication procedure

Endoscopy
- Stretta procedure (see Figure 17-4)

Data from Scott M, Gelhot AR: Gastroesophageal reflux disease: Diagnosis and management, *Am Fam Physician* 59(5):1161-69, 1999; Heitkemper MM: Upper gastrointestinal problem. In Lewis SM, Heitkemper MM, Dirksen SR, editors: *Medical-surgical nursing*, ed 6, St. Louis, 2004, Mosby.

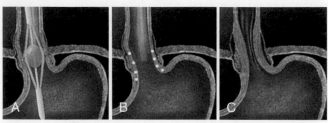

FIG 17-4 Stretta procedure used to treat gastroesophageal reflux disease (GERD). **A**, Catheter positioned. **B**, Multiple sites treated with radiofrequency energy. **C**, Remodeling occurs with collagen formation. (Courtesy Curon Medical, Inc., Freemont, Calif.)

Attention to medical metabolism of these medications and their interaction with other prescribed and over-the-counter medications should be considered, particularly among minority populations (see the *Cultural Considerations* box, Biologic Variations of Medication Metabolism).

CULTURAL CONSIDERATIONS

Biologic Variations of Medication Metabolism

According to research, medications are metabolized differently among ethnic and racial groups. This can result in different therapeutic consequences from what is expected as well as unexpected side effects. Most research has been conducted with antihypertensive and psychotropic drugs. Individuals are referred to as poor or slow metabolizers because the drug-metabolizing enzyme functions are slowed or impaired by deoxyribonucleic acid (DNA) mutations (or differences). Others may be considered extensive metabolizers because they have normally functioning enzymes.

For example, more Asians and African Americans than whites are slow metabolizers in relation to tricyclic antidepressants used to treat the illness of depression. As a result, these individuals achieve a more rapid therapeutic response to the drugs. When prescribing tricyclic antidepressant medications, physicians, primary health care providers, and nurse practitioners can start treatment with lower doses of the drugs in these cases.

Application to nursing: Because the pharmacokinetics of specific drugs have not been studied extensively in minority populations, it is important for health care providers who prescribe medications to be alert to atypical responses and side effects caused by biologic variations of medical metabolism.

Data from Hines SE: Intelligent prescribing in diverse populations, *Patient Care Nurse Pract* 3(5):47, 2000.

Nutrition Therapy

Patients may be able to minimize symptoms of GERD by manipulating the way they eat and by avoiding certain foods, especially those high in fat. The *Teaching Tool* box, Recommendations for Minimizing Heartburn, summarizes nutritional recommendations for GERD.

PEPTIC ULCER DISEASE

Peptic ulcer disease (PUD) is the term used to describe a break or ulceration in the protective mucosal lining of the lower esophagus, stomach, or duodenum. These ulcerations expose the submucosal areas to gastric secretions and autodigestion. Peptic ulcers can be acute or chronic and superficial (erosions) or deep. Deep ulcers can penetrate the muscularis mucosa and damage blood vessels, causing hemorrhage, or perforate the GI wall. Infection with *Helicobacter pylori* and nonsteroidal anti-inflammatory drugs (NSAIDs) are major causes of duodenal ulcers (Figure 17-5). *H. pylori* weakens the protective mucosal layer of the stomach and duodenum, allowing gastric acid to damage epithelial tissues, which leads to ulcerogenesis.[7,9] NSAIDs likely promote mucosal inflammation and ulcer formation through cellular damage, reducing gastric blood flow, reducing mucus and HCO_3 secretion, and decreasing the ability of cells to repair and replicate, leading to breakdown of mucosal defense mechanisms.[9]

Treatment goals focus largely on eradicating *H. pylori*, reducing stomach acidity, relieving symptoms, healing the ulcer, preventing reoccurrence, and avoiding complications. This is accomplished through *triple therapy*, a combination of antibiotics and acid-reducing medications (see Table 17-2) taken for at least 10 to 14 days.[10,11] Triple therapy involves at

TABLE 17-2	MEDICATIONS USED TO TREAT GASTROESOPHAGEAL REFLUX DISEASE	
MEDICATION	**ACTION**	**POTENTIAL ADVERSE EFFECTS**
Antacids Aluminum salts (AlternaGEL, Alu-Cap, Amphojel, Basaljel)	Neutralize gastric acid	Constipation, hypophosphatemia, accumulation in patients with renal impairment
Calcium salts, Tums, Tums E-X, Titralac (Amitone)		Constipation, milk-alkali syndrome with high doses, rebound hyperacidity (depending on dosage)
Magnesium salts (Phillips' Milk of Magnesia, Mygel, Almacone)		Diarrhea
Sodium bicarbonate (Citrocarbonate)		Milk-alkali syndrome with high doses
Magnesium-aluminum combinations (Maalox, Maalox Plus, Mylanta, Mylanta Double Strength, Di-Gel, Gelusil)		Take iron or folic acid supplement separately by 2 hours; take separately from citrus fruit/juice or calcium citrate by 3 hours; minor changes in bowel function Magnesium-containing products may accumulate in patients with renal impairment Magnesium-containing products may cause diarrhea
Over-the-Counter H$_2$-Receptor Blockers	Inhibit histamine stimulation of gastric parietal cells, suppressing gastric acid secretion	
Nizatidine (Axid AR) Famotidine (Pepcid AD) Cimetidine (Tagamet HB)		Take at least 2 hours after iron supplement; take magnesium supplement or magnesium-aluminum antacids separately by at least 2 hours; limit caffeine/xanthine; avoid alcohol Liquid cimetidine precipitates tube feeding
Prokinetic Agents	Increase gastric emptying and lower esophageal sphincter pressure	
Metoclopramide (Reglan) Bethanechol (Urecholine)		Most effective when used in combination with acid-suppression therapy; drowsiness, psychiatric symptoms, and extrapyramidal reactions may occur with long-term use
H$_2$-Receptor Blockers	Inhibit histamine stimulation of gastric parietal cells, suppressing gastric acid secretion	
Cimetidine (Tagamet) Famotidine (Pepcid) Nizatidine (Axid) Ranitidine (Zantac)		Take at least 2 hours after iron supplement; take magnesium supplement or magnesium-aluminum antacids separately by at least 2 hours; limit caffeine/xanthine; avoid alcohol Liquid cimetidine precipitates tube feeding
Proton Pump Inhibitors	Strongly inhibit gastric acid secretion by irreversibly inhibiting the H$^+$-K$^+$ adenosine triphosphatase pump of parietal cells	Uncommon; include diarrhea, nausea, dizziness, and headaches
Lansoprazole (Prevacid) Omeprazole (Prilosec) Pantoprazole (Protonix) Rabeprazole (Aciphex) Esomeprazole (Nexium)		Optimal: take 30-60 minutes before a meal; swallow whole, do not crush; omeprazole only—may open capsule and sprinkle granules on 1 Tbsp applesauce; avoid alcohol

Data from Pronsky ZM, Crowe JP: *Food-medication interactions*, ed 16, Birchrunville, Pa, 2010, Food-Medication Interactions; National Digestive Diseases Information Clearinghouse (NDDIC), National Institute of Diabetes & Digestive & Kidney Diseases (NIDDK): *Heartburn, gastroesophageal reflux (GER), and gastrointestinal reflux disease (GERD)*, NIH Pub. No 07-0882, Bethesda, Md, 2007 (May), National Institutes of Health. Accessed February 28, 2010, from http://digestive.niddk.nih.gov/ddiseases/pubs/gerd/index.htm.

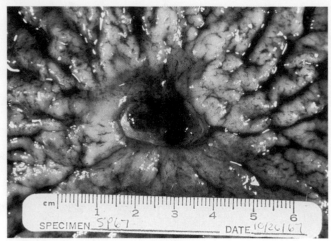

FIG 17-5 Chronic peptic ulcer. (From Damjanov I, Linder J, editors: *Anderson's pathology,* ed 10, vol 2, St. Louis, 1996, Mosby.)

least two antibiotics plus the acid reducers. The acid-reducing medications help relieve pain and help the antibiotics work more effectively.

Nutrition Therapy

Most people still believe ulcers are caused by stress or spicy foods, although hundreds of research studies show that *H. pylori* causes approximately 80% of ulcers, with the remaining 20% generally caused by NSAIDs.[11] Therefore, it should be no surprise there is no evidence that a "bland diet" (or any specific diet for that matter) improves symptoms or promotes ulcer healing. Any dietary modifications must be individualized to include avoidance of foods that a patient can associate with dyspeptic symptoms.[12] From a realistic approach, avoiding red and black pepper, chili pepper, coffee (caffeinated and decaffeinated), caffeine, and alcohol (these foods and spices may cause superficial mucosal damage, worsen existing disease, or interfere with treatment) and eating a good-quality diet are recommended.[12] Regardless of the cause of an ulcer, smoking does aggravate PUD, although the reason is unclear. Therefore cessation of smoking is recommended.[11,12]

DUMPING SYNDROME

One of the functions of the stomach is to control the rate of gastric emptying of nutrients into the small intestine. The rate at which the stomach empties is synchronized by signals from the stomach and duodenum.[13] This process ensures efficient digestion, absorption, and metabolism.

When part or all of the stomach (partial or total gastrectomy) is removed for treatment of PUD or bypassed to control obesity (Figure 17-6), or the pyloric sphincter is removed, dumping syndrome may develop. Impairment of the normal reservoir function of the stomach causes a large volume of abnormally increased osmolarity or hyperosmolar food to be dumped rapidly into the small intestine. These hyperosmolar contents draw water into the lumen and stimulate bowel motility.

Some symptoms occur 10 to 20 minutes postprandially (early phase occurring after a meal) and are characterized by feelings of epigastric fullness, abdominal cramps, nausea, or diarrhea in addition to vasomotor symptoms of tachycardia, postural hypotension, profuse sweating at times, weakness, flushing, or syncope. Some patients experience intestinal symptoms but not vasomotor symptoms and vice versa. The late phase, which occurs less frequently than the early phase, develops about 1 to 3 hours postprandially and is associated with symptoms similar to hypoglycemia: perspiration, hunger, nausea, anxiety, tremors, or weakness.[14]

Nutrition Therapy

Food and meals can be manipulated or restricted to help alleviate patients' symptoms while providing a nutritionally sound diet. Patients who have dumping syndrome often lose weight[14] and should have their nutritional status evaluated regularly by a registered dietitian to detect early deficiencies of iron, vitamin B$_{12}$, protein, and vitamin D.[2] Generally, liquids should be consumed between meals rather than with meals to slow movement of food from the stomach into the duodenum. Simple carbohydrates are limited because they may exacerbate the dumping. Protein, fat, and complex carbohydrates are better tolerated.[2] The *Teaching Tool* box, Recommendations to Alleviate Dumping Syndrome, summarizes medical nutrition therapy.

CELIAC DISEASE (GLUTEN-SENSITIVE ENTEROPATHY)

Celiac disease, also called *gluten-sensitive enteropathy* or *nontropical sprue,* is a chronic autoimmune disorder in which the mucosa of the small intestine, especially the duodenum and proximal jejunum, is damaged by gluten. The gliadin fraction in wheat, secalin in rye, and hordein in barley are the specific prolamins (storage proteins), collectively known as *gluten,* that trigger the toxic reaction in genetically predisposed individuals.[15] This results in malabsorption of nutrients, causing a wide variety of symptoms that can vary greatly depending on the duration and severity of the disease, the person's age, and the presence of extraintestinal conditions.

Although the classic symptoms include diarrhea, abdominal distention, fat malabsorption, and weight loss, among others, many patients do not present with gastrointestinal symptoms and are asymptomatic. However, in severe cases of gluten-sensitive enteropathy, the digestion and absorption of proteins, fats, carbohydrates (especially lactose), calcium, vitamin D, vitamin K, iron, folate, and vitamin B$_{12}$, as well as other nutrients, becomes impaired. These malabsorptions can result in severe nutritional deficiencies such as osteopenia or osteoporosis, inadequate blood coagulation and easy bruising of skin caused by lack of vitamin K, iron deficiency anemia, and macrocytic anemia of the pernicious anemia type as a result of vitamin B$_{12}$ and folate malabsorption.[13]

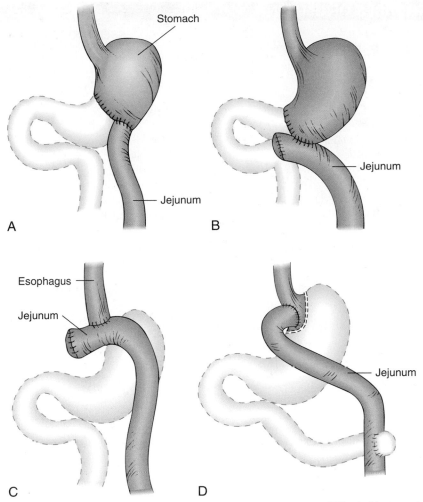

FIG 17-6 Typical gastric surgery resections. **A,** Partial gastrectomy, Billroth I (gastroduodenostomy). **B,** Partial gastrectomy, Billroth II (gastrojejunostomy). **C,** Total gastrectomy. **D,** Roux-en-Y bypass procedure. (**A-C,** From Rolin Graphics.)

✳ **TEACHING TOOL**

Recommendations to Alleviate Dumping Syndrome

Coping with dumping syndrome may seem overwhelming to newly diagnosed clients. Have your clients consider these suggestions to make the disorder more manageable:

- Avoid drinking liquids with meals. Make sure you consume adequate fluids between meals to prevent dehydration. Drink liquids 30 to 60 minutes before or after meals and limit servings to ½ to 1 cup.
- Carbonated beverages may cause excess gas formation and therefore are not recommended.
- Eat small, frequent meals to decrease intestinal distention caused by rapid emptying of large meals. Eat foods slowly, chew them well, and relax while eating.
- Avoid any foods that are not tolerated.
- Keep simple sugars (monosaccharides and disaccharides) to a minimum. Initially avoid sugar, honey, syrup, and other foods high in sugar; they may need long-term limitation.

- Food and liquids should not be at extreme temperatures (i.e., not too hot or too cold).
- Milk and milk products containing lactose may not be tolerated. Establish tolerance by gradually introducing them into the diet. Lactose-reduced milk is usually not tolerated (lactase enzymes result in splitting this disaccharide to monosaccharides, which are just as likely to promote dumping).
- Lie down for 15 to 30 minutes after meals to help decrease symptoms of dumping. If bothered by reflux, recline (at an angle) rather than lie flat.
- Pectin, a dietary fiber, may be helpful in delaying gastric emptying. Pectin can be purchased in powder form in grocery stores and supermarkets. Taking 1 teaspoon of pectin powder three times daily may be effective.

Data from American Dietetic Association: *Nutrition care manual,* Chicago, Author. Accessed February 28, 2010, from www.nutritioncaremanual.org.

TABLE 17-3   SOURCES OF GLUTEN

GRAINS TO INCLUDE	GRAINS TO AVOID	PROCESSED FOODS THAT MAY CONTAIN WHEAT, BARLEY, OR RYE
Rice	Wheat, all varieties including:	Bouillon cubes
Corn	• Einkorn,	Brown rice syrup
Amaranth	• Emmer	Candy
Quinoa	• Spelt	Cold cuts
Teff (or Tef)	• Kamut	Hot dogs
Millet	• Wheat starch	Salami
Finger millet (ragi)	• Wheat bran	Sausage
Sorghum	• Wheat germ	Communion wafers*
Indian rice grass (Montina)	• Cracked wheat	French fries
Arrowroot	• Hydrolyzed wheat protein	Gravy
Buckwheat	Barley	Imitation fish
Flax	Rye	Licorice
Job's tears	Cross-bread varieties such as triticale	Matzo**
Sago	(cross between wheat and rye)	Rice mixes
Potato		Sauces
Soy		Seasoned snack foods (e.g., tortilla chips, potato chips)
Legumes		Seitan
Mesquite		Self-basting turkey
Tapioca		Soups
Wild rice		Soy sauce
Cassava (Manloc)		Vegetables in sauce
Yucca		
Nuts		
Seeds		

*Communion wafers are generally made from wheat, although gluten-free wafers are manufactured by Ener-G Foods (www.ener-g.com). Low-gluten Communion wafers that conform to (Catholic) Canon law have been developed by the Benedictine Sisters of Perpetual Adoration (www.benedictinesisters.org).
**Shemura oat matzos are produced in England by Rabbi E. Kestenbaum.
Data from American Dietetic Association Nutrition Care Manual. *Celiac disease*. Accessed February 28, 2010, from www.nutritioncaremanual.org.

In the early stages of celiac disease, fat malabsorption is more typical than other nutrient malabsorption. This condition is often called idiopathic steatorrhea (fat malabsorption by unknown causes). In more severe cases of gluten-sensitive enteropathy, the digestion and absorption of proteins, carbohydrates, calcium, vitamin K, folate, and vitamin B_{12}, as well as other nutrients, becomes impaired. These malabsorptions can result in severe nutritional deficiencies, weight loss, osteomalacia, inadequate blood coagulation caused by lack of vitamin K, and macrocytic anemia of the pernicious anemia type as a result of vitamin B_{12} and folate malabsorption.[13]

Nutrition Therapy

Once gluten is removed from the diet, symptoms gradually improve during the following weeks and months. Intestinal mucosa subsequently returns to a near normal condition. There is only one catch: maintaining an asymptomatic state depends on lifelong avoidance of gluten.

For individuals with this condition, abstaining from wheat, oats, rye, and barley is not as simple as it may sound. Gluten-containing grains and products made from these grains are staples in the American diet. They are used as emulsifiers, thickeners, and other additives in commercially processed foods. Patients, with the help of registered dietitians and support groups, must become ardent label readers because unintentional ingestion of gluten is the most common cause of recurrence of symptoms. Furthermore, availability of alternatives to wheat-based breads, crackers, and pasta is limited when eating away from home. A diet that restricts these four grains can become monotonous. Table 17-3 summarizes gluten sources.

LACTOSE INTOLERANCE

The most common disaccharidase disorder is a deficiency of lactase, the intestinal brush border enzyme that hydrolyzes lactose into glucose and galactose (see Chapter 4). This lactase deficiency leads to a condition called *lactose intolerance*. Lactose intolerance is prevalent worldwide among African Americans, Asians, and South Americans.

Undigested lactose remaining in the intestine will, through osmotic effect, draw water into the digestive tract, resulting in intestinal symptoms such as abdominal cramping, flatulence, and diarrhea. The severity of these symptoms often depends on the amount of lactose ingested and the degree of intolerance an individual has. Lactase deficiency is sometimes secondary to or accompanied by acute or chronic diseases that damage the intestine, such as gluten-sensitive enteropathy or Crohn's disease; it may also be present in people who have had small bowel or gastric surgery.

Nutrition Therapy

Tolerance for lactose varies from population to population and from person to person. For individuals who have or who are suspected of having lactose intolerance, health care professionals need to establish the patient's tolerance by gradually adding small amounts of lactose-containing foods to a lactose-free diet. Most people can tolerate 6 to 9 g of lactose at a given time, which is the amount in 4 to 6 ounces of milk. Small amounts of lactose within the patient's tolerance level can generally be consumed on several occasions throughout the day. Individuals usually can tolerate lactose if it is consumed along with other foods, rather than alone as a beverage or a snack. Yogurt may be better tolerated than milk, but this varies with brand and processing method. *Lactobacillus acidophilus* milk is probably not better tolerated than regular milk. Cocoa and chocolate milk may be better tolerated. Lactase enzyme is available as Lactaid or Dairy Ease and may be added to milk 24 hours in advance of ingestion. In addition, a tablet form is available that can be ingested just before eating a meal that contains lactose. Depending on the degree of intolerance, patients may use one-half to three tablets.[2]

Restricting lactose-containing foods may place a person at risk for calcium, riboflavin, and vitamin D deficiency, depending on the degree of lactose restriction. These nutrients can be provided at the Recommended Dietary Allowance (RDA) level with lactase enzyme-treated milk and milk products or with supplementation.[2] Calcium is of particular importance to children and women. Vitamin D supplementation is necessary only for those individuals who do not obtain adequate exposure to sunlight[2] and for older adults whose production of vitamin D may be reduced.

INFLAMMATORY BOWEL DISEASE

Inflammatory bowel disease (IBD) refers to two idiopathic chronic inflammatory conditions of the intestines—chronic ulcerative colitis (CUC) and Crohn's disease (also called regional enteritis). CUC is an inflammatory process confined to the mucosa of any or all of the large intestine. Crohn's disease is an inflammatory disorder that involves all layers of the intestinal wall and may include the small or large intestine or both. It is associated with stricture formation, fistulous tracts, and abscesses. Both cause diarrhea, which may be profuse and bloody. The term *colitis* applies only to inflammatory disease of the colon.[9]

Other major symptoms in IBD include abdominal pain, and clinical signs include intestinal bleeding, protein loss, and fever, all of which result in nutritional depletion. Causes of nutritional depletion in IBD include decreased intake, malabsorption, increased nutrient loss, increased nutrient use and thus increased nutrient requirements, and drug-nutrient interactions. Proper management requires persistent attention to nutritional maintenance and repletion along with therapies to facilitate healing of the inflamed bowel, which may include pharmacotherapy, surgery, and nutritional support.[9,15] Surgery is curative in ulcerative colitis, but Crohn's disease tends to recur following surgical resection of affected sections in the majority of patients.[9]

Nutrition Therapy

Goals of nutrition therapy are to replace nutrients lost as a result of the inflammatory process, correct deficits, and provide adequate nutrition to achieve and maintain energy, nitrogen, fluid, and electrolyte balance.[2,15] Attention must be given to intestinal function, including previous intestinal resections, site and extent of disease process (Figure 17-7), and anticipated medical and surgical treatment.

During acute stages of IBD, medical nutrition therapy is individualized based on food tolerance and portion(s) of the GI tract affected.[2,15] Risk for malnutrition is high in patients with IBD because they commonly reduce or restrict food intake in response to association with fullness, pain, and diarrhea. In addition to reduced intake, altered digestion and absorption, increased nutrient losses or requirements, and drug-nutrient interactions may further increase risk for nutrient deficiencies. Precise diet and weight histories are essential to determine risk for malnutrition and potential nutrient deficiencies.[2] The most common nutrients that may be insufficient or malabsorbed include several minerals (iron, calcium, zinc, magnesium, selenium) and numerous vitamins (folate, thiamine, riboflavin, pyridoxine, vitamin B_{12}, and vitamins A, D, and E).[16] A high-kcal, high-protein diet divided into small, frequent meals is suggested for those at risk for malnutrition.[2] During remission, a high-fiber diet (as tolerated) (Box 17-4) is recommended to stimulate peristalsis and improve muscular tone of the walls of the GI tract, especially the colon. To maximize nutrient intake, unwarranted restrictions should be avoided.[2]

For the acute episodes, bowel rest and a low-fiber diet (Table 17-4) are frequently suggested to minimize symptoms.

ILEOSTOMIES AND COLOSTOMIES

Occasionally, when disease or obstruction cannot be resolved, all or a segment of the colon, including the rectum, is removed. Appropriate nutrition therapy depends on which procedure, either an ileostomy or a colostomy, is performed. An ileostomy consists of the removal of the entire colon and rectum. A surgical formation of an opening of the ileum onto the surface of the abdomen is made, through which fecal matter is emptied. A colostomy consists of the surgical creation of an artificial anus on the abdominal wall by incising the colon and bringing it out to the surface. It may be single-barreled (one opening) or double-barreled (distal and proximal loops open onto the abdomen).

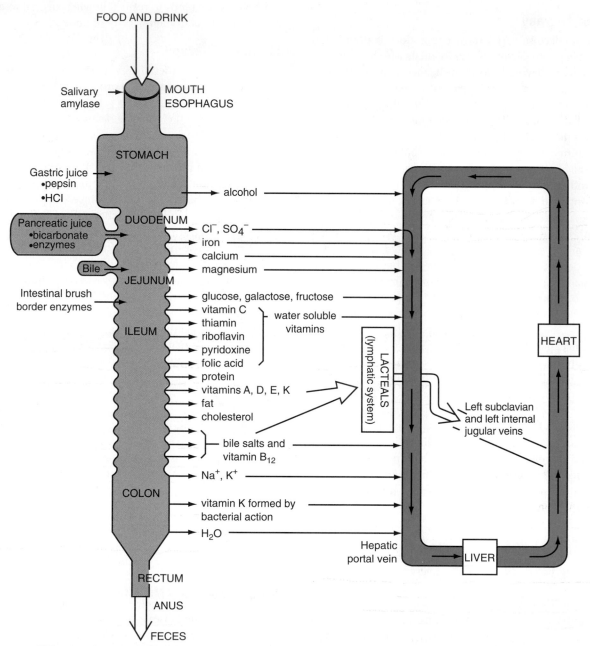

FIG 17-7 Site and extent of disease process and effect on nutrient absorption. (From Mahan LK, Escott-Stump S: *Krause's food & nutrition therapy,* ed 12, Philadelphia, 2008, Saunders.)

BOX 17-4 INCREASING FIBER INTAKE*

EXCELLENT SOURCES	GOOD SOURCES	FAIR SOURCES	POOR SOURCES
All-Bran cereal	Apple with skin	Banana	Celery
Bran Buds cereal	Prunes	Pineapple, canned	Cucumber
Bran Chex cereal	Raisins	Cheerios	Lettuce (iceberg)
Corn Bran cereal	Strawberries, raw	Corn, whole kernel canned	Mushrooms
Raisin Bran cereal	Blueberries	Cauliflower	Onions
Grape Nuts cereal	Broccoli, cooked	Carrots	Grapefruit
Fiber One cereal	Green beans, frozen	Tomato, raw	Fruit juices
Pear, with skin	Peas, cooked	Brown rice	Vegetable juices
Baked beans	Potato with skin		Crisped rice cereal
Kidney beans, cooked	Sweet potato with skin		Corn flakes cereal
Chickpeas (garbanzo)	Black-eyed peas		Refined white flour products (white
	Whole-wheat bread		breads, rolls, bagels, most pastas,
	Shredded wheat cereal		pizza crust, crackers)
	Bran muffin		
	Oatmeal, cooked		
	Graham crackers		

NOTE: Increasing fiber without increasing fluid can lead to more constipation, abdominal pain, bloating, and gas. Fiber intake should be increased gradually, over a period of weeks while simultaneously increasing fluids.

*Current recommendations for Adequate Intake (AI) are for 25-38 g/day. This goal can be met by eating a well-balanced diet containing a variety of foods: 2-4 servings of fruit, 3-5 servings of vegetables, 6-11 servings of whole grain breads or cereals, plenty of fluids.

Data from University Health Center: *A high fiber diet: The best approach to constipation and irritable bowel syndrome,* College Park, Md, 2002, University of Maryland. Accessed May 12, 2006, from www.health.umd.edu; American Dietetic Association: *Nutrition care manual,* Chicago, 2005, Author. Accessed February 28, 2010, from www.nutritioncaremanual.org.

TABLE 17-4 GUIDELINES FOR FIBER-RESTRICTED DIETS

FOOD GROUP	RECOMMENDED FOODS	FOODS NOT RECOMMENDED
Dairy	Buttermilk	Yogurts with nuts or dried fruits
	Evaporated, skim, and low-fat milk	Whole milk
	Soy milk	Half-and-half
	Yogurt with live active cultures	Cream
	Powdered milk	Sour cream
	Cheese	Regular (whole milk) ice cream
Grains	White flour	Whole-wheat or whole grain breads, rolls,
Choose grains with <2 gm dietary fiber/serving	Bread, bagels, rolls, crackers, pasta made from white or refined flour	crackers, or pasta
		Brown or wild rice
	Cold or hot cereals made from white or refined flour	Barley, oats, and other whole grains
		Cereals made from whole grains or bran
		Breads or cereals made with seeds or nuts
		Popcorn
Fruits and vegetables	Fruit juice without pulp, except prune juice	All raw fruits and vegetables (except banana, melons, lettuce)
	Ripe bananas	Dried fruits, including prunes and raisins
	Canned soft fruits	Fruit juice with pulp
	Most well-cooked vegetables without seeds or skins	Canned fruit in heavy syrup
		Any fruits sweetened with sorbitol
	Potatoes without skin	Prune juice
	Lettuce	Fried vegetables
	Strained vegetable juice	Beets
		Cruciferous vegetables (broccoli, Brussels sprouts, cabbage, cauliflower)
		Greens (collard, mustard, turnip)
		Corn
		Potato skins

Continued

TABLE 17-4	GUIDELINES FOR FIBER-RESTRICTED DIETS—cont'd	
FOOD GROUP	**RECOMMENDED FOODS**	**FOODS NOT RECOMMENDED**
Proteins	Tender, well-cooked meat, poultry, fish, eggs, or soy foods made without added fat Smooth nut butters	Fried meat, poultry, or fish Luncheon meats, such as bologna or salami Sausage or bacon Hot dogs Fatty meats Nuts Chunky nut butters
Beverages 8-10 cups of fluid is recommended each day; more may be needed to replace fluids lost to diarrhea	Decaffeinated coffee Caffeine-free teas Soft drinks without caffeine Rehydration beverages	Caffeinated beverages (coffee, tea, colas, energy drinks) Limit beverages containing high fructose corn syrup to 12 oz/day Avoid beverages sweetened with sorbitol Alcoholic beverages
Fats Other foods		Limit to <8 teaspoons/day Sugar alcohol such as xylitol and sorbitol Honey

Modified from American Dietetic Association Nutrition Care Manual. *Fiber-restricted nutrition therapy.* Accessed February 28, 2010, from www.nutritioncaremanual.org.

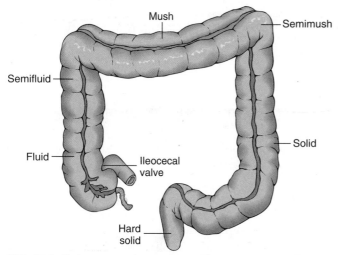

FIG 17-8 Colostomy site and its effect on output. Excess motility causes less absorption and diarrhea or loose feces. Poor motility causes more absorption, resulting in hard feces and constipation. (From Rolin Graphics. Modified from Guyton AC: *Textbook of medical physiology,* ed 11, Philadelphia, 2005, Saunders.)

Nutrition therapy goals are tied to the liquidity of the effluent. In the case of an ileostomy, the effluent is more liquid because the ileocecal valve, which controls rate of movement from the small intestine to the large, is absent. Therefore, water, sodium, and other minerals that would otherwise be absorbed are lost, making fluid and electrolyte replacement an important goal.[17] With a colostomy, the effluent is proportional to the length of the remaining bowel (Figure 17-8). The more liquid the stool, the greater the loss of fluid and electrolytes. Any restrictions placed on the patient should be based solely on individual tolerance in both cases.[2] The *Teaching Tool* box, Eating Well with a Colostomy or Ileostomy, provides nutritional recommendations.

SHORT BOWEL SYNDROME

When large portions of the small intestine must be resected because of illness or injury, short bowel syndrome (SBS) may occur. Symptoms and resulting consequences of SBS depend on the site of resection, extent of small bowel removed, elapsed time since resection, absence or presence of ileocecal valve, condition of the remaining intestine, and whether there is colon continuity.[15] An inadequate absorptive surface results in malabsorption of vitamin B_{12} and other vitamins and less than optimal nutritional status.[9]

Nutrition Therapy

Nutritional management should take into consideration the individual's digestive and absorptive capabilities. If the patient is unable to consume adequate nutrients or if enteral nutrition exacerbates symptoms, then parenteral nutrition support is indicated; however, it is preferable to return to enteral feedings as soon as possible to prevent atrophy of the GI tract. Dietary fat restriction or the use of MCT fat (oil) may be beneficial.[18] **MCT fats (oils)** are specialized modular formulas made of medium-chain triglycerides that do not require pancreatic lipase or bile for digestion and absorption. They are absorbed directly into the portal vein (like amino acids and monosaccharides) rather than the lymphatic system like other lipids.

Frequent monitoring of nutritional status, especially fluid and electrolyte balance, is crucial. If a patient continues to fail on an oral diet, long-term parenteral nutrition at home may be indicated.

DIVERTICULAR DISEASES

When the musculature of the bowel walls weakens, **diverticula** (pouchlike herniations protruding from the muscular layer of the colon) often develop, resulting in the condition

✴ TEACHING TOOL

Eating Well with a Colostomy or Ileostomy

Meals can still be an enjoyable experience for patients with colostomies and ileostomies. Individual experimentation works best to determine the most appropriate dietary restrictions. The following are some strategies that may reduce negative symptoms:

Eating Practices That May Cause Gas

Chewing gum
Use of drinking straws
Carbonated beverages
Smoking
Chewing tobacco
Eating quickly

Eating Practices That May Reduce Discomfort

Take small bites of food.
Chew thoroughly.
Eat foods at regular times each day.
Smaller, more frequent meals may be better tolerated.
Eating largest meal in the middle of the day may help decrease stool output at night.

Foods That May Help Control Odor or Gas

Buttermilk
Parsley
Yogurt
Kefir
Cranberry juice

Foods That May Help Control Diarrhea

Applesauce
Banana or banana flakes
Pectin
Pasta
Potatoes
Rice
Cheese

Recommendations

Eat at least three meals a day at regular intervals.
Chew foods thoroughly.
Drink 8 to 10 cups of fluids each day. May be increased during hot weather.
Eat a small evening meal.
Try new foods one at a time. Do not eliminate a food from your diet without trying it several times.

Data from American Dietetic Association: *Nutrition care manual,* Chicago, Author. Accessed February 28, 2010, from www.nutritioncaremanual.org.

diverticulosis. It is thought to develop as the result of long-term, low-fiber eating habits and increased intracolonic pressure such as that created with straining to have a bowel movement.[15,19] Usually this condition remains undetected unless the diverticula become infected and inflamed from trapped fecal material and colon bacteria. This resulting complication is called **diverticulitis.**

Nutrition Therapy

During periods of inflammation, the medical goal is to rest the bowel, allowing the infection to resolve. Patients are given nothing by mouth, and then progress to liquids. As inflammation abates, a high-fiber diet is recommended to reduce straining during defecation. High-fiber diets increase fiber-rich foods in the general diet by including fruits, vegetables, legumes, whole grain breads, and cereals. Box 17-4 lists foods used to increase fiber intake. Historically, nuts and seeds have been excluded for fear they might become entrapped in diverticula. There is no evidence-based research to suggest that such foods worsen risk of diverticulitis. Conversely, eating high-fiber foods is the only treatment for diverticulosis.[19]

Current fiber recommendations for Adequate Intake (AI) are 25 to 38 g/day. Translating these recommendations into real food, Americans should consume at least five servings or cups of fruits/vegetables and six servings or ounces of whole grain breads/cereals/legumes per day.

Fiber should be added to the diet gradually to allow the intestinal tract to adapt. This minimizes potential adverse side effects such as abdominal distress, bloating, flatulence, cramps, and diarrhea, which are usually temporary and will abate after several days. Care should also be taken to consume adequate amounts of fluid—at least 8 to 12 cups per day.[2]

INTESTINAL GAS AND FLATULENCE

Excessive gas in the GI tract can be the result of several factors. Belching is typically caused by the habit of swallowing air (aerophagia) while eating or drinking. Foods that contain high amounts of air, such as carbonated beverages, may also contribute to this problem. Aerophagia does not usually contribute to the formation of colon gas. Presence of flatus in the colon is the result of gases formed from food ingestion or fermentation of certain foods by intestinal bacteria. Typically, gas is reabsorbed through the colon wall as it passes through the bowel, but if motility is disturbed, bloating and distention may result, causing abdominal pain.

Nutrition Therapy

Because eating habits as well as the type of foods eaten can contribute to excess gas production, a thorough appraisal of the patient's usual eating pattern and habits is necessary. Specific treatment depends on the source of the gas. Gas-forming foods can be avoided on a trial basis to determine if they are a source of discomfort. Remaining upright for 30 minutes after meals may also be beneficial.

CONSTIPATION

Constipation is a symptom, not a disease. There can be many different causes of constipation. Organic causes include intestinal obstruction, spasms of the sigmoid colon, diverticulitis, and tumors. The most common cause of functional constipation is failure to respond to the urge to defecate. Other functional causes include lack of fiber or fluid, prolonged bed rest or lack of regular exercise, or habitual use of laxatives or enemas. When these conditions are untreated, the colon becomes **atonic** (lacking normal muscle tone).[18] Many women experience constipation during the last trimester of pregnancy as the growing fetus impairs the passage of feces.

If constipation becomes severe, bowel movements may diminish in frequency to only once every week or so. This allows tremendous quantities of fecal material to accumulate in the colon, causing it to distend to a diameter as great as 3 to 4 inches. This condition, **megacolon**, can occur because of congenital, toxic, or acquired in nature factors. Congenital megacolon (also called *Hirschsprung's disease*) is the result of lack or deficiency of autonomic ganglion cells in the smooth muscle wall of the colon.[13,20] Consequently, neither defecation reflexes nor peristaltic motility can occur through this area of the large intestine.[13] Toxic megacolon is a complication of ulcerative colitis and may result in perforation of the colon, leading to septicemia and death. The most common treatment for congenital and toxic megacolon is surgery.[20] Acquired megacolon results from chronic refusal to defecate, with the colon becoming dilated and impacted with feces. Laxatives and enemas are often the necessary treatment.[20]

Nutrition Therapy

Although laxatives are commonly chosen for self-treatment, diet is usually the treatment of choice for constipation. Recommendations include consuming adequate fluids and a wide variety of foods that contain ample amounts of fiber (see Box 17-4). Fiber is important in providing bulk in the diet, which stimulates peristalsis. Care should be taken to increase fiber in the diet gradually to avoid any adverse reactions. Although dietary fiber cannot be digested by humans, it can be broken down by bacteria that live in the intestine. Therefore, flatulence and osmotic diarrhea may result. Osmotic diarrhea is diarrhea-associated water retention in the large intestine resulting from an accumulation of nonabsorbable water-soluble solutes.

Some foods high in fiber are also high in phytates and oxalate, which decrease the bioavailability of certain vitamins and minerals—namely, calcium, copper, selenium, zinc, iron, and magnesium.[2] However, nutrient deficiencies are unlikely to occur if an adequate balanced diet from a variety of foods is consumed. The body may adjust to the decreased availability of nutrients by increased absorption of those that are available.[2]

Copious amounts of fiber, particularly wheat bran, may result in the formation of bezoars in some people. **Bezoars** are physical obstacles created by tangles of fibrous material in the GI tract that may cause dangerous GI obstructions. This tends to occur more commonly in individuals who have diabetes and who suffer from gastroparesis.[2] (See Chapter 19 for more information about gastroparesis.)

DIARRHEA

Diarrhea (like constipation) is a symptom, not a disease. It is usually categorized in one of two ways: acute or chronic. Treatment is determined by cause. Acute diarrhea is typically of short duration and is usually the result of enteritis. **Enteritis** is infection of the small intestine caused by a virus, bacteria, or protozoa. Box 2-6 lists common foodborne pathogens that may cause diarrhea. Other causes of acute diarrhea include the intended effect or side effects of medications, change in dietary habits or intake, or emotional stress. Diarrhea that lasts longer than 2 weeks is considered chronic. Long-term diarrhea is usually the result of GI irritation or malabsorption. Both may necessitate permanent dietary changes. Chronic, persistent diarrhea may signify a more serious disease and should be evaluated by a physician.

Nutrition Therapy

Nutrition therapy is based on the cause of diarrhea. In severe cases, the patient may be restricted to nothing by mouth to allow the GI tract to rest; however, it is usually unnecessary to withhold all feedings. Administration of fluids to achieve or maintain hydration is a primary concern. This may be done with enteral or parenteral fluids (carbohydrate and electrolytes). Enteral therapy may consist of oral rehydration solutions or a clear liquid diet for 1 or 2 days before progressing to a low-fat, low-fiber, or low-lactose diet. Small, frequent meals are often better tolerated than three larger meals. After 2 or 3 days, progression to a general or normal diet is usually tolerated.[9] It is also important to educate the patient regarding cause and prevention of subsequent incidences of diarrhea.[9]

SUMMARY

Disorders of the GI tract include those that affect the esophagus, stomach, small intestine, and large intestine. Some disorders affect the muscular action of these sections of the GI tract, thereby affecting flow of sustenance through the GI tract; these include dysphagia and hiatal hernia. Other disorders, such as peptic ulcer and diverticulitis, lead to site-specific tissue inflammation and pain. Several disorders may be caused by inability of the body to produce necessary digestive enzymes (e.g., lactase in lactose intolerance) or inability to metabolize nutrient substances (e.g., gliadin, resulting in severe reactions caused by celiac disease). Most disorders are also influenced by lifestyle behaviors that affect stress levels and alter dietary patterns. All GI disorders require some level of medical nutritional therapy that is individualized to meet the needs of each patient.

THE NURSING APPROACH

Case Study: Dysphagia and Feeding Self-Care Deficit

Pierre, age 80, had a stroke one month ago and is in a rehabilitation center. He has been getting physical therapy for hemiparesis (weakness) in his right arm and leg. Because of aphasia (speech problems) and dysphagia (swallowing difficulties), he was evaluated by a speech therapist and initially received nourishment through a small-bore nasoduodenal feeding tube. Pierre's speech therapy is continuing, related to expressive aphasia. Per doctor's orders, he has advanced to a soft diet.

ASSESSMENT

Subjective (unable to understand Pierre's attempts to speak)

Objective (from physical examination)
- Coughs and chokes frequently when trying to eat or drink
- Fed by nursing staff, does not assist with feeding, eats very slowly
- Can follow directions but has difficulty expressing himself

DIAGNOSES (NURSING)

1. Risk for aspiration related to impaired swallowing
2. Feeding self-care deficit related to weakness of right hand and arm as evidenced by being fed by nurse; does not assist with feeding

PLANNING

Patient Outcomes

Short term (within two weeks):
- Pierre will be able to eat with minimal or no choking.
- Lung sounds will remain clear.
- He will be able to assist with his own feeding.

Long term (by discharge):
- No aspiration pneumonia
- Pierre will be able to feed himself using adaptive equipment and assistance in setting up his food.

Nursing Interventions

1. Implement aspiration precautions.
2. Reinforce rehabilitation efforts by the health care team.

IMPLEMENTATION

1. Met with the health care team to design and implement an individualized rehabilitation care plan.
   - The doctor prescribed the diet and therapies.
   - The dietitian planned nourishment consistent with physical limitations and nutrient needs.
   - The physical therapist strengthened the patient's weak arm to help with self-feeding.
   - The speech therapist taught the patient how to chew and swallow safely and to communicate needs.
   - The occupational therapist provided adaptive equipment for self-feeding and taught the patient how to become more independent.
   - The nurse helped facilitate schedules for the various therapies, helped feed the patient when other disciplines were not there, and reinforced teaching.

   Team efforts enhance rehabilitation measures. Nurses are with the patient 24 hours per day and thus are in a position to coordinate necessary therapies and help implement the plan of care.

2. Tested Pierre's gag reflex and listened to lung sounds every morning before feeding him.
   Presence of the gag reflex reduces risk for aspiration. Assessment should be ongoing for any signs of aspiration pneumonia.
3. Positioned him in an upright position (high Fowler's) during meals and for 30 minutes after the meal.
   Gravity assists the passage of food and reduces the risk of choking and aspiration.
4. Reduced distractions such as television during mealtimes.
   Creating focus for eating helps the patient concentrate on new swallowing and feeding techniques.
5. Assessed Pierre's food preferences by having him point to pictures of foods he likes, within the soft diet prescribed by the physician and at the recommendation of the dietitian.
   When the patient is able to make decisions about what to eat, he may feel some control of his situation. Foods that are easiest to chew and swallow include finely chopped meat and smooth textures. Nuts, tough skins, and dry, crispy, raw, or stringy foods are not allowed.
6. Added a commercial thickening agent to juices and water.
   Thin liquids provoke choking; thicker liquids are easier to swallow.
7. Used custard, gelatin, and liquid nutritional supplements between meals two or three times a day.
   Intake at mealtime is limited by patient tolerance and time. Between-meal snacks provide extra calories and liquids.
8. Instructed Pierre to follow specific steps when swallowing:
   - Take a breath before swallowing
   - Hold breath during swallowing
   - Exhale forcefully after swallowing
   - Swallow again

   This maneuver decreases the potential for aspiration by closing off the trachea.
9. Had suction equipment available during feedings.
   The nurse may need to remove fluids from the patient's mouth and throat by suction in order to prevent aspiration.
10. Provided mouth care before and after meals.
    A fresh mouth encourages appetite. Removal of pocketed food (food remaining in the weak side of the mouth) reduces danger of choking.
11. Encouraged Pierre to feed himself, using special plates and utensils.
    Adaptive equipment may facilitate success of the patient's attempts to feed himself.

EVALUATION

Short term (at the end of two weeks):
- Pierre was still choking occasionally on his food and liquids, but his lungs remained clear.
- He was beginning to feed himself.
- Goals partially met.

Continued

THE NURSING APPROACH—cont'd

Case Study: Dysphagia and Feeding Self-Care Deficit—cont'd

DISCUSSION QUESTIONS

As Pierre started feeding himself, he sometimes left food on the same side of the plate as his weak arm. He also failed to see the nurse when she would come to assist feeding him if the nurse stood at his weak side. The nurse added the nursing diagnosis of "Unilateral neglect."

1. What causes this problem?
2. How could the nurse teach Pierre to compensate for this condition?

NOTE: Periodic swallowing reevaluation is recommended. Swallowing dysfunction is different for every patient and appropriate dietary modifications are determined by speech pathologists and dietetic specialists.

Nursing Diagnoses-Definitions and Classification 2009-2011. Copyright © 2009, 1994-2009 by NANDA International. Used by arrangement with Blackwell Publishing Limited, a company of John Wiley & Sons, Inc.

CRITICAL THINKING

Clinical Applications

Theresa, age 35, is admitted with microcytic anemia. Her medical history indicates that she underwent a total gastrectomy 2 years ago to treat bleeding ulcers. On admission she weighs 120 pounds and she is 5 feet 9 inches tall. She has lost 30 pounds since the surgery. She has been taking ferrous sulfate and monthly injections of vitamin B_{12}. On admission her laboratory findings are as follows: hemoglobin 8 g/dL; hematocrit 26%; serum albumin 2.7 g/dL. Her typical dietary intake is as follows:

Breakfast

1 egg scrambled in 1 teaspoon margarine
½ cup cream of wheat with 1 teaspoon margarine
1 slice white toast with 1 teaspoon margarine
1 cup black coffee

10 AM

6 saltine crackers
12-ounce can diet cola

Lunch

2 baked chicken wings
1 cup cooked carrots
1 medium boiled red potato
1 medium banana
12 ounces diet lemon-lime soda

3 PM

½ bagel with 1 tablespoon cream cheese
8-ounces chocolate milk

Dinner

1 broiled chicken breast
½ cup steamed broccoli
1 cup hot tea with artificial sweetener

9 PM

6 saltine crackers
1 tablespoon peanut butter
1 cup black coffee

1. What are common nutrition problems found in patients who have gastrectomies?
2. Which of these problems were experienced by Theresa?
3. What factors explain iron deficiency anemia that develops after a gastrectomy? What is used to treat this anemia?
4. How do Theresa's laboratory values compare with normal values? What do these values indicate?
5. Why is Theresa receiving monthly injections of vitamin B_{12}? Would you advise her to eat more foods high in B_{12}? Explain your rationale.
6. After reviewing Theresa's usual dietary intake, what food groups and/or nutrients are lacking in her diet?
7. What suggestions would you offer Theresa concerning her dietary habits?
8. Should Theresa continue to consume six smaller meals and snacks? Why or why not?

WEBSITES OF INTEREST

Crohn's Disease/Ulcerative Colitis/Inflammatory Bowel Disease Pages

http://qurlyjoe.bu.edu/cduchome.html
Provides information on several digestive diseases including chat rooms, resources, retail items, and pharmaceutical links.

National Digestive Diseases Information Clearinghouse (NDDIC)

www.niddk.nih.gov/health/digest/nddic.htm
Sponsored by the National Institute of Digestive Diseases, this database contains health promotion and education materials not indexed elsewhere.

National Institute of Diabetes and Digestive and Kidney Diseases (NIDDK)

www.niddk.nih.gov

Contains information, resources, and related links on digestive diseases, diabetes, kidney and urologic diseases, and nutrition.

REFERENCES

1. Beyer PL: Gastrointestinal disorders: roles of nutrition and the dietetics practitioner, *J Am Diet Assoc* 98:272-277, 1998

2. American Dietetic Association: *Nutrition care manual*, Chicago, Author. Accessed February 21, 2010, from www.nutritioncaremanual.org.

3. Agency for Health Care Policy and Research (AHCPR): *Diagnosis and treatment of swallowing disorders (dysphagia) in acute-care stroke patients*, AHCPR Pub No 99-E024, Rockville, Md, 1999, U.S. Department of Health and Human Services. Accessed February 21, 2010, from www.ncbi.nlm.nih.gov/books/bv.fcgi?rid=hstat1.chapter.11701.

4. Milazzo LS, Buchard J, Lund DA: The swallowing process: Effects of aging and stroke. In Erickson RV, editor: Medical management of the elderly stroke patient, *Phys Med Rehabil State Art Rev* 3:489, 1989.

5. Loustau A, Lee KA: Dealing with the dangers of dysphagia, *Nursing* 15:47-50, 1985.

6. Kuthlemeier KV, Palmer JB, Rosenberg D: Effect of liquid bolus consistency and delivery method on aspiration and pharyngeal retention in dysphagia patients, *Dysphagia* 16:119-122, 2001.

7. McCance KL, Huether SE: *Pathophysiology: The biological basis for diseases in adults and children*, ed 5, St. Louis, 2006, Mosby.

8. Lui JY, et al: Determining an appropriate threshold for referral to surgery for gastroesophageal reflux disease, *Surgery* 133:5-12, 2003.

9. Merck & Co, Inc: *The Merck manual of diagnosis and therapy: Helicobacter pylori infection*, Whitehouse Station, NJ, Updated January 2007, Author. Accessed February 28, 2010, from www.merck.com.

10. Ramakrishnan K, Salinas RC. Peptic ulcer disease, *Am Fam Physician* 76(7):1005-12, 2007. Accessed February 28, 2010, from www.aafp.org/afp.

11. American Gastroenterological Association: *Peptic ulcer disease*, Bethesda, Md (no date), Author. Accessed February 28, 2010, from www.gastro.org/patient-center/digestive-conditions/peptic-ulcer-disease.

12. American Dietetic Association Nutrition Care Manual: *Peptic ulcers: nutrition prescription*. Accessed February 28, 2010, from www.nutritioncaremanual.org.

13. Guyton AC: *Textbook of medical physiology*, ed 11, Philadelphia, 2005, Saunders.

14. Beyer PL: Medical nutrition therapy for upper gastrointestinal tract disorders. In Mahan LK, Escott-Stump S, editors: *Krause's food & nutrition therapy*, ed 12, Philadelphia, 2008, Saunders.

15. Beyer PL: Medical nutrition therapy for lower gastrointestinal tract disorders. In Mahan LK, Escott-Stump S, editors: *Krause's food & nutrition therapy*, ed 12, Philadelphia, 2008, Saunders.

16. Moore MC: *Mosby's pocket guide to nutritional assessment and care*, ed 5, St. Louis, 2005, Mosby.

17. Nelms MN, Fraizier C: Immunology. In Nelms MN, et al, editors: *Nutrition therapy and pathophysiology*, ed 2, Belmont, Calif, 2010, Cengage/Thomson.

18. Kirby D, Birkenhauer RS: Gastrointestinal disorders. In Lysen LK, editor: *Quick reference to clinical dietetics*, ed 2, Boston, 2006, Jones and Bartlett.

19. Escott-Stump S: *Nutrition and diagnosis related care*, ed 6, Baltimore, 2007, Lippincott Williams & Wilkins.

20. MedlinePlus: *Medical encyclopedia: Toxic megacolon*, Atlanta (updated May 27, 2008) A.D.A.M., Inc., for Medline Plus. Accessed February 28, 2010, from www.nlm.nih.gov/medlineplus/ency/article/000248.htm.

Nutrition for Disorders of the Liver, Gallbladder, and Pancreas

Although the liver, gallbladder, and pancreas are not part of the digestive tract proper, little digestion, absorption, or metabolism would take place without them.

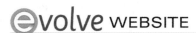 **WEBSITE**
http://evolve.elsevier.com/Grodner/foundations/

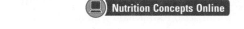 Nutrition Concepts Online

ROLE IN WELLNESS

Although the liver, gallbladder, and pancreas are not part of the digestive tract proper, little digestion, absorption, or metabolism would take place without them. Disease or injury to these ancillary digestive organs can have a devastating effect on nutritional status. Nutrition therapy is part of the treatment for disorders of the liver, gallbladder, and pancreas. It is also necessary to prevent nutritional deficiencies because of the role these organs have on digestive functioning.

Wellness requires well-functioning body organs. In particular, consider how disorders of the liver, gallbladder, and pancreas affect the five dimensions of health. The *physical health* dimension is crucially dependent on these organs. As ancillary digestive organs, their malfunctioning can devastate nutritional status. Reasoning skills, an aspect of *intellectual health,* are required to make lifestyle decisions related to levels of alcohol and fat intake if a person is at risk for cirrhosis or pancreatic disorders. The strain in dealing with chronic life-threatening illness, such as cystic fibrosis (CF), challenges *emotional health.* Because of the relationship of these disorders to digestive functioning, restrictive dietary guidelines may inhibit the ability to easily socialize with others, thereby limiting *social health.* The *spiritual health* dimension, through religious beliefs, may provide patients with comforting perspectives for coping with serious physical disorders.

LIVER DISORDERS

The liver, the largest organ in the body, lies beneath the diaphragm in the right upper quadrant of the abdomen (Figure 18-1) and is responsible for the majority of biochemical functions that take place in the body. The liver's management of bile production and its role in intermediary metabolism of carbohydrates, protein, lipids, and vitamins influence nutritional status. Thus it is easy to understand that impaired liver function can result in major imbalances in metabolism and nutritional status. As with many other diseases, progressive decline of nutritional status can further impair liver function. Figure 18-1 summarizes only a few of the liver's many roles in metabolism and nutritional status.

Fatty Liver

Fatty liver (also called *hepatic steatosis*) is typically a symptom of an underlying problem. Although it is the earliest form of alcoholic liver disease, it can also be caused by excessive kcal intake, obesity, complications of drug therapy (e.g., corticosteroids, tetracyclines), total parenteral nutrition (TPN), pregnancy, diabetes mellitus, inadequate intake of protein (e.g., kwashiorkor), infection, or malignancy.[1] Fatty infiltration of the liver develops when triglycerides build up in the liver tissue, which may eventually produce an enlarged liver. This infiltration is a function of improper fat metabolism. It can be reversed if the causative agent is removed.[1] Therefore, if alcohol abuse occurs, then abstinence from alcohol is necessary as part of the treatment and may lead to reversal of the infiltration and prevent further fibrosis or necrosis. Whatever the cause, proper nutrition in the form of a well-balanced diet is important in reversing fatty infiltration.

Viral Hepatitis

Defined as inflammation of the liver, acute hepatitis can occur as the result of infectious mononucleosis, cirrhosis, toxic chemicals, or viral infection. There are five types of hepatitis that have been characterized, and although symptomatology, clinical signs, and presentation are similar,

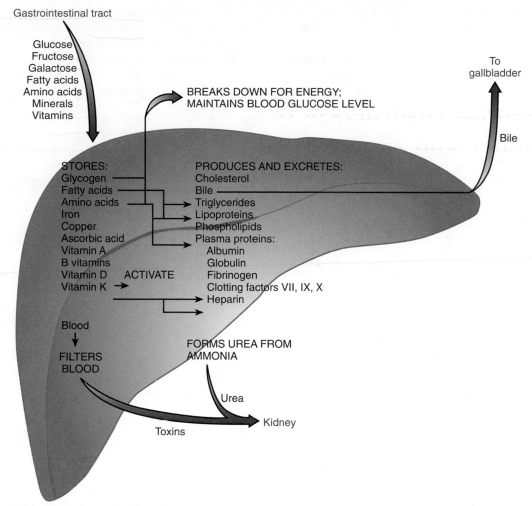

Gastrointestinal tract

Glucose
Fructose
Galactose
Fatty acids
Amino acids
Minerals
Vitamins

BREAKS DOWN FOR ENERGY;
MAINTAINS BLOOD GLUCOSE LEVEL

To gallbladder

Bile

STORES:
Glycogen
Fatty acids
Amino acids
Iron
Copper
Ascorbic acid
Vitamin A
B vitamins
Vitamin D
Vitamin K

ACTIVATE

PRODUCES AND EXCRETES:
Cholesterol
Bile
Triglycerides
Lipoproteins
Phospholipids
Plasma proteins:
    Albumin
    Globulin
    Fibrinogen
    Clotting factors VII, IX, X
    Heparin

Blood

FILTERS
BLOOD

FORMS UREA FROM
AMMONIA

Urea

Kidney

Toxins

FIG 18-1 Role of the liver in metabolism and nutrition. Any damage to the liver may affect nutritional status. (From Rolin Graphics. Modified from Davis J, Sherer K: *Applied nutrition and diet therapy for nurses,* ed 2, Philadelphia, 1994, Saunders.)

immunologic and epidemiologic characteristics are different (Table 18-1).

Hepatitis A virus (HAV) is typically transmitted through the fecal-oral route (contaminated food or water) but occasionally can be spread by transfusion of infected blood.[2,3] It is frequently the result of poor hand washing or stool precautions and is widespread in overcrowded areas with poor sanitation (Box 18-1). Vaccination is recommended for persons at risk for HAV.[4] Onset of HAV is rapid—typically within 4 to 6 weeks[2]—and time to onset of symptoms may be dose related.[5] Occurrence of disease manifestations and severity of symptoms directly correlate with the patient's age.[5] Treatment of acute HAV is generally supportive—usually consisting of bed rest—because no antiviral therapy is available. Hospitalization and intravenous (IV) fluids may be necessary for dehydration caused by nausea and vomiting.[5,6] An adequate diet that excludes alcohol is recommended.[7]

Hepatitis B virus (HBV) is an exceptionally resistant virus capable of surviving extreme temperatures and humidity.[6,8] HBV is transmitted via blood and sexual contact.[6,8] Globally, the vast majority of cases are transmitted perinatally.[6] (See the *Cultural Considerations* box, Hepatitis B Virus Prevalence Rates, for information about the prevalence of HBV among ethnic groups.) HBV transmits more easily than the human immunodeficiency virus (HIV) or hepatitis C, with the virus readily found in serum, semen, vaginal mucus, saliva, and tears. IV drug users, patients with hemophilia, those on renal dialysis, and those who have undergone organ transplantation are at increased risk for HBV (Box 18-2). As a result, routine HBV vaccination is recommended for risk groups of all ages and for children up to age 18.[4] Average incubation time of HBV is approximately 12 weeks.[6,8] As with HAV, the majority of patients are asymptomatic.[8] Those who acquire chronic HBV infection (determined by biopsy) can be healthy, asymptomatic carriers but remain infectious to others through parenteral or sexual transmission.[6] As with acute HAV, no well-established antiviral treatment is available for acute HBV infection.[6] Chronic HBV is treated with interferon alpha and lamivudine to reduce symptoms and prevent or delay progression of chronic hepatitis to cirrhosis or hepatocellular carcinoma (HCC).[6,8] An adequate diet that excludes alcohol is recommended for patients with acute and chronic HBV without cirrhosis.[8]

Hepatitis C virus (HCV) (previously called *non-A, non-B hepatitis*) infection is increasing worldwide and is the major cause of hepatitis in the United States.[7] It is transmitted through contaminated blood, saliva, or semen, although HCV is predominantly associated with blood exposure (e.g., transfusion, IV drug use,[9] acupuncture, tattooing, and sharing razors).[10] Onset is usually slow (i.e., approximately 8 weeks),

can develop into some form of chronic liver disease,[3,6,7] and is a risk factor for liver cancer.[2,6] Most cases of acute HCV are asymptomatic; therefore, it is infrequently detected.[4] Chronic infection develops in 70% to 80% of people infected with HCV.[8] Progression from HCV to cirrhosis may take 10 to 40 years.[6,7] A more rapid disease progression is observed in those infected with HIV or HBV, people with alcoholism, men, and

---

🌐 CULTURAL CONSIDERATIONS

Hepatitis B Virus Prevalence Rates

Hepatitis B virus (HBV) prevalence rates among Asians/Pacific Islanders are the highest of any racial or ethnic group. In China, 90% of people are exposed to the hepatitis virus and 10% are carriers of HBV.

Approximately 50% of women who deliver infants who carry HBV in the United States are foreign-born Asians/Pacific Islanders. Similarly, 85% of men and 60% of women in Korea are exposed to HBV. HBV is a major risk factor for chronic cirrhosis and liver cancer and accounts for up to 80% of liver cancers. The mortality from liver cancer is five times higher among Chinese Americans.

Currently, there are two medications used for immunoprophylaxis against HBV: hepatitis B immunoglobulin (HBIG), which provides passive immunization, and the hepatitis B vaccine. *Healthy People 2010* recommends that by 2010 HBV transmission be reduced through the implementation of vaccination programs targeted to adolescents and adults of high-risk groups.

Application to nursing: Nurses working with clients who are at high risk for HBV can advocate for hepatitis B vaccinations for these individuals. These clients may include foreign-born individuals, individuals with alternative sexual orientation, people with histories of current or past drug abuse, and those exposed to or already diagnosed with HIV.

Data from Tong M: The impact of hepatitis B infection in Asian Americans, *Asian Am Pac Isl J Health* 4(1-3):125-126, 1996; Choe JH, et al: Hepatitis B and liver cancer beliefs among Korean immigrants in Western Washington, *Cancer* 104(12 Suppl):2955-2958, 2005.

TABLE 18-1   COMPARISON OF HEPATITIS VIRUSES

	HEPATITIS A (HAV)	HEPATITIS B (HBV)	HEPATITIS C (HCV)	HEPATITIS D (HDV)	HEPATITIS E (HEV)
Symptoms					
• Jaundice	X	X	X	X	X
• Low-grade fever	X	X	X	X	
• Malaise	X	X	X	X	
• Anorexia	X	X	X	X	
• Dark urine	X	X	X	X	
• Diarrhea	X	X	X	X	
• Pale stools	X	X	X	X	
• Hepatitis B surface antigen (HbsAg) in serum		X	X	X	
• Can be asymptomatic			X	X	
• Flu-like aches & pains					X
Transmission					
• Fecal-oral	X				X
• Foodborne	X				X
• Sexual	X	X		X	
• Parenteral		X		X	
• Perinatal		Rare			
• Contaminated food or water	X				X
• Blood or serum			X		

TABLE 18-1 COMPARISON OF HEPATITIS VIRUSES—cont'd

	HEPATITIS A (HAV)	HEPATITIS B (HBV)	HEPATITIS C (HCV)	HEPATITIS D (HDV)	HEPATITIS E (HEV)
• Sharing contaminated needles, tattooing/piercing equipment			X		
• Co-infected with HBV				X	
Prevention					
• Handwashing	X	X	X	X	
• Good personal hygiene	X	X	X	X	
• Appropriate infection control measures	X	X	X	X	
• Safe sex practices		X	X	X	
• Avoid drinking contaminated water					X

BOX 18-1 RISK FACTORS FOR HEPATITIS A VIRUS

- Travelers to areas where HAV is common
- Homosexual men
- Sexual contact with infected people
- Use of injectable and noninjectable drugs
- Household contact with infected people
- Health care and public safety workers
- People, especially children, living in regions of the United States that have consistently increased rates of HAV

Data from Centers for Disease Control and Prevention: *Viral hepatitis,* Atlanta (reviewed November 18, 2009), Author. Accessed March 10, 2010, from www.cdc.gov/hepatitis/index.htm.

BOX 18-2 RISK FACTORS FOR HEPATITIS B VIRUS

- People with multiple sex partners or partners diagnosed with a sexually transmitted disease
- Homosexual men
- Sexual contact with infected people
- Use of injectable drugs
- Household contact with chronically infected people
- Infants born to infected mothers
- Infants and children of immigrants from areas with high rates of HBV infection
- Health care and public safety workers
- Patients receiving hemodialysis treatments

Data from Centers for Disease Control and Prevention: *Hepatitis B fact sheet,* Atlanta (reviewed November 18, 2009), Author. Accessed March 10, 2010, from www.cdc.gov/hepatitis/index.htm.

those who acquired the infection at an older age.[7] Treatment goals include the following[6,7]:

- Decrease viral replication or eradicate HCV.
- Delay fibrosis and progression to cirrhosis.
- Decrease incidence of HCC.
- Ameliorate symptoms such as fatigue and joint pain.
- Prevent hepatic decompensation and obviate liver transplantation.

Chronic HCV is treated with a combination therapy of interferon alpha and ribavirin.[6,7] No special diet is recommended.

Hepatitis D virus (HDV) can only occur if an individual with HBV is subsequently exposed to HDV (co-infection or superinfection).[2,3,10] The incubation period is 21 to 45 days but may be shorter in cases of superinfection.[10] Clinical course varies, ranging from acute, self-limiting infection to acute fulminant liver failure.[10] HDV is found throughout the world but is prevalent in the Mediterranean basin, Middle East, Amazon basin, Samoa, China, Japan, Taiwan, and Myanmar (formerly Burma).[2,3,10] Of those infected with HDV, 90% are likely to be asymptomatic.[10] Parenteral transmission is understood to be the most common means of infection,[6,10] making IV drug use a risk factor.[10] Treatment is composed of support for the most part.[10] Patients co-infected with HBV and HDV are less responsive to interferon therapy than patients infected with HBV alone.[6] Diet does not need to be restricted.[10]

Hepatitis E virus (HEV) is an enterically transmitted (oral-fecal route), self-limiting infection.[6,11] Prevalence of HEV in the United States is generally attributed to travel in endemic areas[11] (e.g., South, Southeast, and Central Asia; Africa; Mexico[6]; and India[11]). Predominating factors for transmission include tropical climates, inadequate sanitation, and poor personal hygiene. The incubation period ranges from 15 to 60 days, and symptoms include myalgia, anorexia, nausea/vomiting, weight loss (typically 5 to 10 pounds), dehydration, jaundice, dark urine, and light-colored stools.[11] Therapy should be predominantly preventive. Travelers to endemic areas should avoid drinking water or other beverages that may be contaminated. Uncooked fruits or vegetables should not be eaten. No vaccines are available for HEV.[11] Once infection occurs, therapy is limited to support.[6,11] Patients should receive adequate hydration and electrolyte repletion. Hospitalization may be necessary for those unable to maintain an adequate oral intake.[11]

Nutrition Therapy

Treatment for all types of hepatitis is similar. Because there are no medications to treat hepatitis, bed rest and proper nutrition are the major constituents of therapy. During periods of nausea and vomiting, hydration via IV fluids may be necessary.

Oral feedings should be initiated as soon as possible, with frequent feedings high in kcal and in high-quality protein (see Chapter 14), to promote adequate intake and minimize loss of muscle mass. Adequate protein, 1.0-1.2 g/kg body weight, is recommended for most persons. Dietary fats should not be limited unless they are not well tolerated (e.g., steatorrhea). Fat plays an important role in providing concentrated kcal and making food taste better, which is important when trying to get a lot of kcal into a patient who probably doesn't have an appetite. Fluid intake should be adequate to accommodate the high protein intake unless otherwise contraindicated. Supplementation with a multivitamin that includes vitamin B complex (especially thiamine and vitamin B_{12} because of decreased absorption and hepatic uptake of these vitamins), vitamin K (to normalize bleeding tendency), vitamin C, and zinc for poor appetite is recommended.[12] Abstinence from alcohol is imperative.

Cirrhosis

Cirrhosis is a chronic degenerative disease in which liver cells are replaced by the buildup of fibrous connective tissue and fat infiltration (fatty infiltration; Figure 18-2). This damage can be the result of a variety of reasons, including the following:

- Alcoholic cirrhosis (see the *Health Debate* box, Alcohol: Proscribe or Prescribe?)
- Hepatitis (postnecrotic cirrhosis)
- Biliary cirrhosis disorders
- Chronic autoimmune disease
- Metabolic disorders (Wilson's disease or hemochromatosis)
- Chronic hepatotoxic drug use

Such conditions may cause liver cells to die, and the formation of new cells results in scarring that can cause congestion of hepatic circulation (blood backing up in the portal vein), which results in further decline of liver function, portal hypertension, and esophageal varices.

Esophageal varices are usually the result of collateral circulation that develops around the esophagus when normal blood flow through the liver is blocked (Figure 18-3). Blood vessels tend to enlarge and bulge into the lumen of the esophagus, where they may rupture. This bleeding tends to recur and can eventually be fatal. Patients with esophageal varices should eat soft, low-fiber foods. Another complication of cirrhosis, ascites, is the accumulation of fluid in the peritoneal cavity. Body fluid is trapped in a third space from which it cannot escape.[2] This causes the characteristic swollen or distended abdomen often seen in patients with cirrhosis.

To treat patients with ascites, a dietary sodium restriction (2000 mg) is used, sometimes along with a fluid restriction.[10] If diuretics are used, attention should be given to whether the drug depletes or spares potassium. If a potassium-depleting diuretic is used, potassium levels should be monitored.

As liver disease continues to progress, blood is shunted from portal circulation to systemic circulation. This causes blood to bypass the liver and could result in hepatic encephalopathy, which if left untreated can lead to hepatic coma. Hepatic encephalopathy may be best described as a form of "cerebral intoxication" caused by intestinal contents that have not been metabolized by the liver.[3] This results in toxins (e.g., ammonia) not being eliminated from the body, and nutrient metabolism may be compromised. Patients with hepatic encephalopathy have been reported to experience changes in consciousness, changes in behavior, loss of concentration and memory, confusion, apathy, personality changes, and other psychiatric symptoms.[2,3] Neurologic changes include spasticity, muscle spasms, asterixis or flapping (involuntary jerky movements, especially of the hands), athetoid postures, and rigidity of the limbs with flexion withdrawal of the lower limbs.[13]

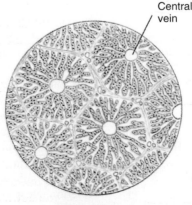 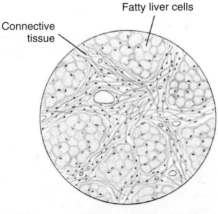

Central vein

Connective tissue

Fatty liver cells

Normal liver tissue structure

Cirrhotic liver tissue with scarring and fatty infiltration

FIG 18-2 Comparison of normal liver tissue structure with cirrhotic liver tissue changes. (Medical and Scientific Illustration. From Williams SR: *Nutrition and diet therapy*, ed 8, St. Louis, 1997, Mosby.)

❧ **HEALTH DEBATE**

Alcohol: Proscribe or Prescribe?

Alcohol is probably the most commonly used hepatotoxic drug. Next to caffeine, it is probably the most socially acceptable drug in the United States. It is legal, but sales are regulated by state-controlled establishments, and advertising on television is limited. The advertisements we see give us the message that if we would just drink a specific brand of beer or wine we would (1) be more athletic, (2) learn to "speak Australian," (3) become irresistible to a gorgeous man/woman, (4) hike through the Rocky Mountains, (5) fulfill a deep desire to become an English bulldog with an attitude, and/or (6) pretend we're jet-setters by drinking imported or microbrewed beer.

However, we get negative messages, too, and rightly so. Alcohol's link to birth defects and traffic accidents is well recognized. Heavy alcohol intake (three or more drinks* daily) causes damage to the liver (e.g., fatty liver and cirrhosis), brain, and heart and increases the risk of cancer. Could any possible good come from such a drug? The answer seems to be yes.

Current research indicates that alcohol may decrease the risk of heart disease. Several population studies have found a lower coronary artery disease mortality risk among moderate drinkers (defined as one or two drinks daily) as compared with nondrinkers. At first it looks as if red wine is the magic elixir, but white wine, beer, and hard liquor seem to be just as beneficial. On the other hand, it appears that the more one drinks, the greater the risk of developing certain cancers. Chronic, heavy drinking is associated with cancers of the mouth, throat, larynx, and liver. Moderate alcohol consumption has been linked to cancers of the breast, colon, and rectum.

So what's a person to do? Don't drink if you do not currently drink, are pregnant or trying to conceive, are taking medication, driving, or unable to control your drinking. The dangers outweigh any possible benefits. If you're concerned about heart disease and drink small quantities of alcohol every day or every other day, you're probably okay. Remember that alcohol is a drug. And like any drug, it is most effective when administered at the appropriate dosage. It may be beneficial to discuss this matter with your personal physician.

*One drink equals 12 oz beer, 5 oz wine, or 1½ oz hard liquor.
Data from Mukamal KJ, et al: Alcohol consumption and risk of coronary heart disease in older adults: The Cardiovascular Health Study, *J Am Geriatr Soc* 54(1):30-37, 2006.

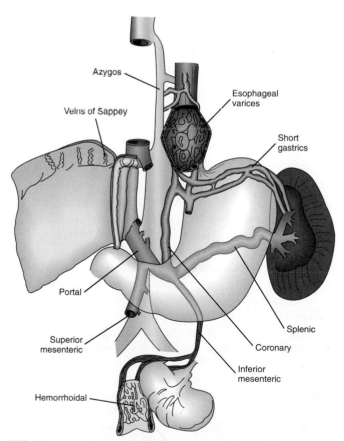

FIG 18-3 Varices related to portal hypertension. Portal vein, its major tributaries, and the most important shunts (collateral veins) between the portal and caval systems. (Redrawn from Kissane JM, editor: *Anderson's pathology*, ed 9, St. Louis, 1990, Mosby.)

Exact cause of encephalopathy has not been identified with certainty,[3] but it probably results from a combination of biochemical alterations that affect neurotransmission.[2] The most hazardous substances appear to be end products of protein metabolism, particularly ammonia.[2]

Several methods are used to lower ammonia levels, but each has potential side effects. Neomycin is an antibiotic used to sterilize the bowel by reducing the numbers of bacteria in the gastrointestinal (GI) tract, thus decreasing the amount of urea that can be converted to ammonia.[2] Plant proteins also produce less ammonia. Neomycin treatment allows more protein to be included in the diet for tissue regeneration, although protein can still be restricted. One disadvantage of neomycin use is that it contributes to malabsorption of most nutrients and can cause nausea, vomiting, diarrhea, and nephrotoxicity.[2] Another method is use of lactulose, a nonabsorbable disaccharide that is metabolized by intestinal bacteria, resulting in a lower pH stool.[3] The lowered pH traps ammonia in the colon; the ammonia is then excreted. It has a laxative action and diarrhea is common.

Nutrition Therapy

The most important aspect of nutrition therapy to keep in mind is that each patient has individual nutritional needs that must be addressed. Protein and energy malnutrition is commonplace in patients with end-stage liver disease who have cirrhosis. A minimum of 0.8 g protein per kg body weight per day is essential. To promote positive nitrogen balance and avert breakdown of endogenous protein stores, 1.2 g protein per kg dry or appropriate body weight is recommended. Protein restriction should be avoided, because it could possibly worsen malnutrition. If a patient appears to be protein sensitive (e.g., increased occurrence of encephalopathy), branched-chain amino acid–based formulas with restricted aromatic amino acids can be used to ensure a sustained level of protein intake. A protein restriction of less than 0.5 g per kg body weight per day may result in endogenous protein breakdown and further nutritional decline.[14]

Energy (basal metabolic rate [BMR] + 20% based on dry weight) intake should be high enough to prevent protein (muscle) catabolism and spare dietary protein that might otherwise be used for anabolism. Adjustments must be made for catabolic stress factors such as infection, trauma, surgery, or loss of nutrients (steatorrhea).[14]

Sodium may need to be restricted to 2000 mg per day if edema or ascites are present.[14] Sometimes it is necessary to restrict sodium to as little as 1000 mg per day for patients whose edema and ascites are resistant to diuretic therapy. Diets this low in sodium are restrictive, unpalatable, difficult to comply with, and possibly deficient in calcium.

Fluids are given in relation to input/output records, daily weights, and electrolyte values.[14] Fluid restrictions are often necessary to prevent or decrease ascites formation.[7] Fluid restrictions usually begin at 1500 mL/day and may decrease to 1000 to 1200 mL/day, depending on the patient's response. The nurse may provide suggestions on how to cope with thirst in an effort to improve compliance with these kinds of fluid restrictions. Sample suggestions are listed in the *Teaching Tool* box, Suggestions for Coping with Fluid Restriction.

Vitamin deficiencies in patients with cirrhosis are common, and often nutrition intake was poor before the onset of liver disorders. If clinical evaluation reveals the presence of deficiencies, water-soluble supplements with emphasis on folate, vitamin B_{12}, and thiamine may be necessary.

Liver Transplantation

Liver transplantation is regarded as an appropriate treatment for end-stage liver disease. Nutritional goals for those awaiting organ transplantation depend on the individual's weight history and current status.[15] Most patients in this condition show some indications of compromised nutritional status and therefore require special attention to nutritional needs.[15] It is often difficult to assess nutritional status in patients with liver disorders because many assessment parameters (e.g., body weight, nitrogen balance studies, total lymphocyte count, serum protein levels) are affected by edema, ascites, and hepatic necrosis seen in end-stage liver failure.[15] Therefore it may be more appropriate to use subjective parameters such as weight changes, appetite, satiety level, taste changes, diet history, and GI symptoms.[15] Weight change, however, is more often a reflection of fluid shifts rather than true weight loss. Physical examination findings such as temporal wasting of muscle and wasting of the upper extremities can be helpful to estimate the degree of malnutrition.

Nutrition Therapy

Each phase of the transplantation procedure dictates specific nutritional requirements (Table 18-2). The primary objective

TEACHING TOOL

Suggestions for Coping with Fluid Restriction

The following simple yet effective suggestions may help patients cope with fluid restrictions while maintaining personal comfort:

1. Drink to quench thirst only. Avoiding high-sodium foods will result in less thirst.
2. Try to avoid drinking from habit or to be sociable.
3. Eat ice-cold fruit between meals.
4. Sliced lemon wedges can stimulate saliva and moisten a dry mouth.
5. Keep the mouth clean by brushing teeth frequently and rinsing mouth with water (do not swallow rinse water).
6. Chew gum, suck hard candy (tart or sour is best), or use mints to stimulate saliva flow.
7. Try sucking on ice; most people find it more satisfying than the same amount of water because it stays in the mouth longer.
8. Limit fluids at mealtime; when appropriate, take medications with mealtime liquids or soft foods like applesauce.
9. Take all medications at one time to decrease amount of total fluid needed.
10. Add lemon juice to ice cubes to suck on; you will use fewer because the tartness of the lemon will make your mouth water. Use about half a lemon per tray of water. Or freeze lemonade into small, individualized popsicles in an ice cube tray.
11. Take a small amount of fluid at one time.
12. If allowable, use high-fat foods to help decrease the desire for fluid with a meal. (Gravies and margarine will moisten foods and make them easier to swallow.)

Modified from Dunning S: *Ideas to control fluid* (Bio-Medical Applications of Carbondale, Dialysis Services Division), Carbondale, Ill, 1995, Fresenius Medical Care.

in pretransplantation nutrition therapy is to provide enough kcal and protein to decrease protein catabolism and correct any nutritional deficiencies. The 4 to 8 weeks following surgery—the immediate posttransplantation period—require individualization of nutrition therapy according to the patient's needs.[16] Ascites, edema, or excess fluid make using the patient's actual weight unreliable for determining kcal and protein needs. Ideal (desirable) weight is a better reference point. Adequate kcal and protein are necessary for the hypercatabolic (but not necessarily hypermetabolic) stresses that result from surgery and high doses of glucocorticoids.[16] TPN may be necessary if nutritional needs cannot be met enterally (feeding by mouth and/or with nasoenteric feeding).[16] When oral intake is initiated, early satiety and altered tastes may prevent adequate intake. In such cases, between-meal feedings or supplements should be used to meet kcal and protein goals. Fluid losses from drains, nasogastric tubes, stool output, and urine should be considered when determining postoperative fluid needs.

For the long-term posttransplantation patient, a healthy, well-balanced diet is the nutrition goal. Because of common

TABLE 18-2	NUTRITION CARE GUIDELINES FOR LIVER TRANSPLANTATION	
	SHORT-TERM POSTTRANSPLANTATION	**LONG-TERM MANAGEMENT**
Energy	1.2-1.5 × BEE (use higher range if patient is severely underweight)	1.2-1.3 × BEE or as adequate to maintain weight
Protein	1.5-2 g/kg/day	0.8-1 g/kg
Carbohydrate		20-30 g dietary fiber/day
Fat		25%-35% kcal
		<10% kcal from saturated fats
		<300 mg cholesterol/day
Vitamins	History of alcoholism could suggest deficiencies in A, B_6, B_{12}, niacin, thiamine, folate	RDA amounts
	History of cholestatic liver disease could suggest preexisting deficiencies of fat-soluble vitamins and B_{12}	Consider supplementation/restriction based on pretransplantation condition and diagnosis or posttransplantation complications
Minerals	Provide RDA in consideration of medical history	RDA
Electrolytes		Sodium <4 g/day
		Monitor potassium, phosphorus, magnesium
		Supplement/restrict as needed
Fluids	30-35 mL/kg, adjusting for increased losses or decreased needs	30-35 mL/kg; requirements higher in hot climates or with fever
Common Complications Long-Term Posttransplantation		
Excessive weight gain	Reduce kcal intake; aerobic exercise 3-5 times/week; reduce corticosteroid dose as able	
Hyperlipidemia	Recommendations as above; change corticosteroid to tacrolimus; lipid-lowering medication with caution	
Diabetes mellitus	Diet and insulin or oral hypoglycemic agent to maintain glycemic control (fasting glucose <125 mg/dL, hemoglobin A_{1C} <7%); blood glucose self-monitoring; aerobic exercise 3-5 times/week; reduce corticosteroid doses as able	
Osteoporosis	1000-1500 mg calcium/day; vitamin D supplements; weight-bearing exercise; discontinue smoking; moderate sodium and protein intake; hormone replacement therapy when appropriate	

BEE, Basal energy expenditure; *RDA,* Recommended Dietary Allowance.
Data from Hasse JM: Adult liver transplantation. In Hasse JM, Blue LS, editors: *Comprehensive guide to transplant nutrition,* Chicago, 2002, American Dietetic Association.

posttransplantation complications (e.g., excessive weight gain, hypertension, hyperlipidemia, diabetes), adjustments in kcal, fat, and concentrated carbohydrates may be necessary.[16]

GALLBLADDER DISORDERS

The gallbladder lies directly beneath the right lobe of the liver, and, along with the hepatic, cystic, and common bile ducts, composes the biliary system (Figure 18-4). Bile is transported from the liver to the gallbladder via the common hepatic duct system where it is concentrated and stored until being released into the duodenum to expedite absorption of fats, fat-soluble vitamins, and certain minerals and to activate release of pancreatic enzymes. The most common disorders of the gallbladder include cholelithiasis, choledocholithiasis, and cholecystitis.

One of the main constituents of bile is cholesterol, which is also a major constituent of gallstones. The amount of cholesterol in bile is determined in part by the amount of dietary fat consumed. As might be expected, chronic intake of high-fat foods increases risk of developing cholelithiasis

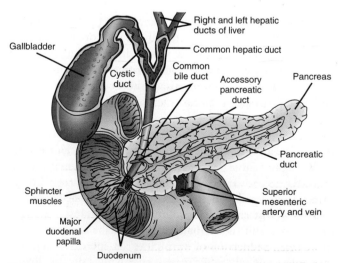

FIG 18-4 Gallbladder and bile ducts. Obstruction of either the hepatic or the common bile duct by stone or spasm prevents bile from being ejected into the duodenum. (From Rolin Graphics.)

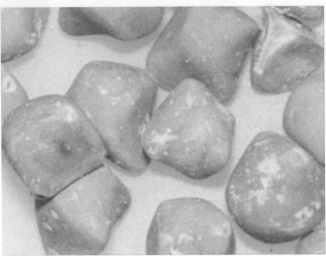

FIG 18-5 Gallstones. (From Stevens A, Lowe J: *Pathology*, London, 1995, Mosby.)

BOX 18-3	SUGGESTED RISK FACTORS IN GALLBLADDER DISEASE

Advanced age
Gender (female)
Obesity with high-fat intake
Hormonal imbalance (estrogen, progestin, insulin)
Certain drugs (oral contraceptives, clofibrate, cholestyramine)
Enzyme defects
Very low-calorie diets (VLCDs, medically supervised, used for weight loss)

Data from Escott-Stump S: *Nutrition and diagnosis-related care*, ed 6, Baltimore, 2007, Lippincott Williams & Wilkins.

(Figure 18-5). Gallstones are commonly found in women who are multiparous, on estrogen therapy, or use oral contraceptives; obese individuals; those with sedentary lifestyles; those who have experienced rapid weight loss; and the aged.[17] Other predisposing conditions to the development of gallstones are diabetes mellitus, regional enteritis, and familial tendencies[3] (Box 18-3).

An interesting phenomenon is that people who lose a great deal of weight rapidly (e.g., through very low-calorie diets [VLCDs] and some commercial weight loss programs) are at a greater risk for developing gallstones than those who are obese. In fact, gallstones are one of the most medically significant complications of voluntary weight loss.[18] Dieting may cause a shift in the balance of bile salts and cholesterol in the gallbladder. Cholesterol level is increased and the amount of bile salts is decreased. Following a diet too low in fat or going for long periods without eating (e.g., skipping breakfast), a common practice among dieters, may also decrease gallbladder contractions. If the gallbladder does not contract often enough to empty out the bile, gallstones may form.[18] People considering losing a significant amount of weight should see a physician to evaluate their medical history, individual circumstances, and the proposed method of weight loss.

If cholelithiasis is asymptomatic, no specific therapy is necessary. Symptoms usually manifest after eating, especially a high-fat meal, and include a mild, aching pain in the midepigastrium that may increase in intensity during a colic attack. The pain may radiate to the right upper quadrant and right subscapular region. Nausea, vomiting, tachycardia, and diaphoresis also may be present.[19]

Cholecystitis occurs when gallstones block the cystic duct or as the result of stasis, bacterial infection, or ischemia of the gallbladder. This inflammation is associated with pain, tenderness, and fever. Fat intolerance may manifest as regurgitation, flatulence, belching, epigastric heaviness, indigestion, heartburn, chronic upper abdominal pain, and nausea. Jaundice and steatorrhea may also be present.[2] Recommended therapy for symptomatic cholelithiasis and cholecystitis is surgical removal of the gallbladder (cholecystectomy).

Nutrition Therapy

Because cholelithiasis and cholecystitis usually produce rather painful symptoms, the main objective of nutritional care is to decrease the patient's discomfort. Most patients become acutely aware of foods that cause discomfort and thus avoid these foods. Low-fat diets are traditionally used to treat cholecystitis. During an acute attack, the hospitalized patient may receive IV fluids with nothing orally. Avoiding fatty foods is often advised, but no good evidence supports this recommendation.[20]

Chronic cholecystitis with inflammation is usually treated with a fat-restricted diet. Individual food intolerances vary widely, but many complain of foods that cause flatulence and bloating.

Following cholecystectomy, bile enters the small intestine continually rather than in response to food in the GI tract. Immediately after an open laparotomy cholecystectomy, patients may receive nothing orally or clear liquids until they can tolerate a regular diet. Some patients need to follow a low-fat diet for several weeks after surgery. Total amount of fat in the diet is more important than the type of fat consumed. Following a laparoscopic cholecystectomy, patients may be on a regular diet immediately after surgery.

PANCREATITIS

In addition to hormonal functions, the pancreas secretes enzymes necessary for protein, carbohydrate, and fat digestion. The pancreas also secretes sodium bicarbonate to neutralize acidic gastric contents as they enter the duodenum, which provides the optimal pH for the activation of these enzymes.

Pancreatitis is an inflammatory process characterized by decreased production of digestive enzymes and bicarbonate and malabsorption of fats and proteins. This acute inflammation causes blood vessels that supply the pancreas to become exceptionally permeable and leak fluid and plasma proteins into spaces between pancreatic cells, causing localized edema and damage. Pancreatic enzymes are ordinarily secreted into the intestinal lumen, where they are activated. However, if the pancreas is damaged, the enzymes are retained and activated within the pancreas, resulting in autodigestion and severe pain.[2,3] When the enzymes amylase and lipase cannot be secreted into the intestine, they enter the bloodstream and levels can become high. In fact, elevated levels of serum amylase are an indication of pancreatitis. In addition to severe pain, patients with pancreatitis often experience nausea and vomiting.[3]

Acute pancreatitis is most commonly caused by excessive alcohol consumption and gallbladder disease. Chronic pancreatitis is usually associated with chronic alcohol consumption and is characterized by chronic pain and exocrine and endocrine insufficiency. Diabetes mellitus can occur as the result of chronic pancreatitis if beta cells are damaged, thus decreasing insulin production.[2]

Nutrition Therapy

The primary goal is to provide for the patient's nutritional needs while minimizing pancreatic secretions.[21,22] Traditionally, gut rest with IV fluids or parenteral nutrition has been standard practice.[22] However, clinical evidence indicates parenteral nutrition administered within 24 hours of admission worsens outcome[23] by increasing the inflammatory response and impairing the immune response.[22] Bowel rest leads to atrophy of intestinal mucosa and bacterial translocation.[22] In contrast, early introduction of enteral nutrition promotes fewer infections, shorter hospital stays, and overall decreased medical costs.[22,23]

Low-fat, elemental formulas are recommended because they tend to reduce pancreatic stimulation.[21] Feeding into the lower small bowel, in the jejunum distal to the ligament of Treitz, allows areas associated with pancreatic stimulation to be bypassed. Patients receiving enteral feedings should be closely monitored for increases in pancreatic enzymes, abdominal pain, or discomfort. Enteral feedings should be terminated if any of these symptoms occur.[21]

Use of parenteral support is recommended when enteral feedings exacerbate abdominal pain. Peripheral parenteral nutrition can be used for nonstressed patients who are expected to receive nothing by mouth for less than 10 days. Central parenteral nutrition may be necessary if the patient will receive nothing by mouth for longer than 5 to 7 days.[21]

Whatever feeding route is chosen, the patient must receive adequate energy and nutrients based on the severity of the pancreatitis. Restricting fat to less than 50 g/day typically prevents symptoms of steatorrhea. A medium-chain triglyceride product such as MCT oil may be used to increase kcal if needed. The rest of the kcal should come from protein (at least 1.5 g protein/day) and carbohydrates. Because patients are usually anorectic, providing meals in six feedings daily may facilitate adequate nutritional intake. In some cases, replacement pancreatic enzymes are taken orally with meals to control maldigestion and malabsorption. Complete abstinence from alcohol is essential but often difficult to achieve.

CYSTIC FIBROSIS

Cystic fibrosis (CF) is an autosomal recessive inherited disease of the mucus-producing exocrine glands that is characterized by high levels of sodium and chloride in saliva and tears; high levels of electrolytes in sweat; and highly viscous secretions in the pancreas, bronchi, bile ducts, and small intestine that may be obstructive.[2] CF occurs in about 1 of every 3300 live births of white infants and 1 in every 15,300 nonwhite births.[24] Mean age of survival in the United States is 37 years.[24] Physical signs such as growth retardation, failure to gain weight, abdominal protuberance, lack of subcutaneous fat, and poor muscle tone are common findings. Frequent pulmonary infections, pancreatic insufficiency, and GI malabsorption put individuals with CF at great nutritional risk.[25] Death most often results from malnutrition, bronchopneumonia, lung collapse, and cor pulmonale.[13] The *Personal Perspectives* box, Ways of Coping, summarizes one young man's experience dealing with CF.

Nutrition Therapy

Nutrition is of prime importance in the treatment of CF.[26] Nutritional requirements vary depending on the age of the patient and severity of disease.[26] Poor nutritional status because of undernutrition contributes to poor growth, pulmonary complications, and susceptibility to infection. The primary goal of nutritional therapy for patients with CF is to exceed the Dietary Reference Intakes (DRI) for kcal and all other nutrients by 1.2 to 2 times.[26] Dietitians estimate individual energy requirements based on basal metabolic rate, activity level, lung function, and fat absorption. Improvements in pancreatic enzyme replacement therapy now allow higher amounts of dietary fats, which were previously prohibited.[26] Because fat provides such a concentrated source of energy, it does not need to be restricted below 30% to 40% of total kcal, and pancreatic enzyme replacement therapy can be individualized according to the patient's intake.[26] Although the sodium requirement may be considerably higher for patients with CF, routine sodium supplementation appears unnecessary because the average American diet contains an overabundance of sodium. Multivitamin supplements should be prescribed for all patients with CF.[26] Additional fat-soluble vitamins may be prescribed as well in a water-miscible form if fat malabsorption is severe.

Infants

Pancreatic enzyme replacement therapy should be used along with all types of milk products, including breast milk.[27] Supplemental fat or carbohydrate may be necessary for some infants to increase kcal density to more than 20 kcal/ounce. Introduction of beikost is not different for infants with CF.[27]

Children and Adolescents

Nutritional adequacy of the diet, compliance with pancreatic enzymes, and growth patterns should be closely monitored because as the child becomes older and more independent, compliance may become questionable.

PERSONAL PERSPECTIVES

Ways of Coping

There are many websites for specific disorders. These sites often reveal another perspective of dealing with illness—the perspective of the patient. By exploring websites, we can read about the experiences of patients and their families and sometimes even enter chat rooms. Following is an Internet essay written in 1995 for a college English course by Jeffrey Mason, a young man with cystic fibrosis. Jeffrey, who was 23 years old, died in 1997 shortly after receiving a double lung transplant, but his words and love of humor live on.

Sick Humor as a Method of Coping

As one who lives daily with the reality of chronic illness, I have found that seemingly "sick" humor may serve as a means of coping with the spectre of death which looms in my own life. Many professionals also agree that "sick" humor is a natural mechanism in helping people cope with tragedy.

Although many people find it offensive and distasteful, "sick" humor is often an essential part of the coping mechanism when one is faced with situations beyond one's control.

During the winter of 1994, I was very ill, and many of the doctors wondered if I would pull through or not. Several months before, in the fall of 1993, I had had to have what is known as a gastrostomy tube, or G-tube, placed in my stomach. This tube went from the outside of my body, through my abdomen wall and into my stomach. Its purpose was to provide extra nutrition by infusing a formula of high calorie liquid nutrition through the tube at night as I slept.

This was still fairly new to me in February, and I was having a hard time adjusting to it. I was hospitalized and my parents and friends came to visit me, we decided to come up with a "Top 10" style list of the Top 10 Reasons Why Having Cystic Fibrosis Is Great. We proceeded to come up with more than ten reasons, one of the best being the ability to throw up (through the G-Tube) without opening my mouth! This, indeed, would be considered vulgar or "sick" by many, but for me, it was a real way of helping me deal with the new appendage that was protruding from my stomach.

Another personal example of "sick" humor as a coping mechanism involves the life expectancy of a patient in my condition. Having a relatively "severe" case of the disease, it is known that without a lung transplant in the near future, this disease will progressively choke the life out of me. To cope with such a reality of death, my family and I participate in what we refer to as Dead Jeff Jokes. These basically take the form of "Jeff, when you die, can I have your . . . ?" where various possessions of mine such as my cassette and compact disc collection or my car are inserted at the end of the sentence. Although this sounds downright mean and nasty, it is, for us, a legitimate way for our family to cope with the gravity of my illness. We have often said, "If you can't laugh at it, what can you do?"

One final personal example of the use of "sick" humor to cope with fears involves a friend of mine named Dottie. Dottie and I were at a meeting of Cystic Fibrosis patients at the home of another friend and patient. During the meeting, we watched a brief segment of the local news in which several Cystic Fibrosis patients, including Dottie, were interviewed. At one point in the segment, the reporter stated, "The average life expectancy of a patient with Cystic Fibrosis is twenty-nine. Dottie is twenty-six." Immediately following this statement, another patient, a good friend of Dottie's, shouted, "Bye, Dottie!" as if to say that the reporter had just stated that she had but three years left to live. The room burst with laughter, and we still joke about it today. By joking about the reality of the death, which surrounds us, we are able to better cope with it and feel we have some semblance of control over it.

Although many people find it outrageous and offensive, "sick" humor offers a very effective and legitimate means of coping with situations that are beyond one's control. Anthropologists, psychologists, and psychiatrists have come to recognize this as a natural means of dealing with tragic and uncontrollable events. In my own life, the "sick" humor which abounds has been an essential element by which I am able to continue to fight the disease which surely seeks to destroy me.

From Mason J: *Sick humor as a method of coping,* July 6, 1998, with permission from Leon C. and Diana M. Mason.

Reevaluation of the patient's diet is important to ascertain whether recommendations are adequate to support growth and maintain nutritional status. As changes occur in the disease process and growth continues, nutritional needs will also change. Weight gain, linear growth, and level of pancreatic enzyme replacement therapy also should be closely monitored and assessed during this time.

SUMMARY

The liver, gallbladder, and pancreas are important ancillary digestive organs. Disorders of the liver include hepatitis, an inflammation of the liver, and cirrhosis, a chronic degenerative disease that causes fibrous connective tissue and fat infiltration of the liver. Nutrition therapy includes bed rest and proper nutrition for hepatitis and individual nutrition plans for cirrhosis that often restricts protein to ease liver function. Meeting nutrition therapy needs while still providing for adequate energy and RDA nutrient levels is challenging. Liver transplantations occur as treatment for end-stage liver disease. Nutrition therapy involves a variety of dietary plans specific to each phase of the procedure.

Gallbladder disorders include cholelithiasis, choledocholithiasis, and cholecystitis; these disorders are characterized by the formation of gallstones within the gallbladder. Nutrition therapy may require low-fat diets, but not all individuals may respond. Chronic cholecystitis with inflammation is usually treated with fat- and kcal-controlled diets until surgery. Moderation of fat is often indicated postoperatively.

Pancreatitis affects production of digestive secretions, resulting in malabsorption of dietary fats and protein. In serious cases, medical nutritional therapy tends to require enteral or parenteral nutrition. Regardless of the feeding route, fat intake is restricted.

Cystic fibrosis is an inherited disease of the mucus-producing exocrine glands. Nutrition therapy is of prime importance, with the goal to exceed the RDA for kcal and all other nutrients, necessitating the use of vitamin supplementation.

THE NURSING APPROACH

Case Study: Cirrhosis of the Liver

Eric, aged 50 years, developed cirrhosis subsequent to chronic hepatitis. As the liver damage progressed, he had frequent hospitalizations. At this admission he is being treated with diuretics because of ascites (fluid in the peritoneal cavity) and peripheral edema. He is receiving lactulose to reduce levels of ammonia because of hepatic encephalopathy. The doctor has prescribed a 2000-kcal, 40-g protein, 1-g sodium diet with fluids restricted to 1200 mL per day.

ASSESSMENT
Subjective (from patient statements)

- "I don't have any appetite. You wouldn't either if you were feeling sick to your stomach and throwing up."
- "I'm thirsty."
- "Just leave me alone. Where am I anyway?"
- "Is it nighttime? I can't remember what I was doing."
- Usual weight 205 pounds when he doesn't have ascites

Objective (from physical examination)

- Present weight 210 pounds
- Dark amber urine, jaundice of skin and sclera
- Abdominal distention, ascites
- Peripheral edema in ankles and lower legs
- Muscle wasting of upper extremities and thighs
- Enlargement of the liver seen on radiograph
- Lab results: Normal blood urea nitrogen, normal hematocrit, low albumin, and elevated liver enzymes
- Disoriented to date, time, and place

DIAGNOSES (NURSING)

1. Imbalanced nutrition: less than body requirements related to anorexia and nausea and vomiting as evidenced by muscle wasting and loss of true body weight
2. Excess fluid volume related to intrahepatic pressure and decreased colloidal osmotic pressure as evidenced by ascites and peripheral edema
3. Acute confusion related to toxicities in the brain as evidenced by agitation; disorientation to date, time, and place; and short-term memory loss

PLANNING
Patient Outcomes

Short term (at the end of one week):
- Eating meals well
- Decrease of jaundice, nausea, and vomiting
- Loss of 1500 mL of body fluids, as evidenced by weight 207 pounds (loss of 3 pounds), output greater than intake on records, decreased abdominal girth and ankle edema
- Slight decrease of liver enzymes, and electrolytes within normal ranges

- No further muscle wasting of extremities
- Oriented to date, time, and place, and calmer

Nursing Interventions

1. Provide 2000-kcal diet with protein, sodium, and water restrictions as ordered.
2. Facilitate loss of excess fluid.
3. Orient Eric frequently.

IMPLEMENTATION

1. Asked the dietitian to assess Eric's nutritional status and food preferences in order to optimally implement the diet of 2000 kcal, 40 g protein, 1 g sodium, with 1200 mL fluid restriction.
   With patient assessment, the dietitian can individualize complex diets.
2. Helped deliver small frequent meals with high kcal, high carbohydrates, moderate fats, and restricted proteins (following the plan of the dietitian).
   Patients with nausea and distended abdomens usually tolerate small, frequent meals better than large meals. High kcal are needed for healing and prevention of catabolism of body proteins. Fat contains high kcal and fat-soluble vitamins but may not be metabolized well, causing steatorrhea (fat in the stools). Protein is needed for healing, but excess could increase ammonia production and make encephalopathy worse.
3. Removed noxious odors and unpleasant objects from the room before meals and gave antiemetic medication as ordered.
   Unpleasant smells and sights can trigger nausea, thus leading to anorexia. Antiemetics are given to prevent vomiting.
4. Restricted sodium to 1 g and planned with Eric how to restrict fluids to 1200 mL per day (300 mL with meals and 300 mL total between meals). Posted the plan on the bulletin board by Eric's bed and taught him, his family, and nursing staff the reasons for the fluid restriction.
   Sodium is limited in order to decrease fluid retention. Fluid restriction is necessary to decrease portal hypertension, ascites, and peripheral edema. Involving the patient in planning encourages commitment and a sense of control. Dietary restrictions are easier to follow when purposes are understood. Written communication of the plan helps coordinate efforts.
5. Gave Eric ice, hard candy, and lemon wedges to reduce thirst.
   Thirst is minimized by spacing out fluid intake and providing treats that can dissolve slowly in the mouth.
6. Allowed no alcohol intake.

Continued

THE NURSING APPROACH—cont'd

Case Study: Cirrhosis of the Liver—cont'd

Alcohol would further damage the liver and add to the patient's confusion.

7. Oriented Eric frequently to date, time, and place and gave him simple instructions and reminders. Wrote the date and name of the nurse on the white board by the patient's bed and clock.

Confused patients become less agitated when told where they are, even if they forget quickly what the nurse just told them.

8. Asked dietary staff for herbs and spices that could be put on Eric's low-sodium food for flavoring.

Low-sodium foods are bland without additional flavoring.

9. Provided supplemental vitamins and liquids (such as Ensure or Ensure Plus).

Nutrient-dense supplements increase nourishment and kcal. Drinking liquid nourishment requires less energy than chewing foods.

10. Gave diuretic medicines as ordered.

Diuretics cause increased urine output, thus reducing body fluids, ascites, and peripheral edema.

11. Gave lactulose as ordered.

Ammonia is produced when intestinal bacteria metabolize protein. Ammonia going to the brain (because the liver cannot detoxify it) contributes to hepatic encephalopathy. Lactulose is a synthetic nonabsorbable disaccharide that is given to reduce ammonia in the intestines. Lactulose is metabolized in the intestines, releasing organic acids and lowering the pH; this enables trapping of ammonia in the stool, where it can be excreted. Lactulose also causes diarrhea, limiting time for intestinal bacteria to produce ammonia.

12. Carefully measured and recorded intake and output each shift; measured and recorded patient weights and abdominal girth daily.

Ongoing assessment of fluid balance helps evaluate effectiveness of treatment.

13. Monitored lab reports for changes.

Diarrhea from lactulose may lead to loss of fluids and electrolytes. Some diuretics cause loss of potassium.

EVALUATION

At the end of one week:

- Eating meals well
- No change in muscle wasting of extremities
- Jaundice, nausea, and vomiting decreased
- Liver enzymes slightly decreased and electrolytes within normal ranges
- Quickly forgot about his water restriction even with frequent reminders
- Exceeded water intake (about 1400 mL rather than 1200 mL per day)
- Body fluids decreased by 1000 mL, as evidenced by weight of 208 pounds (loss of 2 pounds), output greater than intake on records, decreased abdominal girth and ankle edema
- Oriented to place but not date and time
- Goals partially met

DISCUSSION QUESTIONS

During a follow-up appointment with the physician, the nurse asked Eric how he was doing with his diet. His response was "Not very well. I really don't know what foods I am supposed to eat."

1. What other questions should the nurse ask? What nursing diagnosis will the nurse probably identify?
2. Should the nurse suggest to the doctor that he refer Eric to a dietitian? Why?

Nursing Diagnoses-Definitions and Classification 2009-2011. Copyright © 2009, 1994-2009 by NANDA International. Used by arrangement with Blackwell Publishing Limited, a company of John Wiley & Sons, Inc.

CRITICAL THINKING

Clinical Applications

Chronic alcohol abuse is usually the cause of chronic liver disease (cirrhosis and hepatic encephalopathy) and chronic pancreatitis. One way to evaluate the risk of alcohol-related liver disease is to assess the pattern, quantity, and duration of alcohol intake; usual dietary intake; and socioeconomic factors affecting eating habits. Data can be collected from the patient or reliable friend or family member and evaluated to determine amount (grams) and the kcal value of alcohol consumed. When consumed in large quantities, alcohol can provide the majority of the day's kcal intake.

To assess this information, we should review a few basics. Alcohol provides 7 kcal/g.* The average percent alcohol content (based on weight per volume) of various forms of alcoholic beverages is as follows:

Beer = 4% to 6%

Wine = 9% to 12%

Distilled alcohol (whiskey, rum, gin, or brandy) = 35% to 50%

The concentration of alcohol in distilled beverages (hard liquor) is usually referred to as *proof*. One proof equals 0.5% alcohol, which means that 80-proof tequila contains 40% alcohol. Hard liquor is routinely measured in a jigger or shot, which is 1½ ounces or 45 mL.

1. How many grams of alcohol and kcal would two shots of 80-proof tequila provide?
2. What is the best way to obtain information from an individual about his/her alcohol consumption?
3. You obtain the following information from the alcohol intake questionnaire and diet history: Alcohol is con-

*Any beverages used as mixers should be included in the estimated kcal intake.

sumed 7 days/week at home, work, and bars. A typical day's intake consists of a Bloody Mary (1 cup tomato juice, two shots 80-proof vodka) first thing in the morning, followed by 5 cups of black coffee (some at home, some at work). Three more shots of 80-proof vodka are consumed at work. Lunch is usually fast-food double cheeseburger, small fries, and a cup of black coffee. After work, four 12-ounce. bottles of beer (4% alcohol) and pretzels (about 30) are consumed at the local bar with friends. Dinner at home consists of a lunchmeat sandwich (usually two slices white bread, 2 ounces bologna, 1 teaspoon mustard), 10 potato chips, and two more 12-ounce beers. Total intake for the day is approximately 3200 kcal.

How many grams of alcohol are consumed? _____ grams alcohol

How many kcal are provided by the alcohol? _____ kcal from alcohol

What percent of the kcal are provided by alcohol? _____ % energy from alcohol

Alcohol Intake Assessment Tool

1. How many days a week do you drink alcoholic beverages?
   Circle number of days: 0 1 2 3 4 5 6 7
2. Where do you drink?
   Circle all that apply:
   a. At home
   b. At a friend's
   c. At a bar
   d. At work
   e. In the car
   f. Other (specify)
3. Which alcoholic beverages do you consume?
   Circle all that apply:
   a. Beer
   b. White, red, or rosé wine
   c. Sherry or port
   d. Gin
   e. Whiskey
   f. Vodka
   g. Rum
   h. Other (specify)
4. How do you determine how much you drink?
   Circle all that apply:
   a. Count the number of beer cans
   b. Count the number of wine glasses
   c. Count the number of shots poured
   d. Count the number of bottles of wine
   e. Count the number of bottles of liquor used a day or week
   f. I don't know exactly how much I drink
   g. Other method of deciding alcohol intake (specify)
5. On any drinking day, how many drinks do you have?
   Circle letter(s) indicating drinks consumed and number within each category consumed to indicate number of drinks per day:

a. Beer	1	2	3	4	5	>5
b. White, red, or rosé wine	1	2	3	4	5	>5
c. Sherry or port	1	2	3	4	5	>5
d. Gin	1	2	3	4	5	>5
e. Whiskey	1	2	3	4	5	>5
f. Vodka	1	2	3	4	5	>5
g. Rum	1	2	3	4	5	>5
h. Other (specify)	1	2	3	4	5	>5

6. For how long have you been drinking this quantity?
7. Do you drink this amount on a regular basis?

Professionals working with individuals who consume excessive amounts of alcohol advise that self-reported intakes may constitute about half of what is actually consumed. Therefore, double-checking any information obtained from a patient about alcohol intake with a reliable family member or friend is recommended.

Modified from Roe DA, Lasswell AB: Nutritional assessment and tools. In Lasswell AB, et al, editors: *Nutrition for family and primary care practitioners*, Philadelphia, 1986, F. Stickley.

WEBSITES OF INTEREST

Alcoholics Anonymous
www.alcoholics-anonymous.org
Dedicated to the self-help approach for overcoming alcoholism, including links for teenagers, newcomers, health professionals, and the AA Grapevine.

American Liver Foundation
www.liverfoundation.org
Devoted to research, education, and support groups related to hepatitis and all liver diseases.

National Institute on Alcohol Abuse and Alcoholism
www.niaaa.nih.gov
Provides leadership for the national effort to reduce alcohol-related problems through research, collaborative endeavors of agencies and organizations, and educational resources.

REFERENCES

1. Guyton AC, Hall JE: *Textbook of medical physiology*, ed 11, Philadelphia, 2005, Saunders.
2. McCance KL, Huether SE: *Pathophysiology: The biologic basis for disease in adults and children*, ed 6, St. Louis, 2009, Mosby.
3. Price SA, Wilson LM: *Pathophysiology: Clinical concepts of disease processes*, ed 6, St. Louis, 2002, Mosby.
4. Centers for Disease Control and Prevention: *Viral hepatitis*, Atlanta, (reviewed November 18, 2009), Author. Accessed March 11. 2010, from www.cdc.gov/hepatitis/index.htm.
5. Gilroy RK, Mukherjee S: *Hepatitis A*, New York, (updated December 22. 2009), eMedicine/WebMD. Accessed March 10, 2010, from http://emedicine.medscape.com/article/177484-overview.
6. Wolf DC: *Hepatitis, viral*, New York, (updated July 1, 2009), eMedicine/WebMD. Accessed March 10, 2010, from http://emedicine.medscape.com/article/185463-overview.
7. Mukherjee S, Dhawan VK: *Hepatitis C*, New York, (updated June 18, 2009), eMedicine/WebMD. Accessed March 10, 2010, from http://emedicine.medscape.com/article/177792-overview.
8. Pyrsopoulos NT, Reddy KR: *Hepatitis B*, New York, (updated June 19, 2009), eMedicine/WebMD. Accessed March 10, 2010, from http://emedicine.medscape.com/article/177632-overview.
9. Ismail MK, Riely C: *Alcoholic fatty liver*, New York, (updated September 15, 2008), eMedicine/WebMD. Accessed March 10, 2010, from http://emedicine.medscape.com/article/170409-overview.
10. Lacey SR: *Hepatitis D*, New York, (updated January 3, 2010), eMedicine/WebMD. Accessed March 10, 2010, from http://emedicine.medscape.com/article/178038-overview.
11. Schwartz JM, Ingram K, Flora KD: *Hepatitis E*, New York, (updated November 11, 2009), eMedicine/WebMD. Accessed March 10, 2010, from http://emedicine.medscape.com/article/178140-overview.
12. American Dietetic Association Nutrition Care Manual: *Hepatits: nutrition prescription*. Accessed March 10, 2010, from www.nutritioncaremanual.org.
13. Escott-Stump S: *Nutrition and diagnosis-related care*, ed 6, Baltimore, 2007, Lippincott Williams & Wilkins.
14. American Dietetic Association Nutrition Care Manual: *Cirrhosis: nutrition prescription*. Accessed March 12, 2010, from www.nutritioncaremanual.org.
15. Weseman RA, Mukherjee S: *Nutritional requirements of adults before transplantation*, New York, 1996-2006 (updated November 4, 2008), eMedicine/WebMD. Accessed March 12, 2010, from www.emedicine.com/med/topic3504.htm.
16. American Dietetic Association Nutrition Care Manual: *Organ transplant: liver*. Accessed March 12, 2010, from www.nutritioncaremanual.org.
17. Gladden D, et al: *Cholecystitis*, New York, (updated December 11, 2009), eMedicine/WebMD. Accessed March 12, 2010, from www.emedicine.com/med/topic346.htm.
18. Public Health Service, National Institutes of Health, and National Institute of Diabetes & Digestive & Kidney Diseases: *Dieting and gallstones*, NIH Pub No 02-3677, Washington, DC, 2008, National Institutes of Health.
19. Heuman DM, Mihas AA, Allen J: *Cholelithiasis*, New York, (updated August 25, 2009), eMedicine/WebMD. Accessed March 12, 2010, from www.emedicine.com/med/topic836.htm.
20. Hasse JM, Matarese LE: Medical nutrition therapy for liver, biliary system, and exocrine pancreas disorders. In Mahan LK, Escott-Stump S, editors: *Krause's food & nutrition therapy*, ed 12, Philadelphia, 2008, Saunders.
21. Moore MC: *Mosby's pocket guide to nutritional assessment and care*, ed 5, St. Louis, 2005, Mosby.
22. Aranda-Michel J, Mubarak A, Figueroa R: Gastrointestinal and liver diseases. In Heimburger DC, Ard JD, editors: *Handbook of clinical nutrition*, St. Louis, 2006, Mosby.
23. McClave SA, et al: Nutrition support in acute pancreatitis: A systematic review of the literature, *JPEN J Parenter Enteral Nutr* 30(2):143-156, 2006.
24. *The Merck manual: Cystic fibrosis [general]*, Section 19. Pediatrics. Cystic fibrosis, Whitehouse Station, N.J., Updated August 2008, Merck & Co, Inc. Retrieved March 12, 2010, from www.merck.com/mmpe/sec19/ch278/ch278a.html#.
25. American Dietetic Association Nutrition Care Manual: *Cystic fibrosis*. Accessed March 12, 2010, from www.nutritioncaremanual.org.
26. Newton LE, Morgan SL: Pulmonary disease. In Heimburger DC, Ard JD, editors: *Handbook of clinical nutrition*, St. Louis, 2006, Mosby.
27. Ramsey BS, Farrell PM, Pincharz P: Nutritional assessment and management in cystic fibrosis: A consensus report, *Am J Clin Nutr* 55:108-116, 1992.

Nutrition for Diabetes Mellitus

Diabetes mellitus is a group of conditions characterized by either a relative or complete lack of insulin secretion by the beta cells of the pancreas or by defects of cell insulin receptors, which result in disturbances of carbohydrate, protein, and lipid metabolism.

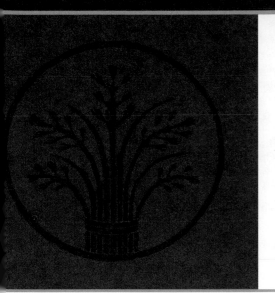

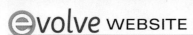

evolve WEBSITE

http://evolve.elsevier.com/Grodner/foundations/

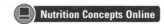

ROLE IN WELLNESS

The number of people diagnosed with diabetes is at epidemic proportions in the United States[1] (Figure 19-1), and it is estimated that more than 6.2 million people with the disease have not been diagnosed (Box 19-1).[2] As a chronic disorder, diabetes mellitus requires long-term lifestyle changes of both dietary intake and physical activity. Approaching this disorder in a proactive manner by maintaining blood glucose levels as near to normal as possible can lessen the negative impact of diabetes and achieve a higher level of wellness (see the *Personal Perspectives* box, A Tale of Diabetes).

A way to achieve a proactive approach is to consider diabetes through the five dimensions of health. Long-term serious physical health complications may be avoided if hyperglycemia is controlled through dietary and lifestyle modifications to maintain the *physical health* dimension. The ability of the individual to understand the condition; to be compliant on a regular basis regarding insulin injections, if required; and to follow dietary and exercise recommendations may depend on the *intellectual health* dimension. *Emotional health* may be tested. Not only must the individual deal with a chronic lifelong condition, but also changes in dietary intake may necessitate the loss of symbolic foods, which may be emotionally upsetting. Support, especially from family members and friends, is crucial. *Social health* may be pivotal in adjustment to this disorder. If one is already secure in social relationships, adaptations in social situations will be easier and more acceptable. People who eat special diets based on their religious or spiritual beliefs may need special adaptations of the diabetic diet to sustain their *spiritual health* dimension.

DIABETES MELLITUS

Diabetes mellitus is a group of conditions characterized by either a relative or complete lack of insulin secretion by the beta cells of the pancreas or by defects of cell insulin receptors, which results in disturbances of carbohydrate, protein, and lipid metabolism and hyperglycemia (Figure 19-2).[3] Diabetes is usually diagnosed and characterized by elevated fasting blood glucose (>126 mg/dL if found on at least two occasions) or hyperglycemia. The main goal of treatment is maintenance of insulin/glucose homeostasis.

In addition to everyday maintenance necessary to control blood glucose levels, diabetes mellitus is associated with disability and premature death because of the disease's effect on structural and functional alterations in many body systems, especially macrovascular and microvascular damage. Ranked as one of the most costly health problems in America,[4] diabetes mellitus is often called a "silent killer." Everyone with diabetes mellitus is vulnerable to long-term complications (Table 19-1) and premature death, which is associated with all types of diabetes. Manifestation of these complications may be preempted with control of hyperglycemia[2,5-7] (Table 19-2). Macrovascular complications increase the risk of coronary artery disease, peripheral vascular disease, and cerebrovascular accidents. Microvascular effects include nephropathy (kidney disorder) and retinopathy (eye disorder from blood vessel changes). As a result of nephropathy, approximately half of all individuals with type 1 diabetes mellitus develop chronic renal failure and chronic kidney disease (CKD). Retinopathy is the leading cause of blindness in North America. In addition, neuropathy complications affect peripheral circulation, causing decreased sensations in extremities that may result in injury without the patient's knowledge. Healing

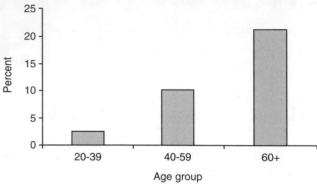

FIG 19-1 Estimated number of new cases of diagnosed diabetes in people aged 20 years or older, by age group, in the United States in 2005. National Health and Nutrition Examination Survey estimates from 1999 through 2002 were projected to the year 2005. (From National Center for Chronic Disease Prevention and Health Promotion, Centers for Disease Control and Prevention: *National estimates on diabetes,* Atlanta, 2007, Author. Accessed March 29, 2010, from www.cdc.gov/diabetes/pubs/estimates05.htm.)

is impaired because of the effects of diabetes on the circulatory system; gangrene may develop, and amputation may be necessary (Figure 19-3). Autonomic effects of diabetes may include orthostatic hypotension, persistent tachycardia, gastroparesis, neurogenic bladder (urinary bladder dysfunction from neurologic damage), impotence, and impaired visceral pain sensation that can obscure symptoms of angina pectoris or myocardial infarction.

Development of these long-term complications is believed to be correlated to the level and frequency of hyperglycemia experiences throughout the life span of a person who has diabetes. Results of the Diabetes Control and Complications Trial[8] indicate intensive therapy is more effective than conventional therapy in delaying and slowing progression of retinopathy by 75%, nephropathy by 50%, and neuropathy by 60% in patients with type 1 DM. Results of the United Kingdom's Prospective Diabetes Study[9] indicate better blood glucose control reduces risk of retinopathy by 25% and nephropathy by 30% and possibly reduces neuropathy in type 2 DM.

Glucose intolerance can be classified into two primary categories: type 1 diabetes mellitus (T1DM)* and type 2 diabetes mellitus (T2DM). Other types include latent autoimmune diabetes of adults (LADA), gestational diabetes mellitus (GDM), impaired glucose tolerance (IGT), and other forms of diabetes.[3,10,11] These classifications, based on etiology, treatment needs, and their symptoms, are summarized in

---

*According to the *Report of the Expert Committee on the Diagnosis and Classification of Diabetes Mellitus*, the terms *insulin-dependent diabetes mellitus* and *non-insulin-dependent diabetes mellitus* and their acronyms, *IDDM* and *NIDDM*, should no longer be used because they are confusing and have frequently resulted in classifying patients based on treatment rather than etiology.

BOX 19-1   INDIVIDUALS AT RISK FOR DIABETES MELLITUS

Generally, people with type 1 diabetes mellitus (T1DM) display acute symptoms and noticeably elevated blood glucose levels. However, type 2 diabetes mellitus (T2DM) is often not diagnosed until complications develop. Roughly one third of all people with T2DM may be undiagnosed. According to the American Diabetes Association, there is sufficient indirect evidence to justify opportunistic screening of individuals at high risk of developing DM. Criteria for testing asymptomatic, undiagnosed adults and children at risk for occurrence or development of T2DM follow:

Adults ≥45 years of age	All
Adults <45 years of age	Overweight (BMI ≥25 kg/m²)
	First-degree relative has diabetes
	Member of a high-risk population (e.g., African American, Hispanic American, Native American, Asian/Pacific Islander)
	Delivered an infant weighing >9 pounds or previously diagnosed with GDM
	Hypertensive (≥140/90 mm Hg)
	HDL cholesterol level ≤35 mg/dL and/or a triglyceride level ≥250 mg/dL
	On previous testing, had IGT
	Other clinical conditions associated with insulin resistance (e.g., PCOS or acanthosis nigricans)
Children (10 years of age or at onset of puberty, if puberty occurs at a younger age)	Overweight (≥85th percentile for age and gender, >85th percentile weight for height, or weight >120% of ideal for height)

Plus any two of the following:
- Family history of T2DM in first- or second-degree relative
- Race/ethnicity (e.g., African American, Hispanic American, Native American, Asian/Pacific Islander)
- Signs of insulin resistance or conditions associated with insulin resistance (acanthosis nigricans, hypertension, dyslipidemia, or PCOS)

BMI, Body mass index; *GDM,* gestational diabetes mellitus; *HDL,* high-density lipoprotein; *IGT,* impaired glucose tolerance; *PCOS,* polycystic ovarian syndrome.
Modified from American Diabetes Association: Standards of medical care for patients with diabetes mellitus, *Diabetes Care* 26(Suppl 1):S33-S50, 2003, with permission from the American Diabetes Association

Table 19-3. More than 90% of people with diabetes have T2DM, whereas 5% to 10% have T1DM.[2,3]

Type 1 Diabetes Mellitus

Onset of T1DM is usually sudden. Cells use glucose for energy, and without endogenous insulin, cells literally begin

Text continued on page 411.

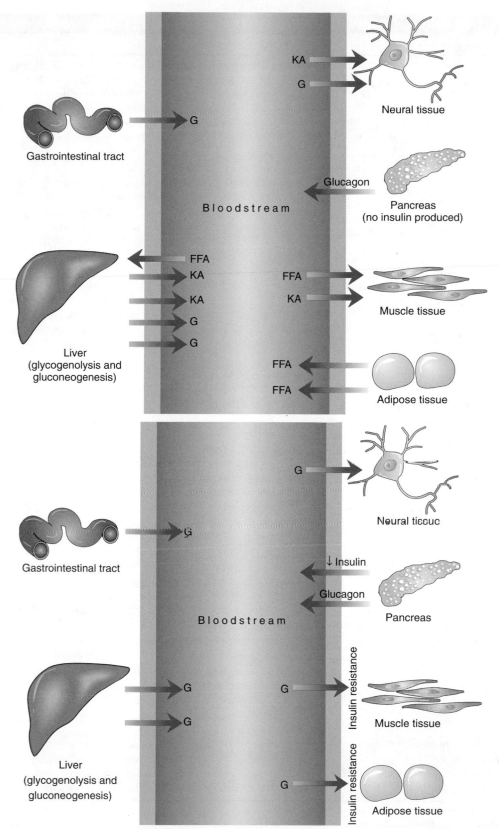

FIG 19-2 Energy metabolism in diabetes. A, Energy metabolism in type 1 diabetes mellitus, **B,** Energy metabolism in type 2 diabetes mellitus. (From Copstead-Kirkhorn L-E, Banasik J: *Pathophysiology,* ed 3, Philadelphia, 2005, Saunders.)

TABLE 19-1 CLINICAL COMPLICATIONS OF DIABETES MELLITUS

COMPLICATION	MANIFESTATION	INCIDENCE
Dental disease	Periodontitis	Those with diabetes are often at twice the risk of those without diabetes. Almost 30% of people with diabetes have severe periodontal disease with loss of attachment of gums to the teeth measuring 5 mm or more.
Pregnancy	Congenital malformations	Poorly controlled diabetes before conception and during the first trimester of pregnancy can cause major birth defects in 5%-10% of pregnancies and spontaneous abortions in 15%-20% of pregnancies. Poorly controlled diabetes during second and third trimesters of pregnancy can result in excessively large newborns.
Microvascular*	Retinopathy	Leading cause of blindness in adults between 20 and 74 years of age
	Nephropathy	More than 30% of people with type 1 diabetes mellitus (T1DM) will develop kidney disease, compared with perhaps 10% of those with T2DM. People with T1DM have 15 times the risk of end-stage renal disease as those with T2DM.
Macrovascular†	Coronary artery disease	Patients with DM are two to four times more likely to have heart disease; heart disease deaths are also two to four times higher than in adults without DM.
	Peripheral vascular disease	
	Cerebrovascular disease	Patients with DM are two to four times more likely to suffer stroke
Neuropathy	Peripheral	Approximately 60% to 70% of people with diabetes have mild to severe forms of nerve damage. Neuropathy is a major contributing factor in foot and leg amputations among people with diabetes. Risk of leg amputation is 15-40 times greater for a person with DM.
	Autonomic (postural hypotension, persistent tachycardia, neurogenic bladder, incontinence, gastroparesis, impotence)	Impotence occurs in approximately 13% of men who have T1DM and 8% of men with T2DM. Some reports indicate men older than 50 years have impotence rates as high as 50% to 60%.
Skin conditions	Atherosclerosis	As blood vessels narrow, the skin changes. It becomes hairless, thin, cool, and shiny. Toes become cold. Toenails thicken and discolor.
	Fungal infections (usually *Candida albicans*)	Common fungal infections are "jock itch," "athlete's foot," ringworm, and vaginal infection that cause itching.
	Bullosis diabeticorum (diabetic blisters)	Rare condition that can occur on backs of hands, fingers, toes, feet, and sometimes legs or forearms. They look like burn blisters, are painless, and have no redness. Often occur in people with neuropathy; only treatment is to bring blood glucose levels under control.
	Diabetic dermopathy	Light brown scaly skin patches often mistaken for age spots; occurs most often on the front of both legs. Patches do not hurt, open up, or itch.
	Necrobiosis lipoidica diabeticorum (NLD)	Rare condition. Similar to diabetic dermopathy; however, spots are fewer but larger and deeper. Often start as dull, red raised area. Sometimes itchy and painful; spots may crack open.
	Eruptive xanthomatosis	Firm, yellow, pealike enlargements in the skin. Occurs most often on backs of hands, feet, arms, legs, and buttocks. Usually occurs in young men with T1DM who have high levels of cholesterol and lipids in their blood. Usually disappear when glucose levels are controlled.
	Digital sclerosis	Tight, thick, waxy skin on backs of hands. Finger joints become stiff. Occurs in about 30% of those with T1DM. Only treatment is to control blood glucose levels.
	Disseminated granuloma annular	Sharply defined ring-shaped or arc-shaped raised areas on skin that can be red, red-brown, or skin colored. Occurs most often on distal parts of the body.
	Acanthosis nigricans	Tan or brown raised areas on sides of the neck, axilla, and groin. May sometimes occur on hands, elbows, and knees. Usually manifests in the obese.

*Compounds effects of macrovascular problems.
†Exacerbated by concurrent hypertension, hypercholesterolemia, smoking, and aging.
Data from Centers for Disease Control and Prevention: *National diabetes fact sheet: general information and national estimates on diabetes in the United States,* Atlanta, 2007, U.S. Department of Health and Human Services, Centers for Disease Control and Prevention, 2008. Accessed March 29, 2010, from www.cdc.gov/diabetes/pubs/pdf/ndfs_2007.pdf; American Diabetes Association: *Skin complications,* Alexandria, Va, Author. Accessed March 29, 2010, from www.diabetes.org/living-with-diabetes/complications/skin-complications.html; National Institute of Diabetes & Digestive & Kidney Disease: *National Diabetes Information Clearinghouse: Diabetes control and complications trial* (DCCT), NIH Pub No. 08-3874, Bethesda, Md, 2008 (May), National Institutes of Health. Accessed March 29, 2010, from http://diabetes.niddk.nih.gov/dm/pubs/control/; National Institute of Diabetes & Digestive & Kidney Diseases: *National diabetes statistics,* NIH Pub No 08-3892, Bethesda, Md, 2008 (June), National Institutes of Health. Accessed March 29, 2010, from http://diabetes.niddk.nih.gov/dm/pubs/statistics/index.htm.

TABLE 19-2 CRITERIA FOR DIAGNOSING DIABETES

DIABETES TYPE	FORMER TERM	ETIOLOGY	CRITERIA
Type 1 diabetes mellitus (T1DM)*: immune mediated or idiopathic	Insulin-dependent diabetes mellitus (IDDM), type I diabetes, juvenile-onset diabetes, ketosis-prone diabetes, brittle diabetes	Beta cell destruction, usually leading to absolute insulin deficiency *Immune-mediated diabetes*: results from cellular-mediated autoimmune destruction of beta cells of the pancreas; markers of immune destruction include islet cell autoantibodies (ICA), autoantibodies to insulin (IAA), autoantibodies to glutamic acid decarboxylase (GADA), insulinoma-associated-2 autoantibodies (IA-2A) *Idiopathic diabetes*: no known etiology, but there is no evidence of autoimmunity	Symptoms† of DM and casual plasma glucose ≥200 mg/dL (casual is defined as any time of day without regard to last meal) *OR* FPG ≥126 mg/dL (fasting is defined as no kcal intake for at least 8 hr) *OR* 2-hr PG ≥200 mg/dL during OGTT (performed as described by WHO using glucose load containing the equivalent of 75 g anhydrous glucose dissolved in water)
Type 2 diabetes mellitus (T2DM) (adults)	Non-insulin-dependent diabetes mellitus (NIDDM), type II diabetes, adult-onset diabetes, maturity-onset diabetes, ketosis-resistant diabetes, stable diabetes	Insulin resistance with insulin secretory defect	
Type 2 diabetes (children)	Maturity-onset of the young (MODY)	Insulin resistance resulting from genetic and familial factors, fetal environment factors, particularly maternal gestational diabetes and intrauterine growth restriction, and lack of physical activity during childhood and adolescence	Overweight (BMI >85th percentile for age and gender, weight for height >85th percentile, or weight >120% of ideal for height) *PLUS* Any two of the following: • Family history of T2DM in first- or second-degree relative • Native American, African American, Hispanic American, Asian/Pacific Islander • Signs of insulin resistance or conditions associated with insulin resistance (acanthosis nigricans, HTN, dyslipidemia, or PCOS)
Latent autoimmune diabetes of adults (LADA)	Type 1.5 diabetes, slowly progressive type 1 diabetes, latent type 1 diabetes, youth-onset diabetes of maturity, LADA-type 1, LADA-type 2	Gradual immune-mediated destruction of islet beta cells, which tends to become insulin dependent at a later stage than individuals with T1DM	Elevated levels of pancreatic autoantibodies in individuals who do not require insulin for glycemic control; GADA appears to be the most sensitive marker

Continued

TABLE 19-2   CRITERIA FOR DIAGNOSING DIABETES—cont'd

DIABETES TYPE	FORMER TERM	ETIOLOGY	CRITERIA
Gestational diabetes (GDM)	Gestational diabetes, type III diabetes	Islet cell function abnormalities or peripheral insulin resistance are thought to decrease insulin secretory response and insulin sensitivity	*One-step approach:* Diagnostic OGTT *Two-step approach:* Initial screening to measure plasma or serum glucose concentration 1 hour after 50-g oral glucose load (GCT) and perform diagnostic OGTT on those women exceeding glucose threshold value on GCT. Glucose threshold ≥140 mg/dL identifies about 80% of women with GDM.
Prediabetes: Impaired glucose tolerance (IGT) Impaired fasting glucose (IFG)	Borderline diabetes, chemical diabetes	These are not clinical entities, but risk factors for future diabetes and cardiovascular disease	FPG levels ≥100 mg/dL but <126 mg/dL Individuals with IGT often manifest hyperglycemia only when challenged with oral glucose load used in OGTT

*Patients with any form of diabetes may require insulin treatment at some stage of their disease. Such use of insulin does not classify the patient as having type 1 DM.
†Symptoms include polyuria, polydipsia, and unexplained weight loss.
BMI, Body mass index; *FPG,* fasting plasma glucose; *GCT,* glucose challenge test; *HTN,* hypertension; *OGTT,* oral glucose tolerance test; *PCOS,* polycystic ovarian syndrome; *PG,* plasma glucose; *WHO,* World Health Organization.
Data from American Diabetes Association: Diagnosis and classification of diabetes mellitus, *Diabetes Care,* 29(Suppl 1):S43-S48, 2006; American Diabetes Association: Standards of medical care in diabetes—2006, *Diabetes Care* 29(Suppl 1):S4-S42, 2006; American Diabetes Association: Youth type 2 diabetes, *Diabetes Care* 28(3):638-644, 2005; American Diabetes Association: Gestational diabetes mellitus, *Diabetes Care* 27(Suppl 1):S88-S90, 2004; American Diabetes Association: Type 2 diabetes in the young, *Diabetes Care* 27(4):998-1010, 2004; Nabhan F, Emanuele MA, Emanuele N: Latent autoimmune diabetes of adulthood, *Postgrad Med Online* 117(3):7-12, 2005. Retrieved March 25, 2006, from www.postgradmed.com/index.php?article=1597; Thomas AM: Pathophysiology of gestational diabetes mellitus. In Thomas AM, Gutierrez YM, editors: *American Dietetic Association guide to gestational diabetes mellitus,* Chicago, 2005, American Dietetic Association.

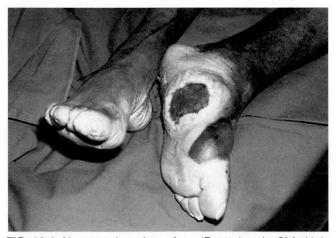

FIG 19-3 Neuropathy ulceration. (From Lewis SM, Heitkemper MM, Dirksen SL: *Medical-surgical nursing: Assessment and management of clinical problems,* ed 6, St. Louis, 2004, Mosby.)

TABLE 19-3   METABOLIC GOALS IN DIABETES MANAGEMENT

GLYCEMIC CONTROL	GOAL
A_{1c}	<7.0%
Preprandial capillary plasma glucose (mg/dL)	90-130
Peak postprandial capillary plasma glucose (mg/dL)*	<180
Cardiovascular	
Blood pressure (mm Hg)	<139/80
Triglycerides (mg/dL)	<150
LDL cholesterol (mg/dL)	<100
Males: HDL cholesterol (mg/dL)	>40
Females: HDL cholesterol (mg/dL)	>50

*Measurement should be made 1 to 2 hours after the beginning of the meal.
Data from American Diabetes Association: Standards of medical care in diabetes: 2010, *Diabetes Care* 33(Suppl 1):S11-S61, 2010.

PERSONAL PERSPECTIVES

A Tale of Diabetes

> **Type 1 Diabetes Mellitus: A Tale of Longevity**
> Childhood diabetes is now aggressively approached with an array of gadgets to assist in controlling the disorder. But imagine trying to maintain blood glucose levels when the pancreas is producing little if any insulin and the means to self-inject insulin is not yet available or still is being refined as treatment. When Robert Cleveland was diagnosed as a young boy and his brother, Gerald, at age 16, his mother could only depend on diet and exercise to treat her sons. Now at 86 years old, Robert has lived with the disease for almost 81 years, and Gerald—at 90—is the oldest known individual with type 1 diabetes mellitus. Robert and Gerald's successful longevity probably has to do with their methodical practice of lifestyle habits. For all these years, they've restricted their intake of simple starches and sweets, exercised, maintained healthy body weights, and continually tracked and recorded their glucose levels, food intake, and insulin dosages, testing their blood glucose many times a day. Such determination plus a positive attitude is reflected by Gerald's comment, "My main reason to stay alive is to prove to young people there's a way to live with diabetes, to live well."

Data from Pérez-Peña R: Diabetic brothers beat odds with grit and luck, *New York Times,* February 5, 2006, section A1, pp 1, 30.

BOX 19-2	SYMPTOMS AND CLINICAL SIGNS OF TYPE 1 DIABETES MELLITUS

Sudden onset of the following:
- Polyphagia
- Polyuria
- Polydipsia
- Weight loss

to starve. The body responds by sending signals to eat because cells are hungry, but because the end product of digestion (glucose) cannot enter cells, glucose builds up in the bloodstream. It is common for the person to experience weight loss while consuming large quantities of food (**polyphagia**). Because glucose cannot enter cells and it builds up in the bloodstream, blood becomes hypertonic and the body tries to get rid of the excess glucose by increasing urine output (**polyuria**). In reaction to increased excretion of urine, the body again responds by increasing thirst (**polydipsia**) to replace lost fluids (Box 19-2). The majority of individuals diagnosed with T1DM are usually 20 years of age or younger, but a growing number of cases are being documented in older individuals.[12]

T1DM is an autoimmune disease resulting in beta-cell destruction.[3,12,13] Causes of the autoimmune destruction of beta cells are not clearly understood, but multiple genetic predispositions and unidentified environmental factors appear to contribute to T1DM.[2] One or more **autoantibodies**

are present in 85% to 89% of individuals diagnosed with T1DM.[12] Rate of beta-cell destruction is variable, being rapid in infants and children and slow in adults. In fact, the first manifestation of T1DM may be diabetic ketoacidosis (DKA). Adults may retain enough residual beta-cell function to prevent ketoacidosis for many years, but when they eventually become dependent on insulin, they also are at risk for DKA.[3]

Some forms of T1DM have no known cause and are referred to as *idiopathic diabetes.* Individuals with idiopathic diabetes produce no insulin and are prone to ketoacidosis, but they have no evidence of autoimmunity. Individuals with T1DM who fall into this category represent a very small minority, and most are of African or Asian ancestry.[3]

Insulin

Everyone with T1DM requires exogenous insulin to maintain normal blood glucose levels and to survive.[14] Some individuals with T2DM may require insulin to optimize blood glucose control. Regardless of the type of diabetes, the goal of insulin therapy, in conjunction with nutrition therapy and physical activity,[15] is to mimic physiologic insulin delivery. Optimal insulin management can be realized only by evaluating blood glucose monitoring records, adjusting food and exercise activities, and proposing insulin adjustments.

Bioengineered human insulin is the only insulin available for use in the United States. Types of insulin are classified into three groups according to duration of their action: rapid or short acting, intermediate acting, and long acting (Table 19-4). Patterns of insulin administration vary with type of diabetes and desired glycemic control (Figure 19-4).

As you can see in Figure 19-4, a single dose of insulin is rarely capable of providing optimal glycemic control in T1DM. There are three basic types of insulin administration regimens: fixed (conventional or standard therapy), flexible (intensive insulin therapy), and continuous subcutaneous insulin infusion (CSII).

Conventional or standard insulin therapy is composed of a constant dose of intermediate-acting insulin combined with short- or rapid-acting insulin, or a mixed dose of insulin. Insulins may be mixed by the patient or purchased premixed (for example 30 units of 70/30 insulin). Administration of their insulin (Figure 19-5) and food intake must be synchronized to avoid hypoglycemia.[15] Nutrition goals are based on overall diabetes management goals: target glycemic goals and nutrition-related behaviors that affect these goals.

Flexible or intensive insulin therapy is composed of multiple daily injections (MDIs) of short- or rapid-acting insulin before meals, as well as intermediate insulin once or twice daily. This allows insulin to be adjusted to correspond with food intake, imitating endogenous insulin secretion in a person without diabetes. Insulin doses can also be adjusted to treat hyperglycemia, inconsistent carbohydrate intake, or modification in usual physical activity.[15] Results of the Diabetes Control and Complications Trial show that intensive insulin therapy (when compared with conventional therapy)

TABLE 19-4 TYPES OF INSULIN

CLASSIFICATION	RAPID ACTING ANALOG (CLEAR)	SHORT ACTING (CLEAR)	INTERMEDIATE ACTING (CLOUDY)	EXTENDED LONG-ACTING ANALOG (CLEAR)	PREMIXED (CLOUDY)	ANTIHYPERGLYCEMIC DRUG (SYNTHETIC ANALOG AMYLIN) (CLEAR)
Insulin type (brand name)	Lispro (Humalog) Aspart (NovoRapid) Glulisine (Apidra) Inhalation powder (Exubera)	Regular (Actrapid, Humulin R, Novolin R)	NPH (Humulin N, Novolin N, Insulatard) Lente (Novolin L)	Insulin glargine (Lantus) Insulin detemir (Levemir)	70/30 (NovoMix 30, Mixtard, Humulin 70/30) [70% NPH, 30% regular] 50/50 (Mixtard 60, Humulin 50/50) [50% NPH, 50% regular] 90/10 (Mixtard 10) [90% NPH, 10% regular] 80/20 (Mixtard 20) [80% NPH, 20% regular] 60/40 (Mixtard 40) [60% NPH, 40% regular]	Pramlintide (Symlin) Slows transit of digesting food through intestine; given at mealtimes to increase efficacy of insulin; should not be mixed with insulin
Onset of action*	5-15 minutes	30-60 minutes	1-3 hours	1 hour	10-60 minutes	
Peak of action*	1-3 hours	1-5 hours	8-15 hours	None	Dual	
Duration of action*	3-5 hours	5-8 hours	20-24 hours	24 hours	10-24 hours	

*Times given are averages of all types of insulin in the category.
Data from Eli Lilly and Company, Indianapolis (www.lilly.com); Novo Nordisk, Denmark (www.novonordisk.com); Aventis Pharmaceuticals Inc. (Sanofi Aventis), Bridgewater, NJ (www.lantus.com); Pfizer Inc., New York (www.pfizer.com); Amylin Pharmaceuticals, Inc., San Diego (www.symlin.com); Rystrom JK: Insulin therapy. In Ross TA, Boucher JL, O'Connell BS, editors: *American Dietetic Association guide to diabetes: Medical nutrition therapy and education,* Chicago, 2005, American Dietetic Association.

postpones onset and slows development of retinopathy, nephropathy, and neuropathy in patients with T1DM.[4]

It is important that the insulin regimen is integrated with the patient's lifestyle.[9] Individuals who use intensive therapy should know their basic insulin doses for both insulins they use. This allows them to fine-tune short- and rapid-acting insulin doses when they deviate from usual meal plans and/or exercise programs. This type of therapy may not be appropriate for everyone.

CSII is a form of intensive therapy. Rapid- or short-acting insulin is pumped continuously in micro-amounts through a subcutaneous catheter and is monitored 24 hours a day (Figure 19-6). Boluses or rapid- or short-acting insulins are given before meals.

Exercise

Along with medical nutrition therapy (discussed later in this chapter) and insulin, exercise is the third component used to treat diabetes. Exercise, like insulin, lowers blood glucose

levels, assists in maintaining normal lipid levels, and increases circulation. For most individuals, consistent and individualized exercise helps reduce the therapeutic dose of insulin. Patients with T1DM should be instructed not to perform exercise at the time insulin is at its peak. Ideally, they should exercise when blood glucose levels are between 100 and 200 mg/dL or about 30 to 60 minutes after meals. They should avoid exercising when blood glucose is greater than 250 mg/dL and ketones are present in the urine.[15] In the case of T1DM, glucose control can be compromised if proper adjustments are not made in food intake or insulin administration. Patients with T2DM who take oral hypoglycemic agents may be at risk of postexercise hypoglycemia.[16]

General guidelines that may assist in regulating the glycemic response to exercise in people with T1DM are summarized as follows:[17]

- *Metabolic control before exercise:* Avoid exercise if fasting glucose levels are greater than or equal to 250 mg/dL and ketosis is present or if glucose levels are

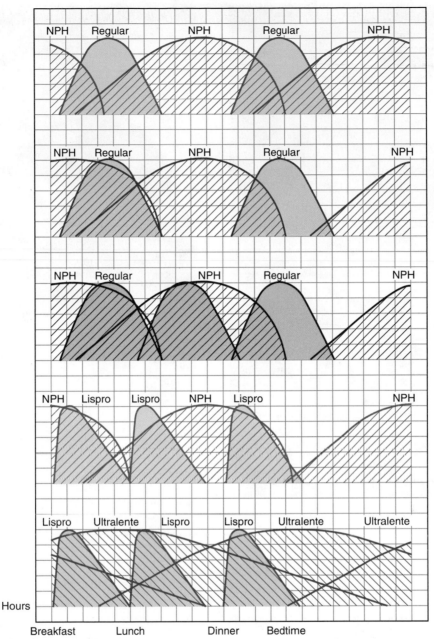

FIG 19-4 Typical patterns of insulin use. (Designed by Lisa Siegel. From Copstead-Kirkhorn L-E, Banasik J: *Pathophysiology*, ed 3, Philadelphia, 2005, Saunders.)

greater than 300 mg/dL, regardless of whether ketosis is present. Ingest added carbohydrate if glucose levels are less than 100 mg/dL.

- *Blood glucose monitoring before and after exercise:* Identify when changes in insulin or food intake are necessary. Learn the blood glucose response to different exercise conditions.
- *Food intake:* Consume added carbohydrate as needed to avoid hypoglycemia. Carbohydrate-based foods should be readily available during and after exercise (Box 19-3).

Hypoglycemia can occur during exercise that lasts longer than 1 hour and for up to 24 hours after unusually strenuous, prolonged, and/or sporadic exercise. Blood glucose levels should be monitored, and carbohydrates should be increased and/or insulin adjustments should be made. People with T1DM who do not have complications and are in good blood glucose control can perform all levels of exercise, including leisure activities, recreational sports, and competitive sports.[17] To do this safely, the patient must possess the ability to collect self-monitored blood glucose data (during exercise) and then use these data to adjust the therapeutic regimen (insulin and medical nutrition therapy).[17]

Type 2 Diabetes Mellitus

Type 2 DM is an insidious disease. People with T2DM rarely have the classic symptoms of diabetes (i.e., polyuria,

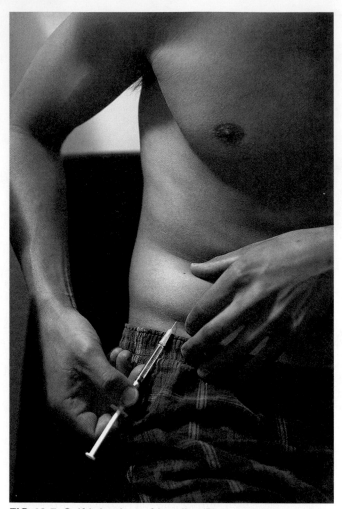

FIG 19-5 Self-injection of insulin. (Photos.com.)

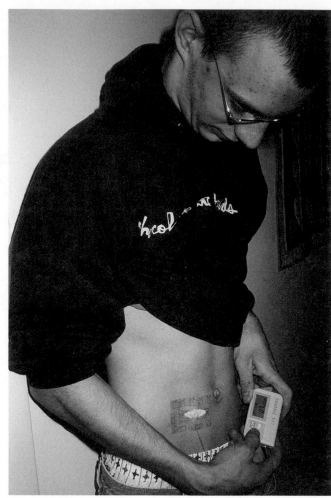

FIG 19-6 Insulin injection using an insulin pump. (From Peckenpaugh NJ: *Nutrition essentials and diet therapy*, ed 9, Philadelphia, 2003, Saunders.)

polyphagia, polydipsia) (Box 19-4). In fact, some of the first symptoms that cause individuals to seek medical attention are the complications (e.g., heart attack, stroke, neuropathic problems) associated with diabetes. It is not uncommon for a person to have T2DM years before diagnosis.

Unlike T1DM, the primary metabolic problem in T2DM is insulin resistance or failure of cells to respond to insulin produced by the body. Eventually the pancreas loses its ability to produce insulin.[18] Family history and obesity are the two strongest risk factors for T2DM. In fact, obesity by itself produces an insulin-resistant state that causes beta cells to produce excessive amounts of insulin. Because not all obese people develop diabetes, there seems to be a genetic tendency for diabetes that leads to beta-cell exhaustion and hyperglycemia in some obese people.[19] Additionally, upper body obesity has been recognized as an even greater risk factor for diabetes than degree of obesity.[20] Upper body obesity, defined as a waist-to-hip ratio greater than 0.8 for women and 0.95 to 1 for men, is a risk factor not only for diabetes but also heart disease and hypertension[2] (see also the *Cultural Considerations* box, Factors of Type 2 Diabetes Mellitus Prevalence).

Oral Glucose-Lowering Medications

Oral glucose-lowering medications are used to treat T2DM when diet and physical activity alone cannot control hyperglycemia. The variety of new drugs for treatment of diabetes has greatly expanded during the past several years. There are seven classes of oral diabetes medications (Table 19-5).[21,22]

Blood Glucose Monitoring

Blood glucose levels are the cornerstone of diabetes management. Prospective randomized clinical trials[5,7] demonstrate improved glycemic control is correlated with sustained reduced rates of retinopathy, nephropathy, and neuropathy.[5] Blood glucose levels can be monitored by **glycosylated hemoglobin (A1C)** or self-monitoring.[5,23] Recommended glycemic goals are outlined in Table 19-3. Self-monitoring of blood glucose (SMBG) and A1C in combination are the best indicators of glycemic control. Table 19-6 shows the correlation between mean plasma glucose levels and A1C levels.

Glycosylated hemoglobin (A1C) is formed through an irreversible process. As red blood cells (RBCs) circulate in the bloodstream, hemoglobin combines with glucose, forming

BOX 19-3	**FOOD PORTIONS CONTAINING 15 GRAMS OF CARBOHYDRATE PER SERVING**

Grains, Breads, Cereals, Starches
1 slice bread
¾ cup dry cereal
½ cup cooked cereal
⅓ cup cooked rice or pasta

Milk and Yogurt
1 cup milk
⅓ cup (6 ounces) unsweetened or sugar-free yogurt

Fruits
1 small fresh fruit
½ cup canned fruit (canned in juice)
1 cup melon or berries
¼ cup dried fruit
½ cup unsweetened fruit juice

Vegetables
½ cup cooked potatoes, peas, or corn
3 cups raw vegetables
1½ cups cooked vegetables
Small portions (½ cup) of nonstarchy vegetables are free

Sweets and Snack Foods
½ cup or ¾ ounce snack food (pretzels, chips)
4 to 6 snack crackers
1 ounce sweet snack (2 small cookies)
½ cup regular ice cream
1 tablespoon sugar

Data from American Diabetes Association, American Dietetic Association: *Choose Your Foods,* Alexandra, Va/Chicago, 2008, Authors.

BOX 19-4	**SYMPTOMS AND CLINICAL SIGNS OF TYPE 2 DIABETES MELLITUS**

- Gradual onset of polyuria and polydipsia
- Easily fatigued
- Frequent infections (especially of the urinary tract)

CULTURAL CONSIDERATIONS
Factors of Type 2 Diabetes Mellitus Prevalence

Type 2 DM poses a major health threat worldwide. According to the Centers for Disease Control and Prevention, at least 18.2 million people in the United States report having diabetes. It is estimated that more than 5.4 million people have undiagnosed diabetes. Although these figures represent diabetes of all types, 90% to 95% of people with diabetes have T2DM. People with diabetes are prone to acute and long-term complications. The prevalence of T2DM has been positively associated with age and minority group status. Diabetes is two to three times more prevalent among those older than 65 years than among those ages 20 to 44 years.

Among ethnic groups significantly at risk for T2DM are African Americans, Hispanic/Latino Americans, Native Americans, Asian Americans, and Pacific Islander Americans. GDM also presents more often in African Americans, Hispanic/Latino Americans, and Native Americans than among others.

According to some researchers, it is possible that a number of African Americans, Hispanic/Latino Americans, Native Americans, Asian Americans, and Pacific Islander Americans were born with a "thrifty gene" that results in more efficient storage of energy from food. This ability was valuable to aid survival for when sustenance was scarce. But now with abundant food year-round, this thrifty gene may be responsible for easier storage of excess energy and increased risk for T2DM.

Other factors influencing preventive and diabetes management care among minority groups in the United States include limited access to health care, cultural attitudes and behaviors related to medicine, and self-care.

Application to nursing: For minority and cultural groups, language barriers, health care access, level of acculturation, practices of diabetes self-care and possible genetic variations may contribute to higher risk of long-term diabetes complications. Nurses are encouraged to understand ethnic and cultural considerations when caring for minority populations.

Data from Centers for Disease Control and Prevention: *Frequently asked questions: Groups especially affected by diabetes,* Atlanta (last reviewed August 9, 2010), Author. Accessed March 29, 2010, from http://www.cdc.gov/diabetes/consumer/groups.htm.

glycohemoglobin. The amount of glycohemoglobin formed depends on the amount of glucose in the bloodstream circulation over the RBCs' 120-day life span. Therefore, the amount of A_{1C} is a reflection of the average blood glucose level for the 100- to 120-day period before the test; the more glucose the RBC was exposed to, the greater the value. This value is not affected by short-term factors such as food intake, exercise, or stress, so the blood sample can be drawn at any time. This is an easier sample to obtain than the fasting blood glucose test.

Self-monitoring can be performed in the individual's home with blood glucose meters, which can be purchased at pharmacies. A droplet of blood is obtained through a finger-stick on a regular basis to monitor glucose levels before and after meals and at bedtime. Self-monitoring and charting is particularly useful in evaluating glycemic control, physical activity, and effectiveness of the meal plan in meeting the goals of medical nutrition therapy.

Records should be kept of SMBG levels for review by the health care team to determine food, insulin, and exercise needs. This allows for individualized treatment, especially with meal plans, and makes indiscriminate, general dietary advice or tear-off diet sheets unjustified. SMBG is recommended three or more times daily for nearly all individuals with T1DM and pregnant women taking insulin. Individuals with T2DM who take insulin usually need to perform SMBG more often than those who do not take insulin.[23]

TABLE 19-5 ORAL HYPOGLYCEMIC AGENTS

DRUG CLASS	DRUG NAME(S)	ACTION	TARGET ORGAN(S)	SIDE EFFECTS	HOW TAKEN
Alpha-glucosidase inhibitor (AGIs)	*Acarbose:* Precose	Delays absorption of glucose from GI tract	Small intestine	Excess flatulence, diarrhea (particularly after high-carbohydrate meal), abdominal pain, may interfere with iron absorption	Must be taken with meals 3 times/day
	Miglitol: Glyset				
Biguanides	*Metformin:* Glucophage	Decreases hepatic glucose production and intestinal glucose absorption; improves insulin sensitivity	Liver, small intestine, and peripheral tissues	Less likely to gain weight; may lose weight; anorexia, nausea, diarrhea, metallic taste, may reduce absorption of vitamin B_{12} and folic acid, rarely suitable for adults <80 yr of age	Take with first main meal
Meglitinides (nonsulfonylurea insulin releasers)	*Nateglinide:* Starlix	Stimulates secretion of insulin	Pancreatic beta cells	Hypoglycemia and weight gain; *repaglinide* has a lightly increased risk for cardiac events	Take with meals
	Repaglinide: Prandin				
Sulfonylureas, First Generation	*Acetohexamide:* Dymelor	Stimulates secretion of insulin	Pancreatic beta-cells	Hypoglycemia and weight gain; *tolbutamide* may be associated with cardiovascular complications; *chlorpropamide* can cause hyponatremia; should not be used by women who are pregnant or nursing, or by individuals allergic to sulfa drugs; sulfonylurea interacts with many other drugs (prescription, OTC, and alternative); *Diabinese:* avoid alcohol	Take before or with meals
	Tolazamide: Tolinase *Tolbutamide:* Orinase *Chlorpropamide:* Diabinese				
Second Generation	*Glimepiride:* Amaryl *Glyburide:* DiaBeta, Micronase, Glynase PresTabs				
Thiazolidinediones (TZDs)	*Pioglitazone:* Actos	Improves insulin sensitivity	Activates genes involved with fat synthesis and carbohydrate metabolism	Possible liver damage, weight gain, mild anemia	Once or twice daily
	Rosiglitazone: Avandia				

Data from Data from Nelms MN, et al: *Nutrition therapy and pathophysiology,* ed 2, Belmont, Calif, 2010, Cengage/Thomson; Mahan LK, Escott-Stump S: *Krause's food and nutrition therapy,* ed 12, Philadelphia, 2008, Saunders; Schenkler E, Roth SL: *William's essentials of nutrition and diet therapy* ed 10, St. Louis, 2011, Mosby.

TABLE 19-6	CORRELATION BETWEEN MEAN PLASMA GLUCOSE LEVELS AND A$_{1C}$ LEVELS	
MEAN PLASMA GLUCOSE (mg/dL)	**A$_{1C}$ (%)**
60	4
90	5
120	6
150	7
180	8
210	9
240	10
270	11
300	12
330	13

Data from Rickheim P, et al: *Insulin basics,* Minneapolis, 2001, International Diabetes Center.

BOX 19-5	SYMPTOMS OF HYPOGLYCEMIA

- Hunger
- Erratic behavior
- Confusion
- Trembling, shaking
- Cool, clammy, pale skin

BOX 19-6	SYMPTOMS AND CLINICAL SIGNS OF DIABETIC KETOACIDOSIS

- Polyuria
- Polyphagia
- Weight loss
- Nausea
- Dry, flushed skin and mucous membranes
- Dehydration and metabolic acidosis
- Polydipsia
- Fruity (acetone) breath
- Generalized weakness
- Vomiting
- Weakness, fatigue

Hypoglycemia

Hypoglycemia (below normal values of blood glucose levels) usually results from too much insulin, skipping meals, or too much exercise without a concomitant increase in food intake. Onset is sudden and can be fatal if left untreated. Usually, hypoglycemia occurs at a time when plasma insulin (or oral hypoglycemic agents) levels peak or during the night when the patient sleeps (fasting). Box 19-5 lists the symptoms of hypoglycemia.

Symptoms usually occur when blood glucose drops below 50 mg/dL or there is a relatively significant drop in blood glucose. For example, if a patient is in a consistent state of hyperglycemia (e.g., 180 to 200 mg/dL) and blood glucose levels are brought down to 90 mg/dL, the patient may experience hypoglycemia even though the blood glucose level is in the normal range. The key is that for this patient, the normal blood glucose is low.

Diabetic Ketoacidosis

Diabetic ketoacidosis (DKA) is a life-threatening condition caused by insulin deficiency. When glucose cannot be used by cells, or when endogenous sources of energy are unavailable, the body breaks down fats and proteins for energy, which can cause ketosis. Ketosis is an abnormal accumulation of ketones caused by metabolism of fatty acids for energy with little carbohydrate metabolism occurring; ketoacidosis may then result. This condition results in hyperglycemia that causes osmotic diuresis, leads to dehydration, and precipitates lactic acidosis. Lowered pH, resulting from the acidosis,

stimulates the respiratory center and produces deep, rapid respirations known as Kussmaul's respirations. Large amounts of ketone bodies in the body also produce a fruity or acetone odor on the breath (a person suffering from DKA could be mistaken for someone who is inebriated). Box 19-6 lists symptoms and clinical signs of DKA. If this condition is not recognized and treated promptly, the acidosis and dehydration may lead to loss of consciousness and possibly coma and death.[17] Common conditions that precipitate DKA include insufficient or interrupted insulin therapy, too much food, infection, or other stresses (e.g., trauma, surgery, emotional stress, myocardial infarction).

HYPERGLYCEMIC HYPEROSMOLAR SYNDROME

Hyperglycemic hyperosmolar nonketotic syndrome (HHNS), like DKA, is a life-threatening emergency caused by a relative or actual insulin deficiency resulting in severe hyperglycemia. Most often HHNS is triggered by stress (trauma, infection) that increases the body's demand for insulin. Although enough insulin may be present in the plasma to prevent formation of ketones, thus preventing acidosis, there may not be enough to prevent hyperglycemia. If hyperglycemia is left untreated, serum becomes hyperosmolar and produces osmotic diuresis and simultaneous significant loss of electrolytes via urine. Mortality for HHNS is 10% to 25%.[20] Symptoms and clinical signs of HHNS are listed in Box 19-7.

NUTRITION THERAPY

Even though the term "ADA diet" has never been clearly defined, there is no one "diabetic diet" or "ADA diet." In the past it typically meant a physician-determined kcal level with specific percentages of carbohydrate, protein, and fat based on the exchange lists. The American Diabetes Association (ADA) urges that the term "ADA diet" not be used given that the ADA no longer endorses any particular meal plan or specific percentages of nutrients.[24] Diet orders such as "no concentrated sweets," "no sugar added," "low sugar," and "liberal diabetic" are not considered suitable because they do not reflect diabetes nutrition recommendations and pointlessly restrict sucrose. Such meal plans propagate the false notion that merely restricting sucrose-sweetened foods will improve blood glucose control.[24]

BOX 19-7 SYMPTOMS AND CLINICAL SIGNS OF HHNS

- Polyuria
- Polyphagia
- Weight loss
- Nausea
- Dry, flushed skin and mucous membranes
- Dehydration secondary to osmotic diuresis
- Polydipsia
- Possible seizures and tremors
- Generalized weakness
- Vomiting
- Fatigue

Nutrition therapy is an essential element of glycemic control and diabetes self-management education (DSME). Individualized nutrition therapy is required to achieve treatment goals.[24] The basis for nutrition therapy and DSME includes a comprehensive nutrition assessment, self-care treatment plan, and the client's health status, learning ability, readiness to change, and current lifestyle. The key is to tailor the meal planning approach to each individual's needs.[25] Individuals using intensive insulin therapy have flexibility in when and what they eat, whereas people using conventional insulin therapy must be consistent with timing of meals and amounts of food consumed.

Recommendations for total fat, saturated fat, cholesterol, fiber, vitamins, and minerals are the same for individuals with diabetes as for the general population. Carbohydrate recommendations are based on the individual's eating habits, blood glucose, and lipid goals (Box 19-8 Carbohydrate Counting). Blood glucose control is not impaired by the use of sucrose in the meal plan, but sucrose-containing

BOX 19-8 CARBOHYDRATE COUNTING

Carbohydrate counting is one of the meal planning approaches used in the Diabetes Control and Complications Trial (DCCT) and allows for greater focus on consistency in food consumption. The proposition of carbohydrate counting gives priority to the total amount of carbohydrates consumed—regardless of whether monosaccharides, disaccharides, or polysaccharides—rather than the source. Scientific evidence indicates that all forms of carbohydrate basically affect blood glucose levels similarly when eaten in the same gram amount: "A carbohydrate is a carbohydrate is a carbohydrate."
One carbohydrate choice = 15 g carbohydrate
1 starch
1 fruit
1 milk
Carbohydrate counting can be used for all types of diabetes and in clients of all age groups. The challenges and advantages of carbohydrate counting are outlined following. Three levels of carbohydrate counting based on increasing levels of complexity and required skills have been jointly developed, organized, and published by the American Dietetic Association and the American Diabetes Association.

Level 1
Getting Started is the basic booklet that introduces the goal of carbohydrate consistency and flexible food choices. This level works well with clients who have T1DM, T2DM, and GDM. It is recommended that one to three client contacts of 30 to 90 minutes each with a registered dietitian or certified diabetes educator be used when teaching Level 1.

Level 2
Moving On is the intermediate booklet that assumes basic understanding and knowledge for the client to adjust medica-

tion, food, and activities based on patterns from daily records. This level works well with people using diet only, oral hypoglycemic agents, or insulin to control their diabetes and who have mastered the basics of carbohydrate counting (Level 1). Level 2 takes one to three client contacts of 30 to 60 minutes each with a registered dietitian or certified diabetes educator.

Level 3
Using Carbohydrate/Insulin Ratios is an advanced booklet for which a client needs understanding and knowledge at the intermediate level to adjust insulin doses based on the client's individual responses to food, medication, and activity. Level 3 is intended for people on intensive insulin therapy and who have mastered insulin adjustment and supplementation. Level 3 takes one to three contacts of 30 to 60 minutes each with a registered dietitian or certified diabetes educator.

Carbohydrate Counting
Advantages
- Focuses on a single nutrient
- Flexibility in food choices
- Potential for improved blood glucose levels
- Clients feel more empowered
- More precise matching of food and insulin

Challenges
- Weighing/measuring foods
- Maintaining food records (initially and periodically)
- Recording blood glucose levels (before/after eating)
- Dealing with numbers and calculations
- Weight management
- Maintenance of healthy eating pattern

Data from Diabetes Control and Complications Trial Research Group: The effect of intensive treatment of diabetes on the development and progression of long-term complications in insulin-dependent diabetes mellitus, *N Engl J Med* 329:977-986, 1993; American Diabetes Association: Nutrition principles and recommendations in diabetes, *Diabetes Care* 27(Suppl 1):S36-S46, 2004; American Diabetes Association, American Dietetic Association: *Carbohydrate counting series: getting started (level 1), moving on (level 2), using carbohydrate/insulin ratios (level 3), information for the health professional*, Chicago, 1995, American Dietetic Association.

TABLE 19-7   HISTORICAL PERSPECTIVE OF NUTRITION RECOMMENDATIONS FOR DIABETES MELLITUS

YEAR	CARBOHYDRATE	FAT	PROTEIN
Pre-1921	Starvation diets		
1921	20% of total energy	70% of total energy	10% of total energy
1950	40% of total energy	40% of total energy	20% of total energy
1971	45% of total energy	35% of total energy	20% of total energy
1986	≤60% of total energy	<30% of total energy	12%-20% of total energy
1994	Based on nutrition assessment and treatment goal	Based on nutrition assessment and treatment goals; less than 10% of energy from saturated fats	10%-20% of total energy
2002	Individuals should receive individualized nutrition therapy as needed to achieve treatment goals, preferably provided by a registered dietitian familiar with components of diabetes nutrition therapy (NT).		
	Whole grains, fruits, vegetables, and low-fat milk should be included in a healthy diet.	<10% of energy from saturated fat ~10% of energy from polyunsaturated fat	Ingested protein is just as potent a stimulant of insulin secretion as carbohydrate
	Total amount of carbohydrate in meals or snacks is more important than source or type of carbohydrate.	Intake of trans fat should be minimized <300 mg cholesterol/day	Protein requirements may be >0.8g/kg/ day for individuals with less-than-optional glycemic control
	Sucrose and sucrose-containing foods should be eaten in the context of a healthy diet (they do not need to be restricted, but should be substituted for other carbohydrate sources or covered with insulin or other glucose-lowering medication).	Fat intake should be individualized and designed to fit ethnic and cultural backgrounds	Usual protein intake (15%-20% of total energy) need not be modified if renal function is normal
	Individuals receiving intensive insulin therapy should adjust their pre-meal insulin dosages based on carbohydrate content of meals		
	Individuals receiving fixed daily insulin dosages should be consistent in day-to-day carbohydrate intake		

Data from American Diabetes Association: Nutrition recommendations and principles for people with diabetes mellitus, *Diabetes Care* 27(Suppl 1):S36-S46, 2004; Franz MJ, et al: Evidence-based nutrition principles and recommendations for the treatment and prevention of diabetes and related complications, *Diabetes Care* 25:148-198, 2002.

foods should be substituted for other carbohydrates and foods, and should not be eaten in addition to a meal plan. Protein intake can range from 15% to 20% of daily kcal from animal and vegetable protein sources. *If* diabetes is well controlled, blood glucose levels are not affected by moderate alcohol use. Alcohol kcal ought to be considered as additional kcal, and no food should be omitted. Alcohol should be consumed with food to reduce the risk of hypoglycemia.[26]

In 2002 the ADA published its sixth set of recommendations since 1950 (Table 19-7). Goals of nutrition therapy that apply to all individuals with diabetes are as follows:[26,27]

1. Attain and maintain optimal metabolic outcomes including:
   a. Glucose level in normal range, or as close to normal range as is safely possible to prevent or reduce risk of complications
   b. Lipid or lipoprotein profile that reduces risk for macrovascular disease
   c. Blood pressure levels that reduce risk for vascular disease (Box 19-9)

BOX 19-9   STRATEGIES FOR METABOLIC CONTROL (TYPE 2 DIABETES MELLITUS)

- Nutritionally adequate meal plan with a reduction of total fat, especially saturated fats
- Meals spaced throughout the day
- Mild to moderate weight loss (5-10 kg [10-20 lb]) even if desirable body weight is not achieved (moderate decrease in energy intake, increase in kcal expenditure)
- Regular exercise
- Monitoring of blood glucose levels, glycosylated hemoglobin, lipids, and blood pressure
- Oral hypoglycemic or insulin if preceding does not work

2. Prevent and treat chronic complications. Modify nutrient intake and lifestyle as appropriate for prevention and treatment of obesity, dyslipidemia, cardiovascular disease, hypertension, and nephropathy.
3. Enhance health using healthy food choices and physical activity.

4. Address individual nutritional needs with regards to personal and cultural preferences and lifestyles while respecting the individual's wishes and willingness to change.

Owing to the complexity of nutrition issues, the ADA[26] recommends a registered dietitian who is knowledgeable and skilled in implementing nutrition therapy into diabetes management and education be the medical team member responsible for providing medical nutrition therapy. It is also essential all health care team members be knowledgeable about nutrition therapy and supportive of the patient with diabetes who needs to make these important lifestyle changes.

Nutrition therapy is an integral component of diabetes management and DSME. It involves conducting a nutrition assessment to evaluate a patient's food intake, metabolic status, lifestyle, and willingness to make changes; goal setting; nutrition education; and evaluation. To enhance compliance, the medical nutrition therapy plan should be individualized and take into consideration the patient's lifestyle, cultural background, and financial situation. Patients with diabetes require an assessment by a registered dietitian to determine an appropriate nutrition prescription and plan for DSME.[23,24]

Nutrition therapy should be individualized, taking into consideration a person's usual eating habits and other lifestyle factors.[27] Consistency within an eating pattern will result in lower glycosylated hemoglobin levels rather than following an arbitrary eating style.[27]

Other related nutrient issues include use of fructose and other nutritive and nonnutritive sweeteners. Although fructose creates a smaller rise in plasma glucose than sucrose and other carbohydrates, large amounts of fructose (up to 20% of daily kcal intake) provide no advantage as a sweetener based on its negative effects on serum cholesterol and low-density lipoprotein (LDL) cholesterol levels. Other nutritive sweeteners such as corn sweeteners, fruit juice or juice concentrate, honey, molasses, dextrose, and maltose affect glycemic response and caloric content in a manner similar to that of sucrose. The sugar alcohols (sorbitol, mannitol, and xylitol) result in lower glycemic responses than other simple and complex carbohydrates, and ingesting large amounts may have a laxative effect. Nonnutritive sweeteners approved for use by the U.S. Food and Drug Administration (FDA), such as saccharin, aspartame, and acesulfame K, are considered safe for consumption by individuals with diabetes. Each product has undergone rigorous testing and scrutiny before approval. All were shown to be safe when consumed by the public, including people with diabetes and during pregnancy.[26]

Role of the Nurse

The role of the nurse in caring for the nutritional needs of patients with diabetes varies depending on setting and age of the client. However, the general approach is to become aware of and help assess the patient's knowledge and understanding and adherence with the prescribed diet. When possible, observing meals and food choices as well as monitoring glucose levels can give important clues to the level of compliance. When compliance is faulty, the nurse needs to determine whether knowledge or motivation is the problem (Box 19-10). Knowledge deficits can be remedied in appropriate areas by the nurse or dietitian; lack of motivation may be harder to handle. For example, (1) adolescents with diabetes may not believe long-term complications are related to diet and may be more motivated by the need to eat like their peers, or (2) older adults with diabetes may be set in longtime food intake patterns and may not want to change them as long as they take medication for hyperglycemia.

When a trusting relationship exists between the nurse and patient, discussions about motivations and concerns can take place. The nurse may then influence the patient to be more concerned about his or her long-term welfare. A care plan that meets the patient's social, psychologic, and physical needs can be developed as a result of collaboration among the nurse, physician or primary health care provider, dietitian, and patient (see the *Teaching Tool* box, Helping Clients Follow Instructions). Additional forms of support may be provided by community agencies and associations. These resources, such as the ADA, are listed in Websites of Interest.

✳ TEACHING TOOL

Helping Clients Follow Instructions

Diabetes is on the rise, particularly among ethnic groups for whom English may be a second language or whose education may be limited (e.g., reading at a fourth- or fifth-grade level). Nearly 50% of Americans have low literacy skills that may affect their ability to understand their disease and to follow treatment instructions; these patients struggle when dealing with the health care system. Because diabetes requires long-term behavioral changes and monitoring, compliance is important. Health professionals working with individuals who have low literacy skills and diabetes mellitus can improve understanding and compliance by (1) using patient education materials that are simple and concise, (2) using culturally appropriate graphics showing step-by-step instructions, and (3) involving family members.

Data from Herdener M, Vezear T: Low literacy in patients: Implications for nurse practitioners, *Am J Nurse Pract* 9(9):21, 2005; and Mayeaux EJ Jr, et al: Improving patient education for patients with low literacy skills, *Am Fam Physician* 53(1):205-211, 1996.

As mentioned, nutrition and diet are considered by both patients and health professionals to be the most difficult problem in the management of diabetes. Every day we are faced with changes in our environments that require some adaptation to the situation. We're late for work, so maybe we skip breakfast or grab something quick along the way. The kids have ball practice tonight, so dinner becomes sandwiches and fruit instead of a full-course meal. Most of us make the required changes in stride, not thinking too much about it. Why should we think life for people with diabetes is any dif-

BOX 19-10 OBSTACLES TO DIETARY ADHERENCE IN DIABETES MELLITUS

Obstacle: Extent to which social, career, recreational, and personal goals create situations within which the person must choose between making appropriate food choices and furthering another important life goal.

Assessment: Does the patient see this as a problem? To what extent? Does the patient feel frustrated about it? How has the patient dealt with it in the past? Does the patient make compromises or give in to the competing goals? Is the conflict anticipated or simply handled when it arises? Does time pressure have any effect on the patient's ability to make appropriate choices?

Obstacle: Tempted to overeat to cope with stress and negative emotions

Assessment: How stressful is the patient's life? How does the patient respond to frustration, stress, anxiety, and depression? Any conflicts with friends, family, supervisors, or other authorities? Is food used as an escape or avoidance strategy? If so, how much and what kinds of foods are eaten? How is boredom handled? Can the patient identify any other coping strategies (to use besides eating)?

Obstacle: Ability to resist temptation when confronted with inappropriate foods or when experiencing specific food cravings

Assessment: Does the patient encounter inappropriate foods in the everyday environment? If so, how often? How does the patient react to seeing other people eat these foods? Does the patient experience specific food cravings? If so, what foods, how often, and how strong are the cravings? Is there family support to reduce the availability of inappropriate foods?

Obstacle: Reaction to eating at restaurants, social events, parties, special occasions, and holidays

Assessment: What are family food traditions? How often does the patient eat socially with peers? Do friends and family eat in moderation, or do they overeat at holidays and social events? How does the patient make food choices when faced with a large array of foods? Can the patient order an appropriate meal from a menu? Does the patient even try to stick to the meal plan or simply give up?

Obstacle: Social support

Assessment: Do family and friends make it easier or harder to eat appropriately? What behaviors from family and friends create obstacles? Do others deliberately sabotage the patient? Are there any supportive behaviors that friends or family could do?

Obstacle: Assessment of patient's history of dietary adherence

Assessment: Does the patient become discouraged and give up altogether? Is there a history of taking vacations from appropriate diabetes care? Does the patient work out compromises, or give up entirely?

Obstacle: Assessment of whether the patient can respond assertively when being pressured to deviate from an appropriate eating pattern

Assessment: Can the patient say no clearly and firmly? How worried is the patient about being different from others?

Modified from Schlundt DG, et al: Situational obstacles to dietary adherence for adults with diabetes, *J Am Diet Assoc* 94:874-876, 879, 1994. With permission from the American Dietetic Association.

---

ferent? Historically, those with diabetes have been taught consistency in everything they do: eat at the same time every day, eat the same number of kcal every day, take the same amount of insulin every day, and so on. The new recommendations for medical nutritional therapy consider these perpetual lifestyle changes.

Wouldn't it also be practical when encouraging dietary adherence with a person who has diabetes to discuss situations that cause the individual problems in maintaining control over his or her eating? Schlundt and colleagues[28] have identified seven situations that provide obstacles to adhering to a prescribed diet (Box 19-10). Comprehensive education for individuals with diabetes should include assessment of these obstacles and situational problem solving.[28]

SPECIAL CONSIDERATIONS

Illness

During periods of illness, blood glucose levels may become elevated and diabetes control may worsen. This is caused by an increase in hepatic production of glucose that has been stimulated by infection, illness, injury, or stress (specifically

by the release of epinephrine, norepinephrine, glucagon, and cortisol). Under such conditions, this hyperglycemia increases insulin requirements.[26]

Often, while illness causes an increased need for insulin, there is also a decreased appetite and food intake. Liquids and soft foods are usually better tolerated and help provide some kcal intake while preventing dehydration. The following guidelines have been used in cases of brief illness on an emergency basis for a maximum of 3 days[23,26,29] (see also the *Teaching Tool* box, Sick Day Guidelines):

- Monitor blood glucose at least four times a day (before each meal and at bedtime).
- Test urine for ketones (if blood glucose is greater than 240 mg/dL).
- Medications to control blood glucose should not be omitted. Dosages may need to be adjusted when food intake is reduced, however.
- If regular foods are not tolerated, replace carbohydrates in the meal plan with liquid, semiliquid, or soft foods. The source of the carbohydrate is not of major concern. Sugar-containing liquids may be the only food source tolerated. More important is what the patient can tolerate. A general rule is to consume every 1 to 2 hours

✳ TEACHING TOOL

Sick Day Guidelines

Colds, fever, flu, nausea, vomiting, and diarrhea can cause special problems for individuals with diabetes. Teach the following guidelines to clients to help them manage common illnesses and maintain control of their diabetes:

1. These guidelines apply only to mild, short-term, 1-day illnesses. Call your physician if any of the following occur:
   - You can't keep any liquids or carbohydrates down for more than 8 hours.
   - You are vomiting or have diarrhea.
   - You are spilling ketones in your urine.
   - You begin to breathe rapidly, become drowsy, or lose consciousness.
   - You have questions or concerns.
2. If you take insulin, you must continue to take your usual dose to prevent ketoacidosis. Your need for insulin continues or may increase during illness. Never omit your insulin.
3. If you take oral hypoglycemic agents (tablets), continue to take your usual dose unless you are vomiting. Resume your medication when you are able to tolerate fluids and food again. If vomiting continues, contact your physician.
4. Monitor your blood glucose and test urine for ketones at least four times per day (i.e., before each meal and at bedtime). If your blood glucose reading is greater than 240 mg/dL and there are moderate to large ketone levels in the urine, call your physician.
5. If you can't eat your regular food, replace it with carbohydrates in the form of liquids or soft foods. Eat at least 50 g of carbohydrates every 3 to 4 hours, especially if your blood sugar is less than 240 mg/dL. If your blood sugar is greater than 240 mg/dL, continue to drink liquids, especially those that don't contain kcal (water, broth, diet soft drinks, tea).

Foods Containing 10 g Carbohydrates
½ cup regular soft drink (ginger ale, cola)
½ frozen fruit bar (twin bar)
2 teaspoons corn syrup or honey
2½ teaspoons granulated sugar
¼ cup regularly sweetened gelatin

Foods Containing 15 g Carbohydrates
½ cup orange or grapefruit juice
⅓ cup grape or apple juice
½ cup ice cream
½ cup cooked cereal
¼ cup sherbet
⅓ cup regularly sweetened gelatin
1 cup broth-based soups (reconstituted with water)
1 cup cream soup
¾ cup regular soft drink (ginger ale, cola)
¼ cup milkshake
1½ cups milk
½ cup eggnog (commercial)
⅓ cup tapioca pudding
½ cup custard
1 cup plain yogurt
1 slice toast
6 saltine crackers

6. Drink a large glass of kcal-free liquid every hour to replace fluids. If you feel nauseated or are vomiting, take small sips (1 to 2 tablespoons) every 15 to 30 minutes. Call your physician.
7. When illness subsides, return to your regular meal plan and usual insulin schedule.

From Franz MJ, Joynes JO: *Diabetes and brief illness,* Minneapolis, 1993, International Diabetes Center.

---

approximately 15 g carbohydrate (e.g., ½ cup juice or ½ cup applesauce), or every 3 to 4 hours, 50 g carbohydrate (e.g., 1 cup juice and ¾ cup applesauce or 10 saltine crackers, 1 cup soup, and ½ cup juice). If blood glucose is greater than 240 mg/dL, the entire amount may not need to be consumed.
- Drink 8 to 12 ounces of fluid (water, broth, tea) each hour. A carbohydrate source may also be the fluid source.
- If vomiting, diarrhea, or fever occurs, consume small amounts of salted foods and liquids more frequently to replace lost electrolytes.

Gastroparesis

Approximately 20% to 30% of individuals with diabetes develop gastroparesis with delayed gastric emptying that can manifest with heartburn, nausea, abdominal pain, vomiting, early satiety, and weight loss. Gastroparesis occurs as a result of vagal autonomic neuropathy and occurs more often in T1DM than in T2DM.[30]

Dietary treatment of gastroparesis involves monitoring intake carefully. Carbohydrates should be replaced with foods of soft or liquid consistency. Six small meals may be better tolerated than three large meals. If constipation or diarrhea occurs, fiber intake is altered according to patient needs. If the patient complains of dry mouth, fluids can be increased and food moistened with broth. A low-fat (40 g) soft or liquid diet may be useful to prevent delay in gastric emptying. If metoclopramide (Reglan) is used to increase gastric contractions and relax the pyloric sphincter, the patient may experience side effects of dry mouth or nausea. Insulin should be matched with meals to regulate delayed absorption and glucose changes. Bezoar formation is common with oranges, coconuts, green beans, apples, figs, potato skins, Brussels sprouts, and sauerkraut. If problems are severe, a temporary jejunostomy tube feeding may be indicated.[30]

Diabetes Management through the Life Span

The role of medical nutrition therapy is crucial for optimal blood glucose control. Various life stages, pregnancy outcome, and growth and development of children can be influenced by nutritional intake.

Pregnancy

Women with preexisting diabetes who become pregnant are vulnerable to fetal complications, and maternal health can be compromised when complications of diabetes occur.[31,32] Occasionally the stress of pregnancy may induce GDM, which is a form of glucose intolerance that has its onset during pregnancy and is resolved on parturition. Whether the mother has preexisting diabetes or GDM, risk of fetal abnormalities and mortality is increased in the presence of hyperglycemia, so every effort should be made to control blood glucose levels.[33] Ideally women with diabetes should achieve excellent glycemic control 3 months before conception.[23,34] All women with GDM should receive nutrition counseling by a registered dietitian when possible.[32]

Changes that take place during pregnancy greatly affect diabetes control and insulin use. Some hormones and enzymes produced by the placenta are antagonistic to insulin, thus reducing its effectiveness. Maternal insulin does not cross the placenta, but glucose does. This will cause the fetus's pancreas to increase insulin production if blood glucose levels get too high. The increased production of insulin causes the most typical characteristic of infants born to women with diabetes: macrosomia. Newborns may also have other problems such as respiratory difficulties, hypocalcemia, hypoglycemia, hypokalemia, or jaundice.[35]

Individualization of medical nutrition therapy contingent on maternal weight and height is recommended.[32] Medical nutrition therapy should include provision of adequate kcal and nutrients to meet the needs of the pregnancy and should be consistent with established maternal blood glucose goals.[26] SMBG presents important information about the impact of food on blood glucose levels.[32,33] At the start, minimal SMBG should be planned four times a day (fasting and 1 or 2 hours after each meal), but it is not uncommon for pregnant women with diabetes to test blood glucose levels eight times per day.[33] Blood glucose goals during pregnancy are the following:[33]

- *Fasting:* ≤95 mg/dL
- *1 hour postprandial:* ≤140 mg/dL
- *2 hours postprandial:* ≤120 mg/dL

Guidelines for all pregnant women can be used because there are no unique weight gain recommendations for women with diabetes.[33] Desired weight gain goals are based on prepregnancy body mass index (BMI) and should be steady and progressive (Table 19-8). Thin women should gain more weight than overweight/obese women.[33] Given that women with GDM are often overweight or obese, a minimum weight gain of 15 pounds (6.8 kg) is recommended.[33]

No kcal adjustments are needed for the first trimester. During the second and third trimesters, an increased energy intake of approximately 100 to 300 kcal/day is recommended.[26] High-quality protein should be increased by 10 g/day[26] and can be met easily with one or two extra glasses of low-fat or skim milk or 1 to 2 ounces of meat or meat substitute. As with any pregnancy, 400 mcg/day of folic acid is recommended for prevention of neural tube defects and

TABLE 19-8	DESIRED WEIGHT GAIN GOALS FOR PREGNANT WOMEN WITH DIABETES
BMI RANGE	**RECOMMENDED WEIGHT GAIN**
Obese (BMI ≥30 kg/m²)	~15 pounds (7 kg)
Overweight (BMI >26-29 kg/m²)	~15 to 20 pounds (6.8-11.3 kg)
Normal weight (BMI 19.8-26 kg/m²)	First trimester: ~3 to 5 pounds/month (1.4-2.3 kg) Second and third trimesters: ~1.1 to 2 pounds/week (0.5-0.9 kg)
Underweight (BMI ≥19.8 kg/m²)	Up to 39.6 pounds (18 kg)

Data from Reader D: Diabetes in pregnancy and lactation. In Ross TA, Boucher JL, O'Connell BS, editors: *American Dietetic Association guide to diabetes: Medical nutrition therapy and education*, Chicago, 2005, American Dietetic Association; Franz MJ, et al: Evidence-based nutrition principles and recommendations for the treatment and prevention of diabetes and related complications, *Diabetes Care* 25(1):148-198, 2002.

other congenital abnormalities. Alcohol consumption is not recommended in any amount.

Kcal restriction must be viewed with caution. A minimum of 1700 to 1800 kcal/day of carefully selected foods has been shown to prevent ketosis. Intakes below this level are not advised.[33] Each patient with GDM should be evaluated individually by a registered dietitian, have her care plans adjusted, and be provided patient education as needed to achieve weight goals.

Pregnancy in overt diabetes. A successful pregnancy for a woman who has diabetes requires planning and commitment. Because most fetal malformations occur during the first trimester of pregnancy, achieving and maintaining excellent glycemic control before conception and during early pregnancy is a must. The optimal period of care for a woman with diabetes is *before* conception. Box 19-11 outlines prenatal nutritional recommendations.

Ideally, preconception counseling should begin during puberty and continue through the childbearing years.[23,33,34] Insulin requirements increase during the second and third trimesters because of increased blood glucose levels caused by increased production of pregnancy-associated hormones that are insulin antagonists.[33] Successful preconception care programs have used the following preprandial and postprandial goals[34]:

- *Before meals:* Capillary whole-blood glucose 70 to 100 mg/dL or capillary plasma glucose 80 to 110 mg/dL
- *2 hours postprandial:* Capillary whole-blood glucose less than 140 mg/dL or capillary plasma glucose less than 155 g/dL

Glycated hemoglobin levels should be normal or as close to normal as possible before conception is attempted.[23,26,33,34]

Pregnancy will require greater attention to medical nutrition therapy on a day-to-day basis. Guidance during early

BOX 19-11 PRENATAL NUTRITIONAL RECOMMENDATIONS

NUTRIENT	RECOMMENDATION
Calories	Sufficient to achieve or maintain desired body weight
Carbohydrates	Individualized based on eating habits, blood glucose records and expected physiological effects of pregnancy
Protein	0.75 g/kg/day + additional 10 g/day
Folate	400 mcg/day
Iron	30 mg/day during second and third trimesters
Zinc	15 mg/day
Vitamins and minerals	Prenatal vitamin and mineral supplements often prescribed
Alcohol	Avoid
Caffeine	Limit to <300 mg/day
Nonnutritive sweeteners	Use in moderation

Data from Franz MJ, et al: Evidence-based nutrition principles and recommendations for the treatment and prevention of diabetes and related complications, *Diabetes Care* 25(1):148-198, 2002.

TABLE 19-9 NUTRITION RECOMMENDATIONS FOR GESTATIONAL DIABETES MELLITUS

NUTRIENT	RECOMMENDATIONS
Energy	Sufficient to promote adequate, but not excessive, weight gain and to avoid ketonuria
Carbohydrate	Based effect of intake on glycemic control; intake should be distributed throughout the day
High-sucrose/ high-energy foods	Intake based on effect on glycemic control, nutritional adequacy of diet, and contribution to total meal plan
Protein	0.8 g/kg (Recommended Dietary Allowance) desirable body weight per day + 25 g/day or 1.1 g/kg desirable body weight
Fat	Limit saturated fat
Sodium	Not routinely restricted
Fiber	Increase intake for relief of constipation
Nonnutritive sweeteners	Use in moderation
Vitamins and minerals	Preconception folate; assess for individual needs; multivitamin throughout pregnancy; iron at 12 weeks; calcium in last trimester and while lactating
Caffeine	Limit to <300 mg/day
Alcohol	Avoid

Data from Reader D: Diabetes in pregnancy and lactation. In Ross TA, Boucher JL, O'Connell BS, editors: *American Dietetic Association guide to diabetes: Medical nutrition therapy and education*, Chicago, 2005, American Dietetic Association.

pregnancy should include special consideration for food cravings and nausea. The meal plan should be individualized and should evolve throughout the pregnancy to meet changing nutritional needs and insulin requirements. Three meals and three snacks are usually recommended. Use of frequent home blood glucose monitoring is necessary to help the patient maintain normal fasting and postprandial glucose levels and avoid frequent or severe hypoglycemic reactions.

Gestational diabetes. GDM will develop in about 5% to 10% of all pregnancies. It occurs more frequently among American Indian, African American, and Hispanic/Latina American women.[2] Women who develop GDM are often obese, but weight reduction should not be attempted at this time.[26] Nutrition recommendations for GDM are outlined in Table 19-9. Good glucose control is usually accomplished by individualization of intake and graphing of weight gain. Often, insulin may be prescribed in addition to medical nutrition therapy to reduce the risks of fetal macrosomia, neonatal hyperglycemia, and perinatal mortality.[33] The FDA has not approved any oral hypoglycemic agents for use during pregnancy.[33] Glucose levels usually revert to normal following delivery, but there is an increased risk for later development of T1DM or T2DM. Nearly 20% to 50% of women with GDM eventually develop T2DM[2] (Box 19-12).

Type 2 Diabetes in the Young

Incidence and prevalence of T2DM in children, especially ethnic minority populations, has increased 30-fold over the past 20 years, causing the term *epidemic* to be used to describe the phenomenon.[32,36] This means the burden of diabetes and

BOX 19-12 POSTPARTUM RECOMMENDATIONS

A woman who has gestational diabetes can decrease her chances of developing T2DM by doing the following:
- Screening 6 or more weeks after delivery
- Having a lipid panel performed 5 months or more after delivery
- Maintaining ideal body weight
- Eating a lower-fat diet
- Exercising regularly
- Breastfeeding, which decreases the incidence of diabetes in the first 3 months after delivery.
- Screening before subsequent pregnancies

From Gutierrez YM VML: The emerging of diabetes: The intergenerational effect, *On the Cutting Edge* 23(2):12-15, 2002, with permission from Diabetes Care and Education, A Dietetic Practice Group of the American Dietetic Association.

BOX 19-13   METABOLIC SYNDROME

The term *metabolic syndrome* refers to a dangerous and deadly group of atherosclerotic risk factors (dyslipidemia, insulin resistance, obesity, and hypertension). It affects approximately 47 million people in the United States. A significant risk factor for the metabolic syndrome is central obesity. Treatment is vital because individuals with the metabolic syndrome quickly develop diabetes, coronary artery disease, and stroke. Treat-

ment is multifaceted, including diet, exercise, and pharmacologic treatment including statins, fibrates, angiotensin-converting enzyme (ACE) inhibitors, and thiazolidinediones.

Metabolic syndrome can be diagnosed using National Cholesterol Education Program (NCEP), Adult Treatment Panel III (ATP III), or International Diabetes Federation (IDF) criteria.

RISK FACTOR	NCEP ATP III CRITERIA	IDF CRITERIA
Central obesity	Men: waist circumference >102 cm (>40 in) Women: waist circumference >88 cm (>35 in)	Europoid, Sub-Saharan, Eastern Mediterranean and Middle East (Arab) men: waist circumference ≥94 cm for men Europoid, Sub-Saharan, Eastern Mediterranean and Middle East (Arab) women: waist circumference ≥80 cm South Asian, Chinese, ethnic South and Central American men: waist circumference ≥90 cm South Asian, Chinese, ethnic South and Central American women: waist circumference ≥80 cm Japanese men: waist circumference ≥85 cm Japanese women: waist circumference ≥90 cm
Triglycerides	≥150 mg/dL (1.7 mmol/L)	>150 mg/dL (1.7 mmol/L) or treatment for this lipid abnormality
High-density lipoprotein-cholesterol	Men: <40 mg/dL (0.9 mmol/L) Women: <50 mg/dL (1.1 mmol/L)	Men: <40 mg/dL (0.9 mmol/L) Women: <50 mg/dL (1.1 mmol/L) or specific treatment for this lipid abnormality
Blood pressure	≥130/≥85 mm Hg	≥130/≥85 mm Hg or treatment of previously diagnosed hypertension
Insulin resistance		Fasting plasma glucose >100 mg/dL (5.6 mmol/L) or previously diagnosed T2DM

Data from Scott CL: Diagnosis, prevention, and intervention for the metabolic syndrome, *Am J Cardiol* 92:35i-42i, 2003; Expert Panel on the Detection, Evaluation, and Treatment of High Blood Cholesterol in Adults: Executive summary of the Third Report of the National Cholesterol Education Program (NCEP) Expert Panel on the Detection, Evaluation, and Treatment of High Blood Cholesterol in Adults (Adult Treatment Panel III), *JAMA* 285:2486-2497, 2001; International Diabetes Federation: The IDF consensus worldwide definition of the metabolic syndrome [press release], Brussels, Belgium, 2005 (April 14), Author. Accessed March 29, 2010, from www.idf.org/webdata/docs/Metabolic_syndrome_definition.pdf.

accompanying complications will affect many more individuals, thus causing an enormous drain on resources. More Americans will be taking potent medications, which have side effects, for most of their lives. What has accompanied this epidemic of T2DM in children across the United States? The answer apparently lies within another epidemic: childhood obesity.[36]

Obesity is the most prominent clinical risk factor for T2DM in children and adolescents. About one-third of children with T2DM have a BMI greater than 40, indicating morbid obesity, and 17% have BMIs greater than 45 (normal BMI range for the pediatric population is 35 to 39).[36] Besides morbid obesity, other clinical signs that may indicate risk for T2DM include the following[36]:

- Acanthosis nigricans (hyperpigmentation and thickening of the skin into velvety irregular folds in the neck and flexural areas), which reflects chronic hyperinsulinemia (Box 19-13)
- Polycystic ovary syndrome (PCOS), which is associated with insulin resistance and obesity (Box 19-14)

- Hypertension, which may occur in 20% to 30% of patients with T2DM

Girls appear to be more susceptible than boys to T2DM, with an overall female-to-male ratio of 1.7:1 regardless of race.[36] In addition, adolescents with T2DM generally have obese parents who themselves tend to have insulin resistance or overt type 2 DM.[22] Reported cases of T2DM showed diagnosis to occur during the usual pubertal age period (ages 12 to 16 years).[36] Although there are currently insufficient data to make definite T2DM screening recommendations for children or adolescents, a panel of experts on children with diabetes developed the recommendations outlined in Box 19-15.

As with T2DM in adults, the ideal treatment goal is normalization of blood glucose values and A_{1C}. Successful control of associated comorbidities, such as hypertension and hyperlipidemia, is also important. The ultimate goal is to decrease risk of acute and chronic complications associated with diabetes. Initial treatment varies depending on clinical symptoms. The range of disease at diagnosis varies from asymptomatic hyperglycemia to DKA and hyperosmolar

BOX 19-14 POLYCYSTIC OVARY SYNDROME

Polycystic ovary syndrome (PCOS) is the most common hormonal reproductive problem a woman of reproductive age can have. It can affect menstrual cycle, fertility, hormones, insulin production, heart, blood vessels, and appearance. Clinical features include the following:

- High level of male hormones (hyperandrogenism)
- Menstrual dysfunction or anovulation
- Possible development of small cysts in ovaries
- Hyperinsulinemia, peripheral insulin resistance, or diabetes
- Luteinizing hormone hypersecretion
- Weight gain or obesity with upper body fat distribution
- Dyslipidemia, hypercholesterolemia
- Infertility or recurrent pregnancy loss
- Hirsutism
- Sleep apnea
- Acanthosis nigricans
- Adult acne

Approximately 5% to 10% of women in the United States have PCOS. Obesity is present in half, and approximately 10% of this group will develop T2DM by age 40. There is no single test to diagnose PCOS and there is no cure. Treatment is based on an individual's symptoms.

Women with PCOS may be at increased risk for endometrial hyperplasia or cancer. They are also at increased risk for diabetes and heart disease,

Data from National Women's Health Information Center: *Frequently asked questions about polycystic ovarian syndrome (PCOS)*, Fairfax, Va, 2010 (December), U.S. Department of Health and Human Services. Accessed March 29, 2010, from www.womenshealth.gov/faq/polycystic-ovary-syndrome.cfm.

BOX 19-15 TESTING FOR TYPE 2 DIABETES MELLITUS IN CHILDREN

Criteria	Overweight (BMI >85th percentile for age and gender, or weight for height >85th percentile, or weight >120% of ideal for height)
	Plus any two of the following risk factors:
	• Family history of T2DM in first- or second-degree relative
	• Race/ethnicity (Native American, African American, Latino, Asian American, Pacific Islander)
	• Signs of insulin resistance or conditions associated with insulin resistance (acanthosis nigricans, hypertension, dyslipidemia, or PCOS)
Age of initiation	10 years or at onset of puberty, if puberty occurs at a younger age
Frequency	Every 2 years
Test preferred	Fasting plasma glucose

Modified from American Diabetes Association: Standards of medical care in diabetes: 2010, *Diabetes Care* 33(Suppl 1):S11-S61, 2010; and Nelms MN, et al: *Nutrition therapy and pathophysiology*, ed 2, Belmont, Calif, 2010, Wadsworth/Cengage.

HHNS. Both DKA and HHNS are associated with high morbidity and mortality in children. Medical nutrition therapy and exercise are obvious first-line treatments, but most children diagnosed with T2DM will require drug therapy.[26] Although insulin is the only FDA-approved drug for treatment of diabetes in children, oral agents are most often used for children with T2DM.

All children with T2DM should receive comprehensive self-management education, including SMBG, referral to a registered dietitian with knowledge and experience in nutritional management of children with diabetes, behavior modification strategies for lifestyle changes, increased daily physical activity, and decreased sedentary activity (e.g., TV viewing and computer use).

Perhaps the relevance of this epidemic is best summed up by Levetan:[37]

Less than one century ago, there were no airplanes, no cars, and no fast-food restaurants. Not surprisingly, this phenomenal technologic growth has come at a price—an expanded girth that has extended not only to adults but also to children. This has resulted in a 70% rise in diabetes among 30- to 40-year-olds and a doubling in the number of children with type 2 diabetes in less than a decade.

SUMMARY

DM is a group of conditions characterized by either a relative or complete lack of insulin secretion by the beta cells of the pancreas or defects of cell insulin receptors, which results in disturbances of carbohydrate, protein, and lipid metabolism and hyperglycemia. Long-term complications often lead to disability and premature death. The complications may be related to the level and frequency of hyperglycemia experiences throughout the life span in addition to genetic and environmental factors.

The two primary categories of glucose intolerance are T1DM and T2DM. T1DM symptoms appear suddenly and include polyphagia, polyuria, polydipsia, and weight loss. Everyone with T1DM requires exogenous insulin to maintain normal blood glucose levels. The primary metabolic problem in T2DM is insulin resistance. Family history and obesity are the two strongest risk factors for T2DM. The gradually occurring symptoms of T2DM are polyuria, polydipsia, fatigue, and frequent infections. Some individuals with T2DM may require insulin to optimize blood glucose control. Additional types of diabetes include GDM, impaired glucose tolerance, and other less common forms of diabetes. Related conditions that may occur are hypoglycemia, DKA, and HHNS.

The main goal of treatment is maintenance of plasma insulin/glucose homeostasis. Treatment may include the use of insulin, medical nutrition therapy, and exercise. Control of blood glucose levels is the cornerstone of diabetes management and can be monitored several ways: (1) fasting blood glucose determination by reputable laboratories, (2) glycosylated hemoglobin determination by reputable laboratories, and (3) self-monitoring with standardized devices.

Medical nutrition therapy is an essential component of successful diabetes management, and the complexity involved requires a team approach to enhance the ability of the patient to obtain good metabolic control. The diabetes management team should include a registered nurse, a physician or primary health care provider, a registered dietitian, and the person

with diabetes. Successful medical nutrition therapy involves the diabetes management team conducting a thorough assessment, encouraging the patient's role in goal setting, implementing nutrition intervention, and regularly evaluating the nutrition care plan.

The current guidelines for medical nutrition therapy for diabetes management include to (1) plan for near normal blood sugar levels and optimal lipid levels; (2) individualize diet plans; (3) reach a reasonable weight; and (4) if desired, consume some sugar and foods that contain sugar if substituted for other carbohydrate foods. Nutrition recommendations for total fat, saturated fat, cholesterol, fiber, vitamins, and minerals are the same for individuals with diabetes as for the general population.

Recommendations are modified for protein, carbohydrates, sucrose, and alcohol because of the nature of diabetes in relation to carbohydrate metabolism or the effects of diabetic complications.

THE NURSING APPROACH

Case Studies: Type 1 and Type 2 Diabetes Mellitus

CASE STUDY #1: TYPE 1 DIABETES MELLITUS
Jason, age 15, has come to diabetes camp this summer for the first time. Diagnosed with type 1 diabetes mellitus (T1DM) two years ago, he is the only one in his family who has diabetes. He lives with his parents, a younger brother, and a younger sister. The camp nurse assessed Jason's situation and created a successful plan of care.

ASSESSMENT
Subjective (information told directly to the camp nurse)
* "My blood sugar has been bouncing all over the place."
* "The nurse practitioner suggested that I come to diabetes camp. I want to control my blood sugar so I can feel better."
* "I have been thinking about getting an insulin pump. I hate checking my blood sugar and giving myself shots. I take four shots a day now. I'd like a pump that will measure my blood sugar and give me insulin automatically."
* "I want to be the same as my friends. They can eat whatever they want whenever they want. I don't want to be different."

Objective (information from his camp admission record)
* Jason injects Lantus insulin (long acting) at bedtime and Humalog insulin (rapid acting) immediately before meals.
* He has not seen a dietitian since he was first diagnosed and does not follow any special meal plan.
* Last hemoglobin A$_{1c}$ was 8% (normal 4.4% to 6.7%)

DIAGNOSES (NURSING)
1. Health-seeking behaviors as evidenced by participation in diabetes camp and "I want to control my blood sugar so I can feel better"
2. Deficient knowledge: insulin pumps related to misinformation as evidenced by "I'd like a pump that will measure my blood sugar and give insulin automatically" and "I hate checking my blood sugar and giving myself shots" four times a day

PLANNING
Patient Outcomes
Short term (by the end of day two at camp):
* Jason will follow camp rules and participate fully in all activities and education sessions.
* He will have minimal or no episodes of hypoglycemia.
* He will observe how some campers use insulin pumps and will express interest in learning more.

Long term (by the end of camp in five days):
* He will make friends and express desire to return to camp next summer.
* He will set a goal to continue at home to follow his meal plan and to check blood glucose and give insulin before each meal and at bedtime.
* He will have minimal or no episodes of hypoglycemia.
* He will recognize that an insulin pump does not measure blood glucose and is not automatic.

Nursing Interventions
1. Set rules for camp and participate with campers in activities.
2. Give a presentation during an education session.
3. Be a role model by following a meal plan.
4. Be on call for emergencies.

IMPLEMENTATION
1. Established the following rules for diabetic campers. Each camper will:
   * Demonstrate to a counselor the correct technique for injecting insulin and using the camper's personal blood glucose meter.
   * Check and record blood glucose before each meal and at bedtime.
   * Follow the meal plan established by the camp dietitian.

Continued

- Follow the prescription for insulin determined by the camp doctor and meet with the camp doctor and nurse daily to discuss possible insulin adjustments.
- Report blood glucose below 60 (mg/dL) to a counselor or the camp nurse and consume crackers and juice as needed.
- Participate in all planned group activities and education sessions.
- Seek treatment for illness and injuries at the camp medical cabin.

Rules are set to create order and safety and a learning environment.

2. Accompanied campers to activities: swimming, boating, hiking, dancing, singing, and skits.

Activities provide fun and opportunities for campers to make friends. Campers learn how to recognize and treat hypoglycemia that may occur following exercise. The nurse is present to treat emergencies and mingle socially with the campers.

3. Taught classes regarding sick day management and recognition and treatment of hypoglycemia.

Camp provides practical diabetes education and prepares campers to recognize and report problems of hyperglycemia and hypoglycemia.

4. Wore a fanny pack containing blood glucose testing equipment, glucose tablets, glucagon, and glucose for intravenous administration.

Quick action is needed to treat hypoglycemia, as follows:

- If blood glucose results are below 60 mg/dL and the camper is alert, a camper can eat glucose tablets or food containing 15 g of carbohydrate. After waiting 15 minutes, the camper should recheck the blood glucose. If it is still low, the camper should again eat 15 g of food.
- When a camper is not responsive enough to eat glucose, glucagon can be given subcutaneously.
- If necessary, a needle can be inserted into a vein for immediate injection of concentrated glucose.

5. Was on call for emergencies each night.

Many episodes of hypoglycemia occur during the night. Sometimes a camper may fall from his or her bed with severe hypoglycemia, and this awakens counselors or other campers so they can seek help.

6. Served as a role model, following a meal plan established by the camp dietitian. Selected foods according to serving sizes and number of carbohydrates in an individualized meal plan. Measured foods, using measuring cups and spoons.

Campers need good role models. They learn serving sizes by measuring foods.

EVALUATION (BY THE CAMP NURSE)

Short term (at the end of two days):

- Jason had made friends and was having fun at activities.
- He checked his blood glucose four times a day, followed his meal plan, and gave himself insulin before each meal and at bedtime, based on his doctor's prescription.
- He had no episodes of hypoglycemia.
- Jason expressed interest in learning more about insulin pumps.
- Goals met.

Long term (at the end of camp on day five:

- Jason stated he wanted to keep in touch with friends from camp and return to camp next summer.
- He said he wanted to continue measuring his blood glucose four times a day, follow his meal plan, and give insulin four times a day at home.
- He learned a lot about insulin pumps from friends at camp. He recognized that a pump does not measure blood glucose and is not automatic. He said he wants to learn more about carbohydrate counting and insulin pumps (See Box 19-8).
- He had one episode of hypoglycemia late at night after hiking and swimming and treated it successfully with juice, crackers, and cheese.
- Goals met.

DISCUSSION QUESTIONS

Risk for Hypoglycemia is another nursing diagnosis that could be added to Jason's care plan. Jason witnessed the nurse giving one of the campers a glucagon injection when the camper's blood sugar was low and he was not alert enough to eat anything.

1. How does a glucagon injection raise blood sugar? After a client becomes more alert, what food should be given? Why?
2. How could Jason begin to learn about carbohydrate servings by reading exchange lists for diabetes?

CASE STUDY #2: TYPE 2 DIABETES MELLITUS

Juanita, age 47, is from Mexico and has been newly diagnosed with type 2 diabetes mellitus (T2DM). She speaks only a few words in English. Juanita's daughter, Maria, has accompanied her to the health clinic because she is bilingual and can act as an interpreter. Maria works as an accountant and is computer literate. Juanita was given a nutrition instruction sheet by the doctor, but she could not read the English words, so she came to the clinic to learn what she should eat. Because the dietitian would not be available to meet with Juanita until two weeks later, the nurse gave initial instructions to Juanita and Maria.

ASSESSMENT

Subjective (directly from Juanita or interpreted by her daughter)

- "My daughter told me what the instruction sheet said, but it doesn't have any of the foods I usually eat. Do I have to change everything I eat?"
- "The doctor said I shouldn't eat sugar anymore."
- "If I eat right, I don't need to take any diabetes medicine."
- "I usually cook tacos or enchiladas or burritos for my family. Can't I just eat what they eat?"
- "I don't go walking very often. I usually stay home."

Objective (from physical exam and Juanita's medical record)

- Height 5 feet, weight 135 pounds
- Blood glucose 160 mg/dL today one hour after eating lunch
- The doctor diagnosed diabetes after treating Juanita for a vaginal yeast infection and obtaining labwork needed for a diagnosis of diabetes.
- No diabetes medicine was prescribed.

THE NURSING APPROACH—cont'd

Case Studies: Type 1 and Type 2 Diabetes Mellitus—cont'd

DIAGNOSES (NURSING)

1. Deficient knowledge: dietary management of diabetes related to new diagnosis as evidenced by desire to know what to eat, "Do I have to change everything I eat?" and "The doctor said I shouldn't eat sugar anymore."
2. Imbalanced nutrition: more than body requirements related to excess food and inadequate exercise as evidenced by 135% ideal body weight

PLANNING

Patient Outcomes

Short term (by the end of this visit):
- Juanita will understand that the main dietary focuses are healthy food choices and weight loss.
- She will agree to read the Spanish resources about diabetes.
- She and her daughter will make an appointment to meet with the dietitian as soon as possible.

Nursing Interventions

1. Stress the importance of healthy food choices and weight loss.
2. Provide resources in Spanish.

IMPLEMENTATION

1. Told Juanita that she could still eat foods she prepares for her family, although it would be healthy for all to limit fat and sugar and salt.

   Meal plans are designed for individuals based on usual eating patterns and preferences. Healthy food choices are applicable to the entire family.
2. Explained that Juanita should focus on small serving sizes in order to lose weight, which would improve diabetes control and general health.

   When an overweight or obese person with T2DM loses weight, glucose resistance is reduced and cardiovascular health is improved.
3. Gave Juanita a Spanish pamphlet "Choose Your Foods: Plan Your Meals" (2009, American Diabetes Association and American Dietetic Association).

   This guide is a good introduction to healthy eating for people with diabetes, preparing the patient to meet with a dietitian. Brochures are generally helpful when written in the patient's language.
4. Informed Maria that the American Diabetes Association has Spanish educational materials at www.diabetes.org.

Authoritative resources are available for Hispanic/Latino patients who are newly diagnosed with diabetes. Many resources at American Diabetes Association are free, and cooking books for Latinos may be purchased.

5. Wrote down government websites for Spanish pamphlets about diabetes:
   - National Diabetes Education Program at www.ndep.nih.gov (e.g., "Tasty Recipes for People With Diabetes and Their Families," 2008, specifically designed for Latin Americans)
   - National Institute of Diabetes & Digestive & Kidney Diseases at www.diabetes.niddk.nih.gov (e.g., "What I Need to Know About Eating and Diabetes," 2008)

   Many free Spanish resources are available from the government to help patients understand diabetes and what to eat.
6. Encouraged Juanita and her daughter to make an appointment to meet with the dietitian as soon as possible.

   The dietitian can design an individualized meal plan for the patient.
7. Suggested that Juanita make an appointment with the doctor for follow-up diabetes management and to ask about safe exercise, such as walking.

   Regular visits to the doctor are important to good diabetes management. The level of exercise should be determined by the doctor who knows about the patient's medical condition.

EVALUATION

Short term (at the end of the visit):
- Juanita and her daughter identified healthy food choices and weight loss as the main focuses for eating
- They agreed to read the Spanish version of "Choose Your Foods: Plan Your Meals."
- Maria indicated that she would visit the websites suggested.
- They made appointments with the dietitian and the doctor.
- Goals met.

DISCUSSION QUESTIONS

1. What are the basic differences between a healthy food pyramid and a diabetes food pyramid?
2. How could you help Maria explain the importance of appropriate serving sizes?

Nursing Diagnoses-Definitions and Classification 2009-2011. Copyright © 2009, 1994-2009 by NANDA International. Used by arrangement with Blackwell Publishing Limited, a company of John Wiley & Sons, Inc.

CRITICAL THINKING

Clinical Applications

Alan, age 75, is a white man admitted to the hospital following a cerebrovascular accident. He has a history of T2DM, hypertension, moderate obesity, and possible alcohol abuse. Medications on admission include furosemide (Lasix), hydrochlorothiazide, propranolol (Inderal), and chlorpropamide (Diabinese) 500 mg bid. Alan comes to the clinic regularly, and at his last visit he complained of blurred vision, polydipsia, polyuria, and a weight loss of 8 pounds in the past 2 weeks. He was admitted to the hospital with a diagnosis of urinary tract infection and hyperglycemic hyperosmolar nonketotic (HHNS) syndrome. Physical examination revealed the following:

- Height: 5 feet 11 inches
- Weight: 215 pounds
- Blood pressure: 160/82

- Cholesterol: 380 mg/dL
- Triglycerides: 300 mg/dL
- Blood sugar: 750 mg/dL
- Family history: Sister has had T2DM for 10 years
1. Explain how Alan's blood glucose level could become so high without producing ketones.
2. If this patient's HHNS is not treated, how would you expect his disease to progress?

3. What are Alan's blood glucose and lipid goals?
4. What is the purpose of the prescribed medications? Are there any possible drug-nutrient interactions?
5. How frequently should blood sugars be monitored?
6. What are possible complications?

WEBSITES OF INTEREST

American Diabetes Association (ADA)

www.diabetes.org

Educates and sponsors community services and research to prevent, cure and manage diabetes.

National Diabetes Information Clearinghouse (NDIC)

http://diabetes.niddk.nih.gov/

Functions as a diabetes information dissemination service of the National Institute of Diabetes and Digestive and Kidney Diseases (NIDDK), National Institutes of Health (NIH).

American Association of Diabetes Educators (AADE)

http://aadenet.org

As the accreditation association for diabetes educators, AADE educates and supports diabetes educators as they lead clients to self-management of diabetes and related chronic conditions.

REFERENCES

1. American Diabetes Association: *Diabetes statistics*, Alexandria, Va, Author. Accessed March 14, 2010, from www.diabetes.org/diabetes-statistics/dangerous-toll.jsp.
2. Centers for Disease Control and Prevention: *National diabetes fact sheet: general information and national estimates on diabetes in the United States*, Atlanta, 2007, U.S. Department of Health and Human Services, Centers for Disease Control and Prevention, 2008. Accessed March 14, 2010, from www.cdc.gov/diabetes/pubs/pdf/ndfs_2007.pdf.
3. American Diabetes Association: Diagnosis and classification of diabetes mellitus, *Diabetes Care* 31:S55-S60, 2008.
4. American Diabetes Association: Economic costs of diabetes in the U.S. in 2007, *Diabetes Care* 31:596-615, 2008.
5. The Oxford Centre for Diabetes, Endocrinology & Metabolism, Diabetes Trials Unit: *UK prospective diabetes study*, Oxford, United Kingdom, Author. Accessed March 29, 2010, from www.dtu.ox.ac.uk/.
6. American Diabetes Association: Implications of the diabetes control and complications trial (position statement), *Diabetes Care* 26(Suppl 1):S25-S27, 2003.
7. Ousman Y, Sharma M: The irrefutable importance of glycemic control, *Clin Diabetes* 19:71-72, 2001.
8. Diabetes Control and Complications Trial Research Group: The effect of intensive treatment of diabetes on the development and progression of long-term complications in insulin-dependent diabetes mellitus, *N Engl J Med* 329:977-986, 1993.
9. American Diabetes Association: Implications of the United Kingdom Prospective Diabetes Study (position statement), *Diabetes Care* 26:S28-S32, 2003.
10. Palmer JP, Hirsch IB: What's in a name: Latent autoimmune diabetes of adults, type 1.5, adult-onset, and type 1 diabetes, *Diabetes Care* 26(2):536-538, 2003.

11. Nabhan F, Emanuele MA, Emanuele N: Latent autoimmune diabetes of adulthood, *Postgrad Med Online* 117(3):7-12, 2005. Accessed March 28, 2010, from www.postgradmed.com.
12. Notkins AL, Lernmark A: Autoimmune type 1 diabetes: resolved and unresolved issues, *J Clin Invest* 108:1247-1252, 2001.
13. Cihakova D, Johns Hopkins Medical Institutions Autoimmune Disease Research Center: *Type 1 diabetes mellitus*, Baltimore, 2000 (modified September 10, 2001), Johns Hopkins University School of Medicine & Johns Hopkins Health System. Accessed March 29, 2010, from http://autoimmune.pathology.jhmi.edu/diseases.cfm?systemID=3&DiseaseID=23.
14. National Institute of Diabetes and Digestive and Kidney Diseases: *National diabetes statistics, 2007 fact sheet*, Bethesda, Md, 2008, U.S. Department of Health and Human Services, National Institutes of Health. Accessed March 29, 2010, from http://diabetes.niddk.nih.gov/dm/pubs/statistics/index.htm.
15. Rystrom JK: Insulin therapy. In Ross TA, Boucher JL, O'Connell BS, editors: *American Dietetic Association guide to diabetes: Medical nutrition therapy and education*, Chicago, 2005, American Dietetic Association.
16. Sigal RJ, et al: Physical activity/exercise and type 2 diabetes, *Diabetes Care* 27:2518-2539, 2004.
17. American Diabetes Association: Physical activity/exercise and diabetes, *Diabetes Care* 27(Suppl 1):S58-S62, 2004.
18. Copstead LC, Banasik JL: *Pathophysiology*, ed 3, St. Louis, 2005, Saunders.
19. National Institute of Diabetes & Digestive & Kidney Diseases: *Diabetes mellitus: Challenges and opportunities. Final report and recommendations. Full report of participants in the Trans-NIH symposium*, Bethesda, Md, 1997, National Institutes of Health.

Accessed March 29, 2010, from http://www2.niddk.nih.gov/AboutNIDDK/ReportsAndStrategicPlanning/Interim_Evaluation_Report_1997.htm.

20. Kissebah AH, et al: Relation of body fat distribution to metabolic complications of obesity, *J Clin Endocrinol Metab* 54:254-260, 1982.

21. Votey SR, Peters AL: Diabetes mellitus, type 2—A review, New York (updated January 29, 2010), eMedicine/WebMD. Accessed March 29, 2010, from http://emedicine.medscape.com/article/766143-overview.

22. Freeman J: Oral diabetes medications. In Ross TA, Boucher JL, O'Connell BS, editors: *American Dietetic Association guide to diabetes: Medical nutrition therapy and education*, Chicago, 2005, American Dietetic Association.

23. American Diabetes Association: Standards of medical care in diabetes: 2010, *Diabetes Care* 33(Suppl 1):S11-S61, 2010.

24. American Diabetes Association: Translation of the diabetes nutrition recommendations for health care institutions, *Diabetes Care* 26(Suppl 1):S70-S72, 2003.

25. Pastors JG, Waslaski J, Gunderson H: Diabetes meal-planning strategies. In Ross TA, Boucher JL, O'Connell BS, editors: *American Dietetic Association guide to diabetes: Medical nutrition therapy and education*, Chicago, 2005, American Dietetic Association.

26. Franz MJ, et al: Evidence-based nutrition principles and recommendations for the treatment and prevention of diabetes and related complications. *Diabetes Care* 25(1):148-198, 2002.

27. American Diabetes Association: Nutrition principles and recommendations in diabetes, *Diabetes Care* 27(Suppl 1):S36-S46, 2004.

28. Schlundt DG, et al: Situational obstacles to dietary adherence for adults with diabetes, *J Am Diet Assoc* 94:874-876, 879, 1994.

29. Franz MJ, Joynes JO: *Diabetes and brief illness*, Minneapolis, 1993, International Diabetes Center.

30. Escott-Stump S: *Nutrition and diagnosis-related care*, ed 6, Baltimore, 2007, Lippincott Williams & Wilkins.

31. Rizzo T, et al: Correlations between antepartum maternal metabolism and child intelligence, *N Engl J Med* 325:911-916, 1991.

32. American Diabetes Association: Gestational diabetes mellitus (position statement), *Diabetes Care* 27(Suppl 1):S88-S90, 2004.

33. Reader D: Diabetes in pregnancy and lactation. In Ross TA, Boucher JL, O'Connell BS, editors: *American Dietetic Association guide to diabetes: Medical nutrition therapy and education*, Chicago, 2005, American Dietetic Association.

34. American Diabetes Association: Preconception care of women with diabetes, *Diabetes Care* 27(Suppl 1):S76-S78, 2004.

35. American Diabetes Association: Type 2 diabetes in children and adolescents, *Pediatrics* 105(3 Pt 1):671-680, 2000.

36. American Diabetes Association: Type 2 diabetes in children and adolescents, *Diabetes Care* 23:381-389, 2000.

37. Levetan C: Into the mouths of babes: The diabetes epidemic in children, *Clin Diabetes* 19:102-104, 2001.

Nutrition for Cardiovascular and Respiratory Diseases

The term cardiovascular disease *encompasses a group of diseases and conditions affecting the heart and blood vessels: coronary artery disease (also referred to as coronary heart disease), hypertension, peripheral vascular disease, congestive heart failure, and congenital heart disease.*

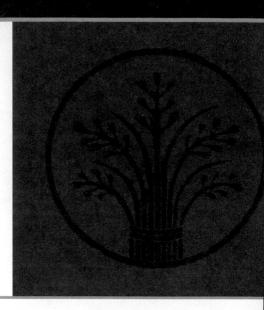

evolve WEBSITE

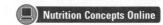
Nutrition Concepts Online

http://evolve.elsevier.com/Grodner/foundations/

ROLE IN WELLNESS

Nurses working in varied settings play a major role in teaching people how to reduce cardiovascular risk factors through lifestyle changes, including reinforcement of dietary modifications. Although dietitians are responsible for developing the medical nutrition plan and for the majority of diet education instruction, nurses reinforce that teaching and answer any additional questions of patients and their families. Therefore, familiarity with diet as it affects cardiovascular disease is essential.

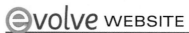
The term *cardiovascular disease (CVD)* encompasses a group of diseases and conditions that affect the heart and blood vessels: coronary artery disease (CAD) (also called *coronary heart disease [CHD]*), hypertension (HTN), *peripheral vascular disease (PVD)*, congestive heart failure (CHF), and congenital heart diseases. CVD has been a public health issue since 1900 and is currently the leading cause of death in the United States for both men and women in all ethnic and racial groups. While death rates from CVD have declined, the burden of the disease remains high. More than 2300 lives are claimed each day by CVD—an average of 1 death every 38 seconds. Cardiovascular disease kills more Americans each year than the next four leading causes of death combined.[1] Most people who have heart attacks die before they ever reach a hospital for treatment, a situation that emphasizes the need for prevention of heart disease.

Although CVD has been a public health concern for decades, health professionals cannot assume that newly diagnosed CAD patients, regardless of education or socioeconomic level, are knowledgeable of the disorder and treatment approaches. Primary prevention is a public health matter. These approaches often include implementing secondary and tertiary preventive strategies. Secondary prevention behaviors reduce the effects of a disease or illness. For CVD, reducing risk factors can minimize negative health effects. The purpose of tertiary prevention is to minimize further complications or to assist in the restoration of health. For CVD, these efforts may involve significant lifestyle changes combined with medication and other medical care. Learning more about the disorder is often helpful for patients and their families (see the *Personal Perspectives* box, Go Red for Women).

Several risk factors for cardiovascular disease are modifiable or altogether preventable; nonetheless, more than 80% of adult Americans have at least one major risk factor. Risk factors are categorized into two groups: modifiable and nonmodifiable (Table 20-1).

A way to understand the far-reaching effects of CVD is to consider this group of diseases and disorders through the five dimensions of health. Of course, the *physical health* dimension is affected as CVD affects the heart, an essential organ; this disease impairs functioning of many body systems. Determining one's own risk factors and devising a program to reduce their effects depends on *intellectual health*. The *emotional health* dimension is stressed because client denial may occur; some individuals view heart problems as something that happens only to other people. Mortality caused by CVD, as well as the many lifestyle modifications necessary, may be frightening—how can we reassure clients and yet still assist them to change behaviors? Because of increased education through the work of health associations and health departments, many restaurants and resorts serve "heart healthy" entrées; with careful selections, socializing can continue unaffected, thereby supporting the *social health* dimension. Ability to cope with physical limitations because of chronic illnesses such as heart disease and diabetes may depend on the *spiritual health* dimension manifested through

Go Red for Women

Go Red for Women is a national campaign of the American Heart Association. The movement encourages women to engage in heart-healthy activities to reduce their personal risk of heart disease, the number one killer of women. The message of the movement, Love Your Heart, spreads awareness that prevention is possible—one heart at a time through the empowerment of women. Go Red for Women local events take place in most communities. The National Wear Red Day, the major event of the campaign, asks everyone to wear something red to highlight ways to reduce risks by simple acts such as the following:

- Seeing a health care provider
- Consuming a healthier diet
- Being more physically active
- Educating others about heart disease

So when everyone—men are welcome to join in—is wearing red blouses, dresses, ties, lipstick, shoes, or jackets, think Love Your Heart! For more information, visit Go Red for Women at www.goredforwomen.org.

Data from American Heart Association: *Go red for women*, Dallas, 2006, Author. Accessed April 7, 2010, from www.goredforwomen.org.

an optimistic attitude and a desire to fight back to achieve the most positive response of the body.

CORONARY ARTERY DISEASE

The underlying pathologic process responsible for coronary artery disease (CAD) is atherosclerosis (Figure 20-1). Beginning in childhood, atherosclerosis may gradually lead to arteriosclerosis.[3] The most common and serious manifestation of atherosclerosis is development of lesions in coronary arteries that can cause angina pectoris if blood flow is partially occluded by a thrombus. If blood flow to the heart is completely occluded, then a myocardial infarction occurs. If thrombosis occurs in a cerebral artery, a cerebrovascular accident (CVA) or stroke occurs. PVD occurs when atherosclerosis in the abdominal aorta, iliac arteries, and femoral arteries produces temporary insufficient blood flow in the arteries on exertion (intermittent claudication) or ischemic necrosis of the extremities, which may lead to gangrene.[4]

The most frequent approach in assessing CAD risk is to measure cholesterol and proportions of the different types of plasma lipoproteins that carry cholesterol in the blood.

TABLE 20-1	MAJOR RISK FACTORS IN CARDIOVASCULAR DISEASE	
LIPID RISK FACTORS	**NONLIPID RISK FACTORS**	
	MODIFIABLE	**NONMODIFIABLE**
LDL cholesterol (>100 mg/dL) ↓ HDL cholesterol (<40 mg/dL)	Tobacco smoke and exposure to tobacco smoke High serum cholesterol (>200 mg/dL) Hypertension (≥140/50 mm Hg) Physical inactivity	Male gender Increasing age (men ≥45 years, women ≥55 years) Heredity (including race) Family history of premature CHD (MI or sudden death <55 years of age in father or other male first-degree relative, or <65 years of age in mother or other female first-degree relatives)
Triglycerides (>150 mg/dL)	Obesity (BMI >30 kg/m²) and overweight (BMI 25-29.9 kg/m²) Diabetes mellitus Atherogenic diet (↑ intakes of saturated fats and cholesterol) Stress and coping Excessive alcohol consumption (>1 drink/day for women and >2 drinks/day for men) Individual response to stress and coping Some illegal drugs (cocaine and IV drug abuse)	

BMI, Body mass index; *CHD*, coronary heart disease; *HDL*, high-density lipoprotein; *LDL*, low-density lipoprotein; *MI*, myocardial infarction. Data from Banasik JL: Alterations in cardiac function. In Copstead LC, Banasik JL, eds: *Pathophysiology*, ed 3, St. Louis, 2005, Saunders; American Heart Association: *Heart and stroke facts*, Dallas, 1992-2003, Author. Accessed April 7, 2010, from www.americanheart.org/presenter.jhtml?identifier=3000333; Grundy SM, et al: Primary prevention of coronary heart disease: guidance from Framingham, *Circulation* 97:1876-1887, 1998; National Cholesterol Education Program (NCEP): *Third report of the NCEP expert panel on detection, evaluation, and treatment of high blood cholesterol in adults (Adult Treatment Panel III): executive summary*, NIH Pub No 01-3670, Washington, DC, 2001 (May), National Institutes of Health, National Heart, Lung, and Blood Institute; National Cholesterol Education Program (NCEP): *Third report of the NCEP expert panel on detection, evaluation, and treatment of high blood cholesterol in adults (Adult Treatment Panel III)*, Washington, DC, 2001, National Institutes of Health, National Heart, Lung, and Blood Institute.

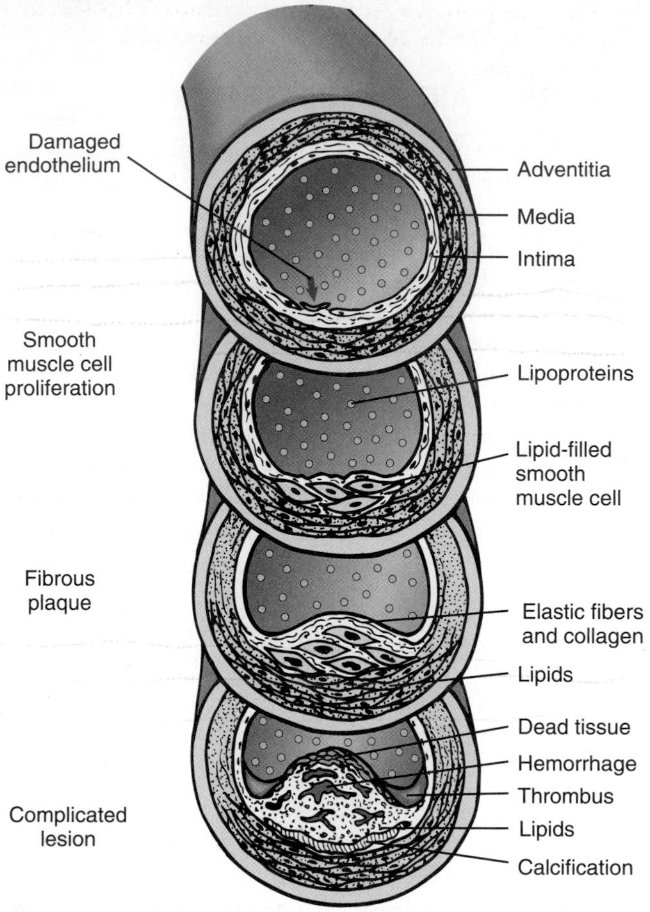
Damaged endothelium
Adventitia
Media
Intima
Smooth muscle cell proliferation
Lipoproteins
Lipid-filled smooth muscle cell
Fibrous plaque
Elastic fibers and collagen
Lipids
Dead tissue
Hemorrhage
Thrombus
Complicated lesion
Lipids
Calcification

FIG 20-1 **Pathogenesis of atherosclerosis.** (From Copstead-Kirkhorn L-E, Banasik JL: *Pathophysiology,* ed 3, St. Louis, 2005, Mosby.)

Cholesterol is a not actually a lipid, but it travels in the bloodstream in spherical particles called *lipoproteins,* which contain lipids and proteins. Cholesterol is an essential component of cell membranes and a precursor of bile acids and steroid hormones and is not required in the diet after weaning. Plasma lipid profile is commonly measured by analyzing the three major classes of lipoproteins in blood from a fasting individual: very low-density lipoproteins (VLDL), low-density lipoproteins (LDL), and high-density lipoproteins (HDL). LDL cholesterol contains approximately 60% to 70% of total serum cholesterol (TC), and high serum levels are causally related to increased risk of CAD. HDLs usually contain 20% to 30% of the total cholesterol, and serum levels are inversely correlated with risk for CAD. VLDLs are largely composed of triglyceride, which contains 10% to 15% of the TC[5] (Box 20-1).

The National Cholesterol Education Program (NCEP) Adult Treatment Panel III (ATP III) report[6] emphasizes LDL cholesterol as the primary target for cholesterol-lowering therapy. The report cites research from laboratory investigations, epidemiologic research, and clinical trials that robustly show LDL-lowering therapy reduces risk for CHD. Therefore, primary goals of therapy are stated in terms of LDL cholesterol (Box 20-2).

Another risk factor for CHD is elevated triglyceride levels.[5,6] Triglyceride is the most common type of fat found in the body. The body gets triglyceride directly from foods and makes it in the liver from carbohydrates, alcohol, and some cholesterol. Serum triglyceride levels range from about 50 to 250 mg/dL.[7] Several factors that may cause triglyceride levels to be elevated are as follows:

- Overweight and obesity
- Physical inactivity
- Cigarette smoking
- Excess alcohol intake
- Very high carbohydrate intake (>60% of total energy)
- Other diseases (e.g., type 2 diabetes mellitus, chronic renal failure, nephrotic syndrome)

BOX 20-1 PLASMA LIPOPROTEINS

- Synthesized primarily in the liver
- Contain varying amounts of triglycerides, cholesterol, phospholipids, and proteins
- Classified according to composition and density
- Kinds of plasma lipoproteins: chylomicrons, high-density lipoproteins (HDLs), low-density lipoproteins (LDLs), and very low-density lipoproteins (VLDLs)

BOX 20-2 ADULT TREATMENT PANEL III CLASSIFICATION OF LDL, TOTAL, AND HDL CHOLESTEROL (MG/DL)

LDL Cholesterol	
<100	Optimal
100-129	Near optimal/above optimal
130-159	Borderline high
160-189	High
≥190	Very high
Total Cholesterol	
<200	Desirable
200-239	Borderline high
≥240	High
HDL Cholesterol	
<40	Low
>60	High

HDL, High-density lipoprotein; *LDL,* low-density lipoprotein.
From National Cholesterol Education Program (NCEP): *Third report of the NCEP expert panel on detection, evaluation, and treatment of high blood cholesterol in adults (Adult Treatment Panel III): Executive summary,* NIH Pub No 01-3670, Washington, DC, 2001 (May), National Institutes of Health, National Heart, Lung, and Blood Institute; National Cholesterol Education Program (NCEP): *Third report of the NCEP expert panel on detection, evaluation, and treatment of high blood cholesterol in adults (Adult Treatment Panel III),* Washington, DC, 2001, National Institutes of Health, National Heart, Lung, and Blood Institute.

TABLE 20-2	CLASSIFICATION OF SERUM TRIGLYCERIDES	
TRIGLYCERIDE CATEGORY	**ATP III LEVELS**	
Normal	<150 mg/dL	
Borderline high	150 to 199 mg/dL	
High	200 to 499 mg/dL	
Very high	≥500 mg/dL	

ATP, Adult Treatment Panel.
From National Cholesterol Education Program (NCEP): *Third report of the NCEP expert panel on detection, evaluation, and treatment of high blood cholesterol in adults (Adult Treatment Panel III)*, Washington, DC, 2001, National Institutes of Health, National Heart, Lung, and Blood Institute.

- Certain drugs (e.g., corticosteroids, protease inhibitors for human immunodeficiency virus [HIV], beta-adrenergic blocking agents, estrogens)
- Genetic factors

After evaluating available research, the ATP III panel concluded that the association between serum triglyceride and CHD is stronger than previously recognized and it considers elevated serum levels as a factor to identify people at risk who are in need of intervention for risk reduction.[5,6] Classifications of triglyceride levels are outlined in Table 20-2.

The ATP III report cites convincing epidemiologic evidence identifying HDL cholesterol as a strong independent and inverse risk factor for increased CHD morbidity and mortality.[6] Low HDL cholesterol is defined as a level of less than 40 mg/dL in both men and women.[6] Factors contributing to low HDL cholesterol levels include the following:

- Elevated serum triglyceride levels
- Overweight and obesity
- Physical inactivity
- Cigarette smoking
- Very high carbohydrate intake (>60% of total energy)
- Type 2 diabetes mellitus
- Certain drugs (e.g., beta blockers, anabolic steroids, progestational agents)
- Genetic factors

Often, a common form of dyslipidemia (atherogenic dyslipidemia) characterized by three lipid abnormalities (elevated triglycerides, small LDL particles, and low HDL cholesterol) is seen in people with premature CHD.[6] Characteristics of individuals with atherogenic dyslipidemia are obesity, abdominal obesity, insulin resistance, and physical inactivity.[8] Because each component of atherogenic dyslipidemia is individually atherogenic, the combination is considered an independent risk factor.[6] Lifestyle modification—weight control and increased physical activity—is the treatment of choice[6] (see the *Cultural Considerations* box, Using T'ai Chi to Reduce Cardiovascular Risk Factors).

Nonlipid Risk Factors

Several nonlipid risk factors are associated with increased CHD risk and are targets for intervention in preventive

efforts. Fixed risk factors (increasing age, male gender, and family history of premature CHD) cannot be modified, and their existence implies need for intensive lowering of LDL cholesterol.[6] Modifiable nonlipid risk factors include hypertension, cigarette smoking, diabetes, obesity, physical inactivity, and atherogenic diet. Table 20-1 summarizes CHD risk factors other than elevated LDL cholesterol.

Nutrition Therapy

The ATP III report[5,6] recommends a comprehensive lifestyle approach to reducing risk for CHD called *Therapeutic Lifestyle Changes (TLC)*, which incorporates the following components:[5,6]

- Reduced intake of saturated fats and cholesterol
- Therapeutic dietary options to enhance lowering of LDL (e.g., plant stanols/sterols and increased soluble fiber)
- Weight reduction
- Increased regular physical activity

TABLE 20-3	ESSENTIAL COMPONENTS OF THERAPEUTIC LIFESTYLE CHANGES (TLC)
COMPONENT	**RECOMMENDATION**
LDL-Raising Nutrients	
Saturated fats	<7% of total energy intake
Dietary cholesterol	<200 mg/day
Therapeutic Options for Lowering LDL	
Plant stanols/sterols	2 g/day
Soluble fiber	10 to 25 g/day
Total energy (kcal)	Adjust total energy intake to maintain desirable body weight and prevent weight gain
Physical activity	Include enough moderate exercise to expend at least 200 kcal/day

LDL, Low-density lipoprotein.
Data from National Cholesterol Education Program (NCEP): *Third report of the NCEP expert panel on detection, evaluation, and treatment of high blood cholesterol in adults (Adult Treatment Panel III),* Washington, DC, 2001, National Institutes of Health, National Heart, Lung, and Blood Institute.

TABLE 20-4	NUTRIENT COMPOSITION OF THE THERAPEUTIC LIFESTYLE CHANGES (TLC) DIET
COMPONENT	**RECOMMENDATION**
Polyunsaturated fat	Up to 10% total energy intake
Monounsaturated fat	Up to 20% total energy intake
Total fat	25% to 35% total energy intake*
Carbohydrate†	50% to 60% total energy intake
Dietary fiber	20 to 30 g/day
Protein	Approximately 15% total energy intake

*ATP III allows for increase of total fat to 35% total energy intake and reduction in carbohydrate to 50% for people with the metabolic syndrome. Any increase in fat intake should be in the form of either polyunsaturated or monounsaturated fat.
†Carbohydrates should come primarily from foods rich in complex carbohydrates including grains—especially whole grains—fruits, and vegetables.
Data from National Cholesterol Education Program (NCEP): *Third report of the NCEP expert panel on detection, evaluation, and treatment of high blood cholesterol in adults (Adult Treatment Panel III): executive summary,* NIH Pub No 01-3670, Washington, DC, 2001 (May), National Institutes of Health, National Heart, Lung, and Blood Institute; National Cholesterol Education Program (NCEP): *Third report of the NCEP expert panel on detection, evaluation, and treatment of high blood cholesterol in adults (Adult Treatment Panel III),* Washington, DC, 2001, National Institutes of Health, National Heart, Lung, and Blood Institute.

Components of TLC are outlined in Table 20-3. ATP III also suggests ranges for other macronutrients in the TLC diet (Table 20-4). Overall, composition of the TLC diet is consistent with recommendations of the *Dietary Guidelines for Americans* (see Chapter 2). Box 20-3 outlines the ATP III's TLC recommendations.

Components and Application of the Therapeutic Lifestyle Changes (TLC) Diet

Saturated fat and cholesterol. Reducing saturated fat (<7% of total energy intake) and cholesterol (<200 mg/day) in the diet is the foundation of the TLC diet.[6] The strongest nutritional influence on serum LDL cholesterol levels is saturated fats. Moreover, there is a "dose response relationship" between saturated fats and LDL cholesterol levels.[6] For every 1% increase in kcal from saturated fats as a percent of total energy, serum LDL cholesterol increases roughly 2%. Conversely, a 1% decrease in saturated fats will lower serum cholesterol by about 2%.[8]

Although weight reduction by itself, even of a few pounds, will reduce LDL cholesterol levels,[6] weight reduction achieved using a kcal-controlled diet low in saturated fats and cholesterol will enhance and maintain LDL cholesterol reductions.[6,8] Although dietary cholesterol does not have the equivalent impact of saturated fat on serum LDL cholesterol levels,[6] high cholesterol intakes increase LDL cholesterol levels.[6,9] Therefore, reducing dietary cholesterol to less than 200 mg per day decreases serum LDL cholesterol in most people.[6]

Monounsaturated fat. Substitution of monounsaturated fat for saturated fats at an intake level of up to 20% of total energy intake is recommended on the TLC diet.[6] Monounsaturated fats lower LDL cholesterol levels relative to saturated fats[6] without decreasing HDL cholesterol or triglyceride levels.[6,11] The best sources of monounsaturated fats are plant oils and nuts.[6] (See Box 5-1 for a listing of plant oils and nuts.)

Polyunsaturated fats. When used instead of saturated fats, polyunsaturated fats, in particular linoleic acid, reduce LDL cholesterol levels. On the other hand they can also bring about small reductions in HDL cholesterol when compared side by side with monounsaturated fats.[6] Liquid vegetables oils, semiliquid margarines, and other margarines low in trans fatty acids are recommended by the TLC diet as the best sources of polyunsaturated fats. Recommended intakes can range up to 10% of total energy intake.[6]

Total fat. Saturated fats and trans fatty acids increase LDL cholesterol levels,[10] whereas serum levels of LDL cholesterol do not appear to be affected by total fat intake.[6] For that reason, the ATP III suggests it is not essential to limit total fat intake for the particular goal of reducing LDL cholesterol levels, provided saturated fats are decreased to goal levels.[6]

Carbohydrate. When saturated fats are replaced with carbohydrates, LDL cholesterol decreases. Then again, very high intakes of carbohydrates (>60% total energy intake) are associated with a reduction in HDL cholesterol and increase in serum triglyceride.[6,11,12] Increasing soluble fiber intake can sometimes reduce these responses.[6] Generally, increasing

BOX 20-3   GUIDE TO THERAPEUTIC LIFESTYLE CHANGES (TLC): HEALTHY LIFESTYLE RECOMMENDATIONS FOR A HEALTHY HEART

Food Items to Choose More Often

Breads and Cereals

≥6 servings per day, adjusted to kcal needs

Breads, cereals, especially whole grains; pasta; rice; potatoes; dry beans and peas; low-fat crackers and cookies

Vegetables

3 to 5 servings per day fresh, frozen, or canned without added fat, sauce, or salt

Fruits

2 to 4 servings per day fresh, frozen, canned, dried

Dairy Products

2 to 3 servings per day fat-free, ½%, 1% milk, buttermilk, yogurt, cottage cheese, fat-free and low-fat cheese

Eggs

2 egg yolks per week

Egg whites or egg substitute

Meat, Poultry, Fish

<5 ounces per day

Lean cuts loin, leg, round, extra-lean hamburger; cold cuts made with lean meat or soy protein; skinless poultry; fish

Fats and Oils

Amount adjusted to kcal level: unsaturated oils; soft or liquid margarines and vegetable oil spreads; salad dressings, seeds, and nuts

TLC Diet Options

Stanol/sterol-containing margarines; soluble-fiber food sources: barley, oats, psyllium, apples, bananas, berries, citrus fruits, nectarines, peaches, pears, plums, prunes, broccoli, Brussels sprouts, carrots, dry beans, soy products (tofu, miso)

Food Items to Choose Less Often

Breads and Cereals

Many baked products, including doughnuts, biscuits, butter rolls, muffins, croissants, sweet rolls, Danish, cakes, pies, coffee cakes, cookies

Many grain-based snacks, including chips, cheese puffs, snack mix, regular crackers, buttered popcorn

Vegetables

Vegetables fried or prepared with butter, cheese, or cream sauce

Fruits

Fruits fried or served with butter or cream

Dairy Products

Whole milk, 2% milk, whole-milk yogurt, ice cream, cream, cheese

Eggs

Egg yolk, whole eggs

Meat, Poultry, Fish

Higher fat meat cuts: ribs, T-bone steak, regular hamburger, bacon, sausage; cold cuts: salami, bologna, hot dogs; organ meats: liver, brains, sweetbreads; poultry with skin; fried meat; fried poultry; fried fish

Fats and Oils

Butter, shortening, stick margarine, chocolate, coconut

Recommendations for Weight Reduction

Weigh Regularly

Record weight, body mass index (BMI), and waist circumferences

Lose Weight Gradually

Goal: lose 10% of body weight in 6 months; lose ½ to 1 pound per week

Develop Healthy Eating Patterns

- Choose healthy foods (see "Food Items to Choose More Often")
- Reduce intake of less healthy foods (see "Food Items to Choose Less Often")
- Limit number of eating occasions
- Avoid second helpings
- Identify and reduce hidden fat by reading food labels to choose products lower in saturated fat and kcal, and ask about ingredients in ready-to-eat foods prepared away from home
- Identify and reduce sources of excess carbohydrates such as fat-free and regular crackers; cookies and other desserts; snacks; and sugar-containing beverages

Recommendations for Increased Physical Activity

Make Physical Activity Part of Daily Routine

- Reduce sedentary time
- Walk, wheel, or bike-ride more; drive less. Take the stairs instead of an elevator. Get off the bus a few stops early and walk the remaining distance. Mow the lawn with a push mower. Rake leaves. Garden. Push a stroller. Clean the house. Do exercises or pedal a stationary bike while watching television. Play actively with children. Take a brisk 10-minute walk or wheel before work, during your work break, and after dinner

Make Physical Activity Part of Exercise or Recreational Activities

Walk, wheel, or jog. Bicycle or use an arm pedal bicycle. Swim or do water aerobics. Play basketball. Join a sport team. Play wheelchair sports. Golf (pull cart or carry clubs). Canoe. Cross-country ski. Dance. Take part in an exercise program at work, home, school, or gym.

From the National Cholesterol Education Program (NCEP): *Third report of the NCEP expert panel on detection, evaluation, and treatment of high blood cholesterol in adults (Adult Treatment Panel III)*, Washington, DC, 2001, National Institutes of Health, National Heart, Lung, and Blood Institute.

soluble fiber to 5 to 10 g per day is accompanied by a roughly 5% reduction in LDL cholesterol.[13]

Protein. Although dietary protein, as a rule, has a negligible effect on serum LDL cholesterol level, substituting plant-based proteins for animal proteins appears to decrease LDL cholesterol. This may be caused by the lack of cholesterol and lower saturated fat content of plant-based protein foods (e.g., legumes, dry beans, nuts, whole grains, and vegetables). This is not to say all animal proteins are high in saturated fat and cholesterol. Fat-free and low-fat dairy products, egg whites, fish, skinless poultry, and lean cuts of beef and pork are low in saturated fat and cholesterol. All foods of animal origin contain cholesterol.

Further dietary options to reduce LDL cholesterol. When 5 to 10 g of soluble fiber (e.g., oats, barley, psyllium, pectin-rich fruit, and beans) is added to the daily diet, there is a roughly 5% reduction in LDL cholesterol.[13] This is considered a therapeutic alternative to augment reduction of LDL cholesterol.[6] Daily intakes of 2 to 3 g plant sterol/sterol esters (isolated from soybean and tall pine tree oils) present an additional therapeutic option because they have been shown to lower LDL cholesterol by 6% to 15%.[6,14-16]

The ATP III[6] recommends patients at risk for CHD or with CHD be referred to registered dietitians or other qualified nutritionists for all stages of medical nutrition therapy. LDL cholesterol should be measured at 6-week intervals to evaluate response to TLC. If the LDL cholesterol target has been realized, or if improvement in LDL lowering has occurred, medical nutrition therapy should be continued. If the goal has not been achieved, several alternatives are available. First, medical nutrition therapy can be reexplained and reinforced. Next, therapeutic dietary options (outlined earlier) can be integrated into TLC. Response to nutrition therapy should be assessed in another 6 weeks. Achievement of the LDL cholesterol target indicates current intensity of medical nutrition therapy should be continued indefinitely. Thought should be given to continuing medical nutrition therapy before adding LDL-lowering medications. If it seems unlikely the LDL target will be realized with medical nutrition therapy, medications should be considered.[6]

Drug Therapy

Use of TLC will attain the LDL cholesterol target goal for many; LDL-lowering medications will be necessary for a segment of the population to achieve the prescribed goal for LDL cholesterol.[6] If treatment with TLC alone is unsuccessful after 3 months, the ATP III recommends initiation of drug treatment. Use of LDL-lowering medications does not negate continued use or need for medical nutrition therapy. Nutrition therapy affords further CHD risk reduction beyond drug efficacy. Suggestions for combined use of TLC and LDL-lowering medications include the following:[6]
- Intensive LDL lowering with TLC, including therapeutic dietary options
  - May prevent need for drugs
  - Can augment LDL-lowering medications
  - May allow for lower doses of medications
- Weight control plus increased physical activity
  - Reduces risk beyond LDL cholesterol lowering
  - Constitutes principal management of metabolic syndrome
  - Raises HDL cholesterol
- Initiating TLC before medication consideration
  - For most people, a trial of medical nutrition therapy of about 3 months is advised before initiating drug therapy
  - Ineffective trials of nutrition therapy exclusive of medications should not be protracted for an indefinite period if goals of therapy are not approached in a reasonable period; medications should not be withheld if they are needed to reach targets in people with a high short-term and/or long-term CHD risk
- Initiating drug therapy simultaneously with TLC
  - For severe hypercholesterolemia in which nutrition therapy alone cannot attain LDL cholesterol targets
  - For those with CHD or CHD risk equivalents in whom nutrition therapy alone will not attain LDL cholesterol targets

The general strategy for initiation and progression of drug therapy is outlined in Figure 20-2. Major drugs used to treat hypercholesterolemia are outlined in Table 20-5.

HYPERTENSION

As many as 65 million Americans age 6 and older have hypertension (HTN) (including one in every three adults).[1] Not only is it a cardiovascular disease itself, but HTN is also a risk factor for CAD. According to the American Heart Association, incidence of HTN is higher in the following groups:[1]
- Until age 45, a higher percentage of men than women have HTN.
- From ages 45 to 54, the percentage of women with HTN is slightly higher.
- For those older than 54, a higher percentage of women have HTN.
- African Americans, Puerto Ricans, Cuban Americans, and Mexican Americans are more likely to have HTN than white Americans.

In about 95% of cases of HTN, cause is not known and is called primary or essential hypertension.[3] Secondary hypertension is the term used when a cause for elevated blood pressure can be identified. Conditions that are possible causes of secondary HTN include renal insufficiency, renovascular diseases, Cushing's syndrome, and primary aldosteronism.[17] Although sometimes called a "silent killer," HTN is easily detected and usually controllable. Classifications of blood pressure are outlined in Table 20-6.

Nutrition Therapy

Prescribed treatment regimens for HTN are individualized and vary because the disease differs in its degree of severity. First line of treatment is usually nonpharmacologic or focused on lifestyle modifications. Modifying dietary intake is a predominant element of nonpharmacologic treatment of existing HTN. Weight loss is the most effective means of lowering

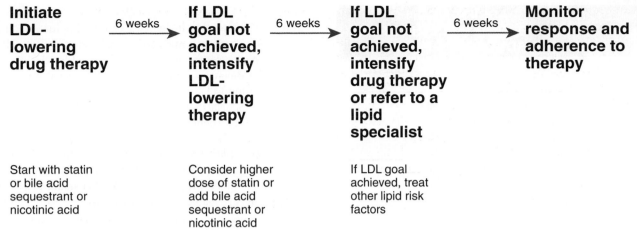

FIG 20-2 Progression of drug therapy. (From National Cholesterol Education Program [NCEP]: *Third report of the NCEP expert panel on detection, evaluation, and treatment of high blood cholesterol in adults [Adult Treatment Panel III]*, Washington, DC, 2001, National Institutes of Health, National Heart, Lung, and Blood Institute.)

TABLE 20-5	MAJOR DRUGS USED TO TREAT HYPERCHOLESTEROLEMIA		
DRUG CLASS	**AVAILABLE DRUGS**	**LIPID/LIPOPROTEIN EFFECTS**	**POTENTIAL NUTRITIONAL SIDE EFFECTS**
Statins (HMG CoA reductase inhibitors)	Lovastatin (Altocor, Mevacor), pravastatin (Pravachol), simvastatin (Zocor), fluvastatin (Lescol), atorvastatin (Lipitor)	↓ LDL cholesterol and triglycerides; moderately ↑ HDL cholesterol	Avoid St. John's wort; avoid grapefruit juice with Lipitor, Zocor, Mevacor Nausea, dyspepsia, abdominal pain, constipation, diarrhea, flatulence; avoid substantial alcohol
Bile acid sequestrants	Cholestyramine (Questran), colestipol (Colestid), colesevelam (WelChol)	↓ LDL cholesterol	Tongue irritation, belching, constipation, dyspepsia, nausea/vomiting, flatulence, diarrhea Fat soluble in water-miscible form and folacin supplement recommended with long-term use
Nicotinic acid (niacin)	A variety of prescription or over-the-counter preparations available in three forms: immediate release, timed release, extended-release nicotinic acid (Niaspan)	↑ HDL cholesterol and ↓ LDL cholesterol and triglycerides	Flushing of face and neck, nausea, vomiting, diarrhea, gout, high blood glucose, peptic ulcers
Fibrates (fibric acid derivatives)	Fenofibrate (Lofibra, Tricor), gemfibrozil (Lopid)	↓ triglycerides and modestly ↑ HDL cholesterol	Take with meals; nausea/vomiting, constipation, flatulence, avoid alcohol
Cholesterol absorption inhibitors	Ezetimibe (Zetia)	↓ LDL cholesterol, slightly ↓ triglycerides and slightly ↑ HDL cholesterol	Diarrhea, stomach pain, fatigue
Combination cholesterol absorption inhibitor and statin	Ezetimibe/simvastatin (Vytorin)	Reduce LDL and triglycerides and moderately increase HDL	Same as statins and cholesterol absorption inhibitors

HDL, High-density lipoprotein; *LDL,* low-density lipoprotein.
Data from Citkowitz E: *Hypercholesterolemia, Familial.* Accessed April 7, 2010, from www.emedicine.com/med/topic1072.htm#section~AuthorsandEditors, (updated August 4, 2009; Pronsky ZM: *Food-medication interactions,* ed 15, Birchrunville, Pa, 2008, Food-Medication Interactions.)

TABLE 20-6	CLASSIFICATION OF BLOOD PRESSURE FOR ADULTS		
CATEGORY	**SYSTOLIC (mm Hg)**		**DIASTOLIC (mm Hg)**
Normal	<120	and	<80
Prehypertensive	120 to 139	or	80 to 89
Stage 1 hypertension	140 to 159	or	90 to 99
Stage 2 hypertension	≥160	or	≥110

Data from *The seventh report of the joint national committee on prevention, detection, evaluation, and treatment of high blood pressure*, NIH Pub No 04-5230, Washington, DC, 2004 (August), National Institutes of Health, National Heart, Lung, and Blood Institute.

BOX 20-4	LIFESTYLE MODIFICATIONS FOR HYPERTENSION PREVENTION AND MANAGEMENT

- Lose weight if overweight. Maintain normal body weight (body mass index 18.5-24.9).
- Limit alcohol intake to no more than 1 ounce (30 mL) ethanol (e.g., 24 oz [720 mL] beer, 10 oz [300 mL] wine, or 2 oz [60 mL] 100-proof whiskey) per day or 0.5 oz (15 mL) ethanol per day for women and lighter-weight people.
- Engage in aerobic physical activity (at least 30 minutes most days of the week).
- Reduce sodium intake to no more than 100 mmol per day (2.4 g sodium or 6 g sodium chloride).
- Adopt DASH eating plan. Consume dietary pattern of fruits, vegetables, and low-fat dairy products and reduce intake of saturated fat and total fat.
- Stop smoking for overall cardiovascular health.

Data from *The Seventh report of the joint national committee on prevention, detection, evaluation, and treatment of high blood pressure*, NIH Pub No. 04-5230, Washington, DC, 2004 (August), National Institutes of Health, National Heart, Lung, and Blood Institute.

blood pressure. Other lifestyle modifications include possible beneficial effects of reducing weight if overweight, decreasing alcohol consumption, increasing physical activity if sedentary, terminating cigarette smoking, decreasing sodium intake, and increasing dietary intake of other minerals such as potassium, magnesium, and calcium. Box 20-4 summarizes lifestyle modifications that help reduce high blood pressure and overall cardiovascular risk.

In addition to being primary treatments for hypertension, weight reduction and sodium restriction augment antihypertensive medications. Weight reduction facilitates lowers blood pressure even when it is only a loss of 10 to 15 pounds. Diet for weight loss and control should include a specific kcal restriction and exercise (aerobic) prescription. Weight loss may be difficult to maintain without a subsequent increase in physical activity (see Appendix D on kcal-controlled diets). Average daily sodium intake in America has been estimated

to be approximately 4 to 6 g (175 to 265 mEq). Most comes from sodium added during processing and manufacturing (Box 8-9). The other main source of dietary sodium is the discretionary use of table salt (sodium chloride). A small portion of dietary sodium also comes from natural sodium content of foods.

The U.S. National High Blood Pressure Education Program recommends trying lifestyle modifications for 3 to 6 months in cases of mild to moderate HTN.[18] A diet rich in fruits, vegetables, and low-fat dairy products along with reduced saturated and total fats has been found to significantly lower blood pressure. The DASH (Dietary Approaches to Stop Hypertension) diet is recommended for prevention and management of HTN.[17,18] The DASH eating plan described in Table 20-7 is based on 2000 kcal/day. The number of daily servings from each group can be modified depending on individual energy needs (see the *Teaching Tool* box, Strategies for Adopting DASH).

An even larger drop in blood pressure is seen when the DASH eating plan is combined with sodium restriction.[17,19] Sodium intake levels of about 3300 mg/day (level consumed by many Americans); an intermediate intake around 2400 mg/day; and a lower intake around 1500 mg/day combined with the DASH eating plan can reduce blood pressure in those with normal blood pressure and HTN (Table 20-8). However, the largest reduction in blood pressure is seen in those using the DASH eating plan at the sodium intake level of 1500 mg/day (see Box 20-5).

For many, a sodium intake of 1500 mg/day would be perceived as a moderately severe restriction. Additionally, maintaining sodium consumption at this level may not currently be realistic, given the amount of sodium added to foods during processing and manufacturing. In fact, if the U.S. food supply were lower in sodium, it would help lower blood pressure in the general population.[20] Salt not only adds its own salty flavor to foods but also seems to alter other tastes and flavors and conceals bitterness without necessarily causing the foods to taste salty. As a result, when salt is reduced or removed from a food, the saltiness as well as other flavors of that food are changed. Although there is currently no acceptable substitute for salt that provides similar taste satisfaction, a salt substitute may be prescribed (Box 20-5). The *Teaching Tool* box, Seven Sneaky Sodium Stowaways, gives tips on helping patients recognize foods potentially high in sodium.

MYOCARDIAL INFARCTION

Myocardial infarctions (MIs), or heart attacks, are the single largest killer of adult men and women in the United States. An American will suffer a heart attack every 20 seconds, and someone dies from one every minute. Disability or death can result after an MI, depending on how much heart muscle is damaged.

Nutrition Therapy

The purpose of nutrition therapy for patients suffering from an MI is to reduce the workload of the heart. This is also a

TABLE 20-7	DASH DIET PATTERN

The DASH diet is based on 2000 kcal/day. The following table indicates the number of recommended daily servings from each food group with examples of food choices. The number of servings may increase or decrease, depending on individual calorie needs.

FOOD GROUP	DAILY SERVING (EXCEPT WHERE NOTED)	SERVING SIZES	EXAMPLES AND NOTES	SIGNIFICANCE TO THE DASH DIET PATTERN
Grains and grain products	7-8	1 slice bread 1 ounce dry cereal* ½ cup cooked rice, pasta, or cereal	Whole-wheat bread, English muffin, pita bread, bagel; cereals; grits; oatmeal	Major source of energy and fiber
Vegetables	4-5	1 cup raw, leafy vegetables ½ cup cooked vegetables 6 ounces vegetable juice	Tomatoes, potatoes, carrots, peas, squash, broccoli, turnip greens, collards, kale, spinach, artichokes, beans, sweet potatoes	Rich sources of potassium, magnesium, and fiber
Fruits	4-5	6 ounces fruit juice 1 medium fruit ¼ cup dried fruit ½ cup fresh, frozen, or canned fruit	Apricots, bananas, dates, grapes, oranges, orange juice, tangerines, strawberries, mangoes, melons, peaches, pineapple, prunes, raisins	Important sources of potassium, magnesium, and fiber
Low-fat or free dairy foods	2-3	8 ounces milk 1 cup yogurt 1½ ounces cheese	Fat-free or 1% milk, fat-free or low-fat buttermilk; nonfat or low-fat yogurt; part-skim mozzarella cheese, nonfat cheese	Major sources of calcium and protein
Meats, poultry, and fish	≥2	3 ounces cooked meats, poultry, or fish	Select only lean meats; trim away visible fats; broil, roast, or boil, instead of frying; remove skin from chicken	Rich sources of protein and magnesium
Nuts, seeds, and legumes	4-5/week	1½ ounces or ½ cup nuts ½ ounce or 2 tablespoons seeds ½ cup cooked legumes	Almonds, filberts, mixed nuts, peanuts, walnuts, sunflower seeds, kidney beans, lentils	Rich sources of energy, magnesium, potassium, protein, and fiber
Fats and oils†	2-3	1 teaspoon soft margarine 1 tablespoon low-fat mayonnaise or salad dressing 2 tablespoons light salad dressing 1 teaspoon vegetable oil	Soft margarine, low-fat mayonnaise, light salad dressing, vegetable oil (e.g., olive, corn, canola, or safflower)	DASH has 27% of kcal as fat, including that in or added to foods
Sweets	5/week	1 tablespoon sugar 1 tablespoon jelly or jam ½ ounce jelly beans 8 ounces lemonade	Maple syrup, sugar, jelly, jam; fruit-flavored gelatin, jelly beans, fruit punch, sorbet, ices, hard candy	Sweets should be low in fat

*Equals ½ to 1¼ cups depending on cereal type. Check the product's nutrition label.
†Fat content changes serving counts for fats and oils. For example, 1 tablespoon of regular salad dressing equals 1 serving; 1 tablespoon of low-fat dressing equals ½ serving; 1 tablespoon of fat-free dressing equals 0 servings.
From U.S. Department of Health and Human Services, Public Health Service, National Institutes of Health, National Heart, Lung, and Blood Institute: *Your guide to lowering your blood pressure with DASH,* NIH Publication No. 06-4082, Bethesda, Md, 2006, Author. Accessed April 7, 2010, from www.nhlbi.nih.gov.

✴ TEACHING TOOL

Strategies for Adopting DASH

Dietary changes are best achieved through small changes in food selections. Use this list of tips as a way to initiate discussion and dietary compliance to reduce hypertension among your clients.

Tips on Eating the DASH Way
Change gradually

- If you now eat one or two vegetables a day, add a serving at lunch and another at dinner.
- If you don't eat fruit now or have only juice at breakfast, add a serving to your meals or have it as a snack.
- Gradually increase your use of fat-free and low-fat dairy products to three servings a day. For example, drink milk with lunch or dinner instead of soda, sugar-sweetened tea, or alcohol. Choose low-fat (1%) or fat-free (skim) dairy products to reduce your intake of saturated fat, total fat, cholesterol, and kcal.
- Read food labels on margarines and salad dressings and choose those lowest in unsaturated fat. Some margarines are now trans fat–free.

Treat meat as one part of the whole meal, instead of the focus.

- Limit meat to 6 ounces a day (two servings)—all that's needed. A serving of 3 to 4 ounces is about the size of a deck of cards.
- If you currently eat large portions of meat, cut portion sizes back gradually—by a half or a third at each meal.
- Include two or more vegetarian-style (meatless) meals each week.
- Increase servings of vegetables, rice, pasta, and dry beans in meals. Try casseroles, pasta, and stir-fry dishes, which have less meat and more vegetables, grains, and dry beans.

Use fruit or other foods low in saturated fat, cholesterol, and kcal as desserts and snacks.

- Fruits and other low-fat foods offer great taste and variety. Use fruits canned in their own juice. Fresh fruits require little or no preparation. Dried fruits are a good choice to carry with you.
- Try these snacks ideas: unsalted pretzels or nuts mixed with raisins; graham crackers; low-fat, fat-free, or frozen yogurt; popcorn with no salt or butter added; and raw vegetables.

Try the following other tips:

- Choose whole grain foods to get added nutrients, such as minerals and fiber. For example, choose whole-wheat bread or whole grain cereals.
- If you have trouble digesting dairy products, try taking lactase enzyme pills or drops (available at drugstores and groceries) before eating dairy foods, or buy lactose-free milk or milk with lactase enzyme added to it.
- Use fresh, frozen, or sodium-free canned vegetables.

From U.S. Department of Health and Human Services, Public Health Service, National Institutes of Health, National Heart, Lung, and Blood Institute: *Your Guide to Lowering Your Blood Pressure with DASH,* NIH Publication No. 06-4082, Bethesda, Md, 2006, Author. Accessed April 7, 2010, from www.nhlbi.nih.gov.

✴ TEACHING TOOL

Seven Sneaky Sodium Stowaways

Provide patients with an easy way to remember categories of foods that may be high in sodium. For most categories, patients on sodium-restricted diets can choose food products that are lower in sodium content; however, label reading becomes an absolute necessity. Review the sodium reduction suggestions in Chapter 8. Also consider that sodium hides in seven categories of foods in the form of salt or as part of an added ingredient. Following are the Seven Sneaky (categories of) Sodium Stowaways:

1. Snacks (corn chips, potato chips, pretzels, peanuts, certain crackers)
2. Seasonings and nonnutritive sweeteners (monosodium glutamate, sodium saccharin)
3. Soups (especially canned and dried mixes)
4. Sauces (dried mixes and bottled, includes ketchup)
5. Smoked meats and fish (smoked ham and lox)
6. Sauerkraut and other pickled foods (pickles, relishes, and pickled herring)
7. Sodium-processed luncheon meats (bologna, salami, ham, corned beef)

good time to initiate education about modification of diet-related cardiac risk factors.

The patient may receive a liquid diet initially (for approximately 24 hours) and progress, as tolerated, to foods of regular consistency. Smaller, frequent meals are usually better tolerated than large meals, which can increase myocardial oxygen demand by increasing splanchnic (visceral) blood flow because approximately 50% of cardiac output is needed for digestion. Caffeine-containing beverages are sometimes restricted to avoid myocardial stimulation. Sodium, cholesterol, fat, and kcal (if weight loss is indicated) are controlled according to the patient's needs.

Consuming omega-3 fatty acids (see Chapter 5) appears to reduce the risk of blood clots that may cause an MI. Sources of omega-3 fatty acids include fish such as tuna, salmon, halibut, sardines, and lake trout.

CARDIAC FAILURE

Cardiac failure is also called **congestive heart failure (CHF),** heart failure, and cardiac decompensation. Location of congestion depends on the ventricle involved. Left ventricle failure produces pulmonary congestion, whereas right ventricular failure results in systemic congestion that causes poor perfusion to all organ systems.[3] Right heart (ventricular) failure has also been reported to result from left heart (ventricular) failure.[4]

Nutrition Therapy

To lessen the workload of the heart, nutrition therapy focuses on restricting dietary sodium. The more severe the heart failure, the more severe the sodium restriction needed to

TABLE 20-8	WHERE'S THE SODIUM?

Only a small amount of sodium occurs naturally in foods. Most sodium is added during processing. The table below gives examples of varying amounts of sodium that occur in foods before and after processing.

FOOD GROUPS	SODIUM (mg)
Grains and Grain Products	
Cooked cereal, rice, pasta, unsalted, ½ cup	0-5
Ready-to-eat cereal, 1 cup	100-360
Bread, 1 slice	110-175
Vegetables	
Fresh or frozen, cooked without salt, ½ cup	1-70
Canned or frozen with sauce, ½ cup	140-460
Tomato juice, canned, ¾ cup	820
Fruit	
Fresh, frozen, canned, ½ cup	0-5
Low-Fat or Fat-Free Dairy Foods	
Milk, 1 cup	120
Yogurt, 8 ounces	160
Natural cheeses, 1½ ounces	110-450
Processed cheeses, 1½ ounces	600
Nuts, Seeds, and Dry Beans	
Peanuts, salted, ⅓ cup	120
Peanuts, unsalted, ⅓ cup	0-5
Beans, cooked from dried or frozen, without salt, ½ cup	0-5
Beans, canned, ½ cup	400
Meats, Fish, and Poultry	
Fresh meat, fish, poultry, 3 ounces	30-90
Tuna canned, water pack, no salt added, 3 ounces	35-45
Tuna canned, water pack, 3 ounces	250-350
Ham, lean, roasted, 3 ounces	1,020

From U.S. Department of Health and Human Services, Public Health Service, National Institutes of Health, National Heart, Lung, and Blood Institute: *Your guide to lowering your blood pressure with DASH*, NIH Publication No. 06-4082, Bethesda, Md, 2006, Author. Accessed April 7, 2010, from www.nhlbi.nih.gov.

reduce extracellular fluids. Patients with mild to moderate heart failure are often prescribed a sodium restriction of 3000 mg/day. People unresponsive to this level or who have severe CHF are more likely to benefit from a 2000 mg/day sodium restriction. Fluid restriction of 1 to 2 L is sometimes indicated in severe heart failure, especially when hyponatremia is present. Fluid requirements depend on medical status and use of diuretics.

Energy requirements may be 20% to 30% above basal needs because of increased cardiac and pulmonary energy demands and increased metabolic rate.[21] Protein and energy intake should be sufficient to maintain body weight. Meeting these increased nutrient and energy requirements could be problematic because of early satiety, gastrointestinal congestion, shortness of breath, anorexia, and nausea. If the patient has cardiac cachexia, additional kcal and protein are needed to prevent further catabolism. Caution must be used when increasing energy, however, so as not to overfeed the patient. Kcal-dense (1.5 to 2 kcal/mL) nutritional supplements may be helpful to increase kcal and protein intake. Enteral or parenteral nutrition (see Chapter 14) may be necessary for patients who cannot meet their nutritional needs through oral intake. If enteral nutrition support is required, continuous rather than bolus feedings are favored because they reduce myocardial oxygen consumption.[22] Concentrated enteral formulas are available if fluid restriction is necessary.

LIFE SPAN IMPLICATIONS

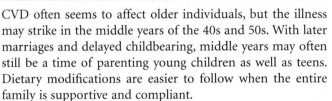

CVD often seems to affect older individuals, but the illness may strike in the middle years of the 40s and 50s. With later marriages and delayed childbearing, middle years may often still be a time of parenting young children as well as teens. Dietary modifications are easier to follow when the entire family is supportive and compliant.

Dietary education should include individuals who buy and prepare meals (and snacks, too) for the patient. Lists of health associations, community hospitals and other organizations offering cooking courses, and bookstores or public libraries with available heart-healthy cookbooks are excellent adjuncts to medical nutrition therapy. By including all family members in the educative process, not only is the health of the individual with CAD enhanced but also primary risk factors for younger family members are decreased. Although children may not need to follow the sometimes extreme restrictions of CAD patients, it is still easier for a 10-year-old to understand that it is heart healthy to have popcorn with little or no butter and salt than to simply blame restrictions on "Daddy's sickness." Lifelong health promotion habits develop early and benefit everyone.

OVERCOMING BARRIERS

Demystifying Labels

Label reading is an important skill for all of us but is especially so for someone with diet-related illnesses, including HTN or CVD. Educating patients about use of food label information helps demystify the process of consuming recommended levels of dietary fat and sodium. Food labels may display two types of messages about packaged food: nutrient content claims and health claims. Federal regulations formulated by the U.S. Food and Drug Administration (FDA) control how certain terms can be used in labeling. Table 20-9 defines terms related to sodium, dietary cholesterol, and fat—nutrients of concern for CVD.

BOX 20-5 DASHING WITH LESS SALT: A SAMPLE MENU

2300-mg SODIUM MENU	SODIUM (mg)	SUBSTITUTIONS TO REDUCE SODIUM TO 1500 MG	SODIUM (mg)
Breakfast			
¾ cup bran flakes	220	¾ cup shredded wheat cereal	1
1 slice whole-wheat bread	149	½ cup fruit yogurt, fat free, no sugar added	86
1 cup low-fat milk	107		
1 teaspoon soft (tub) margarine	26	1 teaspoon soft (tub) margarine, unsalted	0
Lunch			
¾ cup chicken salad (recipe below)	179	Remove salt from recipe	120
2 slices whole-wheat bread	299		
1 tablespoon Dijon mustard	373	1 tablespoon regular mustard	175
½ cup fruit cocktail, juice pack	5		
Salad:			
½ cup fresh cucumber slices	1		
½ cup tomato wedges	5		
1 tablespoon sunflower seeds	0		
1 teaspoon Italian dressing, reduced calorie	43		
Dinner			
3 ounces spicy baked fish (recipe below)	50		
1 cup green beans, cooked from frozen, without salt	12		
1 small baked potato	14		
2 tablespoons fat-free sour cream	21		
1 tablespoon chopped scallions	1		
2 tablespoons grated cheddar cheese, natural, reduced fat	67	2 tablespoons cheddar cheese, natural, reduced fat, low sodium	1
1 small whole-wheat roll	148	1 teaspoon soft margarine, unsalted	0
1 teaspoon soft margarine	26		
1 medium peach	0		
1 cup low-fat milk	107		
Snack			
1 cup orange juice	5		
⅓ cup almonds, unsalted	0		
¼ cup raisins	4		
1 cup fruit yogurt, fat free with no sugar added	173		

This sample menu provides five fruit servings, five vegetable servings, and four dairy servings.

Recipes

Chicken Salad (makes 5 servings)
3 ¼ cup chicken breast, cooked, cubed, skinless
3 tablespoons low-fat mayonnaise
¼ cup celery, chopped
1 tablespoon lemon juice
½ teaspoon onion powder
⅛ teaspoon salt

Steps:
1. Bake chicken, cut into cubes, and refrigerate.
2. Mix all ingredients in a large bowl and serve. Serving size: ¾ cup

Spicy Baked Cod (makes 4 servings)
1 pound cod, or other fish fillet, fresh or thawed from frozen

1 tablespoon olive oil
1 teaspoon spicy seasoning mix (see below)

Steps:
1. Preheat oven to 350° F. Spray small baking dish with cooking oil spray.
2. Wash and dry cod. Place in dish and drizzle with oil and seasoning mix.
3. Bake uncovered for 12 minutes or until fish flakes with fork.
4. Cut into four pieces and serve.

Spicy Seasoning Mix
Mix together the following ingredients and store in airtight container for other recipes: 1½ teaspoons white pepper, ½ teaspoon cayenne pepper, ½ teaspoon black pepper, 1 teaspoon onion powder, 1¼ teaspoons garlic powder, 1 tablespoon dried basil, 1½ teaspoons dried thyme.

From U.S. Department of Health and Human Services, Public Health Service, National Institutes of Health, National Heart, Lung, and Blood Institute: *Your Guide to Lowering Your Blood Pressure with DASH,* NIH Publication No. 06-4082, Bethesda, Md, 2006, Author. Accessed April 7, 2010, from www.nhlbi.nih.gov.

TABLE 20-9	NUTRIENT CONTENT CLAIMS				
TERM	**FAT**	**SATURATED FAT**	**CHOLESTEROL**	**SODIUM**	**KCAL**
Free ("zero," "no," "without," "trivial source of," or "dietarily insignificant source of")	<0.5 g per reference amount*	<0.5 g saturated fat and <0.5 g trans fatty acids per reference amount	<2 mg per reference amount and per labeled serving	<5 mg per reference amount and per labeled amount	<5 kcal per serving
Low ("little," "few" for kcal, "contains a small amount of," "low source of")	≤3 g per serving	≤1 g per serving	≤20 mg per serving	≤140 mg per serving	≤40 kcal per serving
Light or lite	A product has one third fewer kcal than a comparable product or 50% of the fat found in a comparable product, or the sodium content of a low-kcal, low-fat food has been reduced by 50% (light may still be used to describe properties of food such as texture and color).				
Reduced/Less	A nutritionally altered product that contains 25% less of a nutrient or kcal than the regular product (this claim cannot be made on a product if the regular food already meets the requirement for "low").				
Free	A product contains virtually none of one or more of these: fat, saturated fat, cholesterol, sodium, sugars, and kcal.				
Lean[†]	<10 g fat, plus	4 g saturated fat	And <95 mg of cholesterol per serving and per 100 g		
Extra lean[†]	<5 g fat, plus	<2 g saturated fat	And <95 mg of cholesterol per serving and per 100 g		

*"Reference amount" is amount customarily consumed at one seating
†Used to describe the fat content of meat, poultry, seafood, and game meats.
Data from Food and Drug Administration: *Food labeling guide: guidance for industry*, Washington, DC (updated April 2008), Author. Accessed April 7, 2010, from www.fda.gov/Food/GuidanceComplianceRegulatoryInformation/GuidanceDocuments/FoodLabelingNutrition/FoodLabelingGuide/default.htm.

RESPIRATORY DISEASES

Disorders of the pulmonary system are classified into two categories. The first includes disorders that result in chronic long-term changes in respiratory function such as **chronic obstructive pulmonary disease (COPD)**. COPD is a collective phrase for chronic bronchitis, asthma, and emphysema and is the second leading cause of disability in the United States.[23] The goal of nutrition therapy is to maintain respiratory muscle strength and function and to prevent or correct malnutrition. The second category includes disorders that cause acute changes in respiratory function such as **respiratory distress syndrome (RDS)** and **acute respiratory failure (ARF)**. Patients who are critically ill, in shock, severely injured, or who have **sepsis** can develop these disorders.[23] For ARF and RDS, the function of nutrition therapy is to inhibit tissue destruction by providing extra nutrients required for hypermetabolic conditions without contributing to declining respiratory function.

Chronic Obstructive Pulmonary Disease

Energy required for breathing is something most of us often take for granted. Energy needs, however, become evident in patients with respiratory problems. Because of their weakened respiratory system, patients with advanced COPD expend a great deal of energy just breathing and therefore have an increased likelihood of malnutrition. It is common to see significant weight loss from both fat stores and muscle mass (Figure 20-3). Muscle wasting is most evident in the diaphragm and respiratory muscles. Thus, presence of malnutrition contributes to exacerbation of the clinical course.

Malnutrition of these individuals is multifactorial. Contributing factors include altered taste because of chronic mouth breathing and excessive sputum production, fatigue, anxiety, depression, increased energy requirements, frequent infections, and the side effects of multiple medications.

Nutrition Therapy

Preventing malnutrition will not only help preserve muscle strength needed for respiratory function but also maintain the integrity of the immune system. The first step in this prevention is to provide adequate nutrition. Anorexia, early satiety, nausea, and vomiting are all common. Box 20-6 discusses maximizing food intake in COPD. Strategies that are viable options for patients with COPD to assist in maximizing oral intake are in Box 20-7.

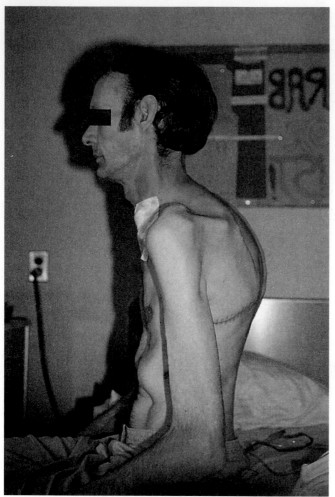

FIG 20-3 Patient with chronic obstructive pulmonary disease. (From Morgan SL, Weinsier RL: *Fundamentals of clinical nutrition,* ed 2, St. Louis, 1998, Mosby.)

BOX 20-6 **MAXIMIZING FOOD INTAKE IN CHRONIC OBSTRUCTIVE PULMONARY DISORDER (COPD)**

Although well-balanced, nutritionally sound meals are provided, it is sometimes difficult for patients with COPD to consume adequate amounts of nutrients, particularly in the home setting. Here are ideas to make mealtimes easier and more nutritious by increasing kcal and protein without increasing the amount of food eaten.

In clinical and home health care settings:
- Eat high-kcal foods first.
- Try more frequent meals and snacks.
- Increase kcal by adding margarine, butter, mayonnaise, sauces, gravies, and peanut butter to foods.
- Limit liquids at mealtimes.
- Try cold foods, which can give a more reduced sense of fullness than hot foods.
- Rest before meals.

In home health care settings:
- Keep favorite foods and snacks on hand.
- Keep ready-prepared meals available for periods of increased shortness of breath.
- Eat larger meals when you are not as tired.
- Avoid foods that you know cause gas.
- Add skim milk powder (2 tablespoons) to regular milk (8 oz) to add protein and kcal.
- Use milk or half-and-half instead of water when making soups, cereals, instant puddings, cocoa, or canned soups.
- Add grated cheese to sauces, vegetables, soups, and casseroles.
- Choose dessert recipes that contain egg, such as sponge cake, angel food cake, egg custard, bread pudding, or rice pudding.

BOX 20-7 **SUGGESTIONS FOR ORAL FEEDING IN CHRONIC OBSTRUCTIVE PULMONARY DISORDER (COPD)**

- Suggest that patients consume small, frequent meals.
- Encourage patients to eat the most when well rested, such as the first meal of the day.
- Encourage the use of high-calorie, high-protein supplements.
- Teach patients to swallow as little air as possible when eating.
- Encourage the use of easily prepared or convenience foods to decrease any fatigue.

Energy expenditure is usually elevated, but it will vary according to a person's level of physical activity.[23,24] Moreover, energy balance and nitrogen balance go hand-in-hand; visceral and somatic proteins can only be conserved if optimal energy balance is maintained.[23] Indirect calorimetry is the most accurate method for determining energy expenditure for hospitalized patients with COPD.[23,24] Adequate protein, but not excessive, is known to stimulate the ventilatory drive. Patients may require 1.2 to 1.9 g protein/kg for maintenance and 1.6 to 2.5 g/kg of body weight for repletion.[23]

Providing nutrients in proper combination is also important to reduce production of carbon dioxide and maintain respiratory function.[23,24] This is particularly crucial for the ventilator-dependent patient. When each type of macronutrient is metabolized, carbon dioxide and water are produced. The **respiratory quotient (RQ)** is the ratio of carbon dioxide produced to the amount of oxygen consumed. Carbohydrate metabolism produces the greatest amount of carbon dioxide and therefore has the highest RQ. Physiologic range for RQ is 0.67 to 1.3. Fat metabolism produces the least amount of carbon dioxide and has the lowest RQ (0.7).[24] An RQ greater

than 1 may indicate carbohydrate is the primary energy source, and it is evidence of accumulating carbon dioxide,[24] which makes respiration that much more difficult for a patient with COPD. Nonprotein kcal should be divided evenly between fat and carbohydrate.[23] The important issue is to provide adequate nutrition without overfeeding the patient. Overfeeding also produces an excessive amount of carbon dioxide and would be reflected in a RQ greater than 1.

Acute Respiratory Failure and Respiratory Distress Syndrome

Almost half of all patients with acute respiratory failure suffer from malnutrition that impairs recovery and prolongs weaning from mechanical ventilation. A diet that minimizes carbon dioxide production while maintaining good nutrition is recommended.[25] Most patients in acute respiratory failure require mechanical ventilation, so in such cases, nutrition support may be provided via enteral or parenteral nutrition.

Nutrition Therapy

Nutrition support should be initiated as soon as possible to help wean the patient from the ventilator[25-27] (see Box 14-4). Nutritional recommendations are similar to those for patients with COPD: high kcal, high protein, moderate to high (50% nonprotein kcal) fat, with moderate (50% nonprotein kcal) carbohydrate.

Enteral nutrition. Commercial formulas that provide 40% to 50% of total kcal from fat are available. Higher-caloric density formulas may be necessary when fluid is restricted in these patients. Low osmolality feedings are started slowly to avoid gastric retention or diarrhea. Continuous administration is recommended unless otherwise contraindicated.[23] Because these patients are at risk for aspiration, special precautions such as elevating the head of the bed or using a tube placed into the duodenum or jejunum are necessary.[23]

Parenteral nutrition. Parenteral nutrition may be needed in treatment of acute respiratory failure. High-glucose concentrations can lead to excess carbon dioxide production, making weaning from the ventilator more difficult; therefore, they should be avoided. The optimal parenteral solution should provide adequate protein to maintain nitrogen balance and 1 to 2 g of lipid per kilogram of body weight.[25] Remaining caloric needs can then be met by carbohydrates. It is additionally recommended to infuse nutrition support for these clients for 24 hours.

Monitoring nutrition support in the critically ill is best managed through a team approach. Daily calorie counts, daily weights, and biochemical parameters are necessary to assess response to nutrition support. Comparison of nutritional intake with indirect calorimetry provides useful guidance to monitor the adequacy of nutrition support.[25] Collaboration with clinical dietitians is best to monitor transition from parenteral to enteral feedings to conventional feeding.

Malnutrition and the method of refeeding have unequivocally been shown to influence outcome in respiratory disease or respiratory failure.[27] Nutrition therapy is important to maintain or replenish nutritional status and can positively or negatively influence weaning from mechanical ventilation. Because a significant number of patients with respiratory disease or failure have clinically relevant malnutrition, nurses and other health care professionals should always be alert to alterations in nutritional status.

SUMMARY

Cardiovascular disease consists of a group of diseases and conditions that affect the heart and blood vessels; they are CAD, HTN, PVD, CHF and CHD. CVD risk factors are categorized into three groups: controllable, noncontrollable, and predisposing. Controllable or lifestyle factors include tobacco use, diet, and physical inactivity. Noncontrollable factors are gender, age, and family history. Predisposing conditions may be diabetes mellitus, hypertension, obesity, and hypercholesterolemia.

CAD begins with atherosclerosis. Atherosclerosis is the development of lesions in coronary arteries that can lead to arteriosclerosis, angina pectoris, or myocardial infarction. If thrombosis occurs in a cerebral artery, a cerebrovascular accident or hemorrhagic stroke occurs. CAD risk is assessed by measuring the total blood cholesterol and the proportions of the different types of lipoproteins that carry cholesterol in the blood. Lowering total cholesterol and LDL cholesterol can be achieved by dietary intervention, including weight loss and exercise. Goals of medical nutrition therapy are to reduce total fat, saturated fat, trans fatty acids, and cholesterol intake in an attempt to reduce plasma total cholesterol, LDL cholesterol, and triglyceride levels.

HTN for which the cause is not known is called *primary* or *essential HTN. Secondary HTN* is when the cause of elevated blood pressure can be identified. Prescribed treatment regimens for HTN are individualized and vary because the disease differs in its degree of severity. First line of treatment is usually nonpharmacologic or focused on lifestyle modifications. Weight reduction and sodium restriction augment antihypertensive medications as well.

MIs are the single largest killer of adults in the United States. The purpose of nutrition therapy is to reduce the workload of the heart. The patient may receive a liquid diet initially and progress to foods of regular consistency as tolerated. Smaller, frequent meals are usually better tolerated than large meals.

CAD, lung disease, complications of hypothyroidism, or damage to the myocardial or cardiac muscle can cause cardiac failure. The condition is characterized by decreased blood flow to the kidneys and retention of sodium and fluid. Patients with CHF often experience edema of the feet and ankles and shortness of breath. To lessen the workload of the heart, nutrition therapy focuses on restricting dietary sodium.

Pulmonary disease is characterized by wasting and malnutrition, largely caused by the effect of the disorder or the secondary consequences of treatment on the GI tract. Medical nutrition therapy focuses on reducing these effects. Two categories of pulmonary disorders cause either chronic changes in respiratory function, such as COPD, or acute changes in respiratory function, such as RDS and ARF. ARF and RDS may develop in patients who are critically ill, in shock, severely injured, or have sepsis. The goal of nutrition therapy for COPD is to maintain respiratory muscle strength and function while preventing or treating existing malnutrition.

As pulmonary disorders progress, nutritional status tends to decline and malnutrition exacerbates declining respiratory muscle function and ventilatory drive. For ARF and RDS, the function of medical nutrition therapy is to inhibit tissue destruction by providing the extra nutrients required for hypermetabolic conditions. Malnutrition and the method of refeeding influence the outcome in respiratory disease or respiratory failure.

THE NURSING APPROACH

Case Study: Hypertension and Heart Failure

The home health nurse visited Reba, a 70-year-old African American woman who had been diagnosed with heart failure and hypertension. Lab tests revealed elevated triglycerides, cholesterol, and LDL. The nurse first became acquainted with Reba when Reba was discharged from the hospital after an acute episode of pulmonary edema. The physician advised Reba to begin a walking program, starting slowly. The physician prescribed a 2-gram-sodium, low-fat, low-calorie diet. Several medications had been prescribed, including digoxin, a diuretic, and a vasodilator. In a previous visit, the nurse instructed Reba to monitor her pulse and blood pressure daily, and to weigh herself daily. The purpose of this follow-up visit was to determine the patient's compliance with the treatment plan and to assess her current health status.

ASSESSMENT

Subjective (from patient statements)

- "Sometimes I forget whether I have taken my medicines."
- "I've kept a record of my pulse, blood pressure, and weight almost every day."
- "Today I weighed 2 pounds more than I did when I was in the hospital."
- "I feel really tired. I get short of breath when I climb stairs (dyspnea). I haven't been going for walks."
- "I have trouble breathing when I lie down at night" (orthopnea).
- "I usually warm up a can of soup or a frozen dinner because I am too tired to cook. I like it when my granddaughter brings me cake and doughnuts."

Objective (from physical examination)

- Height 5 feet 8 inches, weight 182 pounds with truncal obesity
- Blood pressure 162/85, temperature 98° F, pulse 92 irregular; respirations 18, unlabored
- Lung sounds clear
- Pitting edema in ankles
- Jugular venous distention

DIAGNOSES (NURSING)

1. Excess fluid volume related to decreased cardiac output and excess sodium intake as evidenced by blood pressure 162/85, pitting edema of ankles, jugular venous distention, weight 2 pounds more than during hospitalization
2. Decreased cardiac output related to hypertension, weakened cardiac muscles, and obesity as evidenced by pulse 92 irregular, fatigue, shortness of breath with activity, and orthopnea

PLANNING

Patient Outcomes

Short term (at the end of this visit):
- Reba will agree to meet with a dietitian to learn about an individualized nutrition plan and healthy food choices.
- She will commit to read labels and choose foods lower in sodium and fat.
- She will plan to obtain a small medicine organizer.

Long term (at follow-up visit in one month):
- Weight 178 pounds; blood pressure 140/85
- Edema absent or nonpitting, lungs clear
- Report of less fatigue, walking short distances regularly
- Electrolytes within normal range and lipid levels reduced

Nursing Interventions

1. Check Reba's home records of blood pressure, pulse, and weight.
2. Teach her about general dietary measures to reduce her edema.
3. Set up an appointment with a dietitian for an individualized plan.
4. Review her medications and teach her when to notify the doctor.

IMPLEMENTATION (Also see Chapter 5 and Chapter 8.)

1. Measured vital signs, reviewed the log that Reba had recorded, and praised Reba for her conscientious efforts.
   Vital signs help determine the effectiveness of treatments for heart failure and hypertension. Praise often motivates a patient to continue positive behaviors.
   a. Asked Reba to demonstrate how she takes her pulse and blood pressure, using her home blood pressure monitoring equipment.
   b. Compared Reba's results with the nurse's.
   In order to look for valid trends in results, accuracy of measurement technique is needed.

THE NURSING APPROACH—cont'd

Case Study: Hypertension and Heart Failure—cont'd

2. Reviewed Reba's record of daily weights and explained how weight increases with excessive sodium intake.
   a. Taught Reba that sodium causes the body to retain fluid, contributing to weight gain, edema, and dyspnea (difficulty breathing).
   b. Showed Reba how to read labels and choose soups and frozen dinners that are lower in sodium.
   c. Gave her a list of foods that are high in sodium and thus should be limited or avoided.
   d. Told her about herbs that can be used in place of salt to flavor food.
      Patients are more likely to comply with nutrition therapy if they understand the reasons for restrictions and are given practical suggestions as to how to adhere to guidelines.
3. Taught Reba guidelines for making healthy food choices based on fat and calories.
   a. Recommended eating fish and chicken instead of red meat and recommended increasing whole grains, fruits and vegetables, and skim milk (with lactase if needed).
      Omega-3 fatty acids from fish may reduce clot formation, reducing the risk of coronary occlusion. Red meat is a source of cholesterol. Soluble fiber can help reduce LDL cholesterol levels. Lactase additives can be added to milk if necessary because many African Americans have lactose intolerance.
   b. Explained that low-fat, low-cholesterol foods help minimize fatty deposits in the blood vessels and heart.
      A decrease in saturated fats, cholesterol, and trans fats minimizes formation of atherosclerosis.
   c. Recommended nutritious low-calorie foods to help Reba lose weight and thus decrease the workload of the heart.
      Obesity increases peripheral resistance and cardiac workload. Reducing high-fat desserts can help with weight loss and reduction of lipid levels.
   d. Referred Reba to the American Heart Association for additional information and simple recipes.
4. Recommended small, frequent meals rather than large meals, with rest periods before meal preparation and eating.
   Small meals require less energy for eating and digesting food. Rest periods can reduce oxygen consumption, relieve shortness of breath and fatigue, and help increase appetite.
5. Asked Reba to show the nurse her medications, and recommended placing medications in a small weekly organizer.
   Small medicine holders may designate the days of the week, alerting the patient to whether medicine has been taken on a particular day.
   a. Asked Reba to tell the nurse the purpose of each medicine and when each should be taken.
      Verifying a patient's understanding of prescribed medications is important for safety and effectiveness
   b. Informed Reba about special precautions needed when taking her medications.
      Digoxin increases stroke volume by strengthening cardiac muscles, but if doses are excessive, nausea and vomiting may occur and the pulse rate may drop too low. The

patient should withhold the medicine if the pulse is below 60. Diuretics promote loss of sodium and fluid but may also waste potassium. Frequent lab tests are necessary to determine digoxin and potassium levels. Vasodilators decrease peripheral resistance, but they can produce orthostatic hypotension. Patients should be advised to rise slowly from bed to avoid becoming dizzy.

6. Drew blood for the lab to check digoxin levels and electrolyte levels. Told Reba that she may need to eat more foods high in potassium because of the diuretic she was taking.
   Some diuretics waste potassium, but other medicines may conserve potassium. Electrolytes need to be checked regularly because there is danger of death if the potassium levels are too high or too low. Low potassium contributes to digoxin toxicity, so a potassium supplement may be prescribed. Foods high in potassium include fruits (especially bananas and citrus), vegetables (especially green leafy), dairy products, meats, and legumes.
7. Instructed Reba regarding when to call the doctor—for example, when she gains 3 pounds or more in 2 days, when she has difficulty breathing, and when edema gets worse. Also, she should call if her blood pressure is 180/90 or higher and/or her pulse is below 60.
   A gain of 1 kg of weight (2.2 pounds) could indicate retention of 1 L of fluid. Hypertension may lead to a stroke, so medications may need to be adjusted.
8. Set up an appointment with a dietitian for an individualized nutrition plan.
   Because the diet combines several components, it could be confusing to the patient. The DASH (Dietary Approaches to Stop Hypertension) diet focuses on low sodium. The TLC (Therapeutic Lifestyle Changes) diet and low-calorie diets focus on low fat.
9. Encouraged her to begin a walking program for 10 minutes each day, as approved by the doctor.
   Regular exercise strengthens cardiac muscle and increases peripheral vascular blood flow. It also helps with weight reduction.

EVALUATION

Short term (at the end of the visit):
- Reba agreed to meet with a dietitian.
- She said she would read labels and choose foods lower in sodium and fat.
- She planned to ask her granddaughter to buy a small medicine organizer at the drugstore for her.
- Reba made an appointment with the nurse for a visit in 1 month.
- Goals met.

DISCUSSION QUESTIONS

1. Compare and contrast the basic principles of the TLC diet and the DASH diet.
2. Trans fats increase LDL levels and decrease HDL levels, so they should be restricted. Which foods are likely to contain trans fats and thus should be avoided?

CRITICAL THINKING

Clinical Applications

Kevin, age 69, is admitted to the coronary care unit of your hospital. He is 6 feet tall, medium frame, and weighs 210 pounds. He has gained 30 pounds since he retired 4 years ago, which he attributes to boredom and lack of exercise. Three months before admission, Kevin began to experience chest pain that radiated up his neck and down to his stomach. He has a history of hypertension and elevated serum cholesterol levels. After admission to the hospital, Kevin was diagnosed with having had an acute myocardial infarction.

Test results for serum lipids were as follows:

Cholesterol: 300 mg/dL

LDL cholesterol: 200 mg/dL

HDL cholesterol: 30 mg/dL

TG: 600 mg/dL

Medications prescribed after admission: atenolol (Tenormin), diltiazem (Cardizem), nitroglycerin

Diet order: TLC diet

1. What are the risk factors for cardiovascular disease?
2. What are Kevin's risk factors?
3. Define the term *myocardial infarction* and describe what happens when a myocardial infarction occurs.
4. What specific guidelines are included in the National Cholesterol Education Program's (NCEP) TLC diet recommendations?

While caring for Kevin you learn that he snacks on high-fat cheeses, ice cream, potato chips, corn chips, peanuts, and crackers. He also drinks whole milk and eats a lot of butter on his bread at every meal. What characteristics of Kevin's intake contradict the NCEP's TLC diet recommendations? What are some alternative foods that are appealing to Kevin that he could eat for snacks?

WEBSITES OF INTEREST

American Heart Association (AHA)

www.americanheart.org

Contains resources, interactive educational materials, and everyday strategies and support for prevention and treatment of heart disease and stroke.

National Cholesterol Education Program (NCEP)

www.nhlbi.nih.gov/chd

Makes available the wide ranges of educational and research programs of NCEP.

World Hypertension League (WHL)

www.worldhypertensionleague.org

Advocates for the detection, prevention, and treatment of HTN in populations globally through association with the World Health Organization.

REFERENCES

1. Writing Group Members, et al: Heart disease and stroke statistics 2010 update: a report from the American Heart Association, *Circulation* 121:e46-e215, 2010.
2. Centers for Disease Control and Prevention: Declining prevalence of no known major risk factors for heart disease and stroke among adults—United States, 1991-2001, *MMWR Morb Mortal Wkly Rep* 53:4-7, 2004.
3. Price SA, Wilson LM: *Pathophysiology: Clinical concepts of disease processes*, ed 6, St. Louis, 2002, Mosby.
4. McCance KL, Huether SE: *Pathophysiology: The biological basis for disease in adults and children*, ed 5, St. Louis, 2006, Mosby.
5. National Cholesterol Education Program (NCEP): *Third report of the NCEP expert panel on detection, evaluation, and treatment of high blood cholesterol in adults (Adult Treatment Panel III): executive summary*, NIH Pub No 01-3670, Washington, DC, 2001 (May), National Institutes of Health, National Heart, Lung, and Blood Institute.
6. National Cholesterol Education Program (NCEP): *ATP III Update 2004: implications of recent clinical trials for the ATP III Guidelines*, Washington, DC, 2004, National Institutes of Health, National Heart, Lung, and Blood Institute.
7. American Heart Association: *Heart and stroke facts*, Dallas, 1992-2003, Author. Accessed April 7, 2010, from www.americanheart.org/presenter.jhtml?identifier=3000333.
8. Stamler J, et al: Relation of changes in dietary lipids and weight, trial years 1-6, to change in blood lipids in the special intervention and usual care groups in the Multiple Risk Factor Intervention Trial, *Am J Clin Nutr* 65:272S-288S, 1997.
9. Clarke R, et al: Dietary lipids and blood cholesterol: Quantitative meta-analysis of metabolic ward studies, *BMJ* 314:112-117, 1997.
10. Kris-Etherton PM, et al: High-monounsaturated fatty acid diets lower both plasma cholesterol and triacylglycerol concentrations, *Am J Clin Nutr* 70:1009-1015, 1999.
11. Garg A: High-monounsaturated-fat diets for patients with diabetes mellitus: A meta-analysis, *Am J Clin Nutr* 67(Suppl 3):577S-582S, 1998.
12. Knopp RH, et al: Long-term cholesterol-lowering effects of 4 fat-restricted diets in hypercholesterolemic and combined hyperlipidemic men. The Dietary Alternatives Study, *JAMA* 278:1509-1515, 1997.
13. U.S. Department of Health and Human Services, Food and Drug Administration. Food labeling: Health claims: Soluble

fiber from certain foods and coronary heart disease. Final rule, *Fed Reg* 63(32):8103-8121, 1998.

14. Vuorio AF, et al: Stanol ester margarine alone and with simvastatin lowers serum cholesterol in families with familial hypercholesterolemia caused by the FH-North Karelia Mutation, *Arterioscler Thromb Vasc Biol* 20:500-506, 2000.

15. Gylling H, Miettinen TA: Cholesterol reduction by different plant stanol mixtures and with variable fat intake, *Metabolism* 48:575-580, 1999.

16. Hallikainen MA, Uusitupa MI: Effects of 2 low-fat stanol ester-containing margarines on serum cholesterol concentrations as part of a low-fat diet in hypercholesterolemic subjects, *Am J Clin Nutr* 69:403-410, 1999.

17. U.S. Department of Health and Human Services, Public Health Service, National Institutes of Health, National Heart, Lung, and Blood Institute: *Your guide to lowering your blood pressure with DASH*, NIH Publication No. 06-4082, Bethesda, Md, 2006, Author. Accessed April 7, 2010, from www.nhlbi.nih.gov.

18. National High Blood Pressure Program: *The seventh report of the Joint National Committee on prevention, detection, evaluation, and treatment of high blood pressure*, National Institutes of Health, National Heart, Lung, and Blood Institutes, NIH Publication No. 04-5230, Washington, DC, 2004, U.S. Government Printing Office.

19. Sacks FM, et al: Effects on blood pressure of reduced dietary sodium and the dietary approaches to stop hypertension (DASH) diet, *N Engl J Med* 344(1):3-10, 2001.

20. National Institutes of Health: *NIH news release: NHLBI study finds DASH diet and reduced sodium lowers blood pressure for all*, Bethesda, Md, 2001 (December 17), National Institutes of Health. Accessed April 7, 2010, from www.nih.gov/news/pr/dec2001/nhlbi-17.htm.

21. Poehlman, et al: Increased resting metabolic rate in patients with congestive heart failure, *Ann Intern Med* 121:860-862, 1994.

22. Heymsfield SB, et al: Bioenergetic and metabolic response to continuous v intermittent nasoenteric feeding, *Metabolism* 36(6):570-575, 1987.

23. Mueller DH: Medical nutrition therapy for pulmonary disease. In Mahan LK, Escott-Stump S, editors: *Krause's food & nutrition therapy*, ed 12, Philadelphia, 2008, Saunders.

24. American Dietetic Association Nutrition Care Manual: Chronic obstructive pulmonary disease (COPD). Accessed April 7, 2010, from www.nutritioncaremanual.org.

25. American Dietetic Association Nutrition Care Manual: Acute respirator distress syndrome (ARDS). Accessed April 7, 2010, from www.nutritioncaremanual.org.

26. Barber JR, Miller SJ, Sacks G: Parenteral feeding formulations. In Gottschlich M, editor: *The science and practice of nutrition support*, Dubuque, Iowa, 2001, Kendall/Hunt.

Nutrition for Diseases of the Kidneys

The chief life-preserving function of the kidneys is to maintain chemical homeostasis in the body.

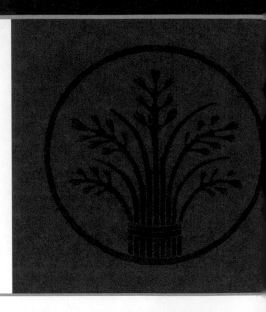

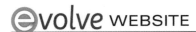 WEBSITE
http://evolve.elsevier.com/Grodner/foundations/

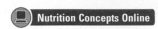

ROLE IN WELLNESS

Although often taken for granted, kidneys filter approximately 1 L of blood per minute to remove excess fluid and more than 200 waste products from the body. In addition, they perform vital metabolic and hormonal functions. Because kidneys play so many roles in wellness, kidney disease has serious consequences. Nutritional needs of patients with kidney disease are complex and ever changing and require constant assessment, monitoring, and counseling. These factors present an ongoing challenge to nursing and other health care team members.

The dimensions of health reveal the challenges in dealing with kidney disorders. Functions of the kidneys affect total physical well-being; implementing nutrition therapy to aid treatment is essential for enhancing the *physical health* dimension. *Intellectual health* dimension is tested because clients need to know (or be taught) anatomy and physiology to fully understand the dysfunction processes that lead to kidney disorders and the necessity to follow a strict diet. The chronic nature and potentially life-threatening aspects of kidney disorders may be emotionally devastating; clients may benefit from psychologic counseling to deal with these illnesses to maintain *emotional health*. The *social health* dimension may be strained by kidney disorders. Significant others may become worn down by the responsibility of caring for loved ones with renal disorders; the ever-present need for dialysis, once initiated, disrupts normal social relationships unless new ways of coping are established. *Spiritual health* may affect physical response to treatment. Individuals participating regularly in religious activities tend to have lower blood pressures compared with those who do not participate.

KIDNEY FUNCTION

The chief life-preserving function of the kidneys is to maintain chemical homeostasis in the body. They do this largely by processing components within the blood to maintain fluid, electrolyte, and acid-base balance and by eliminating wastes in the urine. Each kidney has approximately 1 million "microscopic" workhorses called *nephrons* (Figure 21-1). Each nephron filters and resorbs essential blood constituents, secretes ions as needed for maintaining acid-base balance, and excretes fluid and other substances as urine. Other important functions of kidneys include manufacturing hormones to regulate blood pressure (renin), stimulating production of red blood cells (erythropoietin), and regulating calcium and phosphorus metabolism (final step in vitamin D synthesis). Kidneys also detoxify some drugs and poisons (Box 21-1).

Various inflammatory, obstructive, and degenerative diseases affect kidneys in different ways. These disorders interfere with normal functioning of nephrons to regulate products of body metabolism. Ultimately, kidney failure could lead to homeostatic failure and, if not relieved, death.

NEPHROTIC SYNDROME

Nephrotic syndrome is a term used to describe a complex of symptoms that can occur as a result of damage to the capillary walls of the glomerulus. Glomerular damage results in increased urinary excretion of protein (proteinuria) that leads to decreased serum levels of albumin (hypoalbuminemia), hyperlipidemia, and edema.[1,2] Nephrotic syndrome is often the result of secondary disease processes: primary glomerular disease (**glomerulonephritis**), nephropathy

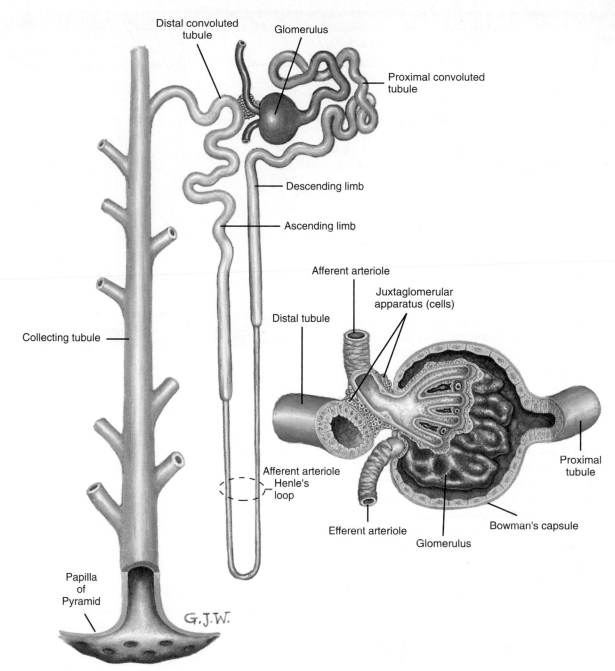

FIG 21-1 The nephron. Blood flows into the glomerulus, and some of its fluid is absorbed into the tubule. Waste products are filtered and passed through the tubule into the bladder. The fluid and dissolved substances needed by the body are resorbed in vessels alongside the tubule. (From Brundage DJ: *Renal disorders, Mosby's clinical nursing series,* St. Louis, 1992, Mosby.)

| BOX 21-1 | **KIDNEY FUNCTIONS** |

- Maintain fluid, electrolyte, and acid-base balance
- Eliminate waste products
- Regulate blood pressure
- Stimulate red blood cell production
- Regulate calcium and phosphorus metabolism
- Eliminate many drugs

secondary to **amyloidosis** (accumulation of waxy starchlike glycoprotein), diabetes mellitus, **systemic lupus erythematosus (SLE)** (a chronic inflammatory disease affecting many body systems), or infectious disease. It may be treated with corticosteroid or immunosuppressive medications, but in some patients, nephrotic syndrome is resistant to treatment and may progress to chronic kidney disease (CKD).[1,2]

It is essential for nursing personnel to monitor patients' weight and intake and output closely. Intake and output

BOX 21-2 FOODS HIGH IN SODIUM

CONDIMENTS	BREADS/ STARCHES	MEATS/MEAT SUBSTITUTES	BEVERAGES	SOUPS	VEGETABLES
Pickles, olives (black and green), salted nuts, meat tenderizers, commercial salad dressings, monosodium glutamate (MSG, Accent), steak sauce, ketchup, soy sauce, Worcestershire sauce, horseradish sauce, chili sauce, commercial mustard, salt, seasoned salts (onion, garlic, celery), butter salt	Salted crackers, potato chips, corn chips, popcorn, pretzels, dehydrated potatoes	Cured, smoked, and processed meats (ham, bacon, corned beef, chipped beef, hot dogs, luncheon meats, bologna, salt pork, canned salmon and tuna); all cheeses except low-sodium and cottage cheese; convenience foods (microwave and TV dinners); peanut butter	Commercial buttermilk, instant hot cocoa mixes	Canned soups, dehydrated soups, bouillon	Sauerkraut, hominy, pork and beans, canned tomato and vegetable juices

should be documented in the medical record every shift.[3] The nurse and dietitian play important roles in developing a nutrition care plan for patients with CKD and in educating them regarding, for example, foods high in sodium (Box 21-2). For the specific sodium content of foods, consult the Food Composition Table on the Evolve website.

Nutrition Therapy

Primary goals of nutrition therapy are to control hypertension, minimize edema, decrease urinary albumin losses, prevent protein malnutrition and muscle catabolism, supply adequate energy, and slow the progression of renal disease.[4,5] Patients need to consume adequate amounts of protein (0.7 to 1 g/kg/day) and energy (35 kcal/kg/day) to prevent catabolism of lean body tissue and avoid malnutrition. Total fat intake should provide less than 30% of total energy needs. Complex carbohydrates should provide the majority of a patient's kcal because protein, and possibly fat intake, should be limited.[5]

Limiting dietary sodium can help control hypertension and edema. Commercial preparation and processing of foods, especially convenience foods, often adds substantial amounts of sodium (see Chapter 8). Patients should also be mindful of possible hidden sources of salt (e.g., water supply, medications). In addition, toothpaste and mouthwash often contain a significant amount of sodium; therefore, patients should be instructed not to swallow these products (Box 21-3).

ACUTE KIDNEY FAILURE

Acute kidney failure (AKF) is characterized by an abrupt loss of renal function that may or may not be accompanied by oliguria or anuria.[1,2,6,7] The most common cause of AKF is acute tubular necrosis (ATN), which is generally described as postischemic (injury after decreased blood supply) or nephrotoxic (toxic to a kidney).[1,7] Although a few patients do not experience any reduction in urine output, two thirds experience the following three stages:[1,2,4,8]

BOX 21-3 HIDDEN SOURCES OF SODIUM

- Baking powder
- Drinking and cooking water
- Medications
  Antacids
  Antibiotics
  Cough medicines
  Laxatives
  Pain relievers
  Sedatives
- Mouthwash
- Toothpaste

1. *Oliguric phase* (usually present within 24 to 48 hours after initial injury, lasting approximately 1 to 3 weeks): This stage is manifested by clinical signs of (retention of excessive amounts of nitrogenous compounds in the blood), acidosis, high serum potassium, high serum phosphorus, hypertension, anorexia, edema, and risk of water intoxication (indicated by low sodium levels).
2. *Diuretic phase* (usually lasts approximately 2 to 3 weeks). The output of urine is gradually increased.
3. *Recovery phase* (usually lasts 3 to 12 months): Kidney function gradually improves, but there may be some residual permanent damage.

Body weight should be taken and recorded daily. When patients do not eat, they may lose approximately 0.5 kg/day.[3] Conversely, any sudden weight gains suggest excessive fluid retention. Monitoring intake, output, and weight will help differentiate whether weight loss or gain is from fluid retention as opposed to lean body mass or adipose tissue. Fluid retention can mask loss of lean body mass.

Nurses and dietitians are the health care professionals who may be called on to assist patients in adhering to prescribed fluid restrictions (see the *Teaching Tool* box, Suggestions for Coping With Fluid Restrictions, in Chapter 18). Nurses work closely with renal dietitians to coordinate meal planning and nutrition education with patients and their significant others.[3] Nutrition education may involve reduced protein, sodium, potassium, and fluid intake. The Food Composition Table on Evolve lists the specific protein, sodium, and potassium content of foods. Nurses should be watchful for constipation as a result of restricted intake of fluids and fresh fruits (most are high in potassium), bed rest, and medication side effects.[3]

Nutrition Therapy

Nutritional needs are partially determined by whether **dialysis** is used for treatment. Dialysis is a procedure that involves diffusion of particles from an area of high to lower concentration, osmosis of fluid across the membrane from an area of lesser to greater concentration of particles, and the ultrafiltration or movement of fluid across the membrane as a result of an artificially created pressure differential. Another determinant of nutrient needs is the underlying cause of the AKF. Patients may be hypermetabolic if renal failure is caused by trauma, burns, septicemia, or infection. These conditions, other underlying medical problems, and renal failure are known to have a negative impact on the patient's appetite, thus increasing concern for nutritional status.

Energy should be provided in sufficient amounts for weight maintenance or to meet the demands of stress accompanying the AKF, usually 30 to 40 kcal/kg.[4,5] Fats, oils, simple carbohydrates, and low-protein starches should provide nonprotein kcal. In cases in which dialysis is not necessary for treatment, 0.6 g of protein per kg body weight (but not less than 40 g per day) for unstressed patients is recommended.[8] This amount can be increased as kidney function improves. When dialysis is used as part of the medical treatment, protein intake can be liberalized to 1 to 1.4 g/kg.[8] In either situation, use of high biologic value or high-quality proteins is recommended.[8] Diets containing less than 60 g of protein per day may be deficient in niacin, riboflavin, thiamine, calcium, iron, vitamin B_{12}, and zinc,[5] and these nutrients may need to be supplemented during convalescence.

During the oliguric stage, sodium may be restricted to 1000 to 2000 mg and potassium to 1000 mg per day. Both sodium and potassium, the principal electrolytes, may be lost during the diuretic phase or during dialysis. Therefore, losses should be replaced as needed depending on urinary volume, serum levels, and frequency of dialysis.[5] Box 21-4 lists foods high in potassium. Fluids are usually restricted to the patient's output (urine, vomitus, and diarrhea) plus 500 mL during the oliguric phase.[5,8] During the diuretic phase, large amounts of fluid may be needed to replace losses.

CHRONIC KIDNEY DISEASE

Progressive, irreversible loss of kidney function[1,2] (excretory endocrine, and metabolic function) can develop over days, months, or years and progress through five stages of chronic kidney disease (CKD).[2,3,7] CKD has many causes; some of the most common are glomerulonephritis, **nephrosclerosis** (necrosis of the renal arterioles, associated with

---

BOX 21-4	FOODS HIGH IN POTASSIUM

Apricots
Avocados
Bananas
Cantaloupes
Carrots, raw
Dried beans, peas
Dried fruits
Melons
Oranges, orange juice
Peanuts (also high in sodium)
Potatoes, white and sweet
Prune juice
Spinach
Swiss chard
Tomatoes, tomato juice, tomato sauce
Winter squash

---

hypertension), obstructive diseases (kidney stones, tumors, congenital birth defects of kidneys and urinary tract), diabetes mellitus, SLE, and illicit use of analgesics or street drugs. Regardless of cause, results will be the same: retention of nitrogenous waste products and fluid and electrolyte imbalances that can affect all body systems.

Management focuses on slowing progression and minimizing complications.[3] Once CKD progresses to stage 5, management centers on replacement, **hemodialysis, peritoneal dialysis (PD)**, and **renal transplantation**.[3]

Nutrition Therapy

Planning diets for CKD, hemodialysis, and PD patients requires the dietitian to calibrate intakes of fluids, energy, protein, lipids, phosphorus, potassium, sodium, and vitamins and other minerals. It is important to design food combinations that not only include necessary nutrients but also that the patient accepts and enjoys. This task can be overwhelming, but there are specialists—renal dietitians—who do this on a daily basis. The National Renal Diet is often used to develop diet guidelines and meal plans (see Appendix F).

Nurses play an important role in helping patients maintain good nutritional status, weight, morale, and appetite by working with renal dietitians to reinforce medical nutrition therapy and nutrition education. Through formal and informal teaching, nurses can help patients appreciate the need for the stringent diet and help them recognize the direct relationship between adherence to the diet and progression or lack of progression of symptoms that reduce their quality of life.

Nutritional management depends on method of treatment in addition to medical and nutritional status of the patient.[9] Table 21-1 provides a comparison of the treatment methods and primary concerns associated with each.

The exact point at which nutrition therapy should begin is highly variable, but conventional wisdom indicates that dietary modifications (Table 21-2) should be initiated as early

TABLE 21-1 **TREATMENTS AND MAJOR CONCERNS FOR PRE-STAGE 1 CHRONIC KIDNEY DISEASE, HEMODIALYSIS, AND PERITONEAL DIALYSIS**

	PRE-STAGE 1 CKD	HEMODIALYSIS	PERITONEAL DIALYSIS
Treatment Modalities	Diet + medication	Diet + medication + hemodialysis Dialysis using vascular access of waste product and fluid removal	Diet + medication + peritoneal dialysis Dialysis using peritoneal membrane of waste product and fluid removal
Duration Concerns	Indefinite Hypertension, glycemic control in patients with diabetes mellitus Glomerular hyperfiltration, rise in BUN, bone disease Anemia, cardiovascular disease	3-4 hours 3 days/week Bone disease, hypertension Amino acid loss, interdialytic electrolyte and fluid changes Anemia, cardiovascular disease	3-5 exchanges 7 days/week Bone disease, weight gain, hyperlipidemia, glycemic control in patients with diabetes mellitus Protein loss into dialysate, glucose absorption from dialysate Anemia, cardiovascular disease

BUN, Blood urea nitrogen; *CKD,* chronic kidney disease.
Data from American Dietetic Association: *National renal diet: Professional guide,* ed 2, Chicago, 2002, American Dietetic Association and K/DOQI clinical practice guidelines for chronic kidney disease: evaluation, classification, and stratification guideline 1. Definition and stages of chronic kidney disease, New York, 2002, National Kidney Foundation.

TABLE 21-2 **NUTRITION GUIDELINES FOR CHRONIC KIDNEY DISEASE WITHOUT DIALYSIS, AND WITH HEMODIALYSIS, AND PERITONEAL DIALYSIS**

NUTRIENT	CKD WITHOUT DIALYSIS	HEMODIALYSIS	PERITONEAL DIALYSIS	COMMENTS
Energy	35 kcal/kg < 60 yrs; 30-35 kcal/kg > 60 yrs	35 kcal/kg < 60 yrs; 30-35 kcal/kg > 60	35 kcal/kg < 60 yrs including dialysate; 30-35 kcal/kg > 60 yrs	
Protein	0.6-0.75 g/kg ≥50% HVB	≥1.2 g/kg ≥50% HVB	≥1.2-1.3 g/kg ≥50% HVB	
Sodium	Individualized, 1-3 g/day	2 g/day	2 g/day	
Potassium	Usually unrestricted unless hyperkalemic	2-3 g/day adjust to serum levels	3-4 g/day adjust to serum levels	
Phosphorus	800-1000 mg/day	800-1000 g/day	800-1000 g/ day	May require phosphate binder
Fluid	As desired	1000 ml+urine output/day	Unrestricted if weight and blood pressure controlled and residual renal function is 2-3 L/day	
Vitamin/mineral supplementation	As appropriate	As appropriate	As appropriate	Supplements designed specially for dialysis patients are available; supplements of vitamin C should not exceed 100 mg/day to prevent hyperoxalemia; vitamin A supplementation is not recommended; in patient receiving rHuEPO, iron supplementation is almost always required; zinc supplementation may be helpful for patients with impaired taste

CKD, Chronic kidney disease; *HBV,* high biological value; *IBW,* ideal body weight.
From National Kidney Foundation Dialysis Outcomes Quality Initiative: *Clinical practice guidelines for nutrition in chronic renal failure, 2000,* New York, 2001, National Kidney Foundation. Accessed April 10, 2010, from www.kidney.org/professionals/kdoqi/guidelines_updates/doqi_nut.html; Wilkens KG, Juneja V: Medical nutrition therapy for renal disorders. In Mahan K, Escott-Stump S, eds: *Krause's food & nutrition therapy,* ed 12, St. Louis, 2008, Saunders.

as possible to minimize **uremic toxicity**, delay progression of renal disease, and prevent wasting and malnutrition.[10,11] This can be accomplished by limiting foods whose metabolic by-products add to buildup of such toxic substances and by providing adequate kcal to prevent body tissue catabolism. Patients often find this diet difficult to follow for a long period; therefore, motivation and encouragement from nursing and other health professionals are crucial.

In view of the fact that malnutrition is so clearly associated with mortality in renal failure, continuing to assess nutritional status and dietary compliance of patients with CRF is important.[12] Because patients may find that foods "don't taste like they used to," encouraging use of spices such as garlic, onions, and oregano to enhance the flavor of allowed foods can be helpful.[3] The National Renal Diet was developed by the Renal Dietitians Practice Group, American Dietetic Association, and National Kidney Foundation Council on Renal Nutrition to provide a renal diet with nationwide applicability. Diet prescription guidelines for pre stage 5 CKD, hemodialysis, and peritoneal dialysis patients were developed over a 5-year period. Because of the national focus of these guidelines, ethnic and geographically unique foods are not included but can be incorporated as part of the individualized diet plan. Vegetarian choices also are not included because high biologic value proteins (eggs, meats, poultry, game, fish, soy, and dairy products) are the preferred protein sources for renal patients, and some foods in vegan diets are of low biologic value. Ovo-vegetarian and lacto-ovovegetarian diets include high biologic value protein sources, but they also tend to be high in phosphorus. One point that requires emphasis is that the National Renal Diet guidelines and food lists are only a starting point for individualized meal plans and education. Patient compliance may be enhanced by designing meal plans to meet the specific needs of each patient. Box 21-5 provides a sample menu for a patient with CKD.

HEMODIALYSIS

During hemodialysis (HD) blood is shunted by way of a special vascular access or shunt (usually in the nondominant forearm), **heparinized**, cleansed of excess fluid and waste products through a semipermeable membrane, and then returned to the patient's circulation (Figure 21-2).[1,7] The **dialysate** (dialysis solution) is an electrolyte solution similar to the composition of normal plasma. Each constituent may be varied according to the patient's needs, the most common being potassium.[3] Average treatment lasts 3 to 6 hours and is usually performed three times per week (Figure 21-3). HD can be performed in a dialysis unit by trained staff. Patients who have received special training may assist in their treatment.

Nutrition Therapy

Individual diet prescriptions (see Table 21-2) are determined by residual kidney function, dialysate components, duration of dialysis, and rate of blood flow through the artificial kidney.[8] The meal plan is designed, monitored,

---

BOX 21-5	SAMPLE RENAL DIET MENU

85 g protein; 2000 mg sodium; 2000 mg potassium; 1000 mg phosphorus; 1000 mL fluid

Breakfast
Apple juice
Oatmeal
Blueberry muffin
Scrambled egg
Low-sodium margarine (2 exchanges)*
2% milk (½ cup)*
Decaffeinated coffee (½ cup)*

Lunch
Lemonade (½ cup)*
Sirloin tips (3 oz) with noodles*
Salad with Italian dressing
Fruit cocktail

Dinner
Fruit punch (½ cup)*
Low-sodium turkey (3 oz) with parsley carrots*
White bread with margarine (2 exchanges)*
Cinnamon applesauce
Hot tea (½ cup)*

*Quantities not exact; for representation only.
Courtesy Memorial Hospital, Carbondale, Ill.

---

and reevaluated by the dietitian. Nurses and others on the medical team are crucial for providing positive reinforcement and encouragement to the patient and family members on an ongoing basis. Objectives for nutrition therapy are to attain or maintain good nutritional status, prevent excessive accumulation of waste products and fluid between treatments, and minimize the effects of metabolic disorders that occur as a result of CKD.[13]

Protein and Energy

Recommendations for protein are intended to counteract protein losses during dialysis, abnormalities in protein metabolism, altered albumin turnover, increased amino acid degradation attributable to metabolic acidosis, inflammation, and infection. The recommended protein intake for patients receiving HD ≥ is 1.2 g protein/kg standard body weight per day with at least 50% of the dietary protein of high biologic value.[13]

Energy expenditure in HD patients is similar to healthy individuals. For adult patients younger than age 60, daily energy intake of 35 kcal/kg of standard body weight is recommended. Obese individuals and adults older than age 60 may benefit from 30 to 35 kcal/kg of body weight.[13]

Fat

Patients receiving HD are at risk for lipid metabolism disorders. As such, less than 30% of total kcal should be from fat, less than 10% of total kcal should be from saturated fat. Dietary cholesterol should be less than 300 mg/day. Restricting cholesterol and energy intake from fats less than these

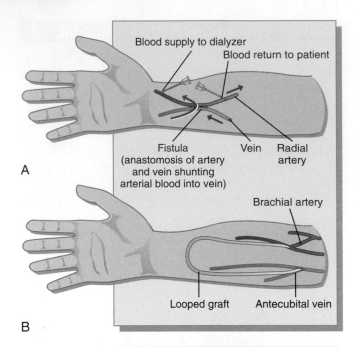

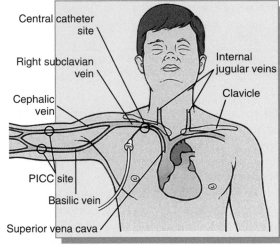

FIG 21-2 Types of access for hemodialysis. A, Arteriovenous fistula (AV); **B,** artificial loop graft; **C,** subclavian catheter (usually temporary). (**A** and **B,** from Mahan LK, Escott-Stump S, editors: *Krause's food & nutrition therapy,* ed 12, Philadelphia, 2008, Elsevier. **C,** from Lewis SM, Heitkemper MM, Dirksen SR: *Medical-surgical nursing: Assessment and management of clinical problems,* ed 5, St. Louis, 2000, Mosby.)

levels may not be beneficial because the decreased energy intake may lead to malnutrition.[13]

Sodium, Potassium, and Fluid

Sodium and fluid restrictions should be individualized to keep in check intradialytic weight gains, blood pressure control, and residual renal function. The recommended intradialytic fluid gains is less than 5% of the patient's dry weight.[13] Corresponding sodium and fluids restrictions are as follows:[13]

- Fluid output >1 L (1000 mL) per day
  2 to 4 g (87 to 174 mEq) sodium per day
  2 L (2000 mL) fluid intake per day

- Fluid output <1 L (1000 mL) per day
  2 grams (87 mEq) sodium per day
  1 to 1.5 L (1000 to 1500 mL) per day
- Anuria
  2 g (87 mEq) sodium per day
- L (1000 mL) per day

Dietary potassium restriction varies depending on urine output. Excretion of potassium increases as glomerular filtration rate (GFR) declines. Generally, 2.5 g of potassium per day is well tolerated. On the other hand, patients with anuria or constipation may experience hyperkalemia. Patients with insulin deficiency, or metabolic acidosis, those in a hypercatabolic state, or those being treated with beta blockers or aldosterone antagonists may require a stricter potassium restriction.

PHOSPHORUS AND CALCIUM

Phosphorus is routinely restricted in patients receiving HD because high levels of serum phosphorus contribute to secondary hyperparathyroidism and raise the calcium-phosphorus product in the plasma.[3,5] Although an intake of 800-1000 mg/kg/day is the usual recommendation, it is often necessary to liberalize this restriction to meet protein needs.[9] Foods high in phosphorus, such as milk, milk products, cheese, beef liver, chocolate, nuts, and legumes, are usually limited or avoided. Medications (phosphate binders) also are used to control serum phosphorus levels. The medications of choice are calcium carbonate, calcium acetate, or sevelamer hydrochloride.[11] They are given at mealtimes to bind phosphate in the food.

Vitamin D

In renal failure, kidneys also lose their endocrine function of producing calcitriol (the active form of vitamin D). Although many forms of vitamin D are available for supplementation, it is this active form that helps prevent bone disease.[3] The active form of vitamin D is available in oral form (e.g., calcitriol [Rocaltrol], doxercalciferol [Hectorol]) and intravenous (IV) form (e.g., calcitriol [Calcijex], paricalcitol [Zemplar], Hectorol), which is given during HD.[11]

Iron

Anemia results from another endocrine function affected by CKD: decreased production of the hormone erythropoietin, which is a hormone that stimulates bone marrow to produce red blood cells. An adequate available iron supply is necessary for normal erythropoiesis to take place. Recombinant erythropoietin (EPO) (e.g., epoetin [Epogen]) can be given during dialysis (by IV) or subcutaneously just after dialysis treatment. Oral or IV iron supplementation is often necessary before administration of recombinant EPO to replenish iron stores.[3,5,11]

Vitamins

Patients treated with HD also are at risk for deficiencies of water-soluble vitamins, particularly vitamin B_6 and folic acid. The reason is twofold: (1) poor intake and loss

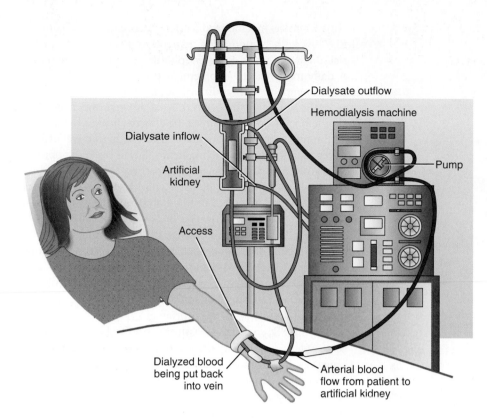

FIG 21-3 Hemodialysis. Treatment is usually for 3 to 6 hours, three times a week. (From Mahan LK, Escott-Stump S, eds: *Krause's food & nutrition therapy,* ed 12, Philadelphia, 2008, Saunders.)

of the nutrients during dialysis.[13,14] Supplementation of the fat-soluble vitamins A, E, and K is usually not necessary. In fact, patients treated with HD have been reported to experience vitamin A toxicity. Supplementation of trace minerals is not necessary unless a deficiency is suspected or documented.[14]

Patients who have a poor dietary intake are at increased risk of nutrient deficiencies and poor nutritional status. Intake can be the result of poor appetite, changes in taste acuity and in food preferences (especially red meat and sweets), nausea and vomiting, or diet limitations. When patients develop changes in taste, foods with sharp, distinct flavors may be useful in stimulating appetite (Box 21-6).

Approximately one third of patients requiring HD each year have diabetes mellitus. Diets for these patients should incorporate nutritional modifications necessary for CKD and provide consistent content and timing of meals and snacks to facilitate glycemic control.[9]

PERITONEAL DIALYSIS

Peritoneal dialysis (PD) removes excess fluid and waste products from blood using the peritoneal membrane as a filter. Dialysate is instilled and removed through a catheter that has been surgically placed into the peritoneal cavity. The peritoneum (i.e., the lining of the abdominal cavity) is used as the dialysis membrane (Figure 21-4). Waste products cross the membrane by passive movement from the peritoneal capillaries into the dialysate in the peritoneal cavity. The dialysate contains dextrose, which increases osmolality of the solution

---

BOX 21-6   SUGGESTIONS FOR PATIENTS WITH ALTERED TASTE

- Brush teeth and tongue 6 to 8 times per day
- Rinse mouth with a chilled mouthwash (commercial product or water mixed with lemon juice or vinegar)
- Suck lemon wedges or hard candy before meals
- Chew gum
- Before meals, drink water with lemon or eat a small amount of sherbet or fruit sorbet

Data from Schatz SR: Helpful hints for common problems. In Byham-Gray L, Wiesen K, editors: *A clinical guide to nutrition care in kidney disease,* Chicago, 2004, American Dietetic Association.

---

and facilitates removal of excess fluid. As the fluid moves from vascular space into the peritoneal cavity, osmolality of the solutions becomes equal. Toxins and excess fluids collected in the peritoneal cavity are then drained from the body through the catheter and discarded.[15] An advantage of PD is that it is usually performed in the home. All forms of PD require special training of the patient and caregiver.

Intermittent Peritoneal Dialysis

Intermittent peritoneal dialysis (IPD) involves infusion of approximately 2 L of dialysate instilled over 20 to 30 minutes. Dialysate is then drained by gravity, and the process is repeated over an 8- to 10-hour period four or five times per week. IPD can be performed manually or mechanically.

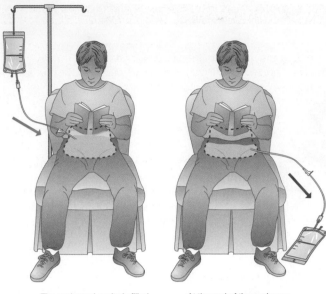

The peritoneal cavity is filled with dialysate, using gravity.

At the end of the exchange, the dialysate is drained into the bag, again using gravity.

FIG 21-4 Continuous ambulatory peritoneal dialysis; 20-minute exchanges usually are given four or five times a day, every day. (From Mahan LK, Escott-Stump S, editors: *Krause's food & nutrition therapy*, ed 12, Philadelphia, 2008, Saunders.)

During the time of dialysis, patients are restricted to a chair or bed.[3] This method is not commonly used as a long-term treatment modality because of the time involvement.

Continuous Ambulatory Peritoneal Dialysis

Continuous ambulatory peritoneal dialysis (CAPD) entails infusion of dialysate four or five "exchanges" within a 24-hour period into the peritoneum. A specific volume of dialysate is infused and allowed to dwell for approximately 4 hours. At the end of the designated time, dialysate containing waste and excess fluid is drained by gravity and a new exchange begins. Dialysate is present 24 hours per day in the peritoneum excluding the 20- to 30-minute exchange when dwelling dialysate is drained and fresh dialysate is instilled.[15] Dialysis exchanges are done continuously, 7 days a week.[3]

Continuous Cycling Peritoneal Dialysis

Continuous cycling peritoneal dialysis (CCPD) is a combination of IPD and CAPD. At night, a cycler (mechanical) performs three dialysate exchanges. During the day, a fourth exchange is infused for the entire day.[3] At bedtime, the fourth exchange is drained, and the process is started again. Although restricted to bed during nighttime infusions, patients are ambulatory during the day.

Nutrition Therapy

Objectives of nutrition therapy (see Table 21-2) are to (1) maintain good nutritional status while replacing albumin lost in the dialysate, (2) minimize complications of fluid imbalance, (3) minimize symptoms of uremic toxicity, and

(4) minimize metabolic disorders secondary to CKD and PD.[15] As with hemodialysis, patients treated with PD are at risk for deficiencies of water-soluble vitamins and minerals. A daily multivitamin supplement that includes folic acid is recommended.[16] In addition, some patients may receive recombinant EPO for correction of anemia and need iron supplementation to maximize the effectiveness of the drug.[3,5]

Energy needs for patients treated with PD are usually lower than for those receiving hemodialysis because approximately 60% of the dialysate is absorbed[16] and needs to be calculated as part of the patient's energy source. Dextrose is used as an osmotic agent in PD dialysate and must be taken into consideration when energy needs are calculated.[3,9]

Protein losses during PD range from 20 to 30 g per day[4,16] and are reflected in higher dietary protein recommendations (see Table 21-2). Serum blood urea nitrogen (BUN) and creatinine levels, uremic symptoms, and weight should be monitored as indicators of sufficient protein intake, and the diet should be adjusted appropriately.[4]

During PD, sodium, potassium, and fluid are continually removed, making severe dietary restrictions unnecessary.[3,4,15] However, it is important to remember that nutrient needs vary among patients and individualized recommendations are necessary. Restriction of dietary phosphorus is critical to prevent development of osteodystrophy (defective bone development). Unfortunately, higher protein requirements for PD consequently provide high amounts of phosphorus. Therefore, severely restricting or eliminating dairy products is necessary to control phosphorus intake, which may result in the need for calcium supplementation.[9] Phosphorus is also controlled by the use of prescribed phosphate binders.

The absorption of glucose from PD dialysate presents challenges in patients with diabetes. Blood glucose levels and hyperlipidemia become more difficult to control.[15] Weight gain caused by increased kcal load of the dialysate may be another common problem with PD. Another condition to watch for is dehydration, which may result from excessive fluid removal and extracellular fluid volume deficits. Careful monitoring of blood glucose, intake and output, and weight are preventive measures.

Although nutritional status is affected by various nondialysis-related causes, anorexia, nausea, and vomiting are key clinical features of uremia and inadequate dialysis. Consequently, nutritional status is an important measure of PD adequacy as well.[17] The National Kidney Foundation[17] suggests ongoing nutritional assessment of PD patients in connection with Kt/V urea and Creatinine clearance (C_{Cr}) measurements using the Protein Equivalent of Nitrogen Appearance (PNA) and Subjective Global Assessment (SGA).

RENAL TRANSPLANTATION

Kidney transplantations are the second most frequent transplant operation in the United States. Approximately 9000 patients receive kidney transplants each year, and in excess of 35,000 are on waiting lists (see the *Cultural Considerations* box, Barriers to Organ Donations). More than 80% of kidneys

🌐 CULTURAL CONSIDERATIONS

Barriers to Organ Donations

In the United States there exists a shortage of organ donations from members of minority groups. This is a concern because successful organ transplantation requires some matching of genetic characteristics. Two studies of African American and Hispanic American communities provide insight about some of the barriers against organ donation.

A study of African American community residents and African American clergy in the greater Houston, Texas, area included focus groups and three cross-sectional surveys. Potential barriers included that community residents tended not to value organ donation; considered donation incompatible with their religion; viewed donation as mutilating a person's body; and felt health care professionals couldn't be trusted to properly declare death before taking organs. In contrast, the African American clergy valued the importance of organ donation in every way.

A telephone-interview survey of Hispanic Americans in Arizona suggested that predictors for willingness to be an organ donor includes participating in a family discussion about organ donation; knowing someone who is willing to be a donor; and disagreeing that carrying a donor card means receiving improper medical care. Barriers consist of organ donation not being discussed; discussion of donation tied to one's mortality (a topic not to be talked about); and putting oneself or family members at risk for inadequate medical care so that the health care professionals have access to organs. Once organ donation is openly discussed, misconceptions can be addressed through educational efforts. Efforts to interact with Hispanic Americans must take into account the diversity and geographic distribution of Hispanic Americans as a cultural group.

Strategies can be implemented to create trust among members of minority groups who are currently less willing to donate organs. The researchers suggest that the medical community develop partnerships with churches and other faith-based organizations to educate people about organ donations.

Application to nursing: Nurses know that organ transplantation of kidneys and livers are lifesaving medical practices. Nurses can educate minority communities by understanding that barriers to organ donations stem from historical and personal experiences with the medical and research community.

Data from Alvaro EM, et al: Predictors of organ donation behavior among Hispanic Americans, *Prog Transplant,*15(2):149-156, 2005; and Davis K et al: Leading the flock: Organ donation feelings, beliefs, and intentions among African American clergy and community residents, *Prog Transplant* 15(3):211-216, 2005.

transplanted from cadavers still function well 1 year after surgery (see also the *Personal Perspectives* box, Organ Donation Helps Family Cope). Outcomes are even better for transplants from living donors.[18] Nutritional care of renal transplant recipients involves continual reassessment of nutritional goals and efficacy of therapy during the different phases of care.[8]

Pretransplantation

Nutritional status is evaluated to identify and correct deficits before surgery. Decreased visceral protein stores and decreased levels of body weight are frequently observed. Vitamin and mineral deficiencies of vitamin B_6, folic acid, vitamins C and D, and iron are common.[1] Poor nutritional status is caused by many different issues,[19] such as the following:

- Blood loss
- Loss of protein and other nutrients during dialysis
- Catabolism caused by chronic illness
- Anorexia caused by altered taste
- Suboptimal oral intake
- Depression

Nutrition therapy usually involves an individualized approach as outlined in Table 21-2.[19]

Immediate and Long-Term Posttransplantation

Kcal needs in the immediate posttransplantation period are high (30 to 35 kcal/kg) because of stress from surgery and catabolism. Energy requirements decline approximately 6 to 8 weeks after transplantation, and kcal should then be provided at a level to achieve and maintain a desirable body weight.[5] Restriction of dietary protein is not necessary. In fact, protein catabolism is increased as the result of surgery and the administration of corticosteroids for immunosuppression.[5]

Steroid therapy may cause glucose intolerance and therefore necessitate restriction of simple carbohydrates.[5] Fats are used to supply energy, but they may need to be limited if hypercholesterolemia or hypertriglyceridemia is present or occurs.[5] Recommendations regarding sodium and potassium should be individualized for each patient.[5] Fluids are generally unrestricted and limited only by graft function. Many drugs used postoperatively and posttransplantation have the potential to influence nutritional needs and status. Careful observation of the patient may prevent problems.

RENAL CALCULI

Renal calculi (kidney stones or urolithiasis) are a common and often recurrent urologic condition. Additionally, it is one of the oldest medical afflictions known to humans.[20] Stone formation is more common among men than women, and approximately half of those who develop renal calculi will suffer recurrence within 10 years.[21] Most calculi are composed of calcium oxalate (70% to 80%), uric acid (10%), struvite (9% to 17%), or cystine (<1%)[1] (Figure 21-5). Formation of kidney stones depends on simultaneous occurrence of the following factors: (1) low urine volume (usually the result of low or inadequate fluid intake); (2) high urine

Organ Donation Helps Family Cope

Being the recipient of an organ donation is both humbling and exhilarating. But what about the organ donor, especially the donor's family if the donor has just died? Majella Lazenby, a former nurse from Australia, shares her experience.

I am a former nurse, but I was still nursing when our family was touched by the transplant experience. My 18-year-old daughter, Alison, suffered a grade five subarachnoid haemorrhage and subsequently became an organ donor.

As is usual in such cases it was a sudden and unexpected catastrophe. She went to bed one night a normal schoolgirl and awoke the next morning in excruciating pain and lost consciousness within 15 minutes. She suffered a respiratory arrest while I called the ambulance. I administered mouth-to-mouth until the ambulance arrived. It was the first time I had ever had to apply resuscitation, but those many years of CPR training obviously came to the fore despite the panic I felt.

She was quickly transported to hospital and placed on a ventilator and the many tests began. Following a CT scan the massive haemorrhage was diagnosed and she was transferred to the intensive care unit. It was totally and utterly shocking to be told quite bluntly by the first doctor I saw in ICU that she "could die in the next hour" or perhaps linger for weeks. I just did not know what to feel, think, or do.

I had great difficulty in processing the fact that she was "brain dead" and I wondered how a normal person without any medical background in the same situation would cope when I had difficulty, even though I had some knowledge. It is especially difficult when there are no outward signs of trauma—she just looked like she was asleep.

The nursing staff who looked after us were integral in making our experience bearable. When I first mentioned organ donation the medical staff would not discuss it but luckily the nursing staff were comfortable in doing so. I was able to talk about the process and have my questions answered. We were able to spend as much time with Alison as we wanted and we were encouraged to touch her and talk to her. The time we had left with her was so precious.

Thirty hours after she lost consciousness and the brain death tests were completed, the donor coordinator was informed and we started the organ donation process. It was so difficult going through the forms and questions required, but it was something I felt very strongly about. In the midst of our horrific pain I just knew this was the only thing to do.

We had briefly discussed organ donation when Alison went for her learner driver's permit and she had affirmed that it was what she would want in the unlikely event that it happened to her. Knowing her wishes made the decision so much easier. Something "good" had to come from the loss of our beautiful girl.

We heard a few weeks later that her organs had helped a toddler, a teenager, two adults with families, and two young women.

Knowing her organs have given others the chance to live a full life has been a great comfort to me as I have struggled to come to terms with her sudden loss.

There is no "getting over it"—you just have to learn to live with the loss and the pain and accept that life is forever changed.

From Lazenby M: Focus: Organ transplant nursing/education. A family's perspective on organ donation, *Aust Nurs J* 13(9):40-41, 2006.

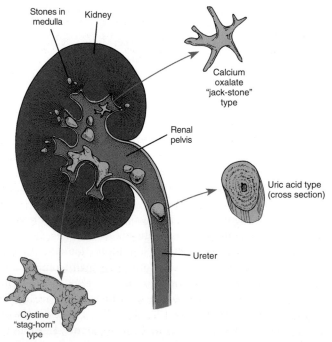

FIG 21-5 Renal calculi. (From Schlenker ED. *Williams' essentials of nutrition & diet therapy,* ed 9, St. Louis, 2007, Mosby.)

pH; (3) excessive urinary excretion of calcium, oxalate, uric acid, or a combination; and (4) decreased levels of substances in urine that normally inhibit stone formation. Dietary oxalate is another possible cause of stone formation.[21] Although calcium is the predominant component of renal calculi, dietary calcium does not appear to play a role in calcium stone formation.[22,23]

Type and cause of stone formation provide impetus for individualization of dietary modifications. A comprehensive diet history is essential to ascertain the extent of dietary modifications required. By and large, dietary interventions include combining restriction of specific dietary components associated with development of the stone in addition to generous fluid intake.[5] Patient education is important in the treatment of renal calculi. Only a motivated and informed patient can be expected to maintain any long-term preventive program.[24] The *Teaching Tool* box, Advice for Preventing Kidney Stones, helps educate patients, and Box 21-7 outlines dietary recommendations for renal calculi.

Calcium Stones

Too much calcium in urine (hypercalciuria) is the most common identifiable cause of calcium renal calculi, which is

✳ TEACHING TOOL

Advice for Preventing Kidney Stones

No immediate "penalty" exists for failing to follow a treatment regimen to prevent formation of kidney stones. The penalty (the next kidney stone) may not become apparent for many months or even years.

Fluids	***Drink fluids … a lot of fluids!*** Simple water is generally the best choice, but ginger ale, lemon-lime soft drinks, and fruit juices may be used. You need to pass at least 2.5 quarts of urine a day to prevent stone formation. To do this, drink 10 to 12 (if not 16) 8-ounce glasses of water daily—more if you live in a hot, dry climate. This is likely the single most important aspect of reducing stone formation.
Calcium	**Do not restrict dietary calcium** (dairy products and calcium-fortified orange juice)—actually don't alter calcium intake unless instructed to do so by your physician. Low-calcium intake increases risk for osteoporosis and oxalic acid kidney stone formation. Higher intake of dietary calcium reduces risk of oxalic acid kidney stone formation. The same protection is not seen with calcium supplementation.
Sodium	**Use fresh or frozen vegetables when possible.** Remove the saltshaker from the kitchen table. Other spices such as pepper or Mrs. Dash can be used instead. Use little or no salt in food preparation or cooking. When following recipes, use half the specified amount of salt. Avoid eating foods with high salt content when possible (most fast foods and packaged foods). Do not add salt to prepared or canned foods (soups, gravies, TV dinners, canned vegetables). The entire family can benefit from this advice.
Protein	**Keep meat (beef and pork) intake to a moderate level.** Six ounces of meat each day provide all the protein needed by the body. Make plans to include at least one meatless (dried beans and peas, legumes) meal per week. A diet low in animal protein and high in vegetable protein decreases the amount of red meat in the diet and increases complex carbohydrates and fiber. A diet with more plant foods is also higher in potassium.
Potassium	**Mom was right! Eat your veggies … and fruits.** A low intake of potassium-rich foods leads to increased risk of kidney stone formation.
Oxalates	**Limit foods high in oxalates.** Oxalates are found primarily in plant foods, but only eight foods—*spinach, rhubarb, beets, nuts, chocolate, tea, wheat bran, and strawberries*—have been found to increase urinary oxalate levels.
Carbohydrates	**Increase intake of complex carbohydrates:** whole grains, and fresh fruits and vegetables. (Gee, does this sound familiar?)
Supplements	**Avoid vitamin C supplements** and calcium-containing antacids (e.g., Tums). If antacids need to be used, magnesium-based antacids (Maalox) are recommended.

Data from No need for kidney stone sufferers to curb calcium, *Environ Nutr* 16:7, 1993; Leslie SW: *Hypercalciuria*, (updated Oct 21, 2009), eMedicine/WebMD. Accessed April 10, 2010, from http://emedicine.medscape.com/article/436343-overview; Craig S: *Renal calculi*, New York, (updated Oct 29, 2009), eMedicine/WebMD. Accessed April 10, 2010, from http://emedicine.medscape.com/article/777705-overview.

responsible for approximately 70% of calcium-combining stones.[24] A variety of mechanisms can cause hypercalciuria, including drugs, medical conditions, and dietary factors. The most common basis of excessive urinary calcium is absorptive hypercalciuria. Approximately 50% of people who form calcium stones have some type of absorptive hypercalciuria, which is caused by increased gastrointestinal absorption of calcium, overly aggressive vitamin D supplementation, or excessive ingestion of calcium-containing foods (milk-alkali syndrome).[24] Increased intestinal calcium absorption creates a subsequent increase in serum calcium levels.[24] Categories and treatment modalities of absorptive hypercalciuria are outlined in Table 21-3.

Conventional wisdom regarding calcium stones has been to limit foods high in calcium (milk, cheeses, yogurt, and green leafy vegetables) and sodium (2 to 3 g/day). But research indicates there is no need to restrict dietary calcium, and in fact a normal calcium intake combined with restricted animal protein and salt appears to protect against calcium stone development.[25] Kidney stone formation is more influenced by the amount of oxalate, not calcium, in the urinary tract. Restricting calcium seems to allow more oxalate to be absorbed and then excreted through the urinary tract. Less oxalate in the urinary tract occurs as higher levels of dietary calcium bind with oxalate so it cannot be absorbed.

In addition to calcium and oxalate, the main dietary contributors include potassium, animal protein, fluid intake,[23,24] sodium, fiber, alcohol, and caffeine.[24] Excessive animal protein (>1.7 g/kg) and high sodium intake make the body more acidic. To bring the body back into homeostasis, the body uses, in part, the body skeleton to buffer this additional acid load. This releases additional calcium into circulation,

BOX 21-7 DIETARY RECOMMENDATIONS FOR RENAL CALCULI

- Tailor diet to specific metabolic disturbance and individual dietary habits (to ensure compliance).
- Calcium restriction should be avoided.
- Calcium (1000-1500 mg/day) and oxalate intakes must be in balance.
- Limit intake of spinach, rhubarb, beets, nuts, chocolate, tea, wheat bran, and strawberries (cause significant increase in urinary oxalate excretion).
- Do not exceed recommended dietary allowance (RDA) for vitamin C (varies for gender and age) (causes significant increase in urinary oxalate excretion).
- Animal protein should be "restricted" to 1 g/kg body weight.
- Salt intake should be restricted to less than 100 mEq/day.
- Potassium intake should be encouraged (5 or more servings of fruits and vegetables/day).
- Include a high fluid intake to produce at least 2 L of urine/day (2-3 L intake/day).

Data from Borghi L et al: Comparison of two diets for the prevention of recurrent stones in idiopathic hypercalciuria, *N Engl J Med* 346(2):77-84, 2002; Goldfarb S: Diet and nephrolithiasis, *Annu Rev Med* 45:235-243, 1994; and Heilbert IP: Update on dietary recommendations and medical treatment of renal stone disease, *Nephrol Dial Transplant* 15:117-123, 2000.

TABLE 21-3 CATEGORIES AND TREATMENT MODALITIES OF ABSORPTIVE HYPERCALCIURIA

CATEGORY	OCCURRENCE	MEDICAL TREATMENT
Type I	Relatively uncommon and most severe	Thiazides and orthophosphates
Type II	Most common and less severe	Thiazides may be prescribed
Type III	Also called *renal phosphate leak;* relatively rare	Oral orthophosphate therapy to correct hypophosphatemia

Data from Leslie SW: *Hypercalciuria* (updated Oct 21, 2009), eMedicine/WebMD. Accessed April 10, 2010, from http://emedicine.medscape.com/article/436343-overview.

which in turn is excreted in urine by the kidneys. Increased acid load also impedes renal calcium reabsorption, resulting in increased urinary calcium excretion. Furthermore, animal proteins are high in purines. Purines are precursors of uric acid, which can form uric acid stones, lower urinary pH, increase overall acid load, contribute to gout, and generally increase urinary calcium excretion and stone formation.[23,24]

Alcohol intake also promotes urinary calcium excretion. Chronic ethanol ingestion creates low serum vitamin D levels, which lead to impaired intestinal calcium absorption and hypercalciuria.

Caffeine has been shown to increase urinary calcium excretion; however, clinical significance is reasonably small unless large amounts of caffeine (34 ounces of caffeine) are ingested.[24] Low fluid intake causes diminished urinary volume, increasing urine concentration and probability of stone formation even if total calcium excretion is unchanged.

Low intake of potassium may be an additional risk factor for stone development. Potassium reduces urinary calcium excretion by induced transient sodium diuresis, resulting in temporary contraction of extracellular fluid volume and increased renal tubular calcium reabsorption. Potassium also increases renal phosphate absorption, thereby raising serum phosphate levels, which reduces serum vitamin D_3, resulting in decreased intestinal calcium absorption.[23,24]

Oxalate Stones

Oxalate is found primarily in foods of plant origin and is the end product of ascorbic acid metabolism. Restriction of dietary oxalate intake has been used to reduce risk of recurrence of calcium oxalate kidney stones. (See Appendix F for a more complete list of oxalate content of foods.) Studies indicate that although oxalate-rich foods enhance excretion of urinary oxalate, the increase is not always proportional to oxalate content of the food.[26] Only eight foods—spinach, rhubarb, beets, nuts, chocolate, tea, wheat bran, and strawberries—caused significant increase in urinary oxalate excretion. Therefore, initial medical nutrition therapy for individuals who form calcium oxalate stones can be limited to restriction of foods definitely shown to increase urinary oxalate.[27] It also may be prudent to instruct patients that vitamin C supplements (>500 mg/day) should be avoided because they may increase urinary oxalate excretion.[28]

Uric Acid Stones

Uric acid is a metabolic product of purines (a nitrogen-containing compound in protein). Uric acid stones are associated with acidic urine (hyperuricosuria).[29] Other causes of hyperuricosuria include gout, certain medications such as aspirin[7] and chemotherapy,[7,29] and high purine intake.[29] Acidic urine appears to be the most significant issue that affects formation of uric acid stones. For this reason, the basis of medical management, an adjunct to fluid ingestion, is to increase the naturally somewhat acidic urine pH to a range of 6 to 6.5.[7] Efficacy of limiting foods high in purines (lean meats, organ meats, legumes, and whole grains) has not been proven (a more complete listing of purine content of foods can be found in Appendix G); protein intake at the level of the recommended dietary allowance (RDA) (0.8 g/kg) will not be counterproductive. Sodium bicarbonate can be used to alkalinize urine, but potassium citrate is the preferred alkalinizing agent because of the availability of slow-release tablets and avoidance of a high sodium load.[21] Allopurinol (Lopurin, Zyloprim), which is effective in reducing high levels of uric acid, also may be given. In view of the fact that allopurinol reduces uric acid quickly, it may bring about an attack of gout.[30] Nonsteroidal anti-inflammatory drugs (NSAIDs), except aspirin (aspirin increases uric acid levels), can be taken for 2 to 3 months to avoid this.

Cystine Stones

Cystine stones form in people with a hereditary disorder that causes the kidneys to excrete excessive amounts of the amino acid cystine (cystinuria).[29] The goal of treatment is to reduce urinary cystine concentration. To do this, urine volume should be greater than 3 L/day, and urine should be alkalinized to a pH in a range of 6.5 to 7.[21,30] If urine becomes too alkaline, however, there is increased risk for calcium phosphate stone formation. Producing urine volume greater than 3 L/day requires an especially high fluid intake of approximately 4 L/day or more. If alkalinization is unsuccessful, medications such as penicillamine can be used, but they are often complicated by side effects such as nephrotoxicity, allergic reactions, and hematologic abnormalities.[30]

Struvite Stones

Struvite stones are caused by urinary tract infections by bacteria that split urea into ammonium in urine. The ammonium then combines with phosphate and magnesium to form stones. Treatment of the infection must be done at the same time as removal of infected stones,[29,30] and for that reason

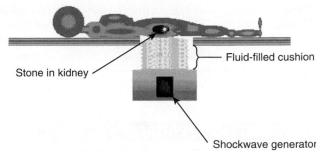

FIG 21-6 Extracorporeal shockwave lithotripsy. (Copyright Dr. Tom Shannon, 2002, Perth, Western Australia. Reprinted with permission from www.tomshannon.com.au/Site/Home.html.)

surgery or lithotripsy is almost always performed. Lithotripsy is extracorporeal shock wave lithotripsy (ESWL), a noninvasive technique whereby high-intensity shock waves cause fragmentation of stones from a device outside the body (Figure 21-6). These stones are often large and a characteristic staghorn shape, which can cause serious damage to the kidneys. Women are twice as likely to have struvite stones. Dietary management has no significant function in this variety of calculi formation.[7]

SUMMARY

The chief life-preserving function of the kidneys is to help maintain chemical homeostasis in the body. Various inflammatory, obstructive, and degenerative diseases affect the kidneys in different ways. These disorders interfere with normal functioning of nephrons that regulate products of metabolism.

Because of glomerular damage, nephrotic syndrome results in increased urinary excretion of protein, decreased serum levels of albumin, hyperlipidemia, and edema. Although treated with corticosteroid or immunosuppressive medications, nephrotic syndrome may resist treatment and progress to CKD. Primary goals of medical nutrition therapy are to control hypertension, minimize edema, decrease urinary albumin losses, prevent protein malnutrition and muscle catabolism, supply adequate energy, and slow the progression of renal disease.

AFK is characterized by an abrupt loss of renal function that may or may not be accompanied by oliguria or anuria. Most common causes are trauma, hemorrhage, shock, nephrotoxic chemicals or drugs, septicemia, and streptococcal infection. Nutritional needs are determined by underlying cause of the condition and whether dialysis is used for treatment. Patients may be hypermetabolic if renal failure was caused by trauma, burns, septicemia, or infection.

CKD is the result of progressive, irreversible loss of kidney function. It can develop over days, months, or years and

progress to CKD. Regardless of cause, results are the same: retention of nitrogenous waste products and fluid and electrolyte imbalances that affect all body systems. Management focuses on slowing progression and minimizing complications. Treatment modalities: include, hemodialysis, CHD, peritoneal dialysis (PD), and transplantation.

Planning diets for CRF, CKD, hemodialysis, and PD patients requires calibrating intakes of fluids, energy, protein, lipids, phosphorus, potassium, sodium, and vitamins and other minerals. Currently, the National Renal Diet is used to develop diet guidelines and meal plans. Individual diet prescriptions are based on residual kidney function, dialysate components, duration of dialysis, and rate of blood flow through the artificial kidney. Medical nutrition therapy objectives are to attain or maintain good nutritional status, prevent or minimize symptoms of uremic toxicity and fluid imbalance between treatments, and minimize effects of metabolic disorders caused by CKD, HD, and PD. Nutritional care of renal transplant recipients involves continual reassessment of nutritional goals and efficacy of therapy during the different phases of care.

Renal calculi are a common, recurrent urologic condition. Most are composed of calcium, oxalate, or phosphorus, with a small proportion made up of cystine or uric acid. Fluid intake has the most significant impact on reducing risk of stone formation. Uric acid is a metabolic product of purines.

Although limiting foods high in purines has not been proven effective, restriction of dietary protein may be effective. Kidney stone formation can be influenced by amount of oxalate in the urinary tract more than by amount of calcium.

Oxalate is found primarily in plant foods and is the end product of ascorbic acid metabolism. Restriction of dietary oxalate intake is used to reduce risk of recurrence of calcium oxalate kidney stone formation.

THE NURSING APPROACH

Case Study: Chronic Kidney Disease

Ian, age 28, developed chronic kidney disease (CKD) a few months ago subsequent to glomerulonephritis. His kidneys produce very little urine or sometimes none at all, requiring Ian to receive hemodialysis treatments three times a week. He hopes for a kidney transplant, but the waiting list is long. The nurse wants to encourage him.

ASSESSMENT

Subjective (From Patient Statements)

- "I don't have any energy. I'm tired all of the time."
- "Food doesn't taste good anymore. I don't have any appetite."
- "I'm sick of trying to follow the diet the dietitian recommended. It's not worth it."
- "Why try? Dialysis will take care of any extra fluid and minerals."
- "I know what I am supposed to eat, but it's too hard. I just eat and drink what I like whenever I want to."

Objective (From Physical Examination)

- Generalized ashen skin color, pale conjunctivae, wasted appearance
- BP 162/105, pulse 92, respirations 20
- Low hemoglobin and hematocrit, high BUN and creatinine
- Weight gain of 6 pounds since last hemodialysis two days ago
- Edema of ankles, crackles (sounds) in both lungs

DIAGNOSES (NURSING)

1. Excess fluid volume related to impaired renal function and excessive intake of fluid and sodium as evidenced by oliguria, weight gain of 6 pounds, ankle edema, crackles in both lungs, and BP 162/105
2. Imbalanced nutrition: less than body requirements related to anorexia, fatigue, and altered taste secondary to impaired renal function as evidenced by ashen skin, pale conjunctivae, wasted appearance, high BUN, and low hemoglobin and hematocrit
3. Noncompliance related to lack of motivation as evidenced by "I'm sick of trying to follow the diet the dietitian recommended," "Why try? Dialysis will take care of any extra fluid and minerals," and "I know what I am supposed to eat, but it's too hard. I just eat and drink what I like whenever I want to."

PLANNING

Patient Outcomes

Short term (by the end of the nurse-patient interaction):
- Commits to meet with the renal dietitian to plan a diet he can follow

- Recognizes the connection between diet, effectiveness of dialysis, and feeling better
- Agrees to take charge of his health by continuing dialysis and taking prescribed medications

Long term (by two weeks):
- Says he is following the renal diet and feels more energetic
- No more than 1 to 2 pounds weight gain per day between dialysis treatments
- BP 130/85, no ankle edema, lungs clear

Nursing Interventions

1. Refer Ian to the renal dietitian.
2. Try to motivate him to adhere to the medical plan, including medical nutrition therapy.
3. Discuss why following the renal diet is necessary and how it can help him feel better.

IMPLEMENTATION

1. Referred Ian to the renal dietitian.
   The renal dietitian can help individualize the complex diet according to the patient's lifestyle, health condition, and food preferences. The dietitian also can teach the patient how to apply general principles of the renal diet.
2. Explained the connection between pathophysiology, diet, and patient problems (signs and symptoms).
   A patient may be motivated to make healthy food choices if he can see a direct positive effect. Failed kidneys cannot remove fluids, electrolytes, and nitrogenous wastes. Restricting certain foods and some fluid intake can help alleviate signs and symptoms of uremia and fluid and electrolyte problems.
   a. Discussed the need to ingest adequate calories (including carbohydrates and unsaturated fats) and high biologic value proteins (soy, lean red meats, fish, chicken, eggs, and milk) to reduce urea formation.
   Nausea, anorexia, and metallic tastes may be reduced by decreasing urea production. Adequate intake of calories decreases protein catabolism, thus decreasing nitrogenous waste. High biologic value proteins produce less urea than low biologic value proteins (e.g., grains and cereals).
   b. Discussed the need to restrict fluids and sodium to reduce fluid retention.
   Hypertension, peripheral edema, and pulmonary edema may result from excessive fluid intake, accentuated by sodium retention. Because the heart has to work harder, heart failure may occur. Dialysis can remove some fluid, but it is more effective and better tolerated by the patient if large accumulations of fluid are not present.

THE NURSING APPROACH—cont'd

Case Study: Chronic Kidney Disease—cont'd

c. Discussed the need to restrict potassium to avoid problems in the heart.

Too much potassium, resulting from decreased excretion by the kidneys, can cause deadly dysrhythmias. Foods high in potassium should be avoided or limited, such as bananas, oranges, potatoes, tomatoes, and milk. Milk is often limited to ½ cup per day because it is high in both potassium and phosphorus.

d. Discussed the need to restrict phosphorus to avoid problems in the bones.

Failed kidneys cannot remove phosphorus, and dialysis does not remove phosphorus well. Phosphorus concentration in the blood is inversely related to serum calcium, so a high level of phosphorus causes decreased absorption of calcium from the intestines. The resultant hypocalcemia stimulates the parathyroid gland to keep the serum calcium in a safe range, and it does so by pulling calcium from the bones. This puts the patient at risk for bone fractures. Foods high in phosphorus should be limited, such as milk, cheese, nuts, legumes, beef liver, and chocolate.

3. Helped Ian plan what he can do to improve his health and nutrition.

Helping the patient take charge of his health provides a sense of control and empowerment.

a. Choose foods from the National Renal Diet.

Foods are grouped into choices by the amount of protein, calories, sodium, phosphorus, and potassium that the foods contain. The dietitian can specify the number of servings in each choice (group), allowing the patient to eat any food within the choice and still follow guidelines of medical nutrition therapy. Choices (groups) include protein, fruits and vegetables, dairy and phosphorus, bread/grains, fluid, and high-kcal foods and flavoring.

b. Download and read the pamphlet "Eat Right to Feel Right on Hemodialysis," 2008, National Institutes of Health, at www.niddk.nih.gov.

The government distributes free publications to educate patients with renal failure. This pamphlet is easy to read, empowering the patient with knowledge.

c. Weigh and measure foods periodically to match recommended serving sizes.

Accuracy is needed to obtain expected results.

d. Eat small, frequent meals, spacing protein foods throughout the day.

Small, frequent meals are usually better tolerated than large meals when the patient has nausea and anorexia. Spreading proteins throughout the day helps control the amount of urea that is in the patient's body at any one time.

e. Brush teeth frequently and chew gum if desired.

Good oral care makes the mouth feel fresher, improving the taste of food. Chewing gum improves taste in the mouth and can stimulate salivary glands, providing moisture in the mouth and possibly decreasing thirst.

f. Set a target range of gaining no more than 1 to 2 pounds per day between hemodialysis treatments. Weigh self every morning and adjust fluid and sodium intake to avoid exceeding the target.

Working toward a goal can provide motivation. Daily fluid allotment is generally 500 to 1000 mL plus the amount of urine output.

g. Make a plan for spacing out allowed fluids throughout the day, including foods that melt at room temperature or are high in water content.

Spreading out fluid intake can help control thirst. Using smaller glasses and freezing some fluids to eat like Popsicles may also reduce thirst.

4. Encouraged Ian to adhere to the medical plan, including hemodialysis three times per week and including medications.

Hemodialysis involves circulating blood through a dialyzer (artificial kidney) to remove urea, metabolic waste products, toxins, and excess fluid. Failed kidneys cannot produce the hormone erythropoietin (necessary for red blood cell production), so anemia is common. Epogen is given to stimulate red blood cell synthesis. In addition, iron, B vitamins, and folic acid are usually prescribed to enhance the erythropoiesis. Failed kidneys cannot produce calcitriol (the active form of vitamin D), so it may be taken orally to promote absorption of calcium and subsequently bone formation. Usually phosphate binders (such as calcium carbonate) are prescribed by a physician and taken with each meal, to facilitate fecal elimination of phosphorus.

5. Suggested involving his family and friends in meal planning.

Family support is extremely helpful. A person with renal failure often lacks energy for grocery shopping and food preparation. Families can eat similar meals with the patient, though serving sizes will probably vary.

a. Recommended purchasing a renal diet cookbook.

Recipes from a renal diet cookbook can add variety to the family meal.

b. Advised Ian to avoid salt and salt substitutes (usually potassium) and add spices such as garlic, onions, and oregano to food.

Adding spices adds flavor to foods.

6. Helped Ian write some short-term goals.

Achievement of small steps provides encouragement.

a. Asked how Ian would reward himself when he achieved each goal.

Positive reinforcement helps establish desirable behaviors.

b. Reminded him that he must stay healthy to be prepared for a possible kidney transplant.

Kidney transplants succeed best when the patient is healthy. Patients are more likely to be considered for a kidney transplant if they are healthy and taking charge of their health.

EVALUATION

Short term (by the end of the nurse-patient interaction):

- Ian stated he was willing to meet with the dietitian at the dialysis center and follow the dietitian's recommendations.
- Ian said he could see how eating the right foods and following the medical plan might make him feel better.

Continued

THE NURSING APPROACH—cont'd

Case Study: Chronic Kidney Disease—cont'd

- He agreed to continue taking prescribed medications and getting hemodialysis.
- Goals met.

The nurse planned to meet with Ian again in two weeks.

DISCUSSION QUESTIONS

Ian met with the nurse for follow-up in two weeks. He kept a record of his weight, his urine output and his fluid intake every day for the two weeks. He gained 1 to 2 pounds per day

between dialysis treatments. He reported that he felt better during the days that he adhered closely to his fluid restrictions. The nurse praised him for his efforts.

1. When assessing Ian, what signs and symptoms would the nurse look for to validate improvement in fluid balance?
2. Ian said he had met with the dietitian but was still having a hard time maintaining his diet. How could the nurse motivate Ian and help him set some small, realistic goals?

CRITICAL THINKING

Clinical Applications

Julia, age 40, works full time in an office and has a sedentary lifestyle. She is 5 feet 6 inches tall, has a medium frame, and weighs 125 pounds (dry weight). Her usual body weight is 132 pounds. Her appetite has not been good for the past 3 months, but it is improving. She is on hemodialysis for 3 hours, three times per week. Her urine output is approximately 500 mL/24 hours.

Her predialysis laboratory results include BUN 57 mg/dL; Na 133 mEq/L; K^+ 4.7 mEq/L; Po_4 6.3 mg/dL; Ca 9.5 mg/dL; serum albumin 3 g/dL; and ferritin 7 mcg/L. Her diet prescription is 2200 kcal, 70 to 80 g protein, 2000 mg Na, 2000 mg K, 1000 mg Po_4, and 1500 mL fluid.

Julia's diet history indicates that she doesn't like meat, but does like cheese and orange juice and will occasionally overindulge on these foods. She admits to having had too much cheese and orange juice when she came in for her last dialysis. The patient is taking Nephro-Vite.

1. What is the purpose of hemodialysis?
2. How are metabolic waste products removed during dialysis?
3. Give two explanations why Julia's serum albumin levels are decreased.
4. Why is the serum ferritin often low in renal patients?
5. Why are high biologic value proteins recommended for patients with renal disease?
6. Why are water-soluble vitamin supplements (Nephro-Vite) usually prescribed for patients with renal disease?

Julia is considering trying a type of peritoneal dialysis so she won't have to go to the kidney dialysis center three times each week.

1. Explain how peritoneal dialysis works.
2. What dietary changes might need to be made if Julia switches to peritoneal dialysis?

Courtesy Kim Dittus, PhD, RD, Syracuse University, Syracuse, N.Y.

WEBSITES OF INTEREST

Life Options Rehabilitation Program

www.lifeoptions.org

Helps individuals live well and long with kidney disease; includes Kidney School™ an interactive, web-based kidney learning center.

National Kidney and Urological Diseases Information Clearinghouse (NKUDIC)

http://kidney.niddk.nih.gov

Functions as an information dissemination service of the National Institute of Diabetes and Digestive and Kidney Diseases (NIDDK).

Renal Support Network (RSN)

http://rsnhope.org

Provides nonmedical services to those affected by chronic kidney disease (CKD) as a nonprofit, patient-focused, patient-run organization.

REFERENCES

1. Huether SE: Alteration of renal and urinary tract function. In McCance KL, Huether SE, editors: *Pathophysiology: The biologic basis for disease in adults and children*, ed 5, St. Louis, 2006, Mosby.
2. Guyton AC: *Textbook of medical physiology*, ed 11, Philadelphia, 2005, Saunders.
3. Swearingen PL, Ross DG: *Manual of medical-surgical nursing care*, ed 4, St. Louis, 1999, Mosby.

4. Wilkens KG, Funeja V: Medical nutrition therapy for renal disorders. In Mahan LK, Escott-Stump S, editors: *Krause's food & nutrition therapy*, ed 12, Philadelphia, 2008, Saunders.

5. American Dietetic Association: *Manual of clinical dietetics*, ed 6, Chicago, 2000, American Dietetic Association.

6. Morgan SL, Weinsier RL: *Fundamentals of clinical nutrition*, ed 2, St. Louis, 1998, Mosby.

7. Wilson LM: Acute renal failure. In Price SA, Wilson LM, editors: *Pathophysiology: Clinical concepts of disease processes*, ed 6, St. Louis, 2002, Mosby.

8. Wiggens KL: *Guidelines for nutrition care of renal patients*, ed 3, Chicago, 2002, American Dietetic Association.

9. Fedje L, Karalis M: Nutrition management in early stages of chronic kidney disease. In Byham-Gray L, Wiesen K: *A clinical guide to nutrition care in kidney disease*, Chicago, 2004, American Dietetic Association.

10. Kopple JD: Nutritional management of nondialyzed patients with chronic renal failure. In Kopple JD, Massry SG, editors: *Nutritional management of renal disease*, ed 2, Baltimore, 2004, Lippincott Williams & Wilkins.

11. Arora P, Verrelli M: *Chronic renal failure*, (updated February 4, 2010), eMedicine/WebMD. Accessed April 10, 2010, from http://emedicine.medscape.com/article/238798-overview.

12. Goldstein DJ, McQuiston B: Nutrition and renal disease. In Coulston AM, Rock CL, Monsen ER: *Nutrition in the prevention and treatment of disease*, San Diego, 2001, Academic Press.

13. Biesecker R, Stuart N: Nutrition management of the adult hemodialysis patient. In Byham-Gray L, Wiesen K: *A clinical guide to nutrition care in kidney disease*, Chicago, 2004, American Dietetic Association.

14. Kalantar-Zedeh K, Kopple JD: Nutrition in maintenance hemodialysis patients. In Kopple JD, Massry SG, editors: *Nutritional management of renal disease*, ed 2, Baltimore, 2004, Lippincott Williams & Wilkins.

15. McCann L: Nutrition management of the adult peritoneal dialysis patient. In Byham-Gray L, Wiesen K: *A clinical guide to nutrition care in kidney disease*, Chicago, 2004, American Dietetic Association.

16. Heimbürger O, et al: Nutritional effects and nutritional management of chronic peritoneal dialysis. In Kopple JD, Massry SG, editors: *Nutritional management of renal disease*, ed 2, Baltimore, 2004, Lippincott Williams & Wilkins.

17. National Kidney Foundation Dialysis Outcomes Quality Initiative: *Clinical practice guidelines for peritoneal dialysis adequacy: Update 2006*, New York, 2006, National Kidney Foundation. Accessed April 10, 2010, from www.kidney.org/professionals/KDOQI/guideline_upHD_PD_VA/pd_intro.htm.

18. National Kidney Foundation: *Answering your questions about living donation*, New York, 2010, Author. Accessed April 10, 2010, from www.kidney.org/atoz/content/answering.cfm.

19. National Kidney Foundation: *Clinical practice guidelines for nutrition in chronic renal failure*, New York, 2000, Author. Accessed April 10, 2010, from www.kidney.org/professionals/kdoqi/guidelines_updates/doqi_nut.html.

20. Weseman RA, Mukherjee S: *Nutritional requirements of adults before transplantation* (updated Nov 4, 2008), eMedicine/WebMD. Accessed April 10, 2010, from http://emedicine.medscape.com/article/431031-overview.

21. Wolf S Jr: *Nephrolithiasis: Treatment & medication* (updated Sept 28, 2009), eMedicine/WebMD. Accessed April 10, 2010, from http://emedicine.medscape.com/article/437096-treatment.

22. Portis AJ, Sundaram CP: Diagnosis and initial management of kidney stones, *Am Fam Physician* 63(7):1329-1338, 2001.

23. Curhan GC, et al: A prospective study of dietary calcium and other nutrients and the risk of symptomatic kidney stones, *N Engl J Med* 328(12):833-838, 1993.

24. Leslie SW: *Hypercalciuria* (updated Oct 21, 2009), eMedicine/WebMD. Accessed April 10, 2010, from http://emedicine.medscape.com/article/436343-overview.

25. Borghi L, et al: Comparison of two diets for the prevention of recurrent stones in idiopathic hypercalciuria, *N Engl J Med* 346(2):77-84, 2002.

26. Brinkley LJ, Gregory J, Pak CY: A further study of oxalate bioavailability in foods, *J Urol* 144:94-96, 1990.

27. Massey LK, Roman-Smith H, Sutton RA: Effect of dietary calcium oxalate and calcium on urinary oxalate and risk of formation of calcium and oxalate kidney stones, *J Am Diet Assoc* 93:901-906, 1993.

28. National Kidney Foundation: *Family history of kidney stones? Watch those megadoses of vitamin C*, New York, 1997 (September 21), Author. Accessed April 10, 2010, from www.kidney.org/news/newsroom/newsitemArchive.cfm?id=150.

29. Craig S: *Renal calculi*, New York, (updated Oct 29, 2009), eMedicine/WebMD. Accessed April 10, 2010, from emedicine.medscape.com/article/777705-overview.

30. Green GB, Coyne DW: Renal diseases. In Green GB, et al, editors: *The Washington manual of medical therapeutics*, ed 31, Philadelphia, 2004, Lippincott Williams & Wilkins.

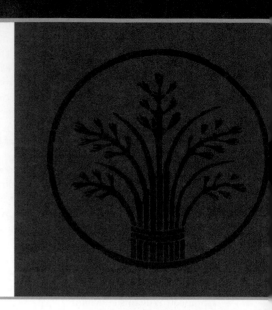

Nutrition in Cancer, AIDS, and Other Special Problems

The nutritional status of patients with cancer, human immunodeficiency virus (HIV), and acquired immunodeficiency syndrome (AIDS) is challenged by manifestations not only of the disease but also by the ramifications of treatment.

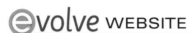 WEBSITE

http://evolve.elsevier.com/Grodner/foundations/

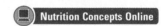 Nutrition Concepts Online

ROLE IN WELLNESS

Wasting and malnutrition, because of the effect of the disease itself or the secondary consequences of treatment, characterize the disorders of this chapter. Consequently, the nutritional status of patients with cancer, human immunodeficiency virus (HIV), and acquired immunodeficiency syndrome (AIDS) is challenged by manifestations not only of the disease but also by the ramifications of treatment. Nutrition therapy focuses on reducing these effects and supporting the nutritional status of patients through the potentially debilitating side effects of treatment. Because these disorders are chronic, nursing care often continues after the patient leaves the hospital setting and returns home. The role of home care and hospice nurses is crucial for providing continued medical care, but also important are the nutritional support and food consumption strategies as patients recover and become acclimated to their conditions. The goal of maintaining good nutritional status is to improve survival rates, reduce treatment side effects, and increase the quality of life.

Consider the effects of these disorders through the health dimensions. The *physical health* dimension challenge is to halt or minimize malnutrition often associated with symptoms or treatments. *Intellectual health* dimension is a factor because these disorders are marked by either their chronic or potentially life-threatening outcomes. For a person to maintain optimal nutrient intake while also dealing with serious illness requires the intellectual capability to comprehend the different aspects of treatment and rehabilitation. Facing death from AIDS or cancer stresses our *emotional health* ability to cope; nurses need to be sensitive to the emotional burden patients and families are experiencing. *Social health* may be compromised because prejudice against (and fear of) clients with HIV/AIDS and cancer affects the potential for

individuals to continue their social and work relations as they did in the past. Dealing with societal and emotional issues may warrant counseling support for clients and their families. *Spirituality* and faith can provide personal insight for gathering strength to heal. (See Personal Perspectives Behind the Cancer Headlines.)

CANCER

Cancer cells differ from normal cells in several ways. These characteristics may involve any or all of the following: (1) uncontrolled cellular reproduction occurs, in which cells become independent of normal growth signals; (2) cells contain abnormal nucleus and cytoplasm; and (3) the mitosis rate generally increases. The nucleus of the cells may be an abnormal shape and have clearly abnormal chromosomes. This process that results in abnormal cell production is called carcinogenesis.[1]

The abnormalities in cell replication occur in several stages: initiation, promotion, and progression. *Initiation* of the process results in a mutation of deoxyribonucleic acid (DNA). Though exact causes are not clear for all malignancies, physical and chemical agents or exposure to microorganisms may initially cause the mutation. The second phase is where the replication of the mutated cell is *promoted* and abnormal cell growth results. Factors that have been identified in some malignancies include estrogen, testosterone, nitrates, cigarette smoke, and alcohol. The third stage is the *progression* of the abnormal cells outside the original location of the cell.

The rate of tumor growth is dependent on characteristics of both the host and tumor. Host factors may include age, sex, nutritional status, the presence of other diseases, hormone production, and immune function. Tumor factors could

BOX 22-1	ESTIMATED NEW CANCER CASES BY SEX, UNITED STATES, 2008

MEN	WOMEN
Prostate	Breast
Lung and bronchus	Lung and bronchus
Colorectal	Colorectal
Urinary bladder	Uterine corpus
	Non-Hodgkin's lymphoma

From American Cancer Society: *Cancer facts and figures 2008,* Atlanta, 2008, American Cancer Society.

include where the tumor is located and its access to adequate blood supply.[1]

Cancer remains a leading cause of mortality in the United States; in 2008, there were an estimated 1.44 million new cases. Cancer is the second leading cause of death, with more than 550,000 deaths each year. Most diagnoses of cancer occur in older individuals, with almost two thirds in people older than age 65. The most common types of cancer include lung, prostate, breast, and colorectal (Box 22-1).[2] Scientists estimate that 50% to 75% of all cancer deaths can be linked to human behaviors and lifestyle factors.

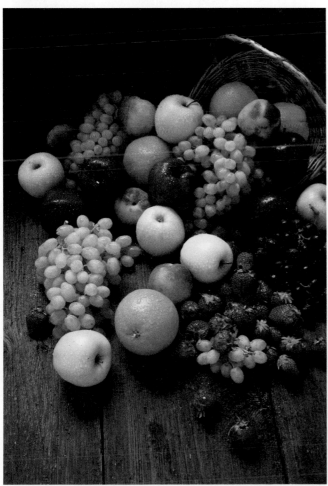

Phytochemicals may play a role in preventing cancer. (Photos.com.)

Nutrition factors are considered one of the important environmental and lifestyle factors in the etiology and prevention of cancer.[3] Nutrition and dietary factors may interact within the process of carcinogenesis in all three stages: initiation, promotion, and progression. Furthermore, nutritional factors may assist in blocking those three stages. For example, antioxidants in the diet may protect the cell from DNA mutation[3] (see the *Health Debate* box, Fact or Fantasy? Food as Pharmaceuticals?). It is important to remember that no one food causes cancer and no one food can prevent it. The National Cancer Institute encourages cancer prevention by encouraging the following guidelines:

- Not smoking cigarettes or using other tobacco products
- Not drinking too much alcohol
- Eating five or more daily servings of fruits and vegetables
- Eating a low-fat diet
- Maintaining or reaching a healthy weight
- Being physically active
- Protecting skin from sunlight

Nutrition and the Diagnosis of Cancer

With more than 100 variations and as the second leading cause of death, cancer affects many individuals in the United States. The physiologic response to malignancy is different for each specific tumor type, but there are general nutrition risk factors that may apply to many cancer patients. Physical impairment because of the location of the tumor or the extent of tumor involvement, metabolic changes, and the use of antineoplastic therapy all place the patient with cancer at increased risk of developing malnutrition or the wasting syndrome of cancer: *cachexia.* Cancer cachexia is a complex syndrome that results in severe wasting of lean body mass and weight loss. Much research has attempted to establish an understanding of this syndrome. Cytokines are proteins that, in small amounts, assist in the communication between cells of the immune system. It is hypothesized that these cytokines, such as lipid mobilizing factor, interleukins, interferons, and proteolysis inducing factor, drive the altered metabolic response in cachexia. Weight loss, anorexia, hypermetabolism, wasting of skeletal muscle mass, and increased levels of lipid breakdown are the result. Cachexia affects almost 50% of all cancer patients and is present even at the beginning stages of tumor development before actual weight loss is observed. Aggressively approaching nutrition support as a major component of medical care can assist with minimizing the nutritional complications of cancer.[4]

Benefits of Nutritional Adequacy

Can adequate nutrition make a difference in those patients with cancer? The answer is yes. Maintenance of nutritional status may accomplish the following:[4-6]

- Decrease the risk of surgical complications.
- Ensure that patients are able to meet increased energy and protein requirements.

෨ HEALTH DEBATE

Fact or Fantasy? Food as Pharmaceuticals?

They are touted as being able to prevent cancer, heart disease, and depression. Some say they can even boost our immune system. There is some opinion that they can even slow down the aging process. They are the foods our mothers tried to make us eat when we were kids. They are fruits and vegetables. What a surprise!

Over the past 20 years, epidemiologic researchers have consistently found that people who eat greater amounts of fruits and vegetables have lower rates of cancer. Fruits and vegetables contain hundreds of compounds such an antioxidants (beta carotene and vitamins C and E), folic acid, fiber, and at least a dozen groups of chemicals called *phytochemicals* (specific chemicals found in plants, primarily in fruits and vegetables) that are not strictly nutrients. Some families of plants have more than others, but none of the phytochemicals are found in animal foods. Following is a list of known phytochemicals, their action in the body, and common food sources.

Most health professionals believe that the whole plant is probably more important than the sum of its nutrients and chemical components. More benefits (some we don't even know yet) are derived from nutrients and phytochemicals by eating foods rather than swallowing supplements. Clients may question why they shouldn't just take specialized supplements of phytochemicals if we know their actions. What do you think? How will you explain your view to clients? Was Mom right? Should we all eat our vegetables?

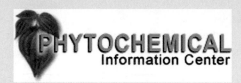

	FLAVONOIDS	CAROTENOIDS	OTHER
BLUE & PURPLE	Anthocyanidins Flavonols Flavan-3-ols Proanthocyanidins		Ellagic acid Resveratrol
GREEN	Flavones Flavanones Flavonols	Beta-carotene Lutein Zeaxanthin	Indoles Isothiocyanates Organosulfur compounds
WHITE	Flavonols Flavanones		Indoles Isothiocyanates Organosulfur compounds
YELLOW/ORANGE	Flavonols Flavanones	Alpha-carotene Beta-carotene Beta-cryptoxanthin Zeaxanthin	
RED	Anthocyanidins Flavonols Flavones Flavan-3-ols Flavanones Proanthocyanidins	Lycopene	Ellagic acid Resveratrol

Data from Webb D: Whole grains boast phytochemicals to fight disease, *Environ Nutr* 24:1, 2001; Phytochemical Information Center, Produce for Better Health Foundation, *Eat your colors, get your phytochemicals*, 2009. Accessed April 8, 2010, from www.pbhfoundation.org/pulse/research/pic/ and www.pbhfoundation.org/pulse/research/pic/phytolist/.

Behind the Cancer Headlines

News about the latest cancer therapies is often in the headlines. Information about cancer and potential therapies is readily available on the Internet. What are not as easily accessible are the experiences of individuals whose lives are touched by cancer. Following is a compilation of comments from individuals of varying ages in my life or people whom I've met.

Michele Grodner
Montclair, NJ

- My mother was in the late stages of a malignant brain tumor, but my brother just couldn't bear the thought of putting "his mother" in a nursing home. Instead, he had her stay with him and his family, setting up a bed in their family room. Within a few days, when she could no longer control her bowels, he found himself sponge bathing his seventy-five-year-old mother who hardly knew where she was. He then understood that he could no longer care for her.

- My friend Karen fought the good fight against breast cancer. For nine years she battled but lost. When she was first diagnosed, she came to see each of us (her neighbors) to tell us in person. I felt honored. I think it was her way of making it real, of announcing it to the world. She learned everything there was to know about every kind of treatment. Several times she traveled to the Dominican Republic for controversial stem cell treatments, riding through the countryside in a rickety van with others in search of medical miracles. The cancer spread, but so did Karen's spirit. Perhaps the miracle of Karen's spirit was to show us how to struggle against disease while still enjoying life.

- Barbara said she didn't want to hold her newborn grandson because she was too weak, but I think it was because she knew that her cancer had spread and she didn't want to become too attached to the baby.

- I was more nervous about choosing a treatment for my prostate cancer than I was when I had lung cancer because I was afraid I would end up incontinent.

- My uncle's case was complicated. What with inoperable bladder and prostate cancer, high blood pressure, anemia, and advancing Parkinson's disease, there was a lot to consider. One day his oncologist told him that "there are no more treatments available for your cancer" and that he (the oncologist) was going on vacation for two weeks. Fortunately, my uncle, guided by my aunt, immediately found a new oncologist who prescribed a different treatment protocol. My uncle is now in remission.

- Help to repair and rebuild normal tissues affected by antineoplastic therapy.
- Promote an increased tolerance to therapy.
- Assist in promoting an enhanced quality of life.

Nutritional Effects of Cancer Treatments

Surgery

Treatment for many malignancies (particularly, solid tumors) includes surgical resection of the tumor.[1] This route of treat-

TABLE 22-1	NUTRITION SIDE EFFECTS OF CANCER SURGERY
SITE OF SURGERY	**SIDE EFFECT**
Head and neck	Impaired chewing and swallowing
Esophagectomy	Diarrhea, steatorrhea, esophageal stenosis
Vagotomy	Gastric stasis, diarrhea, fat malabsorption
Gastrectomy	Dumping syndrome; hypoglycemia; malabsorption; possible deficiencies of iron, calcium, vitamin B_{12}, and fat-soluble vitamins
Pancreatectomy	Type 1 diabetes mellitus, possible malabsorption of fats, protein, fat-soluble vitamins, minerals
Small bowel resection	Possible malabsorption of many nutrients; depends on extent and site of surgery
Ileostomy	Sodium and water losses, vitamin B_{12}, malabsorption, fat malabsorption, bile salt diarrhea

Data from McCallum PD, Polisena CG, editors: *The clinical guide to oncology nutrition,* Chicago, 2002, American Dietetic Association.

ment can allow for diagnosis, resecting a solid tumor, preventing metastasis of the malignancy, or reducing the size of the tumor to alleviate pain. The nutritional consequences related to surgery are dependent on the type and extent of the surgical resection. Resections of any portion of the gastrointestinal (GI) tract can cause alterations in nutrition intake and nutrient absorption.[6] Second, energy and protein requirements may need to be increased to promote optimal wound healing postoperatively. Malabsorption does tend to be the primary nutritional problem with surgeries involving the GI tract; yet unless small bowel resection is extensive, the adaptability of the small intestine may prevent the occurrence of major clinical problems.[6] Many cancer patients enter surgery already experiencing protein-kcal malnutrition that places them at higher risk for complications. For example, more than 60% of patients with malignancies affecting the head and neck enter surgery malnourished.[7] Additionally, any problems associated with surgery (Table 22-1) will be further complicated if the patient receives subsequent radiation therapy and chemotherapy.

Chemotherapy

Most chemotherapy protocols include a combination of chemotherapy agents. Chemotherapy agents include alkylating, antimetabolite agents (folate antagonists), purine/pyrimidine antagonists, anthracyclines, platinum antitumor compounds, antibiotics, nitrosoureas, mitotic inhibitors, cytokines, biologic response modifiers, monoclonal antibodies, immunotherapy, hormones, and enzymes. These agents

TABLE 22-2	NUTRITIONAL IMPLICATIONS OF CHEMOTHERAPEUTIC AGENTS		
DRUG CLASSIFICATION	**SELECTED EXAMPLES**	**ACTIONS**	**NUTRITIONAL IMPLICATIONS**
Alkylating agents	Cisplatin Hexamethylmelamine Dacarbazine	React with susceptible deoxyribonucleic acid (DNA) sites	Anorexia, nausea, vomiting, mucositis/ stomatitis
Antibiotics	Bleomycin Doxorubicin Dactinomycin	Bind to DNA and inhibit cell division, interfere with ribonucleic acid (RNA) transcription	Anorexia, nausea, mucositis/stomatitis, diarrhea; some may cause decreased calcium and iron absorption
Antimetabolites	Methotrexate 5-Fluorodeoxyuridine 5-Fluorouracil	Inhibit a stage of DNA synthesis	Anorexia, nausea, vomiting, diarrhea, mucositis, abdominal pain, intestinal ulceration; some may cause decreased absorption of vitamin B_{12}, fat, and xylose
Hormones	Prednisone Tamoxifen Diethylstilbestrol	Alter cell metabolism to cause unfavorable tumor growth	*Corticosteroids:* sodium and fluid retention, hyperglycemia, gastrointestinal upset, osteoporosis (calcium losses), negative nitrogen balance *Estrogens:* nausea, vomiting, anorexia, hypercalcemia
Enzymes	Asparaginase	Delay DNA and RNA synthesis by inhibiting protein synthesis (deprive cells of asparagine)	Anorexia, nausea, hyperglycemia, pancreatitis, azotemia (uremia), weight loss
Plant alkaloids	Vinblastine Vincristine	Inhibit mitosis	Nausea, vomiting, constipation, diarrhea, abdominal pain
Biologic response modifiers	Interferon Interleukin	Modify host biologic response to tumor	Nausea, vomiting, anorexia, weight change (increase or decrease)

Data from McCallum PD, Polisena CG, editors: *The clinical guide to oncology nutrition,* Chicago, 2002, American Dietetic Association.

act by inhibiting one or more steps of DNA synthesis in rapidly proliferating cells that are characteristic of the malignant cell or by enhancing the host's immune system to allow for improved response to therapy. Using a combination of medications that interrupt the cancer process in different ways allows for maximum effect with the fewest side effects. Cells of the bone marrow and those lining the GI tract tend to be susceptible to damage from chemotherapy because of their rapid turnover rate.[1,4,6]

The effect on these cells accounts for many of the side effects associated with chemotherapy including nausea, vomiting, diarrhea, **mucositis**, hair loss, and immunosuppression.[6,7] The severity and manifestation of the side effects depend on the particular chemotherapy agent, dosage, duration of treatment, rates of metabolism, accompanying drugs, and individual tolerance. These symptoms can lead to malnutrition through a variety of mechanisms: anorexia; nausea; vomiting; mucositis; **stomatitis**; cardiac, renal, and liver injury (toxicity); and learned food aversions.[4-7] Nutritional implications of chemotherapeutic agents are summarized in Table 22-2.

Radiation Therapy

Radiation therapy uses ionizing radiation to kill cells by altering the DNA of the malignant cell. This alteration interferes with the factors controlling replication. Radiation is used to treat tumors sensitive to radiation exposure or tumors that cannot be surgically resected. Radiation also can be used to reduce tumor size so that a successful surgical resection can occur. Though technology has allowed for significant specificity in using radiation therapy some normal cells within the treatment range that are also in that stage of cell replication may also be damaged. This may contribute to the physical side effects, which may include hair loss, mucositis, and vomiting and diarrhea.

Nutritional problems vary according to the region or area of the body radiated, dose, **fractionation**, and whether radiation is used as combination therapy with surgery or chemotherapy.[4-7] Complications may develop during radiation treatment or become chronic and progress even after treatment is completed.[4-7] Primary radiation sites that result in nutrition problems include the head and neck, the abdomen and pelvis (GI tract), and the central nervous system (CNS).[4-7] Radiation at any of the three sites may cause anorexia, nausea, and vomiting. In the head and neck these common effects create problems of food ingestion, such as stomatitis, esophageal mucositis, loss of taste sensation, and changes in the production of saliva. Side effects to the abdomen and pelvis alter the GI tract (radiation enteritis), reducing digestion and absorption of nutrients because of the development of diarrhea and steatorrhea, and possibly, malabsorption, ulceration, and bowel damage or obstruction.

BOX 22-2	COMMON FOODS: SELECT THE LOWER-RISK OPTIONS FOR SAFETY	
TYPE OF FOOD	**HIGHER RISK**	**LOWER RISK**
Meat and Poultry	• Raw or undercooked meat or poultry	• Meat or poultry cooked to a safe minimum internal temperature

Tip: Use a food thermometer to check the internal temperature. See "Food Preparation Strategies" on page 40 for specific safe minimum internal temperature.

Seafood	• Any raw or undercooked fish, e.g., sushi or ceviche	• Smoked fish and precooked seafood heated to 165 °F
	• Refrigerated smoked fish	• Canned fish and seafood
	• Precooked seafood, such as shrimp and crab	• Seafood cooked to 145 °F
Milk	• Unpasteurized milk	• Pasteurized milk
Eggs	Foods that contain raw/undercooked eggs, such as:	*At home:*
	• Caesar salad dressings*	• Use pasteurized eggs/egg products when preparing recipes that call for raw or under-cooked eggs
	• Homemade raw cookie dough*	*When eating out:*
	• Homemade eggnog*	• Ask if pasteurized eggs were used

* Tip: Most pre-made foods from grocery stores, such as Caesar dressing, pre-made cookie dough, or packaged eggnog are made with pasteurized eggs.

Sprouts	• Raw sprouts (alfalfa, bean, or any other sprout)	• Cooked sprouts
Vegetables	• Unwashed fresh vegetables, including lettuce/salads	• Washed fresh vegetables, including salads
Cheese	• Soft cheeses made from unpasteurized milk, such as:	• Hard cheeses
	– Feta	• Processed cheeses
	– Brie	• Cream cheese
	– Camembert	• Mozzarella
	– Blue-veined cheese	• Soft cheeses that are clearly labeled "made from pasteurized milk"
	– Queso fresco	
Hot Dogs and Deli meats	• Hot dogs, deli meats, and luncheon meats that have not been reheated	• Hot dogs, luncheon meats, and deli meats reheated to steaming hot or 165 °F

Tip: You need to reheat hot dogs, deli meats, and luncheon meats before eating them because the bacteria Listeria monocytogenes grows at refrigerated temperatures. This bacteria may cause severe illness, hospitalization, or even death. Reheating these foods destroys this dangerous bacteria, making these foods safe for you to eat.

Pâtés	• Unpasteurized, refrigerated pâtés or meat spreads	• Canned pâtés or meat spreads

Food Safety and Inspection Service, U.S. Department of Agriculture: *Food safety for people with cancer,* September 2006, Author. Accessed April 7, 2010, from www.fsis.usda.gov/PDF/Food_Safety_for_People_with_Cancer.pdf.

Bone Marrow Transplantation

Bone marrow transplantation (BMT) is used to treat certain hematologic malignancies (acute and chronic leukemia and some forms of lymphoma), as well as in adjunct therapy for solid tumors such as breast cancer.[1] Types of transplant include autologous, allogeneic, and syngenic. When using bone marrow transplant as the treatment of a solid tumor, the patient's own bone marrow is harvested and saved before the initiation of chemotherapy or radiation therapy. The patient then receives high-dose chemotherapy and possibly total body irradiation to eradicate the cancer.[4-7] The patient's own bone marrow is then infused as a "rescue" from the effects of both chemotherapy and radiation. For hematologic malignancies, a patient receives bone marrow from a genetically matched donor (allogeneic) or in some cases from a twin (syngenic).

The ability to maintain adequate oral intake is difficult because of the nausea, vomiting, and mucositis that is associated with such high-dose therapies. Parenteral nutrition is a standard component of transplantation protocols, but when possible, recent research indicates that maintaining some oral intake or providing enteral nutrition is important to maintaining the integrity of the small intestine.[8]

Immunosuppression, as a result of the antineoplastic regimens and BMT, places the BMT patient at high risk for infections from bacterial and fungal pathogens. Pathogens can be commonly found in the environment, including fresh fruits and vegetables that ordinarily do not present a hazard to healthy persons (Box 22-2). Therefore, a low-bacterial diet is indicated whenever the plasma neutrophil (a type of white blood cell) count is less than 1000 mm[3,6,7] Standard practice varies between institutions, but in general, food safety guidelines for patients with low immune function or who are neutropenic include avoiding undercooked meats and eggs, ensuring that raw fruits and vegetables are washed well and/or are peeled (including salads and garnishes), and following appropriate sanitation guidelines for food preparation and storage. Frequent monitoring of nutritional intake and encouragement to take in adequate nutrition are essential in the care of these patients (Box 22-3).

A major complication that may occur with an allogeneic BMT is graft versus host disease (GVHD), which is best described as reverse rejection. In this case, the grafted tissue or organ recognizes the host's cells as foreign. GVHD may result in multiple organ damage, but the skin, GI tract, and liver are of particular concern. The nutritional management for GVHD is complicated and may require intense therapy for periods as long as 1 to 2 years posttransplantation.[6,7]

Nutrition Therapy

One of the most important steps in providing nutritional care for the cancer patient is identifying the patient who is at risk.

BOX 22-3   FOOD SAFETY GUIDELINES FOR PROTECTION OF WEAKENED IMMUNE SYSTEMS

Safe food handling can help to decrease a person's risk of foodborne illness. People with weakened immune systems must take extra caution to avoid putting themselves at risk of becoming infected by a foodborne pathogen. It is important to handle food safely, starting with the buying process, through to eating, and on to storing leftovers.

Shopping

- Shop for groceries when you can take food home right away; do not leave food sitting in the car.
- Avoid cans of food that are dented, leaking, or bulging.
- Do not purchase food in cracked glass jars.
- Ensure that safety buttons on metal lids are down and do not make a clicking noise when pushed. Make sure that tamper-resistant safety seals are intact.
- Avoid food in torn or punctured packaging.
- Pick up perishable foods (e.g., meat, eggs, milk) last.
- Place packaged meat, poultry, or fish in separate plastic bags to prevent meat juices from dripping onto other groceries or other meats.
- Make sure the "sell by" or "use by" date has not passed.
- Do not buy any food that has been displayed in any unclean or unsafe manner (e.g., meat allowed to sit outside refrigeration, cooked shrimp displayed next to raw shrimp).
- When ordering in the deli department, make sure the clerk washes his or her hands between handling raw food and cooked food.

Storage

- Keep your refrigerator and freezer clean.
- Use a refrigerator thermometer to make sure the temperature inside is 40° F or below.
- Make sure the temperature inside the freezer is 0° F.
- On arriving home from the store, immediately refrigerate and freeze appropriate foods.
- Leave eggs in their carton; do not place in refrigerator door.
- Store raw meat, poultry, and fish on the bottom shelf of the refrigerator to avoid their juices dripping onto other foods. Raw ground meat, poultry, and fish may be stored for 1 or 2 days; other red meat may be stored for 3 to 5 days.
- Store canned foods and other shelf-stable products in a cool, dry place. Avoid hot garages and damp basements.

Preparation

- Wash hands before, during, and after food preparation and service.

- Use plastic or glass surfaces for cutting raw meat and poultry. Use a separate cutting board for preparing other foods such as fruits, vegetables, and bread.
- Wash cutting boards with hot, soapy water after each use. Cutting boards (except those that are made with laminated wood) can all be washed in the dishwasher.
- After handling raw meat, poultry, and fish, wash hands, work surfaces, and utensils with hot, soapy water.
- Wash all fruits and vegetables before cutting, cooking, or eating them raw.
- Defrost frozen food in a bowl in the refrigerator or microwave. Cook food immediately after thawing.
- Use different utensils and dishes for cooked foods than you used for raw foods.
- Wash kitchen towels and clothes often in hot water in a washing machine.
- A sanitizing solution can be made with one teaspoon of liquid chlorine bleach mixed with one quart of water. Use solution on countertops and other work surfaces. Do not rinse. Allow surface to air-dry.

Cooking

- Keep hot foods hot at 140° F or higher and cold foods cold at 40° F or lower.
- Do not leave perishable foods out for more than 2 hours.
- Promptly refrigerate or freeze leftovers in shallow containers or wrapped tightly in bags.
- Use leftovers within 3 or 4 days.
- When reheating foods in the microwave, cover and rotate or stir foods once or twice during cooking. The food should be steaming hot.
- Do not eat foods past their expiration date.
- Follow the handling and preparation instructions on product labels to ensure top quality and safety.

Meat, Poultry, and Fish

- Do not eat raw or undercooked meat.
- Cook all meat and poultry until it is no longer pink in the middle.
- Fish should be cooked until flaky, not rubbery.
- The temperature inside the meat should be higher than 165° F.
- Cook poultry to an internal temperature of 180° to 185° F.
- Cook fish to 160° F.
- Do not eat stuffing cooked inside poultry. Instead, cook separately to 165° F.
- Cook only shellfish that are closed. Discard any shellfish that do not open during cooking.

BOX 22-3   FOOD SAFETY GUIDELINES FOR PROTECTION OF WEAKENED IMMUNE SYSTEMS—cont'd

Dairy
- Eat or drink only pasteurized milk or dairy products.

Eggs
- Cook eggs until the yolk and white are solid, not runny.
- Do not eat foods that may contain raw eggs, such as Caesar salad dressing or raw cookie dough.
- If eating fried eggs, be sure eggs are fried on both sides.

Fruits and Vegetables
- Raw fruits and vegetables are generally safe to eat if washed carefully first.
- Discard any fruits or vegetables with mold.
- Wash fruits and vegetables under cool running water.
- Do not let cut fruits or vegetables sit unrefrigerated.
- Discard the outermost leaves of a head of lettuce or cabbage.

Water
- Do not drink water straight from lakes, rivers, streams, or springs.
- Always check with your local health department and water company to learn if they have issued any special notices for people with weakened immune systems.
- Water bottles and ice trays should be cleaned with soap and water before use.

Other
- Home canned foods: Use within 1 year of canning. Cook food for 10 minutes before eating.
- Commercially canned foods: Safe to eat without any further cooking.

- Condiments: Use a clean utensil when dipping into jars. Keep jars refrigerated. Do not use homemade mayonnaise.
- Baby food: Use a clean utensil to remove amount needed from jar. Store opened jars in the refrigerator.

Eating Out
- Avoid the same foods when eating out that you would at home (e.g., raw meats, undercooked eggs).
- If the food arrives undercooked, send it back.
- Avoid foods that may contain raw eggs, such as Caesar salad dressing or uncooked hollandaise sauce.
- If you are not sure about the ingredients in a dish, ask your waiter before you order.
- Do not order any raw or lightly steamed fish or shellfish, such as oysters, clams, mussels, sushi, or sashimi.

Traveling
- Do not eat uncooked fruits and vegetables unless you can peel them.
- Avoid salads.
- Eat cooked foods while they are still hot.
- Boil all water before drinking it.
- Drink only canned or bottled drinks or beverages made with boiled water.
- Steaming hot foods, fruits you peel yourself, bottled and canned processed drinks, and hot coffee or tea should be safe.
- Talk with your health care provider about other advice on travel abroad.

From Appendix K: Food safety guidelines for patients with low immune function or who are neutropenic. In Kogut V, Luthringer S: *Nutritional issues in cancer care*, Pittsburgh, 2005, Oncology Nursing Society. Based on data from Centers for Disease Control and Prevention (2005) and the United States Department of Agriculture (2006).

One tool that has been developed for screening for nutritional risk in cancer patients is the Patient-Generated Subjective Global Assessment (PG-SGA).[4,5,8] This screening tool allows for early identification of those patients with a nutritional deficit or who are at risk when treatment is initiated (Figure 22-1).

Cancer patients are at high risk for malnutrition.[4,6] This is in part because of the presence of common symptoms that cancer patients experience. Recognizing clinical signs and treating these symptoms early may assist in the prevention of protein-kcal malnutrition. Table 22-3 summarizes interventions used in treating these symptoms. As with any other disease, nutrition support of cancer patients must be individualized. Staff and patients alike should realize that nutrition is an essential component of the total management of the disease. Prognosis should be considered to appropriately adjust the aggressiveness of the nutritional intervention (supportive, adjunctive, definitive).

Nutritional problems may arise as a result of the cancer itself or the method used to treat it. Nutritional interventions will be tailored to support the energy and protein needs of the patient so that body stores can be maintained, and then as symptoms arise, interventions can be introduced to maximize nutritional intake.

Anorexia Caused by Cancer or Its Treatment

Anorexia is loss of appetite. The etiology of anorexia is generally multifactorial. For cancer patients this may be caused by changes in taste and smell; decreased transit time and subsequent, early satiety; opportunistic infections; therapy and other medication side effects; pain; and emotional and psychologic effects.[4-8]

Treatment Options

Early education of the patient on the role of nutrition is essential to promote adequate nutritional intake. Many cancer patients feel a loss of control after diagnosis of a malignancy. Often, managing their nutritional intake assists in regaining that control. It is essential that the nutrient density of food be stressed. Small, frequent meals; the use of high-kcal supplements; and a pleasant eating environment can help. Medications such as megestrol (Megace) and

Scored Patient-Generated Subjective Global Assessment (PG-SGA)

History (Boxes 1-4 are designed to be completed by the patient.)

Patient ID Information

1. Weight *(See Worksheet 1)*

In summary of my current and recent weight:

I currently weigh about _____ pounds
I am about _____ feet _____ tall

One month ago I weighed about _____ pounds
Six months ago I weighed about _____ pounds

During the past two weeks my weight has:
☐ decreased $_{(1)}$ ☐ not changed $_{(0)}$ ☐ increased $_{(0)}$

Box 1 [____]

2. Food Intake: As compared to my normal intake, I would rate my food intake during the past month as:

☐ unchanged $_{(0)}$
☐ more than usual $_{(0)}$
☐ less than usual $_{(1)}$
I am now taking:
   ☐ *normal food* but less than normal amount $_{(1)}$
   ☐ little solid food $_{(2)}$
   ☐ only liquids $_{(3)}$
   ☐ only nutritional supplements $_{(3)}$
   ☐ very little of anything $_{(4)}$
   ☐ only tube feedings or only nutrition by vein $_{(0)}$

Box 2 [____]

3. Symptoms: I have had the following problems that have kept me from eating enough during the past two weeks (check all that apply):

☐ no problems eating $_{(0)}$

☐ no appetite, just did not feel like eating $_{(3)}$

☐ nausea $_{(1)}$ ☐ vomiting $_{(3)}$
☐ constipation $_{(1)}$ ☐ diarrhea $_{(3)}$
☐ mouth sores $_{(2)}$ ☐ dry mouth $_{(1)}$
☐ things taste funny or have no taste $_{(1)}$ ☐ smells bother me $_{(1)}$
☐ problems swallowing $_{(2)}$ ☐ feel full quickly $_{(1)}$
☐ pain; where? $_{(3)}$ _____
☐ other** $_{(1)}$ _____
   ** Examples: depression, money, or dental problems

Box 3 [____]

4. Activities and Function: Over the past month, I would generally rate my activity as:

☐ normal with no limitations $_{(0)}$

☐ not my normal self, but able to be up and about with fairly normal activities $_{(1)}$

☐ not feeling up to most things, but in bed or chair less than half the day $_{(2)}$

☐ able to do little activity and spend most of the day in bed or chair $_{(3)}$

☐ pretty much bedridden, rarely out of bed $_{(3)}$

Box 4 [____]

Additive Score of the Boxes 1-4 [____] A

The remainder of this form will be completed by your doctor, nurse, or therapist. Thank you.

(Optional for completion by clinicians)

5. Disease and its relation to nutritional requirements *(See Worksheet 2)*

All relevant diagnoses (specify) _____

Primary disease stage (circle if known or appropriate)   I   II   III   IV   Other _____

Age _____

Numerical score from Worksheet 2 [____] B

6. Metabolic Demand *(See Worksheet 3)*

Numerical score from Worksheet 3 [____] C

7. Physical *(See Worksheet 4)*

Numerical score from Worksheet 4 [____] D

Global Assessment *(See Worksheet 5)*

☐ Well-nourished or anabolic (SGA-A)
☐ Moderate or suspected malnutrition (SGA-B)
☐ Severely malnourished (SGA-C)

Total PG-SGA score

(Total numerical score of A+B+C+D above) [____]

(See triage recommendations below)

Clinician Signature _____ RD RN PA MD DO Other ___   Date _____

Nutritional Triage Recommendations: Additive score is used to define specific nutritional interventions including patient & family education, symptom management including pharmacologic intervention, and appropriate nutrient intervention (food, nutritional supplements, enteral, or parenteral triage). First line nutrition intervention includes optimal symptom management.

0-1   No intervention required at this time. Re-assessment on routine and regular basis during treatment.

2-3   Patient & family education by dietitian, nurse, or other clinician with pharmacologic intervention as indicated by symptom survey (Box 3) and laboratory values as appropriate.

4-8   Requires intervention by dietitian, in conjunction with nurse or physician as indicated by symptoms survey (Box 3).

≥ 9   Indicates a critical need for improved symptom management and/or nutrient intervention options.

© FD Ottery, 2001. Used with permission.   email: fdottery@btgc.com or noatpres1@aol.com

Continued

Worksheets for PG-SGA Scoring   © FD Ottery, 2001. Used with permission.

Boxes 1-4 of the PG-SGA are designed to be completed by the patient. The PG-SGA numerical score is determined using
1) the parenthetical points noted in boxes 1-4 and 2) the worksheets below for items not marked with parenthetical points. Scores for
boxes 1 and 3 are additive within each box and scores for boxes 2 and 4 are based on the highest scored item checked off by the patient.

Worksheet 1 - Scoring Weight (Wt) Loss

To determine score, use 1 month weight data if available. Use 6 month
data only if there is no 1 month weight data. Use points below to score
weight change and add one extra point if patient has lost weight during the
past 2 weeks. Enter total point score in Box 1 of the PG-SGA.

Wt loss in 1 month	Points	Wt loss in 6 months
10% or greater	4	20% or greater
5-9.9%	3	10 -19.9%
3-4.9%	2	6 - 9.9%
2-2.9%	1	2 - 5.9%
0-1.9%	0	0 - 1.9%

Score for Worksheet 1 [   ]
Record in Box 1

Worksheet 2 - Scoring Criteria for Condition

Score is derived by adding 1 point for each of the conditions listed below
that pertain to the patient.

Category	Points
Cancer	1
AIDS	1
Pulmonary or cardiac cachexia	1
Presence of decubitus, open wound, or fistula	1
Presence of trauma	1
Age greater than 65 years	1

Score for Worksheet 2 = [   ]
Record in Box B

Worksheet 3 - Scoring Metabolic Stress

Score for metabolic stress is determined by a number of variables known to increase protein & calorie needs. The score is additive so that a patient who has a fever
of > 102 degrees (3 points) and is on 10 mg of prednisone chronically (2 points) would have an additive score for this section of 5 points.

Stress	none (0)	low (1)	moderate (2)	high (3)
Fever	no fever	>99 and <101	≥101 and <102	≥102
Fever duration	no fever	<72 hrs	72 hrs	> 72 hrs
Corticosteroids	no corticosteroids	low dose (<10mg prednisone equivalents/day)	moderate dose (≥10 and <30 mg prednisone equivalents/day)	high dose steroids (≥30 mg prednisone equivalents/day)

Score for Worksheet 3 = [   ]
Record in Box C

Worksheet 4 - Physical Examination

Physical exam includes a subjective evaluation of 3 aspects of body composition: fat, muscle, & fluid status. Since this is subjective, each aspect of the exam is
rated for degree of deficit. Muscle deficit impacts point score more than fat deficit. Definition of categories: 0 = no deficit, 1+ = mild deficit, 2+ = moderate
deficit, 3+ = severe deficit. Rating of deficit in these categories are *not* additive but are used to clinically assess the degree of deficit (or presence of excess fluid).

Fat Stores:

orbital fat pads	0	1+	2+	3+
triceps skin fold	0	1+	2+	3+
fat overlying lower ribs	0	1+	2+	3+
Global fat deficit rating	**0**	**1+**	**2+**	**3+**

Muscle Status:

temples (temporalis muscle)	0	1+	2+	3+
clavicles (pectoralis & deltoids)	0	1+	2+	3+
shoulders (deltoids)	0	1+	2+	3+
interosseous muscles	0	1+	2+	3+
scapula (latissimus dorsi, trapezius, deltoids)	0	1+	2+	3+
thigh (quadriceps)	0	1+	2+	3+
calf (gastrocnemius)	0	1+	2+	3+
Global muscle status rating	**0**	**1+**	**2+**	**3+**

Fluid Status:

ankle edema	0	1+	2+	3+
sacral edema	0	1+	2+	3+
ascites	0	1+	2+	3+
Global fluid status rating	**0**	**1+**	**2+**	**3+**

Point score for the physical exam is determined by the overall
subjective rating of total body deficit.

No deficit	score = 0 points
Mild deficit	score = 1 point
Moderate deficit	score = 2 points
Severe deficit	score = 3 points

Score for Worksheet 4 = [   ]
Record in Box D

Worksheet 5 - PG-SGA Global Assessment Categories

Category	**Stage A** Well-nourished	**Stage B** Moderately malnourished or suspected malnutrition	**Stage C** Severely malnourished
Weight	No wt loss **OR** Recent non-fluid wt gain	~5% wt loss within 1 month (or 10% in 6 months) **OR** No wt stabilization or wt gain (i.e., continued wt loss)	> 5% wt loss in 1 month (or >10% in 6 months) **OR** No wt stabilization or wt gain (i.e., continued wt loss)
Nutrient Intake	No deficit **OR** Significant recent improvement	Definite decrease in intake	Severe deficit in intake
Nutrition Impact Symptoms	None **OR** Significant recent improvement allowing adequate intake	Presence of nutrition impact symptoms (Box 3 of PG-SGA)	Presence of nutrition impact symptoms (Box 3 of PG-SGA)
Functioning	No deficit **OR** Significant recent improvement	Moderate functional deficit **OR** Recent deterioration	Severe functional deficit **OR** recent significant deterioration
Physical Exam	No deficit **OR** Chronic deficit but with recent clinical improvement	Evidence of mild to moderate loss of SQ fat &/or muscle mass &/or muscle tone on palpation	Obvious signs of malnutrition (e.g., severe loss of SQ tissues, possible edema)

Global PG-SGA rating (A, B, or C) = [   ]

FIG 22-1 Patient-Generated Subjective Global Assessment (PG-SGA) of nutritional status.
(Copyright FD Ottery, 2000. Grateful acknowledgment is given to the Society for Nutritional
Oncology Adjuvant Therapy [NOAT] and the Oncology Dietetic Practice Group of the American
Dietetic Association, with special recognition of Suzanne Kasenic, Susan DeBolt, Paula McCallum, and Christine Polisena.)

TABLE 22-3	NUTRITIONAL APPROACHES TO NUTRITION-RELATED PROBLEMS IN CANCER AND CANCER THERAPY
PROBLEM	**RECOMMENDATIONS**
Loss of appetite/early satiety	Eat frequent small meals, increase kcal/protein content of foods, use high-protein/high-kcal supplements, serve foods cool or at room temperature, avoid excess fat, exercise regularly if tolerated, limit liquids at mealtime; appetite may be best in the morning
Diarrhea*	Eat frequent small meals, serve foods cool or at room temperature, increase fluid intake, eat and drink slowly, decrease fiber intake, avoid excess fat, avoid gas-forming foods, limit liquids at mealtime, avoid highly seasoned foods, limit beverages containing caffeine and alcohol; trial avoidance of lactose may be helpful; take antidiarrheal medication per physician
Nausea and vomiting	Eat frequent small meals, avoid strong odors, serve foods cool or room temperature, increase fluid intake, eat and drink slowly, avoid excess fat, limit liquids at mealtime, avoid highly seasoned foods, rest after meals with head elevated, take antiemetic per physician
Chewing and swallowing difficulties	Eat frequent small meals; increase kcal/protein content of foods; use high-protein/high-kcal supplements; serve food cool or at room temperature; increase fluid intake; eat and drink slowly; add sauces and gravy to soften and moisten foods; avoid highly seasoned foods; avoid alcohol, tobacco, and commercial mouthwashes; coarse-textured and acidic foods may irritate
Constipation	Increase fluid intake, increase fiber intake, exercise regularly if tolerated; stool softener and/or laxative may be necessary
Abdominal gas	Eat and drink slowly, decrease fiber intake, avoid excess fat, avoid gas-forming foods, exercise regularly if tolerated, limit lactose if not tolerated
Dry mouth	Increase fluid intake, add sauces and gravy to soften and moisten foods, tart foods or sugar-free hard candy may be used to stimulate saliva, avoid alcohol, tobacco, and commercial mouthwash
Taste/smell alterations	Serve food cool or at room temperature, increase fluid intake, use seasonings to enhance flavors, avoid cooking odors, try alternative protein sources for meat aversion

*Diarrhea secondary to malabsorption, dumping syndrome, or other causes may require different treatment modalities.
Data from McCallum PD, Polisena CG, editors: *The clinical guide to oncology nutrition*, Chicago, 2002, American Dietetic Association.

dronabinol (Marinol) have been used successfully to stimulate appetite in cancer patients.[4-10]

Nausea and Vomiting

Nausea and vomiting may result from (1) delayed transit time; (2) physiologic symptoms such as hypercalcemia or CNS involvement; (3) medications; or (4) simply a result of anticipation on the part of the patient.[4-10]

Treatment Options

The first line of treatment for nausea and vomiting is adequate and aggressive antiemetic therapy. It is essential to give medication 60 to 90 minutes before meals to ensure effectiveness. If nausea and vomiting can be prevented, the risk of developing anticipatory nausea and vomiting will be reduced. Cold foods without odor tend to be best tolerated when the patient experiences nausea and vomiting. Behavioral strategies such as guided imagery and relaxation techniques have also been successful in some environments.[4-10]

Taste Abnormalities

Many cancer patients describe alterations in their ability to taste foods. These alterations may be because of the changes or destruction of the oral mucosa, the presence of tumor by-products systemically, changes in the quantity or quality of saliva, inadequate mouth care, or drug-related taste changes.[4-10]

Treatment Options

It is appropriate for cancer patients to avoid those foods that taste bad to them. However, it is just as important to provide cancer patients with alternate food choices for them to maintain adequate nutrient intake. Foods that are tart or spicy may enhance intake. Additionally, providing guidelines for mouth care is essential.[4-10]

Principles of Nutritional Care

Nutrition should be an essential component of every treatment plan for the cancer patient. The following are expected outcomes for nutrition therapy:
- Weight and lean body mass are maintained within the established goal range through consumption of adequate energy and protein or with appropriate nutritional support.
- Hydration will be adequate as measured by clinical and physical assessment.
- The patient will consume adequate energy and protein to perform activities of daily living.
- The patient will verbalize comprehension of neutropenic precautions.

- The patient will use appropriate and safe complementary nutrition therapies.[10]

ACQUIRED IMMUNODEFICIENCY SYNDROME (AIDS)

In 1983 the retrovirus human immunodeficiency virus (HIV) was isolated as the cause for acquired immunodeficiency syndrome (AIDS). A retrovirus injects its ribonucleic acid (RNA) into the target cell and then transcribes the RNA into DNA using a reverse transcriptase enzyme. Target cells for HIV include the T_4 or CD4 lymphocytes, B-lymphocytes, monocytes, macrophages, and other cells of the immune system.[11,12] Currently there are two major strains of HIV. HIV-1 is commonly found in the United States, whereas HIV-2 is the most common strain found within the African continent.[11]

As many as 1 billion copies of HIV can be made in 1 day, and several generations can exist in just hours. The initial infection with HIV may include symptoms such as fever and malaise. Antibodies are produced against the virus and are detectable within 2 to 4 months after exposure. Screening technology (enzyme-linked immunosorbent assay [ELISA]) allows for more rapid testing for HIV infection but is followed with confirmation tests that include Western blot, modified Western blot, indirect immunofluorescent antibody assay (IFA), and line immunoassay (LIA). These tests confirm the presence of HIV antibodies.[12] The replication of the infected cell results in a steady depletion of the CD4 cell count, causing a severe depression of immune function and increasing the risk for opportunistic infections and malignancies (Table 22-4). The diagnosis of AIDS includes the positive antibody test for HIV; a CD4 cell count of less than 200 mm^3 or less than 14% of the total white blood cell count; and the clinical diagnosis of 1 of 25 AIDS-defining diseases.[12] The progression from HIV to AIDS varies for each individual and may not be evident for several years. The two major prognostic factors for HIV are the CD4 T-cell count and the measurement of plasma HIV RNA (viral load for HIV).

HIV is a bloodborne and sexually transmitted infection. It is transmitted through contact with contaminated blood, semen, vaginal secretions, and breast milk. HIV also crosses the placenta from the mother to the baby. Approximately 40 million people throughout the world have HIV infection, and these are concentrated in southern and eastern African countries. In 2005, new infections were estimated to affect 4.9 million people with an increased number of children and women affected.[13,14] More than 3 million people may have died from complications related to HIV infection during 2005. This is especially true in sub-Saharan Africa where AIDS is the leading cause of death.[13,14] In the United States an estimated 850,000 to 950,000 people live with HIV infection, with an estimated 40,000 new infections each year, primarily in minority populations, women, and youth.

There has been significant progress for treatment of HIV and AIDS over the past decade with the use of drug combinations for highly active antiretroviral therapy (HAART). Until the 1990s treatment for HIV and AIDS focused on treatment with one or two drugs. Today HAART uses combinations of fusion inhibitors, integrase inhibitors, nucleoside/nucleotide reverse transcriptase inhibitors non-nucleoside reverse transcriptase inhibitors, and protease inhibitors.

TABLE 22-4	CLINICAL AND NUTRITIONAL COMPLICATIONS OF AIDS
OPPORTUNISTIC INFECTIONS	**CLINICAL AND NUTRITIONAL PRESENTATION**
Neoplasms	
Kaposi's sarcoma	Oral, esophageal lesions
Lymphoma: Burkitt's immunoblastic	Dependent on primary site—diarrhea and malabsorption possible if GI tract involved
Protozoa/Parasites	
Cryptosporidium spp.	Watery diarrhea, malabsorption, nausea, vomiting, abdominal pain, cholecystitis, pancreatitis
Pneumocystis jiroveci	Pneumonia
Toxoplasmosis	Fever, headache, confusion
Entamoeba histolytica; Entamoeba coli; Giardia lamblia; Acanthamoeba	Diarrhea, nausea, vomiting, loss of appetite
Bacteria	
Mycobacterium avium complex (MAC)	Fever, diarrhea, malabsorption, anorexia
Legionella	Pneumonia
Salmonella	Fever, abdominal pain and cramping, diarrhea
Listeria	Diarrhea, abdominal pain, fever
Shigella	Bloody diarrhea, abdominal pain, fever
Fungi	
Candida albicans	Thrush, stomatitis, esophagitis
Cryptococcus	Meningitis, nausea, vomiting, fever, dementia
Aspergillosis	Pneumonia
Coccidioidomycosis	Pneumonia, fungemia
Histoplasmosis	Fever, pneumonia
Viruses	
Cytomegalovirus (CMV)	Dependent on site of infection—can involve entire gastrointestinal (GI) tract with diarrhea, nausea, and vomiting
Herpes simplex	Painful blisters—symptoms depend on site of infection

Data from Centers for Disease Control and Prevention: 1993 Revised classification system for HIV infection and expanded surveillance case definition for AIDS among adolescents and adults, *MMWR Recomm Rep* 41(RR-17):1-19, 1992. Accessed April 7, 2010, from www.cdc.gov/mmwr/preview/mmwrhtml/00018871.htm.

The goal of these treatment regimens is to maintain a viral load of fewer than 50 copies/mL.[15] Adherence to these regimens is often difficult because of the number and the complexity of medications that must be taken daily. Drug resistance can develop if adherence is not maintained. Other side effects of these medications include nausea, vomiting, diarrhea, and other metabolic changes discussed later in this chapter.

Malnutrition in HIV/AIDS

Malnutrition has been documented in all stages of HIV infection. Most nutritional problems coincide with the incidence of high viral loads, opportunistic infections, and the development of viral resistance. With the evolution of HAART, nutritional problems have shifted to include more chronic disease issues such as hyperlipidemia, insulin resistance, and diabetes mellitus. It is important, though, to realize that much of the world does not have access to these medication regimens and that some people choose not to use them. In these populations, malnutrition is still common.[16,17]

AIDS-related **wasting syndrome** has been included by the Centers for Disease Control and Prevention (CDC) in their classification for AIDS since 1987.[12] This classification defines wasting as an involuntary weight loss of greater than 10% in 1 month with the presence of chronic diarrhea, weakness, or fever for more than 30 days in the absence of a concurrent illness or condition. Research indicates that a 10% weight loss is a strong predictor of survival in HIV infection and that even less than 5% weight loss may be a risk factor for mortality.[17]

The presence of malnutrition and weight loss is still considered an important predictor of both morbidity and mortality from the disease.[16-19] Malnutrition in HIV and AIDS is multifactorial, as shown in Figure 22-2. Altered nutrient intake, weight loss and body composition changes, physical impairment, endocrine disorders, metabolic changes, malabsorption, the presence of opportunistic infections, psychosocial issues, and economic conditions all contribute to malnutrition (see Table 22-4).

Altered Nutrient Intake

Anorexia or loss of appetite is a frequent symptom of altered nutrient intake. A client's lack of appetite may be caused by the HIV infection, the presence of opportunistic infections, fatigue, fever, or medication side effects. Physical impairment from mucositis, esophagitis, pain, nausea, and vomiting affect the client's ability to ingest adequate nutrients. Depression, loneliness, fear, anxiety, or other psychosocial issues can play a significant role in the client's desire to eat. In addition, economic availability of adequate food supplies cannot be forgotten and often may be the most difficult problem to solve.

It is critical to begin interventions early. The first step should be education about the role of nutrition (see the *Teaching Tool* box, Maximizing Food Intake in HIV/AIDS). Nutrition should be considered a crucial element of medical care, not simply as alternative or adjunct therapy. Nutrition is one area in which clients can exert some control over their medical care. Emphasizing the benefits of maintaining nutritional status such as repair and building of tissue, preserving lean body mass and GI function, minimizing fatigue, and improving quality of life are important components of this education. The identification of the contributing factors to anorexia will then guide the client and practitioner in developing strategies to improve oral intake. Strategies for coping with loss of appetite are listed in Table 22-3.

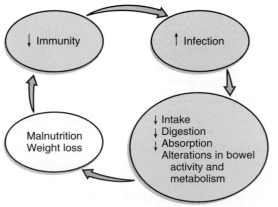

FIG 22-2 Vicious cycle of malnutrition and AIDS. (From Rolin Graphics.)

✺ TEACHING TOOL
Maximizing Food Intake in HIV/AIDS

Clients dealing with the chronic effects of human immuno-deficiency virus/acquired immunodeficiency syndrome (HIV/AIDS) may have difficulty consuming enough kcal to meet physiologic requirements. Home health care nurses can teach the following strategies to increase kcal and protein without necessarily expanding the volume of food:

- Substitute kcal-containing and nutrient-dense foods and beverages for low- or no-kcal foods and beverages: milk or shakes instead of coffee or tea; regular soft drinks for sugar-free drinks.
- Increase the number or size of feedings daily. Offer five or six small meals/snacks.
- Fortify foods with kcal and protein-containing ingredients. Add skim milk powder to milk, shakes, gravies, and hot cereals.
- Use kcal-containing condiments. Add butter/margarine to hot cereals, vegetables, and starches.
- Modify diet according to tolerances. Try cold or room-temperature foods, bland or salty foods; avoid greasy and sweet foods and liquids between meals.
- Add kcal-containing supplements as needed.

Data from Fields-Gardner C, Salamon S, Davis M: *Living well with HIV and AIDS,* Chicago, 2003, American Dietetic Association; and American Dietetic Association: *Manual of clinical dietetics,* ed 6, Chicago, 2000, American Dietetic Association.

Weight Loss and Body Composition Changes

Patients may experience weight loss and changes in body composition. As discussed, weight loss may occur from decreased nutrient intake from physical impairment or as a result of symptoms that impair appetite. Weight loss appears to occur not only from fat stores but also lean body mass. This phenomenon is not as easily explained. Acute weight loss differs from chronic weight loss not only in its etiology but also from the type of energy stores that are depleted. Chronic weight loss, as seen in malnutrition, is often accompanied by a decrease in metabolic rate and a reliance on fat stores for energy. Acute weight loss, such as seen in stress, is accompanied by an increase in metabolic rate, a reliance on glucose as fuel, and a depletion of lean body mass. These changes in body composition and weight loss are commonly seen in the wasting syndrome and often coincide with increases in viral load.[16-19] Body composition changes also have been noted in lipodystrophy or the fat redistribution syndrome.[20] These changes are discussed in detail later in this chapter.

Medications can be prescribed to assist with anorexia and body composition changes. Megestrol acetate (Megace), dronabinol (Marinol), oxandrolone (Oxandrin) or oxymetholone, testosterone, dehydroepiandrosterone (DHEA), and human growth hormone (r-hGH) have all been used with this population.[21] Dronabinol received approval from the U.S. Food and Drug Administration (FDA) in 1985 as an antiemetic for cancer patients and was approved for use as an appetite stimulant in 1992. Studies have shown it offers improvement in appetite, mood, and nausea and has resulted in weight maintenance. Side effects include euphoria, dizziness, and impaired thinking. The FDA initially approved oxandrolone, an oral analog of testosterone, in the 1960s. Clients have experienced an increase in lean body mass, mood elevation, and increased libido with the use of oxandrolone and with testosterone replacement.[22] Both DHEA and r-hGH have been used to improve lean body mass with a decrease in abdominal adiposity.[22-24] DHEA has been used to treat depression in patients with HIV/AIDS as well.[25]

Physical Impairment

Nausea, vomiting, mouth and esophageal lesions, and impaired dentition are all frequent problems for people with AIDS. These may be a result of opportunistic infections such as candidiasis and gingivitis or from side effects of antiretroviral therapy, prophylactic treatment to prevent opportunistic infections, and medication for the management of pain. Determining the causes of impaired intake is crucial to a successful intervention (see Table 22-3 for problem-solving techniques).

Endocrine and Metabolic Disorders

Hypogonadism has been identified in people with HIV and AIDS.[26] This condition is associated with fatigue, decreased libido, loss of muscle mass, muscle weakness, impotence, and loss of body hair. The associated fatigue contributes not only

to decreased appetite but also to impaired ability to prepare and consume meals. Loss of lean body mass is a prominent feature of the malnutrition and wasting syndrome of AIDS. Adrenal insufficiency may contribute to changes in appetite, loss of fuel storage, and changes in metabolism. It is unclear, though, whether any of these abnormalities are causal factors in the development of malnutrition in HIV.

Fat redistribution syndrome (lipodystrophy) has been described as a syndrome of body composition changes and metabolic disturbances. Beginning in the late 1990s, in some patients receiving antiretroviral therapy, shift in adiposity was noted. In many patients, this increase in abdominal obesity was accompanied by an increase in serum triglycerides, cholesterol, glucose, and insulin resistance. The etiology of this syndrome has not been clarified but has been associated with both protease inhibitors and nucleoside analog therapy.[19-21]

Malabsorption

Malabsorption can be a result of (1) opportunistic infections that damage the GI tract, (2) the effects of malnutrition on villus height and enterocyte function, and (3) from the disease itself. In those patients with HIV-related diarrhea, *steatorrhea* has been noted in clients without GI infections. Additionally, other studies have documented abnormal D-xylose tests, which indicates the presence of malabsorption. A significant number of those subjects had diarrhea, and in almost half of those cases, no pathogen could be identified.

Treatment of the underlying cause, if possible, is crucial in reversing the malnutrition caused by malabsorption. To assist with the control of malabsorptive symptoms and diarrhea, the restriction of fat and lactose is common. The use of lactose-free supplements and those supplements containing medium-chain triglycerides such as Advera, Alitraq, Peptamen, or Lipisorb are frequently prescribed. Additionally, probiotics and prebiotics, as well as glutamine and arginine, in enteral products or given separately as a supplement have been used to assist in this malabsorption syndrome and in treating diarrhea.[27] Careful attention must be taken to ensure adequate caloric and protein intake in the face of restricting these important kcal and protein sources. Additionally, fluid losses may be high with the presence of diarrhea. Prevention of dehydration and supplementation with vitamins and minerals are priority considerations as well.

Cycle of Malnutrition and Wasting

Malnutrition and wasting in patients with HIV and AIDS create a vicious cycle that can be fatal. It is unreasonable to expect that the treatment of malnutrition is simple when the causes are so complex. First, interventions must be integrated early. Research has shown promise concerning the efficacy of nutrition interventions. Conducting nutrition assessment and providing counseling have resulted in the ability of patients to maintain or gain weight.[16,21,28] Health care teams can treat the nutritional problems of HIV and AIDS with multiple and complementary modes of therapy (see Box 22-4).

NUTRITION ASSESSMENT IN CANCER AND HIV/AIDS

The initial step in assessing nutritional risk is to evaluate anthropometric data. Body weight compared with the client's usual body weight is much more crucial than comparison with ideal body weight. Any unexplained weight loss should be noted, but weight loss of greater than 10% in 6 months is considered to place the client at risk. Calculation of *body mass index (BMI)* also identifies nutrition risk. A calculated BMI of less than 18 is associated with malnutrition and has been associated with an increased risk of mortality.[29]

Using only weight loss in the assessment may be misleading. Loss of lean body mass is characteristic of the malnutrition of AIDS. Shifts in lean body mass can be noted, although weight may be initially maintained. *Bioelectrical impedance (BIA)* has been successfully used to evaluate changes in lean body mass.[16,21,28] If BIA is not available, a calculation of upper-arm muscle area can be useful in providing a baseline measurement for which the client can be monitored over time.

Biochemical indices include those monitoring disease progression (CD4 or viral load); acute phase proteins that measure inflammatory processes (C-reactive protein) and overall visceral protein stores (serum albumin [Nl 3.5 to 5 g/dL] and prealbumin [Nl 20 to 50 mg/dL]) can be used to monitor more acute changes. Other measures such as transferrin are not applicable because of possible bone marrow suppression in this population.

Dietary assessment may be evaluated by 24-hour recall, food frequency, or food diary. Careful attention should be made to gastrointestinal function, the presence of steatorrhea and diarrhea, and any other physical symptoms that might interfere with adequate oral intake.

Using multiple parameters will allow a more thorough evaluation of the patient's nutritional status and risk for protein-energy malnutrition. The Subjective Global Assessment tool (see Figure 22-1) also serves as an excellent screening tool for HIV and AIDS patients to determine nutritional risk and to assess the need of referral to a registered dietitian. Protocols outlining medical nutrition therapy for people with HIV and AIDS have been established.[16,21,28]

Nutrition Therapy

The following are the overall goals of nutrition management:[16,21,28]

- Preserve lean body mass and gut function
- Prevent development of malnutrition
- Provide adequate levels of all nutrients to maintain daily physical and mental functioning
- Minimize the symptoms of malabsorption
- Prevent nutrition-related immunosuppression
- Improve quality of life

HAART's focus of nutrition therapy includes not only preventing malnutrition but also addressing chronic nutrition problems, such as hyperlipidemia, hyperglycemia, and hypertension. The objectives of the nutrition care plan need to be realistic and individualized. Interventions that are designed should be based on the nutritional assessment and the current medical treatment for that client. After assessment, the first step in planning nutrition therapy is to determine energy and protein requirements. Many clinicians use equations such as the Harris-Benedict equation to determine resting energy expenditure (REE). Using 1.3 to 1.5 X REE should meet most clients' energy requirements for maintenance and weight gain, respectively. The following Mifflin–St. Jeor equation may better predict energy requirements for the hospitalized patient.[30] Protein requirements should be met with the range of 1 to 1.5 g protein/kg of actual body weight depending on the patient's current nutritional status.[30]

Mifflin–St. Jeor Equation

Females: 10 W + 6.25 Ht − 5 Age − 161

Males: 10 W + 6.25 Ht − 5 Age + 5

Where:

W = Weight (in kg)

Ht = Height (in cm)

Age = Age (in years)

Vitamin and mineral status needs to be monitored closely in this population. Deficiencies may evolve not only from suppressed oral intake but also the increased requirements for certain micronutrients. Research has studied the effects of supplementation with beta carotene, vitamin C, vitamin E, selenium, and the amino acids glutamine and arginine but has not provided conclusive information from which to make global supplementation recommendations for the AIDS patient. It is routinely recommended, though, that people with HIV and AIDS take a general multivitamin supplement that meets 100% of the Recommended Dietary Allowance (RDA) for vitamins and minerals. In some individual situations, other supplements may be warranted.[16,21,28]

Antiretroviral therapy requires specific nutrition recommendations. Many of the medications used to treat this condition result in symptoms such as nausea, vomiting, diarrhea, or anorexia that might impair oral intake. Even the number of pills that must be taken can be overwhelming to the patient. Additionally, the ingestion of food along with certain medications may affect the absorption of that drug or vice versa. Examples of these are as follows:[15]

- *Efavirenz (Sustiva):* Avoid taking with high-fat meals.
- *Lopinavir (Kaletra) + ritonavir (Norvir):* Moderate-fat meals increases availability of capsules; it should be taken with food.
- *Saquinavir (Invirase):* Take this protease inhibitor within 2 hours of a meal containing high-fat foods or a large snack containing carbohydrate, protein, or fat.
- *Ritonavir (Norvir):* If this protease inhibitor is consumed with a meal, it may decrease the abdominal cramping and diarrhea that is common when this drug is initially prescribed. These symptoms usually disappear within 8 weeks.
- *Indinavir (Crixivan):* This protease inhibitor should be taken on an empty stomach. A meal can be eaten 1 hour after the drug or 2 hours before the drug. For

---

BOX 22-4   EVALUATION OF COMPLEMENTARY AND ALTERNATIVE THERAPIES

Because currently there are no cures for some cancers and human immunodeficiency virus/acquired immunodeficiency syndrome (HIV/AIDS), patients are potential victims for unproven or fraudulent health and nutrition therapies. Complementary and alternative therapies are being evaluated with long-term research studies, but it is a slow process. Until results are available, it is difficult to evaluate the efficacy of these treatments. For example, the yeast-free diet is commonly recommended to prevent fungal infections. This diet eliminates products containing yeast and simple sugars. Currently, there is no research to support these claims. High doses of vitamins and minerals can actually result in toxicities that are potentially harmful. Complementary and alternative therapies may not only be extremely costly but also interfere with current medical treatments, putting the patient at even more risk. For example, microbial growth in herbal supplements may pose a risk of opportunistic infections in immunosuppressed patients.

The National Center for Complementary and Alternative Medicine (NCCAM) at the National Institutes of Health provides the structure for evaluating complementary and alternative therapies. Presently, a number of clinical studies have been or are being conducted to assess the value of complementary and alternative therapies for such disorders such as cancer and HIV/AIDS. Better sources of data are forthcoming. Questionable practices or products may be reported to the following sources:

- Federal Trade Commission (FTC) Bureau of Consumer Protection; regional FTC office; chief postal inspector, US Postal Service; editor or station manager of media outlet where advertisement appeared; regional Food and Drug Administration (FDA) office; state attorney general; state health department; local Better Business Bureau; congressional representative; local or state professional society; local hospital (if practitioner is a staff member); state licensing board; local district attorney
- National Council Against Health Fraud (www.ncahf.org); Consumer Health Information Research Institute; local, state, or national professional or voluntary health groups

---

some, it may be necessary to eat a small snack with the drug, but fat should be avoided.

Prevention of Foodborne Illness

Prevention of foodborne illness is a crucial component of nutrition therapy and nutrition education for people with HIV and AIDS. As CD4 counts fall, clients are at higher risk for these infections from this source. Nutrition education should focus on safe methods for food purchasing, preparation, and storage. Often a low microbial diet is prescribed that recommends avoidance of undercooked meats and eggs, raw vegetables, and fruits.

Cryptosporidium infections can be life threatening and lead to chronic, debilitating diarrhea. Infectious outbreaks have been linked to water sources. This protozoan is resistant to chlorination, and recent documentation of infections has led to recommendations for those people with AIDS and HIV to monitor their water source.[20,28] Suggestions have been made to avoid all public tap water and to drink only filtered water or water that has been boiled for 1 minute (Box 22-5). Fruits and vegetables can be cleaned with a mixture of 20 drops of 2% iodine in 1 gallon of water to prevent contamination.

Exercise Recommendations

Regular aerobic exercise and resistance training have been suggested to assist with lipid abnormalities, the fat redistribution syndrome, and other body composition changes noted in those patients with HIV and AIDS.[31,32] Recommendations should be individualized and initiated slowly after receiving a physician's approval. Benefits may include the following:

- Increased muscle volume, strength, functional capacity, and quality of life
- Decreased abdominal fat

BOX 22-5   SAFE WATER

To destroy tap water contaminants that may cause illness, the Centers for Disease Control and Prevention recommends that individuals with weakened immune systems boil tap water before consumption. Immune system functioning may be diminished because of the effects of HIV, AIDS, chemotherapy drugs, and immunosuppressive drugs (to prevent organ-transplant rejection).

Data from *Safe food and water: A guide for people with HIV and AIDS*, Atlanta, (updated June 2007), Centers for Disease Control and Prevention. Accessed April 7, 2010, from www.cdc.gov/hiv/pubs/brochure/food.htm.

- Prevention of glucose abnormalities and improved insulin sensitivity
- Improved circulation
- Improved bone metabolism

Multidisciplinary Approach

Malnutrition and wasting associated with the HIV infection/AIDS are multifactorial. Many aspects are not well understood, but that does not negate the fact that nutrition assessment, counseling, and support are critical components of the medical care for HIV and AIDS. Effective treatment requires a multidisciplinary approach based on collaboration of all health care team members, including the nurse and dietitian. Early recognition and intervention for nutritional risk factors are keys to effective nutrition support and related medical therapies (see the *Cultural Considerations* box, AIDS, HIV, and Ethnic Issues of Healing and Medicine: Lessons From Tuskegee).

⊕ CULTURAL CONSIDERATIONS

AIDS, HIV, and Ethnic Issues of Healing and Medicine: Lessons from Tuskegee

As we attempt to heal those experiencing disorders such as AIDS and HIV, which are fairly "new" disorders, we need to understand history to fully comprehend the perspective of the patients with whom we work.

During the middle of the twentieth century (1932-1972), a medical study called the Tuskegee Experiment followed the course of syphilis among African American men from a poor county in Georgia. When the study began, there was no known cure for syphilis, but shortly into the study, penicillin was recognized as an effective drug against the ravages of this sexually transmitted disease. Nonetheless, such treatment was withheld from the men participating in this study, and most were followed to their death, which may or may not have been as a result of syphilis-related causes. The study did not end until the 1970s after the men, their wives, and children were exposed and suffered the consequences of a serious systemic disease that could have been cured with inexpensive penicillin. Because this population was poor and African American, many view this

as the reason such an unethical protocol was allowed to continue.

In 1973, a class-action lawsuit for the individuals and family members affected by the study was filed by the National Association for the Advancement of Colored People (NAACP). A $9 million settlement was awarded and distributed among those affected. In 1997 President Clinton issued a formal apology on behalf of the U.S. government.

Application to nursing: Today, as nurses attempt to encourage and treat ethnic groups for AIDS and HIV, they may not be receptive to treatments and medications because the shadow of deceit of the Tuskegee Experiment makes them leery of the health care system. Knowledge of the past treatment of subgroups provides an understanding of current bias toward accepting government-sponsored medical treatment. By understanding our history, we can provide education about the ethical medical treatments available now.

Data from Chadwick A: *Remembering Tuskegee: Syphilis study still provokes disbelief, sadness,* Washington, D.C., 2002 (July 25), National Public Radio. Accessed April 8, 2010, from www.npr.org/templates/story/story.php?storyId=1147234.

▍SUMMARY

The disorders of cancer and AIDS are characterized by wasting and malnutrition, caused by the effect of the disorders or the secondary consequences of treatment on the GI tract. Nutrition therapy focuses on identifying at-risk patients, preventing malnutrition, and reducing the effects of treatment. Local or systemic effects of the cancer combined with antineoplastic therapy place the patient with cancer at increased risk of developing malnutrition or cancer cachexia through a variety of mechanisms: anorexia, nausea, vomiting, mucositis, organ injury (toxicity), and learned food aversions. Nutrition support must be individualized and is an essential component of the total management of cancer. With the provision of adequate nutritional support, cancer patients may have a decreased risk of surgical complications. They will also

have the nutrients needed to rebuild normal tissues that have been affected by antineoplastic therapy and have an increased tolerance to therapies. Overall, quality of life is enhanced.

AIDS, caused by the retrovirus HIV, leads to the breakdown of the immune system, opportunistic infections, or enteropathy. Malnutrition, a common complication of HIV/AIDS, is multifactorial and includes decreased nutrient (food) intake, malabsorption, and altered metabolism. Goals of nutrition therapy are individualized, and interventions are based on nutritional status, causes of malnutrition, complications that affect nutritional status, and the ability to maintain health as long as possible. Early recognition and intervention for nutritional risk factors and indicators are keys to effective nutrition support and related medical therapies.

▍THE NURSING APPROACH

Case Study: Cancer and Chemotherapy

Sylvia, age 35, is visiting the nurse practitioner for a follow-up visit related to her breast cancer treatment. She has been receiving chemotherapy after a lumpectomy in the right breast and radiation therapy.

ASSESSMENT
Subjective (from patient statements)

- "I've been really sick from the chemo. It makes me feel nauseated all the time, and often I vomit right after the treatment."
- "It's hard to eat very much because my mouth is sore."
- "I'm too tired to do any cooking."

Objective (from physical examination)

- Height 5 feet 6 inches, weight 119 pounds
- Temperature 98.8° F
- Mouth inflamed, tongue appears red and raw; white raised patches on tongue and oral mucosa

DIAGNOSES (NURSING)

1. Risk for imbalanced nutrition: less than body requirements related to nausea, fatigue, and impaired oral mucous membranes
2. Risk for infection related to immunosuppression secondary to chemotherapy

THE NURSING APPROACH—cont'd

Case Study: Cancer and Chemotherapy—cont'd

PLANNING

Patient Outcomes

Short term (by end of this visit):

- Sylvia will describe ways she can increase her overall comfort and food intake.
- She will agree to get resources about coping with chemotherapy from American Cancer Society.

Long term (by follow-up visit in one month):

- Lesions in mouth will be diminished, and Sylvia will be able to eat with less discomfort.
- Sylvia will maintain or increase weight.
- No signs of infection

Nursing Interventions

1. Discuss measures to increase comfort and food intake.
2. Provide Sylvia with resources for information about cancer and chemotherapy.

IMPLEMENTATION

1. Recommended small, frequent meals rather than large meals.

   Small meals are usually easier to tolerate than large meals when the gastrointestinal system is altered. Antineoplastic medications kill cancer cells because they divide rapidly. However, chemotherapy also kills normal cells that divide rapidly, involving the gastrointestinal system, bone marrow, and hair. Commercial nutritional supplements should be consumed between meals rather than with meals, in order to reduce satiety at mealtime.

2. Discussed ways to reduce nausea and vomiting.

   It is best to avoid foods with strong odors. If that is not possible, staying out of the kitchen and having someone else do the cooking may reduce nausea. Room deodorizers also may be helpful. Fried foods are harder to digest, so they should be avoided or minimized.

3. Stressed the importance of eating a well-balanced diet, using nutrient-dense foods. Also suggested eating favorite foods and taking a vitamin supplement.

   A well-balanced diet, including high-protein and high-kcal foods, will provide nourishment and energy to fight cancer, better tolerate chemotherapy, promote healing, and prevent infection. Serving favorite foods may stimulate appetite.

4. Encouraged Sylvia to prioritize her activities and rest before meals.

   When energy is limited, an individual should do the most important activities first. When rested, a patient is more willing to expend energy to eat.

5. Encouraged Sylvia to ask for help with shopping and meal preparation.

   Family members, friends, or church groups may provide assistance so that energy can be conserved and healing can take place.

6. Discussed oral care and treatment for mouth sores.

   Stomatitis (inflammation of the mouth) is a common side effect of chemotherapy. Good oral care with a soft toothbrush and flossing will reduce infection and the likelihood of damage to the oral mucosa. Frequent mouthwashes with baking soda and water help sores heal by shifting the pH to a less acidic environment. Mouthwashes with alcohol should be avoided because they irritate the mucosa.

7. Ordered viscous lidocaine and Nystatin swish-and-swallow.

   Use of viscous lidocaine before eating may numb the sore mouth, decreasing discomfort and allowing the patient to eat. When immunosuppression is present, infection from Candida albicans (yeast infection, called thrush) often occurs; Nystatin swish-and-swallow may be prescribed for treatment.

8. Discussed bacterial precautions regarding food.

   Chemotherapy often causes a low white blood cell count, so hands must be washed thoroughly with soap and water before preparing food and before eating. Cutting boards for meats should be designated and kept separate from cutting boards for other foods.

   No raw fruits and vegetables should be consumed, and commercially bottled water is safer than tap water. Foods need to be well cooked and must be kept hot until eaten. Leftovers need refrigeration and should be eaten within 24 hours.

9. Wrote some suggestions for improving eating while she is receiving chemotherapy.

   When the patient has a sore mouth, provide soft, bland, cool, or lukewarm food and drinks. Avoid tart, salty, acidic (citrus fruits and tomatoes), spicy, coarse, dry, and scratchy foods. Also avoid caffeine, alcohol, and tobacco. Such foods could cause irritation of the mucous membranes, adding to the damage done by the chemotherapy.

10. Encouraged Sylvia to download patient information about Nutrition for the Person with Cancer, 2000, from the American Cancer Society at www.cancer.org.

    Specific information about nutrition before, during, and after treatment is provided free. Especially helpful is the section "When Treatment Causes Eating Problems." Education promotes empowerment.

EVALUATION

Short term (by the end of this visit):

- Sylvia committed to try methods designed to increase her comfort and food intake.
- She agreed to get resources from American Cancer Society.
- Goals met.

DISCUSSION QUESTIONS

At a follow-up visit in one month Sylvia said her mouth was feeling better and she was able to eat somewhat better. She said that she still had problems with nausea and no energy. Her weight was stable and she had no signs of infection. She said the information from American Cancer Society had been very helpful.

1. How could the nurse encourage Sylvia and help her to set some small, realistic goals?
2. What high-calorie and nutrient-dense foods would you recommend for Sylvia?

CRITICAL THINKING

Clinical Applications

Minnie, age 20, is a college student with an uneventful medical history with no significant illness. After finals, she came down with the flu and has felt run-down ever since. She has also had a persistent low-grade fever and cough since the flu. With much insistence by her parents, she went to see her doctor for a physical. She was admitted to the hospital after her chest radiograph indicated a possible malignancy. Following a bone marrow biopsy, chest computed tomography, magnetic resonance imaging, and biopsy of suspect lymph nodes, a diagnosis of non-Hodgkin's lymphoma with positive lymph nodes was made. Bone marrow, as well as other organs, indicated no presence of the disease. Minnie's physicians have determined a chemotherapy regimen using a combination of drugs to be given over 5 days every 4 weeks. Minnie complains of an overall lack of appetite, but she has no nausea, vomiting, constipation, or diarrhea. She is 5 feet 6 inches tall and weighs 120 pounds on admission. Her usual weight is 130 pounds.

1. What are the possible causes of her decreased appetite?
2. What side effects from her chemotherapy might she encounter?
3. How will this affect her nutritional status?

WEBSITES OF INTEREST

American Institute for Cancer Research

http://www.aicr.org

Offers excellent resources and reviews of research regarding nutrition and cancer prevention.

HIV/AIDS Dietetic Practice Group (of the American Dietetic Association)

http://www.hivaidsdpg.org

Provides excellent links for information on HIV/AIDS, caregivers, and organizations offering medical nutrition therapy and food outreach programs.

National Cancer Institute (NCI)

www.cancer.gov

Makes available CancerNet (a cancer data-base on treatment, screening, prevention, and clinical trials), cancerTrials (clinical trials information center), and CANCERLIT (a bibliographic database).

REFERENCES

1. Gould BE: *Pathophysiology for the health professions*, ed 3, St. Louis, 2006, Saunders.
2. American Cancer Society: *Cancer facts and figures 2008*, Atlanta, 2008, Author.
3. World Cancer Research Fund/American Institute for Cancer Research: *Policy and action for cancer prevention. Food, nutrition, and physical activity: a global perspective*, Washington, D.C., 2009, AICR. Accessed April 8, 2010, from www.dietandcancerreport.org.
4. Oncology Nutrition Dietetic Practice Group, Elliott L, et al: *The clinical guide to oncology nutrition*, ed 2, Chicago, 2006, American Dietetic Association.
5. McCallum PD, Polisena CG, editors: *Patient-generated subjective global assessment, training video*, Chicago, 2001, Oncology Nutrition Practice Group of the American Dietetic Association.
6. Grant B: Medical nutrition therapy for cancer. In Mahan LK, Escott-Stump S, editors: *Krause's food & nutrition therapy*, ed 12, Philadelphia, 2008, Saunders.
7. Bloch AS, Charuhas PM: Cancer and cancer therapy. In Gottschlich M, editor: *The science and practice of nutrition support*, Dubuque, Iowa, 2001, Kendall/Hunt.
8. American Society for Parenteral and Enteral Nutrition: Guidelines for the use of parenteral and enteral nutrition in adult and pediatric patients. *JPEN J Parenter Enteral Nutr* 26(Suppl 1):1SA-138SA, 2002.
9. Nahikian-Nelms ML: General feeding problems. In Bloch A, editor: *Nutrition management of the cancer patient*, Rockville, Md, 1990, Aspen.
10. Baileys K, Nahikian-Nelms ML: Lymphoma. In Kogut V, Luthringer SL, editors: *Nutritional issues in cancer care*, Pittsburgh, 2005, Oncology Nursing Society.
11. Wainberg MA: HIV-1 subtype distribution and the problem of drug resistance, *AIDS* 18(Suppl 3):S63-S68, 2004.
12. Centers for Disease Control and Prevention: *Human immunodeficiency virus type 2*, Atlanta, (reviewed July 21, 2006), Author. Accessed April 8, 2010, from www.cdc.gov/hiv/resources/factsheets/hiv2.htm.
13. UNAIDS and World Health Organization: *AIDS epidemic update: December 2005*, Geneva, 2005, Authors. Accessed April 8, 2010, from http://data.unaids.org/Publications/IRC-pub06/epi_update2005_en.pdf.
14. Centers for Disease Control and Prevention: *A glance at the HIV/AIDS epidemic*, Atlanta, 2006 (April), Author.
15. Dybul M, et al: Panel on Clinical Practices for Treatment of HIV. Guidelines for using antiretroviral agents among HIV-infected adults and adolescents, *Ann Intern Med* 137 (5 Pt 2):381-433, 2002.
16. Fenton M, Silverman E: Medical nutrition therapy for human immunodeficiency virus (HIV) disease. In Mahan LK, Escott-Stump S, editors: *Krause's food & nutrition therapy*, ed 12, Philadelphia, 2008, Saunders.

17. Tang AM, et al: Weight loss and survival in HIV-positive patients in the era of highly active antiretroviral therapy, *J Acquir Immune Defic Syndr* 31(2):230-236, 2002.

18. Batterham M, Brown D, Garsia R: Nutritional management of HIV/AIDS in the era of highly active antiretroviral therapy: A review, *Aust J Nutr Diet* 58:211-223, 2001.

19. Wanke C: Pathogenesis and consequences of HIV-associated wasting, *J Acquir Immune Defic Syndr* 37(Suppl 4):S277-S279, 2004.

20. Gerrior J, et al: The fat redistribution syndrome in patients infected with HIV: Measurements of body shape abnormalities, *J Am Diet Assoc* 101(10):1175-1180, 2001.

21. American Dietetic Association: Position of the American Dietetic Association and Dietitians of Canada: Nutrition intervention in the care of persons with human immunodeficiency virus infection, *J Am Diet Assoc* 104(9):1421-1425, 2004.

22. Grunfeld C, et al: Oxandrolone in the treatment of HIV-associated weight loss in men: A randomized, double-blind, placebo-controlled study, *J Acquir Immune Defic Syndr* 41(3):304-314, 2006.

23. Chen CC, Parker CR Jr: Adrenal androgens and the immune system, *Semin Reprod Med* 22(4):369-377, 2004.

24. Koutkia P, et al: Growth hormone secretion among HIV infected patients: Effects of gender, race and fat distribution, *AIDS* 20(6):855-862, 2006.

25. Mwamburi DM, et al: Combination megestrol acetate, oxandrolone, and dietary advice restores weight in human immunodeficiency virus, *Nutr Clin Pract* 19(4):395-402, 2004.

26. Rabkin JG, et al: Placebo-controlled trial of dehydro-epiandrosterone (DHEA) for treatment of nonmajor depression in patients with HIV/AIDS, *Am J Psychiatry* 163(1):59-66, 2006.

27. Heiser CR, et al: Probiotics, soluble fiber, and L-glutamine (GLN) reduce nelfinavir (NFV)- or lopinavir/ritonavir (LPV/r)-related diarrhea, *J Int Assoc Physicians AIDS Care* 3(4):121-129, 2004.

28. Fields-Gardner C, Salamon S, Davis M: *Living well with HIV and AIDS*, Chicago, 2003, American Dietetic Association.

29. Tang AM: Weight loss, wasting and survival in HIV-positive patients: Current strategies. *AIDS Read* 13(12 Suppl):S23-S27, 2003.

30. Frankenfield D, Roth-Yousey L, Compher C: Comparison of predictive equations for resting metabolic rate in healthy nonobese and obese adults: A systematic review, *J Am Diet Assoc* 105(5):775-789, 2005.

31. Detroyer MJ: Exercise recommendations for metabolic complications experienced with HIV/AIDS, *Positive Commun* 6:8, 2001.

32. Yarasheski KE, Roubenoff R: Exercise treatment for HIV-associated metabolic and anthropomorphic complications, *Exerc Sport Sci Rev* 29(4):170-174, 2001.

APPENDIXES

Exchange Lists for Meal Planning

Foods are listed with their serving sizes, which are usually measured after cooking. When you begin, measuring the size of each serving will help you learn to "eyeball" correct serving sizes.

The following chart shows the amount of nutrients in one serving from each list:

GROUPS/ LISTS	CARBOHY- DRATE (g)	PROTEIN (g)	FAT (g)	CALORIES
Carbohydrate Group				
Starch	15	3	0-1	80
Fruit	15	—	—	60
Milk				
Fat-free, low-fat	12	8	0-3	90
Reduced-fat	12	8	5	120
Whole	12	8	8	150
Other carbohy- drates	15	Varies	Varies	Varies
Nonstarchy vegetables	5	2	—	25
Meat and Meat Substitutes Group				
Very lean	—	7	0-1	35
Lean	—	7	3	55
Medium-fat	—	7	5	75
High-fat	—	7	8	100
Fat Group	—	—	5	45

Common Measurements

3 tsp = 1 tbsp   4 oz = ½ cup
4 tbsp = ¼ cup   8 oz = 1 cup
5⅓ tbsp = ⅓ cup   1 cup = ½ pint

STARCH LIST

Cereals, grains, pasta, breads, crackers, snacks, starchy vegetables, and cooked beans, peas, and lentils are starches. In general, 1 starch is as follows:

• ½ cup of cooked cereal, grain, or starchy vegetable
• ⅓ cup of cooked rice or pasta

• 1 oz of a bread product, such as 1 slice of bread
• ¾ to 1 oz of most snack foods (some snack foods may also have added fat)

Nutrition Tips

1. Most starch choices are good sources of B vitamins.
2. Foods made from whole grains are good sources of fiber.
   • A serving from the Bread list, on average, has 1 g of fiber.
   • A serving from the Cereals and Grains list or the Crackers and Snacks list, on average, has 2 g of fiber.
   • A serving from the Starchy Vegetables list, on average, has 3 g of fiber.
3. Beans, peas, and lentils are good sources of protein and fiber.
   • A serving from this group, on average, has 6 g of fiber.

Selection Tips

1. Choose starches made with little fat as often as you can.
2. Starchy vegetables prepared with fat count as one starch and one fat.
3. For many starchy foods (e.g., bagels, muffins, dinner rolls, buns), a general rule of thumb is 1 oz equals one carbohydrate serving. However, bagels or muffins range widely in size. Check the size you eat. Also, use the Nutrition Facts on food labels when available.
4. Beans, peas, and lentils are also found on the Meat and Meat Substitutes list.
5. A waffle or pancake is about the size of a compact disc (CD) and about ¼ inch thick.
6. Because starches often swell in cooking, a small amount of uncooked starch becomes a much larger amount of cooked food.
7. Most of the serving sizes are measured or weighed after cooking.
8. For specific information, check Nutrition Facts on food labels.

One starch exchange equals 15 g carbohydrate, 3 g protein, 0 to 1 g fat, and 80 kcal.

Bread

Bagel, 4 oz	¼ (1 oz)
Bread, reduced-calorie	2 slices (1½ oz)
Bread, white, whole wheat, pumpernickel, rye	1 slice (1 oz)
Bread sticks, crisp, 4 inches × ½ inch	4 (⅔ oz)
English muffin	½
Hot dog or hamburger bun	½ (1 oz)
Naan, 8 × 2 inches	¼
Pancake, 4 inches across, ¼ inch thick	1
Pita, 6 inches across	½
Roll, plain, small	1 (1 oz)
Raisin bread, unfrosted	1 slice (1 oz)
Tortilla, corn, 6 inches across	1
Tortilla, flour, 6 inches across	1
Tortilla, flour, 10 inches across	⅓
Waffle 4½ inches square or across, reduced-fat	1

Cereals and Grains

Bran cereals	½ cup
Bulgur	½ cup
Cereals, cooked	½ cup
Cereals, unsweetened, ready-to-eat	¾ cup
Cornmeal (dry)	3 tbsp
Couscous	⅓ cup
Flour (dry)	3 tbsp
Granola, low-fat	¼ cup
Grape-Nuts	¼ cup
Grits	½ cup
Kasha	½ cup
Millet	⅓ cup
Muesli	¼ cup
Oats	½ cup
Pasta	⅓ cup
Puffed cereal	1½ cups
Rice, white or brown	⅓ cup
Shredded Wheat	½ cup
Sugar-frosted cereal	½ cup
Wheat germ	3 tbsp

Starchy Vegetables

Baked beans	⅓ cup
Corn	½ cup
Corn on the cob, large	½ cob (5 oz)
Mixed vegetables with corn, peas, or pasta	1 cup
Peas, green	½ cup
Plantain	½ cup
Potato, baked with skin	¼ large (3 oz)
Potato, boiled	½ cup or ½ medium (3 oz)
Potato, mashed	½ cup
Squash, winter (acorn, butternut, pumpkin)	1 cup
Yam, sweet potato, plain	½ cup

Crackers and Snacks

Animal crackers	8
Graham crackers, 2½-inch square	3
Matzoh	¾ oz
Melba toast	4 slices
Oyster crackers	24
Popcorn (popped, no fat added, or low-fat microwave)	3 cups
Pretzels	¾ oz
Rice cakes, 4 inches across	2
Saltine-type crackers	6
Snack chips, fat-free or baked (tortilla, potato)	15-20 (¾ oz)
Whole-wheat crackers, no fat added	2-5 (¾ oz)

Beans, Peas, and Lentils (count as 1 starch exchange plus 1 very lean meat exchange)

Beans and peas (garbanzo, pinto, kidney, white, split, black-eyed)	½ cup
Lima beans	⅔ cup
Lentils	½ cup
Miso 🥄	3 tbsp

Starchy Foods Prepared With Fat

(count as 1 starch exchange, plus 1 fat exchange)

Biscuit, 2½ inches across	1
Chow mein noodles	½ cup
Corn bread, 2-inch cube	1 (2 oz)
Crackers, round butter-type	6
Croutons	1 cup
French-fried potatoes, oven-baked (see also the Fast Foods list)	1 cup (2 oz)
Granola	¼ cup
Hummus	⅓ cup
Muffin, 5 oz	⅕ (1 oz)
Popcorn, microwaved	3 cups
Sandwich crackers, cheese or peanut butter filling	3
Snack chips (potato, tortilla)	9-13 (¾ oz)
Stuffing, bread (prepared)	⅓ cup
Taco shell, 6 inches across	2
Waffle, 4 inches square or across	1
Whole-wheat crackers, fat added	4-6 (1 oz)

FRUIT LIST

Fresh, frozen, canned, and dried fruits and fruit juices are on this list. In general, 1 fruit exchange is as follows:

- 1 small fresh fruit (4 oz)
- ½ cup of canned or fresh fruit or unsweetened fruit juice
- ¼ cup of dried fruit

Nutrition Tips

1. Fresh, frozen, and dried fruits have about 2 g of fiber per choice. Fruit juices contain very little fiber.
2. Citrus fruits, berries, and melons are good sources of vitamin C.

Selection Tips

1. Count ½ cup cranberries or rhubarb sweetened with sugar substitutes as free foods.
2. Read the Nutrition Facts on the food label. If 1 serving has more than 15 g of carbohydrate, you will need to adjust the size of the serving you eat or drink.
3. Portion sizes for canned fruits are for the fruit and a small amount of juice.
4. Whole fruit is more filling than fruit juice and may be a better choice.
5. Food labels for fruits may contain the words *no sugar added* or *unsweetened*. This means that no sucrose (table sugar) has been added.
6. Generally, fruit canned in extra-light syrup has the same amount of carbohydrate per serving as the *no sugar added* or the *juice pack*. All canned fruits on the fruit list are based on one of these three types of packaging.

One fruit exchange equals 15 g carbohydrate and 60 kcal. The weight includes skin, core, seeds, and rind.

Fruit

Apple, unpeeled, small	1 (4 oz)
Applesauce, unsweetened	½ cup
Apples, dried	4 rings
Apricots, fresh	4 whole (5½ oz)
Apricots, dried	8 halves
Apricots, canned	½ cup
Banana, small	1 (4 oz)
Blackberries	¾ cup
Blueberries	¾ cup
Cantaloupe, small	⅓ melon (11 oz) or 1 cup cubes
Cherries, sweet, fresh	12 (3 oz)
Cherries, sweet, canned	½ cup
Dates	3

Figs, fresh	3½ large or 2 medium (3½ oz)
Figs, dried	1½
Fruit cocktail	½ cup
Grapefruit, large	½ (11 oz)
Grapefruit sections, canned	¾ cup
Grapes, small	17 (3 oz)
Honeydew melon	1 slice (10 oz) or 1 cup cubes
Kiwifruit	1 (3½ oz)
Mandarin oranges, canned	¾ cup
Mango, small	½ fruit (5½ oz) or ½ cup
Nectarine, small	1 (5 oz)
Orange, small	1 (6½ oz)
Papaya	½ fruit (8 oz) or 1 cup cubes
Peach, medium, fresh	1 (4 oz)
Peaches, canned	½ cup
Pear, large, fresh	½ (4 oz)
Pears, canned	½ cup
Pineapple, fresh	¾ cup
Pineapple, canned	½ cup
Plums, small	2 (5 oz)
Plums, canned	½ cup
Plums, dried (prunes)	3
Raisins	2 tbsp
Raspberries	1 cup
Strawberries	1¼ cups whole berries
Tangerines, small	2 (8 oz)
Watermelon	1 slice (13½ oz) or 1¼ cups cubes

Fruit Juice, Unsweetened

Apple juice/cider	½ cup
Cranberry juice cocktail	⅓ cup
Cranberry juice cocktail, reduced-calorie	1 cup
Fruit juice blends, 100% juice	⅓ cup
Grape juice	⅓ cup
Grapefruit juice	½ cup
Orange juice	½ cup
Pineapple juice	½ cup
Prune juice	⅓ cup

MILK LIST

Different types of milk and milk products are on this list. Cheeses are on the Meat and Meat Substitutes list, and cream and other dairy fats are on the Fat list. Based on the amount of fat they contain, milks are divided into fat-free/low-fat milk, reduced-fat milk, and whole milk. One choice of these includes the following:

TYPE OF MILK	CARBOHYDRATE (g)	PROTEIN (g)	FAT (g)	CALORIES
Fat-free/ low-fat ($\frac{1}{2}$% or 1%)	12	8	0-3	90
Reduced-fat (2%)	12	8	5	120
Whole	12	8	8	150

Nutrition Tips

1. Milk and yogurt are good sources of calcium and protein. Check the Nutrition Facts on the food label.
2. The higher the fat content of milk and yogurt, the greater the amount of saturated fat and cholesterol. Choose lower-fat varieties.
3. For those who are lactose intolerant, look for lactose-reduced or lactose-free varieties of milk. Check the food label for total amount of carbohydrate per serving.

Selection Tips

1. 1 cup equals 8 fluid oz or $\frac{1}{2}$ pint.
2. Look for chocolate milk, rice milk, frozen yogurt, and ice cream on the Sweets, Desserts, and Other Carbohydrates list.
3. Nondairy creamers are on the Free Foods list.
One milk exchange equals 12 g carbohydrate and 8 g protein.

Fat-Free and Low-Fat Milk

(0-3 g fat/serving)
Fat-free milk	1 cup
$\frac{1}{2}$% milk	1 cup
1% milk	1 cup
Buttermilk, low-fat or fat-free	1 cup
Evaporated fat-free milk	$\frac{1}{2}$ cup
Fat-free dry milk	$\frac{1}{3}$ cup dry
Soy milk, low-fat or fat-free	1 cup
Yogurt, fat-free, flavored, sweetened with nonnutritive sweetener and fructose	$\frac{2}{3}$ cup (6 oz)
Yogurt, plain, fat-free	$\frac{2}{3}$ cup (6 oz)

Reduced-Fat

(5 g fat/serving)
2% milk	1 cup
Soy milk	1 cup

Sweet acidophilus milk	1 cup
Yogurt, plain, low-fat	$\frac{3}{4}$ cup

Whole Milk

(8 g fat/serving)
Whole milk	1 cup
Evaporated whole milk	$\frac{1}{2}$ cup
Goat's milk	1 cup
Kefir	1 cup
Yogurt, plain (made from whole milk)	$\frac{3}{4}$ cup

SWEETS, DESSERTS, AND OTHER CARBOHYDRATES LIST

You can substitute food choices from this list for a starch, fruit, or milk choice on your meal plan. Some choices will also count as one or more fat choices.

Nutrition Tips

1. These foods can be substituted for other carbohydrate-containing foods in your meal plan even though they contain added sugars or fat. However, they do not contain as many important vitamins and minerals as the choices on the Starch, Fruit, and Milk lists.
2. When choosing these foods, include foods from the other lists to eat balanced meals.

Selection Tips

1. Because many of these foods are concentrated sources of carbohydrate and fat, saturated fat, and trans fat, the portion sizes are often very small.
2. Look for the words *hydrogenated* or *partially hydrogenated* on the ingredients label. The lower down on the list these words appear, the fewer trans fats there are.
3. Be sure to check the Nutrition Facts on the food label. It is your most accurate source of information.
4. Many fat-free or reduced-fat products made with fat replacers contain carbohydrate. When eaten in large amounts, they may need to be counted. Talk with your dietitian to determine how to count these in your meal plan.
5. Look for fat-free salad dressings in smaller amounts on the Free Foods list.
One carbohydrate exchange equals 15 g carbohydrate, or 1 starch, or 1 fruit, or 1milk.

FOOD	SERVING SIZE	EXCHANGES PER SERVING
Angel food cake, unfrosted	$\frac{1}{12}$ cake (about 2 oz)	2 carbohydrates
Brownie, small, unfrosted	2-inch square (about 1 oz)	1 carbohydrate, 1 fat
Cake, unfrosted	2-inch square (about 1 oz)	1 carbohydrate, 1 fat
Cake, frosted	2-inch square (about 2 oz)	2 carbohydrates, 1 fat
Cookie or sandwich cookie with cream filling	2 small (about $\frac{2}{3}$ oz)	1 carbohydrate, 1 fat
Cookies, sugar-free	3 small or 1 large ($\frac{3}{4}$-1 oz)	1 carbohydrate, 1-2 fats
Cranberry sauce, jellied	$\frac{1}{4}$ cup	1$\frac{1}{2}$ carbohydrates
Cupcake, frosted	1 small (about 2 oz)	2 carbohydrates, 1 fat
Doughnut, plain cake	1 medium (1$\frac{1}{2}$ oz)	1$\frac{1}{2}$ carbohydrates, 2 fats
Doughnut, glazed	3$\frac{3}{4}$ inches across (2 oz)	2 carbohydrates, 2 fats
Energy, sport, or breakfast bar	1 bar (1$\frac{1}{3}$ oz)	1$\frac{1}{2}$ carbohydrates, 0-1 fat
Energy, sport, or breakfast bar	1 bar (2 oz)	2 carbohydrates, 1 fat
Fruit cobbler	$\frac{1}{2}$ cup (3$\frac{1}{2}$ oz)	3 carbohydrates, 1 fat
Fruit juice bars, frozen, 100% juice	1 bar (3 oz)	1 carbohydrate
Fruit snacks, chewy (pureed fruit concentrate)	1 roll ($\frac{3}{4}$ oz)	1 carbohydrate
Fruit spreads, 100% fruit	1$\frac{1}{2}$ tbsp	1 carbohydrate
Gelatin, regular	$\frac{1}{2}$ cup	1 carbohydrate
Gingersnaps	3	1 carbohydrate
Granola or snack bar, regular or low-fat	1 bar (1 oz)	1$\frac{1}{2}$ carbohydrates
Honey	1 tbsp	1 carbohydrate
Ice cream	$\frac{1}{2}$ cup	1 carbohydrate, 2 fats
Ice cream, light	$\frac{1}{2}$ cup	1 carbohydrate, 1 fat
Ice cream, low-fat	$\frac{1}{2}$ cup	1$\frac{1}{2}$ carbohydrates
Ice cream, fat-free, no sugar added	$\frac{1}{2}$ cup	1 carbohydrate
Jam or jelly, regular	1 tbsp	1 carbohydrate
Milk, chocolate, whole	1 cup	2 carbohydrates, 1 fat
Pie, fruit, 2 crusts	$\frac{1}{6}$ of 8-inch commercially prepared pie	3 carbohydrates, 2 fats
Pie, pumpkin or custard	$\frac{1}{8}$ of 8-inch commercially prepared pie	2 carbohydrates, 2 fats
Pudding, regular (made with reduced-fat milk)	$\frac{1}{2}$ cup	2 carbohydrates
Pudding, sugar-free or sugar free and fat-free (made with fat-free milk)	$\frac{1}{2}$ cup	1 carbohydrate
Reduced-calorie meal replacement (shake)	1 can (10-11 oz)	1$\frac{1}{2}$ carbohydrates, 0-1 fat
Rice milk, low-fat or fat-free, plain	1 cup	1 carbohydrate
Rice milk, low-fat, flavored	1 cup	1$\frac{1}{2}$ carbohydrates
Salad dressing, fat-free 🖋	$\frac{1}{4}$ cup	1 carbohydrate
Sherbet, sorbet	$\frac{1}{2}$ cup	2 carbohydrates
Spaghetti sauce or pasta sauce, canned 🖋	$\frac{1}{2}$ cup	1 carbohydrate, 1 fat
Sports drinks	8 oz (1 cup)	1 carbohydrate
Sugar	1 tbsp	1 carbohydrate
Sweet roll or Danish	1 (2$\frac{1}{2}$ oz)	2$\frac{1}{2}$ carbohydrates, 2 fats
Syrup, light	2 tbsp	1 carbohydrate
Syrup, regular	1 tbsp	1 carbohydrate
Syrup, regular	$\frac{1}{4}$ cup	4 carbohydrates
Vanilla wafers	5	1 carbohydrate, 1 fat
Yogurt, frozen	$\frac{1}{2}$ cup	1 carbohydrate, 0-1 fat
Yogurt, frozen, fat-free	$\frac{1}{3}$ cup	1 carbohydrate
Yogurt, low-fat with fruit	1 cup	3 carbohydrates, 0-1 fat

NONSTARCHY VEGETABLE LIST

Vegetables that contain small amounts of carbohydrate and calories are on this list. Vegetables contain important nutrients. Try to eat at least 2 or 3 vegetable choices each day. In general, one vegetable exchange is as follows:
- ½ cup of cooked vegetables or vegetable juice
- 1 cup of raw vegetables

If you eat 3 cups or more of raw vegetables or 1½ cups of cooked vegetables at one meal, count them as 1 carbohydrate choice.

Nutrition Tips

1. Fresh and frozen vegetables have less added salt than canned vegetables. Drain and rinse canned vegetables if you want to remove some salt.
2. Choose more dark green and dark yellow vegetables, such as spinach, broccoli, romaine, carrots, chilies, and peppers.
3. Broccoli, Brussels sprouts, cauliflower, greens, peppers, spinach, and tomatoes are good sources of vitamin C.
4. Vegetables contain 1 to 4 g of fiber per serving.

Selection Tips

1. A 1-cup portion of broccoli is about the size of a light bulb.
2. Tomato sauce is different from spaghetti sauce, which is on the Sweets, Desserts, and Other Carbohydrates list.
3. Canned vegetables and juices are available without added salt.
4. Starchy vegetables such as corn, peas, winter squash, and potatoes that contain larger amounts of calories and carbohydrates are on the Starch list.

One vegetable exchange (½ cup cooked or 1 cup raw) equals 5 g carbohydrate, 2 g protein, 0 g fat, and 25 kcal.

Foods

Artichoke
Artichoke hearts
Asparagus
Bean sprouts
Beans (green, wax, Italian)
Beets
Broccoli
Brussels sprouts
Cabbage
Carrots
Cauliflower
Celery
Cucumber
Eggplant
Green onions or scallions
Greens (collard, kale, mustard, turnip)
Kohlrabi
Leeks
Mixed vegetables (without corn, peas, or pasta)
Mushrooms
Okra
Onions
Pea pods
Peppers (all varieties)
Radishes
Salad greens (endive, escarole, lettuce, romaine, spinach)
Sauerkraut 🧂
Spinach
Summer squash
Tomato
Tomato sauce 🧂
Tomato/vegetable juice 🧂
Tomatoes, canned
Turnips
Water chestnuts
Watercress
Zucchini

MEAT AND MEAT SUBSTITUTES LIST

Meat and meat substitutes that contain both protein and fat are on this list. In general, one meat exchange is as follows:
- 1 oz of meat, fish, poultry, or cheese
- ½ cup of beans, peas, or lentils

Based on the amount of fat they contain, meats are divided into very lean, lean, medium-fat, and high-fat lists. This is done so that you can see which ones contain the least amount of fat. One ounce (one exchange) of each of these includes the following:

TYPE OF MEAT	CARBOHYDRATE (g)	PROTEIN (g)	FAT (g)	CALORIES
Very lean	0	7	0-1	35
Lean	0	7	3	55
Medium-fat	0	7	5	75
High-fat	0	7	8	100

Nutrition Tips

1. Choose very lean and lean meat choices whenever possible. Items from the high-fat group are high in saturated fat, cholesterol, and calories and can raise blood cholesterol levels.
2. Beans, peas, and lentils are good sources of fiber, about 3 g per serving.

🧂 = 400 mg or more of sodium per exchange.

3. Some processed meats, seafood, and soy products may contain carbohydrate when consumed in large amounts. Check the Nutrition Facts on the label to see if the amount is close to 15 g. If so, count it as a carbohydrate choice as well as a meat choice.

Selection Tips

1. Weigh meat after cooking and removing bones and fat; 4 oz of raw meat is equal to 3 oz of cooked meat. Some examples of meat portions are as follows:
   - 1 oz cheese = 1 meat choice and is about the size of a 1-inch cube or 4 cubes the size of dice
   - 2 oz meat = 2 meat choices, such as the following:
     - 1 small chicken leg or thigh
     - ½ cup cottage cheese or tuna
   - 3 oz meat = 3 meat choices and is about the size of a deck of cards, such as the following:
     - 1 medium pork chop
     - 1 small hamburger
     - ½ of a whole chicken breast
     - 1 unbreaded fish fillet
2. Limit your choices from the high-fat group to three times per week or less.
3. Most grocery stores stock Select and Choice grades of meat. The Select grades of meat are the leanest. The Choice grades contain a moderate amount of fat, and Prime cuts of meat have the highest amount of fat.
4. Hamburger may contain added seasoning and fat, but ground beef does not.
5. Read labels to find products that are low in fat and cholesterol (5 g of fat or less per serving).
6. Dried beans, peas, and lentils are also found on the Starch list.
7. Peanut butter, in smaller amounts, is also found on the Fat list.
8. Bacon, in smaller amounts, is also found on the Fat list.
9. Don't be fooled by ground beef packages that say X% lean (e.g., 90% lean). This is the percentage of fat by weight, NOT the percentage of calories from fat. A 3.5-oz patty of this raw ground beef has about half its calories from fat.
10. Meatless burgers are in the Combination Foods list (3 oz of soy-based burger = ½ carbohydrate + 2 very lean meats; 3 oz of carbohydrate vegetable- and starch-based burger = 1 carbohydrate + 1 lean meat).

One exchange equals 0 g carbohydrate, 7 g protein, 0 to 1 g fat, and 35 kcal.

Meal Planning Tips

1. Bake, roast, broil, grill, poach, steam, or boil meat and fish rather than frying.

2. Place meat on a rack so that the fat will drain off during cooking.
3. Use a nonstick spray and a nonstick pan to brown or fry foods.
4. Trim off visible fat or skin before or after cooking.
5. If you add flour, bread crumbs, coating mixes, fat, or marinades when cooking, ask your dietitian how to count it in your meal plan.

One exchange equals 0 g carbohydrate, 7 g protein, 3 g fat, and 55 kcal.

Very Lean Meat and Substitutes List

One very lean meat exchange is equal to any one of the following items:

Poultry: Chicken or turkey (white meat, no skin), Cornish hen (no skin) — 1 oz

Fish: Fresh or frozen cod, flounder, haddock, halibut, trout, lox (smoked salmon); 🧂 tuna, fresh or canned in water — 1 oz

Shellfish: Clams, crab, lobster, scallops, shrimp, imitation shellfish — 1 oz

Game: Duck or pheasant (no skin), venison, buffalo, ostrich — 1 oz

Cheese with 1 g of fat or less per ounce:
Fat-free or low-fat cottage cheese — ¼ cup
Fat-free cheese — 1 oz

Other
Processed sandwich meats with 1 g of fat or less per ounce, such as deli thin, shaved meats, chipped beef, 🧂 turkey ham — 1 oz
Egg whites — 2
Egg substitutes, plain — ¼ cup
Hot dogs with 1 g of fat or less per ounce 🧂 — 1 oz
Kidney (high in cholesterol) — 1 oz
Sausage with 1 g of fat or less per ounce — 1 oz

Count the following items as one very lean meat and one starch exchange:
Beans, peas, lentils (cooked) — ½ cup

Lean Meat and Substitutes List

One lean meat exchange is equal to any one of the following items:

Beef: USDA Select or Choice grades of lean beef trimmed of fat, such as round, sirloin, and flank steak; tenderloin; roast (rib, chuck, rump); steak (T-bone, Porterhouse, cubed); ground round — 1 oz

Pork: Lean pork, such as fresh ham; canned, cured, or boiled ham; Canadian bacon; 🧂 tenderloin, center loin chop — 1 oz

Lamb: Roast, chop, or leg — 1 oz

Veal: Lean chop, roast   1 oz
Poultry: Chicken, turkey (dark meat, no skin),   1 oz
   chicken (white meat, with skin), domestic
   duck or goose (well-drained of fat, no skin)
Fish
   Herring (uncreamed or smoked)   1 oz
   Oysters   6 medium
   Salmon (fresh or canned), catfish   1 oz
   Sardines (canned)   2 medium
   Tuna (canned in oil, drained)   1 oz
Game: Goose (no skin), rabbit   1 oz
Cheese:
   4.5%-fat cottage cheese   ¼ cup
   Grated Parmesan   2 tbsp
   Cheeses with 3 g of fat or less per ounce   *1 oz*
Other
   Hot dogs with 3 g of fat or less per ounce 🖌   1½ oz
   Processed sandwich meat with 3 g of fat or   1 oz
      less per ounce, such as turkey pastrami or
      kielbasa
   Liver, heart (high in cholesterol)   1 oz
One exchange equals 0 g carbohydrate, 7 g protein, 5 g fat, and 75 kcal.

Medium-Fat Meat and Substitutes List

One medium-fat meat exchange is equal to any one of the following items:
Beef: Most beef products fall into this category   1 oz
   (ground beef, meat loaf, corned beef, short
   ribs, Prime grades of meat trimmed of fat,
   such as prime rib)
Pork: Top loin, chop, Boston butt, cutlet   1 oz
Lamb: Rib roast, ground   1 oz
Veal: Cutlet (ground or cubed, unbreaded)   1 oz
Poultry: Chicken (dark meat, with skin),   1 oz
   ground turkey or ground chicken, fried
   chicken (with skin)
Fish: Any fried fish product   1 oz
Cheese with 5 g of fat or less per ounce
   Feta   1 oz
   Mozzarella   1 oz
   Ricotta   ¼ cup (2 oz)
Other
   Egg (high in cholesterol, limit to 3 per week)   1
   Sausage with 5 g of fat or less per ounce   1 oz
   Tempeh   ¼ cup
   Tofu   4 oz or ½ cup
One exchange equals 0 g carbohydrate, 7 g protein, 8 g fat, and 100 kcal.

High-Fat Meat and Substitutes List

Remember that these items are high in saturated fat, cholesterol, and calories and may raise blood cholesterol levels if eaten on a regular basis.

   One high-fat meat exchange is equal to any one of the following items:
Pork: Spareribs, ground pork, pork sausage   1 oz
Cheese: All regular cheeses, such as   1 oz
   American, 🖌 cheddar, Monterey Jack,
   Swiss
Other
   Processed sandwich meats with 8 g of fat   1 oz
      or less per ounce, such as bologna,
      pimento loaf, salami
   Sausage, such as bratwurst, Italian,   1 oz
      knockwurst, Polish, smoked
   Hot dog (turkey or chicken) 🖌   1 (10/lb)
   Bacon   3 slices
       (20 slices/lb)
   Peanut butter (contains unsaturated fat)   1 tbsp
Count the following items as 1 high-fat plus 1 fat exchange:
   Hot dog (beef, pork, or combination) 🖌   1 (10/lb)

FAT LIST

Fats are divided into three groups, based on the main type of fat they contain: monounsaturated, polyunsaturated, and saturated. Monounsaturated and polyunsaturated fats in the foods we eat are linked with good health benefits. Saturated fats and fats called trans fatty acids (or trans unsaturated fatty acids) are linked with heart disease. In general, one fat exchange is as follows:

- 1 tsp of regular margarine or vegetable oil
- 1 tbsp of regular salad dressing

Nutrition Tips

1. All fats are high in calories. Limit serving sizes for good nutrition and health.
2. Nuts and seeds contain small amounts of fiber, protein, and magnesium.
3. If blood pressure is a concern, choose fats in the unsalted form to help lower sodium intake, such as unsalted peanuts.

Selection Tips

1. Check the Nutrition Facts on food labels for serving sizes. One fat exchange is based on a serving size containing 5 g of fat.

---

2. The Nutrition Facts on food labels usually list total fat grams and saturated fat grams per serving. When most of the calories come from saturated fat, the food fits into the Saturated Fats list.

3. Occasionally the Nutrition Facts on food labels list monounsaturated and/or polyunsaturated fats in addition to total and saturated fats. If more than half the total fat is monounsaturated, the food fits into the Monounsaturated Fats list; if more than half is polyunsaturated, the food fits into the Polyunsaturated Fats list.

4. When selecting fats to use with your meal plan, consider replacing saturated fats with monounsaturated fats.

5. When selecting regular margarine, choose those with liquid vegetable oil as the first ingredient. Soft margarines are not as saturated as stick margarines and are healthier choices.

6. Avoid foods on the Fat list (such as margarines) listing hydrogenated or partially hydrogenated fat as the first ingredient because these foods contain higher amounts of trans fatty acids.

7. When selecting reduced- or lower-fat margarines, look for liquid vegetable oil as the second ingredient. Water is usually the first ingredient.

8. When used in smaller amounts, bacon and peanut butter are counted as fat choices. When used in larger amounts, they are counted as high-fat meat choices.

9. Fat-free salad dressings are on the Sweets, Desserts, and Other Carbohydrates list and the Free Foods list.

10. See the Free Foods list for nondairy coffee creamers, whipped topping, and fat-free products, such as margarines, salad dressings, mayonnaise, sour cream, cream cheese, and nonstick cooking spray.

One fat exchange equals 5 g fat and 45 kcal.

Monounsaturated Fats List

Avocado, medium	2 tbsp (1 oz)
Oil (canola, olive, peanut)	1 tsp
Olives	
Ripe (black)	8 large
Green, stuffed 🖋	10 large
Nuts	
Almonds, cashews	6 nuts
Mixed (50% peanuts)	6 nuts
Peanut butter, smooth or crunchy	½ tbsp
Peanuts	10 nuts
Pecans	4 halves
Sesame seeds	1 tbsp
Tahini or sesame paste	2 tsp

Polyunsaturated Fats List

Margarine	
Stick, tub, or squeeze	1 tsp
Lower-fat spread (30%-50% vegetable oil)	1 tbsp
Mayonnaise	
Regular	1 tsp
Reduced-fat	1 tbsp
Nuts: walnuts, English	4 halves
Oil (corn, safflower, soybean)	1 tsp
Salad dressing	
Regular 🖋	1 tbsp
Reduced-fat	2 tbsp
Miracle Whip salad dressing	
Regular	2 tsp
Reduced-fat	1 tbsp
Seeds: pumpkin, sunflower	1 tbsp

Saturated Fats List

Bacon, cooked	1 slice (20 slices/lb)
Bacon, grease	1 tsp
Butter	
Stick	1 tsp
Whipped	2 tsp
Reduced-fat	1 tbsp
Chitterlings, boiled	2 tbsp (½ oz)
Coconut, sweetened, shredded	2 tbsp
Coconut milk	1 tbsp
Cream, half and half	2 tbsp
Cream cheese	
Regular	1 tbsp (½ oz)
Reduced-fat	1½ tbsp (1½ oz)
Fatback or salt pork 🖋	See below*
Shortening or lard	1 tsp
Sour cream	
Regular	2 tbsp
Reduced-fat	3 tbsp

*Use a piece 1 inch × 1 inch × ¼ inch if you plan to eat the fatback cooked with vegetables. Use a piece 2 inches × 1 inch × ½ inch when eating only the vegetables with the fatback removed.

FREE FOODS LIST

A *free food* is any food or drink that contains fewer than 20 calories or less than or equal to 5 g of carbohydrate per serving. Foods with a serving size listed should be limited to 3 servings per day. Be sure to spread them out throughout the day. If you eat all 3 servings at one time, it could raise your blood glucose level. Foods listed without a serving size can be eaten whenever you like.

Fat-Free or Reduced-Fat Foods

Cream cheese, fat-free	1 tbsp (½ oz)
Creamers, nondairy, liquid	1 tbsp
Creamers, nondairy, powdered	2 tsp
Margarine spread, fat-free	4 tbsp
Margarine spread, reduced-fat	1 tsp
Mayonnaise, fat-free	1 tbsp
Mayonnaise, reduced-fat	1 tsp
Miracle Whip, fat-free	1 tbsp
Miracle Whip, reduced-fat	1 tsp
Nonstick cooking spray	
Salad dressing, fat-free or low-fat	1 tbsp
Salad dressing, fat-free, Italian	2 tbsp
Sour cream, fat-free, reduced-fat	1 tbsp
Whipped topping, regular	1 tbsp
Whipped topping, light or fat-free	2 tbsp

Sugar-Free Foods

Candy, hard, sugar-free	1 candy
Gelatin dessert, sugar-free	
Gelatin, unflavored	
Gum, sugar-free	
Jam or jelly, light	2 tsp
Sugar substitutes*	
Syrup, sugar-free	2 tbsp

---

*Sugar substitutes, alternatives, or replacements that are approved by the U.S. Food and Drug Administration (FDA) are safe to use. Common brand names include the following:
Equal (aspartame)
Splenda (sucralose)
Sprinkle Sweet (saccharin)
Sweet One (acesulfame K)
Sweet-10 (saccharin)
Sugar Twin (saccharin)
Sweet 'N Low (saccharin)

Drinks

Bouillon, broth, consommé ✎
Bouillon or broth, low-sodium
Carbonated or mineral water
Club soda

Cocoa powder, unsweetened	1 tbsp
Coffee	
Diet soft drinks, sugar-free	
Drink mixes, sugar-free	
Tea	
Tonic water, sugar-free	

Condiments

Catsup	1 tbsp
Horseradish	
Lemon juice	
Lime juice	
Mustard	
Pickle relish	1 tbsp
Pickles, dill ✎	1½ medium
Pickles, sweet (bread and butter)	2 slices
Pickles, sweet (gherkin)	¾ oz
Salsa	¼ cup
Soy sauce, regular or light ✎	1 tbsp
Taco sauce	1 tbsp
Vinegar	
Yogurt	2 tbsp

Seasonings

Flavoring extracts
Garlic
Herbs, fresh or dried
Pimiento
Spices
Tabasco or hot pepper sauce
Wine, used in cooking
Worcestershire sauce
Be careful with seasonings that contain sodium or are salts, such as garlic or celery salt, and lemon pepper.

COMBINATION FOODS LIST

Many of the foods we eat are mixed together in various combinations that do not fit into any one Exchange List. Often it is hard to tell what is in a casserole dish or prepared food item. This list of exchanges for some typical combination foods helps you fit these foods into your meal plan. Ask your dietitian for information about any other combination foods you would like to eat.

FOOD	SERVING SIZE	EXCHANGES PER SERVING
Entrées		
Tuna noodle casserole, lasagna, spaghetti with meatballs, chili with beans, macaroni and cheese 🖌	1 cup (8 oz)	2 carbohydrates 2 medium-fat meats
Chow mein (without noodles or rice) 🖌	2 cups (16 oz)	1 carbohydrate 2 lean meats
Tuna or chicken salad	½ cup (3 ½ oz)	½ carbohydrate 2 lean meats 1 fat
Frozen Entrées and Meals		
Dinner-type meal 🖌	Generally 14-17 oz	3 carbohydrates 3 medium-fat meats 3 fats
Meatless burger, soy-based	3 oz	½ carbohydrate 2 lean meats
Meatless burger, vegetable- and starch-based	3 oz	1 carbohydrate 1 lean meat
Pizza, cheese, thin crust 🖌	¼ of 12-inch (6 oz)	2 carbohydrates 2 medium-fat meats 1 fat
Pizza, meat topping, thin crust 🖌	¼ of 12-inch (6 oz)	2 carbohydrates 2 medium-fat meats 2 fats
Pot pie 🖌	1 (7 oz)	2 ½ carbohydrates 1 medium-fat meat 3 fats
Entrée or meal with fewer than 340 calories 🖌	About 8-11 oz	2-3 carbohydrates 1-2 lean meats
Soups		
Bean 🖌	1 cup	1 carbohydrate 1 very lean meat
Cream (made with water) 🖌	1 cup (8 oz)	1 carbohydrate 1 fat
Instant 🖌	6 oz prepared	1 carbohydrate
Instant with beans/lentils 🖌	8 oz prepared	2 ½ carbohydrates 1 very lean meat
Split pea (made with water) 🖌	½ cup (4 oz)	1 carbohydrate
Tomato (made with water) 🖌	1 cup (8 oz)	1 carbohydrate
Vegetable beef, chicken noodle, or other broth type 🖌	1 cup (8 oz)	1 carbohydrate

FAST FOODS LIST*

FOOD	SERVING SIZE	EXCHANGES PER SERVING
Burrito with beef ✎	1 (5-7 oz)	3 carbohydrates 1 medium-fat meat 1 fat
Chicken nuggets ✎	6	1 carbohydrate 2 medium-fat meats 1 fat
Chicken breast and wing, breaded and fried ✎	1 each	1 carbohydrate 4 medium-fat meats 2 fats
Chicken sandwich, grilled ✎	1	2 carbohydrates 3 very lean meats
Chicken wings, hot ✎	6 (5 oz)	1 carbohydrate 3 medium-fat meats 4 fats
Fish sandwich/tartar sauce ✎	1	3 carbohydrates 1 medium-fat meat 3 fats
French fries ✎	1 medium serving (5 oz)	4 carbohydrates 4 fats
Hamburger, regular ✎	1	2 carbohydrates 2 medium-fat meats
Hamburger, large ✎	1	2 carbohydrates 3 medium-fat meats 1 fat
Hot dog with bun ✎	1	1 carbohydrate 1 high-fat meat 1 fat
Individual pan pizza ✎	1	5 carbohydrates 3 medium-fat meats 3 fats
Pizza, cheese, thin crust ✎	¼ 12-inch (about 6 oz)	2½ carbohydrates 2 medium-fat meats
Pizza, meat, thin crust ✎	¼ 12-inch (about 6 oz)	2½ carbohydrates 2 medium-fat meats 1 fat
Soft-serve cone ✎	1 small (5 oz)	2½ carbohydrates 1 fat
Submarine sandwich ✎	1 sub (6-inch)	3 carbohydrates 1 vegetable 2 medium-fat meats 1 fat
Submarine sandwich (less than 6 g fat) ✎	1 sub (6-inch)	2½ carbohydrates 2 lean meats
Taco, hard or soft shell ✎	1 (3-3½ oz)	1 carbohydrate 1 medium-fat meat 1 fat

*Ask at your fast-food restaurant for nutrition information about your favorite fast food, or check websites.

PLANNING INDIVIDUALIZED DIETS USING EXCHANGE LISTS

Step 1: Conduct Nutrition History

A 4-hour or 3-day recall (see Chapter 14) can be used to determine usual food intake. Categorize intake into exchanges (or servings) from each list at each meal and snack. Translate into kcal and grams of carbohydrate, protein, and fat from exchanges. Round off kcal level to the nearest 50 or 100.

Calculations of food intake are not precise enough to allow more accuracy, and patients may consume an extra 50 to 60 kcal/day from free foods (see the Exchange Lists). When in doubt, round up instead of down. Determine percentages of carbohydrate, protein, and fat in current intake.

To determine total kcal, add up the number of exchanges actually consumed from each exchange group. Multiply the number of exchanges by the number of kcal in each exchange group.

Number of exchanges from Starch list	=	_____	×	80 kcal	=	_____
Number of exchanges from Fruit list	=	_____	×	60 kcal	=	_____
Number of exchanges from Milk list	=	_____	×	80 kcal (skim)	=	_____
	=	_____	×	120 kcal (low-fat)	=	_____
	=	_____	×	150 kcal (whole)	=	_____
Number of exchanges from Vegetable list	=	_____	×	25 kcal	=	_____
Number of exchanges from Meat list	=	_____	×	35 kcal (very lean)	=	_____
	=	_____	×	55 kcal (lean)	=	_____
	=	_____	×	75 kcal (medium-fat)	=	_____
	=	_____	×	100 kcal (high-fat)	=	_____
Number of exchanges from Fat list	=	_____	×	45 kcal	=	_____
				TOTAL kcal		_____

Using the total number of each exchange group, calculate the grams of carbohydrate (CHO), protein (PRO), and fat (FAT).

	NUMBER OF EXCHANGES CHO			NUMBER OF EXCHANGES PRO			NUMBER OF EXCHANGES FAT		
Bread list	_____ × 15 g	=	_____ g	_____ × 2 g	=	_____ g	_____ × 0-3 g	=	_____ g
Fruit list	_____ × 15 g	=	_____ g	_____ × 0 g	=	_____ g	_____ × 0 g	=	_____ g
Milk list	_____ ×	–	_____ g	_____ ×	=	_____ g	_____ ×	=	_____ g
Skim	_____ × 12 g	=	_____ g	_____ × 8 g	=	_____ g	_____ × 0 g	=	_____ g
Low-fat	_____ × 12 g	=	_____ g	_____ × 8 g	=	_____ g	_____ × 5 g	=	_____ g
Whole	_____ × 12 g	=	_____ g	_____ × 8 g	=	_____ g	_____ × 8 g	=	_____ g
Vegetable list	_____ × 5 g	=	_____ g	_____ × 2 g	=	_____ g	_____ × 0 g	=	_____ g
Meat list	_____ ×	=	_____ g	_____ ×	=	_____ g	_____ ×	=	_____ g
Very lean	_____ × 0 g	=	_____ g	_____ × 7 g	=	_____ g	_____ × 0-1 g	=	_____ g
Lean	_____ × 0 g	=	_____ g	_____ × 7 g	=	_____ g	_____ × 3 g	=	_____ g
Medium-fat	_____ × 0 g	=	_____ g	_____ × 7 g	=	_____ g	_____ × 5 g	=	_____ g
High-fat	_____ × 0 g	=	_____ g	_____ × 7 g	=	_____ g	_____ × 8 g	=	_____ g
Fat group	_____ × 0 g	=	_____ g	_____ × 0 g	=	_____ g	_____ × 5 g	=	_____ g
	TOTAL	=	_____ g	TOTAL	=	_____ g	TOTAL	=	_____ g

Take total kcal from above and determine the percentage of the diet that is carbohydrate, protein, and fat:

A. Multiply total grams CHO × 4 kcal = _____kcal
Multiply total grams PRO × 4 kcal = _____kcal
Multiply total grams FAT × 9 kcal = _____kcal
TOTAL _____kcal

B. Divide each nutrient's total kcal by the total kcal for the day, and multiply by 100 to get the percentage of kcal.

Kcal from CHO × 100 = % kcal from CHO _____ × 100 = _____Total kcal
Kcal from PRO × 100 = % kcal from PRO _____ × 100 = _____Total kcal
Kcal from FAT × 100 = % kcal from FAT _____ × 100 = _____Total kcal

Step 2: Calculate Daily Kilocalorie Requirements

Kcal needs are based on age, weight, and activity level. Use the Harris-Benedict equation to calculate energy needs. Round figure to nearest 100 kcal. Subtract kcal if weight loss is desired. Reducing kcal intake by 500 kcal/day will theoretically produce a 1-pound weight loss per week. Never reduce kcal level to below that required for basal energy needs.

Example: CG is a 62-year-old female with type 2 diabetes. She is 5 feet 5 inches tall (medium frame) and weighs 140 pounds. CG walks 10 to 12 miles per week at the mall.

$$655.1 + [9.6 \times wt \, (kg)] + [1.8 \times ht \, (cm)] - [4.7 \times age \, (yr)]$$

$$655.1 + [9.6 \times 63.6 \, kg] + [1.8 \times 165.1 \, cm] - [4.7 \times 62]$$

$$655.1 + 610.6 + 297.2 - 291.4 = 1271.5 \, kcal$$

$$1271.5 \, kcal \times 1.3 \, (activity \, factor) = 1652.95 \, kcal$$

Round off to 1700 kcal

If weight loss is desired, subtract 500 kcal: 1700 − 500 = 1200 kcal, which is below her basal energy needs of 1271.5 kcal. Adjust to 1300 kcal if weight loss is determined to be a treatment goal.

Step 3: Determine Distribution of Carbohydrate, Protein, and Fat Kilocalories

This should be based on the patient's usual intake, blood glucose levels, blood lipid levels, and treatment goals.

Example: CG's 24-hour recall indicates an intake of approximately 1500 kcal distributed into 17% protein, 30% fat, and 53% carbohydrate. Her pertinent lab values are glycosylated hemoglobin 6%, cholesterol 210 mg/dL, LDL cholesterol 179 mg/dL, HDL cholesterol 55 mg/dL. Although her lipid levels are at the high end of normal or just slightly above normal, her exercise and eating habits appear to be sufficient to control her blood glucose levels. In this case, you would distribute her kcal in the same pattern as found in her diet recall:

Carbohydrate:

$$1500 \, kcal \times 0.53 = 795 \, kcal \div 4 \, kcal/g = 199 \, g$$

Protein:

$$1500 \, kcal \times 0.17 = 255 \, kcal \div 4 \, kcal/g = 64 \, g$$

Fat:

$$1500 \, kcal \times 0.30 = 450 \, kcal \div 9 \, kcal/g = 50 \, g$$

Step 4: Determine Servings from Each Exchange List

These calculations are based on the amount of carbohydrate, protein, and fat in each Exchange List and the patient's preferences for foods within each list or group. The type of milk the patient uses should be calculated into the meal plan. Skim milk and low-fat milks are recommended, but whole milk can be used if the patient will not drink the others. Although lean meats should be encouraged, when calculating fat grams per meat serving, use the fat value that best represents actual intake. People do not need to add or subtract fat exchanges when using different meat categories.

Example: CG's usual eating pattern indicates she uses the following amounts from the milk, vegetable, and fruit exchange groups:

	SERVINGS	CARBO-HYDRATE (g)	PROTEIN (g)	FAT (g)	KCAL
Milk, skim	1	12	8	1	90
Vegetables	4	20	8	0	100
Fruits	4	60	0	0	240
CARBOHYDRATE SUBTOTAL		92	16	1	430

The Starch list is the only group remaining that provides carbohydrates. To determine the number of servings to be used from this group, subtract the total grams of carbohydrate (92 g) from the Milk, Vegetable, and Fruit lists from the total grams of carbohydrate (199 g) in the meal plan. This amount is divided by 15 g carbohydrate/serving in the Starch list.

	SERVINGS	CARBOHYDRATE (g)	PROTEIN (g)	FAT (g)	KCAL
Carbohydrate subtotal		92	16	1	460
Starches	7	105	21	7	560
PROTEIN SUBTOTAL		197	45	8	1020

The Meat list is the only group remaining that provides protein. To determine the number of servings to be used from this group, subtract the total grams of protein (48 g) from the Milk, Vegetable, and Starch lists from the total grams of protein (56 g) in the meal plan. This amount is divided by 7 g protein/serving in the Meat list.

	SERVINGS	CARBOHYDRATE (g)	PROTEIN (g)	FAT (g)	KCAL
Protein subtotal		197	45	8	1020
Meat/lean	4	0	28	12	220
FAT SUBTOTAL		197	73	20	1240

The Fat list is the only group remaining that provides fat. To determine the number of servings to be used from this group, subtract the total grams of fat (20 g) from the milk, starch, and meat lists from the total grams of fat (50 g) in the meal plan. This amount is divided by 5 g fat/serving in the Fat list.

	SERVINGS	CARBOHY- DRATE (g)	PROTEIN (g)	FAT (g)	KCAL
Fat subtotal		197	73	20	1240
Fats	6	0	0	30	270
TOTAL		197	73	50	1510

Note: When calculating the number of servings from each Exchange List, round to the nearest whole number. It is usually impractical to calculate and plan half servings from the lists.

The daily distribution of servings from the Exchange List is as follows. These servings can now be divided into the appropriate number of meals and snacks per day.

	SERVINGS	CARBOHY- DRATE (g)	PROTEIN (g)	FAT (g)	KCAL
Carbohy- drates	12				
Starches	7	105	21	7	560
Fruit	4	60	0	0	240
Milk (skim)	1	0	0	30	270
Vegeta- bles	4	20	8	1	90
Meats/lean	4	0	28	12	220
Fats	6	0	0	30	270

Modified from American Dietetic Association: *Exchange lists for meal planning,* Alexandria, Va, 2003, American Diabetes Association; American Dietetic Association: *Handbook of clinical dietetics,* ed 2, New Haven, Conn, 1992, Yale University Press; Davis JR, Sherer K: *Applied nutrition and diet therapy for nurses,* ed 2, Philadelphia, 1994, Saunders; American Dietetic Association: Nutrition recommendations and principles for people with diabetes mellitus, *J Am Diet Assoc* 94:504-506, 1994; and Tinker LF, Heins JM, Holler HJ: Commentary and translation: 1994 nutrition recommendations for diabetes, *J Am Diet Assoc* 94:507-511, 1994.

B

Eating well with Canada's Food Guide

PDF and other download formats are available at www.hc-sc.gc.ca/fn-an/food-guide-aliment/order-commander/index-eng.php.

Recommended Number of Food Guide Servings per Day

Age in Years	Children			Teens		Adults			
	2-3	4-8	9-13	14-18		19-50		51+	
Sex		Girls and Boys		Females	Males	Females	Males	Females	Males
Vegetables and Fruit	4	5	6	7	8	7-8	8-10	7	7
Grain Products	3	4	6	6	7	6-7	8	6	7
Milk and Alternatives	2	2	3-4	3-4	3-4	2	2	3	3
Meat and Alternatives	1	1	1-2	2	3	2	3	2	3

The chart above shows how many Food Guide Servings you need from each of the four food groups every day.

Having the amount and type of food recommended and following the tips in *Canada's Food Guide* will help:

- Meet your needs for vitamins, minerals and other nutrients.
- Reduce your risk of obesity, type 2 diabetes, heart disease, certain types of cancer and osteoporosis.
- Contribute to your overall health and vitality.

What is One Food Guide Serving?
Look at the examples below.

Vegetables and Fruit

Fresh, frozen or canned vegetables 125 mL (½ cup)

Leafy vegetables Cooked: 125 mL (½ cup) Raw: 250 mL (1 cup)

Fresh, frozen or canned fruits 1 fruit or 125 mL (½ cup)

100% Juice 125 mL (½ cup)

Grain Products

Bread 1 slice (35 g)

Bagel ½ bagel (45 g)

Flat breads ½ pita or ½ tortilla (35 g)

Cooked rice, bulgur or quinoa 125 mL (½ cup)

Cereal Cold: 30 g Hot: 175 mL (¾ cup)

Cooked pasta or couscous 125 mL (½ cup)

Milk and Alternatives

Milk or powdered milk (reconstituted) 250 mL (1 cup)

Canned milk (evaporated) 125 mL (½ cup)

Fortified soy beverage 250 mL (1 cup)

Yogurt 175 g (¾ cup)

Kefir 175 g (¾ cup)

Cheese 50 g (1½ oz.)

Meat and Alternatives

Cooked fish, shellfish, poultry, lean meat 75 g (2 ½ oz.)/125 mL (½ cup)

Cooked legumes 175 mL (¾ cup)

Tofu 150 g / 175 mL (¾ cup)

Eggs 2 eggs

Peanut or nut butters 30 mL (2 Tbsp)

Shelled nuts and seeds 60 mL (¼ cup)

Oils and Fats
- Include a small amount – 30 to 45 mL (2 to 3 Tbsp) – of unsaturated fat each day. This includes oil used for cooking, salad dressings, margarine and mayonnaise.
- Use vegetable oils such as canola, olive and soybean.
- Choose soft margarines that are low in saturated and trans fats.
- Limit butter, hard margarine, lard and shortening.

Make each Food Guide Serving count...
wherever you are – at home, at school, at work or when eating out!

▶ **Eat at least one dark green and one orange vegetable each day.**
Go for dark green vegetables such as broccoli, romaine lettuce and spinach.
Go for orange vegetables such as carrots, sweet potatoes and winter squash.

▶ **Choose vegetables and fruit prepared with little or no added fat, sugar or salt.**
Enjoy vegetables steamed, baked or stir-fried instead of deep-fried.

▶ **Have vegetables and fruit more often than juice.**

▶ **Make at least half of your grain products whole grain each day.**
Eat a variety of whole grains such as barley, brown rice, oats, quinoa and wild rice.
Enjoy whole grain breads, oatmeal or whole wheat pasta.

▶ **Choose grain products that are lower in fat, sugar or salt.**
Compare the Nutrition Facts table on labels to make wise choices.
Enjoy the true taste of grain products. When adding sauces or spreads, use small amounts.

▶ **Drink skim, 1%, or 2% milk each day.**
Have 500 mL (2 cups) of milk every day for adequate vitamin D.
Drink fortified soy beverages if you do not drink milk.

▶ **Select lower fat milk alternatives.**
Compare the Nutrition Facts table on yogurts or cheese to make wise choices.

▶ **Have meat alternatives such as beans, lentils and tofu often.**

▶ **Eat at least two Food Guide Servings of fish each week.**[*]
Choose fish such as char, herring, mackerel, salmon, sardines and trout.

▶ **Select lean meat and alternatives prepared with little or no added fat or salt.**
Trim the visible fat from meats. Remove the skin on poultry.
Use cooking methods such as roasting, baking or poaching that require little or no added fat.
If you eat luncheon meats, sausages or prepackaged meats, choose those lower in salt (sodium) and fat.

Enjoy a variety of foods from the four food groups.

Satisfy your thirst with water!
Drink water regularly. It's a calorie-free way to quench your thirst. Drink more water in hot weather or when you are very active.

[*] Health Canada provides advice for limiting exposure to mercury from certain types of fish. Refer to www.healthcanada.gc.ca for the latest information.

Source: Eating Well With Canada's Food Guide (2007), Health Canada. Reproduced with the permission of the Minister of Public Works and Government Services Canada, 2010.

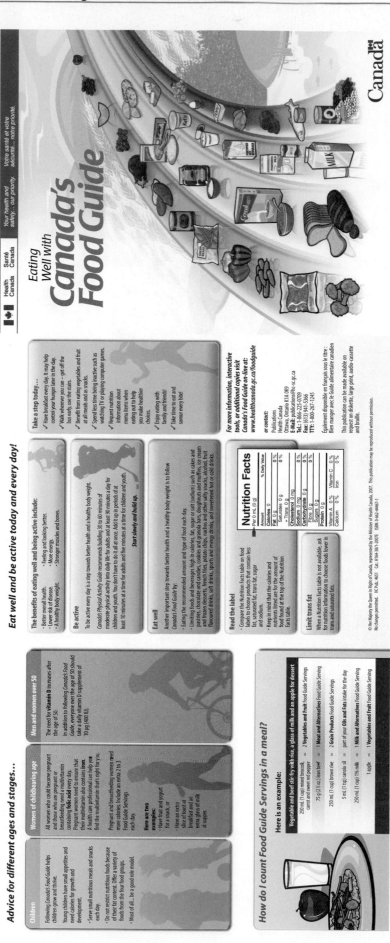

Body Mass Index Table: Obesity Values

For lower body mass indexes, see Table 10-1 in Chapter 10, "Management of Body Composition."

HEIGHT (INCHES)	36	37	38	39	40	41	42	43	44	45	46	47	48	49	50	51	52	53	54
								BODY WEIGHT (POUNDS)											
58	172	177	183	186	191	196	201	205	210	215	220	224	229	234	239	244	248	253	258
59	178	183	188	193	198	203	208	212	217	222	227	232	237	242	247	252	257	262	267
60	184	189	194	199	204	209	215	220	225	230	235	240	245	250	255	261	266	271	276
61	190	195	201	206	211	217	222	227	232	238	243	248	254	259	264	269	275	280	285
62	196	202	207	213	218	224	229	235	240	246	251	256	262	267	273	278	284	289	295
63	203	208	214	220	225	231	237	242	248	254	259	265	270	278	282	287	293	299	304
64	209	215	221	227	232	238	244	250	256	262	267	273	279	285	291	296	302	308	314
65	216	222	228	234	240	246	252	258	264	270	276	282	288	294	300	306	312	318	324
66	223	229	235	241	247	253	260	266	272	278	284	291	297	303	309	315	322	328	334
67	230	236	242	249	255	261	268	274	280	287	293	299	306	312	319	325	331	338	344
68	236	243	249	256	262	269	276	282	289	295	302	308	315	322	328	335	341	348	354
69	243	250	257	263	270	277	284	291	297	304	311	318	324	331	338	345	351	358	365
70	250	257	264	271	278	285	292	299	306	313	320	327	334	341	348	355	362	369	376
71	257	265	272	279	286	293	301	308	315	322	329	338	343	351	358	365	372	379	386
72	265	272	279	287	294	302	309	316	324	331	338	346	353	361	368	375	383	390	397
73	272	280	288	295	302	310	318	325	333	340	348	355	363	371	378	386	393	401	408
74	280	287	295	303	311	319	326	334	342	350	358	365	373	381	389	396	404	412	420
75	287	295	303	311	319	327	335	343	351	359	367	375	383	391	399	407	415	423	431
76	295	304	312	320	328	336	344	353	361	369	377	385	394	402	410	418	426	435	443

From NIH/National Heart, Lung, and Blood Institute: Appendix V: Body mass index chart (chart 2), Clinical guidelines on the identification, evaluation, and treatment of overweight and obesity in adults, Bethesda, Md, June 1998, National Institutes of Health.
To use the Table, find the appropriate height in the left-hand column. Move across to a given weight. The number at the top of the column is the BMI at that height and weight. Pounds have been rounded off.

D

Kilocalorie-Restricted Dietary Patterns

The goal of weight management is weight stabilization through the adoption and maintenance of healthy lifestyle behaviors, including consistent eating patterns. Although these changes in behavior may result in minimal weight changes, health status may improve.

Certain chronic medical conditions are improved by weight loss. Consequently, although physical and psychologic risks of kcal-restricted diets may occur, the benefits outweigh the risks. Following is a guide for comparison of weight loss programs and brief reviews of the primary weight loss formats of these diets. Programs should be contacted directly to determine current fees. New programs may become available through the Internet and should be judged by the following criteria.

COMPARISON OF WEIGHT LOSS PROGRAMS

PROGRAM	APPROACH/METHOD	HEALTHY LIFESTYLE COMPONENTS	COMMENTS (PRO/CON)	AVAILABILITY
Do-It-Yourself Programs				
Overeaters Anonymous (OA)	Nonprofit volunteer support groups for compulsive overeating patterned after the 12-step Alcoholics Anonymous program	Recommends emotional, spiritual, and physical recovery changes. Makes no exercise or food recommendations	Inexpensive. Provides group support. No need to follow a specific diet plan to participate. Minimal organization at the group level, so groups vary in approach. No health care providers on staff	505-903-6008; www.oa.org
Take Off Pounds Sensibly (TOPS)	Nonprofit support organization with weekly group meetings	No official lifestyle or exercise recommendations, but endorses slow, permanent lifestyle changes. Uses award programs for healthy lifestyle changes; special recognition given to best weight losers	Mandatory weigh-in at weekly meetings. Provides peer support. Members must submit written weight goals and diets from a health professional. Inexpensive form of continuing group support. Used as adjunct to professional care. Encourages long-term participation. Lacks professional guidance at chapter level because meetings run by volunteers. Groups vary widely in approach	800-932-8677; www.tops.org
Nonclinical Programs				
Atkins Diet	The original low-carb diet focusing on low glycemic approach (Atkins Glycemic Index) with 3 phases of carb limitations	Presents as a lifestyle approach encouraging education but limited approach	Emphasizes carb counting without focusing on saturated fat intake. High protein intake overstressed. Internet support.	800-6-Atkins; www.atkins.com

PROGRAM	APPROACH/METHOD	HEALTHY LIFESTYLE COMPONENTS	COMMENTS (PRO/CON)	AVAILABILITY
Diet Center	Focus on achieving healthy body composition through diet and personalized exercise plans. Kcal levels individualized to meet client needs and goals. Clients encouraged to visit center daily for weigh-in	One-on-one counseling helps clients design personal solutions to weight control problems; sessions conducted by non–health professionals. Emphasizes body composition, not pounds, as a measure of health. Maintenance program is available	Based on regular supermarket food; Diet Center prepackaged cuisine optional. Lack of professional guidance at client level. Little group support available	800-656-3294; www.dietcenter. com
Jenny Craig	Personal weight management menu plans based on Jenny Craig's cuisine with additional store-bought foods. Diet ranges from 1000 to 2600 kcal, depending on client needs. Mandatory weekly one-to-one counseling; group workshops	Individual consultations; group workshops provide motivation and peer exchange. A separate, 12-month maintenance program addresses issues such as body image and maintaining motivation to exercise	Little food preparation. Vegetarian and kosher meal plans available; also for clients who are diabetic, hypoglycemic, and breastfeeding. Recipes provided. Must rely on Jenny Craig cuisine for participation. Lack of professional guidance at client level Internet support	800-945-3669; www.jennycraig. com
Nutri/System	Menu plans based on Nutri/System's prepared meals with additional grocery foods. Focus on low-glycemic carbs and low-fat foods. Personal counseling and group sessions available	Women's and men's, type 2 diabetes, vegetarian programs	Relatively rigid diet with company foods. Portion-controlled Nutri/System foods deters adjustment to regular food preparation and food related situations. Little contact with health professionals	800-435-4074; www.nutrisystem. com
South Beach Diet	Based on glycemic index through use of "right" carbs of whole grains and certain fruits and vegetables; "right" fats, of olive and canola oil; and lean protein sources	Focus on positive lifestyle changes through consumption of healthy carbs, frequent meals and snacks of whole foods. Emphasis on regular physical activity.	After initial 2 week plan, offers well-balanced diet. Internet support for tracking food intake, recipes, exercise, etc. RDs available on internet site	866-218-2681; www. southbeachdiet. com
Weight Watchers	Emphasis on portion control and healthy lifestyle habits. Weekly group meetings with mandatory weigh-in or Internet memberships	Focus on positive lifestyle changes, including regular exercise. Encourages daily minimum physical activity level	Flexible program offering group and internet support, and well-balanced diet. Vegetarian plan available, plus healthy eating plans for pregnant and breastfeeding women. Encourages long-term participation for members to attain their weight loss goals. Lacks professional guidance at client level. Internet support	800-651-6000; www. weightwatchers. com

Continued

PROGRAM	APPROACH/METHOD	HEALTHY LIFESTYLE COMPONENTS	COMMENTS (PRO/CON)	AVAILABILITY
Clinical Programs				
Health Management Resources (HMR)	Medically supervised very-low-calorie diet (VLCD) of fortified, high-protein liquid meal replacements (520-800 kcal daily) or a low-kcal option consisting of liquid supplements and prepackaged HMR entrées (800-1300 kcal daily). Dieters receive the HMR Risk Factor Profile that measures and displays an individual's medical and lifestyle health risks. Mandatory weekly 90-minute group meetings. Maintenance meetings are 1 hour per week. One-on- one counseling. Need to have BMI >30 for VLCD	Recommends every client burn a minimum of 2000 kcal in physical activity weekly. Advocates consuming a diet with no more than 30% of kcal from fat and at least 3 to 5 servings of fruits and vegetables per week. Emphasizes lifestyle issues in weekly classes and in personal coaching	Each location has at least one physician and health educator on staff. Participants assigned "personal coaches" (i.e., registered dietitians, exercise physiologists, health educators) who help dieters learn and practice weight management skills. Dieters on VLCD see a physician or registered nurse weekly. Few decisions about what to eat. Supervised by a health professional. Requires a strong commitment to physical activity. Side effects of VLCD may include intolerance to cold, constipation, dizziness, dry skin, and headaches. All options include liquid supplement; diet is very high in protein, even at higher-kcal levels	Available at hospitals and medical settings nationwide; 800-418-1367; www.hmrprogram.com
Physicians in a Multidisciplinary Program	The multidisciplinary aspect implies the coordination of services, availability of individual and/or group counseling, and comprehensive medical supervision. May provide food and liquid-based weight loss programs	Varies. All factors in weight management considered	Professional diverse staff coordinate aspects of care and long-term management of obesity and associated medical problems. Often university-based programs, having structured peer-review mechanisms and may conduct research. Costs tend to be high	Very limited
Others				
Registered Dietitians (RDs)	Highly personalized approach to weight loss and maintenance	RDs help clients identify barriers to weight loss and maintenance and provide education about healthy lifestyles. Exercise encouraged as part of safe, sensible weight control program	Personalized approach to clients' health concerns. Trained health professionals address medical history and can account for it in diet therapy. Appropriate for any age-group. Can be expensive	In private practice, outpatient hospital clinics, health maintenance organizations (HMOs), and physicians' practices. ADA headquarters for referral to local RD: 800-877-1600; www.eatright.org
Physicians Practicing Alone	Individualized approach to weight loss and maintenance. Clients able to coordinate the management of weight with concurrent management of associated medical problems. Options include medications and surgery	Varies with physician and weight-loss approach. Should include exercise and nutrition counseling	Appropriate for clients with complex or serious associated medical problems. Physicians often inadequately trained in nutrition and low-kcal physiology. Service costs can be high	Generally available, but some physicians may be reluctant to treat obesity

Moderate Restriction of Kilocalories

Kcal restriction should be at least 500 kcal less than the individual's daily requirement for energy; daily intake should not be lower than about 1200 kcal. Adults, depending on their gender, height, and weight, may lose weight at intakes between 1200 and 1500 kcal. Intake below this level cannot provide sufficient amounts of nutrients unless supplements are prescribed. The diet should still follow general dietary guidelines and provide 45% to 65% kcal from carbohydrates, about 10% to 35% kcal from protein, and 20% to 35% kcal from fat.

The *Exchange Lists for Meal Planning* is often used to implement kcal-restricted diets. By prescribing the number of each exchange allowed, the individual can then design a dietary pattern based on personal taste preference and scheduling. The following exchanges equal about 1200 kcal: 2 carbohydrates as milk, 3 vegetable, 4 fruit, 5 carbohydrate (either as starch, milk, fruit, or vegetables), 5 lean meat, and 3 fat.

VERY-LOW-CALORIE DIETS (VLCD)

VLCDs are intended for use by moderately or severely obese individuals (BMI >30) whose attempts with more traditional methods have been unsuccessful and for individuals with BMI of 27 to 30 or higher whose medical condition depends on weight loss for improvement. Containing only 200 to 800 kcal, a VLCD causes rapid weight loss but increases the risk of gout, gallstones, and other related symptoms, including cardiac complications. Individuals must be under the complete and regular supervision of a physician. The American Dietetic Association (ADA) has developed medical nutrition intervention procedures for the use of VLCD.[1] Maintenance of the weight loss is difficult and depends on nutritional counseling, exercise, and lifestyle changes. Regain of lost weight most often occurs after 5 years even with adjunct support of behavior therapy.[1]

FORMULA DIETS

Developed by pharmaceutical and food manufacturers, these solutions are available in a variety of forms. Designed to replace meals, they may provide a daily total of about 900 kcal and often contain or may be supplemented by vitamins and minerals.[1] Although helpful for quick weight loss, the loss is rarely maintained because boredom with the solution and the lack of learning new eating approaches soon lead to the weight being regained.

PHARMACOTHERAPY

Criteria for pharmacotherapy are a BMI greater than 30 or clients with comorbidities and BMI of 27. The pharmacotherapy should be accompanied by medical nutrition therapy and exercise. Generally, starting weight loss is only 5% to 15% of original weight. Weight loss is regained when drug therapy is discontinued.

The use of pharmacologic drugs for obesity intervention is controversial among health professionals because of the lack of data on long-term effects and the possibility of abuse when prescribed to patients not meeting the criteria for pharmacotherapy.

REFERENCE

1. American Dietetic Association: Weight management, *J Am Diet Assoc* 109:330-346, 2009.

Foods Recommended for Hospital Diet Progressions*

FOOD CATEGORY	CLEAR LIQUID	FULL LIQUID
Soups	Broth or bouillon	Broth or bouillon; regular or high-protein consommé; strained vegetable, meat, or cream soups containing finely homogenized meat
Beverages	Coffee, tea, decaffeinated coffee, carbonated beverages as tolerated	Coffee, tea, decaffeinated coffee, carbonated beverages as tolerated, eggnogs, instant breakfast beverages, yogurt drinks, fruit-flavored drinks
Meat and meat substitutes	None	Clean, fresh eggs cooked to a liquid consistency or in custards; egg substitutes; pasteurized eggs used in eggnogs or cooking; salmonella-free frozen eggs
Fats	None	Butter, margarine, cream, cream substitute
Milk	None	Milk and milk beverages; plain or flavored yogurt without seeds, nuts, or fruit pieces; cocoa
Starches	None	Refined cooked cereals, strained whole grain cereals, high-protein cereals; mashed white potato diluted in cream soups
Vegetables	None	Vegetable juice and vegetable purees that are strained and diluted in cream soups

PURÉED	MECHANICAL SOFT	SOFT	REGULAR
Broth or bouillon, consommé, strained or blenderized cream soup	Soups made with allowed foods	Soups made with allowed foods	All
All	All	All	All
Strained or pureed meat or poultry, cottage cheese, cooked scrambled eggs and egg substitutes pureed as tolerated	Ground or finely diced, moist (gravy or sauces) meats and poultry; flaked fish without bones; eggs; cottage cheese; cheese; creamy peanut butter; soft casseroles	Moist, tender meat, fish, or poultry; eggs; cottage cheese; milk-flavored cheese; creamy peanut butter; soft casserole	All
Butter, margarine, cream, cream substitute, oil, gravy, white sauce, whipped cream, whipped topping	Butter, margarine, cream, cream substitute, oil, gravy, salad dressing, whipped cream, whipped toppings	Butter, margarine, cream, cream substitute, oil, gravy, salad dressing, whipped cream, whipped toppings, crisp bacon	All
Milk and milk beverages; plain or flavored yogurt without seeds, nuts, or fruit pieces; cocoa	Milk and milk beverages, plain or flavored yogurt without seeds or nuts, cocoa	All	All
Refined cooked cereals; mashed potatoes; pureed rice or noodles thinned with sauce or gravy; soft, crustless bread pureed with milk or other liquid if tolerated; bread crumbs may be added to soups, casseroles, and vegetables	Cooked or refined ready-to-eat cereals; potatoes; rice; pasta; white, refined wheat, or light rye breads or rolls; graham crackers as tolerated; pancakes; soft waffles; muffins; plain crackers	Cooked or refined ready-to-eat cereals; potatoes; rice; pasta; white, refined wheat, or light rye breads or rolls; graham crackers as tolerated; pancakes; soft waffles; muffins; plain crackers	All
Vegetable juice and strained or puréed vegetables	Soft, cooked vegetables without hulls or tough skin (peas and corn); juices	Soft, cooked vegetables; lettuce and tomatoes; limit gas-forming vegetables and whole-kernel corn	All

PURÉED	MECHANICAL SOFT	SOFT	REGULAR
Fruits	Clear fruit juices (apple, cranberry, grape) or strained fruit juices	Fruit juices, nectars	
Desserts	Flavored gelatin, high-protein gelatin, Popsicles and fruit ices	Flavored gelatin, puddings, high-protein puddings, custard, regular and high-protein gelatin desserts, plain ice cream, frozen yogurt, sherbet, fruit ices, Popsicles	
Sweets	Sugar, honey, hard candy, sugar substitute	Sugar, honey, hard candy, sugar substitute, syrup	
Miscellaneous	Salt	Salt, pepper, flavorings, chocolate syrup, cinnamon, nutmeg, brewer's yeast	
Supplements	High-protein, high-kcal, low-residue oral supplements; Polycose	Liquid commercially prepared nutritional supplements, Polycose	
Strained or pureed fruit, fruit juice, nectars	Cooked or canned fruit without seeds or skins, banana, fruit juice, nectars, citrus fruit without membrane	Cooked or canned fruit, soft fresh fruit, fruit juice, nectars	All
Flavored gelatin; puddings; custard; plain ice cream without seeds, nuts, or fruit pieces; sherbet; frozen yogurt; fruit ices; Popsicles	Flavored gelatin; puddings; custard; plain ice cream, without nuts, or fruit; sherbet; frozen yogurt; fruit ices; Popsicles	Flavored gelatin; puddings; custard; ice cream without nuts, sherbet, frozen yogurt, fruit ices, Popsicles, cake, cookies without nuts or coconut	All
Sugar, honey, hard candy, sugar substitute, syrup, jelly	Sugar, honey, hard candy, sugar substitute, syrup, jelly	Sugar, honey, candy without nuts or coconut, sugar substitute, syrup, plain chocolate candies, molasses, marshmallows	All
Salt, pepper, flavorings, ground spices, smooth condiments	Salt, pepper, flavorings, ground spices, smooth condiments	Salt, pepper, flavorings, mildly seasoned condiments, herbs, spices, ketchup, mustard, vinegar in moderation	All
Liquid commercially prepared nutritional supplements, Polycose	Liquid commercially prepared nutritional supplements, Polycose	All	All

Data from American Dietetic Association: *Manual of clinical dietetics*, ed 6, Chicago, 2000, ADA.
*Any foods not listed should be excluded from the diet.

National Renal Diet

Milk Choices	Per Day
Average per choice: 4 g protein, 120 kcal, 80 mg sodium, 100 mg phosphorus	
Milk (fat-free, low-fat, whole)	½ cup
Lo Pro	1 cup
Buttermilk, cultured	½ cup
Chocolate milk	½ cup
Light cream or half and half	½ cup
Ice milk or ice cream	½ cup
Yogurt, plain or fruit-flavored	½ cup
Evaporated milk	¼ cup
Sweetened condensed milk	¼ cup
Cream cheese	3 tbsp
Sour cream	4 tbsp
Sherbet	1 cup

Nondairy Milk Substitutes	Per Day
Average per choice: 0.5 g protein, 140 kcal, 40 mg sodium, 30 mg phosphorus	
Dessert, nondairy frozen	½ cup
Dessert topping, nondairy frozen	½ cup
Liquid nondairy creamer, polyunsaturated	½ cup

Meat Choices	Per Day
Average per choice: 7 g protein, 65 kcal, 25 mg sodium, 65 mg phosphorus	
Prepared without added salt	
Beef	
Round, sirloin, flank, cubed, T-bone, and Porterhouse steak; tenderloin, rib, chuck, and rump roast; ground beef or ground chuck	1 oz
Pork	
Fresh ham, tenderloin, chops, loin roast, cutlets	1 oz
Lamb	
Chops, roasts, cutlets	1 oz
Veal	
Chops, roasts, cutlets	1 oz
Poultry	
Chicken, turkey, Cornish hen, domestic duck and goose	1 oz
Fish	
Fresh and frozen fish	1 oz
Lobster, scallops, shrimp, clams	1 oz
Crab, oysters	1½ oz

Canned tuna, canned salmon, (canned without salt)	1 oz
Sardines (canned without salt) ✦	1 oz
Wild game	
Venison, rabbit, squirrel, pheasant, duck, goose	1 oz
Egg	
Whole	1 large
Egg white or yolk	2 large
Low-cholesterol egg product	¼ cup
Chitterlings	2 oz
Organ meats ✦	1 oz

Prepared with Added Salt	
Beef	
Deli-style roast beef ✹	1 oz
Pork	
Boiled or deli-style ham ✹	1 oz
Poultry	
Deli-style chicken or turkey ✹	1 oz
Fish	
Canned tuna, canned salmon ✹	1 oz
Sardines ✹ ✦	1 oz
Cheese	
Cottage ✹	¼ cup

Starch Choices	Per Day
Average per choice: 2 g protein, 90 kcal, 80 mg sodium, 35 mg phosphorus	
Breads and Rolls	
Bagel	½ small
Bread (French, Italian, raisin, light rye, sourdough, white)	1 slice (1 oz)
Bun, hamburger or hot dog type	½
Danish pastry or sweet roll, no nuts	½ small
Dinner roll or hard roll	1 small
Doughnut	1 small
English muffin	½
Muffin, no nuts, bran, or whole wheat	1 small (1 oz)
Pancake ✹ ✦	1 small (1 oz)
Pita or "pocket" bread	½ 6-in diameter
Tortilla, corn	2 6-in diameter
Tortilla, flour	1 6-in diameter
Waffle ✹ ✦	1 small (1 oz)

From American Dietetic Association: *National renal diet: professional guide,* ed 2, Chicago, 2002, American Dietetic Association.

✹ = High sodium. Each serving counts as 1 starch choice and 1 salt choice.

✦ = High phosphorus

Cereals and Grains Prepared Without Added Salt

Cereals, ready-to-eat, most brands	¾ cup
Puffed rice	2 cups
Puffed wheat	1 cup
Cereals, cooked	
Cream of Rice or Wheat, Farina, Malt-O-Meal	½ cup
Oat bran or oatmeal, Ralston	⅓ cup
Cornmeal, cooked	½ cup
Grits, cooked	½ cup
Flour, all-purpose	2½ tbsp
Pasta (noodles, macaroni, spaghetti), cooked	½ cup
Pasta made with egg (egg noodles), cooked	⅓ cup
Rice, white or brown, cooked	½ cup

Starchy Vegetables Prepared or Canned Without Added Salt

Corn	⅓ cup or ½ ear
Green peas	¼ cup
Potatoes, baked, white, or sweet	1 small (3 oz)
Potatoes, boiled or mashed	½ cup
Potatoes, deep fried	½ cup or 10 small
Potatoes, hashed brown	½ cup
Squash, butternut, mashed	½ cup
Squash, winter, baked (all other varieties), cubed	1 cup

Crackers and Snacks

Crackers: saltines, round butter	4 crackers
Graham crackers	3 squares
Melba toast	3 oblong
Popcorn, plain	1½ cups popped
Potato chips	1 oz, 14 chips
Pretzels, sticks or rings 🧂	¾ oz, 10 sticks
Pretzels, sticks or rings, unsalted	¾ oz, 10 sticks
RyKrisp 🧂	3 crackers
Tortilla chips	¾ oz, 9 chips

Cake

Cake, angel food	1/20 cake or 1 oz
Sandwich cookie 🧂	4 cookies
Shortbread cookie	4 cookies
Sugar cookie	4 cookies
Sugar wafer	4 cookies
Vanilla wafer	10 cookies
Fruit pie	⅛ pie
Sweetened gelatin	½ cup

🧂 = High sodium—each serving counts as 1 starch choice and 1 salt choice.

🦴 = High phosphorus.

Vegetable Choices

See Starch Choices for other vegetables. Average per choice: 1 g protein, 25 kcal, 15 mg sodium, 20 mg phosphorus

Prepared or Canned Without Added Salt Unless Otherwise Indicated

1-Cup Serving

Alfalfa sprouts	Escarole
Cabbage	Lettuce, all varieties
Celery	Pepper, green, sweet
Cucumber (or ½ whole)	Radishes, sliced (or 15 small)
Eggplant	Turnips
Endive	Watercress

½-Cup Serving

Artichoke	Onions
Bamboo shoots	Parsnips 🦴
Bean sprouts	Pumpkin
Beans, green or wax	Rutabagas 🦴
Beets	Sauerkraut 🧂🧂🧂
Carrots (or 1 small)	Squash, summer
Cauliflower	Tomato (or 1 medium)
Chard	Tomato juice, unsalted
Chinese cabbage	Tomato juice, canned with salt 🧂🧂🧂
Collards	Tomato puree
Kale	Turnip greens
Kohlrabi	Vegetable juice cocktail, unsalted
Mushrooms, fresh raw (or 4 medium)	Vegetable juice cocktail, canned with salt 🧂🧂🧂

¼-Cup Serving

Asparagus (or 2 spears)	Mushrooms, fresh cooked
Avocado (¼ whole)	Mustard greens
Beet greens	Okra
Broccoli	Snow peas
Brussels sprouts	Spinach
Chili pepper	Tomato sauce
Prepared or Canned with Salt	

Vegetables canned with salt (use serving size listed below) 🧂

🧂 = High sodium—each serving counts as 1 starch choice and 1 salt choice.

🧂🧂 = High sodium—each serving counts as 1 vegetable choice and 2 salt choices.

🧂🧂🧂 = High sodium—each serving counts as 1 vegetable choice and 3 salt choices.

🦴 = High phosphorus.

Fruit Choices

Average per choice: 0.5 g protein, 70 kcal, 15 mg phosphorus

1-Cup Serving

Apple (1 medium)	Papaya nectar
Apple juice	Peach nectar
Apple sauce	Pear nectar
Cranberries	Pear, canned or fresh (1 medium)
Cranberry juice cocktail	Tangerine (1 medium)

½-Cup Serving

Apricot nectar	Lemon (½ medium)

Banana (½ small)
Blueberries
Figs, canned
Fruit cocktail
Grapes (15 small)

Grape juice
Grapefruit (½ medium)

Grapefruit Juice
Gooseberries
Kiwifruit (½ medium)
¼-Cup Serving
Apricots (2 halves)
Apricots, dried (2)
Blackberries
Cantaloupe (⅛ small)
Cherries
Dates (2 tbsp)
Figs, dried (1 whole)

Lemon juice
Mango (½ medium)
Nectarine (½ medium)
Orange (½ medium)
Peach, canned or fresh
    (½ medium)
Pineapple
Plums, canned or fresh (1
    medium)
Rhubarb
Strawberries
Watermelon

Honeydew melon (⅛ small)
Orange juice
Papaya (¼ medium)
Prune juice
Prunes, cooked (5)
Raisins (2 tbsp)
Raspberries

Fat Choices   Per Day

Average per choice: trace protein, 45 kcal, 55 mg sodium,
    5 mg phosphorus

Unsaturated Fats

Margarine	1 tsp
Reduced-calorie margarine	1 tbsp
Mayonnaise	1 tsp
Low-calorie mayonnaise	1 tbsp
Oil (safflower, sunflower, corn, soybean, olive, peanut, canola)	1 tsp
Salad dressing (mayonnaise-type)	2 tsp
Salad dressing (oil-type)	1 tbsp
Low-calorie salad dressing (mayonnaise-type)	2 tbsp
Low-calorie salad dressing (oil-type) ✎	2 tbsp
Tartar sauce	1½ tsp
Saturated Fats	
Butter	1 tsp
Coconut	2 tbsp
Powdered coffee creamer	1 tbsp
Solid shortening	1 tsp

✎ = High sodium—each serving counts as 1 starch choice and 1
salt choice.

High-Calorie Choices

Average per choice: trace protein, 100 kcal, 15 mg sodium,
    5 mg phosphorus
Beverages

Carbonated beverages (fruit flavors, root beer; colas or pepper-type) 🦴	1 cup
Cranberry juice cocktail	1 cup
Fruit-flavored drink	1 cup
Kool-Aid	1 cup
Lemonade	1 cup
Limeade	1 cup
Tang	1 cup

Wine*	½ cup
Frozen Desserts	
Fruit ice	½ cup
Juice bar (3 oz)	1 bar
Popsicle (3 oz)	1 bar
Sorbet	½ cup
Candy and Sweets	
Butter mints	14
Candy corn	20 or 1 oz
Chewy fruit snacks	1 pouch
Cranberry sauce or relish	¼ cup
Fruit chews	4
Fruit roll ups	2
Gumdrops	15 small
Hard candy	4 pieces
Honey	2 tbsp
Jam or jelly	2 tbsp
Jelly beans	10
LifeSavers or cough drops	12
Marmalade	2 tbsp
Marshmallows	5 large
Sugar, brown or white	2 tbsp
Sugar, powdered	3 tbsp
Syrup	2 tbsp
Special Low-Protein Products	

Ask your dietitian for information on how to obtain these
    products.

Low-protein gelled dessert	½ cup
Low-protein bread	1 slice
Low-protein cookies	2
Low-protein pasta	½ cup
Low-protein rusk	2 slices

🦴 = High phosphorus.

*Check with your physician before using alcohol.

Salt Choices

Average per choice: 25 mg sodium

Salt	⅛ tsp
Seasoned salts (onion, garlic, etc.)	⅛ tsp
Accent	½ tsp
Barbecue sauce	2 tbsp
Bouillon	⅓ cup
Chili sauce	1½ tbsp
Dill pickle	⅙ large or ½ oz
Ketchup	1½ tbsp
Mustard	4 tsp
Olives, black	3 large or 1 oz
Olives, green	2 medium or ⅓ oz
Soy sauce	¾ tsp
Light soy sauce	1 tsp
Steak sauce	2½ tbsp
Sweet pickle relish	2½ tbsp
Taco sauce	2 tbsp
Tamari sauce	¾ tsp
Teriyaki sauce	1¼ tsp
Worcestershire sauce	1 tbsp

A HEALTHY FOOD GUIDE: KIDNEY DISEASE

Name: _____   _____   g protein
Date: _____   _____   kcal
Your dietitian is: _____   _____   mg phosphorus
Telephone number: _____   _____   mg sodium

YOUR DAILY MEAL PLAN

BREAKFAST		SAMPLE MENU		SNACK			SAMPLE MENU
Milk	_____	choices	_____		_____	choices	_____
Nondairy milk substitute	_____	choices			_____	choices	_____
Meat	_____	choices	_____	**Dinner**			
Starch	_____	choices		Milk	_____	choices	_____
Fruit	_____	choices		Nondairy milk substitute	_____	choices	_____
Fat	_____	choices	_____	Meat	_____	choices	_____
High-calorie	_____	choices	_____	Starch	_____	choices	_____
Salt	_____	choices	_____	Vegetable	_____	choices	_____
Snack				Fruit	_____	choices	_____
	_____	choices	_____	Fruit	_____	choices	_____
	_____	choices	_____	High-calorie	_____	choices	_____
Lunch				Salt	_____	choices	_____
Milk	_____	choices	_____	**Snack**			
Nondairy milk substitute	_____	choices	_____		_____	choices	_____
Meat	_____	choices	_____		_____	choices	_____
Starch	_____	choices	_____				
Vegetable	_____	choices	_____				
Fruit	_____	choices	_____				
Fat	_____	choices	_____				
High-calorie	_____	choices	_____				
Salt	_____	choices	_____				

G

Foods High in Lactose, Purines, and Oxalates

LACTOSE CONTENT OF FOODS

Lactose contents are approximate, depending on portion size and product preparation. Foods not listed do not usually contain lactose. Most individuals can experiment with different lactose-containing foods to determine their level of tolerance. Although dairy products all contain lactose, processing reduces the lactose in some products.

High-Lactose Foods

Buttermilk
Cheesecake, cream pies
Cold cuts and hot dogs (some may contain varying amounts of lactose)
Cottage cheese (nonfat, low-fat, regular)
Cream
Cream cheese
Cream or milk soups
Creamy sauces (white sauce, Alfredo sauce, vegetables au gratin)
Evaporated milk
Half and half
Ice cream (regular and low-fat), ice milk, frozen yogurt
Milk (nonfat, skim, low-fat, whole)
Milk-related products
Powdered milk
Pudding, custard
Ricotta cheese
Salad dressings with milk
Sour cream
Yogurt

Low-Lactose Foods

Aged cheese (cheddar, Swiss)
Butter/margarine
Commercial bread or cake products (bread, muffins, pancakes, waffles, biscuits)
Drug preparations (tablets) (may contain lactose as filler, but usually tolerated)
Lactose-reduced milk (nonfat, skim, low-fat, whole)
Processed cheese (depending on milk solids added)
Processed foods containing dry milk solids or whey
Ready-to-eat cereals containing milk/lactose
Sherbet
Yogurt (may be tolerated)

PURINE CONTENT OF FOODS

High-Purine Foods: Content 150 to 825 mg/100 g

Fish/Seafood

Anchovies
Herring
Mackerel
Sardines
Scallops

Meats

Brains
Goose
Gravies
Kidney
Liver
Meat extracts
Sweetbreads
Wild game

Moderate-Purine Foods: Content 50 to 150 mg/100 g

Vegetables

Asparagus
Cauliflower
Green peas
Mushrooms
Spinach

Grains and Legumes

Legumes (split peas, beans, lentils)
Oatmeal
Wheat bran and germ
Whole grain breads and cereals

Fish/Seafood

Crabs
Eel
Fish (all kinds)
Lobsters
Oysters

Meats and Related Products

Beef
Lamb
Pork
Veal

Poultry

Chicken
Duck
Turkey

Low-Purine Foods: Content 0 to 50 mg/100 g

Beverages

Carbonated beverages
Coffee
Tea

Grains

Breads and cereals (refined white flour)

Dairy

Cheese
Milk (all fat levels)

Miscellaneous

Eggs
Fats
Fish roe
Fruits, fruit juices
Gelatin
Nuts
Sugars (all types) and sweet foods
Vegetables

OXALATE CONTENT OF FOODS

High-Oxalate Foods: >10 mg/Serving

Vegetables

Beans (wax, green, dried)
Beets
Cassava
Celery
Chives
Collards
Cucumbers
Dandelion greens
Green peppers
Okra
Parsley
Rutabagas
Spinach
Summer squash
Sweet potatoes
Swiss chard

Fruits and Juices

Blackberries
Blueberries
Citrus peel (lemon, lime, orange)
Fruit cocktail
Gooseberries
Grapes (purple/Concord)
Plums
Raspberries (black, red)
Red currants
Rhubarb
Strawberries
Tangerines

Starches/Breads

Amaranth
Bran
Breads
Fruit cake
Grits
Pasta
Soybean crackers
Wheat germ

Meat and Protein Sources

Baked beans (tomato sauce)
Tofu

Fats

Almonds
Cashews
Nut butters
Peanuts
Pecans
Sesame seeds
Tahini
Walnuts

Beverages

Beer
Chocolate milk
Cocoa
Coffee (instant)
Colas
Ovaltine
Tea

Others

Chocolate
Cocoa powder
Tomato soup
Vegetable soup

Data from Nelson JK, et al: *Mayo Clinic diet manual*, ed 7, St Louis, 1994, Mosby; and Dietary Department, University of Iowa Hospital and Clinics, Iowa City: *Recent advances in therapeutic diets*, ed 5, Ames, Iowa, 1996, Iowa State University Press.

Cultural and Religious Dietary Patterns

CULTURAL FOODS

Foods specifically associated with these cultural groups are noted. Individuals may consume typical American foods as well; assumptions of dietary patterns cannot be made, but knowledge of these unique foods provides a common understanding of the range of possible food choices.

ETHNIC GROUP	BREAD, CEREAL, RICE, AND PASTA GROUP	VEGETABLE GROUP	FRUIT GROUP	MILK, YOGURT, AND CHEESE GROUP	MEAT, POULTRY, FISH, DRY BEANS, EGGS, AND NUTS GROUP	FATS, OILS, AND SWEETS
Native American Each tribe may have specific foods; listed here are commonly consumed foods	Blue corn flour (ground dried blue corn kernels) used to make cornbread, mush dumplings; fruit dumplings (walakshi); fry bread (biscuit dough deep fried); ground sweet acorn; tortillas; wheat or rye used to make cornmeal and flours	Cabbage, carrots, cassava, dandelion greens, eggplant, milkweed, onions, pumpkin, squash (all varieties), sweet and white potatoes, turnips, wild tullies (a tuber), yellow corn	Dried wild cherries and grapes; wild banana, berries, and yucca	None	Duck, eggs, fish eggs (roe), geese, groundhog, kidney beans, lentils, nuts (all), peanuts, pine nuts, pinto beans, venison, wild rabbit	None
African American	Biscuits, cornbread as spoon bread, cornpone or hush puppies, grits	Leafy greens including dandelion greens, kale, mustard greens, collard greens, turnips	None	Buttermilk	Pork and pork products, scrapple (cornmeal and pork), chitterlings (pork intestines), bacon, pig's feet, pig ears, souse, pork neck bones, fried meats and poultry, organ meats (kidney, liver, tongue, tripe), venison, rabbit, catfish, buffalo fish, mackerel, legumes (black-eyed peas, kidney, navy, chickpeas)	Lard

ETHNIC GROUP	BREAD, CEREAL, RICE, AND PASTA GROUP	VEGETABLE GROUP	FRUIT GROUP	MILK, YOGURT, AND CHEESE GROUP	MEAT, POULTRY, FISH, DRY BEANS, EGGS, AND NUTS GROUP	FATS, OILS, AND SWEETS
Japanese	Rice and rice products, rice flour (mochiko), noodles (somen/ soba), seaweed around rice with or without fish (sushi)	Bamboo shoots (takenoko), burdock (gobo), cabbage (napa), dried mushrooms (shiitake), eggplant, horseradish (wasabi), Japanese parsley (seri), lotus root (renkon), mustard greens, pickled vegetables, seaweed (laver, nori, wakame, kombu), vegetable soup (mizutaki), white radish (daikon)	Pear-like apple (nasi), persimmons	None	Fish and shellfish including dried fish with bones, raw fish (sashimi), and fish cake (kamaboko); soybeans as soybean curd (tofu), fermented soybean paste (miso), and sprouts; red beans (adzuki)	Soy and rice oil
Chinese	Rice and related products (flour, cakes, and noodles); noodles made from barley, corn, and millet; wheat and related products (breads, noodles, spaghetti, stuffed noodles [wonton] and filled buns [boa])	Bamboo shoots; cabbage (napa); Chinese celery; Chinese parsley (coriander); Chinese turnips (lo bok); dried day lilies; dry fungus (black Judas ear); leafy green vegetables including kale, Chinese cress, Chinese mustard greens (gai choy), Chinese chard (bok choy), amaranth greens (yin choy), wolfberry leaves (gou gay), and Chinese broccoli (gai lan); lotus tubers; okra; snow peas; stir-fried vegetables (chow yuk); taro roots, white radish (daikon)	Kumquat	None	Fish and seafood (all kinds, dried and fresh), hen, legumes, nuts, organ meats, pigeon eggs, pork and pork products, soybean curd (tofu), steamed stuffed dumplings (dim sum)	Peanut, soy, sesame and rice oil; lard

Continued

ETHNIC GROUP	BREAD, CEREAL, RICE, AND PASTA GROUP	VEGETABLE GROUP	FRUIT GROUP	MILK, YOGURT, AND CHEESE GROUP	MEAT, POULTRY, FISH, DRY BEANS, EGGS, AND NUTS GROUP	FATS, OILS, AND SWEETS
Filipino	Noodles, rice, rice flour (mochiko), stuffed noodles (wonton), white bread (pan de sal)	Bamboo shoots, dark green leafy vegetables (malunggay and salvyot), eggplant, sweet potatoes (camotes), okra, palm, peppers, turnips, root crop (gabi)	Avocado, bitter melon (ampalaya), guavas, jackfruit, limes, mango, papaya, pod fruit (tamarind), pomelos, tangelo (naranghita)	Custards	Fish in all forms; dried fish (dilis); egg roll (lumpia); fish sauce (alamang and bagoong); legumes such as mung beans, bean sprouts, chickpeas, organ meats (liver, heart, intestines); pork with chicken in soy sauce (adobo); pork sausage; soybean curd (tofu)	None
Southeastern Asians (Laos, Cambodia, Thailand, Vietnam, the Hmong and the Mien)	Rice (long and short grain) and related products such as noodles; Hmong cornbread or cake	Bamboo shoots, broccoli, Chinese parsley (coriander), mustard greens, pickled vegetables, water chestnuts, Thai chili peppers	Apple pear (Asian pear), bitter melon, coconut cream and milk, guava, jackfruit, mango	Sweetened condensed milk	Beef; chicken; deer; eggs; fish and shellfish (all kinds of freshwater and saltwater); legumes including black-eyed peas, peanuts, kidney beans, and soybeans; organ meats (liver, stomach); pork; rabbit; soybean curd (tofu)	Lard, peanut oil
Mexican	Corn and related products; taco shells (fried corn tortillas); tortillas (corn and flour); white bread	Cactus (nopales), chili peppers, salsa, tomatoes, yambean root (jicama), yucca root (cassava or manioc)	Avocado, guacamole (mashed avocado, onion, cilantro [coriander], chilies), papaya	Cheese, flan, sour cream	Black or pinto beans (frejoles); refried beans (frejoles refritos); flour tortilla stuffed with beef, chicken, eggs, or beans (burrito); corn tortilla stuffed with chicken, cheese, or beef topped with chili sauce (enchilada); Mexican sausage (chorizo)	Bacon fat, lard (manteca), salt pork

ETHNIC GROUP	BREAD, CEREAL, RICE, AND PASTA GROUP	VEGETABLE GROUP	FRUIT GROUP	MILK, YOGURT, AND CHEESE GROUP	MEAT, POULTRY, FISH, DRY BEANS, EGGS, AND NUTS GROUP	FATS, OILS, AND SWEETS
Puerto Rican and Cuban	Rice; starchy green bananas, usually fried (plantain)	Beets, eggplant, tubers (yucca), white yams (boniato)		Flan, hard cheese (queso de mano)	Chicken, fish (all kinds and preparations including smoked, salted, canned, and fresh), legumes (all kinds especially black beans), pork (fried), sausage (chorizo)	Olive and peanut oil, lard
Jewish These foods reflect religious and cultural customs of Jewish people. Adherences to religious dietary patterns by followers of the different forms of Judaism (Orthodox, Conservative, Reform, and Reconstructionist) vary. Generally, Orthodox Jews and many Conservative Jews follow kosher dietary rules when eating at home and dining out. Others may only observe these rules when in their own homes. "Keeping kosher" rules are reviewed in the religious dietary pattern section	Bagel, buckwheat groats (kasha), dumplings made with matzoh meal (matzoh balls or knaidelach), egg bread (challah), noodle or potato pudding (kugel), crepe filled with farmer cheese and/or fruit (blintz), unleavened bread or large cracker made with wheat flour and water (matzoh)	Potato pancakes (latkes); a vegetable stew made with sweet potatoes, carrots, prunes, and sometimes brisket (tzimmes); beet soup (borscht)	None	None	A mixture of fish formed into balls and poached (gefilte fish); smoked salmon (lox)	Chicken fat

RELIGIOUS DIETARY PATTERNS

Beliefs of several major religions include practices that affect or prescribe specific dietary patterns or prohibit consumption of certain foods. Individuals practicing these religions may or may not adhere to all of the prescribed customs. A brief review of some of these practices follows.

Muslim

Pork and pork-related products are not eaten. Meats that are consumed must be slaughtered by a prescribed ritual called halal; these procedures are similar to the Judaic kosher slaughtering of animals, so Muslims may eat kosher meats. Coffee, tea, and alcohol are not consumed. During the month of Ramadan, Muslims fast during the day from dawn to sunset.

Christianity

Some sects may not eat meat on holy days; others prohibit alcohol consumption.

Hinduism and Buddhism

Animal foods of beef, pork, lamb, and poultry are not eaten. Followers are lacto-vegetarians or vegans.

Judaism

No pork or pork-related products or seafood or fish without scales and fins are eaten. Dairy foods are not consumed with meat or animal-related foods (excludes fish). If meat or dairy is eaten, 6 hours must pass for the other to be acceptable for consumption. Animals are slaughtered according to ritual, in which blood is drained and carcass is salted and rinsed; meat prepared this way is kosher. Preparation of processed foods must adhere to guidelines. Because meat and dairy must not mix, two sets of dishes and utensils are used at home and in kosher restaurants. Foods that are neither meat nor dairy are called *pareve* and labeled by food manufacturers. Additional customs affect food consumption on Saturday, the Sabbath, during which no cooking occurs. Fasting (no water or food) for 24 hours occurs during Yom Kippur (Day of Atonement). During Passover, an 8-day holiday, no leavened bread is consumed—only matzoh (made from flour and water) and products made from matzoh flour. Other symbolic food restrictions may be observed.

Mormon

Alcohol and caffeine prohibited or strongly discouraged.

Seventh-day Adventist

General restrictions of pork and pork-related products, shellfish, alcohol, coffee, and tea are followed. Some followers are ovo-lacto vegetarians, whereas others are vegans.

CULTURAL FOODS WEBSITES

Racial and ethnic populations (African American, Alaskan Native, American Indian, Asian American, black, Hispanic, Latino, Native Hawaiian, Pacific Islander, multiracial, and white)
www.cdc.gov/omhd/Populations/populations.htm
Culinary History Timeline (social history, manners, and menus)
www.foodtimeline.org/food1.html

World Food Habits (English-language resources for the anthropology of food and nutrition)
http://lilt.ilstu.edu/RTDIRKS/

ETHNIC GROUP WEBSITES

Native American
Indian Health Service
www.ihs.gov
Native American and Alaskan Native
www.cdc.gov/omhd/Populations/AIAN/AIAN.htm
African American
Black or African American populations
www.cdc.gov/omhd/Populations/BAA/BAA.htm
Asian
Japanese, Chinese, Filipino, Laos, Cambodia, Thailand, Vietnam, the Hmong and the Mien
Asia Society (country profiles, style and living, traditions, religions, and philosophies)
http://asiasociety.org/style-living
Mexican, Puerto Rican, and Cuban countries and their cultures
www.everyculture.com
Jewish
Virtual Library, Kashrut: Jewish Dietary Laws
www.jewishvirtuallibrary.org/jsource/Judaism/kashrut.html
Religious Dietary Patterns
Judaism: Virtual Library, Kashrut: Jewish Dietary Laws
www.jewishvirtuallibrary.org/jsource/Judaism/kashrut.html
Muslim
Islamic Food and Nutrition Council of America
www.ifanca.org/index.php
Christianity
Faithandfood.com
www.faithandfood.com
Hinduism and Buddhism
Faithandfood.com
www.faithandfood.com
Mormon
Official Website of The Church of Jesus Christ of Latter-day Saints
www.mormon.org
Seventh-day Adventist
Health Ministries Department of the Seventh-day Adventist Church World Headquarters
www.health20-20.org

A

absorption the process by which substances pass through the intestinal mucosa into the blood or lymph

acanthosis nigricans hyperpigmentation and thickening of the skin into velvety irregular folds in the neck and flexural areas

Acceptable Macronutrient Distribution Range (AMDR) intake range for an energy source associated with reduced chronic disease risk while supplying adequate essential nutrients

acesulfame K a synthetically produced nonnutritive sweetener

acetyl coenzyme A (acetyl CoA) important intermediate byproduct in metabolism formed from the breakdown of glucose, fatty acids, and certain amino acids

acupuncture the use of fine needles to open blockages of the flow of Qi, or life force, and thus restore balance

acute respiratory failure (ARF) sudden absence of respirations, with confusion or unresponsiveness caused by obstructive airflow or failure of the pulmonary gas exchange mechanism

acute tubular necrosis (ATN) acute death of cells in the small tubules of the kidneys as a result of disease or injury

adaptive thermogenesis energy (or heat released) used by the body to adjust to changing physical and biologic environments

adenosine triphosphate (ATP) an energy-rich compound used for all energy-requiring processes in the body

Adequate Intake (AI) the approximate level of an average nutrient intake determined by observation of or experimentation with a particular group or population that appears to maintain good health

adipocytes cells specialized for storage of fat

adipose tissue stored form of fat (mainly triglycerides) in the body

ADPIE acronym for assessment, diagnosis, planning, implementation, and evaluation

adrenocorticotropic hormone (ACTH) an adrenal cortex hormone that stimulates secretion of more hormones

aerobic glycolysis the conversion of glucose to ATP for energy when oxygen is available

aerobic pathway a form of energy production that depends on oxygen and increases the use of fat

aerophagia swallowing of air, usually the result of eating with the mouth open, followed by belching, gastric distress, or flatulence

alcoholic cirrhosis associated with chronic alcohol abuse; accounts for 50% of all cases; also called Laënnec's cirrhosis

aldosterone a hormone secreted by the adrenal gland in response to sodium levels in kidneys; affects kidneys to balance fluid levels as needed

allogeneic transplant between different individuals of the same species who are not genetically identical; an allogeneic bone marrow transplant

alternative medicine healing practices that replace conventional medical treatment

alternative sweeteners nonnutritive sweeteners (or artificial sweeteners) synthetically produced to be sweet tasting but do not provide nutrients and few, if any, kcal; aspartame, saccharin, acesulfame K, and sucralose are alternative sweeteners

amino acid pool the assortment of amino acids available to cells

amino acid score a simple measure of an amino acid composition of a food as compared with a reference protein; based on the limiting amino acid

amino acids organic compounds containing carbon, hydrogen, oxygen, and nitrogen

aminopeptidase an intestinal peptidase that releases free amino acids from the amino end of short-chain peptides

amyloidosis a disorder characterized by accumulation of waxy starchlike glycoprotein (amyloid) in organs and tissues affecting function

anaerobic glycolysis the conversion of glucose to pyruvate to provide energy in the absence of oxygen

anaerobic pathway a form of energy production that does not require oxygen

anaphylaxis a severe immune system response to an allergen

anencephaly a congenital defect in which the brain does not develop; death may occur shortly after birth

angina pectoris chest pain that often radiates down the left arm and is frequently accompanied by a feeling of suffocation and impending death

anorexia nervosa a mental disorder characterized by self-imposed starvation; may include binge-eating episodes associated with bulimic behaviors

antidiuretic hormone (ADH) a hormone secreted by the pituitary gland in response to low fluid levels; affects kidneys to decrease excretion of water; also called vasopressin

antineoplastic therapy substance, procedure, or measure that prevents the proliferation of malignant cells; usually chemotherapy, radiation therapy, surgery, biologic response modifiers, or bone marrow transplantation

antioxidant a compound that guards other compounds from damaging oxidation

anuria less than 250 mL urine excretion every 24 hours

appetite desire for food

ariboflavinosis a group of symptoms associated with riboflavin deficiency

aromatherapy using extracts or essences of herbs, flowers, and trees in the form of essential oils to support health and well-being

arteriosclerosis thickening, loss of elasticity, and calcification of arterial walls, resulting in decreased blood supply to tissues

ascites abnormal intraperitoneal accumulation of fluid containing large amounts of protein and electrolytes, usually resulting in abdominal swelling, hemodilution, edema, or decreased urinary output

aspartame a nonnutritive sweetener formed by the bonding of the amino acids phenylalanine and aspartic acid

asthma a chronic respiratory disorder characterized by airway obstruction caused by excessive mucus production and respiratory mucosa edema; may be triggered by infection, cold air, vigorous exercise, stress, or inhalation of environmental allergens or pollutants

ataxia muscle weakness and loss of coordination

atherosclerosis development of lesions (also called fatty streaks) in the intima of arteries; during aging the lesions develop into fibrous plaques that project into the vessel lumen and begin to disturb blood flow

athetoid purposeless weaving motions of the body or extremities

atonic lacking normal muscle tone

autoantibodies self-antibodies; in the pancreas, these include islet cell autoantibodies, autoantibodies to insulin, and autoantibodies to glutamic acid decarboxylase (GAD65)

autologous transplantation in which the donor and recipient are the same individual; an autologous bone marrow transplant

Ayurveda a system of healing focusing on diet and herbal remedies that emphasizes the use of body, mind, and spirit to prevent and treat disorders

B

basal metabolism the amount of energy required to maintain life-sustaining activities for a specific period

beikost (BYE-cost) supplemental or weaning foods

beriberi a severe chronic deficiency of thiamine characterized by muscle weakness and pain, anorexia, mental disorientation, and tachycardia

beta cells insulin-producing cells situated in the islets of Langerhans of the pancreas

bezoars physical obstacles created by tangles of fibrous material in the GI tract that may cause dangerous GI obstructions

bile a substance that emulsifies fats to aid the digestion of lipids; produced by the liver and stored in the gallbladder

biliary atresia a congenital condition in which the major bile duct is blocked, limiting the availability of bile for fat digestion

biliary cirrhosis associated with obstruction of biliary drainage or biliary disorders; accounts for 15% of all cases

binge-eating disorder (BED) a mental disorder characterized by frequent binge-eating behaviors, not accompanied by purging or compensatory behaviors; commonly called compulsive overeating

bingeing feeling out of control when eating, resulting in the consumption of excessive amounts of food

bioelectric impedance analysis (BIA) a method using a mild electric charge to estimate lean body mass to determine body fat composition

biofeedback the use of special devices to convey physiologic information to enable a person to learn how to consciously control these medically important functions

biologic value a method to determine the quality of food protein by measuring the amount of nitrogen kept in the body after digestion, absorption, and excretion

body mass index (BMI) a measure that describes relative weight for height and is significantly correlated with total body fat content

bolus a masticated lump or ball of food ready to be swallowed

branched-chain amino acids (BCAA) leucine, isoleucine, and valine

bulimia nervosa a mental disorder characterized as the binge-and-purge syndrome; includes experiencing repetitive food binges accompanied by purging or compensatory behaviors

C

cachexia general ill health and malnutrition, marked by weakness and emaciation

calcitonin a hormone that reacts in response to high blood levels of calcium; released by the Special C cells of the thyroid gland

calcitriol active vitamin D hormone that raises blood calcium levels

calcium rigor a condition of hardness or stiffness of muscles when blood calcium levels are too high

calcium tetany a condition of spasms and nerve excitability when blood calcium levels are too low

cancer uncontrolled growth of cells that tend to invade surrounding tissue and metastasize to distant body sites

carbohydrates organic compounds composed of carbon, hydrogen, and oxygen

carboxypeptidase a pancreatic protease that hydrolyzes polypeptides and dipeptides into amino acids

carcinogenesis the process of cancer production

cardiac decompensation impaired cardiac output (reasons not entirely understood)

cardiovascular endurance the ability of the body to take in, deliver, and use oxygen for physical work

cheilosis inflammation of the mucous membrane of the mouth and lips (angular stomatitis) caused by riboflavin and other B vitamin deficiencies

chemical digestion the chemical altering effects of digestive secretions, gastric juices, and enzymes on food substance composition

chiropractic manipulation a manipulation modality addressing the ties between body structure (particularly of the spine) and function and how those ties affect the maintenance and return to health

cholecystectomy surgical removal of the gallbladder, performed to treat cholelithiasis and cholecystitis

cholecystitis acute inflammation of the gallbladder associated with pain, tenderness, and fever

cholecystokinin (CCK) a hormone secreted by the small intestine that initiates pancreatic exocrine secretions, acts against gastrin, and activates the gallbladder to release bile

choledocholithiasis gallstones in the common bile duct

cholelithiasis presence of stones in the gallbladder

chronic dieting syndrome a lifestyle inhibited or controlled by a constant concern about food intake, body shape, or weight that affects an individual's physical and mental health status

chronic hunger a continual experience of undernutrition

chronic obstructive pulmonary disease (COPD) a progressive and irreversible condition identified by obstruction of airflow, chronic bronchitis, asthma, and emphysema (also called chronic obstructive lung disease)

chronic ulcerative colitis (CUC) an inflammatory process confined to the mucosa of any or all of the large intestine

chylomicrons the first lipoproteins formed after absorption of lipids from food

chyme a semiliquid mixture of food mass

chymotrypsin a pancreatic protease that hydrolyzes polypeptides into dipeptides

cis fatty acids cis indicates the configuration of the double bond in a natural oil

coenzyme a substance that activates an enzyme

colic sharp visceral pain

colostomy surgical creation of an artificial anus on the abdominal wall by incising the colon and bringing it out to the surface; may be single-barreled (one opening) or double-barreled (distal and proximal loops open onto the abdomen)

colostrum the fluid secreted from the breast during late pregnancy and the first few days postpartum; contains immunologic active substances (maternal antibodies) and essential nutrients

complementary and alternative medicine a cluster of medical and health care approaches, methods, and items not associated with conventional medicine

complementary medicine non-Western healing approaches used at the same time as conventional medicine

complete protein proteins containing all nine essential amino acids

complex carbohydrates polysaccharides of starch and fiber

component puréeing each food item is pureed separately (food thickeners may be added to help maintain consistency), then presented in a manner that resembles the original product (e.g., a pork chop can be pureed, then molded into a pork-chop shape and served)

comprehensive nutritional assessment a procedure conducted by dietetic professionals to determine appropriate medical nutrition therapy based on the identified needs of the patient

congestive heart failure (CHF) circulatory congestion resulting in the heart's inability to maintain adequate blood supply to meet oxygen demands

constipation straining to pass hard, dry stools; slow movement of feces through colon

conventional therapy consists of (1) one or two daily injections of insulin, including mixed intermediate and rapid-acting insulins; (2) daily self-monitoring of urine or blood glucose; and (3) education about diet and exercise

cor pulmonale an abnormal cardiac condition characterized by hypertrophy of the right ventricle as a result of hypertension of the pulmonary circulation

coronary artery disease (CAD) term used for several abnormal conditions that may affect the arteries of the heart and produce various pathologic effects, especially the reduced flow of oxygen and nutrients to the cardiac tissue

Crohn's disease an inflammatory disorder that involves all layers of the intestinal wall and may involve the small or large intestine or both; is associated with stricture formation, fistulous tracts, and abscesses

cystic fibrosis a genetic disorder in which excessive mucus is produced, primarily affecting respiratory airways; also limits fat absorption in the digestive system; most common among white populations

D

Daily Values (DVs) a system for food labeling composed of two sets of reference values: reference daily intakes (RDIs) and daily reference values

deamination a process through which an amino acid group breaks off from an amino acid molecule, resulting in molecules of ammonia and keto acid

denatured a change in the shape of protein structures caused by heat, light, acids, alcohol, or mechanical actions

densitometry underwater weighing

diabetes mellitus a disorder of carbohydrate metabolism characterized by hyperglycemia caused by insulin that is either defective or deficient

dialysate dialysis solution

dialysis a procedure that involves diffusion of particles from an area of high to lower concentration, osmosis of fluid across the membrane from an area of lesser to greater concentration of particles, and the ultrafiltration or movement of fluid across the membrane as a result of an artificially created pressure differential

diarrhea frequent passing of loose, watery bowel movements

diet-induced thermogenesis/thermic effect of food (TEF) an increase of cellular activity when food is eaten

diet manual the reference (usually in a three-ring binder or on computer) that describes the rationale and indications for using a specific diet, lists the allowed and restricted foods, and provides sample menus

dietary fiber carbohydrates (polysaccharides) and lignin in plant foods that cannot be digested by humans

Dietary Reference Intakes (DRIs) dietary standards including Estimated Average Requirement (EAR), Recommended Dietary Allowance (RDA), Adequate Intake (AI), and Tolerable Upper Intake Level (UL)

dietary standards a guide to adequate nutrient intake levels against which to compare the nutrient values of foods consumed

dietary supplements substances consumed orally as an addition to dietary intake

digestion the process through which foods are broken down into smaller and smaller units to prepare nutrients for absorption

digestive system a series of organs that functions to prepare ingested nutrients for digestion and absorption

dipeptidase an intestinal peptidase that completes the hydrolysis of proteins to amino acids

disaccharides a sugar formed by two single carbohydrate units bound together; sucrose, maltose, and lactose are disaccharides

disease prevention the recognition of a danger to health that could be reduced or alleviated through specific actions or changes in lifestyle behaviors

diverticula pouchlike herniations protruding from the muscular layer of the colon

diverticulitis inflammation of one or more diverticula

diverticulosis the presence of diverticula

dry beriberi thiamine deficiency affecting the nervous system, producing paralysis and extreme muscle wasting

dumping syndrome contents from the stomach empty too rapidly into the duodenum, causing symptoms of profuse sweating, nausea, dizziness, and weakness

durable power of attorney a legal document in which a competent adult authorizes another competent adult to make decisions for him/her in the event of incapacitation

dysphagia the inability to swallow normally or freely or to transfer liquid or solid foods from the oral cavity to the stomach; may be caused by an underlying central neurologic or isolated mechanical dysfunction

E

eating disorders a group of behaviors fueled by unresolved emotional conflicts, symptomized by altered food consumption

edema excess accumulation of fluid in interstitial spaces caused by seepage from the circulatory system

edentulous toothless

eicosapentaenoic acid (EPA) the main omega-3 fatty acid in fish

elemental formulas solutions that provide ready-to-absorb basic nutrients, requiring minimal digestion

emetics substances that cause vomiting

emulsifier a substance that works by being soluble in water and fat at the same time

endogenous originating from within the body or produced internally

endometrium mucous membrane of the uterus

enrichment returning nutrients that were lost during processing to their original levels in foods

enteral nutrition administration of nourishment via the gastrointestinal (GI) tract

enteritis infection of the small intestine caused by a virus, bacteria, or protozoa

ergogenic aids drugs and dietary regimens believed by some (but not proven) to increase strength, power, and endurance

esophageal varices large and swollen veins at the lower end of the esophagus that are especially vulnerable to ulceration and hemorrhage, usually the result of portal hypertension

esophagitis inflammation of the lower esophagus

essential amino acids (EAAs) amino acids that cannot be manufactured by the human body

essential fat certain components of body fat that are essential for life

essential fatty acids (EFAs) polyunsaturated fatty acids that cannot be made in the body and must be consumed in the diet

essential or primary hypertension elevated blood pressure for which the cause is unknown

Estimated Average Requirement (EAR) the amount of a nutrient needed to meet the basic requirements of half the individuals in a specific group; the basis for setting the RDAs

Estimated Energy Requirement (EER) dietary energy intake predicted to maintain energy balance in a healthy adult of a defined age, weight, and level of physical activity consistent with good health.

exocrine glands glands that secrete chemicals into ducts that release into a cavity or to the surface of the body, such as salivary glands (mouth) and the liver (gallbladder)

exogenous originating outside the body or produced from external sources

extracellular fluid all fluids outside cells including interstitial fluid, plasma, and watery components of body organs and substances

F

faith healing healing by invoking divine intervention without the use of conventional or surgical therapy

fatty infiltration accumulation of fat (triglycerides) in the liver

feeding relationship the interactions or patterns of behaviors that surround food preparation and consumption within a family

fetal alcohol syndrome (FAS)/fetal alcohol spectrum disorder (FASD) a disorder caused by alcohol consumption during pregnancy that produces a range of specific anatomic and central nervous systems defects

flatus intestinal gas

flexibility the ability to move muscles to their full extent without injury

fluid volume deficit (FVD) the state in which a person experiences vascular, cellular, or intracellular dehydration

fluid volume excess the state in which a person experiences increased fluid retention and edema

fluorosis a condition of mottling or brown spotting of the tooth enamel caused by excessive intake of fluoride

food allergy the overreaction to a food protein or other large molecule that produces an immune response

food choice the specific foods that are convenient to choose when we are actually ready to eat

food intolerance an adverse reaction to a food that does not involve the immune system

food liking foods we really like to eat

food preferences the foods we choose to eat when all foods are available at the same time and in the same quantity

fractionation administration of radiation in smaller doses over time rather than in a single large dose; minimizes tissue damage

G

galactosemia an autosomal recessive disorder resulting in an inability to metabolize galactose and lactose milk products

gastrin a hormone secreted by stomach mucosa that increases the release of gastric juices

gastroesophageal reflux (GER) return of gastric contents into the esophagus that results in a severe burning sensation under the sternum; commonly called heartburn

gastroesophageal reflux disease (GERD) a syndrome of chronic or recurrent return of gastric contents into the esophagus that results in a severe burning sensation under the sternum and possibly nausea, belching, cough, or hoarseness

gastrointestinal (GI) tract the main organs of the digestive system that form a tube that runs from the mouth to the anus

gerontology the study of aging

gestational diabetes mellitus (GDM) a form of diabetes occurring most commonly after the 20th week of gestation

glomerulonephritis inflammation of the glomerulus of the kidney, characterized by proteinuria, hematuria, decreased urine production, and edema

glossitis   inflammation of the tongue

glucagon   a pancreatic hormone that releases glycogen from the liver

glucocorticoid   an adrenal cortex hormone that affects food metabolism

gluconeogenesis   the process of producing glucose from fat and protein

glycemic index   the level to which a food raises blood glucose levels compared with a reference food

glycemic load   the total glycemic index effect of a mixed meal or dietary plan; calculated by sum of products of glycemic index for each of the foods multiplied by amount of carbohydrate in each food

glycogen   carbohydrate energy stored in the liver and muscles

glycogenesis   the process of converting glucose to glycogen

glycogenolysis   the process of converting glycogen back to glucose

glycolysis   the conversion of glucose to carbon compounds

glycosylated hemoglobin (A$_{1C}$)   a substance (glycohemoglobin) formed when hemoglobin combines with some of the glucose in the bloodstream

goiter   enlargement of the thyroid gland caused by iodine deficiency

H

hard water   water containing high amounts of minerals such as calcium and magnesium

health   the merging and balancing of five physical and psychologic dimensions of health: physical, mental, emotional, social, and spiritual

health literacy   the ability to understand basic health concepts and apply to one's own health decisions

health promotion   strategies used to increase the level of health of individuals, families, groups, and communities

heme iron   dietary iron found in animal foods of meat, fish, and poultry

hemochromatosis   a hereditary disorder of iron metabolism characterized by excessive dietary iron absorption and deposition of iron in body tissues

hemodialysis   a procedure to remove impurities or wastes from the blood in treating renal insufficiency by shunting the blood from the body through a machine for diffusion and ultrafiltration and then returning it to the patient's circulation

hemodilution   dilution of the blood

hemoglobin   oxygen-transporting protein in red blood cells

hemosiderosis   a condition in which too much iron is stored in the body

heparinized   use of an antithrombin factor to prevent intravascular clotting

hepatic coma   neurophysiologic symptom of extensive liver damage caused by chronic or acute liver disease

hepatic encephalopathy   a type of brain damage caused by liver disease and consequent ammonia intoxication

hepatotoxic   potentially destructive to liver cells

hiatal hernia   herniation of a portion of the stomach into the chest through the esophageal hiatus of the diaphragm

high fructose corn syrup (HFCS)   corn syrup processed to contain an increased proportion of fructose producing similar sweetness or higher than sugar (sucrose)

high-density lipoproteins (HDLs)   lipoproteins that carry fats and cholesterol from body cells to the liver and are made of large proportions of proteins

high-quality protein   a food containing the best balance and assortment of essential and nonessential amino acids for protein synthesis

homeopathic medicine   an alternative medical system through which a small amount of a diluted substance is prescribed to relieve symptoms for which the same substance, given in larger amounts, will cause the same symptoms

homeostasis   a state of physiologic equilibrium produced by a balance of functions and of chemical composition within an organism

hormones   substances that act as messengers between organs to cause the release of needed secretions

hunger   a physiologic need for food

hydrogenation   breaking a double bond on a fatty acid carbon chain and saturating it with hydrogen

hydroxyapatite   a natural mineral structure of bones and teeth

hyperbilirubinemia   a neonatal condition of excessively high levels of bilirubin (red bile pigment) leading to jaundice, in which bile is deposited in tissues throughout the body

hypercaloric   more than 1 kcal/mL

hypercholesterolemia   total blood cholesterol levels greater than 200 mg/dL; greater than normal amounts of cholesterol in the blood; may be reduced or prevented by avoiding saturated fats

hyperemesis gravidarum   severe and unrelenting vomiting in the second trimester of pregnancy or vomiting that severely interferes with the mother's life; a serious condition usually requiring intravenous replacement of nutrients and fluids

hyperglycemia   elevated blood glucose levels (>120 mg/dL)

hyperosmolar   abnormally increased osmolarity

hyperplasia   an increase in the number of cells occurring during the growth spurts accompanying normal development

hypertension (HTN)   an average systolic blood pressure >140 mm Hg or a diastolic pressure >90 mm Hg (or both)

hypertonic   having greater concentration of solute than another solution

hypertrophy   an increase in the size of cells

hypoglycemia   blood glucose levels that are below normal values

hypogonadism   a deficiency in the secretory activity of the ovary or testis

hyponatremia   low blood sodium

hypophosphatemia   low serum phosphorus levels

hyporeflexia   a neurologic condition characterized by weakened reflex reactions

hypoxia   lack of oxygen to the cells

I

iatrogenic   inadvertently caused by treatment or diagnostic procedures

idiopathic steatorrhea   fat malabsorption caused by unknown causes

ileostomy   entire colon and rectum removed; surgical formation of an opening of the ileum onto the surface of the abdomen, through which fecal matter is emptied

incidental (indirect) food additives   substances that inadvertently contaminate processed foods

incomplete protein   proteins lacking one or more of the essential amino acids

insensible perspiration   water lost invisibly through evaporation from the lungs and skin

insoluble dietary fibers   dietary fibers that do not dissolve in fluids

insulin   a hormone produced by the pancreas that regulates blood glucose levels

integrative medicine   merging of conventional medical therapies with CAM modalities for which safety and efficacy, based on scientific data, have been demonstrated

intensive therapy   consists of (1) administration of insulin more than three times daily (injection or pump) with dosage adjusted according to results of self-monitoring of blood glucose performed at least four times daily, (2) dietary intake, and (3) anticipated exercise

intentional (direct) food additives   substances purposely added during manufacturing to food products

interstitial fluid   fluid between the cells containing concentrations of sodium and chloride

intracellular fluid   fluid within the cells composed of water plus concentrations of potassium and phosphates

intrinsic factor   a substance produced by stomach mucosa that is required for vitamin B$_{12}$ absorption

irradiation   a procedure by which food is exposed to radiation that destroys microorganisms, insect growth, and parasites that could spoil food or cause illness

ischemic   deficient supply of blood to a body part (as the heart or brain) that is due to obstruction of the inflow of arterial blood

isotonic   having the same concentration of solute as another solution, therefore exerting the same amount of osmotic pressure as that solution

K

keratomalacia   a condition caused by vitamin A deficiency in which the cornea becomes dry and thickens from the formation of hard protein tissue

ketone bodies a breakdown product of fatty acid catabolism

ketosis a condition in which the absence of plasma glucose results in partial oxidation of fatty acids and the formation of excessive amounts of ketones

Kt/V a measurement of adequacy and protein nutritional status

kwashiorkor malnutrition caused by a lack of protein while consuming adequate energy

L

lactation the production of breast milk

lacto-vegetarian dietary pattern a food plan consisting of only plant foods plus dairy products

lifestyle a pattern of behaviors

limiting amino acid the essential amino acid or amino acids that incomplete proteins lack

linoleic acid an essential polyunsaturated fatty acid with the first double bond located at the sixth carbon atom from the omega end

linolenic acid an essential polyunsaturated fatty acid with the first double bond located at the third carbon atom from the omega end

lipogenesis anabolism (synthesis) of lipids

lithotripsy extracorporeal shock wave lithotripsy (ESWL), a noninvasive technique whereby high-intensity shock waves cause fragmentation of stones from a device outside the body

locus of control the perception of one's ability to control life events and experiences

low birth weight weighing less than 5.5 pounds (2500 g) at birth

low-density lipoproteins (LDLs) lipoproteins that carry fats and cholesterol to body cells and are made of large proportions of cholesterol

M

macrophages cells that are able to surround, engulf, and digest microorganisms and cellular debris; big scavenger cells

macrosomia larger body size

major minerals essential nutrient minerals required daily in amounts of 100 mg or higher

malnutrition an imbalanced nutrient and/or energy intake

marasmus malnutrition caused by a lack of energy (kcal) intake

MCT fat (oil) specialized modular formulas made of medium-chain triglycerides that do not require pancreatic lipase or bile for digestion and absorption; they are absorbed directly into the portal vein (like amino acids and monosaccharides) rather than the lymphatic system like other lipids

mechanical digestion the crushing and twisting effects of teeth and peristalsis that divide foods into smaller pieces

medical nutrition the use of specific nutrition services to treat an illness, injury, or condition

meditation a self-directed technique of relaxing the body and calming the mind

megacolon massive, abnormal dilation of the colon that may be congenital, toxic, or acquired

menopause the end of menstruation because of the cessation of ovarian and follicular function

metabolism a set of processes through which absorbed nutrients are used by the body for energy and to form and maintain body structures and functions

metastasis the spread of malignant cells to other sites from the original tumor location

microcephaly abnormal smallness of head with brain underdevelopment

monosaccharides a sugar composed of a single carbohydrate unit; glucose, fructose, and galactose are monosaccharides

monounsaturated fatty acid a fatty acid containing a carbon chain with one unsaturated double bond

mucosa the inside GI muscle tissue layer composed of mucous membrane

mucositis inflammation of mucous membranes

multifactorial phenotype a characteristic that is the product of numerous genetic and environmental factors

multiple organ dysfunction syndrome (MODS) the progressive failure of two or more organ systems at the same time (e.g., the renal, hepatic, cardiac, or respiratory systems)

muscular strength and endurance the ability of the muscles to perform hard or prolonged work

muscularis a thick layer of muscle tissue surrounding the submucosa

myocardial infarction (MI) occlusion of a coronary artery; sometimes called heart attack

myoglobin oxygen-transporting protein in muscle

N

naturopathic medicine the use of the body's natural healing forces to recover from disease and to achieve wellness; it incorporates techniques from Eastern and Western traditions

nephrosclerosis necrosis of the renal arterioles, associated with hypertension

nephrotoxic toxic or destructive injury to a kidney

night blindness the inability of the eyes to readjust from bright to dim light caused by vitamin A deficiency

nitrogen-balance studies measurement of the amount of nitrogen entering the body compared with the amount excreted

nocturia excessive urination at night

nonessential amino acids (NEAAs) amino acids manufactured by the human body

nonheme iron dietary iron found in plant foods

nutrients substances in foods required by the body for energy, growth, maintenance, and repair

nutrition the study of essential nutrients and the processes by which nutrients are used by the body

nutrition therapy the provision of nutrient, dietary, and nutrition education needs based on a comprehensive nutritional assessment to treat an illness, injury or condition; may also be called medical nutrition therapy; definition may be dictated by state laws licensing registered dietitians (RDs)

nutritional risk the potential to become malnourished because of primary (inadequate intake of nutrients) or secondary (caused by disease or iatrogenic affects) factors

nutritional support although commonly used in reference to enteral and parenteral nutrition delivery systems, it can refer to any nutrition intervention used to minimize patient morbidity, mortality, and complications

nutritionist a professional who has completed a master's or doctorate degree in foods and nutrition

O

oliguria less than 400 mL urine excretion every 24 hours

osmolality concentration of electrically charged particles per kilogram of solution

osmotic diarrhea diarrhea-associated water retention in the large intestine resulting from an accumulation of nonabsorbable water-soluble solutes

osteodystrophy defective bone development associated with disturbances in calcium and phosphorus metabolism and renal insufficiency

osteomalacia an adult disorder caused by vitamin D or calcium deficiency characterized by soft, demineralized bones

osteopathic medicine an approach based on the assumption that the systems of the body function together with disease stemming from the musculoskeletal system

osteoporosis a multifactorial disorder in which bone density is reduced and remaining bone is brittle, breaking easily

overnutrition consumption of too many nutrients and too much energy compared with DRI levels

ovo-lacto vegetarian dietary pattern a food plan consisting of only plant foods plus dairy products and eggs

oxygen debt the amount of oxygen required to clear lactic acid buildup from the body

oxytocin a hormone that initiates uterine contractions of labor and has a role in the ejection of milk in lactation

P

pancreatitis inflammation of the pancreas; may be acute or chronic

parathormone a hormone that raises blood calcium levels; secreted by the parathyroid gland in response to low blood calcium levels

parenteral nutrition administration of nutrients by a route other than the gastrointestinal (GI) tract, usually intravenously

pellagra the deficiency disorder of niacin characterized by diarrhea, dermatitis, and dementia

pepsin a gastric protease

pepsinogen the inactive form of pepsin

percutaneous endoscopic placement (PEG) placing feeding tube into stomach via the esophagus and then drawing it through the abdominal skin using a stab incision

perimenopause the time before menopause during which hormonal, biologic, and clinical changes begin to occur

peripheral vascular disease (PVD) condition affecting blood vessels outside the heart, characterized by a variety of signs and symptoms such as numbness, pain, pallor, elevated blood pressure, and impaired arterial pulsations. Causative factors include obesity, cigarette smoking, stress, sedentary occupations, and numerous metabolic disorders

peristalsis the rhythmic contractions of muscles causing wavelike motions that move food down the GI tract

peritoneal dialysis (PD) a dialysis procedure performed to correct an imbalance of fluid or electrolytes in the blood or other wastes by using the peritoneum as the diffusible membrane

pernicious anemia inadequate red blood cell formation caused by a lack of intrinsic factor in the stomach with which to absorb vitamin B_{12}

phenylketonuria (PKU) a genetic disorder in which the body cannot break down excess phenylalanine

phospholipids lipid compounds that form part of cell walls and act as a fat emulsifier

physical activity any body movement produced by skeletal muscles that results in energy expenditure

physical fitness the limits on the actions that the body is capable of making

phytochemicals nonnutritive substances in plant-based foods that appear to have disease-fighting properties

pica a condition characterized by a hunger and appetite for nonfood substances

plaque deposits of fatty substances, including cholesterol, that attach to arterial walls

polydipsia excessive thirst

polymeric formulas solutions that provide intact nutrients (e.g., whole proteins and long-chain triglycerides) that require a normally functioning gastrointestinal tract (GI) tract

polyphagia excessive hunger and eating

polysaccharide a carbohydrate consisting of many units of monosaccharides joined together; starch and fiber are food sources, and glycogen is a storage form in the liver and muscles

polyunsaturated fatty acid (PUFA) a fatty acid containing two or more double bonds on the carbon chain

polyuria excessive urination

portal hypertension increased blood pressure in the portal circulation caused by compression or occlusion in the portal or hepatic vascular system

postischemic injury after decreased blood supply to a body organ or part

postnecrotic cirrhosis associated with history of viral hepatitis, improperly treated hepatitis, or hepatic damage from toxic chemicals

postprandial occurring after a meal

preeclampsia a sudden rise in arterial blood pressure accompanied by rapid weight gain and marked edema during pregnancy; also known as pregnancy-induced hypertension

primary or essential hypertension elevated blood pressure for which the cause is unknown

prolactin a hormone responsible for milk synthesis

proteases protein enzymes

protein efficiency ratio (PER) a method to determine the quality of food protein by comparing weight gain to protein intake

protein energy malnutrition (PEM) malnutrition caused by the lack of protein, energy, or both

proteins organic compounds formed from chains of amino acids

Q

Qi gong a modality of Traditional Chinese Medicine that merges breathing regulation, movement, and meditation to increase the flow of Qi, or life force, in the body

R

reactant a substance that enters into and is altered during a chemical reaction

recombinant erythropoietin (EPO) recombinant human erythropoietin; drug used to treat anemia by replacing erythropoietin for patients with Chronic Renal Failure who do not produce this hormone in adequate amounts

Recommended Dietary Allowance (RDA) the level of nutrient intake sufficient to meet the needs of almost all healthy individuals of a life stage and gender group

recumbent measures measurements taken while the subject is lying down or reclining

refeeding syndrome physiologic and metabolic complications associated with reintroducing nutrition (refeeding) too rapidly to a person with PEM; these complications can include malabsorption, cardiac insufficiency, congestive heart failure, respiratory distress, convulsions, coma, and perhaps death

refined grains grains that contain only some of the edible kernel

regional enteritis Crohn's disease

registered dietitian (RD) a professional trained in foods and the management of diets (dietetics) who is credentialed by the Commission on Dietetic Registration of the American Dietetic Association; credentialing is based on completing a bachelor of science degree from an approved program, receiving clinical and administrative training, and passing a registration examination

reiki an energy therapy based on the belief that by healing the patient's spirit, the physical body will also heal

renal transplantation the transfer of a kidney from one person to another

respiratory distress syndrome (RDS) a respiratory disorder identified by insufficient respiration and abnormally low levels of circulating oxygen in the blood

respiratory quotient (RQ) ratio of CO_2 exhaled to O_2 inhaled; depending the net metabolic needs of the body, the ratio ranges from 0.7 to 1 and averages around 0.8; carbohydrate metabolism produces an RQ of 1; protein metabolism, an RQ of 0.8; and fat metabolism, an RQ of 0.7.

retrovirus a ribonucleic acid (RNA) virus that becomes integrated into the deoxyribonucleic acid (DNA) of a host cell during replication; human immunodeficiency virus (HIV) is a retrovirus

rickets a childhood disorder caused by vitamin D or calcium deficiency that leads to insufficient mineralization of bone and tooth matrix

S

saccharin a nonnutritive sweetener

saliva the secretions of the salivary glands of the mouth

saturated fatty acid a fatty acid with carbon chains completely saturated or filled with hydrogen

scurvy extreme vitamin C deficiency disorder characterized by inflammation of connective tissues, gingivitis, muscle degeneration, bruising, and hemorrhaging as the vascular system weakens

secondary hypertension elevated blood pressure for which the cause can be identified

secretin a hormone secreted by the small intestine that causes the pancreas to release bicarbonate to the small intestine

segmentation the forward and backward muscular action that assists in controlling food mass movement through the GI tract

senescence older adulthood

sepsis systemic infection

serosa the outermost layer of the GI wall; made of serous membrane

set point a natural level (of some characteristic) that the body regulates or defends

simple carbohydrates monosaccharides and disaccharides

sleep apnea when breathing stops for short periods during sleep

small for gestational age (SGA) having a lower birth weight than expected for the length of gestation

soft water water filtered to replace some of the minerals with sodium

soluble dietary fibers dietary fibers that dissolve in fluids

solute a substance dissolved in another substance

solvent the liquid in which another substance (the solute) is dissolved to form a solution

somatic protein skeletal muscle proteins

somatostatin a hormone produced by the pancreas and hypothalamus that inhibits insulin and glucagons

spina bifida a congenital neural tube defect caused by the incomplete closure of the fetus's spine during early pregnancy; may involve incomplete development of brain, spinal cord, and/or their protective coverings, resulting in a range of disabilities

sterols fatlike class of lipids that serve vital functions in the body

stomatitis inflammation of mucous membranes of the mouth

storage fat layers and cushions of fat providing stored energy and protection from extremes of environmental temperatures; also protects internal organs against physical trauma

submucosa a layer of connective muscle tissue under the mucosa

sucralose a nonnutritive sweetener, suitable for cooking, that provides no energy

sugar alcohols nutritive sweeteners related to carbohydrates that provide 2 to 3 kcal/g; sorbitol, mannitol, and xylitol are sugar alcohols, also called sugar replacers

syngenic transplant from an identical twin

systemic lupus erythematosus (SLE) a chronic inflammatory disease affecting many systems of the body whose cause is unknown; pathophysiology includes severe vasculitis, renal involvement, and lesions of the skin and nervous system

T

tachycardia rapid beating of the heart

TCA cycle cellular reactions that liberate energy from fragments of carbohydrates, fats, and protein; also called the tricarboxylic acid cycle or Krebs cycle

teratogen an agent capable of producing a malformation or a defect in the unborn fetus

therapeutic touch an energy therapy based on facilitating energy flow in and around the body

thermic effect of food (TEF)/diet-induced thermogenesis an increase of cellular activity when food is eaten

third space (also third spacing) a condition in which fluid shifts from the blood into a body cavity or tissue where it is no longer available as circulating fluid

thrombosis an abnormal vascular condition in which a blood clot (thrombus) develops within a blood vessel

thrombus blood clot

thyrotoxicosis iodine-induced goiter

Tolerable Upper Intake Level (UL) the level of nutrient intake that should not be exceeded to prevent adverse health risks

trace minerals essential nutrient minerals required daily in amounts of 20 mg or less

trans fatty acids fatty acids with unusual double-bond structures caused by hydrogenated unsaturated oils

triglycerides the largest class of lipids found in food and body fat; composed of three fatty acids and one glycerol molecule

trypsin the primary pancreatic protease

type 1 diabetes mellitus (DM) a form of diabetes mellitus in which the pancreas produces no insulin at all

type 2 diabetes mellitus (DM) a form of diabetes mellitus in which the pancreas produces some insulin that is defective and unable to serve the complete needs of the body

U

undernutrition consumption of not enough energy or nutrients based on DRI values

unrefined grains grains prepared for consumption containing all edible portions of kernels

urea product of ammonia conversion produced during deamination

uremia excessive amounts of urea and other nitrogenous waste products in the blood

uremic toxicity buildup of toxic waste products (urea and other nitrogenous waste products) in the blood; symptoms include anorexia, nausea, metallic taste in the mouth, irritability, confusion, lethargy, restlessness, and pruritus (itching)

V

vegan dietary pattern a food plan consisting of only plant foods

very low-calorie diets (VLCDs) usually defined as diets containing 800 kcal/day or less

very low-density lipoproteins (VLDLs) lipoproteins that carry fats and cholesterol to body cells and are made of the largest proportions of cholesterol

villi fingerlike projections on the walls of the small intestine that increase the mucosal surface area

visceral fat fat that is within the abdominal cavity

visceral proteins proteins other than muscle tissue; for example, internal organs and blood

vitamins essential organic molecules needed in very small amounts for cellular metabolism

vomiting reverse peristalsis

W

wasting syndrome an involuntary weight loss of more than 10% in 1 month with the presence of either chronic diarrhea, weakness, or fever for more than 30 days in the absence of a concurrent illness or condition

wellness a lifestyle enhancing our level of health

Wernicke-Korsakoff syndrome cerebral form of beriberi that affects the central nervous system

wet beriberi thiamine deficiency with edema affecting cardiac function by weakening of heart muscle and vascular system

whole grain products food items made using unrefined grains

Wilson's disease a rare, inherited disorder of copper metabolism in which copper accumulates slowly in the liver and is then released and taken up in other parts of the body; as copper accumulates in red blood cells, hemolysis and hemolytic anemia occur

X

xerophthalmia a condition caused by vitamin A deficiency ranging from night blindness to keratomalacia; may result in complete blindness

INDEX